Lippincott Williams & Wilkins'

CLINICAL

Medical Assisting

FOURTH EDITION

Lippincott Williams & Wilkins'

CLINICAL
Medical Assisting

FOURTH EDITION

Judy Kronenberger, RN, CMA, PhD

Professor and Program Director, Medical Assistant Technology
Sinclair Community College
Dayton, Ohio

Denise Woodson, MA, MT(ASCP)SC

Academic Coordinator
Health Sciences and Nursing
Smarthinking, Inc.
Richmond, Virginia

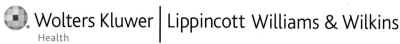

Wolters Kluwer | Lippincott Williams & Wilkins
Health

Philadelphia • Baltimore • New York • London
Buenos Aires • Hong Kong • Sydney • Tokyo

Acquisitions Editor: Kelley Squazzo
Senior Product Manager: Amy Millholen
Design Coordinator: Stephen Druding
Marketing Manager: Shauna Kelley
Compositor: SPi Global
Printer: C & C Offset Printing Co.

Library of Congress Cataloging-in-Publication Data
Kronenberger, Judy.
    Lippincott Williams & Wilkins' clinical medical assisting / Judy Kronenberger, Denise Woodson. — 4th ed.
        p. ; cm.
    Clinical medical assisting
    Lippincott Williams and Wilkins' clinical medical assisting
    Includes index.
    ISBN 978-1-4511-1575-8
  I. Woodson, Denise. II. Title. III. Title: Clinical medical assisting. IV. Title: Lippincott Williams and Wilkins' clinical medical assisting.
    [DNLM: 1. Physician Assistants. 2. Clinical Medicine—methods. W 21.5]
    616.07'5—dc23
                                                                    2012006859

DISCLAIMER
Care has been taken to confirm the accuracy of the information present and to describe generally accepted practices. However, the authors, editors, and publisher are not responsible for errors or omissions or for any consequences from application of the information in this book and make no warranty, expressed or implied, with respect to the currency, completeness, or accuracy of the contents of the publication. Application of this information in a particular situation remains the professional responsibility of the practitioner; the clinical treatments described and recommended may not be considered absolute and universal recommendations.

The authors, editors, and publisher have exerted every effort to ensure that drug selection and dosage set forth in this text are in accordance with the current recommendations and practice at the time of publication. However, in view of ongoing research, changes in government regulations, and the constant flow of information relating to drug therapy and drug reactions, the reader is urged to check the package insert for each drug for any change in indications and dosage and for added warnings and precautions. This is particularly important when the recommended agent is a new or infrequently employed drug.

Some drugs and medical devices presented in this publication have Food and Drug Administration (FDA) clearance for limited use in restricted research settings. It is the responsibility of the health care provider to ascertain the FDA status of each drug or device planned for use in their clinical practice.

The publishers have made every effort to trace the copyright holders for borrowed material. If they have inadvertently overlooked any, they will be pleased to make the necessary arrangements at the first opportunity.

CCS0412

I would like to dedicate this edition of the book to the memory of my dad, Wesley Bitton, who was a fan and cheerleader for all endeavors in my life, including this one. He instilled a love for lifelong learning and a work ethic that make me the person I am today. Although I miss his sense of humor and hugs, I have no doubt that he is looking down and cheering me on with this edition! My other cheerleader is my soul mate and husband, Joe, who provided unconditional love and patience during the many hours I spent sitting at the computer desk. Thank you for understanding! I would also like to thank my children, Brian, Jennifer, Eric, and Brittany for their support of me and for having an "absent" mom on occasion during this project. Also at the top of my list of people to thank are my grandsons, Arthur, Victor, Joseph, and Hayden. They remind me that it is okay to "play" once in a while, and they make me think twice about what is really important in life. Of course, I have to thank the many students I have had the pleasure of teaching who continue to inspire me after many years of educating medical assistants. Lastly, I am very grateful to have Denise Woodson as coauthor and, more importantly, as a friend. We are truly a team!

JUDY KRONENBERGER

To John, the love of my life. In memory of Clarice Connor, my favorite aunt.

DENISE WOODSON

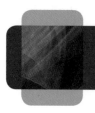

About the Authors

Judy Kronenberger

Judy is currently a Professor and Program Director in the Medical Assistant Technology program at Sinclair Community College in Dayton, Ohio. She is an active member of the American Association of Medical Assistants (AAMA) and enjoys serving this organization as a MAERB/CAAHEP site surveyor (since 2001) for medical assistant programs seeking accreditation or re-accreditation. Judy has served the Ohio State Society of Medical Assistants in various capacities, including her most recent position as the State President (2011–2012). Her education includes an Associate Degree in Nursing (Sinclair Community College), a Bachelor of Arts degree in Human Development (McGregor School at Antioch University), a Master's of Science Degree in Education (University of Dayton), and a PhD in Higher Education (University of Dayton). She is committed to student-centered learning and coordinates a first-year experience course for new students to promote persistence and academic success. Judy resides in Kettering, Ohio, with her husband of 32 years. She enjoys reading and spending time with her four grandsons whenever possible!

Denise Woodson

Denise has a Bachelor of Science degree in Medical Technology from the University of Tennessee at Chattanooga and a Master's degree in Allied Health Education from Central Michigan University. In addition to American Society for Clinical Pathology certification as a medical laboratory scientist (medical technologist), she has a Specialist in Chemistry certification from the American College of Clinical Pathology. In her 30+ years of clinical experience, Denise has supervised three hospital clinical chemistry laboratories. These positions included adjunct faculty appointments for local community college clinical internships in Medical Laboratory Technician programs.

Denise has held the Chief Technologist and Laboratory Manager positions in three hospitals, managing 10–100+ laboratory employees. In addition to clinical and employee management, she has specialized in laboratory accreditation compliance with the College of American Pathologists and Clinical Laboratory Improvement Amendments (CLIA).

On retirement from the clinical laboratory, Denise worked 5 years in a group medical practice to experience that segment of the health care system. She worked in the laboratory, with the physicians, and also mentored medical assisting students in their externship programs.

Denise taught Laboratory Science and other required classes for 4 years in an accredited Medical Assisting program.

Currently, Denise holds the position of Academic Coordinator of Health Sciences and Nursing for Smarthinking, Inc. Smarthinking delivers online tutoring offering one-on-one help when students need assistance. For 8 years, she has managed a staff of approximately 30 health science and nursing tutors, including medical assistants.

In addition, Denise has consulted with physician office laboratories to develop and train employees to maintain CLIA compliance.

Denise currently lives in Richmond, Virginia, with her husband and two cats, Saphy and Little Hoo.

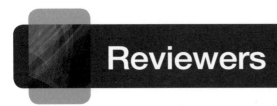
Reviewers

Lenora Binegar, AAS
Medical Program Advisor
Department of Health
Washington County Career Center
Marietta, Ohio

Mindy Brown
Medical Assisting Instructor
Pima Medical Institute
Colorado Springs, Colorado

Patricia Bucho, AS
Instructor
Department of Allied Health
Long Beach City College
Long Beach, California

Estelle Coffino, BS, MPA
Administrator/Chair of Allied Health Programs
Department of Allied Health
The College of Westchester
White Plains, New York

Brandi DeLeon, RT(R), RMA, BS
Medical Insurance Coding Specialist
Fortis Institute
Mulberry, Florida

Jane W. Dumas, MSN, CCMA, CPT, CET
Allied Health Department Chair, MA Program
    Director
Department of Allied Health
Remington College, Cleveland West Campus
Cleveland, Ohio

Donna Guisado, RDA, MSLM
Corporate Director of Education & Compliance
North-West College
West Covina, California

Forrest Heredia, CPC-I
Administrative Assistant Instructor
Medical Administrative Assistant Department
Pima Medical Institute
Tucson, Arizona

Heather Kies, MHA, CMA (AAMA)
Program Director of Medical Assisting
Department of Health & Natural Sciences
Goodwin College
East Hartford, Connecticut

Paul Lucas, AS
Program Director of Medical Assisting
Department of Medical Assisting
Brown Mackie College
Fort Wayne, Indiana

Dona Marotta, CMA (AAMA), BS
Program Director
Department of Medical Assisting
Alegent Health School of Medical Assisting
Omaha, Nebraska

Joyce Minton, MS, EdS
Medical Assisting Director
Department of Advanced Health Technologies
Wilkes Community College
Wilkesboro, North Carolina

Jean L. Mosley, BS, CMA (AAMA)
Medical Assisting Program Director, Instructor
Department of Medical Assisting
Surry Community College
Dobson, North Carolina

Brigitte Niedzwiecki, BSN, MSN
Medical Assistant Program Director, Instructor
Department of Medical Assisting
Chippewa Valley Technical College
Eau Claire, Wisconsin

Wanda Sciambi-Wines, LPN, CMA
National Director of Medical Programs
Department of Education (Corporate Level)
Education Affiliates
Baltimore, Maryland

Sharon Skonieczki, MS, BS, CMA (AAMA)
Program Director
Department of Medical Assisting
Elmira Business Institute
Elmira, New York

Carrie Smith
Instructor
Pima Medical Institute
Tucson, Arizona

Patti Zint, MA, HCA
Program Director
Department of Medical Assisting and Health Care
    Administration
Carrington College
Phoenix, Arizona

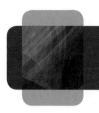

Preface

Health care is changing; however, your role as the most versatile health care member is an important part of the successful physician practice and will continue to be integral as health care changes. Although the skills you perform may vary among medical offices, your education and training in the exciting field of medical assisting will prepare you for a variety of clinical skills, making you an essential part of the health care team.

Lippincott Williams & Wilkins' Clinical Medical Assisting, Fourth Edition, will provide you with the information and skills necessary to perform competently and with confidence. This edition has been updated to include the most current (2008) American Association of Medical Assistants (AAMA) curriculum standards for medical assistants in all three domains: cognitive, psychomotor, and affective. These standards are required for Commission on Accreditation of Allied Health Education Programs (CAAHEP)-accredited programs. This edition also includes the content and skills required by the American Medical Technologists (AMT) for Accrediting Bureau of Health Education Schools (ABHES)-accredited programs. These standards and competencies define your roles and responsibilities as a professional medical assistant and this edition of the textbook and ancillary materials continue to support your education and training to fulfill these role responsibilities.

Organization of the Text

As with previous editions, great care and concern were taken to organize this book in a logical and reader-friendly presentation. Icons have been added to indicate content that is part of the cognitive, psychomotor, and affective learning domains. The fourth edition is divided into two sections:

- Part I, The Clinical Medical Assistant, consists of two units. Unit One provides you with critical information regarding nutrition and wellness, aseptic techniques, infection control, patient assessment, vital signs, and assisting with the physical examination. You will also find an overview of pharmacology as well as information to help you properly prepare and administer medications. The final chapter in this unit will give you the tools to recognize and respond to emergencies in the medical office. Unit Two focuses on specialty examinations, diagnostic tests, and therapeutic procedures for specific areas of medicine. Each chapter provides you with a brief overview of the system, typical therapeutic measures used to treat common disorders, and the role of the medical assistant in assisting the physician with diagnosis and treatment. The last two chapters in this unit focus on duties relating to special populations, including pediatrics and geriatrics.

- Part II, The Clinical Laboratory, introduces you to the physician office laboratory. This section will provide you with detailed information on maintaining a safe laboratory environment that operates in compliance with federal, state, and local regulations, including the Needlestick Safety and Prevention Act. Updated information includes more emphasis on physiology related to hematology, urinalysis, microbiology, immunology, and chemistry. Skills included in this unit include competencies on collecting and processing specimens, handling the specimens in a manner that supports accurate testing, and following quality control protocols to monitor and evaluate testing procedures, supplies, and equipment. In addition, medical terminology related to the clinical laboratory is emphasized in this edition, including procedures to document and maintain a quality assurance program to ensure thorough patient care.

Features

Instructors should find the time invested to "link" the text and ancillary materials with the most current CAAHEP and ABHES standards useful. Our goal is to make this textbook the most student-friendly resource available in the medical assisting field.

A variety of key chapter features are included to spark interest and promote comprehension, including:

- Chapter outline
- Learning outcomes specific to CAAHEP and ABHES standards
- Key terms
- Key points highlighted throughout the text
- Icons to indicate content that is part of the cognitive, psychomotor, and affective learning domains—NEW!
- Step-by-step procedure boxes
- Spanish terminology boxes
- Critical thinking challenges
- Checkpoint questions
- Unique information boxes, tables, and displays
- Video icons next to topics and procedures for which there is a skills video available in the online student resources—NEW!

- Full-color illustrations
- Media Menu, containing information on videos, animations, and Internet resources

This textbook is fully supported with a robust teaching and learning package, each element of which is designed to help you and your instructor get the most out of the textbook. The resource package includes the following:

- A code in each text to access CareTracker, a web-based electronic medical record (EMR) and practice management (PM) software. This fully integrated EMR and PM gives students the experience of documenting and tracking patient encounters from check in to check out for a real-world experience. Case Studies provided on thePoint walk students through the software helping them build proficiency and confidence in an EMR/PM environment and helping instructors meet the CAAHEP and ABHES EHR competency.
- A complete instructor's resource kit accompanying the textbook includes a test generator, image bank, PowerPoint slides, lesson plans, answer keys for the text checkpoint questions and Study Guide, CAAHEP and ABHES competencies mapping spreadsheets linking the text and ancillary content to the competencies, and more.
- Online student resources, including certification exam preparation review questions, games and review activities, competency evaluation forms, work products, animations, videos, key terms audio glossary, and Spanish-English audio glossary.
- A separate student Study Guide is available for purchase to enhance learning and comprehension, with competency evaluation forms for each procedure in the textbook; critical thinking exercises; self-assessment exercises, such as matching and multiple choice; and study and work products.

As medical assisting instructors, we hope these books exceed your expectations. May your career in medical assisting be challenging and fulfilling!

Judy Kronenberger, RN, CMA, PhD
Denise Woodson, MA, MT(ASCP)SC

User's Guide

This User's Guide shows you how to the put the features of *Lippincott Williams & Wilkins' Clinical Medical Assisting, Fourth Edition* to work for you.

Chapter Opening Elements

Each chapter begins with the following elements, which will help orient you to the material:

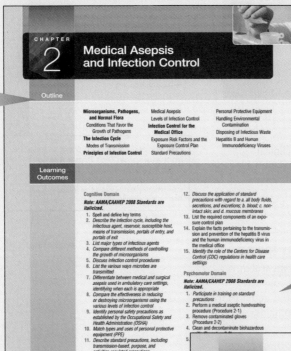

Chapter Outline

This serves as your "roadmap" to the chapter content.

Learning Outcomes

The Learning Outcomes list the skills learned, including the CAAHEP and ABHES Competencies specific to the chapter.

Key Terms

The key terms that are defined in the chapter are listed for quick reference.

Special Features

Unique chapter features will aid readers' comprehension and retention of information—and spark interest in students and faculty:

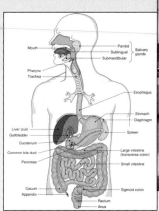 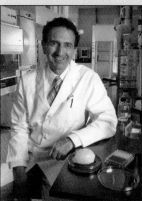

Stunning Art Program

Full-color illustrations and photographs clarify clinical concepts for the learner.

PATIENT EDUCATION
KEGEL EXERCISES

The patient's age, gravidity, and past childbearing take their toll on the muscles of the perineum. Kegel exercises can increase the tone of this area. Stronger perineal support helps eliminate stress incontinence and supports the vaginal walls to avoid uterine prolapse.

These exercises should be performed three times every day for 5 minutes each time. In addition, the exercises should be done in three positions: lying down, sitting, and standing. Explain to the patient that she can do Kegel exercises at any time, such as when standing in the grocery line, waiting at a stop light, or sitting in class. Essentially, the exercises involve tightening the pelvic muscles...

Patient Education Boxes

Contain in-depth information on topics the student needs to know in order to educate patients.

COG Drug Actions and Interactions

PSY Self Boundaries

What kind of person are you? Are you a friendly

9. **AFF** Explain how to respond to a patient who has cultural or religious beliefs who may be uncomfortable about disrobing.

COG
AFF
PSY

Domain Icons

Indicate content that is part of the cognitive, psychomotor, and affective learning domains.

 Waived Tests Based on Immunological Test Principles

There are many immunoassay test kits available today, and the number is growing. This is an area of CLIA-waived testing that is making an increasing number of diagnostic test results available in the physician's office.

Video Icons

Are located next to topics for which there is a skills video available in the online student resources.

---

español español

SPANISH TERMINOLOGY

¿Tiene una buena memoria?
  Is your memory good?
¿Le duele la cabeza?
  Have you any pain in the head?
¿Siente vértigo?
  Do you feel dizzy?
Voltése para el lado izquierdo (derecho).
  Turn on your left (or right) side.

Spanish Terms and Phrases

Assist students communicating with Spanish-speaking patients.

PSY PROCEDURE 7-1:	Opening Sterile Surgical Packs

Purpose: Open sterile packages without contaminating the contents
Equipment: Surgical pack, surgical or Mayo stand

Steps	Reasons
1. Wash your hands.	Handwashing aids in infection control. Your hands should be clean for this procedure.
2. Verify the procedure to be performed and remove the appropriate tray or item from the storage area. Check the label for contents and expiration date. Check the package for tears and moisture.	Packages that have passed the expiration date should not be used. Moist or torn areas contaminate the contents of the package.
3. Place the package, with the label facing up, on a clean, dry, flat surface such as a Mayo or surgical stand.	Although the field will be protected by a barrier undersurface, microorganisms must be kept at a minimum by using an area as free of pathogens as possible. The surgical stand makes it easy to move the field for the physician's convenience.
4. Without tearing the wrapper, carefully remove the sealing tape. With commercial packages, carefully remove the outer protective wrapper.	Many disposable packages are wrapped in clear plastic film that will become the sterile field when properly opened. Packages prepared in the office are sealed with autoclave tape, which should clearly indicate that the package has been through the autoclave.
5. Loosen the first flap of the folded wrapper by pulling it up, out, and away; let it fall over the far side of the table or stand.	This prevents you from having to reach across the sterile field again.

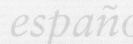

Step 5. Open the first flap away from you.

Procedure Boxes

Break procedures down into steps, demonstrating how to perform essential skills properly. Needed equipment and supplies are listed. Reasons are given for the steps, ensuring greater understanding.

 WHAT IF?

The first Pap smear or gynecologic examination for young women may cause great anxiety. What if an 18-year-old woman is to have her first Pap smear today? How should you handle the situation?

Bring the patient into the room and encourage her to talk about her feelings. Do not have her change into an examining gown until she has had an opportunity to speak with the physician or practitioner about the procedure. The physician may require the presence of another health care worker, like the medical assistant, during the examination; how...

What If Boxes

Present a variety of real-life scenarios that students must be prepared to handle in the medical office. Each situation is clearly defined and explained.

☑ CHECKPOINT QUESTION

2. What is the document the physicians' office prepares to outline its plan for chemical safety?

Checkpoint Questions

Review questions appear throughout the chapter to ensure
student comprehension of the material learned in the section.

Legal Tip Boxes

Contain important
legal information
to help the aspiring
medical assistant
understand the legal
implications associated
with the profession.

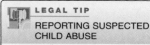

LEGAL TIP

**REPORTING SUSPECTED
CHILD ABUSE**

The Federal Child Abuse Prevention and Treatment
Act mandates that threats to a child's physical
and mental welfare be reported by anyone having
contact with children in a professional or employment setting (e.g., teachers, physicians, nurses,
medical assistants, daycare workers). Health care
workers, teachers, social workers, and others who
work with children are protected against liability if
they report their suspicions in good faith.

ETHICAL TIP

**Common Issues of Laboratory Noncompliance
with CLIA Standards**

Efforts to reduce medical errors, improve health
care quality, and increase patient safety have been
gaining national attention. As a part of the POL survey by a CMS surveyor, the CMS surveyor provides
observations of noncompliance in the CW POL and
to CMS. It is the ethical responsibility of anyone
performing laboratory tests to be informed of what
testing he or she is allowed to perform and the performance requirements of each

Ethical Tip Boxes

Offer guidelines to
help the student learn
and abide by the ethi-
cal standards set forth
by the AAMA.

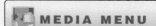

MEDIA MENU

- **Student Resources on thePoint**
  - **Animation: Immune Response**
  - **Video: Collecting a Throat Specimen
    (Procedure 29-1)**
  - **Video: Testing Stool Specimen for Occu
    Blood: Guaiac Method (Procedure 29-8)**
  - **Video: Preparing a Smear for Microscop
    Evaluation (Procedure 29-9)**
  - **Video: HCG Pregnancy Test
    (Procedure 29-1**

Media Menus

Located at the end of
every chapter, the Media
Menu contains infor-
mation on video clips,
animations, and Internet
resources that are avail-
able to the student.

Chapter Closing Elements

Chapter Summary

Reviews key points from
the chapter.

Chapter Summary

Working with children offers many rewards; however,
the special developmental needs and unique physiology of children make these patients challenging and
must always be taken into consideration. This chapter
focuses on:

- The skills necessary to assist with a well-child visit
  including obtaining and recording normal growth
  information. It is important to record this information carefully to assist the physician in detecting problems as early as possible.
- Caring for the child who comes to the office for a
  sick-child visit. This includes maintaining the reception area by separating sick and well children if
  possible and disinfecting any toys to avoid cross-
  contamination in other children.
- Common diseases that may be seen in childhood
  including ear infections, upper respiratory infections,
  and gastrointestinal problems. Although these diseases are common, they are not pleasant for the child

or the caregiver. You will have a role in reassuring
anxious parents while caring for their sick children
competently and professionally.
- Education of the pediatric patient caregiver including vaccine information. Parents should always be
  encouraged to ask questions and should expect to get
  honest and clear answers.
- Legal and ethical issues related to immunizations,
  child abuse, and neglect. You must always be alert for
  signs of neglect and/or abuse and be ready to report
  your suspicions to the physician.
- Your role in preventing disease in the pediatric patient
  and assisting with pediatric procedures. In addition
  to caring for children, you must also provide patient
  education to caregivers and older children to prevent
  the spread of disease. Also, your expertise in working
  with pediatric patients will be appreciated by the physician and the other staff who may find it necessary to
  have you assist with a variety of pediatric procedures.

Warm Ups for Critical Thinking

1. During years of practice, Dr. Hernandez has found
   that many new parents are unfamiliar with basic
   child care needs. He decides to publish a short booklet for his new parents describing various aspects of
   child care. The booklet should be informative and
   professional and show genuine concern for children.
   Using your creativity and your knowledge of child
   care, develop a sample booklet for Dr. Hernandez's
   patients after choosing two of the following topics:
   - General safety tips
   - Types of office visits
   - Immunizations (what they are, why they are
     important, at what ages they are given, side
     effects and adverse effects)
   - What a parent can expect during an office visit
   - Brief explanation of child development
   - Tips for administering oral medications to children
2. You obtained the weight on Lillian Parks, a
   7-month-old girl. She weighs 16½ pounds according

   to your balance [   ]. What percentile
   is this patient according to [   ]
   would you explain a percentile to [   ]
   the infant?
3. The father of a toddler is insistent that you give the
   child an immunization in the arm rather than the
   thigh. How would you handle this situation?
4. Research one of the following conditions that may
   be found in pediatric patients and prepare a poster
   detailing the causes, signs and symptoms, and treatment. Include information for the caregivers or
   school personnel who may have questions about
   these conditions:
   - Strep throat
   - Pediculosis
   - Conjunctivitis
5. Compare the developmental skills of a 3-year-old
   and 5-year-old child. What are the similarities?
   What are the differences?

Warm Ups for
Critical Thinking

Real-life scenarios that
require the student to
develop, create, write,
or search for more
information.

Additional Learning Resources

This powerful learning tool also includes:

• the **Point** Companion Site for Students comes with new review activities and games, animations, videos, certification preparation question bank, competency evaluation forms, an English-to-Spanish audio glossary and key terms glossary, and student work products. The student companion site can be accessed at: http://thepoint.lww.com/kronenbergerclin4e

• Instructor Resources on thePoint include lesson plans, image bank, test generator, PowerPoint lecture slides, answer keys, CAAHEP and ABHES competencies mapping spreadsheets linking the text and ancillary content to the competencies, and more.

Available for purchase separately:

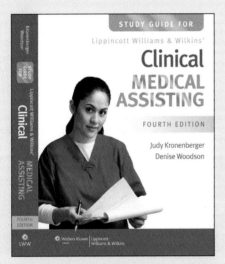

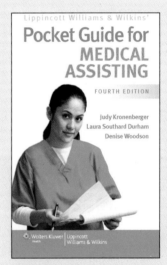

• *Study Guide for Lippincott Williams & Wilkins' Clinical Medical Assisting* comes with procedure skill sheets, case studies for critical thinking, and a variety of question types to meet the needs of different learning styles and to reinforce content and knowledge.

• *Lippincott Williams & Wilkins' Pocket Guide for Medical Assisting* gives step-by-step coverage of medical assisting procedures in both administrative and clinical settings. The small size makes it perfect for clinical and office use.

Acknowledgments

This book would never have been successfully completed without the assistance, persistence, and hard work of many people. At the risk of leaving out others at Lippincott Williams & Wilkins (LWW) who made this book possible (we apologize in advance!), we would like to thank Kelley Squazzo, the Acquisitions Editor, who was there from the beginning to offer support, insight, and guidance whenever needed. A special thank you should also go to Julie Stegman, (Senior Publisher, Health Professions), John Larkin (Product Manager), Rachel Stark (Editorial Assistant), Eric Branger (Product Director), and Kelly Horvath (Copyeditor) for making this book and ancillary materials a reality and supporting the education of medical assistants.

In particular, we owe a huge thank you to Amy Millholen, our Senior Product Manager at LWW, for keeping us focused and the project organized to ensure that the chapter content remained student-centered. We could not have done it without you, Amy! To all the other staff at LWW who helped in this edition of the book but who may not be mentioned specifically, we offer our most sincere gratitude and thanks!

We thank Wake Forest Center for Regenerative Medicine for their help and support in providing photos, materials, and expertise. We also thank Brenda Allen at Orthopedic Specialists of the Carolinas for her help with forms, information, and encouragement.

The authors and staff at LWW thank the administration, staff, and students at Forsyth Technical Community College in Winston-Salem, NC, who provided the location, faces, and skills for the photo and video shoots.

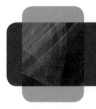

List of Procedures

Contents

PART I

The Clinical Medical Assistant

PART II

The Clinical Laboratory

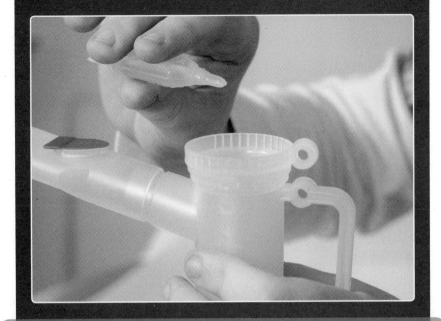

The Clinical Medical Assistant

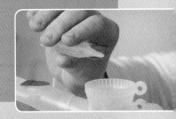

CHAPTER

1

Nutrition and Wellness

Outline

Digestion & Metabolism   Therapeutic Nutrition   Staying Well
Essentials of Nutrition   **Wellness**   Substance Abuse
  Nutrients   Physical Fitness
  Nutritional Guidelines   Weight Management

Learning Outcomes

Cognitive Domain

Note: AAMA/CAAHEP 2008 Standards are italicized.

1. Spell and define the key terms
2. *Describe the normal function of the digestive system*
3. *Analyze charts, graphs, and/or tables (BMI) in the interpretation of health care results*
4. Name all of the essential nutrients
5. Discuss the body's basal metabolic rate and its importance in weight management
6. Explain how to use the food pyramid and MyPlate guides to promote healthy food choices
7. Read and explain the information on food labels

8. Describe therapeutic diets and the patients who need them
9. List the components of physical fitness
10. Discuss suggestions for a healthy lifestyle
11. Explain the importance of disease prevention
12. List and describe the effects of the substances most commonly abused
13. Recognize the dangers of substance abuse

Psychomotor Domain

Note: AAMA/CAAHEP 2008 Standards are italicized.

1. Teach a patient how to read food labels (Procedure 1-1)

2. *Instruct patients according to their needs to promote health maintenance and disease prevention*
3. *Document patient education*
4. *Perform within scope of practice*

Affective Domain

Note: AAMA/CAAHEP 2008 Standards are italicized.

1. *Apply critical thinking skills in performing patient assessment and care*
2. *Use language/verbal skills that enable patients' understanding*
3. *Demonstrate respect for diversity in approaching patients and families*
4. *Apply active listening skills*
5. *Demonstrate empathy in communicating with patients, family, and staff*
6. *Use appropriate body language and other nonverbal skills in communicating with patients, family, and staff*
7. *Demonstrate awareness of the territorial boundaries of the person with whom you are communicating*
8. *Demonstrate sensitivity appropriate to the message being delivered*
9. *Demonstrate recognition of the patient's level of understanding in communications*
10. *Recognize and protect personal boundaries in communicating with others*
11. *Demonstrate respect for individual diversity, incorporating awareness of one's own biases in areas including gender, race, religion, age, and economic status*

ABHES Competencies

1. Comprehend and explain to the patient the importance of diet and nutrition
2. Effectively convey and educate patients regarding the proper diet and nutrition guidelines
3. Identify categories of patients that require special diets or diet modifications
4. Document accurately

Key Terms

anabolism

basal metabolic rate (BMR)

body mass index (BMI)

calories

catabolism

dental cavities

endorphins

essential amino acids

euphoria

guided imagery

homeostasis

metabolism

minerals

predisposed

The human body requires certain things such as regular exercise and a balanced diet to maintain its efficiency. Together, diet and exercise offer important benefits for overall health maintenance and disease prevention for people of all ages. Psychological wellness is also crucial to a balanced, healthy life. Avoiding harmful substances and unhealthy practices is as important to overall health as diet and exercise. As a medical assistant, you should consider yourself a role model for your patients. Throughout your career, you will have many opportunities to teach patients the essentials of good health and disease prevention by knowing how behaviors affect short-term and long-term health.

COG Digestion and Metabolism

Digestion consists of both the physical and chemical breakdown of complex food into simpler substances that the body can use for energy. When you swallow, food travels from the mouth, through the esophagus, into the stomach, and through the small and large intestines. The process of digestion begins in your mouth as the enzymes in your saliva start to break down the food as you chew. As the partly digested food passes through the remainder of the digestive tract, enzymes continue to break down food, and, in the small intestines, the process of absorption allows these nutrients to be absorbed into the bloodstream. Once in the bloodstream, the nutrients are taken to the liver to be further broken down and filtered before making their way to every cell in the body. Any nutrients not needed are eliminated from the body or stored as fat for future energy use. The process whereby food is broken down, absorbed, used by the cells, or stored by the body is known as **metabolism.**

There are two phases in the process of metabolism, **catabolism** and **anabolism.** Catabolism is the destructive phase of metabolism in which larger molecules are converted into smaller molecules. An example of catabolism includes the conversion of glycogen into pyruvic acid. This process releases energy, which is measured in **calories.** This energy is needed for cell growth and heat production. In some cases, nutrients are broken down and reassembled by the body to produce substances needed by the body. This process is known as anabolism, which is considered the constructive phase of metabolism as the smaller molecules are converted to larger molecules. An example of anabolism is the conversion of amino acids into specific proteins. The speed of these metabolic processes are particular to each individual, which explains why some people seem to be able to eat more and maintain a healthy weight, whereas others consume the same amount of food and gain weight.

COG Essentials of Nutrition

Although many factors influence **homeostasis,** making healthy food choices gives you the best chance at maintaining a state of wellness including homeostasis. When the body is working efficiently and in balance, it is considered to be homeostatic. Eating a diet that includes all nutrients in adequate amounts increases your body's ability to maintain wellness.

Nutrients

Nutrients include the elements found in the food we eat that are important for all aspects of health maintainence. Essential nutrients include vitamins, minerals, carbohydrates, proteins, fiber, and certain fats. Micronutrients are elements that are needed in trace amounts. The consumption of water is also important to metabolic processes and general good health.

Carbohydrates

Carbohydrates are chemical substances that are broken down by the body into simple sugars (glucose), which provide energy to all cells of the body. Foods that contain carbohydrates include those made from grain products, fruits, vegetables, legumes, and sugars. Chemically, carbohydrates are made of carbon, hydrogen, and oxygen atoms and, depending on the structure of these elements in the carbohydrate molecule and how easily digested by the body, they are considered *complex* or *simple.* Complex carbohydrates take longer to digest and therefore provide long-term energy to the body. Examples of these types of carbohydrates include starches that are found in grains, legumes, potatoes, and pasta. Simple carbohydrates are unrefined sugars found in fruits and plants, which are easily broken down and absorbed by the body. Refined sugars have a high caloric value but no nutritious value and should be kept to a minimum. Carbohydrates consumed but not used by the body for energy are converted to fat and stored in the adipose tissue of the body.

Proteins

When broken down, proteins are made up of amino acids, which provide energy, build and repair tissue, and assist with antibody production in the body. There are approximately 80 amino acids found in nature, but the human body only needs 20 of them. The body produces 11 of these on its own; the other nine are known as **essential amino acids** and come from your diet. Some animal proteins provide all the necessary amino acids and are called *complete proteins.* Examples of foods that contain complete proteins include milk, cheese, eggs, fish, and meat from animals or poultry. Other proteins do not contain all of the nine essential amino acids and are considered *incomplete proteins.* Plants, such as beans, legumes, nuts, and seeds, are natural sources of incomplete proteins. A combination of both types of proteins, complete and incomplete, will ensure a proper amount of protein in the diet.

Fats

Fats, also known as lipids, serve as a concentrated source of heat production and energy and provide essential fatty acids. Many tissues, including heart and skeletal muscle, derive energy from fatty acids. Chemically, fats are composed of carbon, hydrogen, and oxygen but in different proportions than those found in carbohydrates. Food must supply essential fatty acids that are necessary for nutritional well-being. If the body has inadequate supplies of glucose to break down for energy, it will catabolize, or break down, fats. Fats have important functions within the body including providing a cushion for internal organs, insulation to maintain normal body temperature, and assisting cells to function properly. Because the body can store fat reserves for future energy use in adipose tissue, an excess of fat in the diet will result in weight gain. Although food labels often list information about fats, these labels can be confusing. Table 1-1 lists the types, characteristics, and sources of fats.

Vitamins

Vitamins are organic substances that enhance the breakdown of proteins, carbohydrates, and fats. Some vitamins are used in the formation of blood cells and hormones as well as in the production of neurochemical substances necessary for life. Eating a diet that contains

TABLE **1-1**	The Good and Bad Fats	
Type of Fat	**What Does It Do?**	**Where Is It Found?**
Monounsaturated (MUFA) fat	Does not raise "bad" cholesterol levels	Olive oil and canola oil
Omega-3 fatty acid	May protect against heart disease	Salmon, albacore tuna, mackerel, sardines, herring, and trout
Polyunsaturated (PUFA) fat	Contains some essential fatty acids; does not raise "bad" cholesterol levels	Natural oils found in certain fish and nuts; vegetable oils such as corn oil, soybean oil, and sunflower oil
Saturated fat	Raises "bad" cholesterol levels, increases risk of heart disease	Meat, poultry, dairy products, processed and fast foods
Trans fat or hydrogenated fat[a]	Raises "bad" cholesterol levels, increases risk of heart disease	Cookies, cakes, margarine, crackers, and some fried foods
Triglycerides	Excess amounts increase risk of heart disease when coupled with other risk factors	Main form of fat in foods, produced by the body and stored as fat from excess calories

[a]Trans fats are created by adding hydrogen to vegetable oil. This process, called *hydrogenation*, increases the shelf life of certain products. Hydrogenation turns liquid vegetable oils into solid fats.
Source: http://www.fda.gov/AboutFDA/Transparency/Basics/ucm194310.htm

all of the nutrients usually means that the vitamins necessary to maintain good health are consumed in adequate amounts. However, many people supplement their intake of food with a daily multivitamin to make sure they are getting a proper amount of each vitamin in the appropriate amounts.

Vitamins are categorized as either *fat-soluble* or *water-soluble*. Fat-soluble vitamins include vitamins A, D, E, and K. These vitamins are usually absorbed with foods that contain fat and are stored in the liver, kidneys, and body fat. Bile, which is formed in the liver, breaks down fat-soluble vitamins. The consumption of additional fat-soluble vitamins should be avoided because the body stores these vitamins, and an excess can result in serious illness.

Water-soluble vitamins include vitamin C and the B-complex vitamins such as thiamin (B1), riboflavin (B2), niacin (B3), and folic acid. The body does not store these vitamins, and they must be provided daily through the diet. Any excess water-soluble vitamins taken in will not be stored but excreted by the body.

PATIENT EDUCATION

WOMEN AND FOLIC ACID

Folate, one of the B vitamins, has been found to reduce the risk of neural tube defects in developing fetuses. These types of defects, like spina bifida and anencephaly, affect the fetus's brain and spine during early pregnancy. Neural tube defects can cause paralysis and, in extreme cases, death.

In 1998, the March of Dimes, in its dedication to wiping out birth defects, began a national campaign to get the word about folate out to women of childbearing age who may become pregnant. The March of Dimes joined forces with other agencies to provide education, training, and vitamin distribution to women across the nation. Since that time, women have become more aware of the importance of folic acid, and physicians provide more information and assistance to patients.

A daily intake of 400 µg/day of synthetic folate or folic acid from fortified foods or supplements is recommended for women of childbearing age who may become pregnant. Women are encouraged to eat foods naturally rich in folate including liver; avocado; orange juice; boiled asparagus; spinach; and green, leafy vegetables. Vegetables should be eaten raw or lightly steamed as cooking may destroy the vitamins. Many breakfast cereals and breads are fortified with folic acid. Women of childbearing age are also encouraged to read labels to see if the amount of folic acid in products meets their daily requirement. The March of Dimes campaign has played a significant role in decreasing the occurrence of neural tube defects by 50% to 70%.

 CHECKPOINT QUESTION

1. Why is it important to follow the recommended dosage of a fat-soluble vitamin?

Minerals

Minerals are inorganic substances used in the formation of hard and soft body tissue, muscle contraction, nerve conduction, and blood clotting. As with vitamins, you get minerals from the foods you eat. Examples of minerals necessary for good health include sodium, potassium, calcium, phosphorus, magnesium, iron, and iodine. Because the body uses minerals in differing amounts, those minerals that are only required in small amounts are known as *trace minerals*. Minerals that are only needed in trace amounts include flourine, zinc, copper, cobalt, and chromium.

Cholesterol

All animals produce a substance known as *cholesterol*, which is necessary for the body to function properly. Foods such as meat, poultry, seafood, eggs, and dairy products are considered animal products and therefore contain cholesterol. Egg yolks and organ meats, such as liver, are particularly high in cholesterol. Vegetables and vegetable products do not contain cholesterol; however, they may contain oils and fats.

The body requires cholesterol to maintain good health, and it is manufactured in sufficient amounts by the body. Unfortunately, the consumption of animal products also provides cholesterol and can result in an unhealthy amount of cholesterol in the bloodstream. Any excess cholesterol in the blood can result in plaque buildup inside the blood vessels, eventually causing occlusion or blockage of the blood vessel. According to the National Cholesterol Education Program (NCEP), it is recommended that adults consume fewer than 300 mg of dietary cholesterol each day to avoid this problem.

Lipoproteins

Lipoproteins are substances composed of lipids (fats) and proteins that transport cholesterol between the liver and arterial walls. Food sources do not contain lipoproteins; they are found only in the body. The amounts and types of lipoproteins found in the blood are a good indicator of the risk of heart disease. There are two types of lipoproteins categorized as *low-density lipoproteins (LDLs)* and *high-density lipoproteins (HDLs)*.

LDLs transport cholesterol from the liver to the walls of large- and medium-sized arteries. Excess LDLs in the blood can cause plaques to form, which reduce the flow of blood within the affected artery. Circulation becomes impaired, and, as LDL levels rise above the normal range, the risk of heart disease increases. Due to these risks, LDL is occasionally labeled "bad" cholesterol. Factors that contribute to an unhealthy increase in LDL levels include excess body fat and a diet high in saturated fat and cholesterol. An LDL level above 160 mg/dL indicates an increased risk for heart disease.

HDLs are responsible for carrying cholesterol away from arterial walls back to the liver, which then removes cholesterol from the body. High levels of HDL have been linked to a reduction in the risk of heart disease. For this reason, HDL is sometimes called "good" cholesterol. Regular exercise helps increase HDL levels. An HDL level above 35 mg/dL indicates a lower risk for heart disease.

 CHECKPOINT QUESTION

2. What are complete proteins, and where are they found?

Fiber

Fiber is necessary in the diet to help the body with elimination of waste products in the digestive system. Foods that are high in fiber content include all vegetables, raw and cooked fruits, and whole-grain foods, such as breads, grains, and cereals. Patients with chronic colitis, ileitis, or diverticulitis may be instructed to follow a low-fiber diet, avoiding fresh fruits and vegetables and consuming only broiled, boiled, or baked meats, fish, and poultry; pastas; dairy products; well-cooked vegetables; fruit and vegetable juices; and canned fruit. A high-fiber diet may be recommended for patients with constipation or to regulate bowel movements. These patients would be told to avoid fatty foods and eat whole grain cereals and breads. There are many brands of over-the-counter fiber supplements that can be added to a liquid for daily regularity. When discussing healthy food choices with your patients, do not forget to discuss healthy food preparation (Box 1-1).

BOX 1-1

HEALTHY FOOD PREPARATION TIPS

Here are a few guidelines on how to prepare healthy foods that you can share with your patients:

- Broil, boil, bake, roast, or grill meat, poultry, and fish.
- Trim the fat from beef.
- Use a cooking rack so that fat drips away from the meat.
- Remove the skin from chicken. Use caution with raw chicken. Wash hands and cutting surfaces immediately.
- Cook homemade soups or gravies and then chill them. Skim the fat off and then reheat.
- Use unsaturated oils (canola, corn, safflower).
- Use nonstick spray when possible. Avoid saturated oils (e.g., butter, lard).

Nutritional Guidelines

The United States Department of Health and Human Services (DHHS), the United States Department of Agriculture (USDA), the National Academy of Sciences, and the Food and Nutrition Board are all involved in establishing the guidelines recommended for a healthy diet. All of these organizations have Web sites that can give you more information on nutrition and how to maintain a healthy diet.

MyPyramid and MyPlate Guidelines

The USDA developed a food guidance system in 1992 called MyPyramid, to help people maintain healthy diets and sufficient exercise levels. In 2005, MyPyramid was updated to reflect the Dietary Guidelines for Americans (Fig. 1-1). The categories of food in this guidance system include oil and five main food groups:

1. Grains
2. Vegetables
3. Fruits
4. Milk
5. Meat and beans

Figure 1-2 is a sample food pyramid based on a 2,000 calorie diet. In 2010, the USDA updated the dietary guidelines for Americans, and in 2011, provided a new, simplified visual reference to communicate these guidelines to the public. This concept, known as MyPlate, is based on the same food groups and recommendations for healthy eating as MyPyramid (Fig. 1-3). Although MyPlate does not give specific information about serving sizes, it is a reminder to Americans to choose reduced portions at meals, include a plate of one-half fruits and vegetables, drink fat-free or 1% milk, eat whole grains, decrease dietary sodium by comparing and choosing those with low numbers, and drink water instead sugary drinks.

Grains

Foods in the grain food group include bread, cereal, oatmeal, crackers, rice, and pasta. The USDA recommends choosing whole grains (as opposed to refined

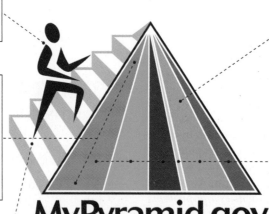

Figure 1-1 Anatomy of MyPyramid.

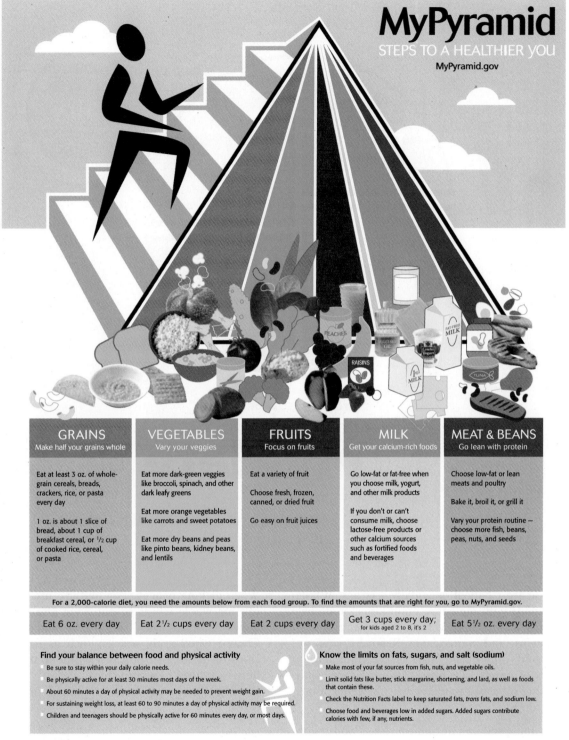

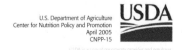

Figure 1-2 MyPyramid guide based on a 2,000-calorie diet.

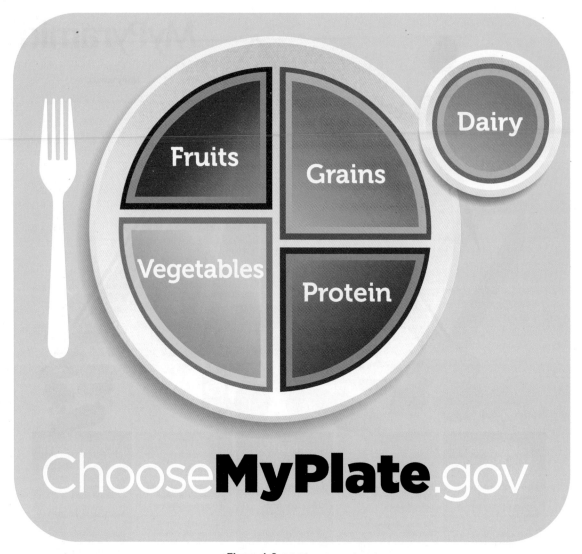

Figure 1-3 MyPlate icon.

grains) for at least half of your daily servings. Whole grains are made with the entire grain kernel and contain nutrients such as fiber, certain vitamins, carbohydrates, proteins, and antioxidants. Refined grains, on the other hand, only include part of the grain kernel. These types of grains lack fiber, iron, and some vitamins. Here are some tips to follow when selecting foods from this group:

- Look at the product's ingredient list. Foods with ingredients such as "whole wheat," "bulgur," "whole-grain corn," "oatmeal," "whole oats," or "wild rice" at the beginning of the list indicate whole grains.
- Look for foods that are high in dietary fiber. Nutrition labels indicate the percentage of the recommended daily value (DV) that is included in one serving.
- Substitute brown rice or whole-wheat pasta for white rice or pasta made from refined grains. Likewise, substitute whole-wheat bread for white bread.

- When making pancakes or muffins, use recipes that call for whole wheat or oat flour. Use whole-grain flour or oatmeal when baking cakes and cookies.
- Choose whole-grain snacks, such as baked tortilla chips or air-popped popcorn (without added salt or butter), instead of potato chips.
- Eat whole-grain cereals, such as muesli or toasted oat cereal.

Vegetables

The vegetables group is subdivided into five categories: dark green vegetables, orange vegetables, dry beans and peas, starchy vegetables, and other vegetables. The key to choosing foods within this group is to select a variety of vegetables from different categories. Other tips include:

- Eat fresh seasonal vegetables. Fresh vegetables have more flavor and generally cost less than processed vegetables (e.g., canned or frozen vegetables). Processed vegetables may also contain sauces or seasonings that add sodium and fat.

- When buying canned vegetables, look for foods without added salt. Choose vegetables labeled "no salt added," or check the sodium content on the nutrition label.
- Choose foods with high levels of potassium, such as sweet potatoes, tomato paste, beet greens, white potatoes, white beans, soybeans, lima beans, and spinach.
- Eat a green salad with lunch or dinner each day. Add only a small amount of salad dressing.
- Prepare vegetable main dish meals, such as soups, stews, and stir-fries. Include potatoes in soups and stews for added texture and nutrients.

Fruits

The fruits food group includes 100% fruit juice as well as fresh, frozen, dried, and canned fruit. Here are some tips for selecting foods from this group:

- Get most of your daily servings from whole fruit instead of juice. Whole or cut-up fruit contains dietary fiber, while most juices do not.
- When buying packaged fruit, look for items that do not contain added sugar. For example, select canned fruit stored in 100% juice or water instead of syrup.
- Eat a wide variety of fruits to obtain the greatest nutritional benefit. Prune juice, bananas, and dried apricots supply potassium. Pears, raspberries, and blackberries provide dietary fiber. Guava, kiwi, and oranges are good sources of vitamin C.
- Add fresh berries, peaches, or bananas to your cereal at breakfast and drink a glass of 100% orange or grapefruit juice.
- Snack on cut-up or dried fruit. Cut-up fruit is often sold in convenient single-serving packages, and dried fruit can be stored in a bag or desk drawer. One-fourth cup of dried fruit is equal to one-half cup of other fruit.
- When baking cakes, substitute applesauce for some of the oil in the recipe.

Milk

Also referred to as the "milk, yogurt, and cheese group," this food group includes all milk and milk products that retain their calcium content. Found in this food group are liquid milk (including lactose-free milk), milk-based desserts (such as pudding and ice cream), hard and soft cheeses, and yogurt. Not included in this group are milk products such as butter and cream cheese, which do not provide calcium. In choosing foods from this group, it's important to select low-fat or nonfat items. Other tips include:

- Drink a glass of low-fat or fat-free milk with meals.
- Have pudding made from low-fat or fat-free milk for dessert.

- When making hot cereals or oatmeal, use low-fat or fat-free milk instead of water. Also substitute milk for water when preparing condensed cream soups.
- Snack on low-fat or fat-free yogurt topped with fresh fruit.
- Add low-fat cheese to soups, stews, and casseroles. Top vegetables with melted low-fat cheese, or add low-fat or fat-free yogurt to baked potatoes.
- For those who are lactose intolerant, choose lactose-free or lower lactose milk products. Although soy milk, orange juice, and other products may be calcium fortified, these foods do not provide all the essential nutrients supplied by foods within the milk group.

Meat and Beans

The meat and beans group includes all foods made from meat, poultry, eggs, dry beans, peas, nuts, and seeds. The high fat and cholesterol content of some foods in this group (such as beef or egg yolks) makes varying your food choices important. It is also crucial to select a variety of foods to obtain the greatest nutritional benefit. For example, sunflower seeds and almonds are high in vitamin E; salmon and trout contain omega-3 fatty acids; clams and oysters provide iron; beef, lamb, pork, poultry, fish, shellfish, and eggs are good sources of protein.

Here are some guidelines to use when choosing foods from the meat and beans group:

- For vegetarians, alternate protein sources include eggs, beans, nuts, peas, and foods made from soybeans, such as tofu.
- Select lean cuts of beef (round steaks, roasts, top loin, top sirloin) and pork (pork loin, tenderloin, ham). When buying ground beef, look for packages labeled "90% lean," "93% lean," or "95% lean."
- Choose boneless skinless chicken breasts and turkey cutlets, or remove the skin from poultry before cooking.
- Prepare meat, poultry, and fish without adding fat. First, trim off any visible fat and then broil, grill, roast, or boil foods, being careful to drain off excess fat during cooking. Add little or no breading, and avoid using gravies or sauces that are high in fat.
- Prepare meatless main dishes containing dry beans or peas. For example, use kidney or pinto beans to make chili, cook split pea soup or minestrone, add chickpeas or garbanzo beans to a salad, or prepare tofu or veggie burgers.
- Eat fish more often than you eat meat or poultry. Salmon, trout, and herring are excellent sources of omega-3 fatty acids.
- Substitute nuts in dishes containing meat or poultry. Add pine nuts instead of chicken to pesto sauce; substitute peanuts or cashews for meat in vegetable stir-fries; and add walnuts, almonds, or pecans to green salads instead of meat or chicken.

Oils

One additional category is oils. Included in this category are fats that maintain a liquid form at room temperature including vegetable oils and oils that come from other natural plant and fish sources. Fats that are solid at room temperature, such as butter, shortening, and beef or chicken fat, are not considered oils. The recommended daily servings for this category are relatively small, usually several teaspoons, depending on a person's age, gender, and level of physical activity. Therefore, the most important guideline to use when choosing foods in this category is to avoid exceeding recommended amounts. Most people consume enough oils in the foods they eat (e.g., olives, avocados, nuts, fish, cooking oils, and salad dressing).

 CHECKPOINT QUESTION

3. Who publishes the MyPyramid and MyPlate food guidance systems and why?

 LEGAL TIP

U.S. GOVERNMENT IS CONCERNED ABOUT AMERICANS' EATING HABITS

The U.S. government is dedicated to improving America's nutritional needs, and this is evident when you consider the many bills passed and programs provided by the agencies of the federal government. Based on data concerning dietary intake and evidence of public health problems, experts say that Americans have formed some poor eating habits. Studies have shown that Americans consume too many calories per day as well as unhealthy amounts of saturated and trans fat, cholesterol, added sugars, and sodium. In addition, most people do not meet the recommended daily intakes for a number of nutrients. The federal government says most manufacturers must list the nutrients and their amounts in food packaging. The U.S. Food and Drug Administration (FDA) mandates the information included on a food label. A recent new mandate requires manufacturers to list the amount of trans fats in their products.

In the 1960s, the federal government instituted the Presidential Physical Fitness Award, which outlined specific physical programs for school physical fitness programs. The USDA regulates the public school lunch programs and requires lunches to satisfy the recommended daily dietary requirements. Head Start is a federal preschool program that has an excellent food program, ensuring that disadvantaged children get at least one nutritious meal a day. Their food programs, along with agricultural extensions across the nation, train parents in proper nutrition and food preparation through regular workshops and training.

Understanding Food Labels

The Nutritional Labeling and Education Act was passed in 1990 to help consumers identify nutritional content in food products. Most food manufacturers (except meat and poultry) are required to list the nutritional information prominently on the package. The FDA regulates this information. Mandatory food labeling was designed to help consumers make informed food choices. Even fast food restaurants are including labeling as consumers become more health conscious.

Currently, food labels must include measurements of calories, fat content, cholesterol, sodium, carbohydrates, dietary fiber, protein, vitamins, calcium, and any other nutrients contained in the product. Foods that only have a few of certain nutrients are not required to list them on the label. It is important to pay attention to the serving size noted on the label because the amount of a particular nutrient noted on the label is specific to that size. In addition to the amount of nutrients, the percentage of the total daily intake is listed on the right side of the label. This information on the food label helps you choose the daily allowances of the good nutrients like fiber, protein, vitamins, and minerals and a minimal amount of the things that are harmful like fats, cholesterol, sodium, and sugar. A DV of 0% is listed for those things that should be kept to a minimum. The calories listed on the label measure how much energy is received from one serving, including how many of those calories are from fat. Calories will be discussed in greater detail later.

To get the full benefit of food labels, patients must understand how to read them. You can help your patients understand how to use this information by becoming familiar with reading food labels and adapting the way you present this information based on the needs of the individual patient. Figure 1-4 is a sample food label with an explanation of each component. Procedure 1-1 outlines the steps in instructing a patient to read food labels.

 CHECKPOINT QUESTION

4. What information is listed on the right side of a food label?

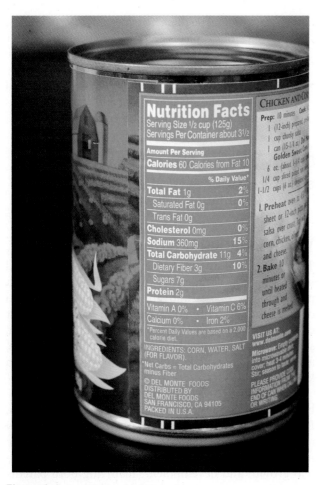

Figure 1-4 Sample food label.

 PATIENT EDUCATION

VEGETARIAN DIETS

Patients may ask you about vegetarian diets. There are three types of vegetarian diets. A lacto-ovo-vegetarian diet means that the diet of vegetables is supplemented with milk, eggs, and cheese. A lacto-vegetarian diet means the diet is supplemented only with milk and cheese. A pure vegetarian diet is only vegetables and excludes all foods of animal origin. It is possible to eat healthily and obtain necessary nutrients with all three vegetarian diets. The USDA provides guidelines educating vegetarians about appropriate foods that provide essential nutrients.

Therapeutic Nutrition

Although each part of the lifespan brings different nutritional needs, sometimes a patient's medical condition or situation will require diet restrictions and special foods. In these situations, the physician will order a therapeutic diet, and you may be responsible for teaching the patient how to follow the guidelines. Chronic conditions that require special diets include diabetes and heart disease. Patients such as those who are confined to bed or those recovering from surgical procedures may also be required to eat certain foods. Regardless of the reason for the therapeutic diet, the purposes include facilitating the healing process, promoting healthy weight, assisting with chewing and swallowing, and/or influencing the components found in blood, such as cholesterol or blood glucose levels. Table 1-2 shows an example of a special diet that may be prescribed to treat high blood pressure. This special diet is referred to as the *Dietary Approaches to Stop Hypertension (DASH)* eating plan.

 CHECKPOINT QUESTION

5. List four possible reasons for a patient's need for a special therapeutic diet.

TABLE **1-2**	Example of a Therapeutic Diet: The DASH Eating Plan	
What Does This Diet Accomplish?	**Who May Follow This Diet?**	**Basic Dietary Guidelines**
• Lowers blood pressure • Reduces the risk of developing hypertension • Lowers "bad" cholesterol levels	• Adults with blood pressure above normal levels	• Consume more servings of grains, vegetables, and fruit. • Limit foods and beverages containing added sugars. • Limit sodium intake to 1,500–2,300 mg per day. • Increase potassium intake from natural sources, such as potatoes, spinach, bananas, apricots, soybeans, and low-fat or nonfat milk.

Source: http://www.nhlbi.nih.gov/hbp/prevent/h_eating/h_eating.htm.

COG **Wellness**

Physical Fitness

Physical fitness is characterized by endurance, flexibility, and strength. Along with a healthy and balanced diet, regular exercise is necessary for maintaining physical fitness. Physical movement helps maintain a healthy musculoskeletal system, a normal weight, and a positive mental attitude. Studies have shown that exercising regularly improves the immune system and causes the production of **endorphins**, the body's "natural painkillers" that tend to produce **euphoria**, or "good feelings."

PATIENT EDUCATION

CALCULATING TARGET HEART RATE

Patients who are starting an exercise program may need to learn how to calculate their target heart rate. Aerobic activities, such as running, bike riding, rowing, and swimming, are most effective when target heart rate is maintained. Target heart rate should be anywhere between 60% and 90% of a patient's maximum heart rate. To find a patient's target heart rate, follow these steps:

1. Subtract the patient's age (in years) from 220 (beats/minute) to calculate the maximum heart rate. For example, a 35-year-old patient would have a maximum heart rate of 185.

$$220 - 35 = 185$$

2. Multiply the maximum heart rate by the desired intensity level (60%–90% of the maximum heart rate) to obtain the target heart rate. A patient with a maximum heart rate of 185 who would like to exercise at 70% intensity would need to maintain a target heart rate of 129.5.

$$185 \times 0.70 = 129.5$$

Components of Physical Fitness

There are several components of physical fitness:

- *Cardiovascular health and endurance.* Regular exercise, particularly aerobic activities, can improve cardiovascular system functioning and endurance. Benefits of a healthy heart include lowered blood pressure, lower cholesterol levels, and a reduced risk for developing conditions such as type 2 diabetes or heart disease.
- *Flexibility.* Stretching exercises give muscles increased flexibility, or a greater range of motion. Calisthenics, yoga, and other stretching activities improve flexibility. Greater flexibility makes everyday physical tasks easier to accomplish; it also helps decrease the risk of muscle injury.
- *Bone and muscle strength.* Exercise can help build strong bones, while weight lifting and resistance training increase muscle strength and endurance.

 CHECKPOINT QUESTION

6. What types of physical activities promote cardiovascular health and endurance?

Weight Management

The rate of obesity in the United States has doubled in the past two decades. Nearly one-third of the adult population is obese, and an estimated 16% of children and adolescents are overweight. Excess body fat can result in a higher risk of certain health conditions, such as hypertension, heart disease, type 2 diabetes, gallbladder disease, respiratory disorders, and certain kinds of cancers.

In the last 20 years, the obesity rate has doubled among children and tripled among adolescents. Because obesity in childhood often leads to obesity in adulthood, it is important to find ways to slow the unhealthy rate of weight gain while maintaining normal growth and development. Involving both parents and children in managing body weight is essential for compliance with any prescribe dietary plan. Simple methods for managing body weight include eating more nutritious, lower calorie foods and increasing physical activity. Even losing a small amount of weight is beneficial to overall health and preventing future weight gain.

Physiologic Issues

Reducing and maintaining a healthy weight depends on a familiar formula—increased physical activity + taking in fewer calories = reduction in body weight. The energy that the body expends burns the calories you consume. Knowing how many calories your body requires based on age and gender is necessary for calculating the amount of calories required to lose or maintain weight. To do this, you must understand the three basic ways the body expends energy. These include:

- **Basal metabolic rate (BMR)** (or how many calories the body uses to perform basic functions, such as respiration and heartbeat, while in a resting state)
- Energy expended during physical activity
- The thermic effect of food (or how much energy the body expends while processing different foods)

The body's daily caloric needs are most accurately determined by taking into account all three of these factors. Each of these is discussed in the following sections.

WHAT IF?

A patient who is a young mother of three says that she would like to stay fit, but she has no time for a fitness plan. What are some ways she can incorporate exercise into her busy schedule?

Remind her that exercise does not have to consist of a 30-minute walk or an hour in the gym. Give her some suggestions for creative ways to be physically active every day. For example, take the stairs instead of the elevator. Take two steps at a time for leg and buttock strengthening. On weekends, take a long walk or run around with the children at the park. Doing yard work is another way to be physically active; mowing the lawn with a push mower and raking leaves are ways to stay active while accomplishing necessary chores. While watching television in the evening, jog in place or do jumping jacks. Do calf raises while waiting in line at the grocery store. While talking on the phone, walk up and down stairs or do leg lifts. A simple trip to the grocery store provides exercise by walking and lifting. While driving in the car, tense up various muscle groups for a few seconds and then release. Do leg lifts with your child sitting across your feet. Even a hearty laugh works the abdominal muscles.

The benefits of regular physical activity go beyond maintaining a healthy level of physical fitness. Being active also helps relieve stress. By taking small steps to be more active every day, you will eventually progress to a point where you will want to engage in more physical activity. Then you can hire a babysitter and go take a kickboxing class. Meanwhile, move more.

Basal Metabolic Rate

As mentioned earlier, metabolism is the process of digesting and processing food consumed into energy to be used by the body or stored in adipose tissue as fat reserves. An individual's BMR refers to the amount of energy used in a unit of time to maintain vital functions by a fasting, resting subject. Approximately 60% to 70% of the body's energy is expended through BMR basic activities, such as respiration, heartbeat, and maintaining body temperature.

Level of Physical Activity

The second way that your body expends energy is through physical activity, which makes up 20% to 30% of the body's total energy expenditure. You have already learned the positive effects of physical activity, one of which is to burn calories and maintain a healthy weight. Box 1-2 shows an appropriate workout schedule.

Calories

The third, and last, factor included in how your body expends energy is known as the *thermic effect*, or the amount of energy required to digest specific foods. The energy used by the body can be measured in calories,

BOX 1-2

SAMPLE WORKOUT SCHEDULE

The following is a sample workout schedule that the average healthy patient can follow to maintain physical fitness.

Note: Patients should not participate in an exercise program without consulting a physician first.

- *Warming up.* Take 5 to 10 minutes to warm up your muscles. Walk or jog at a slow pace to prepare your body for the workout.
- *Stretching exercises.* It's important to stretch your muscles when they are warm; this prevents muscle injury. Spend 10 to 12 minutes on stretching exercises, being careful to move slowly and avoid bouncing. Stretching each day also improves flexibility.
- *Strength training.* To increase muscle strength, lift weights at least twice a week for 20 minutes at a time. Also incorporate resistance exercises such as pull-ups, push-ups, and sit-ups into your workout. These exercises should be done at least three times a week for 30 minutes and should include all major muscle groups.
- *Cardiovascular endurance exercises.* Aerobic activities, including running, bike riding, jumping rope, swimming, and hiking, increase your cardiovascular endurance. Devote 30 minutes or more to aerobic activity at least three times a week.
- *Cooling down.* After each workout, take 5 to 10 minutes to cool down. Several minutes of walking or other low-intensity movement will allow your heart rate to return to normal. It is also important to stretch the muscles that have just been used.

Source: http://www.fitness.gov/fitness.htm.

and four different sources contribute calories to a person's diet. These sources include carbohydrates, fats, proteins, and alcohol.

Together, the three factors (BMR, level of physical activity, and the thermic effect of food) determine how many calories your body needs each day. If you take in fewer calories than you need, you lose weight. If you take in more calories than you need, you gain weight. The combination of these three components can be calculated as follows:

- For those who are not physically active: weight (lbs) × 14 = estimated calories/day
- For those who are moderately active: weight (lbs) × 17 = estimated calories/day
- For active individuals: weight (lbs) × 20 = estimated calories/day

Body Mass Index

Body mass index (BMI) measures an individual's ratio of fat to lean body mass. It can be calculated by using the following formula: [weight (pounds) ÷ height (inches)^2] × 703. With the increased incidence of obesity, physicians are turning to BMI for assessing patients' risk for obesity. For adults who are 20 years of age or older, the condition of being overweight or obese is based on their BMI level only (i.e., regardless of age or gender). For children and adolescents, however, weight status is determined by taking into account not only BMI level, but also age and gender.

Because BMI takes into account both weight and height, it is a more accurate way to measure body fat than by measuring weight alone. It is important to note, however, that BMI is not the sole method used to determine obesity. It does have limitations; BMI can overestimate body fat in someone who is very muscular or underestimate body fat in an individual with decreased muscle mass. Other factors, including age, gender, and ethnicity, also cause variations in the relationship between BMI and body fat. Slightly reducing caloric intake for children who are overweight will decrease their body fat, which will improve their BMI over the course of time.

A BMI over 30 is considered obese. The Centers for Disease Control and Prevention offer a body mass calculator on their Web site. By going to http://www.cdc.gov, you can search for the BMI calculator, enter the patient's requested information, and print a graph and information about the patient. There are also growth charts available to track BMI (Fig. 1-5).

 CHECKPOINT QUESTION

7. What is meant by BMR?

 WHAT IF?

You are assisting your physician-employer in the exam room one afternoon when the two of you see a patient who has gained 30 pounds in a year. She appears depressed and complains of leg pain and increased difficulty getting around. The physician explains that she needs to make some changes in her diet (low calorie, low fat) and asks you to assist the patient in getting started. Where should you begin?

You should refer to the *Dietary Guidelines for Americans, 2010* from the USDA and go over the following points:

- *Monitor calories and nutrients.* Eat foods with more nutrients per calorie, and limit saturated and trans fats, added sugars, cholesterol, sodium, and alcohol.
- *Manage your weight.* To prevent weight gain, slightly decrease calories consumed and increase daily physical activity. To maintain a healthy weight, find a balance between the number of calories consumed each day and an appropriate amount of exercise.
- *Exercise regularly.* To prevent unhealthy weight gain, exercise for 60 minutes (moderate to vigorous activity) most days of the week. Include cardiovascular training, flexibility exercises, and weight training to receive the full benefits of physical fitness.
- *Make healthy food choices.* Eat a variety of fruits and vegetables every day, being sure to consume the recommended amount of servings based on energy needs. When selecting foods from the grains food group, choose whole-grain products. Be sure to include the recommended daily servings of milk or milk products in your diet as well.
- *Limit fats.* Try to consume no more than 20% to 35% of calories from fat each day. Most fats in your diet should come from natural sources, such as nuts, vegetable oils, and fish. Limit other fats by selecting foods that are designated as low-fat, nonfat, or lean, and avoid trans fats.
- *Choose healthy sources of carbohydrates.* Select carbohydrate sources that are also high in fiber, such as fruits, vegetables, and whole-grain products. Avoid foods and beverages that contain added sugars or sweeteners.
- *Monitor sodium and potassium intake.* Limit sodium to less than 2,300 mg per day. Select foods that are high in potassium, such as fruits and vegetables.

(box continues on page 18)

Body Mass Index Table

	Normal						Overweight					Obese										Extreme Obesity														
BMI	19	20	21	22	23	24	25	26	27	28	29	30	31	32	33	34	35	36	37	38	39	40	41	42	43	44	45	46	47	48	49	50	51	52	53	54
Height (inches)																		Body Weight (pounds)																		
58	91	96	100	105	110	115	119	124	129	134	138	143	148	153	158	162	167	172	177	181	186	191	196	201	205	210	215	220	224	229	234	239	244	248	253	258
59	94	99	104	109	114	119	124	128	133	138	143	148	153	158	163	168	173	178	183	188	193	198	203	208	212	217	222	227	232	237	242	247	252	257	262	267
60	97	102	107	112	118	123	128	133	138	143	148	153	158	163	168	174	179	184	189	194	199	204	209	215	220	225	230	235	240	245	250	255	261	266	271	276
61	100	106	111	116	122	127	132	137	143	148	153	158	164	169	174	180	185	190	195	201	206	211	217	222	227	232	238	243	248	254	259	264	269	275	280	285
62	104	109	115	120	126	131	136	142	147	153	158	164	169	175	180	186	191	196	202	207	213	218	224	229	235	240	246	251	256	262	267	273	278	284	289	295
63	107	113	118	124	130	135	141	146	152	158	163	169	175	180	186	191	197	203	208	214	220	225	231	237	242	248	254	259	265	270	278	282	287	293	299	304
64	110	116	122	128	134	140	145	151	157	163	169	174	180	186	192	197	204	209	215	221	227	232	238	244	250	256	262	267	273	279	285	291	296	302	308	314
65	114	120	126	132	138	144	150	156	162	168	174	180	186	192	198	204	210	216	222	228	234	240	246	252	258	264	270	276	282	288	294	300	306	312	318	324
66	118	124	130	136	142	148	155	161	167	173	179	186	192	198	204	210	216	223	229	235	241	247	253	260	266	272	278	284	291	297	303	309	315	322	328	334
67	121	127	134	140	146	153	159	166	172	178	185	191	198	204	211	217	223	230	236	242	249	255	261	268	274	280	287	293	299	306	312	319	325	331	338	344
68	125	131	138	144	151	158	164	171	177	184	190	197	203	210	216	223	230	236	243	249	256	262	269	276	282	289	295	302	308	315	322	328	335	341	348	354
69	128	135	142	149	155	162	169	176	182	189	196	203	209	216	223	230	236	243	250	257	263	270	277	284	291	297	304	311	318	324	331	338	345	351	358	365
70	132	139	146	153	160	167	174	181	188	195	202	209	216	222	229	236	243	250	257	264	271	278	285	292	299	306	313	320	327	334	341	348	355	362	369	376
71	136	143	150	157	165	172	179	186	193	200	208	215	222	229	236	243	250	257	265	272	279	286	293	301	308	315	322	329	338	343	351	358	365	372	379	386
72	140	147	154	162	169	177	184	191	199	206	213	221	228	235	242	250	258	265	272	279	287	294	302	309	316	324	331	338	346	353	361	368	375	383	390	397
73	144	151	159	166	174	182	189	197	204	212	219	227	235	242	250	257	265	272	280	288	295	302	310	318	325	333	340	348	355	363	371	378	386	393	401	408
74	148	155	163	171	179	186	194	202	210	218	225	233	241	249	256	264	272	280	287	295	303	311	319	326	334	342	350	358	365	373	381	389	396	404	412	420
75	152	160	168	176	184	192	200	208	216	224	232	240	248	256	264	272	279	287	295	303	311	319	327	335	343	351	359	367	375	383	391	399	407	415	423	431
76	156	164	172	180	189	197	205	213	221	230	238	246	254	263	271	279	287	295	304	312	320	328	336	344	353	361	369	377	385	394	402	410	418	426	435	443

Source: Adapted from *Clinical Guidelines on the Identification, Evaluation, and Treatment of Overweight and Obesity in Adults: The Evidence Report.*

Figure 1-5 Body Mass Index (BMI) Table.

- *Limit alcohol consumption.* Consume alcohol in moderation; women should not exceed one drink per day, and men should not exceed two drinks per day. Those who should avoid alcohol include: pregnant or lactating women, women who may become pregnant, children, adolescents, individuals taking medication that should not be mixed with alcohol, and people who have certain medical conditions.
- *Prevent food-borne illness.* Wash hands, food preparation surfaces, and fruits and vegetables. Cook foods long enough and at high enough temperatures to kill dangerous microorganisms. Properly store perishable items and avoid unpasteurized milk products, raw eggs, undercooked meat or poultry, and raw sprouts.

Remember to document all instructions, verbal and written, in the medical record.

Sociologic and Psychological Issues

Almost every social event you attend centers around food. Food is a part of many of our traditions, such as birthdays, holidays, and family gatherings for any occasion. Eating has become entertainment for many people in our culture.

In addition to these social events, the consumption of food can also be psychological. Perhaps you remember having snacks prepared by your mother and ready for you after school or a treat such as a lollipop when you scraped your knee. Many people are what researchers call "emotional eaters." Instead of facing the stresses of everyday life, emotional eaters use food to cope. Others eat when they are happy as a form of celebration or as a reward for an accomplishment.

Food is everywhere; it is necessary for life. Experts warn that we must make some major lifestyle changes, make better food choices, and become more active to stop the growing epidemic of obesity. This starts with changing bad habits. Your role as a professional medical assistant begins with examining your own eating habits, making better choices, and becoming an example for patients who want or need to make better choices for a healthier life. Of course, understanding why people eat and how food plays a part in our social and psychological well-being is important to making any changes for better health, both for yourself and your patients.

 CHECKPOINT QUESTION

8. What are the ill effects of excess body fat?

Staying Well

Maintaining the proper body weight and consuming the right nutrients in the right amounts are necessary for good health. But, in our busy world, it is difficult to follow a rigid diet or a confining exercise regimen. With some planning and determination, though, you can make even subtle changes to improve your health and quality of life. Eating more slowly, sleeping more, and taking the stairs instead of an elevator are just a few of the things that you can do every day to make you feel better. A healthy body has a better immune system.

Stress

Although a certain amount of good stress is needed to function and thrive in everyday life, too much stress can be harmful. High stress levels are known to cause a long list of health problems. Everything from headaches to leg cramps can be indicators of too much stress. Keep lists of suggestions to manage stress in a central patient education area or waiting area of the office. During waiting times in the examination room, talk to patients about their stress levels. To lessen stress, try using some of the following techniques:

- Think positively. Look for the good in each situation instead of focusing on the bad.
- Devote at least 30 minutes of each day to an activity you truly enjoy, such as spending time with friends, reading, or pursuing a favorite hobby.
- Take a moment to calm your thoughts when faced with a situation that causes you to become angry or agitated.
- Know your limits and don't take on too many obligations.
- Get a good night's sleep.

Even leisure activity reduces stress by providing a temporary break from the everyday pressures and obligations that can make life stressful. Not only will you be better equipped to handle life's daily challenges, but you will also reduce your physical symptoms of stress. High levels of stress and its effects on the body can contribute to heart disease, ulcers, and other conditions in individuals who are **predisposed**, or genetically programmed, for such problems. Stress can also exacerbate chronic conditions, like diabetes, and have a negative impact on a person's emotional health and interpersonal relationships.

Relaxation exercises can calm you down in times of high stress. Sitting or lying comfortably with your eyes closed while imagining a quiet, peaceful place is a self-relaxation technique called **guided imagery**. Meditation is a relaxation technique that calms the mind and the body, relieving physical and emotional stress.

Pollution

Air pollution can negatively affect health. Those who live in areas with high levels of pollution might suffer from respiratory problems and general discomfort due to burning eyes or irritated throats. A number of chemicals detected in polluted air have been linked to birth defects, certain cancers, respiratory disorders, and brain damage. Accidental releases of some chemicals have been known to cause serious injury or even death.

The effects of air pollution on the environment are also problematic. Examples of harm to the environment include the destruction of trees and plants, the pollution of water, and the killing of fish and other animals. Environmental changes may result from damage to the ozone layer, increasing instances of skin cancer and eye damage.

The Clean Air Act of 1990 is a federal law that limits the amounts of certain pollutants that may be released into the air in the United States. This act is designed to provide the same basic health and environmental protection to all Americans; however, it is up to the states to regulate these levels. States may set up stricter laws concerning pollution, but they may not adopt weaker pollution controls than the federal law mandates. A federal agency, the Environmental Protection Agency (EPA), is in place to help the states meet federal regulations. The EPA conducts research and provides funding to support state programs designed to reduce air pollution.

To minimize the harmful effects of pollution, experts suggest that you avoid secondhand smoke, areas with heavy traffic, and inhaling highway fumes. When exercising outdoors, try to avoid busy roads or high-pollution areas when smog levels are high. Check air quality levels that are monitored and reported by your local news stations. Shrubbery in your yard is recommended because it protects you from breathing in pollution and dirt from the street.

Seat Belt Use and Airbags

According to the National Highway Traffic Safety Administration, it is estimated that more than 30,000 people die each year in motor vehicle accidents. Thankfully, proper seat belt use can prevent up to half of these deaths. When the front of a vehicle hits an unmoving object in an automobile accident, the car stops abruptly, but the driver and passengers do not. Momentum keeps moving their bodies forward at the same speed the vehicle was traveling until they are stopped by unmoving objects inside the vehicle, such as the dashboard, steering wheel, or windshield. The impact can cause serious, and sometimes fatal, injuries. However, properly worn seat belts prevent that second crash. Seat belts should fit snugly so the hips and shoulders suffer the greatest impact. These areas of the body can best withstand the impact of a crash. Both the lap belt and shoulder restraint are necessary for the greatest protection. The lap belt keeps the body from moving forward, and the shoulder restraint protects the head and face from coming into contact with the vehicle's dashboard or windshield.

Because a large percentage of motor vehicle deaths result from frontal impact crashes, air bags are engineered to protect passengers and drivers involved in these types of accidents. Although air bags can reduce injuries to the head and chest, they are not intended to replace seat belts. In fact, air bags make seat belts even more effective. When air bags are used in addition to lap belts and shoulder restraints, the risk of injury to the head is greatly reduced.

Distraction on the part of the driver can also be a cause of motor vehicle accidents. According to a U.S. Department of Transportation Web site that focuses on distracted drivers (http://www.distraction.gov), almost 20% of all crashes in 2008 involved a distracted driver. Distractions can occur in three forms: visual (taking your eyes off of the road), manual (taking your hands off of the steering wheel), and cognitive (taking your mind off of the task of driving). Sending text messages, for example, is one of the most dangerous activities listed because it involves all three types of distractions. Other activities that can be distracting include talking on a cell phone; eating or drinking; using a PDA (personal digital assistant) or navigation device such as a GPS (global positioning system); watching a video; or changing the radio station, CD, or MP3 player.

 CHECKPOINT QUESTION

9. What human health effects are thought to be caused by air pollution?

Dental Health

Dental health is an important part of a person's overall health (Fig. 1-6). Flossing removes plaque between and around the individual teeth reducing **dental cavities** (holes in the teeth) and promoting healthy gums. Unattended cavities have a profound effect on the gums as well as on the sinuses and the throat. There are many affordable dental products that make dental

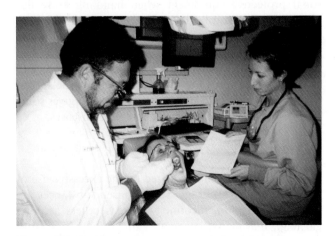

Figure 1-6 Healthy teeth promote general good health.

health simple for patients, including battery-powered toothbrushes, plastic floss holders, and tongue cleaners. Keeping teeth in good repair with regular dental check-ups promotes better general health.

Positive Mental Outlook

Having a positive mental outlook can benefit your health and well-being and possibly even prolong life. Experts say that genetics may play a part in mental attitude, but you also have control over your feelings and emotions. Maybe you cannot control certain events, but you can control your reactions to them or how you let the events affect your daily activities or interactions with others. There have been many instances of terminally ill patients who fared better than expected because they maintained a positive outlook. In almost every situation, you can identify positive and negative aspects. If you pay attention to the positive and downplay the negative, you can train your brain to have a positive attitude.

Genetics

It is undeniable that genetics determine a great deal in regard to your health. However, even if your parents suffered from ill health, there are ways of reducing your own health risks. Studies have shown that genetics play a large role in what diseases a person contracts, but patients should not use this as an excuse to ignore risk factors. Even if there has been no lung cancer in a family, tobacco use would still increase the risk. In other words, good genes can be negated by bad health habits.

Infectious Disease Prevention

Fortunately, the body is equipped with a remarkable immune system that protects a healthy person from illness or injury from most germs or pathogens. However, you can control how many of these germs enter the body by taking a few precautions. Proper handwashing is known to be the best defense against illness. Because germs must enter the body to make you sick, the hands are usually the mode of transportation. Wearing personal protective equipment when handling body fluids will protect you in the workplace. As a health care worker, you are trained to stay safe from blood-borne pathogens. These same actions should be taken at home. Using safe practices in the kitchen and bathroom will also reduce the spread of disease. Preventing the spread of infection takes care and attention. Box 1-3 gives some tips for avoiding infectious or contagious diseases.

Substance Abuse

Substance abuse is characterized by the excessive use of and dependency on drugs. Some abused substances are legal (e.g., alcohol, nicotine), whereas others are illegal (e.g., marijuana, cocaine). Patients with substance

BOX 1-3

THINGS TO DO TO PREVENT INFECTIOUS DISEASES

1. Keep immunizations up to date:
   - Follow recommended immunizations for children and adults.
   - Immunize your pets.
2. Wash your hands often, especially during cold and flu season. Be sure to wash hands:
   - After using the bathroom
   - Before preparing or eating food
   - After changing a diaper
   - After blowing your nose or sneezing or coughing
   - After caring for a sick person
   - After playing with a pet
3. Prepare and handle food carefully:
   - Keep hot foods hot and cold foods cold until eaten or cooked
   - Be sure temperature controls in refrigerators and freezers are working properly
   - Wash counters, cutting boards, and utensils frequently with soap and hot water, especially after preparing poultry and other meats
   - Wash fresh fruits and vegetables before eating
   - Cook ground beef until you can no longer see any pink
4. Use antibiotics only for infections caused by bacteria:
   - Take antibiotics exactly as prescribed and complete the full course of treatment.
   - Never self-medicate with antibiotics or share them with family or friends.
   - Report to your doctor any quickly worsening infection or any infection that does not get better after you finish a prescribed antibiotic.
5. Avoid insect bites:
   - Use insect repellents on skin and clothing when in areas where ticks or mosquitoes are common.
   - If you have visited wooded or wilderness areas and become sick, tell your doctor all the details in order to help diagnose both rare and common illnesses quickly.
6. Stay alert to disease threats when you travel or visit developing countries:
   - Get all recommended immunizations.
   - Use protective medications for travel, especially to areas with malaria.
   - Do not drink untreated water while hiking or camping.
   - If you become ill when you return home, tell your doctor where you've been.

7. Develop healthy habits:

- Eat well, get enough sleep, exercise, and avoid tobacco and illegal drug use.
- When sick, allow yourself time to heal and recover.
- Be courteous to others: wash your hands frequently, and cover your mouth when you sneeze or cough.

Source: Epidemiology and Disease Control and Prevention http://www.edcp.org/factsheets/prevent.cfm.

abuse problems may seek help from trained specialists or counselors or they may come to the physician office seeking help with their dependency issue. Because substance abuse can be highly detrimental to your patients' health, it is important that you have information available about substance abuse available for patients who may have a substance abuse problem. Although many national organizations can provide information, your medical office should also have information available for patients on any local chapters or organizations that may help these patients.

Alcohol

Alcohol is one of the most commonly abused legal substances. Although there have been studies done that link a daily glass of red wine to a potential reduced risk for heart disease, overconsumption of alcohol can contribute to certain health problems. These problems include high blood pressure, cardiomyopathy, fetal alcohol syndrome, and, in some cases of long-term alcohol abuse, possible liver damage.

Some people can drink in moderation. Others are prone to addiction, which is an illness and should be treated as such. Because alcohol contains ethanol, it is considered a mind-altering substance. Ethanol works as a depressant within the central nervous system. The effects of alcohol intoxication include a lack of coordination, slurred speech, blurred vision, and impaired brain function. Large quantities of alcohol can have a negative effect on such basic functions as breathing and heart rate. The long-term effects of excessive alcohol use can include cirrhosis of the liver, certain cancers, an increased risk of stroke, and nutritional deficiencies.

Drugs

Some drugs, like marijuana and hashish, impair short-term memory and comprehension. In addition to altering the user's sense of time and reducing the ability to perform tasks requiring concentration and coordination, these drugs also increase the heart rate and appetite. Long-term users may develop psychological dependence. Because these drugs are inhaled as unfiltered smoke, users take in more cancer-causing agents and do more damage to the respiratory system than with regular filtered tobacco smoke.

Cocaine and crack cocaine are extremely addictive. These illegal drugs stimulate the central nervous system. Crack cocaine is particularly dangerous because this pure form of cocaine is usually smoked and absorbed rapidly in the bloodstream. Use of these drugs can result in psychological and physical dependency and may even cause sudden death. The physical effects of using these substances include dilated pupils, increased pulse rate, elevated blood pressure, insomnia, loss of appetite, paranoia, and seizures. It can also cause death by disrupting the brain's control of the heart and respiration.

Stimulants and amphetamines can have the same effect as cocaine, causing increased heart rate and blood pressure. Symptoms of stimulant use include dizziness, sleeplessness, anxiety, psychosis, hallucinations, paranoia, and even physical collapse. The long-term effects of these substances include hypertension, heart disease, stroke, and renal and liver failure.

Depressants and barbiturates can also cause physical and psychological dependence. Abuse of these drugs can lead to respiratory depression, coma, and death, especially when they are taken with alcohol. Withdrawal can lead to restlessness, insomnia, convulsions, and death.

Hallucinogens, such as lysergic acid diethylamide (LSD), phencyclidine ("angel dust" or PCP), mescaline, and peyote, all interrupt brain messages that control the intellect and keep instincts in check. Large doses can produce seizures, coma, and heart and lung failure. Chronic users complain of persistent memory problems and speech difficulties for up to a year after discontinuing use. Because hallucinogens stop the brain's pain sensors, drug experiences may result in severe self-inflicted injuries.

Narcotics, such as heroin, codeine, morphine, and opium, are addictive drugs. These drugs can produce euphoria, drowsiness, and blood pressure and pulse fluctuations. An overdose can lead to seizures, coma, cardiac arrest, and death.

It is important to teach all pregnant women the damage substance abuse may do to their unborn child and to refer pregnant patients to support services. The most important role of the medical assistant in educating patients about any type of substance abuse is to be supportive and have a list of community resources available to assist patients who need them. Provide positive reinforcements as appropriate and offer services to patients for cessation programs.

Smoking Cessation

The health risks associated with smoking have been well documented for many years. Nicotine is highly addictive whether ingested by inhaling or chewing. This drug reaches the brain in 6 seconds, damages the blood vessels, decreases heart strength, and is associated with many cancers. The withdrawal symptoms include anxiety, progressive restlessness, irritability, and sleep disturbances. There are numerous methods to try to stop smoking; however, the methods vary greatly. Some programs have the patient gradually stop, while other programs seek a total, abrupt stoppage. There are research data to support both methods.

PATIENT EDUCATION

SMOKING CESSATION REQUIRES HELP

Here are some suggestions to help patients stop smoking:

- Find local smoking cessation support groups. Provide phone numbers and contact names of these groups to your patients.
- If there are no local support groups, the American Heart Association, American Lung Association, or American Cancer Society may help.
- Discuss with the physician the options of prescribing various patches, gums, or other interventions for the patient. Some products have side effects, and the physician may opt not to order them based on the patient's age or other medical illnesses.

MEDIA MENU

- **Student Resources on thePoint**
  - **CMA/RMA Certification Exam Review**
- **Internet Resources**

  Fitness and Health Tips Today
  http://fitnesshealthtoday.com

  Body Mass Index and Other Charts
  http://www.cdc.gov/growthcharts

  Dietary Guidelines
  http://www.health.gov/dietaryguidelines

  U.S. Department of Agriculture's MyPlate Website
  http://www.ChooseMyPlate.gov

  American Running and Fitness Association
  http://www.americanrunning.org

  President's Council on Fitness, Sports & Nutrition
  http://www.fitness.gov

  American Alliance for Health, Physical Education, Recreation and Dance
  http://www.aahperd.org

  March of Dimes
  http://www.marchofdimes.com

  American Heart Association
  http://www.heart.org/HEARTORG

  American Lung Association
  http://www.lungusa.org

  Information on Alcoholism
  http://www.cdc.gov/alcohol/faqs.htm

español SPANISH TERMINOLOGY

Debes llevar una dieta balanceada. Utiliza la pirámide de alimentos como guía para ayudarte a escojer los mejores alimentos.

You should have a balanced diet. Using the food guide pyramid helps you to choose the right foods.

Voy a circular los alimentos en estas fotos que puede comer.

Using these pictures, I'll circle the foods you can have.

Estos son los alimentos que debe evitar.

These are the foods you should avoid.

Debe hacer ejercicios por lo menos tres veces a la semana.

You should exercise at least three times a week.

Asegúrese de cuidar de sus dientes.

Be sure and take care of your teeth.

PSY PROCEDURE 1-1: Teach a Patient How to Read Food Labels

Purpose: To instruct a patient in how to read a food label so that he or she may make better food choices
Equipment: Two boxes of the same item, one low calorie or "lite" and the other regular; measuring cup; two bowls; refer to Figure 1-4 for reference

Steps	Reasons
1. Identify the patient.	Correctly identifying the patient prevents errors.
2. Introduce yourself and explain the procedure.	Explaining procedures may reduce patient anxiety.
3. Have the patient look at the labels, briefly comparing the two.	Taking an overall look at the label will show the patient the types of items listed.
4. Ask the patient to pour out a normal serving into a bowl.	The patient's perception of a normal serving size may be wrong.
5. Measure the exact serving size printed on the label. Compare the two. Discuss the difference, if any. **Step 5.** Measure the exact serving size.	Using a measuring cup will show the patient the accuracy of the serving size. Serving sizes noted on package labels are often lesser amounts than what a patient might naturally consume without measuring, which would result in more calories.
6. Explain to the patient each section of the label: a. Serving size and servings per package b. Column for amount in serving c. Column for % daily value (formerly called the *recommended daily allowance [RDA]*)	The patient may be surprised that his or her servings are more or less than on the label, which changes the weights and daily values.
7. Explain calories and calories from fat. Have the patient calculate the percentage of fat calories by multiplying the grams of fat by 9 and dividing that number by the total calories per serving as listed on the label. Multiply the answer by 100. This number is the percentage of calories from fat.	Although manufacturers are required to list this information, patients should know how this is calculated.
8. Read down the label and discuss each nutrient, pointing out the amounts and percentages.	Seeing the labels will help the patient understand.
9. Have the patient compare the two labels and tell you how many total carbohydrates, sugars, and amounts of protein, etc. are on each label.	This will ensure that the patient understands how to determine the types and amounts of ingredients.
10. **AFF** Explain how to respond to a patient who has a religious or personal belief against specific food groups such as meats.	Patients with religious or personal beliefs that eliminate specific foods or food groups may need to be referred to a registered dietician as directed by the physician. Always make sure the physician is aware of any food preferences or allergies.
11. Ask the patient if he or she has any questions.	Having the patient answer your questions and giving him or her an opportunity to ask you questions will ensure the patient's comprehension of the information.

(continued)

PSY PROCEDURE 1-1:   Teach a Patient How to Read Food Labels (continued)

Steps	Reasons
12. Chart the verbal and written instructions given to the patient.	The physician and other workers in the office may need to know what the patient has been taught. Remember, if it's not in the chart, it did not happen.

Charting Example:

9/25/12 Pt. given instructions on reading a food label. Pt. verbalized understanding and eagerness to make healthier

food choices. Instructed to call the office for any questions or concerns. ———————————————— C. Parent, CMA

Note: The medical assistant may sign his/her name in the patient record using only the "CMA" credential if the office has a signature log denoting the entire credential as "CMA(AAMA)."

- Good nutrition and a healthy lifestyle are important to everyone. Knowing the guidelines for a healthy and safe life is important, but practicing those guidelines is essential.
- There is a growing trend in the United States toward obesity, especially among children and young people. The federal government is working to reverse this trend.
- Following the recommendations of the physician will give your patients a better chance at good health and longevity.
- There are ways to stay as safe and healthy, even during daily activities like driving a car. Medical assistants should be prepared to teach these safe and healthy living habits.

- The same safe practices for reducing the spread of disease in the health care workplace, such as handwashing, can be used at home to keep you, your family, and your patients safe from pathogens and infectious diseases.
- To increase chances of good health, patients should be encouraged to limit or avoid harmful substances such as nicotine, alcohol, and drugs.
- Knowing the benefits of good nutrition, physical fitness, and applying suggestions for staying safe and healthy will give patients a good foundation for making the right choices in life.

Warm Ups for Critical Thinking

1. The physician asks you to assist a 65-year-old patient with a low-cholesterol diet. Write a plan for the instruction. Help her plan several sample meals to help get her started. What would you say to her?
2. A 12-year-old boy presents for his routine yearly physical. His current weight is 150 pounds, and his growth chart indicates a steady increase in body weight. Explain the dangers of obesity to the patient's mother. Go to http://www.cdc.gov, search for body mass index, and click on the BMI calculator. Enter the information to complete a BMI chart for the patient with the following measurements: 5 feet, 5 inches tall, 150 pounds, date of birth 5/28/1994.
3. Keep track of all of the food that you consume over a 24-hour period. Calculate your total fat and total carbohydrate intake. Do your meals follow the MyPlate guidelines? If not, what do you need to do to improve your nutritional status? Using pictures from magazines, create well-balanced breakfast, lunch, and dinner plates. Hint: Your plate should be colorful.

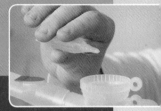

 CHAPTER

2 Medical Asepsis and Infection Control

Outline

Microorganisms, Pathogens, and Normal Flora
Conditions That Favor the Growth of Pathogens
The Infection Cycle
Modes of Transmission
Principles of Infection Control

Medical Asepsis
Levels of Infection Control
Infection Control for the Medical Office
Exposure Risk Factors and the Exposure Control Plan
Standard Precautions

Personal Protective Equipment
Handling Environmental Contamination
Disposing of Infectious Waste
Hepatitis B and Human Immunodeficiency Viruses

Learning Outcomes

Cognitive Domain

Note: AAMA/CAAHEP 2008 Standards are italicized.

1. Spell and define key terms
2. *Describe the infection cycle, including the infectious agent, reservoir, susceptible host, means of transmission, portals of entry, and portals of exit*
3. *List major types of infectious agents*
4. *Compare different methods of controlling the growth of microorganisms*
5. *Discuss infection control procedures*
6. *List the various ways microbes are transmitted*
7. *Differentiate between medical and surgical asepsis used in ambulatory care settings, identifying when each is appropriate*
8. *Compare the effectiveness in reducing or destroying microorganisms using the various levels of infection control*
9. *Identify personal safety precautions as established by the Occupational Safety and Health Administration (OSHA)*
10. *Match types and uses of personal protective equipment (PPE)*
11. *Describe standard precautions, including transmission-based, purpose, and activities-regulated precautions*

12. *Discuss the application of standard precautions with regard to a. all body fluids, secretions, and excretions; b. blood; c. non-intact skin; and d. mucous membranes*
13. List the required components of an exposure control plan
14. Explain the facts pertaining to the transmission and prevention of the hepatitis B virus and the human immunodeficiency virus in the medical office
15. *Identify the role of the Centers for Disease Control (CDC) regulations in health care settings*

Psychomotor Domain

Note: AAMA/CAAHEP 2008 Standards are italicized.

1. *Participate in training on standard precautions*
2. Perform a medical aseptic handwashing procedure (Procedure 2-1)
3. Remove contaminated gloves (Procedure 2-2)
4. Clean and decontaminate biohazardous spills (Procedure 2-3)
5. *Apply local, state, and federal health care legislation and regulations appropriate to the medical assisting practice setting*

6. *Select appropriate barriers/PPE for potentially infectious situations*

Affective Domain

Note: AAMA/CAAHEP 2008 Standards are italicized.

1. *Explain the rationale for performance of a procedure to the patient*

2. *Apply critical thinking skills in performing patient assessment and care*

ABHES Competencies

1. Apply principles of aseptic techniques and infection control
2. Use standard precautions
3. Dispose of biohazardous materials

Key Terms

aerobe	disinfection	Occupational Safety and Health Administration (OSHA)	sanitation
anaerobe	exposure control plan		sanitization
asymptomatic	exposure risk factor		spores
bactericidal	germicide		standard precautions
biohazardous	immunization	pathogens	sterilization
carriers	infection	personal protective equipment (PPE)	transient flora
Centers for Disease Control and Prevention (CDC)	medical asepsis	postexposure testing	vector
	microorganisms	resident flora	viable
disease	normal flora	resistance	virulent

Many patients are seen daily in the medical office for a variety of reasons, including physical examinations for employment, reassurance about a current health problem, and follow-up care for a chronic condition or surgical procedure. In addition, many patients request appointments because of illness. It is important for you to protect patients from each other with regard to contagious diseases and for you to protect yourself from acquiring the many microorganisms with which you will come into contact every day.

To prevent the spread of **disease** in the medical office, medical assistants must meet two goals. First, you must understand and practice **medical asepsis** at all times, using specific practices and procedures to prevent disease transmission. These practices and procedures also allow you to work with ill patients while reducing the chances that you will spread disease to other patients or become infected yourself. Second, you must teach the patients and their families about techniques to use at home to prevent the transmission of disease. Handwashing, the cornerstone of infection control, is discussed in this chapter and is emphasized in all subsequent chapters wherever contact with infectious material might be expected.

In addition, this chapter describes how disease is transmitted and, most important, how to prevent the spread of disease.

COG Microorganisms, Pathogens, and Normal Flora

Microorganisms, living organisms that can be seen only with a microscope, are part of our normal environment. In addition to our physical environment, many microorganisms can be found on your skin and throughout your gastrointestinal, genitourinary, and respiratory systems, and some of these are required for good health. These microorganisms are normal and are referred to as **normal flora** or **resident flora**. Some microorganisms, however, are not part of the normal flora and may cause disease or **infection**. Disease-producing microorganisms are referred to as **pathogens** and are classified as bacteria, viruses, fungi, or protozoa. (Refer to Chapter 29 for a more detailed discussion of microorganisms.)

When normal flora become too many in number or are transmitted to an area of the body in which they are not normally found, they are referred to as transient flora, which can become pathogens under the right conditions. For example, *Staphylococcus aureus*, a microorganism commonly found on the skin, may get into underlying tissue if the skin is broken. In this situation, the normal flora of the skin has become transient flora and may cause disease. Decreased **resistance** in the host is one condition that may allow transient flora to become pathogenic. Individuals who are elderly, receiving certain drugs to treat cancer, or under unusual stress may have a lowered resistance and be particularly susceptible to infections.

Although the body is protected by many nonspecific defenses against disease, infection or illness may occur if the natural barriers are overpowered or breached. The following are some of the body's natural defenses that may prevent the invasion of pathogens into various body organs:

- Skin. As long as the skin is kept clean and remains intact or unbroken, staphylococcal (Staph) bacteria are not considered dangerous. Washing the skin frequently will flush away many of these bacteria along with any other microorganisms.
- Eyes. The eyelashes act as a barrier by trapping dust that may carry microorganisms before they have an opportunity to enter the eye. If any microorganisms do enter the eye, the enzyme lysozyme normally found in tears will destroy some microorganisms, including bacteria.
- Mouth. The greatest variety of microorganisms in the body is in the mouth. Saliva is slightly **bactericidal**, and good oral hygiene will remove or prevent the growth of many of the pathogens in the mouth.
- Gastrointestinal tract. Hydrochloric acid normally found in the stomach destroys most of the disease-producing pathogens that enter the gastrointestinal system. One bacterium, *Escherichia coli*, is resident flora found in the large intestine and is necessary for digestion. It does not usually cause disease as long it remains within the gastrointestinal tract. *Helicobacter pylori* also reside in the digestive tracts of some individuals and may cause gastric ulcers.
- Respiratory tract. Hairs and cilia on the membrane lining of the nostrils are early defenses against airborne microorganisms. If these physical barriers do not stop an invasion, mucus from the membranes lining the respiratory tract should trap the microorganisms and facilitate their removal from the respiratory system as the person swallows, coughs, or sneezes.
- Genitourinary tract. The reproductive and urinary systems provide a less hospitable environment for microorganisms. The slightly acidic environment of these body systems reduces the ability of many microorganisms to survive. In addition, frequent urination flushes the urinary tract and removes many transient microorganisms.

Although these systems have protective mechanisms to prevent infection, any of them may be overpowered by a particularly **virulent** organism. Transient flora is not usually pathogenic unless the person's defenses are compromised by a decrease in resistance.

 CHECKPOINT QUESTION

1. What are pathogenic microorganisms? How does the body prevent an invasion and subsequent infection naturally?

Conditions That Favor the Growth of Pathogens

All microorganisms require certain conditions to grow and reproduce. To reduce the number of microorganisms and potential pathogens in a clinical setting, you must eliminate as many of their life requirements as possible. These requirements include the following:

- Moisture. Few microorganisms can survive with little water or moisture. However, some microorganisms form **spores** and remain dormant until moisture is available.
- Nutrients. Microorganisms depend on their environment for nourishment. Surfaces (tables, counters, equipment, etc.) that are contaminated with organic matter (food products, body fluids, or tissue) promote the growth of microorganisms.
- Temperature. Although some microorganisms can survive even in freezing or boiling temperatures, those that thrive at a normal body temperature of 98.6°F are most likely to be pathogenic to humans. Many microorganisms that leave an infected person can survive for awhile at room temperature; therefore, surfaces that are contaminated with dried organic material should be considered possibly pathogenic.
- Darkness. Many pathogenic bacteria are destroyed by bright light, including sunlight.
- Neutral pH. The pH of a solution refers to the measurement of its acid-base balance on a scale of 1 to 14, with 7 being neutral. Many microorganisms are destroyed in an environment that is not neutral. The pH of blood (7.35–7.45) is preferred by microorganisms that thrive in the human body.
- Oxygen. Microorganisms that need oxygen to survive are called **aerobes**. A few, however, do not require oxygen; these are called **anaerobes**. Although most pathogens are aerobic, the microbes that cause tetanus and botulism are anaerobic.

If any one of these conditions is altered in any way, the growth and reproduction of the pathogen will be affected. Your role as a professional medical assistant in a medical office includes using this knowledge of microbial growth to inhibit the growth and reproduction of microorganisms in the office.

 CHECKPOINT QUESTION

2. Given the six conditions that favor the growth of pathogens, explain how you can alter the growth and reproduction of microorganisms by changing these factors.

COG The Infection Cycle

The infection cycle is often thought of as a series of specific links of a chain involving a causative agent or invading microorganism (Fig. 2-1). The first link in the chain is the reservoir host; this is the person who is infected with the microorganism. Although this person may or may not show signs of infection, his or her body is serving as a source of nutrients and an incubator in which the pathogen can grow and reproduce. These persons are also called **carriers**, or reservoirs, of disease.

The reservoir host may transmit disease only when the pathogen has a means of exit. The second link in the chain is the manner in which the pathogen leaves the reservoir host. Means of exit include the mucous membranes of the nose and mouth, the openings of the gastrointestinal system (mouth or rectum), and an open wound.

In addition to the means of exit, the microbe must have a vehicle in which to leave the host. This next link in the chain, the means of transmission, involves the vehicle that is used by the pathogen when it leaves the reservoir host and spreads through the environment. Vehicles include mucus or air droplets from the oral or nasal cavities and direct contact between an unclean hand and another person or object. Sneezing and coughing without covering the nose and mouth are excellent methods of transmitting microorganisms into the environment and potential hosts.

The fourth link in the chain of the infectious process cycle is the portal of entry. This is the route by which the pathogen enters the next host. With inhalation of contaminated air droplets, the respiratory system is the portal of entry. Another portal of entry is the gastrointestinal system: the pathogen enters the body in contaminated food or drink. Any break in the skin or mucous membranes can be a portal of entry for pathogenic microorganisms.

The final link in the infectious process cycle is the susceptible host (Box 2-1). This host is one to whom the pathogen is transmitted after leaving the reservoir host. If the conditions in the susceptible host are conducive to reproduction of the pathogen, the susceptible host becomes a reservoir host and the cycle repeats.

 CHECKPOINT QUESTION

3. How are the first and fifth links of the infection cycle related?

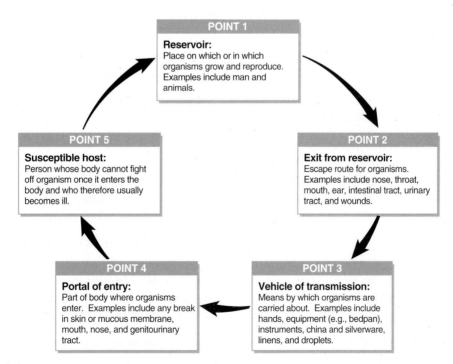

Figure 2-1 The infectious process cycle. Infections and infectious diseases are spread by starting from the reservoir (point 1) and moving in a circle to the susceptible host (point 5). Microorganisms can be controlled by interfering at any point in the cycle.

BOX 2-1

THE SUSCEPTIBLE HOST

The susceptible host is unable to resist the invading pathogens for a variety of reasons:

- *Age.* As the body ages, defense mechanisms begin to lose their effectiveness. The immune system is no longer as active or as efficient as in youth. The immune system may also not be fully functional in the very young.
- *Existing disease.* The stress of an existing illness may deplete the immune system and allow microorganisms to cause illness in someone who might otherwise be able to fight it naturally.
- *Poor nutrition.* A diet deficient in nutrients such as proteins, carbohydrates, fats, vitamins, or minerals will not allow cells of the body to repair or reproduce as they are weakened by disease.
- *Poor hygiene.* Although multitudes of microbes exist on our skin, keeping the numbers down by practicing good hygiene will reduce the numbers of pathogens.

Modes of Transmission

In the third link of the infectious process cycle, the vehicle that spreads the microorganism is often called the mode of transmission. It is important for you to understand the mode of transmission used by various pathogens so that you can break this link in the infectious cycle and prevent the spread of disease.

Direct Transmission

Direct contact between the infected reservoir host and the susceptible host produces direct transmission. Direct transmission may occur when one touches contaminated blood or body fluids, shakes hands with someone who has contaminated hands, inhales infected air droplets, or has intimate contact, such as kissing or sexual intercourse, with someone who is contaminated.

Indirect Transmission

Indirect transmission may occur through contact with a vehicle known as a **vector**. Vectors include contaminated food or water, disease-carrying insects, and inanimate objects such as soil, drinking glasses, wound drainage, and infected or improperly disinfected medical instruments. While visible blood and body fluids are obvious sources of infection, many infectious organisms remain **viable** for long periods on inanimate surfaces that are not visibly contaminated.

Sources of Transmission

Most reservoir hosts are humans, animals, and insects. Human hosts include people who are ill with an infectious disease, people who are carriers of an infectious disease, and people who are incubating an infectious disease but are not exhibiting symptoms. This last group can transmit disease even though they are ambulatory and **asymptomatic** (have no symptoms). Animal sources, which are less common, include infected dogs, cats, birds, cattle, rodents, and animals that live in the wild. Diseases that may be transmitted to humans from infected animals include anthrax and rabies.

In addition to flies and roaches, which carry many diseases, other insect sources feed on the blood of an infected reservoir host and then pass the disease to another victim or susceptible host. Ticks and mosquitoes may transmit diseases, including Lyme disease (ticks) and malaria (mosquitoes). Table 2-1 lists some common diseases and their methods of transmission.

 CHECKPOINT QUESTION

4. The medical office where you work has a policy about not opening windows that do not have screens in examination rooms and the reception area. Why do you think this policy is or is not important?

COG Principles of Infection Control

Most transmission of infectious disease in the medical office can be prevented by strict adherence to guidelines issued by the **Occupational Safety and Health Administration (OSHA)** and the **Centers for Disease Control and Prevention (CDC)**. While most medical assistants take extraordinary precautions when dealing with patients who are known carriers of infectious microorganisms, you may also treat an estimated five unknown carriers for each patient known to be infectious. Therefore, knowledge and use of effective infection control in relation to all patients is essential.

Medical Asepsis

Medical asepsis does not mean that an object or area is free from all microorganisms. It refers to practices that render an object or area free from pathogenic microorganisms. Commonly known as clean technique, medical asepsis prevents the transmission of microorganisms from one person or area to any other within the medical office (Box 2-2).

Handwashing is the most important medical aseptic technique to prevent the transmission of pathogens.

TABLE 2-1	Common Communicable Diseases
Disease	**Method of Transmission**
AIDS	Contact, or contact with contaminated sharps
Chicken pox (varicella)	Direct contact or droplets
Cholera	Ingestion of contaminated food or water
Diphtheria	Airborne droplets, infected carriers
Hepatitis B	Direct contact with infectious body fluid
Influenza	Airborne droplets, infected carriers or direct contact with contaminated articles such as used tissues
Measles (rubeola)	Airborne droplets, infected carriers
Meningitis	Airborne droplets
Mononucleosis	Airborne droplets or contact with infected saliva
Mumps	Airborne droplets, infected carriers, or direct contact with materials contaminated with infected saliva
Pneumonia	Airborne droplets or direct contact with infected mucus
Rabies	Direct contact with saliva of infected animal such as an animal bite
Rubella (German measles)	Airborne droplets, infected carriers
Tetanus	Direct contact with spores or contaminated animal feces
Tuberculosis	Airborne droplets, infected carriers

The proper procedure for washing your hands is detailed in Procedure 2-1. Always wash your hands:

- Before and after every patient contact
- After coming into contact with any blood or body fluids
- After coming into contact with contaminated material
- After handling specimens
- After coughing, sneezing, or blowing your nose
- After using the restroom
- Before and after going to lunch, taking breaks, and leaving for the day

Because you should always assume that blood and body fluids are contaminated with pathogens, you should wear gloves when handling any specimens or when contact with contaminated material is anticipated. However, wearing gloves does not replace handwashing! In fact, your hands should be washed before you apply gloves and after you remove them in all situations to prevent disease transmission.

Other medical aseptic techniques include general cleaning of the office, including the examination and treatment rooms, waiting or reception area, and clinical work areas. Floors are always considered contaminated, and dust and dirt are vehicles for transmission of microorganisms and should be regularly cleaned from all surfaces, including the floor. In addition, you should teach patients and their caregivers proper medical aseptic techniques for use in the home to prevent the spread of disease.

BOX 2-2

GUIDELINES FOR MAINTAINING MEDICAL ASEPSIS

- Avoid touching your clothing with soiled linen, table paper, supplies, or instruments. Roll used table paper or linens inward with the clean surface outward.
- Always consider the floor to be contaminated. Any item dropped onto the floor must be considered dirty and be discarded or cleaned to its former level of asepsis before being used.
- Clean tables, counters, and other surfaces frequently and immediately after contamination. Clean areas are less likely than dirty ones to harbor microorganisms or encourage their growth.
- Always presume that blood and body fluids from any source are contaminated. Follow the guidelines published by OSHA and the CDC to protect yourself and to prevent the transmission of disease.

 CHECKPOINT QUESTION

5. Explain why wearing examination gloves does not replace handwashing.

AFF PATIENT EDUCATION

BASIC ASEPTIC TECHNIQUE

While performing procedures, take the opportunity to instruct your patients in basic aseptic techniques they can use at home to reduce the spread of disease.

- *Handwashing*. This routine aseptic technique is particularly important for patients and families in preventing the spread of disease. Instruct patients to wash their hands before and after eating meals; after sneezing, coughing, or blowing the nose; after using the bathroom; before and after changing a dressing; and after changing diapers.
- *Use tissue*. Explain to patients with respiratory symptoms that using a disposable tissue to cover the mouth and nose when coughing and sneezing decreases the potential to transmit the illness throughout the household. In addition, immediate and proper disposal of the used tissue is essential to prevent the spread of infection.
- *Changing bandages*. Patients and family members who change dressings on wounds should be instructed in the proper procedure for using sterile dressings and clean bandages. Always demonstrate the procedure for the patient and have the patient or family member return the demonstration to ensure their understanding.
- *Sanitation*. Explain the proper techniques for disposing of waste from members of the household with communicable diseases. If in doubt, consult the local public health department for guidelines.

Levels of Infection Control

Sterilization, the highest level of infection control, destroys all forms of microorganisms, including spores, on inanimate surfaces. Sterilization methods include exposing the articles to various conditions, including steam under pressure in an autoclave; specific gases, such as ethylene oxide; dry heat ovens; and immersion in an approved chemical sterilizing agent (see Chapter 6 for a more complete discussion of sterilization techniques). Instruments or devices that penetrate the skin or come into contact with areas of the body considered sterile, such as the urinary bladder, must be sterilized using one of these methods. To save time, many medical offices use disposable sterile supplies and equipment to eliminate the need for manual sterilization (Fig. 2-2).

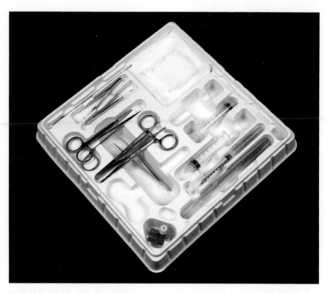

Figure 2-2 Equipment that must be sterile includes items that will penetrate the skin or come into contact with surgical incisions, such as surgical instruments. These items are disposable and meant for one-time use only.

The next highest level of infection control is **disinfection**. Disinfectants or germicides inactivate virtually all recognized pathogenic microorganisms except spores on inanimate objects. There are three levels of disinfection—high, intermediate, and low. Each is described in more detail in the following section.

The lowest level of infection control is **sanitization**, which is cleaning any visible contaminants from the item using soap or detergent, water, and manual friction.

Sanitation

Most instruments, equipment, and supplies used in medical offices must be sanitized regularly according to the recommendations of the manufacturer. **Sanitation** is the maintenance of a healthful, disease-free, and hazard-free environment. Sanitation often involves sanitization procedures that reduce the number of microorganisms on an inanimate object to a safe or relatively safe level. This is accomplished by thoroughly cleaning items such as instruments and equipment with warm, soapy water with mechanical action to remove organic matter and other residue. Cleaning or sanitizing must precede disinfection and sterilization.

Disinfection

Disinfectants, or germicides, inactivate virtually all recognized pathogenic microorganisms but not necessarily all microbial forms, including spores, on inanimate objects. The following factors may affect disinfection:

- Prior cleaning of the object. Equipment and supplies that have been sanitized first are more effectively disinfected.

- The amount of organic material on the object. The more organic matter, such as blood or body tissues, on the item, the more disinfectant agent you must use.
- The type of microbial contamination. All blood and body fluids should be considered contaminated with blood-borne pathogens such as hepatitis B virus (HBV) and human immunodeficiency virus (HIV).
- The concentration of the **germicide** or chemical disinfectant that kills pathogens. Disinfectants diluted with water are relatively ineffective at killing microbes.
- The length of exposure to the germicide. The longer the disinfectant comes into contact with the contaminated object, the more thorough disinfection is likely to be.
- The shape or complexity of the object being disinfected. Objects that have rough edges, corners, or otherwise difficult-to-clean areas may require special techniques to disinfect all surfaces.
- The temperature of the process. Most disinfectants work adequately at room temperature.

Disinfection is categorized into three levels—high, intermediate, and low. High-level disinfection destroys most forms of microbial life except certain bacterial spores. This level of infection control, which is slightly less effective than sterilization, is commonly used to clean reusable instruments that come into contact with mucous membrane–lined body cavities that are not considered sterile, such as the vagina and the rectum. Methods of high-level disinfection include immersion in boiling water for 30 minutes (rarely used in the medical office) and immersion in an approved disinfecting chemical, such as glutaraldehyde or isopropyl alcohol for 45 minutes or according to the guidelines in the disinfectant label.

Intermediate-level disinfection destroys many viruses, fungi, and some bacteria, including *Mycobacterium tuberculosis*, the bacterium that causes tuberculosis. However, intermediate disinfection does not kill bacterial spores. Intermediate disinfection is used for surfaces and instruments that come into contact with unbroken skin surfaces, including stethoscopes, blood pressure cuffs, and splints. Commercial chemical germicides that kill *M. tuberculosis* and solutions containing a 1:10 dilution of household bleach (2 oz of chlorine bleach per quart of tap water) are effective intermediate disinfectants.

Low-level disinfection destroys many bacteria and some viruses, but not *M. tuberculosis* or bacterial spores. This type of disinfection is adequate in the medical office for routine cleaning and removing surface debris when no visible blood or body fluids are on the items being disinfected. Disinfectants without tuberculocidal properties are used for low-level disinfection (Fig. 2-3). Table 2-2 describes disinfection methods, uses, and precautions of various chemicals.

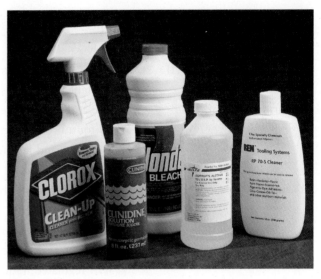

Figure 2-3 These products destroy many pathogenic microorganisms if used correctly.

 CHECKPOINT QUESTION

6. What level of disinfection would you use to clean a reusable instrument that comes into contact with the vaginal mucosa, such as a vaginal speculum? Why?

COG Infection Control for the Medical Office

OSHA is the federal agency responsible for ensuring the safety of all workers, including those in health care. OSHA promulgates and enforces federal regulations that must be followed by all medical offices. The practices of individual offices regarding employees' health and safety must be either put into a policy and procedure manual or compiled separately as an infection control manual. Regardless of where the office policies are kept, however, they must be readily available to both employees of the medical office and OSHA representatives.

Exposure Risk Factors and the Exposure Control Plan

Medical offices must provide clear instructions in the policy or infection control manual for preventing employee exposure and reducing the danger of exposure to biohazardous materials. The **exposure risk factor** for each worker by job description must be included in the written policy. It is based on the employee's risk of exposure to communicable disease. Administrative medical assistants have a low exposure risk and require

TABLE 2-2	Disinfection Methods
Method	**Uses and Precautions**
Alcohol (70% isopropyl)	Used for noncritical items (countertops, glass thermometers, stethoscopes)
	Flammable; damages some rubber, plastic, and lenses
Chlorine (sodium hypochlorite or bleach)	Dilute 1:10 (1 part bleach to 10 parts water)
	Used for a broad spectrum of microbes
	Inexpensive and fast acting
	Corrosive, inactivated by organic matter, relatively unstable
Formaldehyde	Disinfectant and sterilant
	Regulated by OSHA
	Warnings must be marked on all containers and storage areas
Glutaraldehyde	Alkaline or acid. Effective against bacteria, viruses, fungi, and some spores
	OSHA regulated; requires adequate ventilation, covered pans, gloves, masks; must display biohazard or chemical label
Hydrogen peroxide	Stable and effective when used on inanimate objects
	Attacks membrane lipids, DNA, and other essential cell components
	Can damage plastic, rubber, and some metals
Iodine or iodophors	Bacteriostatic agent
	Not to be used on instruments
	May cause staining
Phenols (tuberculocidal)	Used for environmental items and equipment
	Requires gloves and eye protection
	Can cause skin irritation and burns

DNA, deoxyribonucleic acid.

only minimal protection to perform the duties associated with that position. However, clinical medical assistants have a higher exposure risk and require access to a variety of **personal protective equipment (PPE)**, such as gloves, goggles, and/or face shields depending on the task at hand, and **immunization** against hepatitis B at no charge to the employee. The medical office must provide the appropriate equipment and supplies as outlined in this office policy according to OSHA.

Another written policy required by OSHA for offices with 10 or more employees is the **exposure control plan**. The medical office must have a written plan of action for all employees and visitors who may be exposed to **biohazardous** material despite all precautions. In the event of an exposure, you must first apply the principles of first aid and notify your immediate supervisor, office manager, or the office physician. The physician or supervisor should provide guidance regarding **post-exposure testing** and follow-up procedures. Next, you should complete and file an incident report (or exposure report) form explaining the circumstances surrounding the exposure. This report form not only documents

the incident, but also allows management to establish a policy to prevent this type of exposure in the future. In addition, the employer must record the exposure on an OSHA 300 log (Fig. 2-4) and report the exposure to OSHA if one or more of the following criteria are present:

- The work-related exposure resulted in loss of consciousness or necessitated a transfer to another job.
- The exposure resulted in a recommendation for medical treatment, such as vaccination or medication to prevent complications.
- The exposure resulted in the conversion of a negative blood test for a contagious disease into a positive blood test in the employee who was exposed.

Box 2-3 describes biohazard and safety equipment commonly used in medical offices.

 CHECKPOINT QUESTION

7. Explain the difference between exposure risk factors and the exposure control plan.

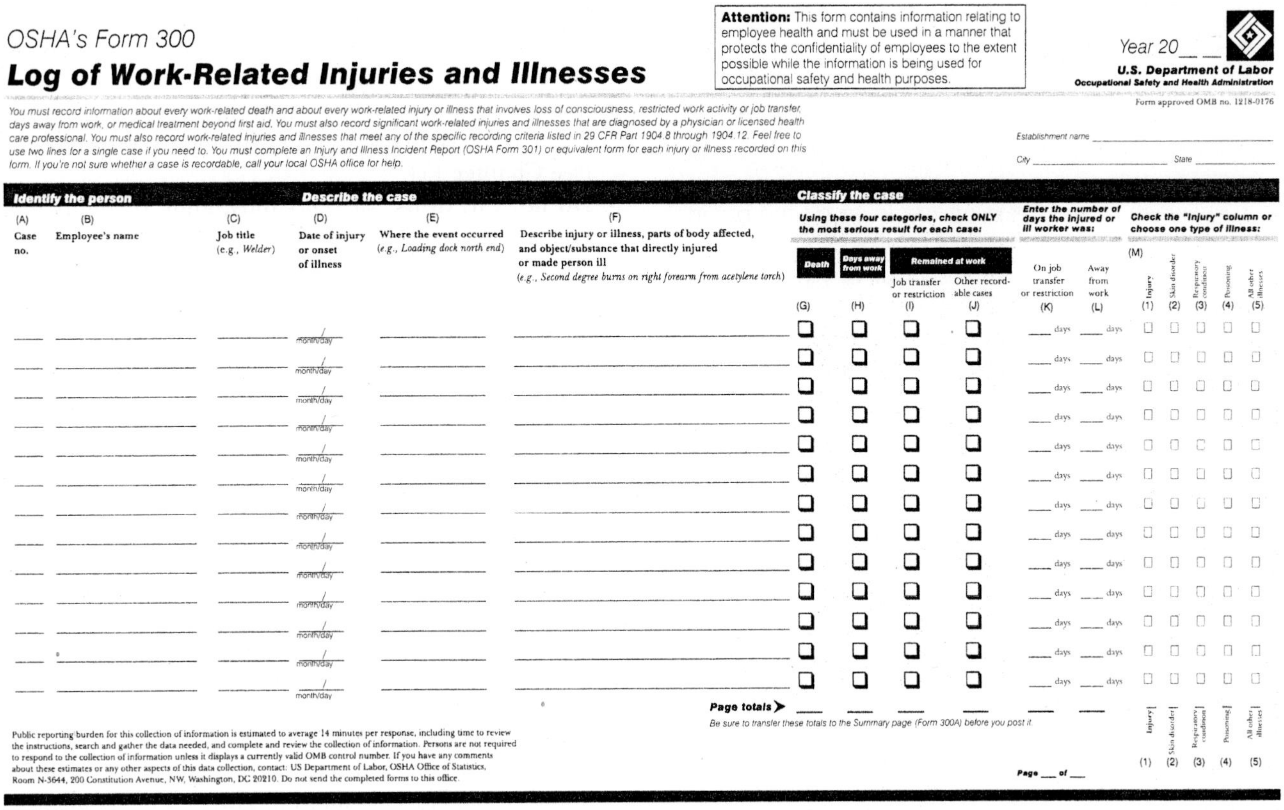

OSHA's Form 300

Log of Work-Related Injuries and Illnesses

Attention: This form contains information relating to employee health and must be used in a manner that protects the confidentiality of employees to the extent possible while the information is being used for occupational safety and health purposes.

Year 20___

U.S. Department of Labor
Occupational Safety and Health Administration

Form approved OMB no. 1218-0176

You must record information about every work-related death and about every work-related injury or illness that involves loss of consciousness, restricted work activity or job transfer, days away from work, or medical treatment beyond first aid. You must also record significant work-related injuries and illnesses that are diagnosed by a physician or licensed health care professional. You must also record work-related injuries and illnesses that meet any of the specific recording criteria listed in 29 CFR Part 1904.8 through 1904.12. Feel free to use two lines for a single case if you need to. You must complete an Injury and Illness Incident Report (OSHA Form 301) or equivalent form for each injury or illness recorded on this form. If you're not sure whether a case is recordable, call your local OSHA office for help.

Establishment name ____________

City ____________ State ____________

Identify the person | **Describe the case** | **Classify the case**

(A) Case no.

(B) Employee's name

(C) Job title (e.g., *Welder*)

(D) Date of injury or onset of illness — month/day

(E) Where the event occurred (*e.g., Loading dock north end*)

(F) Describe injury or illness, parts of body affected, and object/substance that directly injured or made person ill (*e.g., Second degree burns on right forearm from acetylene torch*)

Using these four categories, check ONLY the most serious result for each case:

(G) Death

(H) Days away from work

Remained at work: (I) Job transfer or restriction; (J) Other recordable cases

Enter the number of days the injured or ill worker was:

(K) On job transfer or restriction ___ days

(L) Away from work ___ days

Check the "Injury" column or choose one type of illness:

(M) (1) Injury (2) Skin disorder (3) Respiratory condition (4) Poisoning (5) All other illnesses

Page totals ➤

Be sure to transfer these totals to the Summary page (Form 300A) before you post it.

Injury (1) Skin disorder (2) Respiratory condition (3) Poisoning (4) All other illnesses (5)

Page ___ of ___

Public reporting burden for this collection of information is estimated to average 14 minutes per response, including time to review the instructions, search and gather the data needed, and complete and review the collection of information. Persons are not required to respond to the collection of information unless it displays a currently valid OMB control number. If you have any comments about these estimates or any other aspects of this data collection, contact: US Department of Labor, OSHA Office of Statistics, Room N-3644, 200 Constitution Avenue, NW, Washington, DC 20210. Do not send the completed forms to this office.

Figure 2-4 The OSHA 300 Log form. (Courtesy of the U.S. Department of Labor.)

LEGAL TIP

BLOOD-BORNE PATHOGEN STANDARD TRAINING

According to OSHA, health care facilities, including physician offices, must provide training to newly hired employees who will be exposed to blood or other possibly infectious material while caring for patients. This training must be repeated yearly and include any new issues or policies recommended by OSHA, the CDC, the Department of Health and Human Services, or the U.S. Public Health Service. The following items must be included in the training:

- A description of blood-borne diseases, including the transmission and symptoms
- PPE available to the employee and the location of the PPE in the medical office
- Information about the risks of contracting hepatitis B and about the HBV vaccine
- The exposure control plan and postexposure procedures, including follow-up care, in the event of an exposure

BOX 2-3

BIOHAZARD AND SAFETY EQUIPMENT IN THE MEDICAL OFFICE

- *MSDS binder.* Material safety data sheets (MSDS) are forms prepared by the manufacturers of all chemical substances used in the medical office. The binder should contain sheets for all chemicals used in the office. Each sheet describes how to handle and dispose of the chemical and, most important, the health hazards of the chemical and safety equipment needed when using it.
- *Biohazard waste containers.* Only waste contaminated with blood or body fluids or other potentially infectious material (OPIM) should be placed in biohazard waste containers. Sharps containers are used for disposal of items that have the potential to puncture or cut the skin.
- *Personal protective equipment.* Employers are required to provide PPE appropriate to the risk of exposure. For example, employees who may come into contact with blood, such as the clinical medical assistant giving an injection, need to

(continued)

BOX 2-3 *(continued)*

be protected only by wearing gloves. However, situations that may cause a splash or splatter of blood require full coverage of the skin, eyes, and clothing.

- *Eyewash basin.* Pressing the lever on the basin and turning on the faucets produces a stream of water that forces open the caps of the eyewash basin. To remove contaminants or chemicals from the eyes, lower your face into the stream and continue to wash the area until the eyes are clear or for the amount of time recommended on the MSDS.
- *Immunization.* Employers are required by OSHA to provide immunization against blood-borne pathogens if vaccines are available.

Standard Precautions

Standard precautions are a set of procedures recognized by the CDC to reduce the chance of transmitting infectious microorganisms in any health care setting, including medical offices. By presuming that all blood and body fluids, except perspiration, are contaminated and by following these precautions, you can protect yourself and prevent the spread of disease. Specifically, these precautions pertain to contact with blood, all body fluids except sweat, damaged skin, and mucous membranes and require that you:

- Wash your hands with soap and water after touching blood, body fluids, secretions, and other contaminated items, whether you have worn gloves or not.
- Use an alcohol-based hand rub (foam, lotion, or gel) to decontaminate the hands if the hands are not visibly dirty or contaminated.
- Wear clean nonsterile examination gloves when contact with blood, body fluids, secretions, mucous membranes, damaged skin, and contaminated items is anticipated.
- Change gloves between procedures on the same patient after exposure to potentially infective material.
- Wear equipment to protect your eyes, nose, and mouth and avoid soiling your clothes by wearing a disposable gown or apron when performing procedures that may splash or spray blood, body fluids, or secretions.
- Dispose of single-use items appropriately; do not disinfect, sterilize, and reuse.
- Take precautions to avoid injuries before, during, and after procedures in which needles, scalpels, or other sharp instruments have been used on a patient.
- Do not recap used needles or otherwise manipulate them by bending or breaking. If recapping is necessary to carry a used needle to a sharps container, use a one-handed scoop technique or a device for holding the needle sheath (see Chapter 9).

- Place used disposable syringes and needles and other sharps in a puncture-resistant container (sharps) as close as possible to the area of use.
- Use barrier devices (e.g., mouthpieces, resuscitation bags) as alternatives to mouth-to-mouth resuscitation (see Chapter 11).
- Do not eat, drink, or put candy, gum, or mints into your mouth while working in the clinical area.

 CHECKPOINT QUESTION

8. How will following standard precautions help to protect you against contracting an infection or communicable disease?

Personal Protective Equipment

In any area of the medical office where exposure to biohazardous materials might occur, PPE must be made available and used by all health care workers, including medical assistants. For instance:

- Gloves must be available and accessible throughout the office. If you or a patient is sensitive to the latex found in regular examination gloves, proper alternatives such as vinyl gloves must be available (Box 2-4).
- Disposable gowns, goggles, and face shields must be available in areas where splattering or splashing of airborne particles may occur (Fig. 2-5).
- You must wear gloves when performing any procedure that carries any risk of exposure, such as surgical procedures or drawing blood specimens, disposing of biohazardous waste, or touching or handling surfaces that have been contaminated with biohazardous materials, or if there is any chance at all, no matter how remote, that you may come into contact with blood or body fluids.

Employers who do not make this equipment available are not in compliance with OSHA regulations and may face significant fines. However, employees are responsible for using the PPE correctly and appropriately and washing their hands frequently throughout the day. Remember, pathogens may be carried home to family members and to other persons who come into contact with you or the patient. When removing PPE after a procedure, remove all protective barriers before removing your gloves. Once you have removed all PPE, including your contaminated gloves (Procedure 2-2), always wash your hands (see Procedure 2-1).

 CHECKPOINT QUESTION

9. What PPE should you wear when assisting the physician with a wound irrigation?

BOX 2-4

LATEX ALLERGY AND PREVENTION

The incidence among health care workers of allergic reactions to proteins in latex has increased in recent years. The proteins in latex, a product of the rubber tree that is used to make many products including examination gloves, may cause allergic reactions, especially with repeated exposure. The reactions can be mild (skin redness or rash, itching, or hives) or severe (difficulty breathing, coughing, or wheezing). Respiratory reactions often result when the powder in the gloves becomes airborne and is inhaled as the gloves are removed after use. To protect yourself from exposure and allergy to latex, the following guidelines may be useful:

- Use gloves that are not latex for tasks that do not involve contact or potential contact with blood or body fluids.
- When contact with blood or body fluids is possible, wear powder-free latex gloves. Powder-free gloves contain less protein than the powdered ones, reducing the risk of allergy.
- Avoid wearing oil-based lotions or hand creams before applying latex gloves. The oil in these products can break down the latex, releasing the proteins that cause the allergic reactions.
- Wash your hands thoroughly after removing latex gloves.
- Recognize the symptoms of latex allergy in yourself, your coworkers, and your patients.

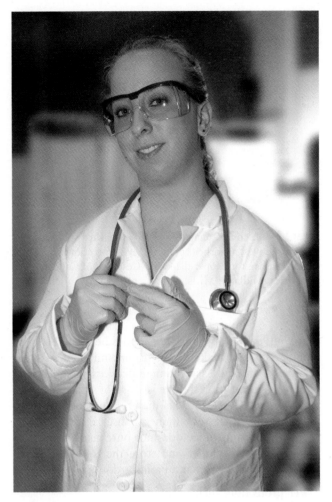

Figure 2-5 Personal protective equipment that must be provided for employees who may come into contact with contaminated materials includes gloves, goggles, face shields, and gowns or aprons to protect clothing.

AFF **WHAT IF?**

What if your patient is offended that you are wearing gloves when drawing a blood specimen?

Sometimes patients become defensive and make statements to the effect that they are "disease free." If this happens to you, reassure the patient by saying that wearing gloves is a standard practice and is used for the protection of the patient also. Use this occasion to teach the patient about standard precautions and the importance of following these guidelines in preventing the spread of disease.

Handling Environmental Contamination

Although not all equipment or surfaces in the medical office must be sterile (free from all microorganisms), all equipment and areas must be clean. Sanitization is cleaning or washing equipment or surfaces by removing all visible soil. Any detergent or low-level disinfectant can be used to clean and disinfect areas such as floors, examination tables, cabinets, and countertops. Because you may be expected to perform cleaning tasks routinely or when these surfaces become soiled with visible blood or body fluids, you should understand how these procedures are correctly performed.

Any surface contaminated with biohazardous materials should be promptly cleaned using an approved germicide or a dilute bleach solution. OSHA requires

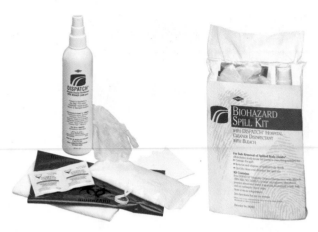

Figure 2-6 A commercially prepared biohazard spill kit contains gloves, absorbent material, eye protection, and a biohazard bag for proper disposal. (Courtesy of Caltech Industries, Midland, MI.)

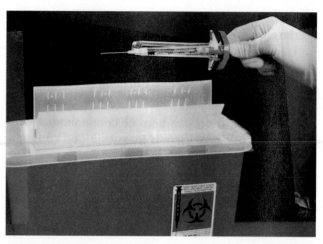

Figure 2-7 All sharps should be disposed of properly by placing them in a plastic puncture-resistant sharps container like the one shown here. Note the biohazard symbol on the sharps container.

that spill kits or appropriate supplies be available, and commercial kits make cleaning contaminated surfaces relatively safe and easy. Commercial kits include clean gloves, eye protection if there is a risk of splashing, a gel to absorb the biohazardous material, a scoop, towels, and a biohazard waste container to discard all used items (Fig. 2-6). If your office does not purchase commercial kits, you should gather and store the following items together in the event that a biohazardous spill occurs:

* Eye protection, such as goggles
* Clean examination gloves
* Absorbent powder, crystals, or gel
* Paper towels
* A disposable scoop
* At least one biohazard waste bag
* A chemical disinfectant

In some cases, you may need a sharps container (Fig. 2-7) and spill control barriers. If there is a large amount of contamination on the floor, you should put on disposable shoe coverings to avoid transmitting microorganisms on your shoes. All gloves, paper towels, eye protection, and shoe coverings should be discarded in the biohazardous waste bags, which must be disposed of properly. Procedure 2-3 outlines the procedure for an area contaminated with blood or body fluids.

Although most medical offices use disposable patient gowns and drapes, some offices continue to use cloth. Hygienic storage of clean linens is recommended, and proper handling of soiled linens, disposable or not, is required. After applying clean examination gloves, handle soiled linen, including examination table paper, as little as possible by folding it carefully so that the most contaminated surface is turned inward to prevent contamination of the air. Contaminated linen should

be placed in a biohazard bag in the examination room where the contamination occurred rather than carried through the hallways of the medical office. Some offices using cloth linens contract with an outside company for the laundering. If linen materials are laundered at the office, use normal laundry cycles following the recommendations of the washer, detergent, and fabric.

 CHECKPOINT QUESTION

10. How would you respond to an employee in the medical office who is unsure about how to clean up a spilled urine specimen? Is this biohazardous?

 AFF TRIAGE

The following three situations occur at the same time in the office where you are employed:

A. You have just finished changing the dressing on a wound that is draining a moderate amount of blood. You still have your gloves on, but you need to document the procedure in the patient's medical record and instruct the patient regarding wound care.

B. As you are cleaning up the materials used to irrigate the wound, you spill the basin used to collect the irrigating solution and blood obtained from the procedure.

C. Another staff member knocks on the door of the examination room and informs you that you have a phone call.

How do you sort these tasks? What do you do first? Second? Third?

Tell the staff member in situation C that you cannot take a phone call now and ask him or her to take a message or refer the call to another medical assistant. The spill in situation B is a biohazardous spill and should be cleaned up and the area decontaminated immediately. You should be familiar with the policy and procedures of the medical office and clean the spill accordingly. Once the spill is cleaned and decontaminated, remove your gloves and wash your hands. Document the wound irrigation, dressing change, and patient education in situation A only after removing your gloves and washing your hands. To prevent the spread of microorganisms to the medical record, you should never handle the medical record while wearing contaminated gloves.

Disposing of Infectious Waste

Federal regulations from the Environmental Protection Agency (EPA) and OSHA set the policies and guidelines for disposing of hazardous materials, but individual states determine policies based on these guidelines. As a result, policies vary widely, and you should review your state and local regulations before making waste disposal decisions. Most medical offices are considered small generators of waste because they produce less than 50 pounds of waste each month. Facilities such as hospitals and large clinics that generate more than 50 pounds are considered large generators and must obtain a certificate of registration from the EPA and maintain a record of the quantity of waste and disposal procedures.

To remain compliant with any state and federal laws, facilities that are considered large generators of infectious waste and some smaller medical offices use an infectious waste service to dispose of biohazardous waste appropriately and safely. These services supply the office with appropriate waste containers and pick up filled containers regularly (Box 2-5). Once the filled containers are picked up by the waste service, the infectious waste is disposed of according to EPA and OSHA guidelines. The service maintains a tracking record listing the type of waste, its weight in pounds, and the disposal destination. When the waste has been destroyed, a tracking form documenting the disposal is sent to the medical office and should be retained in the office records for 3 years. This documentation must be provided to the EPA should an audit be performed to assess compliance. States impose stiff penalties, including fines and/or imprisonment, for violations of regulations involving biohazardous waste.

BOX 2-5

BIOHAZARD WASTE DISPOSAL

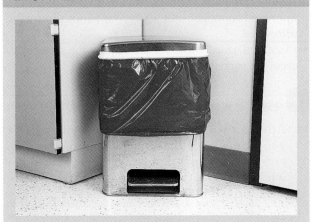

A regular waste container should be used only for disposal of waste that is not biohazardous, such as paper, plastic, disposable tray wrappers, packaging material, unused gauze, and examination table paper. To prevent leakage and mess, nonbiohazardous liquids should be discarded in a sink or other washbasin, not in the plastic bag inside the waste can. Biohazard liquid spills (any waste containing blood or other body fluids) should be cleaned according to the office policy using the guidelines noted in Procedure 2-3. **Never discard sharps of any kind in plastic bags; these are not puncture resistant, and injury may result even with careful handling.** Regardless of the type of waste container used (biohazard or nonbiohazard), bags should not be filled to capacity. When the plastic bag is about two-thirds full, it should be removed from the waste can, with the top edges brought together and secured by tying or with a twist tie. Remove the bag from the area and follow the office policy and procedures for disposal. Put a fresh plastic bag into the waste can.

Because the fee charged by an infectious waste service is based on the type and amount of waste generated, you should follow these guidelines to help keep the cost down while maintaining safety:

- Use separate containers for each type of waste. Don't put bandages in sharps containers (puncture-resistant containers for needles or other sharp items) or paper towels used for routine handwashing in a biohazard bag.
- Fill sharps containers two-thirds full before disposing of them. Most containers have fill lines that must not be exceeded.
- Use only approved biohazard containers.

- When moving filled biohazard containers, secure the bag or top with a closure for that specific container.
- If the container is contaminated on the outside, wear clean examination gloves, secure it within another approved container, and wash your hands thoroughly afterward.
- Place biohazard waste for pick up by the service in a secure, designated area.

 CHECKPOINT QUESTION

11. After drawing a blood specimen from a patient, you notice that the tube of blood is leaking onto the examination table where you put it while finishing the procedure. How do you clean up the blood spill?

Hepatitis B and Human Immunodeficiency Viruses

One of the most persistent health care concerns in the medical office is the transmission of HBV and HIV. Although HIV is the most visible public concern, HBV has been an occupational hazard for health care professionals for many years. HBV is more viable than HIV and may survive in a dried state on clinical equipment and counter surfaces at room temperature for more than a week. In this dried state, HBV may be passed through the medical setting by way of contact with contaminated hands, gloves, or other means of direct transmission. Fortunately, HBV can be contained by the proper use of standard precautions, and it can be killed easily by cleaning with a dilute bleach solution.

HBV and HIV are both transmitted through exposure to contaminated blood and body fluids. Accidental punctures with sharp objects contaminated with blood are one way to become infected, but the viruses may also enter the body through broken skin. Disorders of the skin, including dry cracked skin, dermatitis, eczema, and psoriasis, also allow entrance into the body if contact with contaminated surfaces or equipment occurs.

While there is no vaccine to prevent infection with HIV, employers whose workers, including clinical medical assistants, are at risk for HBV exposure are mandated by OSHA to provide the vaccine to prevent HBV at no cost to the employee. This vaccine is given in a series of three injections that normally produce immunity to the disease. It is recommended that a blood sample be drawn 6 months after the third injection of HBV vaccine to determine whether the person has developed immunity. The blood test can detect the presence, or titer, of antibodies against hepatitis B. The series is repeated if HBV immunity is not found, but the vaccine has been found to be very effective. The immunity may last as long as 10 years. Employees who choose not to receive the vaccine must sign a waiver or release form stating that they are aware of the risks associated with HBV. Individuals who contract hepatitis B may develop cirrhosis (destruction of the cells of the liver) and are at increased risk for developing liver cancer.

In the event of exposure to blood or body fluids infected with HBV, the postexposure plan should include an immediate blood test of the employee. Repeat blood titers should be obtained at specific intervals, usually 6 weeks, 3 months, 6 months, 9 months, and 1 year, as a comparison. If you have been immunized against HBV, usually no further treatment is required. However, if you waive the HBV series, hepatitis B immunoglobulin can be given by injection for immediate short-term protection, and the general series of three immunizations should be started.

The same schedule of evaluation is required after HIV exposure. Again, there is no vaccine to prevent HIV, but other HIV treatments for preventing transmission are being tested.

 CHECKPOINT QUESTION

12. Which virus is more of a threat to the clinical medical assistant: HIV or HBV? Why?

---

español
SPANISH TERMINOLOGY

Lávese las manos frecuentemente.
  Wash your hands frequently.

Cúbrase la boca al toser.
  Cover your mouth when coughing.

¿Es alérgico/alergica al latex?
  Are you allergic to latex?

¿Tiene fiebre?
  Do you have a fever?

¿Qué síntomas tiene?
  What symptoms do you have?

MEDIA MENU

- **Student Resources on thePoint**
  - **Video: Handwashing (Procedure 2-1)**
  - **Video: Removing Contaminated Gloves (Procedure 2-2)**
  - **CMA/RMA Certification Exam Review**
- **Internet Resources**

  Occupational Safety and Health Administration
  http://www.osha.gov

  Latex Allergy Prevention
  http://www.cdc.gov/niosh/docs/98-113/

  Healthcare Associated Infections
  http://www.cdc.gov/hai/

  Food and Drug Administration
  http://www.fda.gov

PSY **PROCEDURE 2-1:** **Handwashing for Medical Asepsis**

Purpose: To prevent the growth and spread of pathogens
Equipment: Liquid soap, disposable paper towels, an orangewood manicure stick, a waste can
Standard: This task should take 2–3 minutes.

Steps	Purpose
1. Remove all rings and your wristwatch if it cannot be pushed up onto the forearm.	Rings and watches may harbor pathogens that may not be easily washed away. Ideally, rings should not be worn when working with material that may be infectious.
2. Stand close to the sink without touching it.	The sink is considered contaminated, and standing too close may contaminate your clothing.
3. Turn on the faucet and adjust the temperature of the water to warm.	Water that is too hot or too cold will crack or chap the skin on the hands, which will break the natural protective barrier that prevents infection.
4. Wet your hands and wrists under the warm running water, apply liquid soap, and work the soap into a lather by rubbing your palms together and rubbing the soap between your fingers at least 10 times.	This motion dislodges microorganisms from between the fingers and removes transient and some resident organisms.

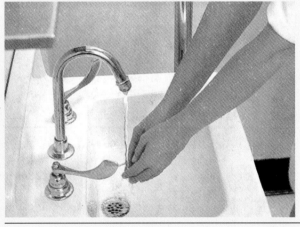

Step 4. Wet hands and wrists.

5. Scrub the palm of one hand with the fingertips of the other hand to work the soap under the nails of that hand; then reverse the procedure and scrub the other hand. Also scrub each wrist.	Friction helps remove microorganisms.

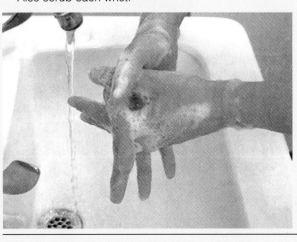

Step 5. Wash hands and wrists with firm rubbing and circular motions.

PSY PROCEDURE 2-1: **Handwashing for Medical Asepsis**
(continued)

Steps	Purpose
6. Rinse hands and wrists thoroughly under running warm water, holding hands lower than elbows; do not touch the inside of the sink.	Holding the hands lower than the elbows and wrists allows microorganisms to flow off the hands and fingers rather than back up the arms.

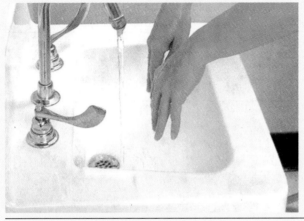

Step 6. Rinse hands thoroughly.

Steps	Purpose
7. Clean under the nails using an orangewood stick *or* scrape the fingernails of one hand against the soapy palm of the other hand for 10 seconds. Repeat with other hand.	Nails may harbor microorganisms. Metal files and pointed instruments may break the skin and make an opening for microorganisms. Do this at the beginning of the day, before leaving for the day, or after coming into contact with potentially infectious material.
8. Reapply liquid soap and rewash hands and wrists.	Rewashing the hands after cleaning the nails washes away any microorganisms that may have been loosened and/or removed.
9. Rinse hands thoroughly again while holding hands lower than wrists and elbows.	
10. Gently dry hands with a paper towel. Discard the paper towel and the orangewood stick if used to clean the nails.	Hands must be dried thoroughly and completely to prevent drying and cracking.

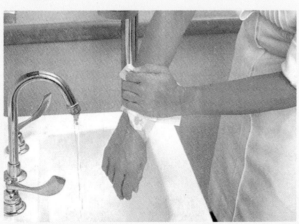

Step 10. Dry hands gently with a paper towel.

Steps	Purpose
11. Use a dry paper towel to turn off the faucets, and discard the paper towel.	Your hands are clean and should not touch the contaminated faucet handles.

PSY PROCEDURE 2-2: **Removing Contaminated Gloves**

Purpose: To remove contaminated gloves to prevent the spread of pathogenic microorganisms
Equipment: Clean examination gloves; biohazard waste container
Standard: This task should take 1–2 minutes.

Steps	Purpose
1. Choose the appropriate size gloves for your hands and put them on.	Gloves should fit comfortably, not too loose and not too tight.
2. To remove gloves, grasp the glove of your nondominant hand at the palm and pull the glove away.	To avoid transferring contaminants to the wrist, be sure not to grasp the glove at the wrist.

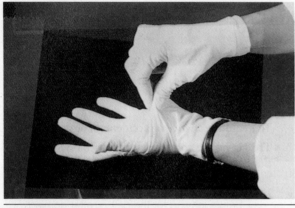

Step 2. Grasp the palm of the glove on your nondominant gloved hand.

Steps	Purpose
3. Slide your hand out of the glove, rolling the glove into the palm of the gloved dominant hand.	You should avoid touching either glove with your ungloved hand.

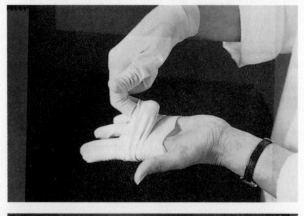

Step 3A. Carefully remove the glove and avoid contaminating your bare skin.

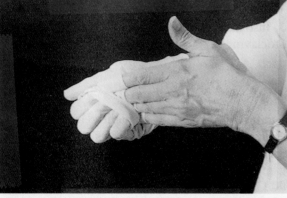

Step 3B. Grasp the soiled glove with your gloved dominant hand.

PSY PROCEDURE 2-2: **Removing Contaminated Gloves**
(continued)

Steps	Purpose
4. Holding the soiled glove in the palm of your gloved hand, slip your ungloved fingers under the cuff of the glove you are still wearing, being careful not to touch the outside of the glove.	Skin should touch skin but never the soiled part of the glove.

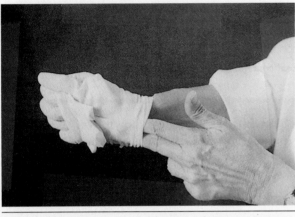

Step 4. Slip your free hand under the cuff of the remaining glove.

Steps	Purpose
5. Stretch the glove of the dominant hand up and away from your hand while turning it inside out, with the already removed glove balled up inside.	Turning it inside out ensures that the soiled surfaces of the gloves are enclosed.

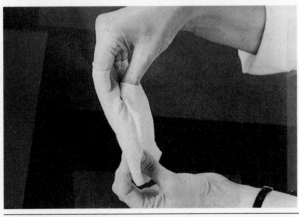

Step 5. Remove the glove by turning it inside out over the previously removed glove.

Steps	Purpose
6. Both gloves should now be removed, with the first glove inside the second glove and the second glove inside out.	
7. Discard both gloves as one unit into a biohazard waste receptacle.	
8. Wash your hands.	Wearing gloves is *not* a substitute for washing your hands!

PSY PROCEDURE 2-3: Cleaning Biohazardous Spills

Purpose: To safely clean contaminated surfaces.
Equipment: Commercially prepared germicide *or* 1:10 bleach solution, gloves, disposable towels, chemical absorbent, biohazardous waste bag, protective eye wear (goggles or mask and face shield), disposable shoe coverings, disposable gown or apron made of plastic or other material that is impervious to soaking up contaminated fluids
Standard: This task should take 3–5 minutes.

Steps	Purpose
1. Put on gloves. Wear protective eyewear, gown or apron, and shoe coverings if you anticipate any splashing.	A plastic gown or apron will protect your clothing from contaminants.
2. Apply chemical absorbent material to the spill as indicated by office policy. Clean up the spill with disposable paper towels, being careful not to splash. 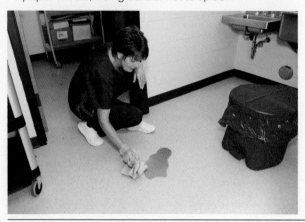	**Step 2.** Wearing PPE, carefully clean up biohazardous spills immediately after they occur.
3. Dispose of paper towels and absorbent material in a biohazard waste bag.	The bag will alert anyone handling the waste that it contains biohazardous material.
4. Spray the area with commercial germicide or bleach solution and wipe with disposable paper towels. Discard towels in a biohazard bag. 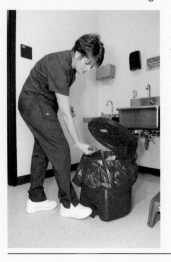	**Step 4.** Place contaminated materials into a biohazard bag.

PSY PROCEDURE 2-3: | **Cleaning Biohazardous Spills (continued)**

Steps	Purpose
5. With your gloves on, remove the protective eyewear and discard or disinfect per office policy. Remove the gown or apron and shoe coverings and put in the biohazard bag if disposable or the biohazard laundry bag for reusable linens.	
6. Place the biohazard bag in an appropriate waste receptacle for removal according to your facility's policy.	
7. Remove your gloves and wash your hands thoroughly.	Wearing gloves does *not* replace proper handwashing.

- Following the principles of medical asepsis and infection control helps ensure a safe environment for patients and health care providers in the medical office. If you fail to follow these principles consistently, you will place yourself and others at risk for infection that may impair patients' recovery and affect health care workers' performance.
- Although avoiding contact with microorganisms in the environment is impossible, sanitation and disinfection will reduce the numbers of microorganisms and potential pathogens, making the environment clean and as disease free as possible.
- OSHA and the CDC issue regulations and standards for health care workers who work with blood and body fluids, and you must always follow them, including wearing PPE. In case of exposure, your office must have an exposure control plan and a post-exposure plan to assist you in receiving appropriate medical attention and follow-up care.
- *Remember*: Handwashing is the single most effective measure to prevent the spread of infection. Wearing gloves does *not* replace handwashing. Hands must *always* be washed after removing gloves.

Warm Ups for Critical Thinking

1. Review Table 2-1 on common communicable diseases. Create a patient education brochure that focuses on the spread of these diseases.
2. A patient who comes into your office has a leg wound that must be cared for at home. When asked about caring for the wound, he tells you that he knows how to do it, but you think he may be confused about the importance of using medical asepsis. How do you handle this situation?
3. On a busy morning in the medical office, you accidently spill a small amount of urine from a specimen container onto the counter. Your coworker needs you to assist with a pediatric injection in the examination room down the hall. Would it be acceptable to clean up the urine spill after you help your coworker? Why or why not?
4. Develop a written policy for new employees regarding disinfecting individual examination rooms in the medical office. Be specific and include issues related to safety.

Medical History and Patient Assessment

Outline

The Medical History
Methods of Collecting Information
Elements of the Medical History

Conducting the Patient Interview
Preparing for the Interview
Introducing Yourself
Barriers to Communication

Assessing the Patient
Signs and Symptoms
Chief Complaint and Present Illness

Learning Outcomes

Cognitive Domain

Note: AAMA/CAAHEP 2008 Standards are italicized.

1. Spell and define key terms
2. *Recognize communication barriers*
3. *Identify techniques for overcoming communication barriers*
4. Give examples of the type of information included in each section of the patient history
5. Identify guidelines for conducting a patient interview using principles of verbal and nonverbal communication
6. *Differentiate between subjective and objective information*
7. Discuss open-ended and closed-ended questions and explain when to use each type during the patient interview

Psychomotor Domain

Note: AAMA/CAAHEP 2008 Standards are italicized.

1. Obtain and record a patient history (Procedure 3-1)
2. *Practice within the standard of care for a medical assistant*
3. *Use reflection, restatement, and clarification techniques to obtain a patient history*
4. *Use medical terminology, pronouncing medical terms correctly, to communicate information, patient history, data, and observations*

5. *Apply local, state, and federal health care legislation and regulations appropriate to the medical assisting practice setting*
6. Accurately document a chief complaint and present illness (Procedure 3-2)

Affective Domain

Note: AAMA/CAAHEP 2008 Standards are italicized.

1. *Demonstrate empathy in communicating with patients, family, and staff*
2. *Apply active listening skills*
3. *Use appropriate body language and other nonverbal skills in communicating with patients, family, and staff*
4. *Demonstrate sensitivity to patients rights*
5. *Demonstrate awareness of the territorial boundaries of the person with whom you are communicating*
6. *Demonstrate sensitivity appropriate to the message being delivered*
7. *Demonstrate recognition of the patient's level of understanding in communications*
8. *Recognize and protect personal boundaries in communicating with others*
9. *Demonstrate respect for individual diversity, incorporating awareness of one's own biases in areas including gender, race, religion, age, and economic status*
10. *Apply critical thinking skills in performing patient assessment and care*

Learning Outcomes *(continued)*

ABHES Competencies

1. Be impartial and show empathy when dealing with patients
2. Interview effectively
3. Recognize and respond to verbal and nonverbal communication
4. Obtain chief complaint, recording patient history

Key Terms

assessment
chief complaint (CC)
demographic
familial

hereditary
Health Insurance Portability and Accountability Act

(HIPAA)
homeopathic medication
medical history

over-the-counter medication
signs
symptoms

To diagnose a patient's present illness, the physician needs the patient's past and current health information. As a professional medical assistant, you are often responsible for obtaining this information as part of the **medical history** and **assessment**. The medical history is a record containing information about a patient's past and present health status, the health status of related family members, and relevant information about a patient's social habits. Assessment begins with gathering information to determine the patient's problem or reason for seeking medical care. Typically, you ask standard questions and document the patient's responses during the assessment on preprinted forms or in a manner decided by the physician and outlined in the medical office policy and procedure manual.

COG The Medical History

 AFF PATIENT EDUCATION

GENERAL TOPICS

While assessing a patient, you can also teach. Your teaching may include information about a specific disease or general care. For example, a diabetic patient may need instruction on glucose testing or diet control. General topics for all patients can include the following:

- Blood pressure management
- Stress management
- Diet or weight control tips
- The importance of exercise
- The effects of alcohol and tobacco
- Instructions for conducting breast or testicular self-examinations
- The importance of proper immunizations
- Cancer warning signs and prevention tips

COG Methods of Collecting Information

To complete the patient's medical history, you and the physician work cooperatively with the patient. In some medical practices, medical assistants gather initial patient information by interviewing the patient using a printed list of questions. Other medical offices ask the patient to fill out a standard form before or during the first appointment. Patients who receive the form in the mail are instructed to bring the completed document to the office at the initial visit. In either case, you must check the form for completeness because the physician uses this information as the basis for more extensive questioning during the examination.

In other practices, the physician may prefer to complete the medical history form during the initial patient interview and examination. In this situation, you should be familiar with the form and ready to assist the physician if needed or asked to do so.

LEGAL TIP

SAFEGUARDING PATIENT INFORMATION

You are responsible for ensuring that information in the patient's medical history is kept confidential. Legally and ethically, the patient has a right to privacy concerning his or her medical records, which includes storage in a secure place. Only health care providers directly involved in the patient's care should be allowed access to the records.

COG Elements of the Medical History

The medical history forms used by the office may vary with the practice specialty, but most forms are composed of these common elements: identifying data (database), past history (PH), review of systems (ROS), family history (FH), and social history. Figure 3-1 shows a medical history form. This information is confidential and protected by the **Health Insurance Portability and Accountability Act (HIPAA)**, a federal law that protects the privacy of health information. No one except those directly involved in the patient's care may have access to it without the patient's permission.

The following are the main elements of the medical history:

- Identifying data (database). The **demographic** information in this section, required for administrative purposes, always includes the patient's name, address, and phone number. It also includes the name, address, and phone number of the patient's employer and insurance carrier and the patient's health insurance policy number, social security number, marital status, gender, and race.
- Past history (PH). This section addresses the patient's prior health status and helps the physician plan appropriate care for any present illness. Information in this section typically includes allergies, immunizations, childhood diseases, current and past medications, and previous illnesses, surgeries, and hospitalizations.
- Review of systems (ROS). A thorough review of each body system may elicit information that the patient forgot to mention earlier or thought was irrelevant. Specific questions, such as symptoms or known diseases, related to each system of the body are included in this section.
- Family history (FH). This section contains the health status of the patient's parents, siblings, and grandparents. This information is important because certain diseases or disorders have **familial** or **hereditary** tendencies. Familial diseases tend to occur often in

a particular family, whereas hereditary diseases are transmitted from parent to offspring. If any immediate family member is deceased, the cause of death should be documented.
- Social history. The social history covers the patient's lifestyle, such as marital status, occupation, education, and hobbies. It may also include information about the patient's diet, use of alcohol or tobacco, and sexual history. This information may help the physician understand how present illness, including any treatment, may affect the lifestyle or how the lifestyle may affect the illness. The social history may also provide a guide for patient education, since some behaviors, such as tobacco use or a diet high in fat, may not yet be causing illness but can cause illness in the future.

CHECKPOINT QUESTION

1. What is the difference between the past history and the family history?

COG Conducting the Patient Interview

PATIENT EDUCATION

GENETIC DISEASES

The patient's family history can provide you with many teaching opportunities. If a patient indicates that previous members of his or her family had certain diseases, then there may be a genetic link. A genetic disease is noted by a mark on the DNA (genetic material) for a specific illness or disease. The patient receives this mark from either or both parents. Some common examples include some forms of high blood pressure, diabetes, heart disease, obesity, and certain cancers. Examples of less common genetic disorders are Tay-Sachs disease, Marfan syndrome, and Huntington disease. Great strides have been made in genetic testing. This allows the patient to have the DNA examined for potential markers of diseases. For example, color blindness is a genetic disorder that can easily be seen on a DNA chain. Patients can have genetic testing done to see whether they carry a particular disease marker. Genetic counseling may also be appropriate depending on the type of genetic disorder. Some insurance plans will pay for genetic testing and counseling. Advise the patient to contact his or her insurance company directly for specific coverage guidelines.

Professional Medical Associates – History Form

NAME: _____ DATE OF BIRTH: _____

What is the main reason for your visit to the doctor? _____

_____

Were you referred? _____ if so, by whom? _____

PAST MEDICAL HISTORY:

Are you allergic to any medication? _____

If so, list medications: _____

List current medications, dosage, and how many times a day you take them:

Medication   Dose   Times A Day

_____

_____

Alcohol Consumption: What type? _____ Amount _____ How Often? _____

                        History of Alcoholism? _____

When was your last TB or Tine test? _____

Have you ever had a positive test for tuberculosis? _____

When was your last Tetanus shot? _____

List all surgeries you have had in the past:

Date   Type of Surgery

_____

_____

List all past hospitalizations (not involving surgeries above):

Date   Reason For Hospital Stay

_____

_____

List all past problems with trauma (broken bones, lacerations, etc.):

_____

REVIEW OF SYSTEMS, PAST MEDICAL PROBLEMS:
If you have been told you have any of the problems listed below, or are having any of the problems listed below, please CIRCLE:

1. <u>GENERAL:</u> Weight loss, weight gain, fever, chills, night sweats, hot flashes, tire easily, problems with sleep, crying spells, history of cancer.

2. <u>SKIN:</u> Rash, sores that won't heal, moles that are new or changing, history of skin problems.

3. <u>HEENT:</u> Headache, eye problems, hearing problems, sinus problems, hay fever, dizziness, hoarseness, sores in your mouth that won't heal, dental problems.

    Do you chew tobacco or dip snuff? _____

4. <u>METABOLIC/ENDOCRINE:</u> Thyroid problems, diabetes or sugar problems, high cholesterol.

Figure 3-1 A sample medical history form, front and back.

5. <u>RESPIRATORY:</u> Cough, wheezing, breathing problems, history of asthma, history of lung problems.

Do you smoke cigarettes or pipe? _____

How much? _____ For how long? _____

6. <u>BREAST (WOMEN):</u> Breast lumps, changes in nipples, nipple discharge, breast problems, family history of breast cancer. When was your last mammogram? _____

7. <u>CARDIOVASCULAR:</u> Heart murmur, rheumatic fever, high blood pressure, angina, heart problems, heart attack, abnormal heart rhythm, chest pain, palpitations, leg swelling, history of phlebitis or blood clots.

8. <u>GI:</u> Problems with appetite, swallowing, heartburn, nausea, vomiting, pain in the abdomen, constipation, diarrhea, blood in stool, history of ulcers, liver problems, hepatitis, jaundice, pancreas problems, gallbladder problems, or colon problems.

9. <u>REPRODUCTIVE (WOMEN):</u> Problems with irregular menstrual cycles, abnormal vaginal bleeding or discharge, history of sexually transmitted diseases, sexual problems.

AGE OF FIRST MENSES (PERIOD) _____ AGE OF MENOPAUSE _____

LAST PAP SMEAR _____ METHOD OF CONTRACEPTION _____

Obstetric History (Women)

NUMBER OF PREGNANCIES _____ PLEASE LIST AS FOLLOWS:

Delivery Date   Pregnancy Complications   Type Delivery   Baby's Weight

_____

_____

<u>MEN:</u> Problems with genital discharge, history of venereal diseases, sexual problems, prostate problems.

METHOD OF CONTRACEPTION _____

10. <u>UROLOGIC:</u> Problems with painful urination, urinary frequency, blood in urine, weak urinary stream, history of bladder or kidney infections, or kidney stones.

11. <u>MUSCULOSKELETAL:</u> Arthritis, back pain, cramps in legs.

12. <u>NEUROLOGIC:</u> Seizures, stroke, arm or leg weakness or numbness, black-out spells, memory or thinking problems, depression, anxiety, psychiatric problems.

13. <u>HEMATOLOGIC:</u> Anemia, bleeding problems, enlarged lymph nodes.

HAVE YOU EVER HAD A BLOOD TRANSFUSION? _____ DATE _____

FAMILY HISTORY:

List any medical problems that run in your family and which family members have these problems.

_____

_____

SOCIAL HISTORY:

MARITAL STATUS: _____

OCCUPATION: _____

EDUCATION: _____

HOBBIES: _____

WHAT DO YOU DO FOR ENJOYMENT? _____

Figure 3-1 *(continued).*

Preparing for the Interview

As a medical assistant, your primary goal during a patient interview is to obtain accurate and pertinent information. To do this, you need to understand the basic components of communication and to use active listening skills. You should also use a variety of interviewing techniques, including reflecting, paraphrasing, asking for examples, asking questions, summarizing, and allowing silence. Communication also includes observation. Specifically, any objective or observable information concerning the patient's physical or mental status should be noted and documented in the patient's record as appropriate. Examples of observations about a patient's physical status include the general appearance (bruising or injury, pale or flushed skin). The mental or emotional condition of the patient includes observations such as lethargy, crying, tearfulness, and confusion. Judgments made about these observations should not be documented in the patient's record because the terminology used (depressed, abused) may be diagnostic, which is out of the scope of training for the medical assistant. In the case of suspected abuse, you should document the observable information in the medical record and alert the physician regarding your suspicions. Procedure 3-1 outlines the process for conducting a successful patient interview.

Before you start interviewing the patient, make sure you are familiar with the medical history form and any previous medical history provided by the patient. Shuffling papers while the patient is talking or asking questions out of order may distract the patient and disrupt the flow of the interview. If the patient is new to the medical practice, review the new patient questionnaire before beginning. Review the chart of any established patient, and update information as indicated.

To safeguard confidential patient information and allow for open communication, conduct the interview in a private and comfortable place. Avoid public areas, such as the reception area, where distractions are likely and where others may hear the patient's answers. Interview the patient alone unless he or she wishes to have family members or significant others present (Fig. 3-2).

AFF **PATIENT EDUCATION**

PREVENTATIVE MEDICINE

While interviewing the patient about his or her chief complaint, you may have an opportunity to teach the patient about various topics. Emphasize to the patient that illnesses can often be treated easier and quicker if prompt medical attention is received. This is a very important point to stress to older patients with chronic medical problems such as diabetes. For example, a diabetic patient who presents with a small foot ulcer in its early stages may be able to be treated with medicated dressings. However, if the ulcer goes untreated and gets bigger, the patient may need surgery to clean the wound and may even require hospitalization for antibiotics. While interviewing the patient about their chief complaint, take the opportunity to stress the importance of preventative medicine.

COG Introducing Yourself

Always begin the interview with new or established patients by identifying yourself, your title, and the purpose of the interview. For example, you might say, "Good morning, Mr. Frank. My name is Angela, and I'm Dr. Martin's medical assistant. I would like to ask you a few questions that will help the doctor diagnose and treat you appropriately. Please be assured that your responses will be kept in strict confidence." Under no circumstance should you identify yourself as a nurse because it is unethical and illegal to give the patient a false impression of your credentials.

The initial impression you make will be a lasting one, so be sure that your demeanor and words communicate genuine respect and concern. By developing professional rapport, you will gain the patient's confidence and trust in you, the physician, and the office staff. Some patients may be reluctant to share private information with you until a sense of trust has been established. This makes the professional role of the medical assistant as a caring and empathic health care worker even more important.

COG Barriers to Communication

As you begin speaking with the patient, you must assess any barriers to communication, such as unfamiliarity with English, hearing impairment, or cognitive impairment. Note the patient's verbal and nonverbal behavior

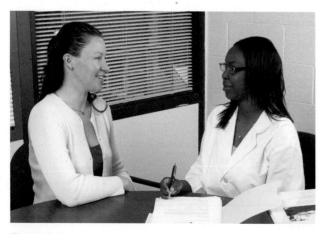

Figure 3-2 Conduct the patient interview in a private office or exam room.

during the interview and adjust your questioning if necessary. Avoid using highly technical or medical terminology when conversing with most patients. If the patient has impaired hearing or vision or difficulty understanding or speaking English, adjust your interviewing techniques to fit the patient's needs; however, remember that raising your voice is not necessary and will not improve communication or understanding with these patients. Instead, it is best to face the patient and maintain eye contact when speaking and use physical cues as appropriate.

 CHECKPOINT QUESTIONS

2. Why is it important for the medical assistant to review the medical history form before beginning the interview?

3. Why should you let the patient know that any information shared during the interview will be kept confidential?

Assessing the Patient

Signs and Symptoms

During the interview, listen carefully as the patient describes current medical problems to identify **signs** and **symptoms**. Signs are objective information that can be observed or perceived by someone other than the patient. Signs include such things as rash, bleeding, coughing, and vital sign measurements. Signs may also be found during the physician's examination.

Symptoms, or subjective information, are indications of disease or changes in the body as sensed by the patient. Usually, symptoms are not discernible by anyone other than the patient. They include complaints such as leg pain, headache, nausea, and dizziness. Observable signs that may indicate that a patient is having these symptoms include facial expressions, such as wincing during pain, holding onto rails or furniture for balance when walking, and gagging.

 AFF WHAT IF?

What if the patient appears highly anxious or intimidated about procedures that seem routine?

You can help put patients at ease by following these steps:

• Treat each patient as an individual with unique needs. Help elderly or disabled patients onto the examination table. If they are unsteady, keep them seated in a regular chair.

• When weighing patients, do not announce their weight aloud, since they may be embarrassed. Instead, ask them in the privacy of the examination room if they want to know their weight.

• Always offer a sheet or blanket to a patient who must change into an examination gown.

• When preparing a patient for a gynecologic examination, have her sit on the examination table until the physician is ready.

• If the physician is delayed, let the patient know. Explain generally the reason for the delay (e.g., an emergency), and let the patient know the approximate length of the delay.

Chief Complaint and Present Illness

After recording the patient's medical history and reviewing the information for accuracy and clarity, you must find out exactly why the patient has come to see the physician for this appointment (Procedure 3-2). Ask an open-ended question to encourage the patient to describe the chain of events leading to this visit. Open-ended questions allow the patient to answer with more than one or two words. For example, you might ask, "What is the reason for your appointment today?" or "Can you describe what has been going on?" Such questions require the patient to explain the visit by giving additional information. In contrast, answers to closed-ended questions usually necessitate only one or two words. Examples of closed-ended questions are "Do you have pain?" and "Are you able to sleep?" These questions can be answered with a simple yes or no and are not going to elicit responses that will be useful to the physician attempting to make a diagnosis.

When open-ended questions are used to determine the reason for the visit, the patient's answer will reveal the **chief complaint** (CC). The CC, which is one statement describing the signs and symptoms that led the patient to seek medical care, is documented in the patient's medical record at each visit. Examples of a CC might include "I've had a headache for the past 3 days" or "Yesterday I lifted a heavy crate and hurt my back." You should document the CC on the progress report form in the patient's record, using the patient's own words in quotation marks whenever possible. The entry should include the date (day, month, and year) and the time of day.

Once you have obtained the CC, continue to probe for more details to further define the patient's present illness (PI). The PI includes a chronologic order of events, including dates of onset and any home remedies or other self-care activities, including **over-the-counter** and **homeopathic medications**. Over-the-counter medications are those that are available without prescriptions. They include natural drugs, such as herbs, vitamins, and some homeopathic agents. Homeopathic medications include small doses of agents that cause similar symptoms in healthy individuals and are given to a person who is ill to help cure the disease causing the symptoms. The following questions could be used to obtain the PI:

- Chronology. How did this first begin?
- Location. Can you explain or show me exactly where the pain is?
- Severity. Can you describe the pain? Is the pain constant?
- Self-treatment. What medications have you taken for the pain? Do they help?
- Quality. Does anything that you do make the symptoms better or worse?
- Duration. Have you had these symptoms before?

Avoid suggesting answers with questions such as "Is the pain sharp?" or "Is the pain worse when you walk?" Many patients will agree or answer positively because they think this must be the expected answer. In addition, do not coax patients by making suggestions of symptoms you might expect them to have based on the chief complaint. Some patients may agree to have the symptoms you describe if they feel that you are suggesting those that "should" be present.

After asking several open-ended questions, it may be appropriate to ask closed-ended questions to obtain specific data. For example, you might ask the patient, "How long have you had this pain?" This kind of question requires only a short answer, not a lengthy description.

Of course, not all patients visit the doctor because they are ill. Some appointments are for routine examinations or tests. In this case, the CC will include a statement about the reason for the visit (e.g., annual physical examination, employment examination); however, you should obtain any additional PI information as appropriate.

 CHECKPOINT QUESTION

4. Explain the difference between a sign and a symptom, and give one example of each.

 AFF **TRIAGE**

While working in the medical office, you begin the day by placing the following three patients into examination rooms:

A. Patient A, a new patient, arrives on time and was given the two-page medical history form to complete.
B. Patient B is an established patient who is scheduled to have his blood pressure checked today because he started a new antihypertensive medication last month.
C. Patient C is a 1-year-old baby who is scheduled to be seen today for a well-child checkup and immunizations.

How would you sort these patients? Who should be seen first? Second? Third?

Patient B should be called back first, since he will probably take the least amount of time. Unless this patient's blood pressure is not responding to the antihypertensive medication or he has unanticipated problems, this type of visit is typically conducted in a timely manner as a convenience to the patient. Patient C should be seen next, since infant checkups usually require additional procedures that may require more time from the medical assistant and physician. Patient A should be given an adequate amount of time to complete the medical history forms, since this information will be necessary for the physician to understand the patient's current and future health problems. The patient should not be rushed to complete this paperwork. If necessary, you may call the patient back and assist with completion of the form, especially if the patient is having difficulty due to a physical disability, such as visual impairment, deformity, or trouble holding a pen or pencil because of arthritis.

español SPANISH TERMINOLOGY

Mi nombre es _____.
My name is _____.

¿Cuál es su nombre?
What is your name?

¿Dónde nació?
When were you born?

¿Dónde vive?
Where do you live?

¿Usted toma algún medicamento?
Do you take medications?

¿Le han hecho alguna cirugía?
Have you had surgery?

¿Uste fuma o bebe alcohol?
Do you smoke? Drink alcohol?

MEDIA MENU

- **Student Resources on thePoint**
  - **CMA/RMA Certification Exam Review**
- **Internet Resources**

  The Health Insurance Portability and Accountability Act
  http://www.cms.gov/HIPAAGenInfo

  American Autoimmune Related Diseases Association
  http://www.aarda.org

  March of Dimes
  http://www.marchofdimes.com

  Genetic Alliance
  http://www.geneticalliance.org

PSY PROCEDURE 3-1:   Interviewing the Patient to Obtain a Medical History

Purpose: Complete the various sections of a medical history form while interviewing a patient
Equipment: Medical history form or questionnaire, black or blue pen
Standard: This task should take 10 minutes.

Steps	Reasons
1. Gather the supplies.	You have everything you need before you begin.
2. Review the medical history form.	Be familiar with the order of the questions and the type of information required to allow for smooth communication with the patient.
3. Take the patient to a private and comfortable area of the office.	A private place prevents distractions and ensures confidentiality.
4. Sit across from the patient at eye level and maintain frequent eye contact.	Standing above the patient may be perceived as threatening and may result in poor communication.
5. Introduce yourself and explain the purpose of the interview.	This helps to establish a professional rapport with the patient.
6. Using language the patient can understand, ask the appropriate questions, and document the patient's responses. Be sure to determine the patient's CC and PI.	You must obtain accurate and complete data for the physician.
7. Listen actively by looking at the patient from time to time while he or she is speaking.	Patients can sense when the interviewer is not listening, so be sure that you show interest in what the patient is saying.
8. Regardless of the confidences shared by the patient, avoid projecting a judgmental attitude with words or actions.	Maintain professionalism, and ensure the patient's trust.
9. **AFF** Explain how to respond to a patient who has English as a second language.	Solicit assistance from anyone who may be with the patient or a staff member who speaks the patient's native language to interpret if available. If no interpreter is available, use hand gestures or pictures to explain procedure to the patient.
10. If appropriate, explain to the patient what to expect during examinations or procedures at that visit.	Keeping the patient informed about his or her care may decrease anxiety.
11. Review the history form for completion and accuracy.	The patient record is a legal document and information placed in the record must be accurate.
12. Thank the patient for cooperating during the interview, and offer to answer any questions.	Courtesy encourages the patient to have a positive attitude about the physician's office.
13. Describe examples of applying local, state, and federal health care legislation and regulation in the medical office.	Local regulations include required reporting of communicable diseases or injuries involving violence. State and federal regulations may include issues related to reimbursement, collection of fees, and privacy (HIPAA).

Charting Example:

10/14/2012 11:00 AM CC: New pt. checkup. Medical hx form complete, pt. indicates no physical or health problems at this time. Family history of colon cancer and hypertension noted. ——————————— E. Parker, CMA

Note: The medical assistant may sign his/her name in the patient record using only the "CMA" credential if the office has a signature log denoting the entire credential as "CMA(AAMA)."

PSY PROCEDURE 3-2:

Document a Chief Complaint (CC) and Present Illness (PI)

Purpose: Accurately record a CC and PI using open-ended and closed-ended questions while interviewing the patient

Equipment: A cumulative problem list or progress notes form, black or blue ink pen

Standard: This procedure should take 10 minutes or less.

Steps	Reasons
1. Gather the supplies, including the medical record containing the cumulative problem list or progress note form.	You have everything you need before you start.
2. Review new or established patient's medical history form.	Be as familiar as possible with the patient to help you obtain a complete CC and PI.

Professional Medical Associates – History Form

NAME: _Fred Smart_   DATE OF BIRTH: _09-15-1945_

What is the main reason for your visit to the doctor? _Physical Exam_

Were you referred? _No_   if so, by whom? _____

PAST MEDICAL HISTORY:

Are you allergic to any medication? _Yes_

If so, list medications: _Penicillin_

List current medications, dosage, and how many times a day you take them:

Medication	**Dose**	**Times A Day**
Multivitamin	_1 tablet_	_every day_

Alcohol Consumption: What type? _Beer_   Amount _2-3_   How Often? _Every week_

History of Alcoholism? _No_

When was your last TB or Tine test? _I can't remember_

Have you ever had a positive test for tuberculosis? _No_

When was your last Tetanus shot? _Last year, I cut my finger when fishing._

List all surgeries you have had in the past:

Date	**Type of Surgery**
1952-childhood?	_Tonsillectomy_

List all past hospitalizations (not involving surgeries above):

Date	**Reason For Hospital Stay**
Spring, 1999	_Pneumonia_

List all past problems with trauma (broken bones, lacerations, etc.):

Cut my finger while fishing last year. I had a broken leg from a car accident in 1984.

REVIEW OF SYSTEMS, PAST MEDICAL PROBLEMS:

If you have been told you have any of the problems listed below, or are having any of the problems listed below, please CIRCLE:

1. GENERAL: Weight loss, weight gain, fever, chills, night sweats, hot flashes, tire easily, problems with sleep, crying spells, history of cancer.

2. SKIN: Rash, sores that won't heal, moles that are new or changing, history of skin problems.

3. HEENT: Headache, eye problems, hearing problems, sinus problems, hay fever, dizziness, hoarseness, sores in your mouth that won't heal, dental problems.

   Do you chew tobacco or dip snuff? _No_

4. METABOLIC/ENDOCRINE: Thyroid problems, diabetes or sugar problems, high cholesterol.

Step 2A. Completed Medical History Form–Front.

(continued)

PSY PROCEDURE 3-2: **Document a Chief Complaint (CC) and Present Illness (PI) (continued)**

Steps	Reasons

5. <u>RESPIRATORY:</u> (Cough,) wheezing, breathing problems, history of asthma, history of lung problems.

Do you smoke cigarettes or pipe? *Cigarettes*

How much? *1 pack a day*   For how long? *20 years*

6. <u>BREAST (WOMEN):</u> Breast lumps, changes in nipples, nipple discharge, breast problems, family history of breast cancer. When was your last mammogram?

7. <u>CARDIOVASCULAR:</u> Heart murmur, rheumatic fever, high blood pressure, angina, heart problems, heart attack, abnormal heart rhythm, chest pain, palpitations, leg swelling, history of phlebitis or blood clots.

8. <u>GI:</u> Problems with appetite, swallowing, heartburn, nausea, vomiting, pain in the abdomen, constipation, diarrhea, blood in stool, history of ulcers, liver problems, hepatitis, jaundice, pancreas problems, gallbladder problems, or colon problems.

9. <u>REPRODUCTIVE (WOMEN):</u> Problems with irregular menstrual cycles, abnormal vaginal bleeding or discharge, history of sexually transmitted diseases, sexual problems.

AGE OF FIRST MENSES (PERIOD) _____   AGE OF MENOPAUSE _____

LAST PAP SMEAR _____   METHOD OF CONTRACEPTION _____

Obstetric History (Women)

NUMBER OF PREGNANCIES _____   PLEASE LIST AS FOLLOWS:

Delivery Date   Pregnancy Complications   Type Delivery   Baby's Weight

<u>MEN:</u> Problems with genital discharge, history of venereal diseases, sexual problems, prostate problems.

METHOD OF CONTRACEPTION _____

10. <u>UROLOGIC:</u> Problems with painful urination, urinary frequency, blood in urine, weak urinary stream, history of bladder or kidney infections, or kidney stones.

11. <u>MUSCULOSKELETAL:</u> Arthritis, back pain, cramps in legs.

12. <u>NEUROLOGIC:</u> Seizures, stroke, arm or leg weakness or numbness, black-out spells, memory or thinking problems, depression, anxiety, psychiatric problems.

13. <u>HEMATOLOGIC:</u> Anemia, bleeding problems, enlarged lymph nodes.

HAVE YOU EVER HAD A BLOOD TRANSFUSION? _____   DATE _____

FAMILY HISTORY:

List any medical problems that run in your family and which family members have these problems.

Grandmother had colon cancer; Father has high blood pressure

SOCIAL HISTORY:

MARITAL STATUS: *Married for 30 years*

OCCUPATION: *Mail Carrier*

EDUCATION: *Graduated high school 1963*

HOBBIES: *Fishing, camping*

WHAT DO YOU DO FOR ENJOYMENT? _____

Step 2B. Completed Medical History Form–Back.

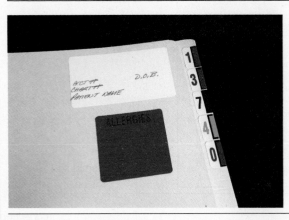

Step 2C. A complete medical record.

(continued)

PSY PROCEDURE 3-2: Document a Chief Complaint (CC) and Present Illness (PI) (continued)

Steps	Reasons
3. Greet and identify the patient while escorting him or her to the examination room.	Greeting the patient by name helps develop a professional rapport and eases patient's anxiety. Correctly identifying the patient may help to prevent errors.

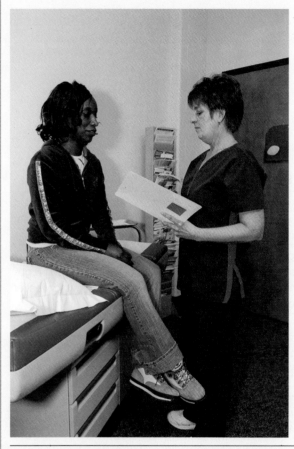

Step 3. Always check patient identification information with what is recorded in the medical record.

Steps	Reasons
4. Using open-ended questions, find out why the patient is seeking medical care; maintain eye contact.	Maintaining eye contact demonstrates that you are actively listening.
5. **AFF** Explain how to respond to a patient who has dementia.	Solicit assistance from caregiver or other staff member to help during the procedure. Give simple directions to the patient about what he/she should do. Speak clearly, not loudly.
6. Determine the PI using open-ended and closed-ended questions.	Use closed-ended questions to obtain specific data only after the patient has responded to open-ended questions.
7. Document the CC and PI correctly on the cumulative problem list or progress report form.	Documentation should include the date, time, CC, PI, and your signature (first initial, last name, and title). Use only correct medical terminology and approved abbreviations.

(continued)

PSY **PROCEDURE 3-2:** **Document a Chief Complaint (CC) and Present Illness (PI)** *(continued)*

Steps	Reasons
09/15/2011 *9:45 a.m. CC: Pt. c/o headache and nausea x3 days. Has taken ibuprofen for the pain with "some relief." The pain is a "dull ache" in the frontal area of the head and face. Denies emesis. Face flushed, skin warm and dry. T 98.9°F, P88, R24, BP 190/110 (L) sitting.* *S. Vincer, CMA*	
	Step 7. Sample documentation in the patient record.
8. Thank the patient for cooperating, and explain that the physician will soon be in to examine the patient.	Courtesy encourages a positive attitude about the physician's office. If you indicate a time frame in reference to the physician coming into the examination room, be honest.
9. Describe examples of applying local, state, and federal health care legislation and regulation in the medical office.	Local regulations include required reporting of communicable diseases or injuries involving violence. State and federal regulations may include issues related to reimbursement, collection of fees, and privacy (HIPAA).

Charting Example:

09/15/2012 9:45 AM CC: Pt. c/o headache and nausea ×3 days Has taken ibuprofen for the pain with "some relief."
The pain is a "dull ache" in the frontal area of the head and face. Denies emesis. Face flushed, skin warm and dry.
T 98.8°F, P 88, R 24, BP 190/110 (L) sitting ————————————————————— S. Vincer, CMA

Note: The medical assistant may sign his/her name in the patient record using only the "CMA" credential if the office has a signature log denoting the entire credential as "CMA(AAMA)."

- In every medical practice, a history is taken from each patient.
- As a professional medical assistant, you need to know the components of a standard medical history form. You may be required to obtain and document the information on the history form and to interview the patient to elicit the chief complaint and present illness.
- The physician relies on the information that you gather and document for diagnosing and treating patients, so it is essential that you question the patient carefully and document accurately.

Warm Ups for Critical Thinking

1. Mrs. Smythe has always been impeccably groomed, articulate, and punctual for her monthly blood pressure checks. Today, she was 15 minutes late, her hair was not combed, she wore no makeup, and her clothes did not match. Are any of these observations worth noting on her chart?

2. After reviewing the following items, determine in which section of the medical history the information should be included and explain why. Identify any items that are irrelevant.
   - Sister died of breast cancer.
   - Son had chicken pox last year.
   - Patient has many allergies.
   - Father died of heart disease.
   - Mother is alive and well.
   - Brother works in real estate.
   - Patient smokes three packs of cigarettes a day.
   - Patient works in a cotton mill.
   - Patient is a runner and teaches aerobics.
   - Patient has recently lost 60 pounds.
   - Patient had an angioplasty last year.

3. Determine which of the following are signs and which are symptoms.
   - Nausea
   - Vomiting
   - Itching
   - Rash
   - Dizziness
   - Abdominal pain
   - Pallor
   - Tingling fingers and toes
   - Ringing in the ears
   - Fever
   - Edema

4. Provide open-ended questions for obtaining additional information from patients with the following complaints:
   - "I am tired; I don't sleep well at night."
   - "I have pain in the bottom of my foot when I walk."
   - "My stomach hurts, and I threw up yesterday."
   - "I have indigestion every day."

5. An elderly patient, Mr. Barnes, comes into the office and is given the medical history form, a pen, and a clipboard. He is unable to hold the pen due to arthritic deformities of his hands. Would it be appropriate to sit with Mr. Barnes in the waiting room and complete the form for him? Why or why not?

Anthropometric Measurements and Vital Signs

Learning Outcomes

Cognitive Domain

Note: AAMA/CAAHEP 2008 Standards are italicized.

1. Spell and define key terms
2. Explain the procedures for measuring a patient's height and weight
3. Identify and describe the types of thermometers
4. Compare the procedures for measuring a patient's temperature using the oral, rectal, axillary, and tympanic methods
5. List the fever process, including the stages of fever
6. Describe the procedure for measuring a patient's pulse and respiratory rates
7. Identify the various sites on the body used for palpating a pulse
8. Define Korotkoff sounds and the five phases of blood pressure
9. Identify factors that may influence the blood pressure
10. Explain the factors to consider when choosing the correct blood pressure cuff size
11. *Discuss implications for disease and disability when homeostasis is not maintained*

Psychomotor Domain

Note: AAMA/CAAHEP 2008 Standards are italicized.

1. Measure and record a patient's weight (Procedure 4-1)
2. Measure and record a patient's height (Procedure 4-2)
3. Measure and record a patient's oral temperature using a glass mercury thermometer (Procedure 4-3)
4. Measure and record a patient's rectal temperature (Procedure 4-4)
5. Measure and record a patient's axillary temperature (Procedure 4-5)
6. Measure and record a patient's temperature using an electronic thermometer (Procedure 4-6)
7. Measure and record a patient's temperature using a tympanic thermometer (Procedure 4-7)
8. Measure and record a patient's temperature using a temporal artery thermometer (Procedure 4-8)
9. Measure and record a patient's radial pulse (Procedure 4-9)
10. Measure and record a patient's respirations (Procedure 4-10)
11. Measure and record a patient's blood pressure (Procedure 4-11)
12. *Obtain vital signs*
13. *Practice standard precautions*
14. *Document accurately in the patient record*

Affective Domain

Note: AAMA/CAAHEP 2008 Standards are italicized.

1. *Apply critical thinking skills in performing patient assessment and care*
2. *Demonstrate respect for diversity in approaching patients and families*

3. *Explain rationale for performance of a procedure to the patient*
4. *Apply active listening skills*
5. *Demonstrate empathy in communicating with patients, family, and staff*
6. *Use appropriate body language and other nonverbal skills in communicating with patients, family, and staff*
7. *Demonstrate awareness of the territorial boundaries of the person with whom you are communicating*
8. *Demonstrate sensitivity appropriate to the message being delivered*
9. *Demonstrate recognition of the patient's level of understanding in communications*
10. *Recognize and protect personal boundaries in communicating with others*
11. *Demonstrate respect for individual diversity, incorporating awareness of one's own biases in areas including gender, race, religion, age, and economic status*

ABHES Competencies

1. Take vital signs
2. Document accurately

Key Terms

afebrile	cardinal signs	hypertension	pyrexia
anthropometric measurements	diaphoresis	hyperventilation	relapsing fever
apnea	diastole	hypopnea	remittent fever
baseline data	dyspnea	intermittent fever	sphygmomanometer
calibrated	febrile	orthopnea	sustained fever
cardiac cycle	hyperpnea	palpation	systole
cardiac output	hyperpyrexia	postural hypotension	tympanic

Vital signs, also known as **cardinal signs,** are measurements of bodily functions essential to maintaining life processes. Vital signs frequently measured and recorded by the medical assistant include the temperature (T), pulse rate (P), respiratory rate (R), and blood pressure (BP). In addition, medical assistants take **anthropometric measurements,** or the height and weight, of patients and document them in the medical record. This information is essential for the physician to diagnose, treat, and prevent many disorders.

Measurements taken at the first visit are recorded as **baseline data** and are used as reference points for comparison during subsequent visits. After the first office visit, the height is usually not taken; however, the vital signs and weight are taken and recorded for each adult patient at each visit to the medical office.

COG Anthropometric Measurements

Weight

An accurate weight is always required for pregnant patients, infants, children, and the elderly. In addition, weight monitoring may be required if the patient has been prescribed medications that must be carefully calculated according to body weight or for a patient who is attempting to gain or lose weight.

Since most medical practices have only one scale, placement of the scale is important. Many patients are uncomfortable if they are weighed in a place that is not private. Types of scales used to measure weight include balance beam scales, digital scales, and dial scales (Fig. 4-1). Weight may be measured in pounds or kilograms, depending upon the preference of the physician and the type of scale in the medical office. Procedure 4-1 describes how to measure and record a patient's weight.

Height

Height can be measured using the movable ruler on the back of most balance beam scales. Some offices use a graph ruler mounted on a wall (Fig. 4-2), but more accurate measures can be made with a parallel bar moved down against the top of the patient's head. Height is measured in inches or centimeters, depending upon the physician's preference. Procedure 4-2 describes how to measure an adult patient's height. Refer to Chapter 22

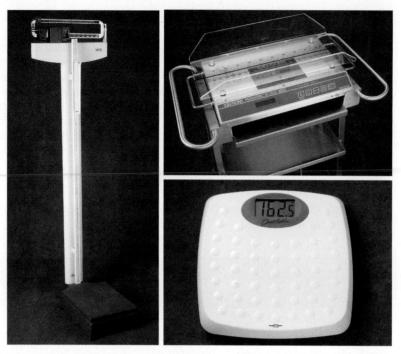

Figure 4-1 The three types of scales used in medical offices include the digital, dial, and balance beam scale.

for the procedure for measuring the height and weight of infants and children.

 CHECKPOINT QUESTION

1. Why is it important to accurately measure vital signs at every patient visit?

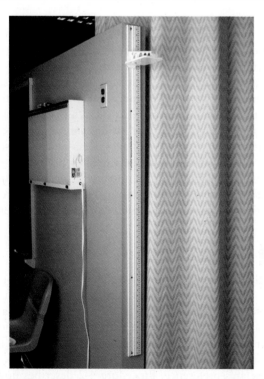

Figure 4-2 A wall-mounted device to measure height and the sliding bar on the balance beam scale.

COG **Vital Signs**

Temperature

Body temperature reflects a balance between heat produced and heat lost by the body (Fig. 4-3). Heat is produced during normal internal physical and chemical processes called *metabolism* and through muscle movement. Heat is normally lost through several processes, including respiration, elimination, and conduction through the skin (Table 4-1). Normally, the body maintains a constant internal temperature of around 98.6° Fahrenheit (F) or 37.0° Celsius (C) (centigrade). A patient whose temperature is within normal limits is said to be **afebrile**, whereas a patient with a temperature above normal is considered **febrile** (has a fever).

Thermometers are used to measure body temperature using either the Fahrenheit or Celsius scale. Box 4-1

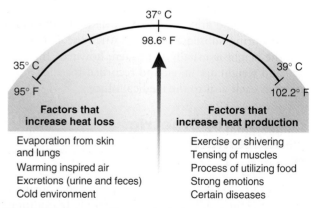

Factors that increase heat loss	Factors that increase heat production
Evaporation from skin and lungs	Exercise or shivering
Warming inspired air	Tensing of muscles
Excretions (urine and feces)	Process of utilizing food
Cold environment	Strong emotions
	Certain diseases

37° C
98.6° F
35° C   39° C
95° F   102.2° F

Figure 4-3 Factors affecting the balance between heat loss and heat production.

TABLE **4-1**	**Mechanisms of Heat Transfer**	
Mechanism	**Definition**	**Example**
Radiation	Diffusion or dissemination of heat by electromagnetic waves.	The body gives off waves of heat from uncovered surfaces.
Convection	Dissemination of heat by motion between areas of unequal density.	An oscillating fan blows cool air across the surface of a warm body.
Evaporation	Conversion of liquid to vapor.	Body fluid (perspiration and insensible loss) evaporates from the skin.
Conduction	Transfer of heat during direct contact between two objects. The body gives off waves of heat from uncovered surfaces.	The body transfers heat to an ice pack, melting the ice.

compares temperatures taken a variety of ways in Celsius and in Fahrenheit. Since glass or electronic thermometers used in the medical office may be in either scale, you should be able to convert from one scale to another (see Appendix G). The patient's temperature can be measured using the oral, rectal, axillary, or **tympanic**

method. The oral method is most commonly used, but use of the tympanic thermometer is also becoming more prevalent, especially in pediatric offices. A newer type of thermometer that you may see is the temporal artery thermometer (Fig. 4-4). This device measures the temperature of the blood within the temporal artery through the skin. If used accurately, both the tympanic thermometer and the temporal artery thermometer give readings that are comparable to the oral temperature.

A reading of 98.6°F orally is considered a normal average for body temperature, with the normal range being 97°F to 99°F. Rectal and axillary readings will vary slightly. Generally, rectal temperatures are 1°F higher than the oral temperatures because of the vascularity and tightly closed environment of the rectum. Axillary temperatures are usually 1°F lower because of lower vascularity and difficulty in keeping the axilla tightly closed. When recording the body temperature, you must

---

BOX 4-1

TEMPERATURE COMPARISONS

	Fahrenheit	Centigrade
Oral	98.6°	37.0°
Rectal	99.6°	37.6°
Axillary	97.6°	36.4°
Tympanic	98.6°	37.0°

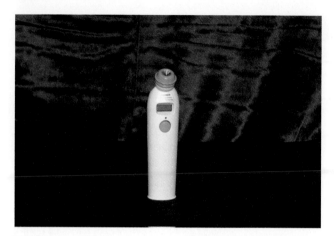

Figure 4-4 A temporal artery scanning thermometer.

indicate the temperature reading and the method used to obtain it, such as oral, rectal, axillary, tympanic, or temporal artery. A rectal temperature reading of 101°F is equivalent to 100°F orally, and an axillary reading of 101°F is equivalent to 102°F orally.

 CHECKPOINT QUESTION

2. How does an oral temperature measurement differ from a rectal measurement? Why?

Fever Processes

Although a patient's temperature is influenced by heat lost or produced by the body, it is regulated by the hypothalamus in the brain. When the hypothalamus senses that the body is too warm, it initiates peripheral vasodilation to carry core heat to the body surface via the blood and increases perspiration to cool the body by evaporation. If the temperature registers too low, vasoconstriction to conserve heat and shivering to generate more heat will usually maintain a fairly normal core temperature. Temperature elevations and variations are often a *sign* of disease but are not diseases in themselves. The following factors may cause the temperature to vary:

* *Age.* Children usually have a higher metabolism and therefore a higher body temperature than adults. The elderly, who have slower metabolisms, usually have lower readings than younger adults. Temperatures of both the very young and the elderly are easily affected by the environment.
* *Gender.* Women usually have a slightly higher temperature than men, especially at the time of ovulation and during pregnancy.
* *Exercise.* Activity causes the body to burn more calories for energy, which raises the body temperature.
* *Time of day.* The body temperature is usually lowest in the early morning before physical activity has begun.
* *Emotions.* Temperature tends to rise during times of stress and fall with depression.

* *Illness.* High or low body temperatures may result from a disease process.

Stages of Fever

An elevated temperature, or fever, usually results from a disease process, such as a bacterial or viral infection. Body temperature may also rise during intense exercise, anxiety, or dehydration unrelated to a disease process, but these elevations are not considered fevers. **Pyrexia** refers to a fever of 102°F or higher rectally or 101°F or higher orally. An extremely high temperature, 105° to 106°F, is **hyperpyrexia** and is considered dangerous because the intense internal body heat may damage or destroy cells of the brain and other vital organs. The fever process has several clearly defined stages:

1. The *onset* may be abrupt or gradual.
2. The *course* may range from a day or so to several weeks. Fever may be **sustained** (constant), **remittent** (fluctuating), **intermittent** (occurring at intervals), or **relapsing** (returning after an extended period of normal readings). Table 4-2 describes and illustrates these courses of fever.

TABLE **4-2**	**Variations in Fever Patterns: Temperature Comparisons**	
	Fahrenheit	**Celsius**
Oral	98.6	37.0
Rectal	99.6	37.6
Axillary	97.6	36.4
Tympanic	98.6	37.0

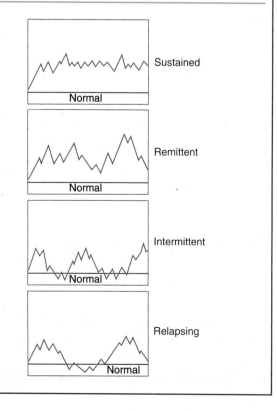

3. The *resolution*, or return to normal, may occur as either a *crisis* (abrupt return to normal) or *lysis* (gradual return to normal).

PATIENT EDUCATION
FEVER

When instructing patients about fever, explain that temperature elevations are usually a natural response to disease and that efforts to bring the temperature back to normal may be counterproductive. However, if the patient is uncomfortable or the temperature is abnormally high, it should be brought down to about 101°F; the body's natural defenses may still be able to destroy the pathogen without extreme discomfort to the patient.

After consulting with the physician, instruct all patients regarding the following comfort measures:

- Consume clear fluids by mouth as tolerated to rehydrate the tissues if nausea and vomiting are not present.
- Keep clothing and bedding clean and dry, especially after **diaphoresis** (sweating).
- Avoid chilling. Chills cause shivering, which raises the body temperature.
- Rest and eat a light diet as tolerated.
- Use antipyretics to keep comfortable, but *do not* give aspirin products to children under 18 years of age. Aspirin has been associated with Reye syndrome, a potentially fatal disorder, following cases of viral illnesses and varicella zoster (chicken pox).

CHECKPOINT QUESTION

3. Explain why the body temperature of a young child may be different from that of an adult.

Types of Thermometers

Glass Mercury Thermometers

In the past, oral, rectal, and axillary temperatures have been measured using a mercury glass thermometer.

Because mercury is a hazardous chemical if exposure occurs, a mercury spill kit must be available should a mercury thermometer break. The exposed mercury must be cleaned using proper procedures according to the office policy and procedure manual. Never allow anyone to touch or manipulate the mercury from a broken thermometer.

Although most medical offices today do not use mercury filled glass thermometers, glass thermometers are available that contain a non-mercury substance. Some offices may use these thermometers or have some available for use in the event the elctronic thermometers malfunction. These thermometers are similar in appearance to mercury thermometers. Both the mercury and non-mercury glass thermometers consists of a glass tube divided into two major parts. The bulb end is filled with mercury or the non-mercury substance and may have a round or a slender tip. Glass thermometers have different shapes for oral and rectal use. Rectal thermometers have a rounded, or stubbed, end and are usually color-coded red on the opposite flat end of the thermometer. Thermometers with a long, slender bulb are used for axillary or oral temperatures and are color-coded blue (Fig. 4-5). When the glass thermometer is placed in position for a specified period, body heat expands the chemical in the bulb, which rises up the glass column and remains there until it is physically shaken back into the bulb.

The long stem of the Fahrenheit thermometer is **calibrated** with lines designating temperature in even degrees: 94°, 96°, 98°, 100°, and so on. Uneven numbers are marked only with a longer line. Between these longer lines, four smaller lines designate temperature in 0.2° increments. The thermometer is read by noting the level of the mercury or non-mercury substance in the glass column. For example, if the level of the chemical falls on the second smaller line past the large line marked 100, the reading is 100.4°F. Celsius thermometers are marked for each degree (35°, 36°, 37°, and so on), with 10 markings between the whole numbers (Fig. 4-6). If the mercury falls on the third small line past the line marked 37, the temperature reading is recorded as 37.3°C.

Glass thermometers may be reused if properly disinfected between patients. Also, before using a glass

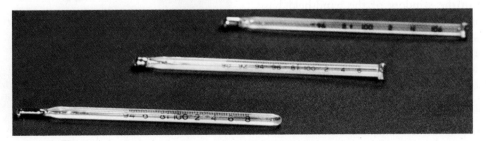
Figure 4-5 Glass mercury thermometers. *Front:* Slender bulb, oral. *Center:* Rounded bulb, red tip, rectal. *Back:* Blue tip, oral.

Centigrade

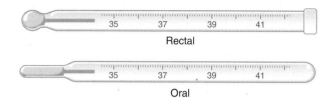

Fahrenheit

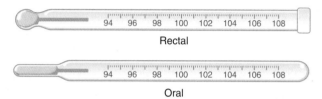

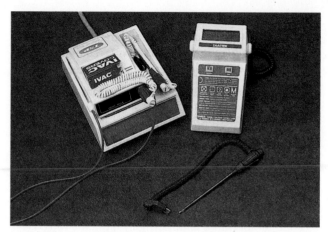

Figure 4-7 Two types of electronic thermometers and probes.

Figure 4-6 The two glass thermometers on the top are calibrated in the Celsius (centigrade) scale, and the two on the bottom use the Fahrenheit scale. Note the blunt bulb on the rectal thermometers and the long thin bulb on the oral thermometers.

thermometer, place it in a disposable clear plastic sheath. When you take the thermometer from the patient, remove the sheath by pulling the thermometer out, which turns the sheath inside out and traps the saliva inside it. Dispose of the sheath in a biohazard container, sanitize, and disinfect the thermometer according to the office policy. Usually, washing the thermometers with warm—not hot—soapy water and soaking in a solution of 70% isopropyl alcohol is sufficient for disinfection.

The procedure for measuring an oral temperature using a glass thermometer is described in Procedure 4-3. The procedures for measuring a rectal or axillary temperature using either the glass thermometer or the electronic thermometer are described in Procedures 4-4 and 4-5.

Electronic Thermometers

Electronic thermometers are portable battery-operated units with interchangeable probes (Fig. 4-7). The base unit of the thermometer is battery operated, and the interchangeable probes are color-coded blue for oral or axillary and red for rectal. When the probe is properly positioned, the temperature is sensed, and a digital readout shows in the window of the hand-held base. Electronic thermometers are usually kept in a charging unit between uses to ensure that the batteries are operative at all times. The procedure for taking and recording an oral temperature using an electronic thermometer is described in Procedure 4-6.

Tympanic Thermometers

Another type of thermometer used in medical offices today is the tympanic, or aural, thermometer. This device is usually battery powered. The end is fitted with a disposable cover that is inserted into the ear much like an otoscope (Fig. 4-8). With the end of the thermometer in place, a button is pressed, and infrared light bounces off the tympanic membrane, or eardrum. When correctly positioned in the ear, the sensor in the thermometer determines the temperature of the blood in the tympanic membrane. The temperature reading is displayed on the unit's digital screen within 2 seconds. This device is considered highly reliable for temperature measurement. Procedure 4-7 describes the complete process for obtaining a body temperature with a tympanic thermometer.

Temporal Artery Thermometer

The temporal artery thermometer measures actual blood temperature by placing the unit on the front of the forehead, pressing the "on/off" button, and sliding the probe scanner over the forehead and down to the temporal artery area of the forehead. Upon releasing the "on/off" button, the temperature is immediately

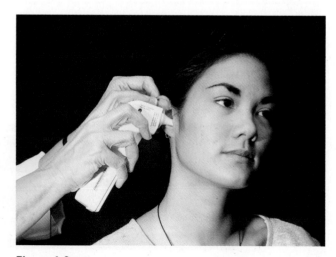

Figure 4-8 The tympanic thermometer in use.

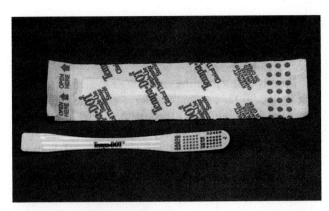

Figure 4-9 Disposable paper thermometer. The dots change color to indicate the body temperature.

recorded in the digital display box located on the front of the thermometer. Depending on the brand and type of temporal artery thermometer purchased, you should read the manufacturer's instructions carefully for proper use and care of the unit. Procedure 4-8 describes the steps for taking a temperature for taking a temperature using the temporal artery thermometer.

Disposable Thermometers

Single-use disposable thermometers are fairly accurate but are not considered as reliable as electronic, tympanic, or glass thermometers. These thermometers register quickly by indicating color changes on a strip. They are not reliable for definitive measurement, but they are acceptable for screening in settings such as day care centers and schools (Fig. 4-9). Other disposable thermometers are available for pediatric use in the form of sucking devices, or pacifiers, but these are not used in the medical office setting.

 CHECKPOINT QUESTION

4. How is the reading displayed on an electronic, tympanic, and temporal artery thermometer?

 Pulse

As the heart beats, blood is forced through the arteries, expanding them. With relaxation of the heart, the arteries relax also. This expansion and relaxation of the arteries can be felt at various points on the body where you can press an artery against a bone or other underlying firm surface. These areas are known as pulse points. With **palpation**, each expansion of the artery can be felt and is counted as one heartbeat. A pulse in specific arteries supplying blood to the extremities also indicates that oxygenated blood is flowing to that extremity.

The heartbeat can be palpated (felt) or auscultated (heard) at several pulse points. The arteries most commonly used are the carotid, apical, brachial, radial, femoral, popliteal, posterior tibial, and dorsalis pedis (Fig. 4-10). Palpation of the pulse is performed by placing the index and middle fingers, the middle and ring fingers, or all three fingers over a pulse point (Fig. 4-11). The thumb is not used to palpate a pulse. The apical pulse is auscultated using a stethoscope with the bell placed over the apex of the heart (Fig. 4-12). A Doppler unit may be used to amplify the sound of peripheral pulses that are difficult to palpate (Fig. 4-13). This unit is a small battery-powered or electric device that consists of a main box with control switches, a probe, and an earpiece unit that plugs into the main box and resembles the earpieces to a stethoscope. The earpiece may be detached so the sounds can be heard by everyone in the room if desired. Follow the following steps to use a Doppler device:

1. Apply a coupling or transmission gel on the pulse point before placing the end of the probe, or transducer, on the area. This gel creates an airtight seal between the probe and the skin and facilitates transmission of the sound.
2. With the machine on, hold the probe at a 90-degree angle with light pressure to ensure contact. Move the probe as necessary in small circles in the gel until you hear the pulse. When contact with the artery is made, the Doppler will emit a loud pumping sound with each heartbeat. Adjust the volume control on the Doppler unit as necessary.
3. After assessing the rate and rhythm of the pulse, clean the patient's skin and the probe with a tissue or soft cloth. Do not clean the probe with water or alcohol, as this may damage the transducer.

Pulse Characteristics

While palpating the pulse, you also assess the rate, rhythm, and volume as the artery wall expands with each heartbeat. The *rate* is the number of heartbeats in 1 minute. This number can be determined by palpating the pulse and counting each heartbeat while watching the second hand of your watch either for 30 seconds and then multiplying that number by 2 or for 1 minute. In healthy adults, the average pulse rate is 60 to 100 beats per minute. At other ages, there is a large variance of pulse rates, as shown in Table 4-3.

The *rhythm* is the interval between each heartbeat or the pattern of beats. Normally, this pattern is regular, with each heartbeat occurring at a regular, consistent rate. An irregular rhythm should be counted for 1 full minute to determine the rate, and the irregular rhythm should be documented with the pulse rate.

Volume, the strength or force of the heartbeat, can be described as soft, bounding, weak, thready, strong, or full. Usually the volume of the pulse is recorded only if it is weak, thready, or bounding.

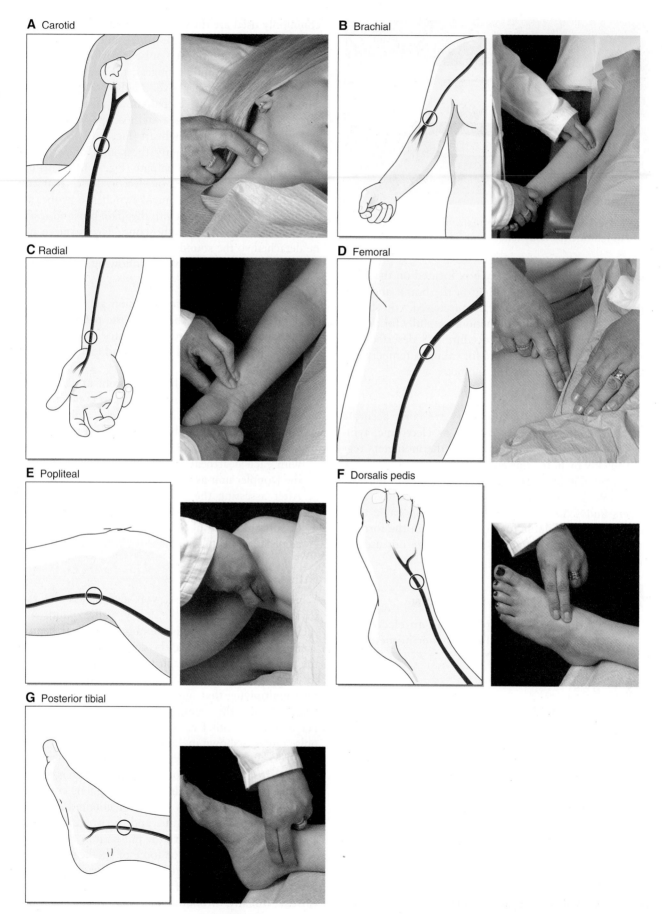

Figure 4-10 Sites for palpation of peripheral pulses.

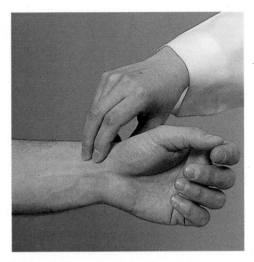

Figure 4-11 Measuring a radial pulse.

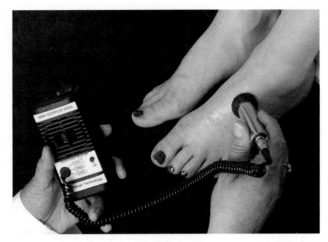

Figure 4-13 The dorsalis pedis pulse being auscultated using a Doppler device.

Factors Affecting Pulse Rates

Many factors affect the force, speed, and rhythm of the heart. Young children and infants have a much faster heart rate than adults. A conditioned athlete may have a normal heart rate below 60 beats per minute. Older adults may have a faster heart rate, as the myocardium compensates for decreased efficiency. Other factors that affect pulse rates are listed in Table 4-4.

The radial artery is most often used to determine pulse rate because it is convenient for both the medical assistant and the patient (Procedure 4-9). If the radial pulse is irregular or hard to palpate, then the apical pulse is the site of choice (Fig. 4-14). To assess the flow of blood into the extremities, you may be asked to palpate peripheral pulses such as the dorsalis pedis. Peripheral pulses that are difficult to palpate may be auscultated with a Doppler unit to check for the presence of blood flow.

 CHECKPOINT QUESTION

5. What characteristics of a patient's pulse should be assessed, and how should they be recorded in the medical record?

 Respiration

Respiration is the exchange of gases between the atmosphere and the blood in the body. With respiration, the body expels carbon dioxide (CO_2) and takes in oxygen (O_2). External respiration is inhalation and exhalation, during which air travels through the respiratory tract to the alveoli so that oxygen can be absorbed into the bloodstream. Internal respiration is the exchange of gases between the blood and the tissue cells. Respiration is controlled by the respiratory center in the brainstem and by feedback from chemosensors in the carotid arteries that monitor the CO_2 content in the blood.

As the patient breathes in (inspiration), oxygen flows into the lungs, and the diaphragm contracts and flattens out, lifting and expanding the rib cage. During expiration, air in the lungs flows out of the chest cavity as

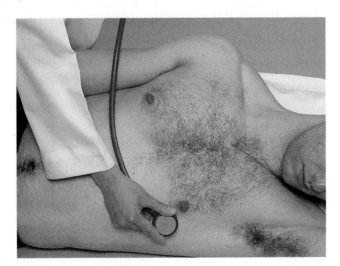

Figure 4-12 Measuring an apical pulse.

TABLE **4-3**	Variations in Pulse Rate by Age
Age	**Beats per Minute**
Birth to 1 year	110–170
1–10 years	90–110
10–16 years	80–95
16 years to midlife	70–80
Elderly adult	55–70

TABLE 4-4	Factors Affecting Pulse Rates
Factor	**Effect**
Time of day	The pulse is usually lower early in the morning than later in the day.
Gender	Women have a slightly higher pulse rate than men.
Body type and size	Tall, thin people usually have a lower pulse rate than shorter, stockier people.
Exercise	The heart rate increases with the need for increased **cardiac output** (the amount of blood ejected from either ventricle in 1 minute).
Stress or emotions	Anger, fear, excitement, and stress will raise the pulse; depression will lower it.
Fever	The increased need for cell metabolism in the presence of fever raises the cardiac output to supply oxygen and nutrients; the pulse may rise as much as 10 beats/minute per degree of fever.
Medications	Many medications raise or lower the pulse as a desired effect or as an undesirable side effect.
Blood volume	Loss of blood volume to hemorrhage or dehydration will increase the need for cellular metabolism and will increase the cardiac output to supply the need.

the diaphragm relaxes, moves upward into a dome-like shape, and allows the rib cage to contract. Each respiration is counted as one full inspiration and one full expiration.

Observing the rise and fall of the chest to count respirations is usually performed as a part of the pulse measurement. Generally, you should not make the patient aware that you are counting respirations because patients often change the voluntary action of breathing if they are aware that they are being watched. Respirations can be counted for a full minute or for 30 seconds with the number multiplied by 2. When appropriate, a stethoscope may be used to auscultate respirations.

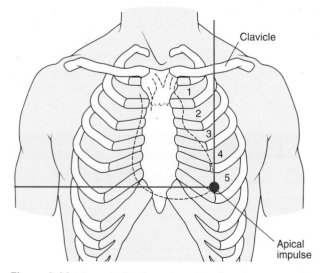

Figure 4-14 The apical pulse is found at the 5th intercostal space at the midclavicular line.

Respiration Characteristics

The characteristics of respirations include rate, rhythm, and depth. *Rate* is the number of respirations occurring in 1 minute. *Rhythm* is the time, or spacing, between each respiration. This pattern is equal and regular in patients with normal respirations. Any abnormal rhythm is described as irregular and recorded as such in the patient's record after the rate.

Depth is the volume of air being inhaled and exhaled. When a person is at rest, the depth should be regular and consistent. There are normally no noticeable sounds other than the regular exchange of air. Respirations that are abnormally deep or shallow are documented in addition to the rate. Abnormal sounds during inspiration or expiration are usually a sign of a disease process. These abnormal sounds are usually recorded as crackles (wet or dry sounds) or wheezes (high-pitched sounds) heard during inspiration or expiration.

Factors Affecting Respiration

In healthy adults, the average respiratory rate is 14 to 20 breaths per minute. Table 4-5 shows the normal variations in respiratory rates according to age. Patients with an elevated body temperature usually also have

TABLE 4-5	Variations in Respiration Ranges by Age
Age	**Respirations per Minute**
Infant	20+
Child	18–20
Adult	12–20

TABLE 4-6	Blood Pressure Readings			
	Systolic BP		**Diastolic BP**	
Normal	<120 mm Hg	and	<80 mm Hg	
Prehypertension	120–139 mm Hg	or	80–89 mm Hg	
Hypertension, stage I	140–159 mm Hg	or	90–99 mm Hg	
Hypertension stage II	≥160 mm Hg	or	≥100 mm Hg	

Source: U.S. Department of Health and Human Services, National Institutes of Health, National Heart, Lung, and Blood Institute

increased pulse and respiratory rates. A respiratory rate that is much faster than average is called tachypnea, and a respiratory rate that is slower than usual is referred to as bradypnea. Further descriptions of abnormal or unusual respirations include the following:

- **Dyspnea:** difficult or labored breathing
- **Apnea:** no respiration
- **Hyperpnea:** abnormally deep, gasping breaths
- **Hyperventilation:** a respiratory rate that greatly exceeds the body's oxygen demand
- **Hypopnea:** shallow respirations
- **Orthopnea:** inability to breathe lying down; the patient usually has to sit upright to breathe

Procedure 4-10 lists the steps for counting and recording respirations.

 CHECKPOINT QUESTION

6. What happens within the chest cavity when the diaphragm contracts?

 Blood Pressure

Blood pressure is a measurement of the pressure of the blood in an artery as it is forced against the arterial walls. Pressure is measured in the contraction and relaxation phases of the **cardiac cycle,** or heartbeat. When the heart contracts, it forces blood from the atria and ventricles in the phase known as **systole.** This highest pressure level during contraction is recorded as the systolic pressure and is heard as the first sound in taking blood pressure.

As the heart pauses briefly to rest and refill, the arterial pressure drops. This phase is known as **diastole,** and the pressure is recorded as the diastolic pressure. Systolic and diastolic pressure result from the two parts of the cardiac cycle, the period from the beginning of one heartbeat to the beginning of the next. When measured using a stethoscope and **sphygmomanometer,** or blood

pressure cuff, these two pressures constitute the blood pressure and are written as a fraction, with the systolic pressure over the diastolic pressure. Table 4-6 describes the classification of blood pressure readings for adults with normal, prehypertension, and hypertension blood pressures. A lower pressure may be normal for athletes with exceptionally well-conditioned cardiovascular systems. Blood pressure that drops suddenly when the patient stands from a sitting or lying position is **postural hypotension,** or *orthostatic hypotension*; it may cause symptoms including vertigo. Some patients with postural hypotension may faint. Extra precautions should be taken when assessing patients going from lying down to sitting or standing.

Two basic types of sphygmomanometers are used to measure blood pressure: the aneroid, which has a circular dial for the readings, and the mercury, which has a mercury-filled glass tube for the readings (Fig. 4-15). Although only one type actually contains mercury, both types are calibrated and measure blood pressure in

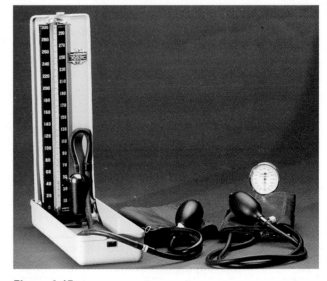

Figure 4-15 A mercury column sphygmomanometer and an aneroid sphygmomanometer.

millimeters of mercury (mm Hg). A blood pressure of 120/80 indicates the force needed to raise a column of mercury to the 120 calibration mark on the glass tube during diastole and to 80 during diastole. The elasticity of the person's arterial walls, the strength of the heart muscle, and the quantity and viscosity (thickness) of the blood all affect the blood pressure.

The sphygmomanometer is attached to a cuff by a rubber tube. A second rubber tube is attached to a hand pump with a screw valve. This device is used to pump air into the rubber bladder in the cuff. When the screw valve is turned clockwise, the bladder in the cuff around the patient's arm is inflated by multiple compressions of the pump. As the bladder inflates, the pressure created against the artery at some point prohibits blood from passing through the vessel. When the screw valve is slowly opened by turning it counterclockwise, the blood pressure can be determined by listening carefully with the stethoscope placed on the artery to the sounds produced as the blood begins to flow through the vessel. Procedure 4-11 describes the steps for correctly obtaining a patient's blood pressure using the radial artery.

 CHECKPOINT QUESTION

7. What is happening to the heart during systole? During diastole?

Korotkoff Sounds

Korotkoff sounds can be classified into five phases of sounds heard while auscultating the blood pressure as described by the Russian neurologist Nicolai Korotkoff. Only the sounds heard during phase I (represented by the first sound heard) and phase V (represented by the last sound heard) are recorded as blood pressure. You may hear other Korotkoff sounds during the procedure, but it is not necessary to record them. Table 4-7 describes the five phases of Korotkoff sounds that may be heard when auscultating blood pressure.

TABLE **4-7**	**Five Phases of Blood Pressure**
Phase	**Sounds**
I	Faint tapping heard as the cuff deflates (systolic blood pressure)
II	Soft swishing
III	Rhythmic, sharp, distinct tapping
IV	Soft tapping that becomes faint
V	Last sound (diastolic blood pressure)

 WHAT IF?

What if a patient has a dialysis shunt (a surgically made venous access port that allows a patient with little or no kidney function to be connected to a dialysis machine) in his left arm? Should you use that arm to take his blood pressure?

No! By taking a blood pressure in that arm, you could cause the shunt to be permanently damaged, and the patient would not be able to receive dialysis until another shunt was prepared by a surgeon. The patient's chart should be clearly marked indicating that a shunt is in place and which arm it is located in. Most dialysis patients are keenly aware of the importance of this shunt and will alert you to the location of their shunt. Also, you should not draw blood from this arm.

Pulse Pressure

The difference between the systolic and diastolic readings is known as the pulse pressure. For example, with the average adult blood pressure of 120/80, the difference between the numbers 120 and 80 is 40. The average normal range for pulse pressure is 30 to 50 mm Hg. Generally, the pulse pressure should be no more than one-third of the systolic reading. If the pulse pressure is more or less than these parameters, the physician should be notified.

Auscultatory Gap

Patients with a history of **hypertension**, or elevated blood pressure, may have an auscultatory gap heard during phase II of the Korotkoff sounds. An auscultatory gap is the loss of any sounds for a drop of up to 30 mm Hg (sometimes more) during the release of air from the blood pressure cuff after the first sound is heard. If the last sound heard at the beginning of the gap is recorded as the diastolic blood pressure, the documented blood pressure is inaccurate and may result in misdiagnosis and treatment of a condition that the patient does not have. As a result, it is important for you to listen and watch carefully as the dial or column of mercury falls until you are certain that you have heard the last sound, or diastolic pressure.

Factors Influencing Blood Pressure

Atherosclerosis and arteriosclerosis are two disease processes that greatly influence blood pressure. These diseases affect the size and elasticity of the artery lumen. The general health of the patient is also a major factor and includes dietary habits, alcohol and tobacco use, the amount and type of exercise, previous heart conditions such as myocardial infarctions, and family history for cardiac disease. Other factors that may affect blood pressure include:

- *Age.* As the body ages, vessels begin to lose elasticity and will require more force to expand the arterial wall. The buildup of atherosclerotic patches inside the artery will also increase the force needed for blood flow.
- *Activity.* Exercise raises the blood pressure temporarily, while inactivity or rest will usually lower the pressure.
- *Stress.* The sympathetic nervous system stimulates the release of the hormone epinephrine, which raises the pressure in response to the fight or flight syndrome.
- *Body Position.* Blood pressure will normally be lower in the supine position.
- *Medications.* Some medications will lower the pressure, while others may cause an elevation.

 PATIENT EDUCATION

HYPERTENSION

After taking a patient's blood pressure, you should tell the patient what you obtained for the blood pressure reading. Patients with hypertension, or high blood pressure, should be encouraged to keep a personal log of their readings and bring this to each physician office appointment. Because the freestanding blood pressure machines found in pharmacies and supermarkets are not always reliable, you should teach patients with hypertension how to take their blood pressure at home.

Blood Pressure Cuff Size

Before beginning to take a patient's blood pressure, assess the size of the patient's arm, and choose the

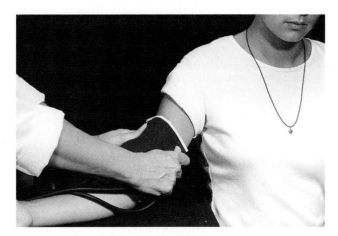

Figure 4-16 Choosing the right blood pressure cuff.

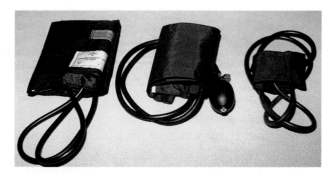

Figure 4-17 Three sizes of blood pressure cuffs (from left): a large cuff for obese adults, a normal adult cuff, and a pediatric cuff.

correct size accordingly. The width of the cuff should be 40% to 50% of the circumference of the arm. To determine the correct size, hold the narrow edge of the cuff at the midpoint of the upper arm. Wrap the width, not the length, around the arm. The cuff width should reach not quite halfway around the arm (Fig. 4-16). Varying widths of cuffs are available, from about 1 inch for infants to 8 inches for obese adults (Fig. 4-17). The blood pressure measurement may be inaccurate by as much as 30 mm Hg if the cuff size is incorrect. Box 4-2 lists causes of errors in blood pressure readings.

 CHECKPOINT QUESTION

8. How are the pulse pressure and the auscultatory gap different?

BOX 4-2

CAUSES OF ERRORS IN BLOOD PRESSURE READINGS

- Wrapping the cuff improperly
- Failing to keep the patient's arm at the level of the heart while taking the blood pressure
- Failing to support the patient's arm on a stable surface while taking the blood pressure
- Recording the auscultatory gap for the diastolic pressure
- Failing to maintain the gauge at eye level
- Applying the cuff around the patient's clothing and attempting to listen through the clothing
- Allowing the cuff to deflate too rapidly or too slowly
- Failing to wait 1–2 minutes before rechecking using the same arm

AFF TRIAGE

While working in a medical office, you have just taken the following three patients' vital signs:

A. A 52-year-old woman complaining of dyspnea. Her respiratory rate is 38, her pulse is 112 and irregular, and her blood pressure is 150/86.

B. A 43-year-old man with a pulse of 54 and blood pressure of 98/52. He denies any shortness of breath, chest pain, or dizziness.

C. A 65-year-old man who had open-heart surgery 2 weeks ago. He states that yellow drainage is coming from the surgical wound on his chest. His temperature is 101.8°F orally, his blood pressure is 188/62, and his pulse is 118 and regular.

How do you sort these patients? Who should be seen first? Second? Third?

Patient A should be seen first. The physician should immediately see any patient complaining of trouble breathing. Her respiratory and pulse rates are faster than normal for an adult. Patient C should be seen second because of his temperature and pulse rate. Patient B should be seen last. A pulse rate of 52 and blood pressure of 98/52 are low, but the patient is not complaining of any symptoms. If he is physically fit, his vital signs may normally be lower than average. If he were complaining of dizziness or feeling faint, he would need to be seen sooner.

 MEDIA MENU

- **Student Resources on thePoint**
  - **Video: Measuring an Adult Height and Weight (Procedures 4-1 and 4-2)**
  - **Video: Measuring Temperature with a Digital, Tympanic, and Temporal Artery Thermometer (Procedures 4-4, 4-5, 4-6, 4-7, and 4-8)**
  - **Video: Measuring a Patient's Pulse and Respirations (Procedures 4-9 and 4-10)**
  - **Video: Measuring a Patient's Blood Pressure (Procedure 4-11)**
  - **Animation: Breathing Sounds**
  - **Animation: Cardiac Cycle**
  - **Animation: Hypertension**
  - **CMA/RMA Certification Exam Review**

Internet Resources

National Reye's Syndrome Foundation
http://www.reyessyndrome.org
American Society of Hypertension
http://www.ash-us.org
American Lung Association
http://www.lungusa.org
National Heart Lung and Blood Institute
http://www.nhlbi.nih.gov
American Heart Association
http://www.heart.org

español **SPANISH TERMINOLOGY**

Voy a tomarle el su pulso radial.
  I am going to take your radial pulse.

Voy a tomarle la su presion sanguínea.
  I am going to take your blood pressure.

Voy a tomarle la temperature.
  I am going to take your temperatura.

¿(Tiene) fiebre?
  Fever?

PSY PROCEDURE 4-1: **Measuring Weight**

Purpose: Accurately measure and record a patient's weight
Equipment: Calibrated balance beam scale, digital scale, or dial scale; paper towel
Standard: This procedure should take 5 minutes.

Steps	Reasons
1. Wash your hands.	Handwashing before contact with patients aids in infection control.
2. Ensure that the scale is properly balanced at zero.	This helps prevent an error in measurement.

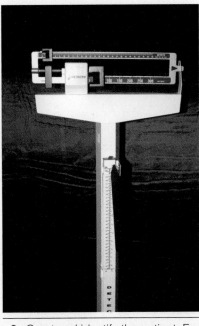

Step 2. A balance beam scale with the weights at zero.

Steps	Reasons
3. Greet and identify the patient. Explain the procedure.	Identifying the patient prevents errors; explaining the procedure promotes cooperation.
4. Escort the patient to the scale, and place a paper towel on the scale.	Since the patient will be standing in bare feet or stockings, the paper towel minimizes microorganism transmission.
5. Have the patient remove shoes and heavy outerwear and put down purse.	Unnecessary items must be removed to get an accurate reading.
6. Assist patient onto the scale facing forward and standing on paper towel without touching or holding on to anything if possible, while watching for difficulties with balance.	Some patients may feel unsteady as the plate of the scale settles.

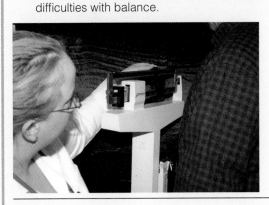

Step 6. The patient should stand erect on the scale.

(continued)

PSY PROCEDURE 4-1:   **Measuring Weight *(continued)***

Steps	Reasons

7. Weigh the patient:
   A. Balance beam scale: Slide counterweights on bottom and top bars (start with heavier bars) from zero to approximate weight. Each counterweight should rest securely in the notch with indicator mark at proper calibration. To obtain measurement, balance bar must hang freely at exact midpoint. To calculate weight, add top reading to bottom one. (Example: If bottom counterweight reads 100 and lighter one reads 16 plus three small lines, record weight as 116 3/4 lb).
   B. Digital scale: Read and record weight displayed on digital screen.
   C. Dial scale: Indicator arrow rests at patient's weight. Read this number directly above the dial.
	If the counterweight is not resting in the notch, the weight will not be accurate. The weight noted on a digital scale may include decimals such as 155.3 pounds. Reading at an angle will result in an incorrect measurement.

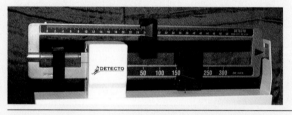

Step 7. The weight of this patient using the balance beam scale is 175 pounds.

Steps	Reasons
8. Return the bars on the top and bottom to zero.	A balance beam scale should be returned to zero after each use.
9. Assist the patient from the scale if necessary, and discard the paper towel.	Patients may lose balance and fall when stepping down from the scale; they should be observed and assisted as necessary. The paper towel may be left in place on the balance beam scale if the height is going to be obtained using this scale.
10. Record the weight.	If the weight and height are measured at the same time, they will be recorded together (see example in Procedure 4-2).
11. **AFF** Explain how to respond to a patient who is visually impaired.	Observe patients carefully to prevent injury and always ask before offering assistance or taking hold of their arm to guide. Make sure path to scales is clear from items that could trip or cause patient to fall. Assist onto the scales and off of the scales as needed.

PSY PROCEDURE 4-2: | **Measuring Height**

Purpose: Accurately measure and record a patient's height
Equipment: A scale with a ruler
Standard: This procedure should take less than 5 minutes.

Steps	Reasons
1. Wash your hands if this procedure is not done at the same time as the weight.	Typically, height is obtained with weight; your hands are already washed.
2. Have the patient remove shoes and stand straight and erect on the scale, with heels together and eyes straight ahead. (Patient may face the ruler, but a better measurement is made with the patient's back to the ruler.)	The posture of the patient must be erect for an accurate measurement.
3. With the measuring bar perpendicular to the ruler, slowly lower it until it firmly touches the patient's head. Press lightly if the hair is full or high.	Hair that is full should not be included in the height measurement.

Step 3. Measure where the bar slides out of the scale (or point of movement). This measure reads 63 inches, or 5 feet 3 inches.

Steps	Reasons
4. Read the measurement at the point of movement on the ruler. If measurements are in inches, convert to feet and inches (e.g., if the bar reads 65 plus two smaller lines, read it at 65 1/2. Remember that 12 inches equals 1 foot; therefore, the patient is 5 feet, 5 1/2 inches tall).	
5. Assist the patient from the scale if necessary; watch for signs of difficulty with balance.	Elderly or ill patients may be unsteady.
6. Record the weight and height measurements in the medical record.	Procedures not recorded are considered not to have been done.
7. **AFF** Explain how to respond to a patient who has dementia.	Solicit assistance from caregiver or other staff member to help patient off and on the scale. Give simple directions to the patient about what he or she should do. Speak clearly, not loudly.

Charting Example:

10/14/2012 9:15 am Ht. 5 ft, 5 1/2 inches, Wt. 136 1/4 lb ——————————— Y. Torres, CMA

Note: The medical assistant may sign his or her name in the patient record using only the "CMA" credential if the office has a signature log denoting the entire credential as "CMA(AAMA)."

PSY **PROCEDURE 4-3:**   **Measuring Oral Temperature Using a Glass Thermometer**

Purpose: Accurately measure and record a patient's oral temperature using a glass thermometer
Equipment: Glass oral thermometer; tissues or cotton balls; disposable plastic sheaths; biohazard waste container; cool, soapy water; disinfectant solution
Standard: This task should take 10 minutes.

Steps	Reasons
1. Wash your hands and assemble all the necessary supplies	Handwashing aids infection control.
2. Dry the thermometer if it has been stored in a disinfectant solution by wiping it from the bulb and going up the stem with a tissue or cotton ball. 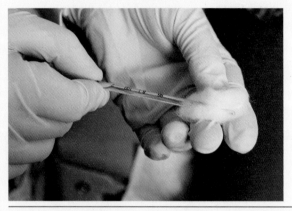 **Step 2.** Dry the glass thermometer beginning at the bulb and moving up the stem.	Removing the wet disinfectant will allow the thermometer to slip easily into the sheath.
3. Carefully check the thermometer for chips or cracks.	A chipped or cracked thermometer could injure the patient.
4. Check the reading by holding the stem horizontally at eye level and turning it slowly	It is easiest to see the column in this position.
5. If the reading is above 94°F, shake down the thermometer by securely grasping it at the end of the stem with your thumb and forefinger and snapping your wrist several times. Avoid hitting the thermometer against anything while snapping your wrist.	The reading must be below 94°F to provide an accurate temperature reading. The reading will never decrease in the thermometer unless the mercury or non-mercury substance is physically forced into the bulb.
6. Insert the thermometer into the plastic sheath. 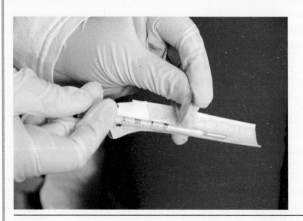 **Step 6.** Place the thermometer into a disposable sheath before using.	Follow the package instructions for placing the thermometer correctly into the sheath.

PSY PROCEDURE 4-3: **Measuring Oral Temperature Using a Glass Thermometer (continued)**

Steps	Reasons
7. Greet and identify the patient. Explain the procedure and ask about any eating, drinking of hot or cold fluids, gum chewing, or smoking within the past 15 minutes.	Eating, drinking, gum chewing, or smoking may alter the oral reading. If the patient has done any of these within 15 minutes, wait 15 minutes or select another route.
8. Place the thermometer under the patient's tongue to either side of the frenulum. **Step 8.** Place the thermometer to one side of the frenulum.	This is the area of highest vascularity and will give the most accurate reading.
9. Tell the patient to keep the mouth and lips closed without biting down on the thermometer.	Keeping the mouth and lips closed prevents air from entering the mouth and causing an inaccurate reading. Biting down on the thermometer may break it.
10. Leave the thermometer in place for 3–5 minutes. Note: The pulse, respirations, and blood pressure may be taken during this time (see Procedures 4-9 to 4-11).	The thermometer may be left in place for 3 minutes if there is no evidence of fever and the patient is compliant. It should be left in place for 5 minutes if the patient is febrile or noncompliant (talks or opens mouth frequently).
11. At the appropriate time, remove the thermometer from the patient's mouth while wearing gloves. Remove the sheath by holding the very edge of the sheath with your thumb and forefinger and pulling down from the open edge over the length of the thermometer to the bulb. Discard the sheath into a biohazard container.	Once removed, the soiled area should be inside the sheath.
12. Hold the thermometer horizontal at eye level and note the level of chemical that has risen into the column.	Holding the thermometer below or above eye level may interfere with seeing the column of chemical and accurately reading the measurement.
13. Sanitize and disinfect the thermometer according to the office policy and wash your hands. **Step 13.** Store clean thermometers in a covered instrument tray padded with gauze to prevent chipping or cracking the glass.	Wash the thermometer with cool or tepid soapy water, rinse with cool water, and dry well. Place the thermometer in a disinfectant solution, such as 70% isopropyl alcohol, according to office policy.

(continued)

PSY PROCEDURE 4-3: **Measuring Oral Temperature Using a Glass Thermometer** *(continued)*

Steps	Reasons
14. Record the patient's temperature in the medical record.	Procedures are considered not done if they are not recorded. The vital signs (temperature, pulse, respirations, and blood pressure) are usually recorded together.
15. **AFF** Explain how to respond to a patient who has English as a second language (ESL).	Solicit assistance from anyone who may be with the patient or a staff member who speaks the language to interpret if available. If no interpreter is available, use hand gestures or pictures to explain procedure to the patient.

Charting Example:

09/10/12 8:50 am T 100.6°F (O) ——————————————————————————————L. Ervin, CMA

Note: The medical assistant may sign his or her name in the patient record using only the "CMA" credential if the office has a signature log denoting the entire credential as "CMA(AAMA)."

PSY PROCEDURE 4-4: **Measuring a Rectal Temperature**

Purpose: Accurately measure and record a rectal temperature using either a glass rectal thermometer or electronic thermometer with a rectal probe attached
Equipment: Glass rectal thermometer or electronic thermometer with rectal probe; tissues or cotton balls; disposable plastic sheaths; surgical lubricant; biohazard waste container; cool, soapy water; disinfectant solution; gloves
Standard: This procedure should take 5 minutes.

Steps	Reasons
1. Wash your hands and assemble the necessary supplies.	Handwashing aids infection control.
2. Insert the thermometer into a plastic sheath.	Follow the package instructions for placing the sheath correctly onto the thermometer. If a glass rectal thermometer is used, follow Steps 2 through 5 in Procedure 4-3 to prepare the thermometer. If an electronic thermometer is used, attach the rectal probe if necessary.

Step 2. Rectal thermometers are noted by the red tip.

PSY **PROCEDURE 4-4:** **Measuring a Rectal Temperature (continued)**

Steps	Reasons
3. Spread lubricant onto a tissue and then from the tissue onto the sheath of the thermometer.	When using a tube of lubricant, avoid cross-contamination by not applying lubricant directly to the thermometer. A lubricant should always be used for rectal insertion to prevent patient discomfort.

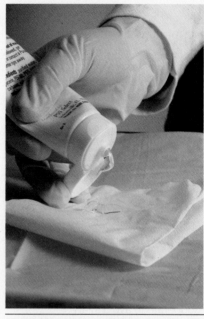

Step 3. Place lubricant onto a tissue first.

Steps	Reasons
4. Greet and identify the patient and explain the procedure.	
5. Ensure the patient's privacy by placing the patient in a side-lying position facing the examination room door and draping appropriately.	If the examination room door is opened, a patient facing the door is less likely to be exposed. The side-lying position facilitates exposure of the anus.

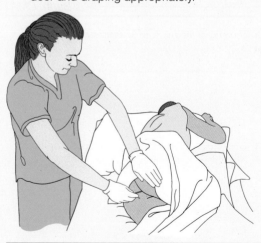

Step 5. The patient is in a side-lying position and draped appropriately.

Steps	Reasons
6. Apply gloves and visualize the anus by lifting the top buttock with your nondominant hand.	Never insert the thermometer without first having a clear view of the anus.
7. Gently insert the thermometer past the sphincter muscle about 1 1/2 inches for an adult, 1 inch for a child, and 1/2 inch for an infant.	Inserting the thermometer at these depths helps prevent perforating the anal canal.

(continued)

PSY PROCEDURE 4-4:   **Measuring a Rectal Temperature (continued)**

Steps	Reasons
8. Release the upper buttock and hold the thermometer in place with your dominant hand for 3 minutes. Replace the drape without moving the dominant hand.	The thermometer will not stay in place if it is not held. Replacing the drape will ensure the patient's privacy.
9. After 3 minutes, remove the glass thermometer and the sheath. The electronic thermometer will signal when the reading is obtained. Discard the sheath into an appropriate waste container and note the reading.	The lubricant or sheath may obscure the column in a glass thermometer and should be removed before you read the thermometer. The electronic thermometer will have a digital display of the reading (see Procedure 4-6).
10. Sanitize and disinfect the glass thermometer according to the office policy. Replace the electronic thermometer into the charger as necessary.	Always make sure thermometers are ready for the next patient.
11. Remove your gloves and wash your hands.	This prevents the spread of microorganisms.
12. Record the procedure and mark the letter R next to the reading, indicating that the temperature was taken rectally.	Temperature readings are presumed to have been taken orally unless otherwise noted in the medical record. The vital signs (temperature, pulse, respirations, and blood pressure) are usually recorded together.
13. **AFF** Explain how to respond to a patient who is developmentally challenged.	To avoid injury, do not use this method to obtain a temperature on an adult when there is the possibility that the patient may not cooperate to avoid injury.

Note: Infants and very small children may be held in the lap or over the knees for this procedure. Hold the thermometer and the buttocks with the dominant hand while securing the child with the nondominant hand. If the child moves, the thermometer and the hand will move together, avoiding injury to the anal canal.

Charting Example:

09/11/2012 8:30 am T 100.2°F (R) ———————————————— J. Barth, CMA

Note: The medical assistant may sign his or her name in the patient record using only the "CMA" credential if the office has a signature log denoting the entire credential as "CMA(AAMA)."

▶ PSY PROCEDURE 4-5: Measuring an Axillary Temperature

Purpose: Accurately measure and record an axillary temperature using a glass thermometer or an electronic thermometer

Equipment: Glass thermometer or electronic thermometer (oral or rectal); tissues or cotton balls; disposable plastic sheaths; biohazard waste container; cool, soapy water; disinfectant solution

Standard: This procedure should take 15 minutes.

Steps	Reasons
1. Wash your hands and assemble the necessary supplies.	Handwashing aids infection control.
2. Insert the thermometer into a plastic sheath.	Follow the package instructions for placing the sheath correctly onto the thermometer. If a glass thermometer is used, follow Steps 2 through 5 in Procedure 4-3 to prepare the thermometer.
3. Expose the patient's axilla without exposing more of the chest or upper body than is necessary.	The patient's privacy must be protected at all times.
4. Place the tip of the thermometer deep in the axilla and bring the patient's arm down, crossing the forearm over the chest. Drape the patient as appropriate for privacy. 	This position offers the best skin contact with the thermometer and maintains a closed environment. **Step 4.** With the thermometer in the axilla, the arm should be down, and the forearm should be crossed across the chest.
5. After 10 minutes, remove the glass thermometer and the sheath. The electronic thermometer will signal when the reading is obtained. Discard the sheath into an appropriate waste container and note the reading.	Axillary temperatures using a glass thermometer take longer than oral or rectal ones. The sheath may obscure the column in a glass thermometer and should be removed before you read the thermometer. The electronic thermometer will have a digital display of the reading (see Procedure 4-6).
6. Sanitize and disinfect the glass thermometer according to the office policy. Replace the electronic thermometer into the charger as necessary.	Always make sure thermometers are ready for the next patient.
7. Wash your hands.	This prevents the spread of microorganisms.
8. Record the procedure and mark a letter A next to the reading, indicating that the reading is axillary.	Temperature readings are presumed to have been taken orally unless otherwise noted in the medical record. The vital signs (temperature, pulse, respirations, and blood pressure) are usually recorded together.
9. **AFF** Explain how to respond to a patient who is from a different generation.	Refer to an elderly patient by their correct title (Mr., Mrs., Miss, etc.). Be respectful to the patient by only using their first name after they have given you permission to do so and do not assume the patient is hearing or cognitively impaired.

(continued)

PSY PROCEDURE 4-5: **Measuring an Axillary Temperature (continued)**

Steps	Reasons

Charting Example:

02/01/2012 3:45 pm T 97.8°F (A) ———————————————————— B. DeMarcus, CMA

Note: The medical assistant may sign his or her name in the patient record using only the "CMA" credential if the office has a signature log denoting the entire credential as "CMA(AAMA)."

 PSY PROCEDURE 4-6: **Measuring Temperature Using an Electronic Thermometer**

Purpose: Accurately measure and record a patient's temperature using an electronic thermometer
Equipment: Electronic thermometer with oral or rectal probe, disposable probe covers, biohazard waste container, gloves for taking a rectal temperature
Standard: This task should take 5 minutes.

Steps	Reasons
1. Wash your hands and assemble the necessary supplies.	Handwashing aids infection control.
2. Greet and identify the patient and explain the procedure.	Identifying the patient prevents errors.
3. Choose the most appropriate method (oral, axillary, or rectal) and attach the appropriate probe to the battery-powered unit.	Many electronic thermometers come with an oral probe and a rectal probe.
4. Insert the probe into a probe cover. Covers are usually carried with the unit in a specially fitted box attached to the back or top of the unit.	All probes fit into one size probe cover. If using the last probe cover, be sure to attach a new box of covers onto the unit to be ready for the next patient.
5. Position the thermometer appropriately for the method.	If measuring the temperature rectally, be sure to wear gloves, apply lubricant to the probe cover, and hold the probe in place.
6. Wait for the electronic thermometer unit to "beep" when it senses no signs of the temperature rising further. This usually occurs within 20–30 seconds.	Removing the thermometer before it signals may result in the recording of an inaccurate temperature.
7. After the beep, remove the probe and note the reading on the digital display screen on the unit before replacing the probe into the unit.	Most units automatically shut off when the probe is reinserted into the unit.
8. Discard the probe cover by pressing a button, usually on the end of the probe, while holding the probe over a biohazard container. After noting the temperature, replace the probe into the unit.	Probe covers should be discarded appropriately. Placing the probe back in the unit often turns the unit off in most models of electronic thermometers.
9. Remove your gloves, if used, wash your hands, and record the procedure.	Be sure to indicate whether the temperature was taken rectally or axillary by placing an R or an A next to the reading in the documentation. The vital signs (temperature, pulse, respirations, and blood pressure) are usually recorded together.

PSY PROCEDURE 4-6: **Measuring Temperature Using an Electronic Thermometer (continued)**

Steps	Reasons
10. Return the unit and probe to the charging base.	Although the unit is battery powered, it should be kept in the charging base so that the battery is adequately charged.
11. **AFF** Explain how to respond to a patient who is hearing impaired.	Make sure the patient can see your face as you are speaking. Speak clearly, not loudly.

Charting Example:

11/28/2012 10:15 am T 101°F (O) ——————————————————————————— D. Shaper, CMA

Note: The medical assistant may sign his or her name in the patient record using only the "CMA" credential if the office has a signature log denoting the entire credential as "CMA(AAMA)."

 PSY PROCEDURE 4-7: **Measuring Temperature Using a Tympanic Thermometer**

Purpose: Accurately measure and record a patient's temperature using a tympanic thermometer
Equipment: Tympanic thermometer, disposable probe covers, biohazard waste container
Standard: This task should take 5 minutes.

Steps	Reasons
1. Wash your hands and assemble the necessary supplies.	Handwashing aids infection control.
2. Greet and identify the patient and explain the procedure.	Identifying the patient prevents errors.
3. Insert the ear probe into a probe cover.	Always put a clean probe cover on the ear probe before inserting it.
4. Place the end of the ear probe into the patient's ear canal with your dominant hand while straightening out the ear canal with your nondominant hand.	Straighten the ear canal of most patients by pulling the top, posterior part of the outer ear up and back. For children under 3 years of age, pull the outer ear down and back.
	Step 4: Place the probe into the ear canal while straightening the ear canal.
5. With the ear probe properly placed in the ear canal, press the button on the thermometer. The reading is displayed on the digital display screen in about 2 seconds.	Pressing the button on the thermometer before the probe is properly placed in the ear will result in an inaccurate reading.
6. Remove the probe and note the reading. Discard the probe cover into an appropriate waste container.	The probe covers are for one patient use only.

(continued)

PSY PROCEDURE 4-7: **Measuring Temperature Using a Tympanic Thermometer** *(continued)*

Steps	Reasons
7. Wash your hands and record the procedure.	Be sure to indicate that the tympanic temperature was taken. The vital signs (temperature, pulse, respirations, and blood pressure) are usually recorded together.
8. Return the unit to the charging base.	The unit should be kept in the charging base so that the battery is always adequately charged.
9. **AFF** Explain how to respond to a patient who is deaf.	Solicit assistance from anyone who may be with the patient or a staff member who knows sign language to interpret if available. If no interpreter is available, use hand gestures or pictures to explain procedure to the patient.

Charting Example:

04/13/2012 2:00 pm T 99.4°F tympanic ———————————————————— M. Smythe, CMA

Note: The medical assistant may sign his or her name in the patient record using only the "CMA" credential if the office has a signature log denoting the entire credential as "CMA(AAMA)."

 PSY PROCEDURE 4-8: **Measuring Temperature Using a Temporal Artery Thermometer**

Purpose: Accurately measure and record a patient's temperature using a temporal artery thermometer
Equipment: Temporal artery thermometer, alcohol wipe
Standard: This task should take less than 5 minutes.

Steps	Reasons
1. Wash your hands and assemble the necessary supplies.	Handwashing aids infection control.
2. Greet and identify the patient and explain the procedure.	Identifying the patient prevents errors.
3. Place the probe end of the hand-held unit on the forehead of the patient. Make sure the patient's skin is dry.	If the patient is diaphoretic, dry the skin with a towel first or take the temperature using another method.

Step 3. The temporal artery thermometer is placed flat against the forehead.

PSY PROCEDURE 4-8: **Measuring Temperature Using a Temporal Artery Thermometer (continued)**

Steps	Reasons
4. With the thermometer against the forehead, depress the on/off button, move the thermometer across and down the forehead, and release the on/off button with the unit over the temporal artery.	Some units may indicate that you should lift the thermometer from the temporal artery and place it behind the ear before releasing the on/off button.

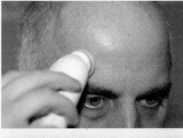

Step 4A. Slide the unit across the forehead.

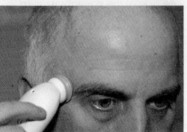

Step 4B. Stop over the temporal artery before releasing the on/off button.

Steps	Reasons
5. The reading is displayed on the digital display screen in 1–2 seconds.	
6. Properly disinfect the end of the thermometer according to manufacturer instructions.	Thermometers must be disinfected between patients.
7. Wash your hands and record the procedure.	Be sure to indicate that a temporal artery temperature was taken. The vital signs (temperature, pulse, respirations, and blood pressure) are usually recorded together.
8. Return the unit to the charging base.	The unit should be kept in the charging base so that the battery is always adequately charged.
9. **AFF** Explain how to respond to a patient who is visually impaired.	Observe patients carefully to prevent injury and always ask before offering assistance or taking hold of their arm to guide. Face the patient when speaking and always let them know what you are going to do before touching them.

Charting Example:

09/22/2012 9:30 am T 98.6°F temporal artery ———————————————— N. Hoffman, CMA

Note: The medical assistant may sign his or her name in the patient record using only the "CMA" credential if the office has a signature log denoting the entire credential as "CMA(AAMA)."

PSY PROCEDURE 4-9: | **Measuring the Radial Pulse**

Purpose: Accurately measure and record a patient's radial pulse
Equipment: A watch with a sweeping second hand
Standard: This procedure should take 3–5 minutes.

Steps	Reasons
1. Wash your hands.	Handwashing is an infection control technique and should be performed before and after any patient contact.
2. Greet and identify the patient and explain the procedure.	In most cases, the pulse is taken at the same time as the other vital signs.
3. Position the patient with the arm relaxed and supported either on the lap of the patient or on a table.	If the arm is not supported or the patient is uncomfortable, the pulse may be difficult to find and the count may be affected.
4. With the index, middle, and ring fingers of your dominant hand, press with your fingertips firmly enough to feel the pulse but gently enough not to obliterate it (see Fig. 4-11).	Do not use your thumb; it has a pulse of its own that may be confused as the patient's. You may place your thumb on the opposite side of the patient's wrist to steady your hand.
5. If the pulse is regular, count it for 30 seconds, watching the second hand of your watch. Multiply the number of pulsations by 2 since the pulse is always recorded as beats per minute. If the pulse is irregular, count it for a full 60 seconds.	Counting an irregular pulse for less than 60 seconds will give an inaccurate measurement.
6. Record the rate in the medical record with the other vital signs. Also note the rhythm if irregular and the volume if thready or bounding.	Procedures are considered not to have been done if they are not recorded. The vital signs (temperature, pulse, respirations, and blood pressure) are usually recorded together.
7. **AFF** Explain how to respond to a patient who is developmentally challenged.	To avoid injury to the patient, assess for safety before completing a procedure when there is the possibility that the patient may not cooperate.

Charting Example:

06/12/2012 11:30 am Pulse 78 and irregular ———————————————— E. Kramer, CMA

Note: The medical assistant may sign his or her name in the patient record using only the "CMA" credential if the office has a signature log denoting the entire credential as "CMA(AAMA)."

PSY PROCEDURE 4-10: **Measuring Respirations**

Purpose: Accurately measure and record a patient's respirations
Equipment: A watch with a sweeping second hand
Standard: This procedure should take 3–5 minutes.

Steps	Reasons
1. Wash your hands.	Handwashing aids in infection control.
2. Greet and identify the patient and explain the procedure.	In most cases, the respirations are counted at the same time as the pulse.
3. After counting the radial pulse and still watching your second hand, count a complete rise and fall of the chest as one respiration. Note: Some patients have abdominal movement rather than chest movement during respirations. Observe carefully for the easiest area to assess for the most accurate reading.	A patient who is aware that you are observing respirations may alter the breathing pattern. It is best to begin counting respirations immediately after counting the pulse without informing the patient.
	Step 3. Continue holding the wrist after taking the pulse and begin counting the respirations.
4. If the breathing pattern is regular, count the respiratory rate for 30 seconds and multiply by 2. If the pattern is irregular, count for a full 60 seconds.	Counting an irregular respiratory pattern for less than 60 seconds may give an inaccurate measurement.
5. Record the respiratory rate in the medical record with the other vital signs. Also, note whether the rhythm is irregular, along with any unusual or abnormal sounds such as wheezing.	Procedures are considered not to have been done if they are not recorded. The vital signs (temperature, pulse, respirations, and blood pressure) are usually recorded together.
6. **AFF** Explain how to respond to a patient who has dementia.	Solicit assistance from caregiver or other staff member to help during the procedure. Give simple directions to the patient about what he or she should do. Speak clearly, not loudly.

Charting Example:

09/15/2012 8:45 am Resp 16 ———————————————————————— J. Thompson, CMA

Note: The medical assistant may sign his or her name in the patient record using only the "CMA" credential if the office has a signature log denoting the entire credential as "CMA(AAMA)."

PSY **PROCEDURE 4-11:**   **Measuring Blood Pressure**

Purpose: Accurately measure and record a patient's blood pressure
Equipment: Sphygmomanometer, stethoscope
Standard: This procedure should take 5 minutes.

Steps	Reasons
1. Wash your hands and assemble your equipment.	Handwashing aids infection control.
2. Greet and identify the patient and explain the procedure.	Identifying the patient prevents errors and explaining the procedure eases anxiety.
3. Position the patient with the arm to be used supported with the forearm on the lap or a table and slightly flexed, with the palm upward. The upper arm should be level with the patient's heart. **Step 3.** Support the arm on the patient's lap, slightly flexed with the palm upward.	Positioning the arm with the palm upward facilitates finding and palpating the brachial artery. If the upper arm is higher or lower than the heart, an inaccurate reading may result.
4. Expose the patient's arm.	Any clothing over the area may obscure the sounds. If the sleeve is pulled up, it may become tight and act as a tourniquet, decreasing the flow of blood and causing an inaccurate blood pressure reading.
5. Palpate the brachial pulse in the antecubital area and center the deflated cuff directly over the brachial artery. The lower edge of the cuff should be 1–2 inches above the antecubital area. **Steps 5 and 6.** Center the cuff over the brachial artery.	If the cuff is placed too low, it may interfere with the placement of the stethoscope and cause noises that obscure the Korotkoff sounds.
6. Wrap the cuff smoothly and snugly around the arm and secure it with the Velcro edges.	If the cuff does not fit smoothly and snugly around the arm, the blood pressure reading may be inaccurate.

PSY PROCEDURE 4-11: **Measuring Blood Pressure (continued)**

Steps	Reasons
7. With the air pump in your dominant hand and the valve between your thumb and the forefinger, turn the screw clockwise to tighten. Do not tighten it to the point that it will be difficult to release. 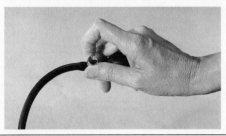	The cuff will not inflate with the valve open. If the valve is too tightly closed, it will be difficult to loosen with one hand after the cuff is inflated. **Step 7.** Holding the bulb and the screw valve properly allows you to inflate and deflate the cuff easily.
8. While palpating the brachial pulse with your nondominant hand, inflate the cuff and note the point or number on the dial or mercury column at which you no longer feel the brachial pulse. 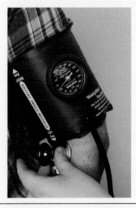	The dial or mercury column should be at eye level. Noting this number gives you a reference point for reinflating the cuff when taking the blood pressure. **Step 8.** Palpate the brachial pulse and place the stethoscope diaphragm bell over this artery.
9. Deflate the cuff by turning the valve counterclockwise. Wait at least 30 seconds before reinflating the cuff.	Always wait at least 30 seconds after deflating the cuff to allow circulation to return to the extremity.
10. Place the stethoscope earpieces in your ears with the openings pointed slightly forward. Stand about 3 feet from the manometer with the gauge at eye level. Your stethoscope tubing should hang freely without touching or rubbing against any part of the cuff.	With the earpieces pointing forward in the ear canals, the openings follow the natural opening of the ear canal. The manometer should be at eye level to decrease any chance of error when it is read. If the stethoscope rubs against other objects, environmental sounds may obscure the Korotkoff sounds.
11. Place the diaphragm of the stethoscope against the brachial artery and hold it in place with the nondominant hand without pressing too hard. 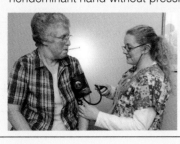	If not pressed firmly enough, you may not hear the sounds. Pressing too firmly may obliterate the pulse. **Step 11.** Hold the stethoscope diaphragm firmly against the brachial artery while taking the blood pressure and listening carefully.

(continued)

PSY **PROCEDURE 4-11:**   **Measuring Blood Pressure**
(continued)

Steps	Reasons
12. With your dominant hand, turn the screw on the valve just enough to close the valve; inflate the cuff. Pump the valve bulb to about 30 mm Hg above the number felt during Step 8.	Inflating more than 30 mm Hg above baseline is uncomfortable for the patient and unnecessary; inflating less may produce an inaccurate systolic reading.
13. Once the cuff is appropriately inflated, turn the valve counterclockwise to release air at about 2–4 mm Hg per second.	Releasing the air too fast will cause missed beats, and releasing it too slowly will interfere with circulation.
14. Listening carefully, note the point on the gauge at which you hear the first clear tapping sound. This is the systolic sound, or Korotkoff I.	Aneroid and mercury measurements are always made as even numbers because of the way the manometer is calibrated.

Step 14A. The meniscus on the mercury column in this example reads 120 mm Hg.

Step 14B. The gauge on the aneroid manometer reads 80 mm Hg.

Steps	Reasons
15. Maintaining control of the valve screw, continue to listen and deflate the cuff. When you hear the last sound, note the reading and quickly deflate the cuff. *Note:* Never immediately reinflate the cuff if you are unsure of the reading. Totally deflate the cuff and wait 1–2 minutes before repeating the procedure.	The last sound heard is Korotkoff V and is recorded as the bottom number or diastolic blood pressure.
16. Remove the cuff and press the air from the bladder of the cuff.	Removing the remaining air from the bladder of the cuff will allow for better storage.
17. If this is the first recording or a new patient, the physician may also want a reading in the other arm or in another position.	Blood pressure varies in some patients between the arms or in different positions such as lying or standing.

PSY PROCEDURE 4-11: **Measuring Blood Pressure** *(continued)*

Steps	Reasons
18. Put the equipment away and wash your hands.	Handwashing should be done after any patient encounter.
4. Record the reading with the systolic over the diastolic pressure, noting which arm was used (120/80 LA). Also, record the patient's position if other than sitting.	Procedures are considered not done if they are not recorded. The vital signs (temperature, pulse, respirations, and blood pressure) are usually recorded together.
20. **AFF** Explain how to respond to a patient who is from a different culture.	Be respectful of the cultural differences by explaining why procedures are important. Provide additional privacy if necessary.

Charting Example:

11/08/2012 3:30 pm T 98.6°F O, P 78, R 16, BP 130/90 LA sitting, 110/78 LA standing —————— Y.Torres,CMA

Note: The medical assistant may sign his or her name in the patient record using only the "CMA" credential if the office has a signature log denoting the entire credential as "CMA(AAMA)."

- Anthropometric measurements include height and weight. Vital signs include:
  - temperature (T)
  - pulse (P)
  - respirations (R)
  - blood pressure (BP)

- When a patient first visits the medical office, these measurements are recorded as a baseline and used as a comparison for data collected at subsequent visits. These measurements, which provide important data for the physician to use in diagnosing and treating illnesses, are very frequently performed by medical assistants.

Warm Ups for Critical Thinking

1. You are asked to teach a patient, Mr. Stone, how to take his blood pressure at home once in the morning and once at night and record these readings for 1 month. Create a patient education brochure that explains the procedure in understandable terms and design a sheet that Mr. Stone can easily use to record these readings.

2. Ms. Black arrived at the office late for her appointment; she was frantic and explained that she had experienced car trouble on the way to the office, could not find a parking place, and just locked her keys inside her car. How would you expect these events to affect her vital signs? Explain why.

3. What size of cuff would you choose for Mrs. Cooper, an elderly female patient who is 5 feet 3 inches tall and weighs approximately 90 pounds? Why?

4. How would you respond to a patient who asks you to give advice on what type of thermometer to buy for use at home? Would the age of the patient be relevant with regard to the type of thermometer you might suggest?

5. An elderly male patient tells you that he is considering stopping the blood pressure medication the physician ordered at the previous visit. He further explains that he has "read all about this drug on the Internet," and he informs you that "it has side effects," although he denies experiencing any at this time. Describe how you would handle this situation.

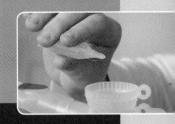

CHAPTER 5

Assisting with the Physical Examination

Learning Outcomes

Cognitive Domain

Note: AAMA/CAAHEP 2008 Standards are italicized.

1. Spell and define the key terms
2. Identify and state the use of the basic and specialized instruments and supplies used in the physical examination
3. Describe the four methods used to examine the patient
4. State your responsibilities before, during, and after the physical examination
5. List the basic sequence of the physical examination

6. *Describe the normal function of each body system*

Psychomotor Domain

Note: AAMA/CAAHEP 2008 Standards are italicized.

1. Assist with the adult physical examination (Procedure 5-1)
2. *Assist the physician with patient care*
3. *Practice standard precautions*
4. *Document accurately in the patient record*
5. *Practice within the standard of care for a medical assistant*

Affective Domain

Note: AAMA/CAAHEP 2008 Standards are italicized.

1. *Apply critical thinking skills in performing patient assessment and care*
2. *Demonstrate awareness of diversity in providing patient care*
3. *Explain rationale for performance of a procedure to the patient*
4. *Apply active listening skills*
5. *Demonstrate sensitivity to patient's rights*
6. *Demonstrate empathy in communicating with patients, family, and staff*
7. *Use appropriate body language and other nonverbal skills in communicating with patients, family, and staff*
8. *Demonstrate awareness of the territorial boundaries of the person with whom you are communicating*
9. *Demonstrate sensitivity appropriate to the message being delivered*
10. *Demonstrate recognition of the patient's level of understanding in communications*
11. *Recognize and protect personal boundaries in communicating with others*
12. *Demonstrate respect for individual diversity, incorporating awareness of one's own biases in areas including gender, race, religion, age, and economic status*

ABHES Competencies

1. Prepare and maintain examination and treatment area
2. Prepare patient for examinations and treatments
3. Assist physician with routine and specialty examinations and treatments

Key Terms

asymmetry	extraocular	palpation	range of motion (ROM)
auscultation	gait	Papanicolaou (Pap) smear	rectovaginal
Babinski reflex	hernia	percussion	sclera
bimanual	inguinal	peripheral vision	speculum
bruit	inspection	PERRLA (pupils, equal, round, reactive to light and accommodation)	symmetry
cerumen	lubricant		transillumination
clinical diagnosis	manipulation		tympanic membrane
diagnosis	nasal septum		
differential diagnosis	occult blood		

The purpose of the complete physical examination is to assess the patient's general state of health and detect signs and symptoms of disease. New patients usually receive a complete physical examination, which gives the physician baseline information about the patient. This baseline information is valuable for future comparison and can aid the physician in **diagnosis** (identifying a disease or condition). Routine examinations are performed thereafter at regular intervals to help maintain the patient's health and prevent disease.

When a patient comes into the office, the physician can make a **clinical diagnosis** based only on the patient's symptoms. At other times, symptoms are vague and could be caused by one of several diseases. In this situation, a **differential diagnosis** is made by comparing symptoms of several diseases. To make any diagnosis, the physician will rely on three basic components: the medical history, the physical examination, and any laboratory and diagnostic tests. Once the data from these three components are collected and evaluated, the physician will make a judgment about the patient's condition and devise a plan of care including appropriate treatment. As a medical assistant, you are responsible for assisting with taking the medical history, preparing the patient for the examination, and assisting the physician during the examination so that a clinical or differential diagnosis can be made as accurately as possible. In addition, you may collect specimens for diagnostic testing.

During the examination, you must anticipate the needs of the physician and patient and be prepared to assist as necessary.

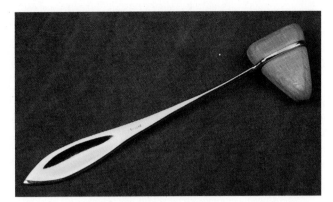

Figure 5-2 A reflex hammer.

COG **Basic Instruments and Supplies**

Instruments used during the physical examination enable the examiner to see, hear, or feel areas of the body being assessed. In most cases, it is the physician who uses these instruments, but you must be familiar with instruments and supplies. These instruments should be kept in a special tray or drawer in a convenient location in each examination room. The exact equipment used varies among medical offices according to physicians' preferences and the specialty. Supplies that should be available in the examination room include a tape measure, gloves, tongue depressors, and cotton-tipped applicators (Fig. 5-1). The purpose of the most common instruments used in the physical examination is described in the following sections.

 CHECKPOINT QUESTION

1. Why is there variation in the types of instruments and supplies used in each medical office?

Percussion Hammer

The percussion hammer is used to test neurologic reflexes. Also called a *reflex hammer*, this instrument has a stainless steel handle and a hard rubber head (Fig. 5-2). The head is used to test reflexes by striking

the tendons of the ankle, knee, wrist, and elbow. The tip of the handle may be used to stroke the sole of the foot to assess the **Babinski reflex** (a reflex noted by extension of the great toe and abduction of the other toes). Some hammers have a brush and needle in the handle specifically used to test sensory perception.

Tuning Fork

The tuning fork is used to test hearing. It is a stainless steel instrument with a handle at one end and two prongs at the other end (Fig. 5-3). The examiner strikes the prongs against his or her hand, which causes them to vibrate and produce a humming sound. While vibrating, the handle is placed against a bony area of the skull near one of the ears, and the patient is asked to describe what, if anything, is heard in that ear. Depending on the results of this hearing test, the physician may order additional auditory tests.

Nasal Speculum

The nasal **speculum** is a stainless steel instrument that is inserted into the nostril to assist in the visual inspection of the lining of the nose, nasal membranes, and septum. The tip of the instrument is inserted into the nose, and the handles are squeezed, opening the end and allowing for visualization (Fig. 5-4). Nasal specula are also available in a disposable form.

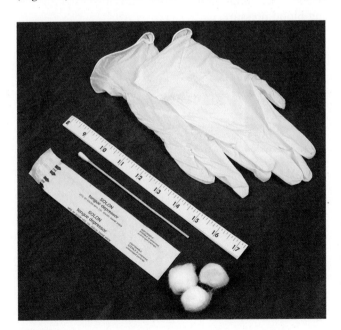

Figure 5-1 Common supplies used in the adult physical examination: tape measure, gloves, tongue depressor, and cotton-tipped applicator.

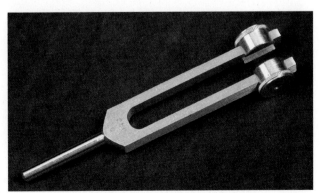

Figure 5-3 A tuning fork.

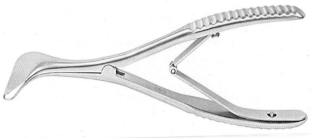

Figure 5-4 A nasal speculum.

Otoscope and Audioscope

The otoscope permits visualization of the ear canal and tympanic membrane. The **tympanic membrane**, or eardrum, is a thin, oval membrane between the outer and middle ear that transmits sound vibrations to the inner ear. The otoscope has a stainless steel handle at one end and a head with a light, a magnifying lens, and a cone-shaped hollow speculum at the other end. A portable otoscope has batteries in the handle to operate the light in the head; other otoscopes are part of a unit attached to the wall and plugged into an electrical outlet (Fig. 5-5A,B). In both types, the hollow speculum is covered with a disposable speculum cover before it is placed in the ear canal. An otoscope with a specialized nasal speculum tip may be used to examine the nose.

The audioscope is used to screen patients for hearing loss. Although it looks like an otoscope, the audioscope's handle has a variety of indicators and selection buttons that can be used to adjust its tones (Fig. 5-6). The examiner places the tip of the audioscope in the patient's ear and asks the patient to respond to each of the tones that is produced. The results are recorded in the patient's medical record.

Ophthalmoscope

The ophthalmoscope is used to examine the interior structures of the eyes. Like the otoscope, it may have a stainless steel handle that contains batteries or may be mounted on the wall (Fig. 5-7). The head of the ophthalmoscope also has a light source, magnifying lens, and opening through which to view the eye. Portable units may have a common base handle with various otoscope or ophthalmoscope tips that can be attached for different examinations.

Examination Light and Gooseneck Lamp

Some offices are equipped with an adjustable overhead examination light for better visualization during the examination. The gooseneck lamp is a floor lamp with a movable stand that bends at the neck for use when the overhead lighting is not adequate (Fig. 5-8). You have the responsibility to make sure all examination lights are in proper working order and to direct the light toward the area of the body as indicated by the physician.

Stethoscope

The stethoscope is used for listening to body sounds. The bell or diaphragm is at one end and is placed on the patient's body. This end is connected to two earpieces by flexible rubber or vinyl tubing (Fig. 5-9). The two earpieces have plastic or rubber tips that must be adjusted and directed outward before being placed in the examiner's ears. The stethoscope is used to listen to the sounds of the heart, lungs, and intestines. It is also used for taking blood pressure.

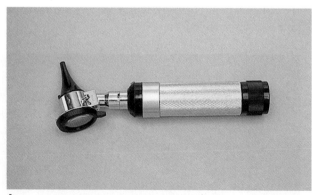

A

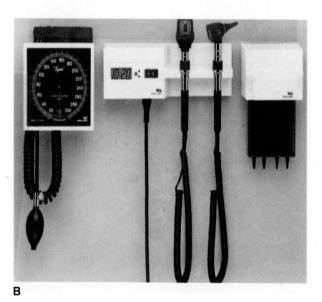

B

Figure 5-5 **(A)** A portable otoscope. **(B)** Wall-mounted examination instruments. From left: sphygmomanometer with cuff, ophthalmoscope, otoscope, and dispenser for disposable otoscope speculum covers.

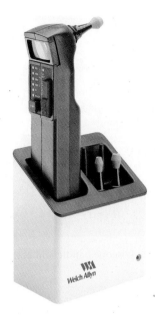

Figure 5-6 An audioscope.

Penlight or Flashlight

A penlight or flashlight provides additional light to a specific area during the examination. The penlight is the shape and size of a ballpoint pen and is easily carried in the examiner's pocket (Fig. 5-10). A common flashlight may be used if a penlight is not available. The penlight is often used to examine the eyes, nose, and throat.

 CHECKPOINT QUESTION

2. Which instruments are used to test the ears and hearing?

COG Instruments and Supplies Used in Specialized Examinations

In addition to the basic instruments described previously, specialized equipment may be used during the physical examination. This chapter introduces the specialized examinations and equipment. A more detailed

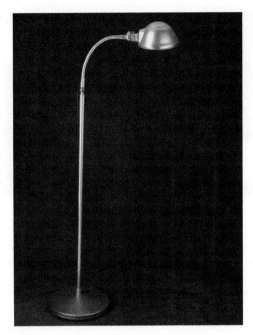

Figure 5-8 An examination light.

description of specialty examinations is provided in Unit Five.

Head Light or Mirror

An ear, nose, and throat specialist (otorhinolaryngologist) may wear a headlight or head mirror during the examination of these structures. This instrument consists of a light or mirror attached to a headband that fits over the examiner's head (Fig. 5-11). A head light provides direct light on the area being examined; the mirror reflects light from the examination light into the area.

Laryngeal Mirror and Laryngoscope

The laryngeal mirror is a stainless steel instrument with a long, slender handle and a small, round mirror. It is used to examine areas of the patient's throat and larynx that may not be directly visible.

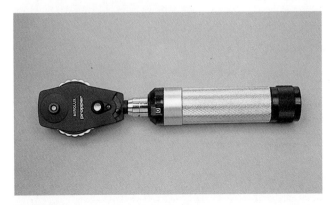

Figure 5-7 A portable ophthalmoscope.

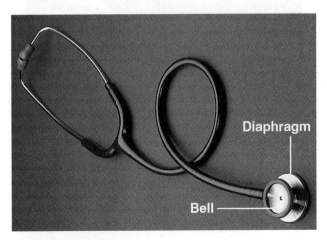

Figure 5-9 A stethoscope.

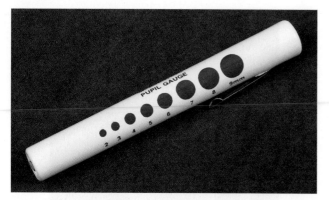

Figure 5-10 A penlight.

The laryngoscope handle is similar to the battery handle of a portable otoscope or ophthalmoscope, but the head allows attachment of curved or straight laryngoscope stainless steel blades and a small light source (Fig. 5-12). The examiner places the blade in the patient's throat to visualize the larynx or vocal cords, which cannot be seen by simply looking down the patient's throat.

Vaginal Speculum

The general physical examination of female patients may include a pelvic examination and **Papanicolaou (Pap) smear**. This is a simple test in which cells obtained from the cervix or vagina are examined microscopically for abnormalities including cancer. To obtain the cells for a Pap smear, or to visually examine internal female reproductive structures, the vaginal speculum is inserted into the vagina to expand the opening (Fig. 5-13). This instrument is made of stainless steel or disposable plastic.

To obtain vaginal or cervical cells, the physician may use the Ayre spatula or cervical scraper (Fig. 5-14). This scraper is about 6 inches long and made of plastic or wood. One tip has an irregular shape that is placed in the

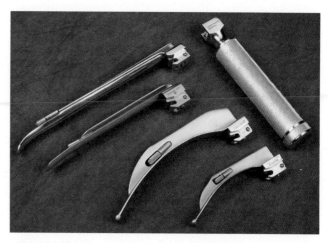

Figure 5-12 A laryngoscope handle and blades (straight and curved).

cervical opening and rotated to collect the specimen; the other end is rounded and may be used to collect cells from the vaginal cul-de-sac. A histobrush may also be used to obtain cells for a Pap smear; it is made of nylon or plastic with soft bristles at one end. The collected cells are transferred to either a glass slide or a liquid preservative and sent to a laboratory for analysis. Chapter 20 has additional information about the gynecologic examination and the role of the medical assistant.

Lubricant

Lubricant is a water-soluble gel used to reduce friction and provide easy insertion of an instrument in the physical examination. After cells are obtained for a Pap smear, lubricant may also be used for a **bimanual** examination. This examination allows the examiner to palpate internal structures of the pelvic cavity with one hand on the abdomen and with two fingers of the other gloved hand inserted into the vagina. Lubricant may also be used for rectal examinations.

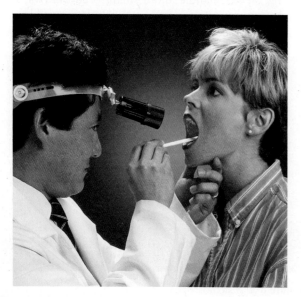

Figure 5-11 A head light.

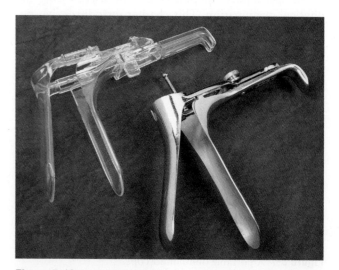

Figure 5-13 Vaginal specula.

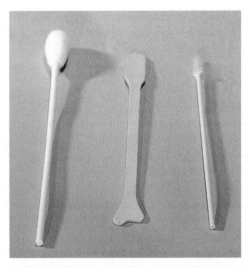

Figure 5-14 Cotton-tipped applicator (*left*), Ayre spatula (*center*), and histobrush (*right*). Cotton-tipped applicators of this size are frequently used to remove excess vaginal secretions or to apply medications during the gynecologic examination.

Anoscope, Proctoscope, and Sigmoidoscope

The instruments used for examination of the rectum and colon vary in length as appropriate for the structure to be examined. The anoscope is a short stainless steel or plastic speculum that is inserted into the rectum to inspect the anal canal. An obturator with a rounded tip extends beyond the anoscope to allow the instrument to be easily inserted into the rectum (Fig. 5-15). After the anoscope is inserted, the obturator is removed for visualization of the internal lining of the rectum.

The proctoscope is another type of speculum that is used to visualize the rectum and the anus. It is longer than the anoscope and allows the examiner to inspect more areas of the rectum. While it also consists of an obturator that is removed after the instrument is inserted, a fiberoptic light handle and magnifying lens are attached. The tubular part of the scope is marked in centimeters so that the depth of abnormalities in the anal canal can be noted.

A longer instrument used to visualize the rectum and the sigmoid colon is the sigmoidoscope. This instrument consists of a tube with an obturator, fiberoptic light handle, and magnifying lens (Fig. 5-16). It may be rigid and

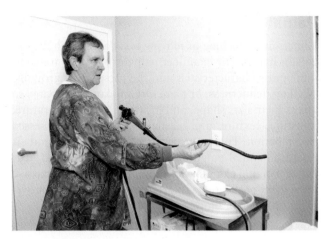

Figure 5-16 A flexible sigmoidoscope.

made of stainless steel, or it may be flexible. The advantages of the flexible sigmoidoscope include a smaller diameter, greater depth during the examination, better visualization of the intestinal mucosa, and less discomfort for the patient.

During all rectal examinations, you need a suction machine, cotton-tipped applicators, glass microscope slides, specimen containers, and laboratory request slips available. Tissue or stool specimens obtained during any rectal procedure must be properly preserved and protected for transport to the laboratory for analysis. More information regarding examinations of the colon is found in Chapter 17.

 CHECKPOINT QUESTION

3. What are the uses of the anoscope, proctoscope, and sigmoidoscope? What is the function of an obturator?

COG Examination Techniques

While performing the physical examination, the physician uses four basic techniques to gather information. These include **inspection**, **palpation**, **percussion**, and **auscultation**. Each technique is described in more detail in the following sections.

Inspection

Inspection is looking at areas of the body to observe physical features. The examiner inspects the patient's general appearance, including movements, skin and membrane color, contour, and **symmetry** or **asymmetry**, which is equality or inequality in size and shape. Inspection is done both with the naked eye and with instruments, using either room lighting or a special light source. In some cases, inspection includes use of the sense of smell to note any unusual odors of the breath (such as a fruity smell in a diabetic patient) or foul odors from infected wounds or lesions.

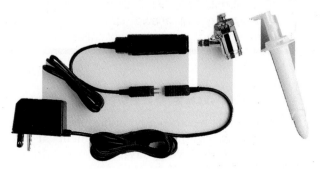

Figure 5-15 The anoscope with the obturator.

Palpation

Palpation is touching or moving body areas with the fingers or hands. The examiner palpates the body to determine pulse characteristics and the presence of growths, swelling, tenderness, or pain. Organs can be palpated to assess their size, shape, and location. Skin temperature, moisture, texture, and elasticity may also be assessed by palpation. Palpation performed with both hands is called bimanual palpation; if the fingers are used, it is called a digital examination. **Manipulation** is the passive movement of the joints to determine the extent of movement or **range of motion (ROM)**.

Percussion

Percussion is tapping or striking the body with the hand or an instrument to produce sounds. Direct percussion is performed by striking the body with a finger. Indirect percussion is done by placing a finger on the area and then striking this finger with a finger of the other hand while listening to the sounds and feeling the vibrations. This allows the examiner to determine the position, size, and density of air or fluid within a body cavity or organ.

Auscultation

Auscultation is listening to the sounds of the body. This examination method uses a stethoscope or the ear placed directly on the patient's body. Areas of the body that can be auscultated include the heart, lungs, abdomen, and blood vessels. In the abdominal examination, auscultation is performed before palpation and percussion, which can affect normal bowel sounds.

 CHECKPOINT QUESTION

4. Which of the examination techniques requires the use of the hands and fingers to feel organs or structures?

COG Responsibilities of the Medical Assistant

Room Preparation

Medical assistants are usually responsible for preparing the examination rooms, equipment, and supplies in the clinical area. The examination room should be clean, well lighted, well ventilated, and at a comfortable temperature for the patient. The examination table is decontaminated with an appropriate disinfectant between patients, and the paper on the table is removed and replaced with clean paper. At the beginning of each day, you are responsible for checking each examination room for adequate supplies and equipment, including the working condition of equipment. Batteries in otoscopes, ophthalmoscopes, and laryngoscopes are to be checked daily and replaced as needed.

Patient Preparation

Once the examination room is ready, you will call the patient back by name from the waiting room and escort him or her to the treatment room. It is important that you develop rapport with your patients and practice good interpersonal skills. This helps put your patients at ease and increases their confidence in you and the physician. Your goal is to create a positive, supportive, caring, and friendly atmosphere. Treat each patient as an individual, and speak clearly with a confident tone of voice as you explain any procedures.

Before the physician sees the patient, it may be your responsibility to obtain and record the patient's history, chief complaint, and vital signs. If a urine specimen is needed, explain how to obtain the specimen, direct the patient to the bathroom, and explain what to do with the specimen.

Once in the examination room, give the patient instructions for disrobing and putting on the examination gown. Depending on the type of examination to be performed, the patient may wear the gown with the opening in the front or in the back. Leave the room while the patient undresses unless the patient needs help. Then ask the patient to sit on the examination table, helping if needed, and cover the legs with a drape. Place the chart outside the examining room door and notify the physician that the patient is ready.

 PATIENT EDUCATION

VITAMINS, HERBS, AND NATURAL REMEDIES

When obtaining the patient's history, it is important to ask about medications and treatments that the patient may be using on a regular basis but may not mention. Many times, patients think that vitamins, herbs, and other over-the-counter products are not medications; however, these should be noted in the medical record because they may interact with prescription drugs that the physician has ordered. Although patients may have specific questions about their medications, advise them that the physician will answer specific questions about drug interactions and complications.

 CHECKPOINT QUESTION

5. What would be the advantage of checking the working condition of equipment at the beginning of each work day?

Assisting the Physician

During the physical examination, you may assist the physician by handing him or her instruments or supplies and directing the light appropriately. Procedure 5-1 describes the steps for assisting the physician with the physical examination.

Depending on the examination and the physical condition of the patient, you may also assist the patient into an appropriate position and adjust the drape to expose only the body area being examined (Fig. 5-17A–K). Be supportive and offer reassurance to the patient during the examination. Always assess the patient's facial

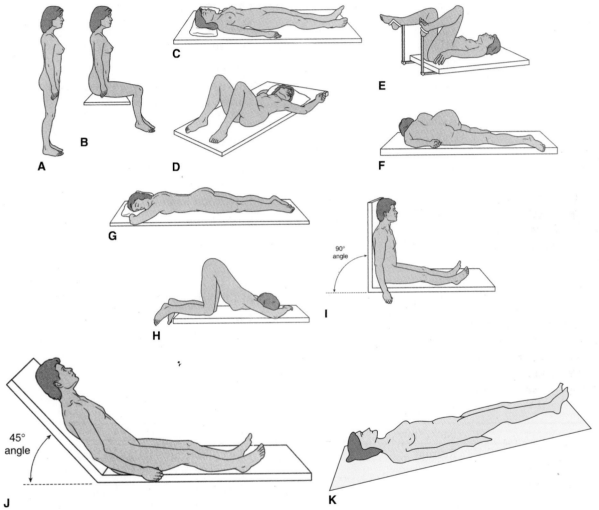

Figure 5-17 Patient examination positions. (**A**) The erect or standing position. The patient stands erect facing forward with the arms at the sides. (**B**) The sitting position. The patient sits erect at the end of the examination table with the feet supported on a footrest or stool. (**C**) The supine position. The patient lies on the back with arms at the sides. A pillow may be placed under the head for comfort. (**D**) The dorsal recumbent position. The patient is supine with the legs separated, knees bent, and feet flat on the table. (**E**) The lithotomy position is similar to the dorsal recumbent position but with the patient's feet in stirrups rather than flat on the table. The stirrups should be level with each other and about 1 foot out from the edge of the table. The patient's feet are moved into or out of the stirrups at the same time to prevent back strain. (**F**) The Sims position. The patient lies on the left side with the left arm and shoulder behind the body, right leg and arm sharply flexed on the table, and left knee slightly flexed. (**G**) The prone position. The patient lies on the abdomen with the head supported and turned to one side. The arms may be under the head or by the sides, whichever is more comfortable. (**H**) Knee-chest position. The patient kneels on the table with the arms and chest on the table, hips in the air, and back straight. (**I**) Fowler position. The patient is half-sitting with the head of the examination table elevated 80°–90°. (**J**) Semi-Fowler position. The patient is in a half-sitting position with the head of the table elevated 30°–45° and the knees slightly bent. (**K**) Trendelenburg position. The patient lies on the back with arms straight at either side, and the head of the bed is lowered with the head lower than the hips; the legs are elevated at approximately 45°.

TABLE 5-1 Examination Positions and Their Uses		
Position	**Body Parts**	**Instruments Needed**
Sitting	General Appearance	
	Head, neck	Stethoscope
	Eyes	Ophthalmoscope, penlight
	Ears	Otoscope, tuning fork
	Nose	Nasal speculum, penlight, substances to smell
	Sinuses	Penlight
	Mouth	Glove, tongue blade, penlight
	Throat	Glove, tongue blade, penlight, laryngeal mirror, laryngoscope
	Axilla, arms	
	Chest	Stethoscope
	Breasts	
	Upper back	Stethoscope
	Reflexes	Percussion hammer
Supine	Chest	Stethoscope
	Abdomen	Stethoscope
	Breasts	
Lithotomy, dorsal recumbent, Sims	Female genitalia and internal organs	Gloves, vaginal speculum, Ayre spatula, histobrush, lubricant
Standing, dorsal recumbent, Sims	Male genitalia and hernia	Gloves
	Male rectum	Gloves, lubricant, fecal occult blood test
	Prostate	Gloves, lubricant
	Legs	Percussion hammer
	Spine, posture, gait, coordination, balance, strength, flexibility	
Prone	Back, spine, legs	
Knee-chest	Rectum	Glove, lubricant, anoscope, proctoscope, or sigmoidoscope, fecal occult blood test
	Female genitalia	Glove, lubricant, vaginal speculum, Ayre spatula, histobrush
	Prostate	Glove, lubricant
Fowler	Head, neck, chest	Stethoscope

expression and level of anxiety by noting verbal and nonverbal behavior during the examination. Table 5-1 lists standard examination positions, the body parts usually examined in these positions, and the instruments needed by the physician for these examinations.

Postexamination Duties

After the physical examination, you should perform any follow-up treatments and procedures as necessary or as ordered by the physician. Always offer the patient help

returning to a sitting position after the examination. Ask the patient to dress, and leave the room unless the patient needs your assistance. Tell the patient what to do after getting dressed. In many offices, the patient gets dressed and remains in the examining room until the medical assistant gives further instructions; in other offices, patients are told to go to the front desk to schedule future appointments or receive further instructions or prescriptions. In either situation, you are responsible for reinforcing any instructions given by the physician and providing appropriate patient education. Unless the patient was advised to wait in the examination room for instructions after dressing, escort the patient to the front desk for scheduling future appointments and addressing billing issues while maintaining confidentiality. Check the medical record to be sure that all data have been accurately documented before releasing the record to the billing department.

Clean all reusable equipment, and properly dispose of any disposable supplies or equipment used during the examination. Cover the examination table with clean paper, and prepare the room for the next patient.

 CHECKPOINT QUESTION

6. What are your four basic responsibilities in the performance of the physical examination?

COG Physical Examination Format

The physical examination of the patient begins with the patient seated on the examining table with a drape sheet over the lap and covering the legs. The physician usually progresses through the examination in an orderly, methodical sequence. The patient's general appearance, behavior, speech, posture, nutritional status, hair distribution, and skin are observed throughout the examination. The next sections describe the areas of the body examined, including normal and abnormal findings.

Head and Neck

The patient's skull, scalp, hair, and face are inspected and palpated for size, shape, and symmetry. The examiner looks for nodules, masses, and local trauma. The patient may be asked to roll the head in all directions to assess range of motion and to check for any limitations of movement. The trachea and lymph nodes on the anterior neck are palpated for size and symmetry.

The thyroid gland, also on the anterior neck, is palpated for size and symmetry. The patient may be asked to swallow to facilitate palpating this gland. The carotid arteries are palpated and auscultated on both sides of the neck to check for any **bruit** (abnormal sound) caused by abnormal blockage.

Eyes and Ears

Usually you perform the visual acuity test before the physician's examination (see Chapter 14). The physician also inspects the **sclera**, or fibrous tissue covering the eye, for normal color. The pupils are inspected with a light to see if they are equal in size, round, and normally reactive to light and accommodation (adjustment). Normal pupil reaction is recorded as **PERRLA**, which means the **p**upils are **e**qual, **r**ound, and **r**eactive to **l**ight and **a**ccommodation. Eye movement is assessed by

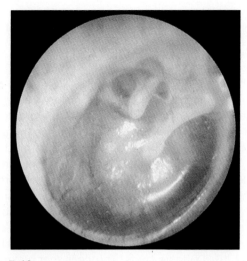

Figure 5-18 A normal tympanic membrane. Reprinted with permission from Moore KL, Agur AM, Dalley AF. Essential Clinical Anatomy, 4th Ed. Baltimore: Lippincott Williams & Wilkins, 2011.)

asking the patient to follow the examiner's fingers. Normal movement may be documented as "EOM intact," which means **extraocular** (outside the eye) movement intact. **Peripheral vision**, or side vision while looking straight ahead, may also be assessed. Using the ophthalmoscope, the physician visualizes the interior of the eye and evaluates the condition of the retina and any pathology of the interlobular blood vessels.

The ears are inspected and palpated for size, symmetry, lesions, and nodules. The otoscope is used to examine the interior of the ear canal, including any **cerumen**, or ear wax. The tympanic membrane is checked for color and intact or broken condition. Normally the tympanic membrane is pearly gray and concave (Fig. 5-18). However, infection may cause discoloration, and fluids behind the eardrum may cause the membrane to bulge outward. Auditory acuity is tested with the tuning fork or the audioscope (see Chapter 14).

Nose and Sinuses

The external nose is palpated for abnormalities and inspected using a nasal speculum and light. The position of the **nasal septum** is noted for any deviation to the right or left. Each nostril is inspected for color of the mucosa, discharge, lesions, obstructions, polyps, swelling, or tenderness. The sense of smell may be assessed by having the patient close the eyes and identify a common substance such as alcohol, lemon, strawberry, or peppermint.

The paranasal sinuses are also inspected and palpated. With the technique of **transillumination** to visualize the sinuses, the room is darkened and a penlight or flashlight is placed against the upper cheek or periorbital ridge.

AFF PATIENT EDUCATION

THE SENSE OF TASTE AND SMELL

When obtaining the medical history, ask the patient whether he or she has had any problems with tasting or smelling. A sudden loss in the ability to taste or smell can be the result of medication, sinus infection, and certain types of tumor. Lack of taste sensation can be the result of normal aging. Normally, the tongue is covered with small bumps called papillae. Each papilla holds about 100 taste buds that allow sweet, salty, sour, and bitter tastes to be identified. The average adult has about 10,000 taste buds. The cells that make up the taste buds are replaced about every 2 weeks. Scientists estimate that, by 80 years of age, most people have lost 60% to 80% of their taste buds, and unfortunately, the remaining taste buds are less sensitive than earlier in life. Sweet and salty taste buds tend to be the most affected.

Mouth and Throat

The physician inspects the mucous membranes of the mouth, gums, teeth, tongue, tonsils, and throat using clean gloves, a light source, and a tongue blade. A laryngeal mirror may also be used. The examiner assesses general dental hygiene and salivary gland function and looks for any abnormalities in the oral cavity, including color, ulcerations, and nodules.

CHECKPOINT QUESTION

7. What is the tympanic membrane, and how does infection affect its appearance?

Chest, Breasts, and Abdomen

The anterior chest is examined with the gown removed to the waist. The physician observes the general appearance and symmetry of the chest and breast area, the respiratory rate and pattern, and any obvious masses or swelling. Palpation includes the axillary lymph nodes and the area over the heart. Underlying structures may also be percussed. Using a stethoscope, the examiner auscultates the lungs for abnormal sounds, at which time the patient may be asked to take deep breaths. The heart sounds and apical pulse are also assessed.

Inspection and palpation of the posterior chest include the muscles of the back and spine. This is followed by percussion of the back to assess lung fields.

With a stethoscope, the examiner listens to posterior lung sounds, again with the patient asked to take deep breaths.

The breasts may be palpated in both male and female patients. The supine position is preferred for palpation of the breasts because the breast tissue flattens out, making any abnormalities easier to feel. The tissue subject to breast examination includes not only the breast and nipple, but the tissue extending up to the clavicle, under the axilla, and down to the bottom of the rib cage.

After the breasts are examined, the drape is lowered to expose the abdomen to the pubic area. The patient's chest is draped or gowned to just below the breasts. The abdomen is inspected for contour, symmetry, and pulsations from the aorta, a large artery that extends from the heart down the center of the thoracic and abdominal cavities. The examiner uses the stethoscope to auscultate the bowel sounds. Percussion may be used to determine the outlines of the abdominal organs, and palpation is used to assess any organ enlargement, masses, pain, or tenderness.

The lower abdomen and groin are palpated to assess enlargement of **inguinal** lymph nodes and detect any **hernia**. A hernia is protrusion of an organ, such as the intestines, through a weakened muscle wall. The femoral arteries, which pass through each groin, may also be palpated and auscultated.

CHECKPOINT QUESTION

8. Why is the patient supine for palpation of the breasts?

LEGAL TIP

ASSISTING DURING EXAMS

During the physical examination, it is recommended that you remain in the examination room if the physician is examining a patient of the opposite gender. For example, if a male physician is performing a gynecologic examination, the medical assistant should remain in the room to protect the physician from being accused of inappropriate behavior. A female physician should also ask the medical assistant to remain present during the examination of a male patient for similar reasons. Although physicians perform these examinations routinely and medical assistants are often busy performing many tasks at once, taking the time to be present during these examinations will provide legal protection for the physician should an accusation of impropriety arise at a later date.

Genitalia and Rectum

The physician puts on clean gloves to examine the external male genitalia and then the rectum. The male genitalia are inspected to note symmetry, lesions, swelling, masses, and hair distribution. The scrotal contents may be visualized using transillumination in a darkened room. In addition, the scrotum is palpated for testicular size, contour, and consistency. The male patient is then asked to stand and bear down as if having a bowel movement while the examiner places a gloved index finger upward along the side of the scrotum in the inguinal ring to assess for a hernia.

The physician asks the patient either to bend over the examination table or to assume the Sims position to inspect the anus for lesions and hemorrhoids. The examiner inserts a gloved and lubricated finger into the rectum to palpate the rectal sphincter muscle and prostate gland for size, consistency, and any masses. An **occult blood** (hidden blood) stool test may be obtained on any stool obtained from the gloved finger. (Chapter 17 describes the procedure for processing the occult blood stool specimen.)

The female genitalia and rectum are usually examined with the patient in the lithotomy position and with one corner of the drape extending over the genitalia and the other corner covering the patient's chest. A gooseneck lamp is adjusted to direct light on the vaginal area, and the external genitalia are inspected for lesions, edema, cysts, discharge, and hair distribution. With clean gloves, the examiner inserts the vaginal speculum and inspects the condition of the vaginal mucosa and cervix. A Pap smear sample from the cervix is obtained, and the speculum is removed. At this time, the examiner performs a bimanual examination to palpate the internal reproductive organs for size, contour, consistency, and any masses. Two fingers of the gloved dominant hand are inserted into the vagina while the gloved nondominant hand is placed on the lower abdomen to compress the internal organs. (See Chapter 20 for a complete description of the procedure for assisting with a gynecologic examination.)

Sometimes a **rectovaginal** examination is necessary to palpate the posterior uterus and vaginal wall. The examiner places a gloved index finger in the vagina and the middle finger of the same hand in the rectum at the same time. The rectum is usually inspected and palpated for lesions, hemorrhoids, and sphincter tone. A stool specimen may be obtained from the gloved finger to test for occult blood.

 WHAT IF?

What if you are assisting the physician during a genital and pelvic examination on a disabled female patient who cannot be placed into the lithotomy position?

Both genital and rectal examinations may be performed with the patient in the dorsal recumbent or Sims position for patients who cannot comfortably assume the usual positions, including the lithotomy position.

Legs

The legs are inspected and the peripheral pulse sites palpated with the patient supine. The patient stands, with assistance if needed, and the peripheral pulse sites may be palpated again and the legs observed for varicose veins.

Reflexes

The examiner uses the percussion hammer to test the patient's reflexes by striking the biceps, triceps, patellar, Achilles, and plantar tendons. The patient is usually sitting when these reflexes are checked but may move to supine for checking the plantar reflexes.

Posture, Gait, Coordination, Balance, and Strength

The general posture of the patient and the spine may be inspected with the patient standing. The patient may be asked to walk and perform other movements so that **gait** and coordination can be observed. A balance test may be done by having the patient stand with the feet together and eyes closed. Range of motion and strength of arms and legs are assessed.

 CHECKPOINT QUESTION

9. What is the function of the rectovaginal and bimanual pelvic examinations?

 TRIAGE

While working in a family practice office, you have to complete the following three tasks:

A. A patient was just discharged, and the examination room has to be cleaned and restocked.
B. The physician states that she is ready to perform a gynecologic examination and needs your assistance.
C. A suture tray has to be set up for a 3-year-old child with a facial laceration.

(continued)

How do you sort these tasks? What do you do first? Second? Third?

First, assist the physician with the examination. When possible, limit the waiting time for female patients to have their gynecologic examination. Next, set up the suture tray. Third, clean and restock the examination room.

COG General Health Guidelines and Checkups

Physicians vary as to how often they recommend a complete physical examination. For patients aged 20 to 40 years, physical examinations are scheduled about every 1 to 3 years. Annual examinations are typically performed on patients over age 40 unless a medical condition requires more frequent visits.

For women, the American Cancer Society recommends the first Pap smear when sexual activity occurs, but no later than 21 years of age. This test should be done annually for conventional testing or every 2 years if the practitioner uses a liquid-based Pap test. A breast examination by a physician is recommended every 3 years for women aged 20 to 40 to detect lumps and thickenings that could be malignancies, but breast self-examinations (BSEs) should be performed monthly to allow the patient to detect and report any abnormalities in breast tissue between visits to the physician (see Chapter 20). As with most cancers, early detection of breast cancer is the key to survival. A baseline mammogram is recommended for those aged 35 and yearly after 40. If the patient is at risk for developing breast cancer, the physician may recommend mammograms earlier and more often.

The American Cancer Society also recommends that male patients have the prostate-specific antigen (PSA) blood test and digital rectal examination (DRE) yearly beginning at age 50 to detect early signs of prostate cancer. Men who are high risk for developing prostate cancer should have these tests starting at age 45. Risk factors include African-American men and those with close family members (father, brothers, or sons) who were diagnosed with prostate cancer before the age of 65. Again, early detection is important for early treatment, which saves lives.

All patients should have a baseline electrocardiogram (ECG) at age 40 and follow-up ECGs as necessary. In addition, a rectal examination and fecal occult blood test are recommended annually beginning at age 40. At age 50, a proctoscopic examination (colonoscopy) is recommended, and if the results are negative, this exam should be performed every 3 to 5 years thereafter.

The Center for Disease Control and Prevention recommends the following immunizations for all adults:

- Tetanus booster every 10 years, or sooner if the patient has an open wound.
- Measles, mumps, rubella (MMR) one or two doses between the ages of 19 and 49 years for patients who do not have documentation of having the vaccine or for those who have never had the disease.
- The varicella vaccine (chicken pox) should be given in two doses between the ages of 19 and 49 years for patients who do not have documentation of having the vaccine or for those who have never had the disease.
- One injection of pneumococcal vaccine should be given at age 65 years.
- After age 50, an annual influenza vaccine should be given.
- Some doctors also recommend a series of three hepatitis B injections for any adult patient who has not received this immunization.

You should take every opportunity to educate patients regarding the signs and symptoms that may signal health problems and when to call the physician.

 PATIENT EDUCATION

THE BODY'S WARNING SIGNALS

Teach patients the CAUTION acronym to recognize these early warning signs of cancer:

C   Change in bowel or bladder habits
A   A sore that does not heal
U   Unusual bleeding or discharge
T   Thickening, lumps, or changes in the shape of the breasts or testicles
I   Indigestion or difficulty swallowing
O   Obvious change in a wart or mole
N   Nagging cough or hoarseness of the voice

Frequent, severe headaches and persistent abdominal pain are other signals that should not be ignored. Instruct patients not to overlook the following signs in their children:

- Continual crying for no obvious reason
- Unexplained nausea and vomiting
- General failure to thrive
- Spontaneous bleeding or bleeding that does not stop in the normal amount of time
- Bumps, lumps, masses, or swelling anywhere on the body
- Frequent stumbling for no apparent reason

 CHECKPOINT QUESTION

10. Why are monthly breast self-examinations important for women aged 20 to 40 years?

español SPANISH TERMINOLOGY

Voy a examinarlo/la.
  I am going to examine you.

Voy a examinar sus oídos.
  I am going to check your ears.

Voy a examinar su nariz.
  I am going to check your nose.

Saque la lengua.
  Stick out your tongue.

Voy a examinar su piel.
  I am going to examine your skin.

Voy a examinar su abdomen (vientre).
  I am going to examine your abdomen.

Voy a examinar su espalda.
  I am going to examine your back.

MEDIA MENU

- **Student Resources on thePoint**
  - **CMA/RMA Certification Exam Review**

- **Internet Resources**

  American Academy of Family Physicians
  http://www.aafp.org/online/en/home.html

  Family Doctor
  http://www.familydoctor.org/online/famdocen/home.html

  American College of Physicians—Internal Medicine
  http://www.acponline.org

  CDC Screen for Life: National Colorectal Cancer Action Campaign
  http://www.cdc.gov/cancer/colorectal/sfl

  American Cancer Society
  http://www.cancer.org

  National Breast Cancer Foundation
  http://www.nationalbreastcancer.org

PSY PROCEDURE 5-1:   Assisting with the Adult Physical Examination

Purpose: Prepare the room and patient for the general physical examination, assist the physician during the examination, assist the patient as needed after the examination, and clean up the examination room
Equipment: A variety of instruments and supplies, including the stethoscope, ophthalmoscope, otoscope, penlight, tuning fork, nasal speculum, tongue blade, percussion hammer, gloves, water-soluble lubricant, an examinations light, and patient gown and draping supplies
Standard: This procedure should take 15 minutes.

Steps	Reasons
1. Wash your hands.	Handwashing aids infection control.
2. Prepare the examination room and assemble the equipment.	A clean room that is free of contamination prevents transfer of microorganisms.
Step 2. The examination room should be clean, neat, and orderly.	
3. Greet the patient by name and escort him or her to the examining room.	Identifying the patient by name prevents errors.
Step 3. Identify the patient and escort him or her to the exam room.	
4. Explain the procedure.	Explaining the procedure reduces anxiety and may help to ensure compliance.
5. Obtain and record the medical history and chief complaint.	Documenting the chief complaint supports the physician and creates a legal document for the visit.
6. Take and record the vital signs, height, weight, and visual acuity.	The vital signs and other measurements give the physician an overall picture of the patient's health.
Step 6. Taking the patient's vital signs is an important part of the physical exam.	

PSY PROCEDURE 5-1: **Assisting with the Adult Physical Examination** *(continued)*

Steps	Reasons
7. If the physician requires it, instruct the patient to obtain a urine specimen and escort him or her to the bathroom (refer to Chapter 28 for more information on obtaining a urine specimen).	Even if a urine specimen is not part of the physical examination, an empty bladder makes abdominal and/or pelvic examinations more comfortable.
8. Once inside the examination room, instruct the patient in disrobing including directions on how to put the gown on (open in the front or back). Leave the room unless the patient needs assistance.	The gown must open in the direction that provides accessibility for the examination. Elderly and disabled persons may need help disrobing and putting on the gown.
9. **AFF** Explain how to respond to a patient who has cultural or religious beliefs who may be uncomfortable about disrobing.	Being respectful of the cultural or religious differences by explaining why procedures are needed is important. Provide additional privacy if necessary.
10. Help the patient sit on the edge of the examination table and cover the lap and legs with a drape.	The sitting position is often the first position used by the physician.

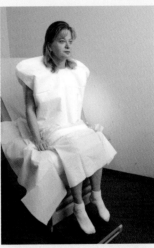

Step 10. The patient should be draped appropriately.

11. Place the medical record outside the examination room and notify the physician that the patient is ready.	Make sure the patient's name on the medical record is facing inward to maintain confidentiality from anyone passing by the room. Alerting the physician helps prevent delays.

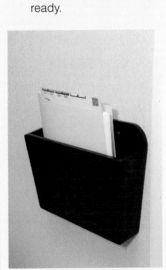

Step 11. Place the medical record with identifying information turned away from the hallway.

(continued)

PSY PROCEDURE 5-1: **Assisting with the Adult Physical Examination** *(continued)*

Steps	Reasons
12. Assist the physician by handing him or her the instruments as needed and positioning the patient appropriately.	Anticipating the physician's needs promotes efficiency and saves time. Only the parts of the body being examined should be exposed. Always preserve patients' privacy and keep them covered as much as possible.

12. Assist the physician by handing him or her the instruments as needed and positioning the patient appropriately.

    A. Begin by handing the physician the instruments necessary for examining the following:
- Head and neck Stethoscope
- Eyes Ophthalmoscope, penlight
- Ears Otoscope, tuning fork
- Nose Penlight, nasal speculum
- Sinuses Penlight
- Mouth Tongue blade, penlight. Hand the tongue blade to the physician by holding it in the middle. When it is returned to you, grasp it in the middle again so that you do not touch the end that was in the patient's mouth.
- Throat Glove, tongue blade, laryngeal mirror, penlight

    B. Help the patient drop the gown to the waist for examination of the chest and upper back. Hand the physician the stethoscope.

    C. Help the patient pull the gown up and remove the drape from the legs so that the physician can test the reflexes. Hand the physician the percussion hammer.

    D. Help the patient to lie supine, opening the gown at the top to expose the chest again. Place the drape to cover the waist, abdomen, and legs. Hand the physician the stethoscope.

    E. Cover the patient's chest and lower the drape to expose the abdomen. Hand the physician the stethoscope.

    F. Assist with the genital and rectal examinations. Hand the patient tissues following these examinations.

        Reason: Tissues may be used to wipe off excess lubricant.

For females:
- Assist the patient to the lithotomy position and drape appropriately.
- For examination of the genitalia and internal reproductive organs, provide a glove, lubricant, speculum, microscope slides or liquid prep solution, and Ayres spatula or brush.
- For the rectal examination, provide a glove lubricant, and fecal occult blood test slide.

PSY PROCEDURE 5-1: | **Assisting with the Adult Physical Examination** *(continued)*

Steps	Reasons
For males: • Help the patient stand and have him bend over the examination table for a rectal and prostate examination. • For a hernia examination, provide a glove. • For a rectal examination, provide a glove, lubricant, and fecal occult blood test slide. • For a prostate examination, provide a glove and lubricant. G. With the patient standing, the physician can assess the legs, gait, coordination, and balance.	
13. Help the patient sit at the edge of the examination table.	The physician often discusses findings with the patient at this time and may provide instructions.
14. Perform any follow-up procedures or treatments.	After the physician examines the patient, there may be additional procedures such as preparing specimens that were obtained.
15. Leave the room while the patient dresses unless he or she needs assistance.	Leaving the room provides privacy for the patient.
16. Return to the examination room when the patient has dressed to answer any questions, reinforce physician instructions, and provide patient education.	Compliance depends on full understanding of the treatment plan. Patient education is the responsibility of all health care workers, including the medical assistant.
17. Escort the patient to the front desk.	You can clarify appointment scheduling or billing issues.
18. Properly clean or dispose of all used equipment and supplies. Clean the room with a disinfectant and prepare for the next patient.	All instruments, supplies, and equipment that came into direct contact with the patient must be appropriately decontaminated or disposed of.
19. Wash your hands and record any instructions from the physician. Also note any specimens and indicate the results of the test or the laboratory where the specimens are being sent for testing.	Procedures and instructions are considered not to have been done if they are not recorded.

Charting Example:

01/19/12 1:30 pm CC: Annual physical exam complete per Dr. Smith. ECG done; results given to Dr. Smith. Blood drawn and sent to Acme lab for CBC, electrolytes, and liver panel. Pt. instructed to return to office in 2 weeks to discuss laboratory results. Pt. given written and verbal instructions for 1,800-calorie, low-sodium diet as ordered. Pt. verbalized understanding ———————————————————————— *J. Bohr, CMA*

Note: The medical assistant may sign his or her name in the patient record using only the "CMA" credential if the office has a signature log denoting the entire credential as "CMA(AAMA)."

Chapter Summary

- Your role as a medical assistant during the physical examination is to assist both the physician and the patient.
- Efficiency, accuracy, and attention to detail are crucial as you assist the physician and anticipate what will be needed in the examination.

- Assessing the patient's needs, developing a good interpersonal relationship, and providing support to the patient are important to help the patient have a pleasant office visit.

Warm Ups for Critical Thinking

1. During the physical examination, the physician asks the patient to walk across the room. What can be determined about the patient's health from observing the patient's gait?
2. After the physical examination, a patient asks you, "Why did the physician hit my chest with his fingers while listening?" How do you explain to the patient what the doctor was doing?
3. Why is it possible for the physician to assess vascular health by checking the interior eye with the ophthalmoscope?
4. How can you anticipate what instruments or supplies the physician may need during the physical examination? Why is this important?
5. When checking the ophthalmoscope for working condition, you discover that it is not working. What do you think might be the problem? How would you handle this situation?

CHAPTER 6

Sterilization and Surgical Instruments

Learning Outcomes

Cognitive Domain

Note: AAMA/CAAHEP 2008 Standards are italicized.

1. Spell and define the key terms
2. *Differentiate between medical and surgical asepsis used in ambulatory care settings, identifying when each is appropriate*
3. Describe several methods of sterilization
4. Categorize surgical instruments based on use and identify each by its characteristics
5. Identify surgical instruments specific to designated specialties
6. State the difference between reusable and disposable instruments
7. Explain how to handle and store instruments, equipment, and supplies
8. Describe the necessity and steps for maintaining documents and records of maintenance for instruments and equipment

Psychomotor Domain

Note: AAMA/CAAHEP 2008 Standards are italicized.

1. Sanitize equipment and instruments (Procedure 6-1)

2. *Prepare items for autoclaving*
3. Properly wrap instruments for autoclaving (Procedure 6-2)
4. *Perform sterilization procedures*
5. Perform sterilization technique and operate an autoclave (Procedure 6-3)
6. *Practice standard precautions*

Affective Domain

Note: AAMA/CAAHEP 2008 Standards are italicized.

1. *Apply ethical behaviors, including honesty and integrity in performance of medical assisting practice*

ABHES Competencies

1. Wrap items for autoclaving
2. Practice quality control
3. Use standard precautions
4. Perform sterilization techniques

Key Terms

autoclave	hemostat	Administration (OSHA)	scissors
disinfection	needle holder		serrations
ethylene oxide	obturator	ratchet	sound
forceps	Occupational Safety and Health	sanitation	sterilization
		scalpels	

The goal of surgical asepsis is to free an item or area from all microorganisms, including pathogens and other microorganisms (see Chapter 2). The practice of surgical asepsis, also known as sterile technique, should be used during any office surgical procedure, when handling sterile instruments to be used for incisions and excisions into body tissue, and when changing wound dressings. Surgical asepsis prevents microorganisms from entering the patient's environment; medical asepsis prevents microbes from spreading to or from patients.

In a medical office, your responsibilities may include assisting with minor surgical procedures while maintaining surgical asepsis. To manage this responsibility, you must do the following:

- Become familiar with many types of surgical instruments
- Understand the principles and practices of surgical asepsis
- Understand and use **disinfection** and **sterilization** techniques
- Use equipment designed for sterilization, treatment, and diagnostic purposes
- Maintain accurate records and inventory of purchases related to surgical equipment and supplies

The physician expects you to understand sterile technique and to be able to maintain sterility throughout procedures. Any break in sterile technique, no matter how small, can lead to infection the body cannot fight.

Even small infections can delay the patient's recovery and are physically, mentally, and financially costly to the patient. Your attention to detail and professional integrity during any surgical aseptic procedure is essential in preventing serious patient complications.

COG Principles and Practices of Surgical Asepsis

As a medical assistant, you are responsible for preventing infection in accordance with the principles and practices of asepsis as it relates to items used during minor office surgical procedures. Surgical asepsis requires the *absence of microorganisms, infection, and infectious material on instruments, equipment, and supplies*. Disinfection, or medical asepsis, is different from sterilization (Table 6-1). By becoming familiar with the manufacturer's recommendations for processing instruments according to the purposes for which the items will be used, you will be able to determine the appropriate level of asepsis.

Sterilization

While **sanitation** and disinfection are adequate for maintaining medical asepsis in the medical office, these practices are not sufficient to process instruments and equipment used during sterile procedures (see Chapter 2). Objects requiring surgical asepsis must be sanitized first and sterilized by either a physical or

TABLE 6-1	Comparison of Medical and Surgical Asepsis	
	Medical Asepsis	**Surgical Asepsis**
Definition	Destroys microorganisms after they leave the body	Destroys microorganisms before they enter the body
Purpose	Prevents transmission of microbes from one person to another	Prevents entry of microbes into the body during invasive procedures
When Used	During contact with a body part that is not normally sterile	During contact with a normally sterile part of the body
Differences in Handwashing Technique	Hands and wrists are washed for 1–2 minutes	Hands and forearms are washed for 5–10 minutes with a brush

120

TABLE 6-2	Sterilization Methods
Methods	**Concentration or Level**
Heat	
Moist heat (steam under pressure)	250°F or 121°C for 30 min
Boiling	212°F or 100°C for ≥30 min
Dry heat	340°F or 171°C for 1 hour
	320°F or 160°C for 2 hours
Liquids	
Glutaraldehyde	Follow manufacturer's recommendations or OSHA requirements and guidelines
Formaldehyde	Follow manufacturer's recommendations or OSHA requirements and guidelines
Gas	
Ethylene oxide	450–500 mg/L 50°C

OSHA, Occupational Safety and Health Administration.

chemical process. Procedure 6-1 describes the procedure for sanitizing instruments in preparation for sterilization. Sterilization is the complete elimination or destruction of all forms of microbial life, including spore forms. Steam under pressure, dry heat, **ethylene oxide** gas, and liquid chemicals are principle sterilizing agents. Although steam under pressure is the most frequently used method of sterilization in the medical office, the method depends on the nature of the material to be sterilized and the type of microorganism to be destroyed. Table 6-2 describes the various methods of sterilization and the temperatures and time of exposure if applicable.

 CHECKPOINT QUESTION

1. How do sanitization, disinfection, and sterilization differ?

 LEGAL TIP

THE RIGHT TO KNOW

Occupational Safety and Health Administration (OSHA) and state regulations have defined a specific law to protect you from hazardous materials. The law, The Right to Know, requires that all companies, including medical offices, using hazardous materials have material safety data sheets (MSDS) available to their employees. MSDS are prepared by the chemical manufacturer and clearly state how to handle and dispose of the chemical. These forms also include a list of possible health hazards to workers and identify the safety equipment needed for using the chemical. Never handle any type of chemical spill without first reading the MSDS. You are required to add to the MSDS binder any MSDS that accompany any supplies or equipment containing hazardous materials. This notebook should be placed in a stationary area where it can be easily consulted in case of an emergency involving hazardous materials.

Sterilization Equipment

Several types of sterilization equipment are used in clinics and medical offices. As a clinical medical assistant, it is your responsibility to do the following:

- Become familiar with the uses and operation of each piece of equipment
- Schedule periodic preventive maintenance or servicing of the equipment
- Maintain adequate supplies for general operational needs

The Autoclave

The most frequently used piece of equipment for sterilizing instruments today is the **autoclave** (Fig. 6-1A,B). The autoclave has two chambers: an outer one where pressure builds and an inner one where the sterilization occurs. Distilled water is added to a reservoir, where it is converted to steam as the preset temperature is reached. The steam is forced into the inner chamber, increasing the pressure and raising the temperature of the steam to 250°F or higher, well above the ordinary boiling temperature of water (212°F or 100°C). The pressure has no effect

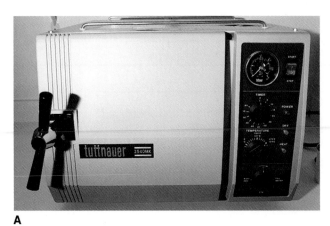

A

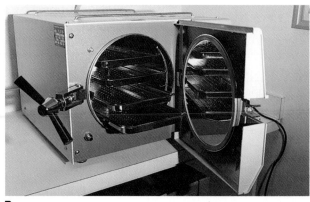

B

Figure 6-1 (A) An autoclave that may be found in the medical office. (B) The interior of the autoclave.

on sterilization other than to increase the temperature of the steam. The high temperature allows for destruction of all microorganisms, including viruses and spores.

An air exhaust vent on the bottom of the autoclave allows the air in the chamber to be pushed out and replaced by the pressurized steam. When no air is present, the chamber seals and the temperature gauge begins to rise. Most automatic autoclaves can be set to vent, time, turn off, and exhaust at preset times and levels. Older models may require that the steps be advanced manually. All manufacturers provide instructions for operating the machine and recommendations for the times necessary to sterilize different types of loads. These instructions should be posted in a prominent place near the machine.

Sterilization is required for surgical instruments and equipment that will come into contact with internal body tissues or cavities that are considered sterile. The autoclave is commonly used to sterilize minor surgical instruments, surgical storage trays and containers, and some surgical equipment, such as bowls for holding sterile solutions. Instruments or equipment subject to damage by water should not be sterilized in the autoclave. These items can be sterilized with gas. Items that are not subject to water damage but may be destroyed by heat can be cold-sterilized or soaked for a prescribed amount of time in a liquid such as glutaraldehyde or formaldehyde. Always follow the manufacturer's recommendations for sterilizing instruments or equipment and for using any chemical products for sterilization. Procedure 6-2 describes preparation of instruments for sterilization in the autoclave.

 CHECKPOINT QUESTION

2. Why is the properly working autoclave more effective at sterilizing equipment compared to boiling water?

Sterilization Indicators

Tape applied to the outside of the material used to wrap instruments or supplies for the autoclave indicates that the items have been exposed to steam, but *the tape cannot ensure the sterility of the contents* (Box 6-1). This special tape (Fig. 6-2) is used to close and label the contents of wrapped packages before placing items in the autoclave. The stripes on the tape become dark upon exposure to steam and allow you to easily determine whether or not a pack has been placed in the autoclave.

Because microorganisms are not visible to the naked eye, sterilization indicators must be placed inside each pack that are designed to register that the proper pressure, temperature, and time were attained in the autoclave to assure destruction of all microbial life (Fig. 6-3). Improper wrapping, loading, or operation of the autoclave may prevent the indicator from registering properly, and the sterility of the contents cannot be assured. Various types of sterilization indicators are available, including those that change colors at high temperatures and those that contain wax pellets, which indicate that the required temperature was reached evidenced by the melted wax. Although most types of sterilization indicators work well, the best method for determining effectiveness of sterilization is the culture test. Strips impregnated with heat-resistant spores are wrapped and placed in the center of the autoclave between the

---

BOX 6-1

AUTOCLAVE INDICATOR TAPE

Autoclave tape is designed to change color in the presence of heat and steam. In extreme instances, the tape may change appearance when stored too close to heat sources. Most tapes have imprinted lines that darken after exposure, but *sterilization of the package contents is not ensured by a color change on the autoclave tape.* Proper sterilization can be assumed only if accompanying sterilization indicators have registered that all elements of the sterilization process (time and temperature) have been achieved.

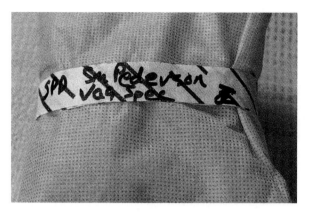

Figure 6-2 The stripes on autoclave tape change color, indicating that the pack has been exposed to steam.

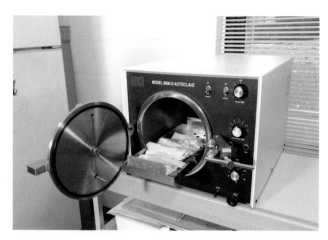

Figure 6-4 Properly loaded autoclave.

packages in a designated load, such as the first load of the day. The strips are removed from their packets and placed in a broth culture to be incubated according to the instructions of the manufacturer. At the end of the incubation period, the culture is compared to a control to determine that all spores have been killed. If sterilization was not achieved, the load must be reprocessed before the items put through the sterilization process can be used in surgical procedures.

 CHECKPOINT QUESTION

3. What is the difference between a sterilization indicator and autoclave tape?

Loading the Autoclave

Improper loading of the autoclave will prevent steam from penetrating the items inside the packs completely, compromising the sterility of the contents. Load the autoclave loosely to allow steam to circulate. Place empty wrapped containers or bowls on their sides with the lids wrapped separately. If containers are upright in the autoclave, air, which is heavier than steam, will settle into the interior of

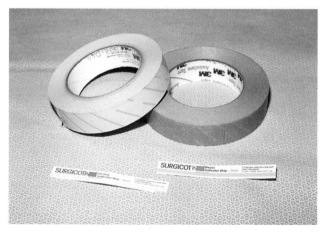

Figure 6-3 Autoclave tape (*top*: steam and gas tape) and sterilization indicators (*bottom left and right*).

the container and keep steam from circulating to the inner surfaces. Place all packs on their sides to allow for the maximum steam circulation and penetration (Fig. 6-4).

Operating the Autoclave

All components of autoclaving—temperature, pressure, steam, and time—must be correct for the items to reach sterility. Follow the instruction manual carefully. All machines use the same principles, but operation varies. Become familiar with the function of the machine in your facility. Instructions may be covered in plastic or laminated and posted beside the machine for easy reference.

The autoclave has a reservoir tank that should be filled with distilled water only. Tap water contains chemicals and minerals that would coat the interior chamber, clog the exhaust valves, and hinder the overall operation of the autoclave. When filling the internal chamber of the autoclave with distilled water from the reservoir, be sure the water level is at the fill line. If too much water is added to the chamber, the steam will be saturated and may not be efficient, and too little water will not produce the required amount of steam. Procedure 6-3 outlines the general steps for operating an autoclave.

The temperature, pressure, and time required vary with the items being sterilized. In most cases, 250°F at 15 pounds of pressure for 20 to 30 minutes will be sufficient, but you should follow the manufacturer's instructions for the load content. Solid or metal loads take slightly less time than soft, bulky loads. The timer should not be set until the proper temperature has been attained. Some microorganisms, such as spores, are killed only if exposed to high enough temperature for a specific amount of time.

When the items have been in the autoclave at the right temperature for enough time, the timer will sound, indicating that the cycle is finished. Be sure to vent the autoclave to allow the pressure to drop safely. After the pressure has dropped to a safe level, open the door of the autoclave slightly to allow the temperature to drop and the load to cool and dry. Newer autoclaves vent automatically. Do not handle or remove items from the autoclave until they are dry because bacteria from your hands would be drawn through the moist coverings and contaminate the items inside the wrapping. Once the items are dry, remove the packages and store them in a clean, dry, dust-free area. Packs that are sterilized on site in the autoclave are considered sterile for 30 days and must be sterilized again after this period. Always store recently autoclaved items toward the back of the cabinet, rotating the previously autoclaved items to the front. In addition, you are responsible for performing maintenance on the autoclave at regular intervals. Post a schedule for this maintenance near the machine; allow for cleaning the lint trap, washing out the interior of the chamber with a cloth or soft brush, and checking the function of all components. This schedule can remind and document the service with space for initialing or signing after the maintenance has been done.

 CHECKPOINT QUESTION

4. Why is it important to set the timer on the autoclave during a cycle only after the correct temperature has been reached?

 AFF TRIAGE

While you are working in a medical office, the following three situations arise:

A. You need to wrap instruments for the autoclave that were sanitized earlier in the day.
B. A 45-year-old woman who just had a mole removed needs postoperative instructions before discharge, and the treatment room where the procedure was done is in need of cleaning for the next patient.
C. A load in the autoclave that ran earlier is finished. The sterilized packs have to be put away.

How do you sort these tasks? What do you do first? Second? Third?

The patient in situation B should be taken care of first. You should take time to explain any postoperative instructions and follow-up care clearly as indicated by the physician. Once the patient is discharged, the treatment room should be cleaned, and any used surgical equipment should be discarded appropriately or prepared for sanitation according to appropriate standard precautions. The next task includes wrapping the sanitized instruments in preparation for the autoclave. After unloading the autoclave and putting the sterilized packs away, the clean wrapped instruments can be placed in the autoclave for sterilization.

COG Surgical Instruments

You must be able to identify surgical instruments according to their design and function. A surgical instrument is a tool or device designed to perform a specific function, such as cutting, dissecting, grasping, holding, retracting, or suturing. Surgical instruments are designed to perform specific tasks based on their shape; they may be curved, straight, sharp, blunt, serrated, toothed, or smooth. Many are made of stainless steel and are reusable; others are disposable. It is your responsibility to know the proper use and care of the surgical instruments in your clinical setting.

Most instruments used in office procedures can be identified by carefully examining the instrument. The most widely used surgical instruments are **forceps, scissors, scalpels,** and **clamps.** Table 6-3 shows the most commonly used instruments and equipment by specialty.

 WHAT IF?

Your medical office has one designated room for minor office surgical procedures, and two physicians in your office have scheduled minor office procedures for the same day and time. What should you do?

It is your responsibility to anticipate what the physician needs and address any concerns immediately. Upon discovering that two patients are scheduled for procedures on the same day and time, you should advise both physicians of the situation immediately. In some cases, the patient may have been told not to eat or drink anything (NPO, or nil per os, which is Latin for "nothing by mouth") on the morning of the procedure, and if this is the case and it is agreeable with both physicians, it would be most appropriate to schedule the patient who is NPO earliest in the day. Once the physicians determine who should use the room first, you should then call the patient who will need to be scheduled at a later time, using this opportunity to remind them of any preoperative orders if necessary. Always allow plenty of time between procedures for disinfecting the room, restocking the room with equipment and supplies, and sanitizing and sterilizing any equipment that was used and may be needed for the following procedure.

TABLE **6-3**	Commonly Used Instruments and Equipment by Specialty	
	Instrument	**Use**
Obstetrics, Gynecology	Vaginal speculum	Open vagina to view vaginal walls, cervical os; perform procedures; sized; may be reusable metal or disposable plastic
	Tenaculum	Grasping and holding tissue with hooklike tips
	Uterine **sound**	Assess depth of uterus; graduated in inches or centimeters
	Uterine dilator	Widens cervical os; usually 3–18 mm
	Curet	Blunt or sharp; for scraping endometrium
	Biopsy forceps	Secure pieces of tissue for microscopic study

Gynecology instruments: (**A**) Graves vaginal speculum. (**B**) Pederson vaginal speculum. (**C**) Duplay tenaculum forceps. (**D**) Schroeder tenaculum forceps. (**E**) Sims uterine sound. (**F**) Simpson uterine sound, malleable. (**G**) Hand uterine dilator. (**H**) Hegar uterine dilator. (**I**) Thomas uterine curets. (**J**) Sims uterine curets.

Orthopedics	Cast saw	Remove cast
	Cutters or spreaders	Cutters are scissor-like instruments used to cut casting material; spreaders are used to separate the edges of a cast that has been cut

Orthopedic instruments: (**A**) Oscillating plaster saw. (**B**) Stille plaster shears. (**C**) Hennig plaster spreader.

(continued)

TABLE 6-3 Commonly Used Instruments and Equipment by Specialty *(continued)*

	Instrument	Use
Urology	Urethral sounds	Explore bladder depth, direction; dilate urethral meatus in stenosis; sized Fr 8–26
	Prostate biopsy	Removes tissue for microscopic study

Urology instruments: (**A**) Otis-Dittel urethral sound. (**B**) Dittel urethral sound.

	Instrument	Use
Proctology	Anoscopes, proctoscopes	Visualize lower intestinal tract; most have **obturator** for ease of insertion
	Sigmoidoscope	Visualize lower sigmoid colon; rigid or flexible, with fiber optic light; some have suction device
	Punch biopsy	Remove small piece of tissue via small circular hole
	Alligator biopsy	Jaws grasp and excise tissue

Proctology instruments: (**A**) Ives rectal speculum (Fansler). (**B**) Pratt rectal speculum. (**C**) Hirschman anoscope.

	Instrument	Use
Otology, Rhinology	Nasal or ear forceps	Insert or remove materials from nose or ear canal
	Nasal speculum	Opens, extends nostrils for visualization of nasal passages
	Curet	Remove cerumen from deep ear canal

Otology and rhinology instruments: (**A**) Wilde ear forceps. (**B**) Lucae bayonet forceps. (**C**) Buck ear curet. (**D**) Vienna nasal speculum.

TABLE 6-3	Commonly Used Instruments and Equipment by Specialty (continued)	
	Instrument	**Use**

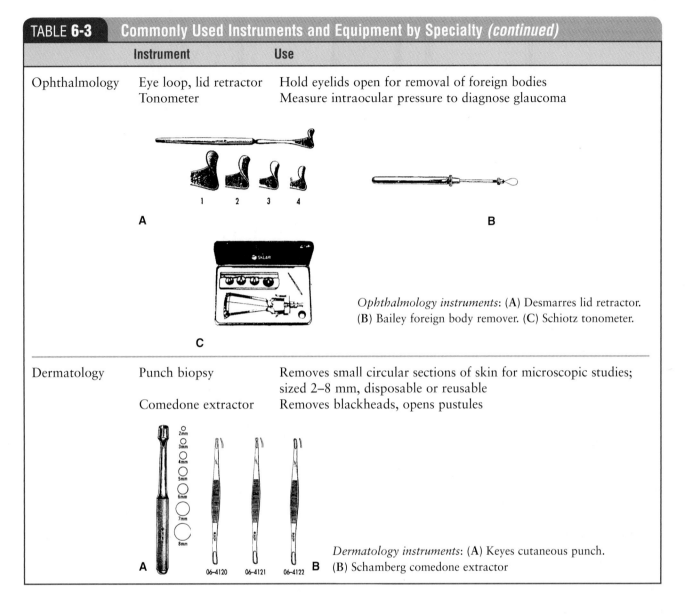

| Ophthalmology | Eye loop, lid retractor | Hold eyelids open for removal of foreign bodies |
| | Tonometer | Measure intraocular pressure to diagnose glaucoma |

Ophthalmology instruments: (**A**) Desmarres lid retractor. (**B**) Bailey foreign body remover. (**C**) Schiotz tonometer.

| Dermatology | Punch biopsy | Removes small circular sections of skin for microscopic studies; sized 2–8 mm, disposable or reusable |
| | Comedone extractor | Removes blackheads, opens pustules |

Dermatology instruments: (**A**) Keyes cutaneous punch. (**B**) Schamberg comedone extractor

Forceps

Forceps are surgical instruments used to grasp, handle, compress, pull, or join tissue, equipment, or supplies. The types of forceps include the following:

- **Hemostat:** A surgical instrument with slender jaws used for grasping blood vessels and establishing hemostasis.
- **Kelly clamp:** A curved or straight forceps or hemostat; those with long handles are widely used in gynecologic procedures.
- **Sterilizer forceps:** Used to transfer sterile supplies, equipment, and other surgical instruments to a sterile field. May also be called sterile transfer forceps.
- **Needle holder:** Used to hold and pass a needle through tissue during suturing.
- **Spring or thumb forceps:** Used for grasping tissue for dissection or suturing, such as tissue forceps and splinter forceps.

A variety of forceps can be seen in Figure 6-5A–Q. All forceps are available in many sizes, with or without **serrations** or teeth, with curved or straight blades, and with ring tips, blunt tips, or sharp tips. Many have **ratchets** in the handles to hold the tips tightly together; these are notched mechanisms that click into position to maintain tension. Some have spring handles that are compressed between the thumb and index finger to grasp objects.

Physicians use a variety of forceps. You should study the names and purposes of each type to assist the physician when a specific instrument is requested.

CHECKPOINT QUESTION

5. What are the most common instruments used in a medical office?

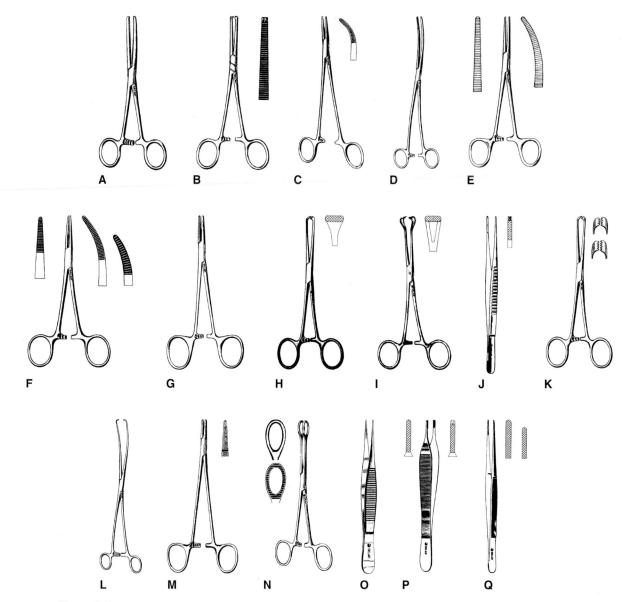

Figure 6-5 Forceps: **(A)** Rochester-Pean forceps. **(B)** Rochester-Ochsner forceps. **(C)** Adson forceps. **(D)** Bozeman forceps. **(E)** Crile hemostat. **(F)** Kelly hemostat. **(G)** Halsted mosquito hemostat. **(H)** Allis forceps. **(I)** Babcock forceps. **(J)** DeBakey forceps. **(K)** Allis tissue forceps. **(L)** Duplay tenaculum forceps. **(M)** Crile-Wood needle holder. **(N)** Ballenger sponge forceps. **(O)** Fine-point splinter forceps. **(P)** Adson dressing forceps. **(Q)** Potts-Smith dressing forceps. (Courtesy of Sklar Instruments, West Chester, PA.)

Scissors

Scissors are sharp instruments composed of two opposing cutting blades held together by a central pin at the pivot. Scissors are used for dissecting superficial, deep, or delicate tissues and for cutting sutures and bandages. Scissors have blade points that are blunt, sharp, or both, depending on the use of the instrument. The types of scissors include the following:

- Straight scissors cut deep or delicate tissue and sutures.
- Curved scissors dissect superficial and delicate tissues.
- Suture scissors cut sutures; they have straight top blades and curved-out, or hooked, blunt bottom blades to fit under, lift, and grasp sutures for snipping.

- Bandage scissors remove bandages; this type has a flattened blunt tip on the bottom longer blade that safely fits under bandages; most common type is the Lister bandage scissors.

Figure 6-6A–C shows various types of scissors.

Scalpels and Blades

A scalpel is a small surgical knife with a straight handle and a straight or curved blade. A reusable steel scalpel handle can hold different blades for different surgical procedures. Straight or pointed blades are used for incision and drainage procedures, while curved blades

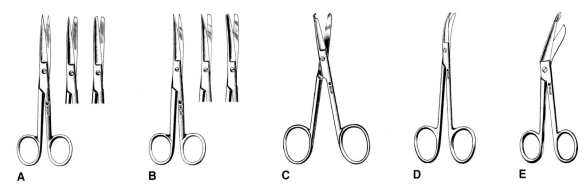

Figure 6-6 Scissors: (**A**) Straight-blade operating scissors. *Left to right:* S/S, S/B, B/B. (**B**) Curved-blade operating scissors. *Left to right:* S/S, S/B, B/B. (**C**) Spencer stitch scissors. (**D**) Suture scissors. (**E**) Lister bandage scissors. S/S, sharp/sharp; S/B, sharp/blunt; B/B, blunt/blunt. (Courtesy of Sklar Instruments, West Chester, PA.)

are used to excise tissue. Reusable handles are used only with disposable blades. Many offices use disposable handles and blades packaged as one sterile unit. Figure 6-7A–C shows various scalpels and blades.

Towel Clamps

Towel clamps are used to maintain the integrity of the sterile field by holding the sterile drapes in place, allowing exposure of the operative site (Fig. 6-8A,B). A sterile field is a specific area that is considered free of all microorganisms.

Probes and Directors

Before entering a cavity or site for a procedure, the physician may first probe the depth and direction of the operative area. A probe shows the angle and depth of the operative area, and a director guides the knife or instrument once the procedure has begun (Fig. 6-9A–C).

Retractors

Retractors hold open layers of tissue, exposing the areas beneath. They may be plain or toothed; the toothed

retractor may be sharp or blunt. Retractors may be designed to be held by an assistant or screwed open to be self-retaining. Figure 6-10A–C shows several types of retractors.

 CHECKPOINT QUESTION

6. What types of instruments are used to remove tissue during a biopsy?

COG Care and Handling of Surgical Instruments

To ensure that surgical instruments always function properly, follow these guidelines:

1. Do not toss or drop instruments into a basin or sink. Surgical instruments are delicate, and the blade or tip is easily damaged by improper handling. Should you drop an instrument accidentally, carefully inspect it for damage. Damaged instruments can usually be repaired and should not be discarded unless repair is not feasible.

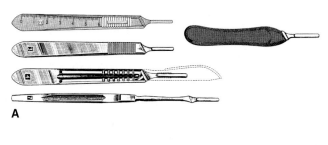

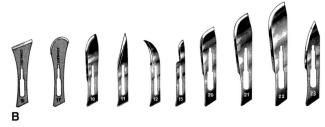

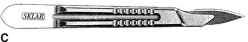

Figure 6-7 Scalpels: (**A**) Scalpel handles. (**B**) Surgical blades. (**C**) Complete sterile disposable scalpel. (Courtesy of Sklar Instruments, West Chester, PA.)

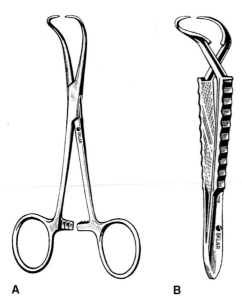

Figure 6-8 Towel clamps: (**A**) Backhaus towel clamp. (**B**) Jones cross-action towel clamp. (Courtesy of Sklar Instruments, West Chester, PA.)

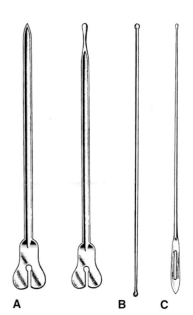

Figure 6-9 Probes: (**A**) Director and tongue tie. (**B**) Double-ended probe. (**C**) Probe with eye. (Courtesy of Sklar Instruments, West Chester, PA.)

2. Avoid stacking instruments in a pile. They may tangle and be damaged when separated.
3. Always store sharp instruments separately to prevent dulling or damaging the sharp edges and to prevent accidental injury. Disposable scalpel blades should be removed from reusable handles and placed in puncture-proof sharps biohazard containers. If a disposable scalpel is used, the whole unit is discarded into the sharps container. Syringes with needles attached and suture needles should also be discarded in a sharps container and never in the trash or with other instruments for processing. Delicate instruments, such as scissors or tissue forceps or those with lenses, are kept separate to be sanitized and sterilized appropriately.
4. Keep ratcheted instruments open when not in use to avoid damage to the ratchet mechanism.

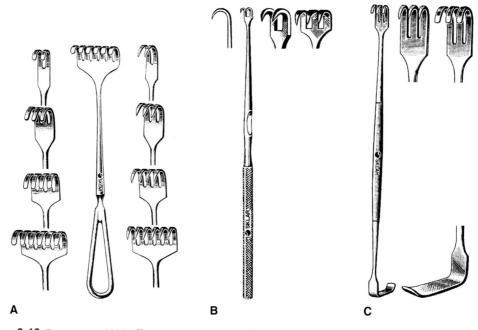

Figure 6-10 Retractors: (**A**) Volkman retractor. (**B**) Lahey retractor. (**C**) Senn retractor. (Courtesy of Sklar Instruments, West Chester, PA.)

5. Rinse gross contamination from instruments as soon as possible to prevent drying and hardening, which makes cleaning more difficult. Always wear gloves and follow OSHA standards to prevent contact with possibly infected blood or body fluids.

6. Check instruments before sterilization to ensure that they are in good working order, and identify instruments in need of repair.

    A. Blades or points should be free of bends and nicks.

    B. Tips should close evenly and tightly.

    C. Instruments with box locks should move freely but should not be too loose.

    D. Instruments with spring handles should have enough tension to grasp objects tightly.

    E. Scissors should close in a smooth, even manner with no nicks or snags. (Scissors may be checked by cutting through gauze or cotton to be sure there are no rough areas).

    F. Screws should be flush with the instrument surface. They should be freely workable but not loose.

7. Use instruments only for the purpose for which they were designed. For instance, never use surgical scissors to cut paper or open packages, because this may damage the cutting edges.

8. Sanitize instruments before they are sterilized so that sterilization will work effectively.

 CHECKPOINT QUESTION

7. What should you do if you drop a surgical instrument accidentally?

COG Storage and Record Keeping

When using and maintaining sterile instruments, equipment, and supplies, staff are responsible for correctly storing these items, keeping accurate records of warranties and maintenance agreements, and keeping reordering information on hand. You should be familiar with the manufacturer's recommendations for each instrument or piece of equipment. Most offices have specific storage or supply areas for keeping sterile and other instruments and equipment. This area should be kept clean and dust free and should be close to the area of need. Clean and sterile supplies and equipment must be separated from soiled items and waste.

Medical assistants are also responsible for keeping accurate records of sterilized items and equipment. Information that must be recorded includes maintenance records and load or sterilization records. These records should include the following:

- Date and time of the sterilization cycle
- General description of the load

- Exposure time and temperature
- Name or initials of the operator
- Results of the sterilization indicator
- Expiration date of the load (usually 30 days)

The maintenance records include service provided by the manufacturer's representative and daily or recommended maintenance to keep the equipment in optimum working condition.

 CHECKPOINT QUESTION

8. What six items should be included on a sterilization record?

COG Maintaining Surgical Supplies

As a clinical medical assistant, you should keep an up-to-date master list of all supplies, including purchases and replacements. Generally, one person is responsible for maintaining inventory, keeping maintenance schedules, and placing orders. If too many staff are involved, these tasks may be overlooked, or efforts may be duplicated. Instruction manuals for all equipment should be kept on file and consulted when ordering supplies for replacement or maintenance. Equipment records for each item should include the following:

- Date of purchase
- Model and serial numbers of the equipment
- Time of recommended service
- Date service was requested
- Name of the person requesting the service
- Reason for the service request
- Description of the service performed and any parts replaced
- Name of the person performing the service and the date the work was completed
- Signature and title of the person who acknowledged completion of the work

Warranties and guarantees should be kept with the equipment records, along with the name of the manufacturer's contact person. A file should be kept to remind the staff of the need for manufacturer service and concurrent or periodic maintenance by the staff.

Parts and supplies for items that are vital to the operation of the facility should always be kept on hand. The shelf life of the item, the storage space available, and the time required to order and receive an item should be considered when deciding what items to keep in inventory. If a piece of equipment cannot function without all of its components or if some of those components have a short life, replacements must be readily available. For example, an ophthalmoscope without a light is virtually useless.

español SPANISH TERMINOLOGY

No toque esta bandeja.
Do not touch this tray.

El doctor estará con usted pronto.
The doctor will be in shortly.

¿Tiene alguna pregunta?
Do you have any questions?

Voy a quitarle el vendaje en estos momentos.
I will take off the bandage now.

¿Está cómodo/cómoda?
Are you comfortable?

MEDIA MENU

- **Student Resources on thePoint**
  - **CMA/RMA Certification Exam Review**
- **Internet Resources**

  Medical Resources New and Reconditioned Equipment: Midmark and Ritter Autoclaves
  http://www.medicalresources.com

  Amsco Autoclaves and Sterilizers: Alfa Medical
  http://www.sterilizers.com

  Sklar Surgical Instruments
  http://www.sklarcorp.com

  Glutaraldehyde Guidelines for Safe Use and Handling in Health Care Facilities
  http://www.nj.gov/health/surv/documents/glutar.pdf

  Occupational Safety and Health Administration
  http://www.osha.gov

PSY **PROCEDURE 6-1:** **Sanitizing Equipment for Disinfection or Sterilization**

Purpose: Properly sanitize instruments in preparation for disinfection or sterilization
Equipment: Instruments or equipment to be sanitized, gloves, eye protection, impervious gown, soap and water, small hand-held scrub brush

Steps	Reasons
1. Put on gloves, gown, and eye protection.	These devices protect against splattering and prevent contamination of your clothes.

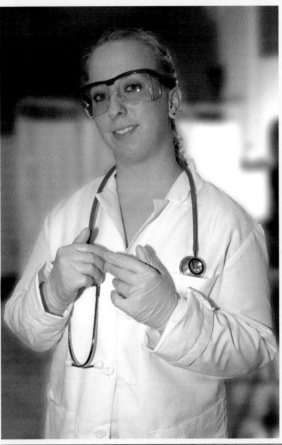

Step 1. Always wear personal protective equipment when a splash may occur.

Steps	Reasons
2. Take any removable sections apart. If cleaning is not possible immediately, soak the instrument or equipment to prevent the parts from sticking together.	
3. Check for operation and integrity of the equipment. Defective equipment should be repaired or discarded appropriately according to office policy.	
4. Rinse the instrument with cool water.	Hot water cooks proteins on, making the contaminants more difficult to remove.
5. After the initial rinse, force streams of soapy water through any tubular or grooved instruments to clean the inside as well as the outside.	
6. Use a hot, soapy solution to dissolve fats or lubricants on the surface. Use the soaking solution indicated by office policy.	

(continued)

PSY PROCEDURE 6-1: **Sanitizing Equipment for Disinfection or Sterilization (continued)**

Steps	Reasons
7. After soaking for 5–10 minutes, use friction with a soft brush or gauze to wipe down the instrument and loosen transient microorganisms. Abrasive materials should not be used on delicate instruments and equipment. Brushes work well on grooves and joints. Open and close the jaws of scissors or forceps several times to ensure that all material has been removed.	These devices protect against splattering and prevent contamination of your clothes.

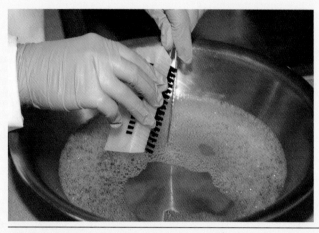

Step 7. Use a brush to loosen microorganisms on instruments.

Steps	Reasons
8. Rinse well.	Proper rinsing removes soap or detergent residue and any remaining microorganisms.
9. Dry well before autoclaving or soaking in disinfectant.	Excess moisture decreases the effectiveness of the autoclave by delaying drying, and it dilutes the disinfectant.
10. Any items (brushes, gauze, solution) used in sanitation are considered grossly contaminated and must be properly disinfected or discarded.	

PSY PROCEDURE 6-2:

Wrapping Instruments for Sterilization in an Autoclave

Purpose: Properly prepare and wrap instruments for sterilization in the autoclave
Equipment: Instruments or equipment to be sterilized, wrapping material, autoclave tape, sterilization indicator, black or blue ink pen

Steps	Reasons
1. Assemble the equipment and supplies. Check the instruments being wrapped for working order.	Any instruments found to be defective, broken, or otherwise needing repair should not be wrapped or autoclaved.
2. Be sure that the wrapping material has these properties: • Permeable to steam but not contaminants • Resists tearing and puncturing during normal handling • Allows for easy opening to prevent contamination of the contents • Maintains sterility of the contents during storage	The wrap may be double layers of cotton muslin, special paper, or appropriately sized instrument pouches.

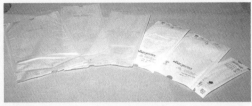

A

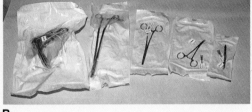

B

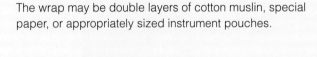

Step 2. (A and B) Autoclave pouches are convenient and come in a variety of sizes.

Steps	Reasons
3. Tear off one or two pieces of autoclave tape. On one piece, indicate in ink the contents of the pack or the name of the instrument that will be wrapped, the date, and your initials.	After the item is wrapped, the contents cannot be seen. Also, dating the package allows the user to determine the quality of the contents based on the amount of time (usually 30 days) that sterilized contents are considered sterile.
4. When using autoclave wrapping material made of cotton muslin or special paper, begin by laying the material diagonally on a flat, clean, dry surface. Place the instrument in the center of the wrapping material with the ratchets or handles open. Include a sterilization indicator.	The ratchets should be left open during autoclaving to allow steam to penetrate and sterilize all surfaces.

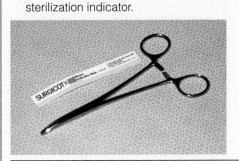

Step 4. The ratchets are open.

(continued)

PSY PROCEDURE 6-2: **Wrapping Instruments for Sterilization in an Autoclave (continued)**

Steps	Reasons
5. Fold the first flap at the bottom of the diagonal wrap up and fold back the corner, making a tab.	Making a tab allows for easier opening of the pack without contaminating the contents.

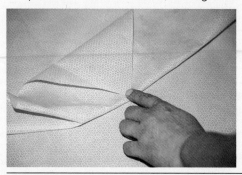

Step 5. Make a tab with the corner.

Steps	Reasons
6. Fold the left corner of the wrap and then the right corner, each making a tab for opening the package. Secure the package with autoclave tape.	If the package is not secured with autoclave tape, the contents could become contaminated.

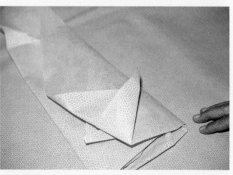

Step 6. The bottom, left, and right corners of the wrap are folded.

Steps	Reasons
7. Fold the top corner down, making the tab tucked under the material.	Tucking the tab prevents the material from coming loose and contaminating the contents.

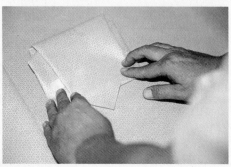

A

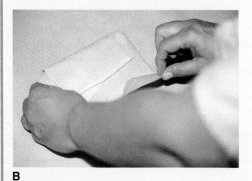

B

Step 7. **(A)** The top corner is folded down. **(B)** Secure the wrapped instrument package with autoclave tape.

PSY PROCEDURE 6-3:   Operating an Autoclave

Purpose: Safely sterilize instruments or equipment using an autoclave
Equipment: Sanitized and wrapped instruments or equipment, distilled water, autoclave operating manual

Steps	Reasons
1. Assemble the equipment, including the wrapped articles with a sterilization indicator in each package according to office policy.	Some offices want a separately wrapped indicator autoclaved with the load for checking that the procedure was performed properly without opening a pack.

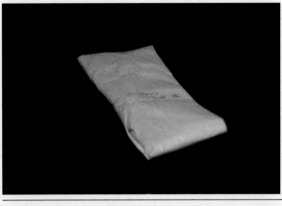

Step 1. Properly wrapped items.

Steps	Reasons
2. Check the water level of the autoclave reservoir and add more if needed.	Use only distilled water in the reservoir tank.
3. Add water to the internal chamber of the autoclave to the fill line.	The ratchets should be left open during autoclaving to allow steam to penetrate and sterilize all surfaces.
4. Load the autoclave: A. Place trays and packs on their sides 1–3 inches apart. B. Put containers on their side with the lid off. C. In mixed loads, place hard objects on the bottom shelf and softer packs on the top racks.	Air circulation is not possible if items are tightly packed. Vertical placement forces out heavier air rather than pooling in the containers. Air can circulate in containers on their side with the lid off. Hard objects may form condensation that will drip onto softer items and wet them.
5. Read the instructions and close the machine. Most machines follow the same protocol: A. Close the door and secure or lock it. B. Turn the machine on. C. When the temperature gauge reaches the point required for the contents of the load (usually 250°F), set the timer. Many autoclaves can be programmed for the required time. D. When the timer indicates that the cycle is over, vent the chamber. E. After releasing the pressure to a safe level, crack the door of the autoclave to allow additional drying. Most loads dry in 5–20 minutes. Hard items dry faster than soft ones.	You should be familiar with the autoclave and how to operate it safely.
6. When the load has cooled, remove the items.	When the load is finished, the contents will be hot to touch.
7. Check the separately wrapped sterilization indicator, if used, for proper sterilization.	If the indicator registers that the load was properly processed, the items in the additional packs are considered sterile; if not, the items should be considered not sterile, and the load must be reprocessed.

(continued)

PSY PROCEDURE 6-3: **Operating an Autoclave** *(continued)*

Steps	Reasons
8. Store the items in a clean, dry, dust-free area for 30 days.	After 30 days, reprocessing is necessary. The pack need not be rewrapped, but the autoclave tape should be replaced with new tape with the current date.
9. Clean the autoclave per manufacturer's suggestions, usually by scrubbing the interior chamber with a mild detergent and a soft brush. Attention to the exhaust valve will prevent lint from occluding the outlet. Rinse the machine thoroughly and allow it to dry.	Always follow the manufacturer's recommendations for cleaning the autoclave.

- Most areas of the medical office require medical asepsis to maintain cleanliness and prevent the spread of infection to the patients and staff.
- When body tissues need repair or must be opened surgically, sterile technique or surgical asepsis is required.
- You are responsible for maintaining surgical asepsis, which necessitates that you understand the principles and practices of medical and surgical asepsis.

- You will need to know disinfection and sterilization techniques commonly used in the medical office including the equipment used to sterilize and disinfect items.
- It will be your responsibility to keep accurate records and adequate supplies on hand.
- In addition, your responsibilities include being familiar with instruments used in office surgical procedures, which is the content of the next chapter.

Warm Ups   for Critical Thinking

1. As the clinical medical assistant at Dr. Will's office, you have been asked to orient new employees to various aspects of the practice and develop an orientation booklet for all staff members. Design a booklet that contains the following information:
   - A basic explanation of the surgical equipment commonly used in the practice
   - The procedures for sanitizing, disinfecting, and sterilizing instruments
   - The operating instructions for the autoclave
2. Create a record that can be used to document sterilization using the autoclave.
3. Research the various types of commercial cold chemical sterilization solutions. Design a step-by-step procedure for using the solution to disinfect and sterilize. Note any hazards or safety precautions that should be followed when working with the chemical.

4. The physician is scheduled to perform a minor office surgical procedure this afternoon, and you realize the instrument she needs for the procedure is broken. How would you handle this situation? What can you do to prevent this situation in the future?
5. When checking the biologic sterilization indicator as required to be done weekly by your office policy, you discover that the autoclave has not been reaching the appropriate temperature sufficient to kill all microorganisms and their spores. The logbook indicated that the check last week found the autoclave to be in good working order. Can you be sure that all items autoclaved this past week are sterilized? What would you do?

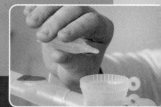

Assisting with Minor Office Surgery

Learning Outcomes

Cognitive Domain

Note: AAMA/CAAHEP 2008 Standards are italicized.

1. Spell and define key terms
2. List your responsibilities before, during, and after minor office surgery
3. Identify the guidelines for preparing and maintaining sterility of the field and surgical equipment during a minor office procedure
4. State your responsibility in relation to informed consent and patient preparation
5. Explain the purpose of local anesthetics and list three commonly used in the medical office
6. Describe the types of needles and sutures and the uses of each
7. Describe the various methods of skin closure used in the medical office
8. Explain your responsibility during surgical specimen collection
9. List the types of laser surgery and electrosurgery used in the medical office and explain the precautions for each
10. Describe the guidelines for applying a sterile dressing

11. *Describe implications for treatment related to pathology*

Psychomotor Domain

Note: AAMA/CAAHEP 2008 Standards are italicized.

1. *Practice standard precautions*
2. Open sterile surgical packs (Procedure 7-1)
3. Use sterile transfer forceps (Procedure 7-2)
4. Add sterile solution to a sterile field (Procedure 7-3)
5. *Prepare a patient for procedures and/or treatments*
6. *Document accurately in the patient record*
7. Perform skin preparation and hair removal (Procedure 7-4)
8. Apply sterile gloves (Procedure 7-5)
9. Apply a sterile dressing (Procedure 7-6)
10. Change an existing sterile dressing (Procedure 7-7)
11. *Assist physician with patient care*
12. Assist with excisional surgery (Procedure 7-8)
13. Assist with incision and drainage (Procedure 7-9)

14. Remove sutures (Procedure 7-10)
15. Remove staples (Procedure 7-11)

Affective Domain

Note: AAMA/CAAHEP 2008 Standards are italicized.

1. *Apply ethical behaviors, including honesty and integrity in performance of medical assisting practice*
2. *Apply critical thinking skills in performing patient assessment and care*
3. *Demonstrate empathy in communicating with patients, family, and staff*
4. *Apply active listening skills*
5. *Use appropriate body language and other nonverbal skills in communicating with patients, family, and staff*
6. *Demonstrate awareness of the territorial boundaries of the person with whom you are communicating*
7. *Demonstrate sensitivity appropriate to the message being delivered*
8. *Demonstrate recognition of the patient's level of understanding in communications*
9. *Recognize and protect personal boundaries in communicating with others*
10. *Demonstrate respect for individual diversity, incorporating awareness of one's own biases in areas including gender, race, religion, age, and economic status*

ABHES Competencies

1. Prepare patients for examinations and treatments
2. Assist physician with minor office surgical procedures
3. Dispose of biohazardous materials
4. Use standard precautions
5. Document accurately

Key Terms

approximate	coagulate	electrode	preservative
atraumatic	cryosurgery	fulguration	purulent
bandage	dehiscence	keratosis	swaged needle
cautery	dressing	lentigines	traumatic

As a clinical medical assistant, you will have many responsibilities when minor surgery is performed in the physician's office. These include the following:

1. Reinforcing the physician's instructions to the patient regarding preparation for surgery, including at-home skin preparation as directed, fasting from food or fluids, bowel preparation, and other preparations that may be ordered.
2. Identifying the patient and gathering the proper equipment and supplies before the physician is ready to do the procedure.
3. Obtaining and witnessing the informed consent document if instructed to do so by the physician.
4. Preparing the treatment room, instruments, supplies, and equipment.
5. Assisting the physician during the procedure.
6. Applying a **dressing** and **bandage** to the surgical wound.
7. Instructing the patient about postoperative wound care, including observing the wound for changes that indicate infection or problems with healing.
8. Assisting the patient as needed before, during, and after the procedure.
9. Assisting with postoperative instructions such as prescriptions, medications, and scheduling return visits.
10. Removing and caring for instruments, equipment, and supplies, including properly disposing of disposable items, sharps, and contaminated or unused supplies.
11. Preparing the room for the next patient.

Although the types of surgery performed in the medical office vary with the type of medical specialty, the procedure for preparing the patient and setting up the supplies and equipment will require the same process, known as sterile technique. Procedures performed in many general practice offices include suture insertion and removal, incision and drainage, and sebaceous cystectomy. Some gynecologic procedures and urinary procedures also require sterile technique.

COG Preparing and Maintaining a Sterile Field

Minor office surgery involves procedures that penetrate the body's normally intact surface. Whenever a patient has an open wound, surgical asepsis must be maintained to prevent pathogens from entering the body tissues and causing an infection. Follow the following guidelines to maintain sterility before and during a sterile procedure:

1. Do not let sterile packages get damp or wet. Microorganisms can be drawn into the package by wicking, or absorption of the liquid along with the pathogens in it. If a package sterilized in the medical office gets moist, it must be repackaged in a clean, dry wrapper and sterilized again. Damp or wet disposable packages must be discarded.
2. Always face a sterile field to ensure that the area has not been contaminated. If you must leave the area or work with your back to the sterile field, the field must be covered with a sterile drape using sterile technique.
3. Hold all sterile items above waist level. When sterile items are not in your field of vision, you must presume that they have become contaminated.
4. Place sterile items in the middle of the sterile field. A 1-inch border around the field is considered contaminated.
5. Do not spill any liquids, even sterile liquids, onto the sterile field. Remember, the surface below the field is not sterile, and moisture will allow microorganisms to be wicked up into the surgical field.
6. Do not cough, sneeze, or talk over the sterile field. Microorganisms from the respiratory tract can contaminate the field.
7. Never reach over the sterile field. Dust or lint from clothing can contaminate the sterile field.
8. Do not pass soiled supplies, such as gauze or instruments, over the sterile field.
9. If you know or suspect that the sterile field has been contaminated, alert the physician. Sterility must be re-established before the procedure can continue.

Sterile Surgical Packs

Preparing the treatment or examination room for a surgical procedure is usually the responsibility of the medical assistant. Many medical offices keep a box with index cards or a loose-leaf binder listing the surgical procedures that are commonly performed in the office, including the items needed for setup. Some medical

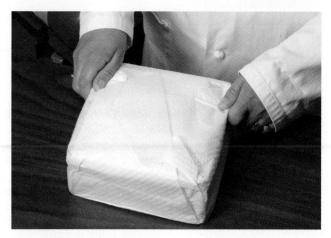

Figure 7-1 A wrapped sterile surgical package.

offices prepackage sterile setups in a suitable wrapper and prepare them in the office by autoclave sterilization (Fig. 7-1). These setups are labeled according to the type of procedure (e.g., lesion removal, suture setup) and contain the general instruments for that procedure. Some basic supplies (e.g., gauze sponges, cotton balls, and towels) may also be included before autoclaving.

To reduce the time and effort of sterilizing packs on site, many offices use commercially packaged disposable surgical packs. Disposable surgical packs have become increasingly popular because they are convenient and come with an almost infinite variety of contents. They may contain one sterile article (such as a 4 × 4 sterile dressing) or a complete sterile surgical setup. Many of the supplies are packaged in peel-apart wrappers with two loose flaps that can be pulled apart, and the sterile items can be dropped carefully onto the operative field. The insides of the wrappers may be opened out and used as a sterile field. Some packages are enclosed in plastic and wrapped inside a barrier material that can be used as a sterile field.

Directions for opening are clearly marked on the outside of sterile packs and should be read carefully before opening. If the surgical pack is opened improperly, the contents will be contaminated and cannot be used. Commercially prepared sterile packs are generally more expensive than packages prepared at the medical office, so care must be taken to avoid waste. Labels on commercially prepared packs list the contents in the pack item by item; site-prepared packs usually only state the type of setup. You should check the expiration date on the package; if the pack has expired, it must not be used because sterility is in question. Procedure 7-1 describes the steps for opening sterile surgical packs.

As discussed in Chapter 6, a sterilization indicator should be put inside each surgical package to show that it has been properly sterilized. Tapes, strips, and packaging with indicator stripes or dots on the outside of the packs do not guarantee sterility. In the autoclave, sterility is achieved only by the right combination of temperature, pressure, steam, and time. In addition, improperly packing the autoclave can impede steam penetration to the articles. Therefore, sterilization indicators should be packaged within each pack and must be checked before beginning the surgical procedure. When you open a package of sterile objects, the procedure is the same whether the items are sterilized at the office or commercially prepared. For all sterile packs or supplies, keep the following in mind:

1. Clean hands are used to open the sterile items or packages. The unsterile area is the outside surface of the outside wrapper.
2. The sterile area includes the inside surface of the outside wrapper, the inside wrapper if any, and the contents of the package. These areas or items must not come into contact with any surface, including the hands, or they are considered contaminated and must be replaced.
3. Items are considered contaminated and should be repackaged and sterilized again:
   A. When moisture is present on the pack
   B. If the items are dropped outside the sterile field
   C. If the date on the outside of the package is beyond 30 days for site-prepared packages or it is past the posted expiration date on commercially prepared packages
   D. If the sterilization indicator inside the pack has not changed color
   E. If the wrapper is torn, damaged, or wet
   F. When any area is known or thought to have been touched by a contaminated item

 CHECKPOINT QUESTION

1. What are the nine guidelines that must be followed to maintain a sterile field?

Sterile Transfer Forceps

Setting up the sterile field requires clean hands and careful technique to avoid contaminating the contents inside the sterile area or field. In the event that sterile items must be manipulated or placed on the sterile field, sterile transfer forceps or sterile gloved hands must be used, since the hands can never be sterilized. The tips of the forceps and the articles being transferred must both remain sterile (Fig. 7-2). The handles, however, are considered medically aseptic, not sterile, because these are touched by the bare hands of the person using them. Sterile transfer forceps are stored in a dry sterile container, in a wrapped sterile package, or in a sterile solution in a closed container system, such as the Bard Parker, which helps protect the tips of the forceps from contamination. In a closed dry container system, the forceps and

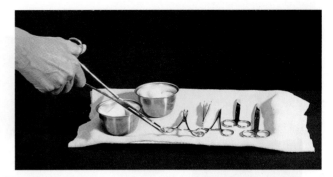

Figure 7-2 Sterile transfer forceps may be used to add or move items on the sterile field.

container must be sanitized and autoclaved daily. In a closed sterile solution system, the forceps and the container are sterilized at least every day, and fresh sterilization solution is added daily. Only one forceps should be stored in a container to decrease the chance of contamination. After using the sterile transfer forceps without contaminating, place the forceps back in the container for use throughout the procedure or in other procedures scheduled that day. Follow office policy for sterilizing the forceps. Proper use of sterile transfer forceps requires that certain guidelines be followed (Procedure 7-2).

Adding Peel-Back Packages and Pouring Sterile Solutions

Procedure packages are frequently prepared with supplies (e.g., cotton balls and gauze squares) to eliminate the need to add more at the time of setup. However, patient assessment at the time of surgery may suggest the need for additional items. These small supplies are usually provided commercially in peel-apart packages. These packages may contain small or single items to be added to the surgical field. The package has an upper edge with two flaps that are used to open the package in a manner that maintains the sterility of the contents. To properly open a package, use both hands with the thumbs just inside the tops of the edges. Separate the flaps using a slow, outward motion of the thumbs and flaps (Fig. 7-3A,B). Keep in mind that the inside of the sealed package and the contents are sterile but will be contaminated if touched by anything that is not sterile, such as your fingers, or if talking, coughing, or sneezing occurs as you open the package. There are three ways to add the contents of peel-back packages to the sterile field:

1. *Sterile transfer forceps.* Peel the edges apart with a rolling motion as described earlier. Holding down the two edges, lift the contents up and away with the forceps (Fig. 7-4).
2. *Sterile gloved hand.* This method requires two persons, usually the medical assistant, who opens the package, and the physician, who removes the contents with a

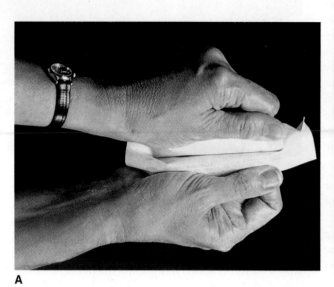

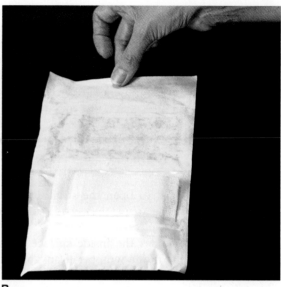

A

B

Figure 7-3 (**A**) Open sterile packets by grasping the edges and rolling the thumbs outward. (**B**) Opening the packet properly forms a sterile field.

sterile gloved hand. You must carefully hold the edges to avoid contaminating the physician's gloves (Fig. 7-5).

3. *Flip of the contents onto a sterile field.* To do this, you step back from the sterile field to prevent your hands and the outer wrapper, which is not sterile, from crossing it. Pull the edges down and away from the package contents and carefully toss or flip the item onto the middle of the sterile field without touching the 1-inch border around the sterile field. This 1-inch area is considered not sterile.

In most cases, items in presterilized peel-back envelopes cannot be sterilized after being opened and must be discarded even if not used. Because such items are relatively expensive, they should not be opened unnecessarily. A supply of items that might be needed during the procedure should be placed conveniently close to the area and added only if needed.

Whether site prepared or commercially prepared, trays are not processed or stored with liquids in open containers. Solutions must be added as needed at the time of setup. Some procedures require sterile water or saline, while others require an antiseptic solution, such as Betadine. These will be poured into sterile containers added to the sterile field with sterile transfer forceps (Procedure 7-3).

 CHECKPOINT QUESTION

2. What are three ways that contents of peel-back packages can be added to the sterile field?

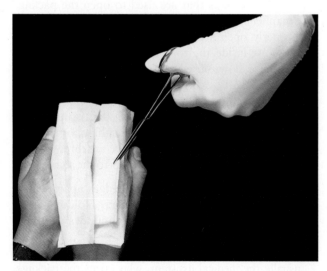

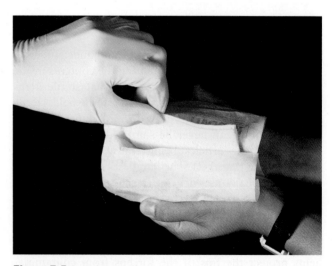

Figure 7-4 The physician may use sterile forceps to remove small supplies from peel-back packages.

Figure 7-5 Sterile gloved hands may be used to remove sterile items.

COG **Preparing the Patient for Minor Office Surgery**

Patient Instructions and Consent

Many of the minor surgical procedures that are performed in the medical office require a full explanation of the procedure and informed consent (Fig. 7-6). Either the patient agrees and the procedure is performed or the patient refuses and the procedure is not done. The informed consent document must state the procedure and its purpose and expected results along with possible side effects, risks, and complications. Although the physician is responsible for informing the patient of the details of the procedure and any risks involved, the patient may ask questions, including how long the procedure will last,

what preparations will be needed, or whether fasting will be necessary. You may answer these questions after verifying the information with the physician.

It is always a good practice to give specific written instructions to the patient for any preparations to be made before arriving at the office so that the procedure can be done on schedule and with no preventable risk to the patient. The physician may prescribe medication for the patient to take at home before the procedure. As with any patient instructions, you should notify the physician if the patient seems confused or does not understand the instructions. Encourage the patient to call the office if questions arise later. Of course, the instructions should be documented in the medical record.

SPECIAL CONSENT TO OPERATION OR OTHER PROCEDURE(S)

PATIENT _____   PATIENT NUMBER _____

DATE _____   TIME _____

1. I HEREBY AUTHORIZE DOCTOR _____ AND/OR SUCH ASSISTANTS AS MAY BE SELECTED BY HIM, TO PERFORM THE FOLLOWING PROCEDURE(S):

   _____

   ON _____
      (NAME OF PATIENT OR MYSELF)

2. THE PROCEDURE(S) LISTED ABOVE HAVE BEEN EXPLAINED TO ME BY DR. _____
   AND I UNDERSTAND THE NATURE AND THE CONSEQUENCES OF THE PROCEDURE(S).

3. I RECOGNIZE THAT, DURING THE COURSE OF THE OPERATION, UNFORESEEN CONDITIONS MAY NECESSITATE ADDITIONAL OR DIFFERENT PROCEDURES THAN THOSE SET FORTH. I FURTHER AUTHORIZE AND REQUEST THAT THE ABOVE NAMED SURGEON, HIS ASSISTANTS, OR HIS DESIGNEES PERFORM SUCH PROCEDURES AS ARE IN HIS PROFESSIONAL JUDGMENT NECESSARY AND DESIRABLE, INCLUDING, BUT NOT LIMITED TO, PROCEDURES INVOLVING PATHOLOGY AND RADIOLOGY. THE AUTHORITY GRANTED UNDER THIS PARAGRAPH SHALL EXTEND TO REMEDYING CONDITIONS NOT KNOWN TO DR. _____ AT THE TIME THE OPERATION IS COMMENCED.

4. I AM AWARE THAT THE PRACTICE OF MEDICINE AND SURGERY IS NOT AN EXACT SCIENCE AND I ACKNOWLEDGE THAT NO GUARANTEES HAVE BEEN MADE TO ME AS TO THE RESULTS OF THE OPERATION OR PROCEDURE.

5. TISSUE REMOVED DURING SURGERY SHALL BE SENT TO PATHOLOGY TO BE EXAMINED AND DISPOSED OF IN ACCORDANCE WITH THE RULES AND REGULATIONS OF THE MEDICAL STAFF OF THE SURGERY CENTER.

_____   _____
Procedure has been discussed with patient. (Surgeon's Signature)   SIGNATURE OF PATIENT

PATIENT IS UNABLE TO SIGN BECAUSE   ☐ HE (SHE) IS A MINOR _____ YEARS OF AGE

    ☐ OTHER (SPECIFY) _____

_____   _____
WITNESS   PERSON AUTHORIZED TO SIGN FOR PATIENT

    _____
    RELATIONSHIP OF ABOVE TO PATIENT

Figure 7-6 Sample consent form.

Positioning and Draping

Before positioning the patient for a minor surgical procedure, ask the patient to void; this helps prevent discomfort during the procedure. Offer to help the patient remove whatever clothing is necessary to expose the operative site. Expose only the area necessary for the procedure to ensure the patient's privacy. An air-conditioned office may be uncomfortably cool for patients. You may provide additional sheets or a blanket for comfort.

Assist the patient to assume a comfortable position on the examining table that offers exposure of and access to the operative site. Provide pillows for comfort and support. Do not make the patient maintain an uncomfortable position, such as the lithotomy or knee-chest, while waiting for the physician. Position the patient only when the physician is ready to begin the procedure. At the end of the procedure, assist the patient from the table, allowing as much time as needed. Often patients who did not need help removing clothing will require help dressing following minor office surgery. Be aware of this and assist as necessary.

The type of procedure and the patient's position determine the type of drapes used to expose the operative site and cover the patient. Disposable paper drapes are most commonly used in the medical office. They come in many sizes and shapes, each suited for specific uses. Paper drapes can be used alone, in combination, or with separate drape sheets and towels. Fenestrated drapes have an opening to expose the operative site while covering adjacent areas. Fenestrated drapes may be small, such as those used for suture insertion, or large, such as those used to cover the legs and lower abdomen but expose the perineal area. Some sterile drapes are combined with adhesive-backed clear plastic, which sticks to the patient's skin and eliminates the need for towel clamps. Sterile drapes are applied by picking

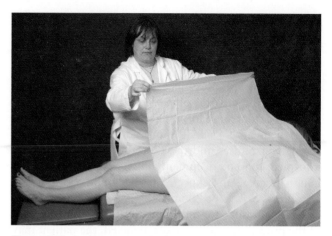

Figure 7-7 Applying a sterile drape.

up the drape on the 1-inch border (no gloves needed), lifting over the surgical area without contaminating the drape, and laying the drape on the patient from farthest away to closest (Fig. 7-7). This ensures that you do not reach over the drape after it is placed on the patient.

When removing contaminated drapes from the patient following a procedure, put on clean examination gloves and carefully roll the items away from the body, keeping the contaminated areas innermost (Fig. 7-8). This helps to surround the dirtier areas of the sheet with the cleaner area and helps prevent contaminating your clothing. Because the sheets, towels, or drapes may be contaminated with blood or other body fluids, follow standard precautions (see Chapter 2).

Preparing the Patient's Skin

The goal of preoperative skin preparation is to remove as many microorganisms as possible from the skin to decrease the chance of wound contamination. Skin preparation may be simply applying an antiseptic solution to the area or may include removing gross contaminants and hair from the operative area. Hair can be removed with depilatory creams but often requires shaving the skin (Procedure 7-4).

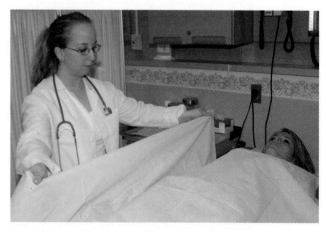

Figure 7-8 Removing a contaminated drape.

CHECKPOINT QUESTION

3. What is a fenestrated drape?

COG Assisting the Physician

Local Anesthetics

When office surgery of any kind is performed, the site is first anesthetized (numbed) with a local anesthetic to minimize the pain and discomfort felt by the patient. Occasionally, when a wound contains embedded debris that must be removed prior to repair, the local anesthetic will be injected before preparing the wound site to facilitate wound cleaning. Lidocaine and lidocaine with epinephrine (0.5%–2%) are two of the many local anesthetics commonly used in medical offices. Others are mepivacaine (Carbocaine™) and bupivacaine (Marcaine™). Epinephrine is added to local anesthetics to cause vasoconstriction and to slow absorption by the body and lengthen the anesthetic's effectiveness. It may be used when the physician anticipates a long procedure, but anesthesia with epinephrine should never be used on the tips of the fingers, toes, nose, or penis, since the vasoconstriction may cause death of tissue in these distal areas.

One of two methods may be used to administer local anesthesia. In one method, you draw the anesthetic for the physician into a syringe, keeping the vial beside the syringe for the physician's approval. In this case, the anesthetic is usually given to the patient before the physician puts on sterile gloves because the outside of the syringe and needle unit are not sterile.

The second method is used if the physician puts on sterile gloves before administering the anesthetic. In this case, a sterile syringe and needle are included on the sterile field setup. When the physician is ready to administer the anesthetic, you show the physician the label on the vial, clean the rubber stopper of the vial with an alcohol swab, and hold the vial while the physician draws the required amount into the syringe. There are many methods of holding the vial securely while the physician withdraws the medication; however, the most common way is for you to hold the vial with one hand while supporting your wrist with the other hand (Fig. 7-9). You and the physician together develop a method to maintain surgical asepsis.

Wound Closure

Many types of wounds require closure to ensure rapid healing with minimal scarring. This is accomplished by bringing the edges of the wound as close together as possible in their original position (approximation). Sutures are used to close wounds and incisions and to bring tissue layers into close approximation. Skin closures are performed after cyst or tissue sample removal, to close lacerations, or any time skin surfaces require assistance for healing. Supplies used to suture skin include needles and suture material. Skin staples are sometimes used to

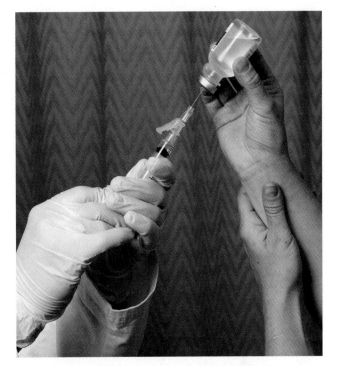
Figure 7-9 Hold the vial containing the anesthetic downward, supporting that wrist with the other hand.

close large incisions over areas where **dehiscence** can occur, such as the knee, hip, or abdomen, but these are not usually inserted in the medical office.

Needles and Sutures

Needles used in minor office surgery are chosen for the type of surgery to be performed. Needles are classified as follows:

- By shape: curved or straight
- By point: tapered or cutting
- By eye: **atraumatic** (swaged) or **traumatic** (with an eye)

Round straight needles are called *domestic needles*, and straight cutting needles are called *Keith needles*. Curved needles used in surgical procedures are usually clamped in a needle holder before being handed to or used by the physician. Straight needles are not clamped in a needle holder but are handed to the physician with the point up. Straight needles are rarely used in medical offices.

Cutting needles are used on tough tissues, such as skin. Round or tapered (noncutting) needles are used on subcutaneous tissue, peritoneum, and muscle. Atraumatic needles, or **swaged needles**, have suture material that has been mechanically attached to the needle by the manufacturer and do not require threading. These are called atraumatic because they cause less trauma than threaded needles as they pass through the tissues. Unlike atraumatic or swaged needles, threaded needles have an eye with a double thickness of suture that must be pulled through tissues. The double thickness of this suture makes a larger and therefore more traumatic opening in the tissues than a swaged suture.

In medical offices, curved swaged needles are used far more often than any other type. Swaged needles are selected for a procedure according to the size and length of the suture material and the attached needle gauge clearly marked on the packaging material. When a suture must be threaded through an eyed needle, both needle gauge and suture size must be selected. The physician usually selects the suture and needle, but you should know your physician's preferences and anticipate needs whenever possible. Sutures, needles, and suture–needle combinations are contained in peel-apart packages that are sterile on the inside so that they can be added to the sterile field (Fig. 7-10). This may be done by sterile transfer forceps, by a sterile gloved hand, or by carefully flipping them onto the sterile field.

Sutures come in various gauges (diameters) and lengths. Very thick sutures are numbered 1 to 5, with 5 being the thickest. Sutures smaller than size 1 are expressed with added zeros. Small sutures, which become progressively smaller, range from 1-0 to 10-0 or smaller (i.e., 1-0, 2-0, 3-0, and so forth). A very fine 10-0 suture, which is about the diameter of a human hair, is generally used in microsurgery. When a fine suture is needed, such as on the face and neck, 23-0 and 24-0 sutures are commonly used. A very fine suture decreases scarring and gives a better cosmetic result.

Sutures also come in absorbable and nonabsorbable forms. Absorbable sutures, or catgut (made from the intestines of sheep or cattle), are readily broken down in the body and usually do not have to be removed. The two forms of absorbable gut suture are chromic, which is chemically treated to delay absorption for several days, and plain, which is not treated and is more quickly absorbed. Absorbable sutures are used most frequently in hospitals during surgery on deep tissues.

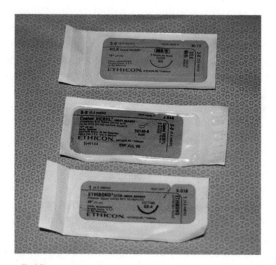

Figure 7-10 Suture material and needles are supplied in see-through packages with the size of the suture material and the type of needle listed on the packet. The inside of the packet is sterile.

Nonabsorbable sutures are available in a great variety of brands, sizes, lengths, and swaged needles; they are the most versatile. Nonabsorbable sutures either remain in the body permanently or are removed after healing. Nonabsorbable sutures are used on the skin, intestines, or bone; to ligate larger vessels; and to attach heart valves and various artificial and natural grafts. Nonabsorbable sutures are made of fibers such as silk, nylon, Dacron, or cotton or stainless steel wire.

Skin Staples

Another form of nonabsorbable suture is the metal skin clip or staple. These are commonly made of stainless steel, but some very specialized types are made of sterling silver for use in neurosurgery and other procedures. When nonabsorbable sutures or staples are used to close skin wounds, they must be removed when the wound has healed completely. Depending on the location of the skin wound, nonabsorbable sutures or staples remain in place for varying lengths of time; the head and neck may require 3 to 5 days due to increased blood supply to these areas. Sutures in the arms and legs may require 7 to 10 days.

 CHECKPOINT QUESTION

4. How do swaged needles differ from threaded ones?

Adhesive Skin Closures

Adhesive skin closures are used to **approximate** the edges of a small wound if sutures are not needed. They are appropriate where there is little tension on the skin edges. The strips are placed transversely across the line of the wound to bring the wound edges in close approximation (Fig. 7-11A,B). In most instances, the strips are left in place until they fall off. However, in some cases, the physician may want them removed or replaced if soiled with drainage. When removing these strips, carefully lift the edges distal to the wound and pull gently toward the wound. Never pull the strips away from the wound because tension on the wound site may disrupt the healing process.

Specimen Collection

Many minor office surgical procedures yield specimens that must be sent to a laboratory to be examined by a pathologist. Specimens include samples of tissue, wound exudate, foreign bodies, and so on. The medical assistant must choose the proper container with the appropriate **preservative** (substance that delays decomposition) for the type of procedure being performed. The laboratory where the specimen is sent usually provides the appropriate containers with preservative, and you should have a stock of them on hand. Hold the open container steady to avoid touching the sides as the physician drops the specimen into the preservative (Fig. 7-12).

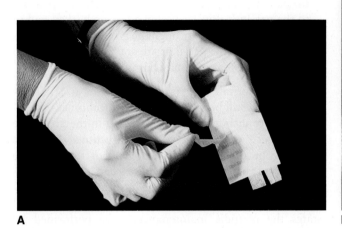

A

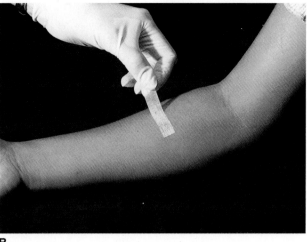

B

Figure 7-11 Adhesive skin closures. (**A**) These lightweight lengths of porous tape are used for closing small wounds. (**B**) Strips are placed transversely across a wound.

You are responsible for attaching a label to the specimen container with the patient's name and the date written clearly on the label, and you must complete a laboratory request form to send with the specimen. These forms require information such as the patient's name, age, sex, and identification number or social security number; date; type of specimen; type of examination; and the physician's name or laboratory contract number. Specimens obtained during a minor surgical procedure must be transported to the pathology laboratory as quickly as possible.

Electrosurgery

Electrosurgery uses high-frequency alternating electric current to destroy or cut and remove tissue. It is used to **coagulate**, or clot, small bleeding vessels. Electrosurgery is considered an alternative to traditional office surgery and is rapidly gaining favor for many procedures. An advantage of electrical surgery is the **cautery** produced by the electricity that seals small bleeding vessels and coagulates nearby cells to reduce bleeding and loss of cell fluid. Electrosurgical units use disposable **electrodes** with tips of various sizes and shapes to deliver the desired amount of electric current to the tissues (Fig. 7-13). The following procedures are considered electrosurgery:

- *Fulguration* destroys tissue with controlled electric sparks. As the physician holds the electrode tip 1 to 2 mm from the site, a series of sparks destroys the superficial cells at the site.

![TRIAGE]

The physician has just performed a needle biopsy for a lesion on Mr. Smith's lower back. You have to do the following three tasks:

A. Label the specimen and complete the laboratory requisition form.
B. Apply a dressing to Mr. Smith's lower back.
C. Help Mr. Smith get dressed and into a wheelchair.

How do you sort these tasks? What do you do first? Second? Third?

The correct order is A, B, C. All specimens must be immediately labeled. Incorrectly labeled specimens or poorly completed requisition forms may result in the laboratory not being able to test the specimen. It is appropriate to apply a dressing to the wound and then assist the patient to get dressed and into a wheelchair.

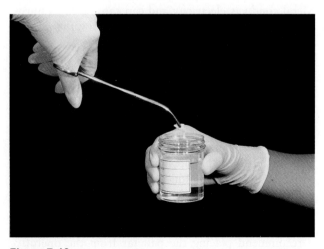

Figure 7-12 • Tissue samples are placed in the preservative by the physician.

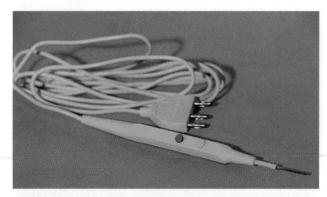

Figure 7-13 A disposable electrosurgical unit. The blade is designed either to cut or to cauterize.

- *Electrodesiccation* dries and separates tissue with an electric current. The electrode is placed directly on the site.
- *Electrocautery* causes quick coagulation of small blood vessels with the heat created by the electric current. Electrocautery is commonly referred to as electrocoagulation.
- *Electrosection* is used for incision or excision of tissue. Bleeding is minimal with this type of procedure, but more damage can occur to surrounding tissues.

Medical offices frequently use electrosurgery to remove moles, cysts, warts, and certain types of skin and cervical cancers. Electrosurgical equipment includes various electrode tips, such as blades, needles, loops, and balls, each with specific uses.

During electrosurgery, your responsibilities are to ensure the safety and comfort of the patient and to pass the electrode to the physician as needed. As with all instruments, the electrode must be passed in its functional position. The electrode is handed to the physician with the tip down.

Because electric current is delivered to the tip by the electrosurgical machine, great care should be exercised to prevent injuries. Although the physician activates the device, it is possible to cause injury to the patient, physician, or yourself by careless handling of the device. Take care to ground the patient before electrosurgery. Metal conducts electricity and can cause serious burns. When assisting with electrosurgery, follow these safety measures:

- Ensure that all working parts are in good repair. The electrical current is carefully regulated; if the machine is defective, serious injury to the patient may occur.
- Ensure that all metal is removed from the patient. The patient must be asked about any metal implants or a cardiac pacemaker. Metal conducts electricity and can cause burns. Metal implants may become very hot, and pacemakers may malfunction during the procedure.
- Ensure that the patient is grounded with a pad supplied by the manufacturer. Attach it to the patient at a site recommended by the manufacturer (some recommend placing the pad far from the operative site; others suggest placing it near the site). Improper placement can result in injury.

- Place the grounding pad firmly and completely against the patient's skin. Apply a conducting gel to the pad and to the patient's skin, or use an adhesive-backed pad to facilitate conduction through the grounding pad. Areas of skin against the pad that are not well connected will result in hot spots and may burn the patient.

Although disposable tips are usually used today, reusable tips may still be used in some medical offices. Reusable tips are disinfected and processed in the autoclave according to the manufacturer's directions. Reusable tips may be polished with steel wool if they become dull. Disposable tips should be discarded after use. Electrosurgical machines should be inspected periodically to ensure proper working order. The operating manual states the periodic maintenance to be performed by office staff and routine inspections to be performed by trained technicians. Surfaces should be kept clean and dry; machines should be kept covered when not in use.

 CHECKPOINT QUESTION

5. Which type of electrosurgery is used for incision or excision of tissue?

Laser Surgery

Lasers are devices that focus high-intensity light in a narrow beam to create extreme heat and energy. In medicine, lasers can be used to cut tissue and coagulate small bleeding vessels. There are many types of lasers, each with fairly specific applications in medicine. The following are the most common types of lasers encountered in the medical office:

- Argon laser: used for coagulation
- Carbon dioxide laser: used for cutting tissue
- Nd:YAG laser: used for coagulation and to separate warts and moles from surrounding tissues

Light from the laser is not usually visible. Colored filters are used to illuminate the laser's target, enabling the physician to direct the laser beam to the affected area. As with other electronic devices, attention to care and handling of the laser helps ensure that it is in good working order when it is needed. It is important to read and follow the manufacturer's recommended maintenance procedures as described in the instruction manual.

Everyone who is in the room, including the patient, during the laser procedure is required to wear goggles for eye protection. Health care workers are recommended to complete a training program before assisting with laser procedures to ensure that safety precautions are followed.

 CHECKPOINT QUESTION

6. What is one important safety feature worth noting when assisting with a laser procedure?

PATIENT EDUCATION

POSTOPERATIVE INSTRUCTIONS

After any surgical procedure, the patient should receive written and verbal discharge instructions, including how to care for the postoperative wound, taking prescribed medications correctly, and returning to the office for follow-up visits, dressing changes, and suture removal as ordered by the physician. The patient should be informed of the signs and symptoms of infection and should be instructed to report the following conditions:

- Excessive bleeding from the wound (additional teaching should include how to stop any excessive bleeding by applying direct pressure or elevating the body area).
- Redness, red streaks, or excessive swelling around the surgical site.
- Fever.

Tell the patient to call the office if these symptoms arise. In addition, you will tell the patient the following:

- When to return to the office to have the dressing or bandage changed or how and when to change the bandage or dressing at home.
- The need for follow-up visits. Have the patient schedule the appointment or appointments before leaving and provide an appointment card for each appointment.
- After speaking with the physician, tell the patient when he or she can take a shower or bath and whether the surgical wound can get wet. (Whether the wound may get wet depends on location and depth of the wound and the surgeon's preference.)
- If a specimen was taken for a pathology test, tell the patient when the results will be available.
- Answer any questions about postoperative experience and always encourage patients to call the office at any time if a problem or concern arises.

 COG Postsurgical Procedures

Sterile Dressings

Sterile dressings are items such as 4 × 4-inch absorbent gauze sponges and nonadhering dressings that have been processed for use on open wounds. Sterile dressings are generally prepackaged in small numbers but may come in bulk containers. They are manufactured in various sizes and shapes, each for a specific use and chosen according to the size of the wound and the amount of drainage. Dressings should be handled with sterile

technique. A sterile dressing may be secured by various bandages (sling, cravat, roller, tubular gauze) to hold the dressing in place, protect the injured part, or restrict movement. Chapter 12 describes bandaging techniques. Procedure 7-5 describes putting on sterile gloves, Procedure 7-6 describes applying a sterile dressing to a surgical wound, and Procedure 7-7 describes changing an existing dressing on a wound.

A sterile dressing is considered contaminated if it is damp or outdated, if its wrapper is damaged, or if it is improperly removed from its wrapper. Sterile dressings are used directly over a wound for the following reasons:

1. To cover and protect from contamination
2. To absorb drainage such as blood, serum, or pus
3. To exert pressure on an open wound to control bleeding
4. To hide disfigurement during healing
5. To hold medications against a wound to facilitate healing

When you remove a dressing, always wear clean examination gloves and carefully observe the wound for any drainage or exudates, noting this in the patient's chart. The terminology for describing wound drainage is outlined in Box 7-1. Immediately following the closure of a wound, it is normal to see serous or serosanguineous drainage in scant or moderate amounts, depending on the extent of the wound or incision. **Purulent** drainage, or drainage with color other than pink, is a sign of infection. Notify the physician when the wound is uncovered so that it can be examined and a decision can be made regarding how well healing is progressing. Box 7-2 describes the types and phases of wound healing.

BOX 7-1

WOUND DRAINAGE

When observing wound drainage, be sure to note:

Color
- Serous (clear)
- Sanguineous (blood tinged)
- Serosanguineous (pinkish or clear and red mixed)
- Purulent (white, green, or yellow-tinged drainage; usually accompanied by an unpleasant odor characteristic of infection)

Amount
- Copious (large amount)
- Medium (moderate amount)
- Scant (small amount)

The amount can also be quantified by indicating the size of the drainage (e.g., 2-inch diameter, entire 4 × 4 dressing saturated) or the size of the dressing.

BOX 7-2

THE HEALING PROCESS

Healing by Primary Intention: This simplest form of healing occurs in wounds whose edges are closely approximated, allowing the entrance of little or no bacteria to complicate the process. The edges of the wound lie closely together, new cells form quickly to bind the site, and capillaries expand themselves across the tissue break to restore circulation to the tissues. Scarring is usually minimal.

Healing by Secondary Intention: Granulation of tissue is present in the wound, and the edges of the wound join indirectly. Because the skin edges are not closely approximated, additional new cells are required to fill spaces in the lesion. Capillaries may not be able to reach across the gap to restore full circulation. Nerves may not rejoin, which results in diminished nerve stimulus through the area. A large scab forms to protect the area while healing goes on below it. Scarring is more severe than with primary intention healing.

Healing by Tertiary Intention: The wound initially is left open if there is the possibility that the wound may already be contaminated with microorganisms and closing it would only trap the microorganisms, increasing the potential for an infection. The wound is left open to fill in with granular tissue. There is considerable scar formation.

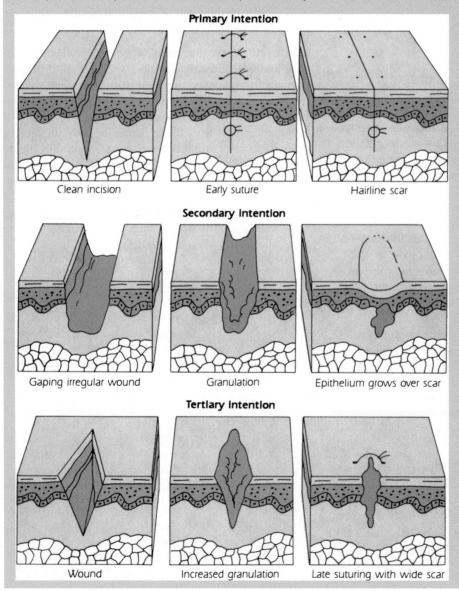

Primary Intention
Clean incision   Early suture   Hairline scar

Secondary Intention
Gaping irregular wound   Granulation   Epithelium grows over scar

Tertiary Intention
Wound   Increased granulation   Late suturing with wide scar

Types of wound healing. (*Top*) Primary intention. *Left to right:* Clean incision; early suture; hairline scar. (*Center*) Secondary intention. *Left to right:* Gaping irregular wound; granulation; epithelium grows over scar. (*Bottom*) Tertiary intention. *Left to right:* Wound; increased granulation; late suturing with wide scar.

BOX 7-2 *(continued)*

Phases of Wound Healing

Phase I (inflammatory, lag, or exudative phase): This phase usually lasts from 1 to 4 days. The body attempts to heal itself by increasing the circulation to the part and by beginning to reroute or repair the supplying vessels. The increased circulation brings with it more white blood cells to mount a defense against pathogens. Serum and red blood cells brought by the additional blood form a glue-like fibrin to plug the wound. As the fibrin dries, it pulls the edges of the wound closer together and forms a scab. Signs that this phase is working are edema from the tissue fluid, warmth from the extra blood, redness from the vasodilation, and pain from the pressure on the nerve endings caused by the edema.

Phase II (proliferative, healing, or granulation phase): This phase may last from several days to several weeks. The vessels continue to repair themselves and may reroute if damage is severe. The scab from phase I continues to dry and to pull the edges of the wound as closely together as possible.

Phase III (remodeling, maturation, or scarring phase): This phase may take from weeks to years, depending upon the severity of the wound. Fibroblasts build scar tissue to guard the area.

CHECKPOINT QUESTION

7. What is the difference between a dressing and a bandage?

LEGAL TIP

PROTECTED HEALTH INFORMATION

Often, patients who are seen in the medical office for minor surgical procedures must have a note from the physician in order to return back to work or to school. Some offices have a standard form that can be filled out and signed by the physician indicating very generally that the patient has had a procedure and should return back to school or work on a specific day. Unless you have the patient's written consent, you should never indicate the type of procedure on these notes or answer specific questions via the telephone should employers or school personnel call the office for information. Giving information without the patient's written consent would be a violation of the privacy laws included in HIPAA (Health Insurance and Portability Act of 1996).

Cleaning the Examination Table and Operative Area

In preparation for the next patient, all used equipment must be discarded properly or transported to the equipment room for sanitizing before sterilization.

The examination room must be cleaned as part of the procedure using standard precautions. Because of the possibility of biohazardous materials, you should remove papers and sheets in a rolling movement so outside surfaces cover the interior of the bundle. Do not let table covers and sheets come into contact with your clothing. Discard the sheets and covers appropriately. After applying gloves, wipe down the examination table, surgical stand, sink, counter, and other surfaces used during the procedure with an approved disinfectant or dilute bleach solution and allow them to dry. Replace the table sheet paper for the next patient.

WHAT IF?

What if you accidentally cut your finger while cleaning up after a minor office surgical procedure?

Remove your gloves and immediately wash your hands with an antiseptic solution. Then have the physician evaluate the wound. The physician will suggest that you wash the wound by performing a handwashing procedure, and antibiotics may be prescribed. The patient should be asked for permission to take a blood sample to test for hepatitis B, hepatitis C, and HIV. State laws vary regarding the legality of health care workers demanding a blood sample for testing. After blood from the patient is examined for the hepatitis B surface antigen, you may be given hepatitis B immunoglobulin (HBIG) and/or hepatitis B vaccine. You should consider obtaining the vaccine for hepatitis now. Many states require that health care workers be

(continued)

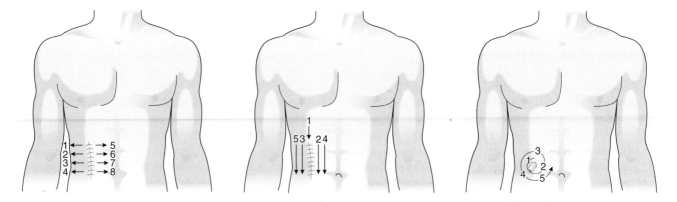

Figure 7-14 Clean a wound outward from the site following any of the numbered patterns shown here.

immunized at their employer's expense. Finally, be sure to notify your supervisor of any work-related injury so that it may be appropriately documented. The Needlestick Safety and Prevention Act requires that a sharps injury log be maintained and that it include the type and brand of device involved in the incident, the area in which the incident occurred, and a description of the incident. The name of the employee should not be recorded in the injury log. Preventing accidental exposure to contaminated blood or body fluids requires being alert and working without distractions.

COG Commonly Performed Office Surgical Procedures

Two of the most frequently performed minor surgeries in the general medical office are excision of skin lesions (moles, **lentigines**, **keratoses**, and skin tags) and incision and drainage of abscesses. Always use sterile technique and follow standard precautions when assisting with these surgical procedures.

Excision of a Lesion

Physicians may excise lesions with electrocautery, laser, **cryosurgery**, or standard surgical equipment. Procedure 7-8 describes the steps for assisting the physician during the excision of a skin lesion using standard equipment. Some lesions are desiccated or fulgurated; however, many lesions are sent to pathology for diagnosis after excision.

Incision and Drainage

An abscess is a local collection of pus in a cavity surrounded by inflamed tissue. It results from the body's response to an infectious process when pathogens

have entered through a break in the skin. Abscesses may be referred to as boils, furuncles (one lesion), or carbuncles (several lesions grouped closely together) and are very painful. The site must be incised and the infected material drained before healing can take place (Procedure 7-9).

COG Assisting with Suture and Staple Removal

In many instances, you will be required to remove sutures from a wound. Patients should understand that they might feel a pulling sensation during suture removal but should not feel pain. First, cleanse the area with an antiseptic solution. Either wearing sterile gloves or using sterile transfer forceps with clean hands, clean the area in a circular motion away from the wound or in straight wipes away from the suture line (Fig. 7-14). The wipe is discarded after each sweep, and a new one is used for the next sweep across the area. Either a sterile disposable suture removal kit, which contains all of the equipment needed for suture removal (Fig. 7-15, or sterile reusable equipment may be used (Procedure 7-10).

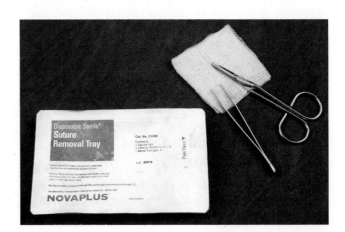

Figure 7-15 A disposable suture removal kit.

Following hospital surgery, some incisions are closed with metal staples rather than sutures. Patients often leave the hospital before the staples can be removed safely and return later to the physician's office to have them removed. Frequently, it will be your responsibility to remove the staples. Most offices use staple removal kits similar to the kits supplied for suture removal. Included in the staple removal kit is a special instrument for removing the staples instead of suture scissors. Procedure 7-11 describes the process for removing staples.

 CHECKPOINT QUESTION

8. What methods may be used to excise lesions in the medical office?

español SPANISH TERMINOLOGY

¿Es alergico/a a la Novcaina u otro tipo de anestesia?
  Are you allergic to Novocaine or other anesthetics?

Tiene que firmar este formulario.
  You need to sign this form.

Usted tiene tres puntos.
  You have three stitches.

¿Le duelen los puntos?
  Do your stitches hurt?

Regrese a la oficina el lunes.
  Return to the office on Monday.

 MEDIA MENU

Student Resources on thePoint

- **CMA/RMA Certification Exam Review**
- **Video: Applying Sterile Gloves (Procedure 7-5)**
- **Video: Applying a Sterile Dressing (Procedure 7-6)**
- **Video: Changing an Existing Sterile Dressing (Procedure 7-7)**
- **Video: Removing Sutures and Staples (Procedures 7-10 and 7-11)**

Internet Resources

American Society of Plastic Surgeons
http://www.plasticsurgery.org
American Society for Dermatologic Surgery
http://www.asds.net
Center for Laser Surgery
http://www.lasersurgery.com
The Association for the Advancement of Wound Care
http://www.aawconline.org

PSY PROCEDURE 7-1:   **Opening Sterile Surgical Packs**

Purpose: Open sterile packages without contaminating the contents
Equipment: Surgical pack, surgical or Mayo stand

Steps	Reasons
1. Wash your hands.	Handwashing aids in infection control. Your hands should be clean for this procedure.
2. Verify the procedure to be performed and remove the appropriate tray or item from the storage area. Check the label for contents and expiration date. Check the package for tears and moisture.	Packages that have passed the expiration date should not be used. Moist or torn areas contaminate the contents of the package.
3. Place the package, with the label facing up, on a clean, dry, flat surface such as a Mayo or surgical stand.	Although the field will be protected by a barrier undersurface, microorganisms must be kept at a minimum by using an area as free of pathogens as possible. The surgical stand makes it easy to move the field for the physician's convenience.
4. Without tearing the wrapper, carefully remove the sealing tape. With commercial packages, carefully remove the outer protective wrapper.	Many disposable packages are wrapped in clear plastic film that will become the sterile field when properly opened. Packages prepared in the office are sealed with autoclave tape, which should clearly indicate that the package has been through the autoclave.
5. Loosen the first flap of the folded wrapper by pulling it up, out, and away; let it fall over the far side of the table or stand.	This prevents you from having to reach across the sterile field again.

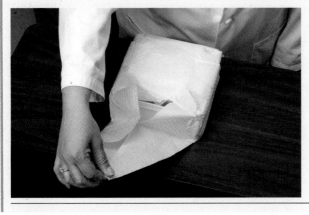

Step 5. Open the first flap away from you.

PSY PROCEDURE 7-1:   **Opening Sterile Surgical Packs (continued)**

Steps	Reasons
6. Open the side flaps in a similar manner, using your left hand for the left flap and your right hand for the right flap. Touch only the unsterile outer surface; do not touch the sterile inner surface.	This method minimizes your movement over the sterile areas of the package.

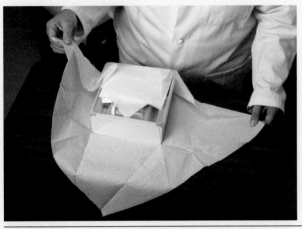

Step 6. Open the side flaps.

Steps	Reasons
7. Pull the remaining flap down and toward you by grasping the outside surface only. The outer surface of the wrapper is now against the surgical stand; the sterile inside of the wrapper forms the sterile field.	

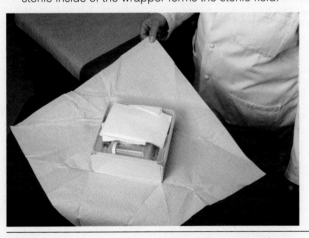

Step 7. Pull the remaining flap down and toward you.

8. Repeat Steps 5 to 7 for packages with a second or inside wrapper. This wrapper also provides a sterile field upon which to work. The field is now ready for the procedure to begin.

(continued)

PSY PROCEDURE 7-1: **Opening Sterile Surgical Packs** *(continued)*

Steps	Reasons
9. If you must leave the area after opening the field, cover the tray and its contents with a sterile drape. Without leaving or turning your back on the sterile setup area, open the sterile drape and carefully lift it out of the package by the edges without contaminating it. Carefully lay the drape over the sterile field, working from your body out so that your arms do not cross the uncovered sterile field but do cross the drape that has been placed over the tray.	Leaving or turning your back on a sterile field makes the sterile field contaminated.

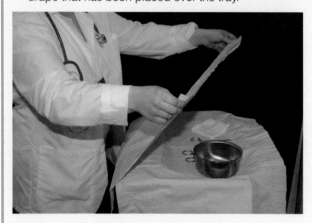

Step 9. Place the drape over the sterile tray without putting your arms over the uncovered tray.

PSY PROCEDURE 7-2: **Using Sterile Transfer Forceps**

Purpose: Use sterile transfer forceps without contamination during a sterile setup
Equipment: Sterile transfer forceps in a container with sterilization solution, a sterile field, sterile items to be transferred

Steps	Reasons
1. Slowly lift the forceps straight up and out of the container without touching the outside of the container or its inside above the level of the solution.	The area above the soaking solution and the rim are considered not sterile.
2. Hold the forceps with the tips down at all times.	This prevents the solution from running toward the unsterile handles and then back to the grasping blades and tips, which would contaminate them.

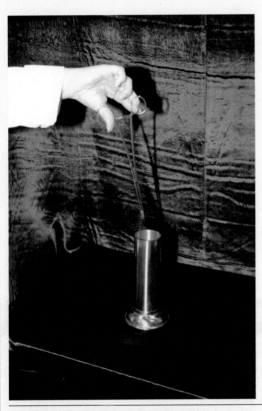

Step 2. The tips of the forceps should be held in a downward position.

Steps	Reasons
3. Keep the forceps above waist level.	This prevents accidental and unnoticed contamination.
4. With the forceps, pick up the articles to be transferred and drop them onto the sterile field, but do not let the forceps come into contact with the sterile field.	The forceps may be moist from the soaking solution, which may wick microorganisms from the surface below onto the sterile field. Note: Transfer forceps that have been wrapped and autoclaved may be placed with tips on the sterile field and handles extending beyond the 1-inch border that is considered contaminated. Doing this allows you to move objects around the field for the physician's convenience.
5. Carefully place the forceps back in the sterilization solution.	The sterilization solution in the forceps container keeps the tips of the forceps sterile for future use. The solution should be changed at least daily or according to office policy.

(continued)

PSY **PROCEDURE 7-2:** **Using Sterile Transfer Forceps** *(continued)*

Steps	Reasons
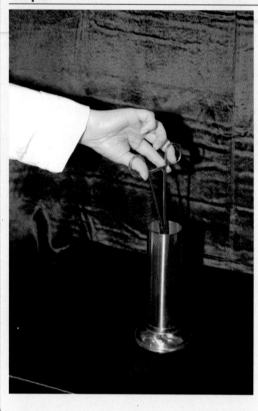	**Step 5.** Put the forceps into the container without contaminating them.

PSY **PROCEDURE 7-3:** **Adding Sterile Solution to a Sterile Field**

Purpose: Pour a sterile solution into a container on the sterile field without contamination
Equipment: Sterile setup, container of sterile solution, sterile bowl or cup

Steps	Reasons
1. As with any drug or medication, identify the correct solution by carefully reading the label. If necessary, use the sterile transfer forceps and place the sterile bowl or cup on the sterile field.	The label should be checked three times to prevent errors: when taking the container from the shelf, before pouring the solution, and when returning the container to the shelf.
2. Check the expiration date on the label; do not use the solution if it is out of date, if the label cannot be read, or if the solution appears abnormal. Sterile water and saline bottles must be dated when opened and must be discarded if not used within 48 hours.	Out-of-date solutions may have changed chemically or deteriorated and are not considered sterile.
3. If you are adding medication, such as lidocaine, to the solution, show the medication label to the physician now.	This allows for verification of the contents.

Steps	Reasons
4. Remove the cap or stopper. Hold the cap with your fingertips, with the cap opening down to prevent contamination of the inside of the cap. If you must put the cap down, place it on a side table (not the sterile field) with the open end up. If you are pouring the entire contents onto the sterile field, discard the cap. Retain the bottle to keep track of the amount added to the field and for charting later. It can then be discarded.	If the cap becomes contaminated and is returned to the bottle, the contents are considered contaminated. Placing the cap on a surface with the opening up prevents contamination of the interior of the cap.
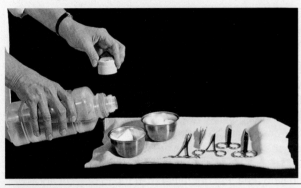	
	Step 4. Hold the cap facing downward to prevent contamination of the inside.
5. Grasp the container with the label against the palm of your hand (known as palming the label).	If solution runs down the side of the bottle in this position, it will not obscure the label.
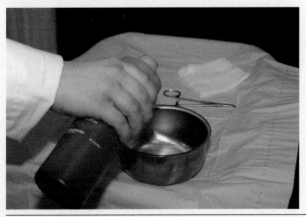	
	Step 5. Hold the bottle of sterile solution with the label in your palm.
6. Pour a small amount of the solution into a separate container or waste receptacle.	The lip of the bottle is considered contaminated; pouring off this small amount cleanses the lip.
7. Without reaching across the sterile field, carefully and slowly pour the desired amount of solution into the sterile container from not less than 4 and not more than 6 inches above the container. The bottle of solution should never touch the sterile container or tray, as this will cause contamination.	Pouring the solution slowly reduces the chance of splashing and overfilling. Solution poured too fast or from an improper height may splash. Touching the container to objects on the sterile field contaminates the field. If the solution splashes onto the field, wicking will cause contamination from the surface below.
8. After pouring the desired amount of solution into the sterile container, recheck the label for the contents and expiration date and replace the cap carefully, without touching the bottle rim with any unsterile surface of the cap.	This ensures accuracy. Careful replacement of the cap ensures that the contents remain sterile.
9. Return the solution to its proper storage area or discard the container after checking the label again.	You will have checked the solution label a total of three times to avoid errors.

PSY PROCEDURE 7-4: **Performing Hair Removal and Skin Preparation**

Purpose: Prepare the skin by removing any hair and applying an antiseptic solution before a surgical procedure
Equipment: Nonsterile gloves; shave cream, lotion, or soap; new disposable razor; gauze or cotton balls; warm water; antiseptic; sponge forceps

Steps	Reasons
1. Wash your hands.	Handwashing aids infection control.
2. Assemble the equipment.	This ensures that all supplies are available. A new razor must be used for each patient to prevent the transmission of pathogens and to ensure the closest possible shave.
3. Greet and identify the patient. Explain the procedure and answer any questions.	This prevents errors in treatment, helps gain compliance, and eases anxiety.
4. Put on gloves and prepare the patient's skin: **A.** For shaving, apply shaving cream or soapy lather to the area. Pull the skin taut and shave by pulling the razor across the skin in the direction of hair growth. Repeat this procedure until all hair is removed from the operative area. Rinse and thoroughly pat the shaved area dry with a gauze square. **B.** If the patient's skin is not to be shaved, wash and rinse the skin with soap and water and dry the skin thoroughly.	Gloves must be worn when contact with blood or body fluids is possible. Shaving cream or soapy lather on the skin reduces friction and helps prevent scratching. Shaving in the direction of hair growth gives the closest shave while reducing the chance of nicking the skin. Rinsing removes soap residue and hair from the shaved area. Pat dry rather than rub to prevent abrasions. Using gauze squares for drying picks up stray hairs that might have been left behind during rinsing.
5. Apply antiseptic solution of the physician's choice to the skin surrounding the operative area using sterile gauze sponges, sterile cotton balls, or antiseptic wipes. Holding the gauze or cotton ball in the sterile sponge forceps, wipe the skin in circular motions starting at the operative site and working outward. Discard each sponge after a complete sweep has been made. If the area is large or circles are not appropriate, the sponge may be wiped straight outward from the operative site, then discarded and the procedure repeated until the entire area has been thoroughly cleaned. At no time should a wipe that has passed over the skin be returned to the cleaned area or to the antiseptic solution.	Discarding sponges after each stroke prevents contamination of the wound by microorganisms brought back to the area from the surrounding skin.
6. Holding dry sterile gauze sponges in the sponge forceps, thoroughly pat the area dry. In some instances, the area may be allowed to air dry.	Moist skin may moisten the sterile drapes, causing wicking and contaminating the site.
7. Instruct the patient not to touch or cover the prepared area.	This avoids contaminating the operative site, which would require repeating the procedure.
8. **AFF** Explain how to respond to a patient who is developmentally challenged.	To avoid injury to the patient, assess for safety before completing a procedure when there is the possibility that the patient may not cooperate.
9. Inform the physician that the patient is ready for the procedure. Drape the prepared area with a sterile drape if the physician will be delayed for more than 10 or 15 minutes or if the sterile tray will be unattended for any length of time.	

PSY PROCEDURE 7-5: | **Applying Sterile Gloves**

Purpose: Apply prepackaged sterile gloves without contamination
Equipment: One package of sterile gloves in the appropriate size

Steps	Reasons
1. Remove rings and other jewelry.	Rings may pierce the gloves and contaminate the procedure.
2. Wash your hands.	Wearing gloves is not a substitute for handwashing but must be done in addition to it.
3. Place the prepackaged gloves on a clean, dry, flat, surface with the cuffed end toward you.	Sterile gloves are packaged for ease of application in this fashion.

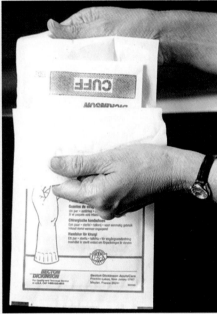

A

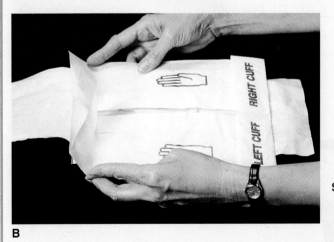

B

Step 3. (A) Pull the outer wrapping apart to expose the sterile inner wrap. (B) With the cuffs toward you, fold back the inner wrap to expose the gloves.

(continued)

PSY PROCEDURE 7-5: **Applying Sterile Gloves (continued)**

Steps

4. Grasping the edges of the outer paper, open the package out to its fullest.

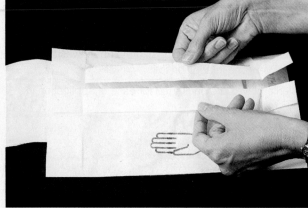

A

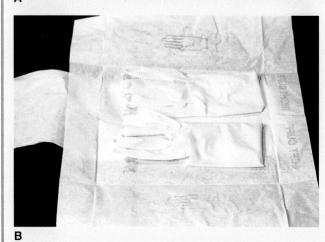

B

5. Using your nondominant hand, pick up the dominant hand glove by grasping the folded edge of the cuff and lifting it up and away from the paper. The folded edge of the cuff is contaminated as soon as it is touched with the ungloved hand. Be very careful not to touch the outside surface of the sterile glove with your ungloved hand.

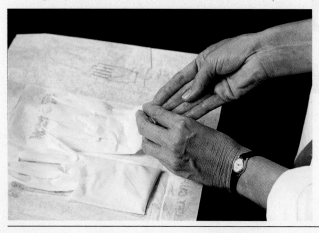

Reasons

The inner surface of the package is a sterile field.

Step 4. (A and B) Grasp the edges and open the packages.

Lift it up and away to avoid letting the fingers of the glove brush an unsterile surface.

Step 5. Using your nondominant hand, lift the cuff of the glove for the dominant hand, touching only the inner surface of the cuff. Curl your thumb inward as you insert your hand.

PSY PROCEDURE 7-5:   **Applying Sterile Gloves (continued)**

Steps	Reasons
6. Curl your fingers and thumb together and insert them into the glove. Then straighten your fingers and pull the glove on with your nondominant hand still grasping the cuff.	This prevents accidental touching of the outside surface of the glove.
7. Unfold the cuff by pinching the inside surface that will be against your wrist and pulling it toward the wrist.	This ensures that only the unsterile portions are touched by the hands.

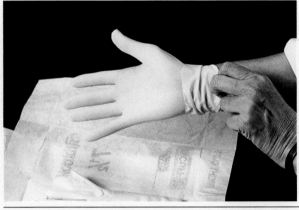

Step 7. Pull the glove snugly into place, touching only the inside surface of the cuff.

Steps	Reasons
8. Place the fingers of your gloved hand under the cuff of the remaining glove, lift the glove up and away from the wrapper, and slide your ungloved hand carefully into the glove with your fingers and thumb curled together.	This prevents the sterile glove from accidentally touching an unsterile surface and ensures that the fingers will not brush the sterile surface of the glove.

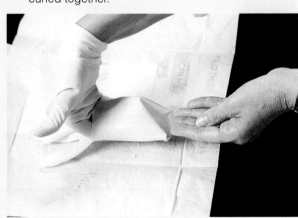

Step 8. With your thumb curled, slip the gloved dominant hand into the cuff of the remaining glove.

(continued)

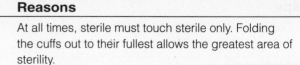

PSY PROCEDURE 7-5: **Applying Sterile Gloves *(continued)***

Steps	Reasons
9. Straighten your fingers and pull the glove up and over your wrist by carefully unfolding the cuff.	At all times, sterile must touch sterile only. Folding the cuffs out to their fullest allows the greatest area of sterility.

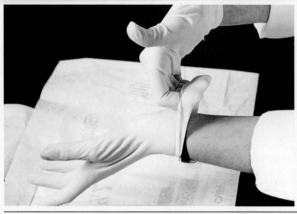

Step 9. Unfold the cuff and pull the glove on snugly.

Steps	Reasons
10. Settle the gloves comfortably onto your fingers by lacing your fingers together and adjusting the tension over your hands.	The gloves should fit snugly without wrinkles or areas that bind the fingers.

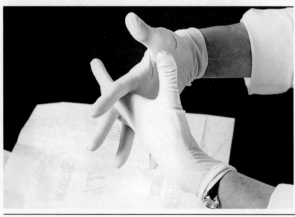

Step 10. Adjust the fingers for a comfortable fit.

Steps	Reasons
11. Remove contaminated sterile gloves exactly as you would remove contaminated nonsterile gloves and discard them appropriately.	If removed correctly, one glove will be balled into the other with no opportunity to touch the soiled area of either glove.

PSY PROCEDURE 7-6:   **Applying a Sterile Dressing**

Purpose: Using sterile dressings and sterile technique, apply a sterile dressing to a surgical wound without contamination

Equipment: Sterile gloves, sterile gauze dressings, scissors, bandage tape, any medication to be applied to the wound if ordered by the physician

Steps	Reasons
1. Wash your hands and assemble the necessary supplies.	Handwashing aids infection control.
2. Assemble the equipment and supplies.	This ensures that all of the supplies are available before beginning the procedure.
3. Greet and identify the patient. Ask about any allergies before selecting tape. With the size the dressing in mind, cut or tear lengths of to secure the dressing. Set the tape aside in a convenient place.	Patients must be identified to prevent errors in tape treatment. Some patients are sensitive to certain of tape adhesives. Many types of hypoallergenic tape are available. Having tape cut and prepared saves time and may prevent the dressing from slipping while tape is cut after the dressing is applied.
4. Explain the procedure and instruct the patient to remain still during the procedure and to avoid coughing, sneezing, and talking until the procedure is complete.	Unexpected movements by the patient may result in contamination of the sterile supplies and the wound. Talking, coughing, and sneezing release droplets of moisture containing microorganisms from the respiratory tract that may contaminate the sterile field and the wound.
5. Open the dressing pack to create a sterile field, leaving the sterile dressing on the inside of the opened package. Observe the principles of surgical asepsis. Many packets are designed to be peeled apart.	Sterile technique ensures sterility of the dressing after it is open. Packages of dressings are sterile on the inside; if opened properly, the inner surface may be used as a sterile field.

Step 5. Open the sterile dressing pack or packs.

Steps	Reasons
6. To maintain sterility: **A.** If sterile gloves are to be used, open the appropriate package of gloves. Using sterile technique, put on the gloves before touching any sterile items. **B.** If using sterile transfer forceps to apply the dressing (the no-touch method), use sterile technique to arrange the dressing on the wound, and do not touch the dressing or the site with the hands.	Sterile items may only be touched with sterile gloves *or* sterile transfer forceps.
7. If ordered by the physician, apply topical medication to the sterile dressing that will directly cover the wound, being careful not to touch the end of the medication bottle or tube to the dressing.	The outside end of the medication bottle or tube may not be sterile.

(continued)

PSY **PROCEDURE 7-6:**   **Applying a Sterile Dressing** *(continued)*

Steps	Reasons

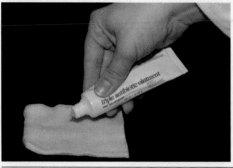

Step 7. Apply medication if ordered without touching the end of the container to the dressing.

8. Using the already opened sterile dressings and sterile technique, apply the number of dressings necessary to cover and protect the wound. Sterile dressings must be carefully placed on the wound and not allowed to drag over the skin.

If the dressing is dragged over the skin, it will be contaminated by microorganisms from the surrounding skin and may cause infection.

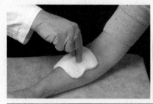 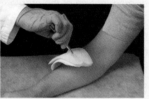

Step 8. Using sterile gloves (*left*). Using sterile forceps (*right*).

9. Apply the previously cut lengths of tape over the dressing to secure it, but avoid overuse of tape. When the wound is completely covered, you may remove your gloves or keep them on while you tape the dressing. Discard the gloves in the proper receptacle.

Tape is used only to keep the dressing in place. It should allow observation of any bleeding or drainage. Too much tape can cause perspiration that will dampen the dressing and compromise sterility. Tape should not obstruct blood circulation. Excessive tape also must later be removed, which may hurt. A bandage may be applied over the dressing to hold it in place, add support, or immobilize the area.

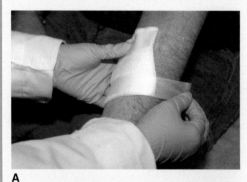

A

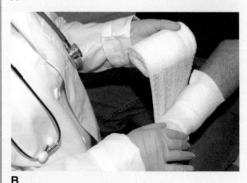

B

Step 9. (A) Securing a dressing with tape.
(B) Securing a dressing with a bandage.

PSY PROCEDURE 7-6: **Applying a Sterile Dressing (continued)**

Steps	Reasons
10. When the patient is to change dressings at home, provide appropriate instructions. Dressings should be kept clean and dry and changed when wet or soiled. Otherwise, dressings should be changed as instructed by the physician. Make sure patients understand the signs of infection, such as redness, swelling, pain, or undue warmth at the site, and instruct them to call the office at once if these appear. Also say what to do in case of excessive bleeding or drainage and how to manage any drains.	Microorganisms may be transported to the wound by capillary action if the dressing is wet or soiled.
11. **AFF** Explain how to respond to a patient who is visually impaired.	Face the patient when speaking and always let him or her know what you are going to do before touching him or her. Give the patient written and oral instructions. Confirm instructions with caregiver.
12. Wearing clean examination gloves, properly dispose of or care for equipment and supplies. Disposable articles contaminated with wound drainage or blood go into a biohazard container. Clean the work area, remove your gloves, and wash your hands.	Follow standard precautions.
13. Return reusable supplies (unopened sterile gloves or dressings, tape) to their appropriate storage areas; all others should be discarded correctly.	Unopened supplies should be returned to the appropriate storage areas for reuse. Discarding uncontaminated reusables is wasteful.
14. Record the procedure.	Procedures are considered not to have been done if they are not recorded in the patient's medical record.

Charting Example:

10/14/2012 4:45 pm DSD applied to surgical wound (L) anterior forearm. No bleeding from incision, edges well approximated with 4 sutures intact. Pt. given verbal and written instructions on dressing change and wound care at home. To RTO in 5 days for suture removal ——————————————— L. Hicks, CMA

Note: The medical assistant may sign his or her name in the patient record using only the "CMA" credential if the office has a signature log denoting the entire credential as "CMA(AAMA)."

PSY PROCEDURE 7-7: **Changing an Existing Sterile Dressing**

Purpose: Carefully remove an existing dressing from a wound and cover it with a sterile dressing using sterile technique
Equipment: Sterile gloves; nonsterile gloves; sterile dressing; prepackaged skin antiseptic swabs or sterile antiseptic solution in a sterile basin and sterile cotton balls or gauze; tape; approved biohazard container

Steps	Reasons
1. Wash your hands and assemble the necessary supplies.	Handwashing aids infection control.
2. Assemble the equipment and supplies.	This ensures that all supplies are available before you begin the procedure.
3. Greet and identify the patient. Explain the procedure and answer any questions.	This prevents errors in treatment, helps gain compliance, and eases anxiety.
4. Prepare a sterile field, including opening sterile dressings. If using a sterile container and solution, open the package containing the sterile basin and use the inside of the wrapper as the sterile field for the basin. Flip the sterile gauze or cotton balls into the basin and appropriately pour in the antiseptic solution. If using prepackaged antiseptic swabs, carefully open an adequate number for the size of the wound and set them aside without contaminating them.	Opening sterile supplies after applying sterile gloves will cause contamination of your gloves and your supplies.
5. Instruct the patient not to talk, cough, sneeze, laugh, or move during the procedure.	Respiratory droplets may contaminate the sterile field. Movement may cause accidental contamination of the field.
6. Wearing clean gloves, carefully remove the tape from the wound dressing by pulling it toward the wound. Remove the old dressing. Note: If the dressing is difficult to remove because of dried blood, it may be soaked with sterile water or saline for a few minutes to loosen it. Gently pull the edges of the dressing toward the center. Never pull on a dressing that does not come off easily. If this procedure does not sufficiently loosen the dressing or causes undue discomfort to the patient, immediately notify the physician.	Tape pulled away from the direction of the wound may pull the healing edges of the wound apart.

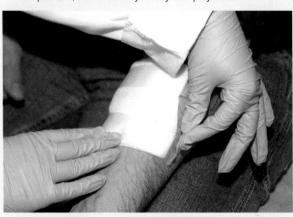

Step 6. Pull the tape toward the wound.

PSY **PROCEDURE 7-7:** **Changing an Existing Sterile Dressing (continued)**

Steps	Reasons
7. Discard the soiled dressing into a biohazard container. Do not pass it over the sterile field.	The dressing will be soiled with blood and body fluids and must be considered hazardous. Dressings passed over the sterile field will shed microorganisms and contaminate the area.
8. Inspect the wound for degree of healing, amount and type of drainage, appearance of wound edges, and so on.	The wound is inspected now because wound cleaning removes most exudate. Make a mental note for charting when the procedure is complete.
9. Observing medical asepsis, remove and discard your gloves. The physician may want to inspect the wound before you remove exudate or drainage to determine whether healing is proceeding as expected. If a culture is ordered, the specimen must be taken before the wound is cleaned to ensure the most reliable findings.	
10. Using proper technique, put on sterile gloves. Clean the wound with the antiseptic solution ordered by the physician. Clean in a straight motion with the cotton or gauze or the prepackaged antiseptic swab. Discard the wipe (cotton ball, swab) after each stroke and use a fresh sterile one to continue. Never return the wipe to the antiseptic solution or to the skin after one sweep across the area.	The wound must be cleaned before fresh dressings are applied. Returning the wipe to the wound area or solution brings microorganisms from the surrounding skin to the open lesion.
11. Remove your gloves and wash your hands.	Your hands must be washed before you apply the sterile dressing with sterile gloves or sterile forceps.
12. Change the dressing using the procedure for sterile dressing application and using sterile gloves or sterile transfer forceps (Procedure 7-6).	The old dressing is removed with clean gloves but sterile technique must be used when applying a new sterile dressing.
13. **AFF** Explain how to respond to a patient who has dementia.	Solicit assistance from a caregiver or other staff member to help during the procedure. Give simple directions to the patient about what he or she should do. Speak clearly, not loudly.
14. Record the procedure.	Procedures are considered not to have been done if they are not recorded.

Charting Example:

11/23/2012 11:30 am Dressing to (R) lower leg changed, small amount of yellow purulent drainage noted—
Dr. Blake aware. Wound culture for C&S obtained and sent to Acme laboratory. Wound cleansed with Betadine
as ordered; DSD reapplied. Moderate amount of redness and swelling at wound site; edges well approximated.
Instructed to RTO in 2 days for C&S results and dressing change ———————— B. Lamont, CMA

Note: The medical assistant may sign his or her name in the patient record using only the "CMA" credential if the office has a signature log denoting the entire credential as "CMA(AAMA)."

PSY PROCEDURE 7-8:   Assisting with Excisional Surgery

Purpose: Prepare for and assist with excisional surgery while maintaining sterile technique
Equipment: At the side: sterile gloves, local anesthetic, antiseptic wipes, adhesive tape, specimen container with completed laboratory request. On the field: basin for solutions, gauze sponges and cotton balls, antiseptic solution, sterile drape, dissecting scissors, disposable scalpel, blade of physician's choice, mosquito forceps, tissue forceps, needle holder, suture and needle of physician's choice.

Steps	Reasons
1. Wash your hands and assemble the necessary supplies.	Handwashing aids infection control.
2. Assemble the equipment.	This ensures that all supplies are available.
3. Greet and identify the patient. Explain the procedure and answer any questions.	This prevents errors in treatment, helps gain compliance, and eases anxiety.
4. Set up a sterile field on a surgical stand with the at-the-side equipment close at hand. Cover the field with a sterile drape until the physician arrives.	Covering the sterile field with a sterile drape will prevent the sterile field from becoming contaminated.
5. Position the patient appropriately.	The required position depends on the location of the lesion.
6. Put on sterile gloves or use sterile transfer forceps and cleanse the patient's skin as described in Procedure 9-4. Some physicians prefer to do this themselves after gloving, using supplies on the field. The physician's preference always takes precedence over any outlined procedure.	The antiseptic discourages the entrance of microorganisms into the wound. After cleansing the skin, remove the gloves, if used, and wash your hands.
7. The physician will perform the procedure; you may be asked to assist. This usually involves adding supplies as needed, watching closely for opportunities to assist the physician, and comforting the patient.	It is not necessary for you to wear sterile gloves during the procedure unless the physician requires you to handle sterile instruments or supplies.
8. If the lesion is to be referred to pathology for analysis, you will be required to assist with collecting the specimen in an appropriate container.	Always follow standard precautions, wearing examination gloves when handling specimens. Have the container ready to receive the specimen.
9. At the end of the procedure, wash your hands and dress the wound using sterile technique (Procedure 7-6).	The wound must be covered to protect the incision from contamination.
10. **AFF** Explain how to respond to a patient who is hearing impaired.	Make sure the patient can see your face as you are speaking. Speak clearly, not loudly.
11. Thank the patient and give appropriate instructions for care of the operative site, changing the dressing, postoperative medications, and follow-up visits as ordered by the physician.	Courtesy encourages the patient to have a positive attitude about the physician's office.

PSY PROCEDURE 7-8:   **Assisting with Excisional Surgery (continued)**

Steps	Reasons
12. Wearing gloves, clean the examining room in preparation for the next patient. Discard all used disposables in appropriate biohazard containers. Return unused items to their proper places. Remove your gloves and wash your hands.	Standard precautions must be followed.

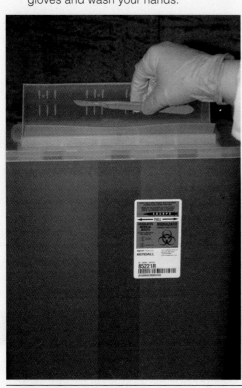

Step 11. Discard any disposable sharp items, such as a scalpel, into the appropriate biohazard container.

Steps	Reasons
13. Record the procedure.	Procedures not recorded in the patient record are not considered to have been done.

Charting Example:

09/19/2012 8:45 am Mole to posterior (L) shoulder removed per Dr. Snider. Specimen sent to Acme lab. T 98.4 (O),
P 96, R 20, BP 134/78 (R) sitting. 4 × 4 DSD applied to surgical incision; minimal sanguineous drainage noted.
Pt. given verbal and written instructions on wound care, postop antibiotics, pain medication, and follow-up visits.
Verbalized understanding. To RTO ×2 days for drsg change ———————————————— B. Cole, CMA

Note: The medical assistant may sign his or her name in the patient record using only the "CMA" credential if the office has a signature log denoting the entire credential as "CMA(AAMA)."

PSY PROCEDURE 7-9:   Assisting with Incision and Drainage (I&D)

Purpose: Prepare for and assist with an incision and drainage procedure while maintaining sterile technique
Equipment: At the side: sterile gloves; local anesthetic; needle and syringe if not placed on sterile field; antiseptic wipes; adhesive tape; sterile dressings; packing gauze; culture tube if the wound may be cultured. On the field: basin for solutions; gauze sponges and cotton balls; antiseptic solution; sterile drape; syringes and needles for local anesthetic; commercial I&D sterile setup or scalpel, dissecting scissors, hemostats, tissue forceps; sterile 4 × 4 gauze sponges; sterile probe (optional).

Steps

The steps for this procedure are similar to those in Procedure 7-8. Specifically, you are expected to prepare the surgical field and the patient's surgical area as instructed or preferred by the physician. After the procedure, the wound must be covered to avoid further contamination and to absorb drainage. The exudate is a hazardous body fluid requiring standard precautions. Although a culture and sensitivity may be ordered on the drainage from the infected area, no other specimen is usually collected.

Charting Example:

04/15/2012 11:30 am Postop VS T 100.4 (O), P 88, R 24, BP 128/88 (R) sitting. 4 × 4 DSD applied to surgical wound
on (L) posterior neck. Given verbal and written instructions on wound care, dressing changes, and followup.
Verbalized understanding ———————————————————————————— E. Black, CMA

Note: The medical assistant may sign his or her name in the patient record using only the "CMA" credential if the office has a signature log denoting the entire credential as "CMA(AAMA)."

PSY PROCEDURE 7-10:   Removing Sutures

Purpose: Using aseptic technique, remove sutures from a wound
Equipment: Skin antiseptic; clean exam gloves; sterile gloves; prepackaged suture removal kit *or* thumb forceps, suture scissors, and 2 × 2 gauze

Steps	Reasons
1. Wash your hands and apply clean examination gloves.	Handwashing aids infection control.
2. Assemble the equipment.	This ensures that all supplies are available.
3. Greet and identify the patient. Explain the procedure and answer any questions.	This prevents errors in treatment, helps gain compliance, and eases anxiety.
4. If dressings have not been removed, remove them and properly dispose of them in the biohazard container. Remove your gloves and wash your hands if a soiled dressing was removed.	Always wash your hands after removing gloves.
5. Put on clean examination gloves and cleanse the wound with an antiseptic, such as Betadine, using a new antiseptic gauze for each swipe down the wound and removing any old drainage or blood.	The wound must be as free of pathogens as possible before removal of the sutures to prevent contamination of the wound.
6. Open the suture removal packet using sterile asepsis or set up a field for on-site sterile equipment. Put on sterile gloves.	Suture removal is a sterile procedure.

PSY PROCEDURE 7-10: **Removing Sutures (continued)**

Steps	Reasons
7. The knots will be tied so that one tail of the knot is very close to the surface of the skin; the other will be closer to the area of suture that is looped over the incision.	

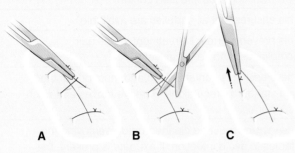

A   B   C

Step 7. (A) With the hemostat or thumb forceps, lift the stitch up and away from the skin. **(B)** Cut the stitch near the skin. **(C)** Using the forceps, pull the freed stitch up and out.

Steps	Reasons
A. With the thumb forceps, grasp the end of the knot closest to the skin and lift it slightly and gently up from the skin.	
B. Cut the suture below the knot as close to the skin as possible.	**B.** Cutting below the knot and close to the skin frees the knot at an area that has not been exposed to the outside surface of the body. The only part of the suture that will pull through the tissues will be the suture that was under the skin surface.
C. Use the thumb forceps to pull the suture out of the skin with a smooth, continuous motion, at a slight angle in the direction of the wound.	**C.** This prevents tension on the healing tissue.
8. Place the suture on the gauze sponge. Repeat the procedure for each suture to be removed.	This helps in counting the number removed; if six sutures were inserted and are now to be removed, there should be six sutures on the gauze sponge at the end of the procedure.
9. Clean the site with an antiseptic solution, and if the physician has so indicated, cover it with a sterile dressing.	Some wounds still need to be protected; some have healed well enough to be left uncovered.
10. **AFF** Explain how to respond to a patient who is developmentally challenged.	To avoid injury to the patient, assess for safety before completing a procedure when there is the possibility that the patient may not cooperate.
11. Thank the patient and properly dispose of the equipment and supplies. Clean the work area, remove your gloves, and wash your hands.	Standard precautions must be followed. Courtesy encourages a positive attitude about the physician's office.
12. Record the procedure, including the time, location of sutures, number removed, and condition of the wound.	Procedures are considered not to have been done if they are not recorded.

Charting Example:

06/26/2012 3:30 pm ×6 sutures removed from (L) ring finger. Wound well approximated,
no drainage ——————————————————————————— J. Rose, RMA

Note: The medical assistant may sign his or her name in the patient record using only the "CMA" credential if the office has a signature log denoting the entire credential as "CMA(AAMA)."

PSY **PROCEDURE 7-11:** **Removing Staples**

Purpose: Using aseptic technique, remove staples from a wound
Equipment: Antiseptic solution or wipes, gauze squares, sponge forceps, prepackaged sterile staple removal instrument, examination gloves, sterile gloves

Steps	Reasons
1. Wash your hands.	Handwashing aids infection control.
2. Assemble the equipment.	This ensures that all supplies are available.
3. Greet and identify the patient. Explain the procedure and answer any questions.	This prevents errors in treatment, helps gain compliance, and eases anxiety.
4. If the dressing is still in place, put on clean examination gloves and remove it. Dispose of the dressing in a biohazard container.	The dressing is contaminated and must be handled with standard precautions. Remove gloves and wash your hands.
5. Clean the incision with antiseptic solution. Pat dry with sterile gauze sponges.	The incision must be cleaned before removing the staples to avoid infection. If exudate is present, the staples may not be easy to see.
6. Put on sterile gloves.	Staple removal is a sterile procedure.
7. Gently slide the end of the staple remover under each staple to be removed. Press the handles together to lift the ends of the staple out of the skin.	The remover is designed to open the staple so that the ends will lift free and minimize discomfort.

Step 7. Slide the end of the staple remover under each staple. Press the handles together to lift the ends of the staple out of the skin.

Steps	Reasons
8. Place each staple on a gauze square as it is removed.	This helps in counting the staples at the end of the procedure.
9. When all staples are removed, gently clean the incision as instructed for all procedures. Pat dry and dress the site if ordered to do so by the physician.	The area should be cleaned and dried before any new dressing is applied to avoid wicking microorganisms. Healing may be far enough along to allow the wound to remain uncovered.
10. **AFF** Explain how to respond to a patient who is visually impaired.	Face the patient when speaking and always let him or her know what you are going to do before touching him or her.
11. Thank the patient and properly care for or dispose of all equipment and supplies. Clean the work area, remove your gloves, and wash your hands.	Standard precautions must be followed.
12. Record the procedure.	Procedures are not considered to have been done if they are not recorded.

Charting Example:

3/17/2012 10:30 am ×15 staples removed from (L) knee incision; edges well approximated, no redness or drainage

noted. Wound left open to air as ordered by Dr. Perez ———————————— *B. Daniels, CMA*

Note: The medical assistant may sign his or her name in the patient record using only the "CMA" credential if the office has a signature log denoting the entire credential as "CMA(AAMA)."

- With the spiraling costs of health care, many procedures that were once performed only in hospitals are now being performed in medical offices.
- As a medical assistant, you will be required to become more proficient in minor surgical procedures as offices change to meet the needs of the patients. Continuing education, research, and on-the-job training will keep you current on the changes in the field of surgery and in the new equipment that is used during minor office surgical procedures.
- No matter how technical or sophisticated the surgical procedure or equipment, you must not forget the feelings of apprehension many patients have. Although it is your responsibility to prepare the treatment room and assist the physician, you are also obligated to instruct the patient accurately on any presurgical preparations, obtain third-party authorization if necessary, reassure the patient during the procedure, and give the patient accurate information about postsurgical care as ordered by the physician.
- After the procedure, you must disinfect the examination room and prepare it for future patients.

Warm Ups | for Critical Thinking

1. Dr. Brown has just informed Mrs. Levine that she should return tomorrow for office surgery. While you are alone with the patient, Mrs. Levine begins to cry and expresses great concern about the procedure. What should you do?
2. Refer to an anatomy book and review the anatomy of a hair follicle. Why are skin nicks more likely if the hair is shaved in the opposite direction of its natural growth?
3. Why is it preferable for infected wounds to heal with delayed or unclosed surface edges?
4. Prepare a patient education sheet outlining postoperative wound care.
5. This morning, you are assisting Dr. Patrick with an ingrown toenail removal. When the patient arrives, you notice that the consent form has not been signed. The patient agrees to sign the consent form but indicates that he has some questions about the risks involved. Should you let him sign the consent? Why or why not? What would you do?

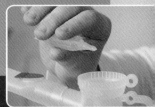

Outline

Medication Names
Legal Regulations
  Food and Drug Administration
  Drug Enforcement Agency
  Inventory, Storage,
    Dispensation, and Disposal
    of Medications

Sources of Drugs
Drug Actions
  Pharmacodynamics
  Pharmacokinetics
  Drug Interactions
  Side Effects and Allergies

Sources of Information
Prescriptions
  Refilling Prescriptions

Learning Outcomes

Cognitive Domain

Note: AAMA/CAAHEP 2008 Standards are italicized.

1. Spell and define key terms
2. *Describe the relationship between anatomy and physiology of all body systems and medications used for treatment in each*
3. Identify chemical, trade, and generic drug names
4. *Discuss all levels of governmental legislation and regulation as they apply to medical assisting practice, including FDA and DEA regulations*
5. Explain the various drug actions and interactions including pharmacodynamics and pharmacokinetics
6. *Identify the classifications of medications, including desired effects, side effects, and adverse reactions*

7. Name the sources for locating information on pharmacology

Affective Domain

Note: AAMA/CAAHEP 2008 Standards are italicized.

1. *Apply critical thinking skills in performing patient assessment and care*
2. *Demonstrate sensitivity to patient rights*

ABHES Competencies

1. Properly utilize PDR, drug handbook, and other drug references to identify a drug's classification, usual dosage, usual side effects, and contradictions
2. Identify and define common abbreviations that are accepted in prescription writing
3. Understand legal aspects of writing prescriptions, including federal and state laws

Key Terms

allergy	contraindications	pharmacodynamics	side effect
anaphylaxis	drug	pharmacokinetics	synergism
antagonism	generic name	pharmacology	trade name
chemical name	interactions	potentiation	

As a clinical medical assistant, you may be responsible for administering medications under the supervision of the physician. It is important that you acquire knowledge of medications, their uses and potential abuses, range of dosages, methods of administration, and adverse effects. **Pharmacology** is the term given to the study of drugs and their actions, dosages, and side effects. A **drug** is a chemical substance that affects body function or functions. Medications are available in many forms and are administered in various ways to produce therapeutic effects.

COG Medication Names

Most medications have a **chemical name**, a **generic name**, and a **trade name** (Box 8-1). The chemical name is the first name given to any medication. It identifies the chemical components of the drug. The generic name is assigned to the medication during research and development. When the drug is available for commercial use and distribution by the original manufacturer, it is given a brand, or trade, name. The trade name is registered by the U.S. Patent Office and has the official trademark symbol (™) after its name. After the patent expires, any other company that manufactures the medication may assign its own trade name to the generic equivalent. The first letter of a trade name is always capitalized; generic names begin with lowercase letters.

Drugs can be classified according to their actions and effects on the body. Table 8-1 lists some commonly used drugs, prescription and nonprescription, and their classifications.

CHECKPOINT QUESTION

1. What is the difference between a drug's chemical name and trade name?

COG Legal Regulations

Food and Drug Administration

Consumers in the United States are protected by federal regulations regarding the production, prescribing, or dispensing of medications. In 1906, the Pure Food and Drug Act was passed. After being amended in 1938, it required that the safety of a drug be proved before distribution to the public. The amended law was renamed the Federal Food, Drug, and Cosmetic Act. In 1952, the Durham-Humphrey Amendment banned many drugs from being dispensed without a prescription. The Kefauver-Harris Amendment of 1962 required testing of prescription and nonprescription medications for effectiveness before their release for sale. The U.S. Food and Drug Administration (FDA) was established to regulate the manufacture and distribution of drugs and food products and to ensure accuracy in the ingredients listed on the labels of food and drug products.

Drug Enforcement Agency

In 1970, the Controlled Substances Act was passed to regulate the manufacture and distribution of drugs whose use may result in dependency or abuse. This act also requires that anyone who manufactures, prescribes, administers, or dispenses controlled substances register with the United States Attorney General under the Bureau of Narcotics and Dangerous Drugs (BNDD). The Drug Enforcement Agency (DEA) is a branch of the

BOX 8-1

DRUG NAMES

Chemical Name	7-chloro-1,3-dihydro-1-methyl-5-phenyl-2H-1,4-benzodiaxe-pin-2-one
Trade Name	Valium™
Generic Name	Diazepam

TABLE 8-1	Classifications of Drugs	
Therapeutic Classification	**Effect or Action/Uses**	**Common Examples**
Adrenergic blocking agents	Affect the alpha receptors of adrenergic nerves	Metoprolol tartrate (Lopressor™), propranolol hydrochloride (Inderal™)
Adrenergics	Mimic the activity of the sympathetic nervous system	Epinephrine (Adrenaline™), ephedrine sulfate
Analgesics	Used to relieve pain	Aspirin, acetaminophen (Tylenol™), codeine
Antacids	Neutralize or reduce the acidity of the stomach	Magnesium (Milk of Magnesia™), calcium carbonate (Tums™)
Anthelmintics	Kills parasitic worms	Piperazine citrate, mebendazole (Vermox™)
Antianginal agents	Promote vasodilation hydrochloride	Nitroglycerine, diltiazem (Cardizem™)
Antianxiety agents	Act on subcortical areas of the brain to relieve symptoms of anxiety	Alprazolam (Xanax™), chlordiazepoxide (Librium™), diazepam (Valium™)
Antiarrhythmics	Various actions and effects	Disopyramide (Norpace™), procainamide hydrochloride (Pronestyl™), esmolol (Brevibloc™)
Antibiotics	Destroy, interrupt, or interfere with the growth of microorganisms	Penicillin, ampicillin, cefaclor, tetracycline
Anticoagulants and thrombolytics	Used to prevent the formation of blood clots or dissolve blood clots	Heparin sodium, streptokinase (Streptase™)
Anticonvulsants	Reduce the excitability of the brain	Phenobarbital, phenytoin (Dilantin™)
Antidepressants	Various actions	Amitriptyline hydrochloride (Elavil™), fluoxetine hydrochloride (Prozac™)
Antidiarrheals	Decrease intestinal peristalsis	Loperamide hydrochloride (Imodium A-D™)
Antiemetic agents	Prevents nausea and vomiting	Dimenhydrinate (Dramamine™), promethazine hydrochloride (Phenergan™)
Antifungals	Destroy or retard the growth of fungi	Ketoconazole (Nizoral™), miconazole nitrate (Monistat 3™ or 7™)
Antihistamines	Counteracts the effects of histamine on body organs and structures	Chlorpheniramine maleate (Chlor-Trimeton™), diphenhydramine hydrochloride (Benadryl™)
Antihypertensives	Increase the size of arterial blood vessels	Chlorpheniramine maleate (Aldomet™), prazosin (Minipres™)
Anti-inflammatory agents	Reduce irritation and swelling of tissues	Aspirin, ibuprofen (Motrin™), naproxen (Naprosyn™)
Antineoplastic agents	Slow the rate of tumor growth	Cyclophosphamide (Cytoxan™)
Antipsychotics	Exact mechanism not understood; used to treat psychoses	Thorazine, Haldol
Antipyretics	Decrease body temperature	Aspirin, acetaminophen (Tylenol™)
Antitussives, mucolytics, and expectorants	Relieve coughing, loosen respiratory secretions, or aid in the removal of thick secretions	Codeine sulfate, Benylin, Entex
Antivirals	Inhibit viral replication	Acyclovir (Zovirax™), AZT
Bronchodilators	Dilate the bronchi	Albuterol sulfate (Ventolin™), metaproterenol (Alupent™)

TABLE 8-1	Classifications of Drugs *(continued)*	
Therapeutic Classification	**Effect or Action/Uses**	**Common Examples**
Cardiotonics	Increase the force of the myocardium	Digoxin (Lanoxin™), milrinone (Primacor™)
Cholinergic blocking agents	Affect the autonomic nervous system	Atropine sulfate, scopolamine hydrobromide
Cholinergics	Mimic the activity of the parasympathetic nervous system	Neostigmine (Prostigmin™), pilocarpine hydrochloride
Decongestants	Reduce swelling of nasal passages	Pseudoephedrine hydrochloride (Sudafed™)
Diuretics	Increase the secretion of urine by the kidneys	Furosemide (Lasix™), chlorothiazide (Diuril™)
Emetics	Promote vomiting	Ipecac syrup
Histamine H_2 antagonists	Inhibit the action of histamine at the H_2 receptor cells of the stomach	Cimetidine (Tagamet™), ranitidine (Zantac™)
Hormones, female	Used to prevent symptoms of menopause	Estradiol (Estraderm™), medroxyprogesterone acetate (Provera™)
Hormones, male	Androgen therapy to treat testosterone deficiency	Fluoxymesterone (Halotestin™)
Immunologic agents (vaccines)	Stimulate the immune response to create protection against disease	Pneumococcal vaccine, influenza virus vaccine, diphtheria and tetanus toxoid
Insulin and oral hypoglycemics	Used to control diabetes	NPH and ultralente insulin, tolbutamide (Orinase™), glipizide (Glucotrol™)
Sedatives and hypnotics	Sedatives relax and calm; hypnotics induce sleep	Butabarbital sodium, temazepam (Restoril™)
Stimulants	Increase activity of the central nervous system	Doxapram hydrochloride (Dopram™), amphetamine sulfate
Thyroid and antithyroid agents	Used to increase or decrease the amount of thyroid hormone produced	Levothyroxine sodium (T_4; Levothroid™)

Summarized from Scherer JC, Roach SS. Introductory Clinical Pharmacology, 5th ed. Philadelphia: Lippincott-Raven Publishers, 1996.

Department of Justice (DOJ) and is designated to exercise strong regulatory control over all drugs listed by the BNDD. This authority extends to prescribing, refilling, and storing controlled substances in the medical office. The DEA is concerned with controlled substances only; medications not subject to abuse are not regulated by this agency.

As a medical assistant, you may be responsible for maintaining or reminding the physician about professional records and licensure, including registration with the DEA. When the physician registers with the U.S. Attorney General under the BNDD, a registration number (DEA number) is issued. Physicians are registered for 3 years after application and acceptance. The DEA does not take responsibility if the physician's registration expires. The registration retires with the physician; it does not stay with the medical office.

The DEA is also responsible for revising the list of drugs in the Schedule of Controlled Substances (Table 8-2). These substances have been identified as having a potential for abuse and dependency. Drug dependence, sometimes referred to as addiction, can be either psychological, physical, or both. A patient who has developed physical dependence on a drug will have mild to severe physiologic symptoms that gradually decrease in intensity after the drug is stopped. Patients who are psychologically dependent have acquired a need for the feeling brought on by the drug. Patients who are prescribed controlled substances must be monitored closely for signs of physical or psychological dependence.

Controlled substances in Schedule II are received from suppliers using a Federal Triplicate Order Form DEA 222. Schedules III, IV, and V do not require triplicate

TABLE 8-2	Controlled Substances	
Schedule	**Description**	**Examples**
I	These drugs have the highest potential for abuse and have no currently accepted medicinal use in the U.S. There are no accepted safety standards for use of these drugs or substances even under medical supervision, although some are used experimentally in carefully controlled research projects.	*Opium, marijuana, lysergic acid diethylamide (LSD), peyote, mescaline*
II	These drugs have a high potential for abuse. They have a current accepted medicinal use in the U.S., but with severe restrictions. Abuse of these drugs can lead to dependence, either psychological or physiologic. Schedule II drugs require a written prescription and cannot be refilled or called into the pharmacy by the medical office. Only in extreme emergencies may the physician call in the prescription. A handwritten prescription must be presented to the pharmacist within 72 hours.	*Morphine, codeine, cocaine, Seconal™, amphetamines, Dilaudid™, Ritalin™*
III	These drugs have a limited potential for psychological or physiologic dependence. The prescription may be called in to the pharmacist by the physician and refilled up to five times in a 6-month period.	*Paregoric, Tylenol with codeine™, Fiorinal™*
IV	These drugs have a lower potential for abuse than those in Schedules II and III. They can be called into the pharmacist by a medical office employee and may be filled up to five times in a 6-month period.	*Librium™, Valium™, phenobarbital*
V	These drugs have a lower potential for abuse than those in schedules I, II, III, and IV.	*Lomotil™, Dimetane™, Expectorant DC™, Robitussin-DAC™*

Five schedules, or categories, of controlled substances were established by the Bureau of Narcotics and Dangerous Drugs. Medications in the five schedules may be revised periodically after review.

forms, but invoices for receipts of the substances must be maintained for 2 years. Box 8-2 describes how to handle inventory of controlled substances.

If controlled substances are prescribed and not administered at the office, ssome states require only that the information be recorded in the patient's chart; others require a separate file of prescription copies of controlled substances. Law enforcement officials recommend that the DEA number not be preprinted on the prescription. Officials at regional DEA offices are available to answer any questions regarding the drugs under its control. As a medical assistant, you should make sure the physician's office is on the DEA's periodic mailing list to keep abreast of changes.

 CHECKPOINT QUESTION

2. What information must be documented when a controlled substance is administered in the medical office?

BOX 8-2

HANDLING INVENTORY OF CONTROLLED SUBSTANCES

1. When you receive controlled substances, make sure that both you and a second employee sign the receipt.
2. List all controlled substances on the appropriate inventory form (see Fig. 8-1).
3. When a controlled substance leaves the medical office inventory, record the following information: drug name, patient, dose, date, ordering physician, and employee who handled the procedure.
4. Keep all controlled substance inventory forms for 2 years.
5. Ensure that controlled substances are kept in a locked safe or in a secure locked box.
6. Notify the local law enforcement agency immediately if these drugs are lost or stolen.

AFF WHAT IF?

Bob Sandler, a 38-year-old accountant, was first seen in the office 2 weeks ago for a back injury that occurred after doing some home repair work the previous weekend. At the initial visit, the physician prescribed an opioid pain medication and a muscle relaxant. Today, Mr. Sandler tells you that his medications were stolen, and he would like a refill for both. What if both drugs had a high potential for abuse and were often purchased illegally on the street? Would you suspect that the patient was selling his medication? How could you be sure that this was not occurring?

Although the medical assistant must be an advocate for the patient, he or she must also be vigilant about the possibility of drug abuse in the patient population and the community at large. It is imperative that the medical assistant gather as much information as possible about "lost" or "stolen" medications and report any illegal activities to the proper authorities. Patients who have had medications stolen that have a high abuse potential will want to report the theft to the police. Some physicians want to see a police report before issuing another prescription.

Inventory, Storage, Dispensation, and Disposal of Medications

Most medical offices store medications in the office for use during office hours or to give to patients for use at home. Often, pharmaceutical company sales representatives will leave medication samples specifically for you to dispense at the direction of the physician. In either situation, it will be your responsibility to maintain an inventory of these medications, including the amount of each drug being stored and a written record of medications taken for administration in the office or dispensed to the patient for use at home (Fig. 8-1). Medications kept in the medical office should be stored away from patients or other visitors who may come to the office. Ideally, the medication area should be locked and accessible only by authorized clinical staff. It will be your responsibility to keep this medication area clean, neat, and organized.

When disposing of medications other than controlled substances, you should follow the office policy and procedure manual. In some cases, the appropriate pharmaceutical representative may need to be notified and may advise you to place any expired medications into a container to be picked up and disposed of by the company. Never dispose of expired medications in regular trash containers. For controlled substances that need to be disposed, a witness should watch the disposal, and both parties will be required to sign appropriate DEA forms noting the name of the drug and the amount disposed.

| Controlled Substance: | Meperidine (Demerol) 50 mg Injection | | | | |
| Amount Ordered: _____ 50 mg vials/ampules | | | | | Date: _____ |

Date	Patient Name	Ordering Physician	Dose Given	Amount Discarded	Employee Signature

Figure 8-1 Controlled substance inventory form.

LEGAL TIP

REPORTING SUSPECTED ABUSE OF CONTROLLED SUBSTANCES IN THE MEDICAL OFFICE

If you suspect that a physician or any other health care professional is illegally diverting controlled substances, you have a legal and ethical responsibility to report this suspicion. Gather and document evidence and the reasons you suspect diversion of substances. You should have a clear and compelling case to present to the proper authorities, usually the local police. In addition, if a physician is involved, report this evidence to the Drug Enforcement Agency and the American Medical Association (AMA). You should also notify the state medical society. If the suspected health care worker is not a physician, report it to the appropriate supervisor or superior. Most states have programs to assist health care professionals in obtaining appropriate psychological help to deal with addiction or dependency issues. In most instances, you will remain anonymous.

COG Sources of Drugs

Drugs are available from numerous natural sources, such as plants, minerals, and animals. They may also be synthetic (prepared in the laboratory by artificial means). Table 8-3 lists a number of commonly prescribed drugs and their sources.

COG Drug Actions and Interactions

Pharmacodynamics

Pharmacodynamics is the study of the ways drugs act on the body, including the actions on specific cells, tissues, and organs. All drugs cause cellular change (drug action) and some degree of physiologic change (drug effect). An action of a local drug, such as an ointment or lotion applied to the skin, is limited to the area where it is administered. A drug administered for a systemic effect is absorbed into the blood and carried to the organ or tissue on which it will act. An example of this is antibiotic therapy for a urinary tract infection. The antibiotic tablets are taken orally, but once they are absorbed, the action takes place in the urinary bladder, where the drug destroys any microorganisms. A systemic effect can

TABLE 8-3	Common Drugs and Their Sources	
Source	**Drug**	**Use**
Plants		
Cinchona bark	Quinidine	Antiarrhythmic
Purple foxglove	Digitalis	Cardiotonic
Opium poppy	Paregoric	Antidiarrheal
	Morphine	Analgesic
	Codeine	Antitussive, analgesic
Minerals		
Magnesium	Milk of Magnesia™	Antacid, laxative
Silver	Silver nitrate	Placed in eyes of newborns to kill *Neisseria gonorrhoeae*; chemical cautery of lesions
Gold	Solganal™	Arthritis treatment
Animal Proteins		
Porcine or bovine	Insulin	Antidiabetic hormone pancreas
Porcine or bovine stomach acids	Pepsin	Digestive hormone
Animal thyroid glands	Thyroid, USP	Hypothyroidism
Synthetics		
	Demerol™	Analgesic
	Lomotil™	Antidiarrheal
	Gantrisin™	Sulfonamide
Semisynthetic		
Escherichia coli bacteria and altered DNA molecules	Humulin™	Antidiabetic hormone

be produced by administering drugs orally (by mouth), sublingually (under the tongue), rectally, by injection, transdermally (through the skin), or by inhalation (through the lungs). A number of factors can influence a drug's action in the body including:

- *Age*: Elderly people have slower metabolic processes. Age-related kidney and liver dysfunctions also extend the break down and excretion times in these patients, so it is necessary to monitor the cumulative effects of drugs in the elderly. Children may have a more immediate response to drugs and, therefore, must be assessed frequently.
- *Weight*: Many drug dosages are calculated and administered according to the patient's weight. As a general rule, the larger the patient, the greater the dose; however, individual sensitivity to the effects of drugs should be taken into consideration.
- *Sex*: Women may react differently to certain drugs than men because of the ratio of fat to body mass or fluctuating hormone levels.
- *Existing pathology*: If the body is compromised by a disease process, absorption, distribution, metabolism, and excretion may be altered.
- *Tolerance*: Some medications given over a long period of time may cause the body to become resistant to their effects, requiring larger doses to achieve the desired response.

Medical assistants should always administer medications under the direct order of a physician. Under no circumstance should the dosage be adjusted or altered unless specifically instructed to do so by the physician.

Pharmacokinetics

Pharmacokinetics is the study of the action of drugs within the body based on the route of administration, rate of absorption, duration of action, and elimination from the body. Specifically, the processes included in pharmacokinetics include absorption (getting the drug into the bloodstream), distribution (movement of the drug from the bloodstream into the cells and tissues), metabolism (the physical and chemical breakdown of drugs by the body, including the liver), and excretion (byproducts sent to the kidneys to be removed from the body). In the presence of hepatic disease, the liver may not be able to break down the drug properly, and the patient may undergo toxic effects caused by an accumulation of the drug in the liver or the bloodstream. In this situation, the drug may be noted as contraindicated by the manufacturer, or not recommended for use, in patients with a history of liver disease. Some drugs reach the kidneys relatively unchanged; these drugs can be detected in the urine during excretion, when the waste products of drug metabolism are eliminated from the body. However, if the kidneys are compromised by

disease, medication may not be properly eliminated, adding to the danger of a cumulative, or building, effect and possible toxicity or poisoning.

 CHECKPOINT QUESTION

3. Why should pharmacokinetics be taken into consideration before administering medications?

Drug Interactions

When two or more drugs are taken simultaneously, one drug may increase, decrease, or cancel the effects of the other. These **interactions** may occur with prescribed drugs, over-the-counter medications, herbal or other natural supplements, and alcohol consumption. These interactions must always be taken into account when prescribing medications, administering medications, obtaining a medication history, or educating a patient about taking medications. Types of interactions include **synergism** (two drugs working together), **antagonism** (an effect in which one drug decreases the effect of another), and **potentiation** (occurs when one drug prolongs or multiplies the effect of another drug). Physicians prescribing two or more drugs may be using these drug interactions to cause a desired effect. An example of this is use of a muscle relaxant and a pain medication to reduce the pain associated with an injury to a muscle or muscle group. However, some drug interactions produce undesirable effects. For example, antacids taken to relieve symptoms of indigestion may prevent absorption of antibiotics, such as tetracycline (antagonism), while sedatives and barbiturates taken together can cause central nervous system depression (synergism). Table 8-4 lists other important drug-related terms you should know.

 PATIENT EDUCATION

FOOD–DRUG INTERACTION

Many medications interact with food. Some medications are best absorbed when taken on an empty stomach. Two such medications are the antibiotics ampicillin and nafcillin (Unipen™). Other medications should be taken with food to decrease the potential for stomach upset. These include ibuprofen (Motrin™), an analgesic and anti-inflammatory); amoxicillin, an antibiotic; and verapamil (Calan™), a heart medication. Certain medications interact with specific types of food. For example, green leafy vegetables can interact with Coumadin, an anticoagulant, and make the patient's bleeding time increase. Also, grapefruit juice interacts with atorvastatin (Lipitor™), a medication used to lower

(continued)

TABLE 8-4	Drug-Related Terms to Know
Term	**Meaning**
Therapeutic classification	States purpose for the drug's use (e.g., cardiotonic, anti-infective, antiarrthymic).
Teratogenic category	Relates the level of risk to fetal or maternal health. These rank from Category A through D, with increasing danger at each level. Category X indicates that the particular drug should never be given during pregnancy.
Indications	Gives diseases for which the particular drug would be prescribed.
Contraindications	Indicates conditions or instances for which the particular drug should not be used.
Adverse reactions	Refers to undesirable side effects of a particular drug.
Hypersensitivity	Refers to an excessive reaction to a particular drug; also known as a drug allergy. The body must build this response; the first exposures may or may not indicate that a problem is developing.
Idiosyncratic reaction	Refers to an abnormal or unexpected reaction to a drug peculiar to the individual patient; not technically an allergy.

blood cholesterol levels, to reduce its efficacy. It is important for patients to know about any food–drug interaction that may affect them. Information about food and drug interactions can be found in most pharmacology books. You will need to learn as much as you can about the medications that are commonly prescribed by the physician with whom you are working.

Side Effects and Allergies

When gathering a patient's medical history, you must always ask about allergies of any sort, particularly allergies to medications. A drug **allergy** is a reaction such as hives, dyspnea, or wheezing. In addition, the allergic reaction **anaphylaxis** can be life threatening. Allergic reactions can be immediate or delayed 2 hours or longer, depending on the route of administration; however, many allergic reactions occur within minutes if the medication is administered by injection. The medical assistant must interview the patient carefully about symptoms of allergies and note in the medical record the names of any medications that produce true allergic symptoms. Drug allergies should always be noted prominently on the front of the patient's medical record and on each page of the medication record. Because of the possibility of an anaphylactic reaction, patients should never be given medications that they have had an allergic reaction to in the past. You should always check the chart and ask the patient before administering any medications in the medical office as an additional safety measure.

Many patients state that they have an allergy to certain medications when in fact the reaction was a **side effect.**

Side effects are reactions to medications that are predictable (as noted by the manufacturer of the medication) and that occur in some patients who take the medication. For example, some medications may cause nausea unless taken with food, and in this case, nausea may be listed by the manufacturer as a side effect. Other medications may cause drowsiness or dryness of the mouth. While side effects are often annoying, they are not life threatening and should not be noted on the patient's allergy list.

If a patient is receiving allergy medications or any medication that has a high incidence of allergic reactions (e.g., penicillin), the patient should wait for 20 to 30 minutes and be rechecked before leaving the office. Some offices require all patients receiving injections to wait for a specific amount of time (15 to 20 minutes) before leaving the office. Always follow the policies of the medical office with regard to administering medications.

 CHECKPOINT QUESTION

4. How does synergism differ from antagonism?

COG Sources of Information

The *Physician's Desk Reference* (PDR) is widely used as a reference for drugs in current use. It is intended for physicians, but since the medical assistant must know about various medications administered in the office, the PDR is a valuable resource for anyone, including the medical assistant, to use before administering medications (Fig. 8-2). This resource is clearly written to identify a drug's chemical name, brand name or names, and generic name. It also lists the properties, indications, side effects, **contraindications,** dosages, and so on.

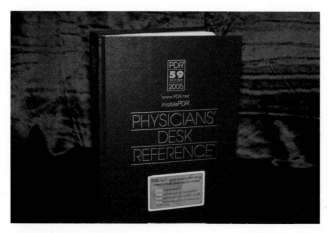

Figure 8-2 The PDR.

One section of the PDR contains pictures of various medications. This book is sometimes distributed to physicians free of charge; however, it is also available for use in libraries and for purchase in bookstores.

The *United States Pharmacopeia Dispensing Information* (USPDI) consists of two paperback volumes providing drug information for the health care provider. It defines drug sources, chemistry, physical properties, tests for identity, storage, and dosage. The USPDI does not contain photographs of the medications and must be purchased by the physician.

The *American Hospital Formulary Service* (AHFS), which is distributed to practicing physicians, contains concise information arranged according to drug classifications. The *Compendium of Drug Therapy* is published annually and is also distributed to physicians. It includes photographs of the drugs and phone numbers of major pharmaceutical companies and poison control centers.

COG Prescriptions

Medications may be administered (given in the office), dispensed (a supply given for later use), or prescribed (a

written order to be filled by a pharmacist). You may be permitted to complete the prescription form and obtain the physician's signature if directed to do so by the physician. An established protocol and traditional form must be followed when filling out prescriptions:

Line 1. *Date.* Prescriptions must be filled within 6 months of the date of issuance.

Line 2. *Patient's name and address.* The pharmacist needs this information to fill the prescription.

Line 3. *Superscription.* The symbol R_x is found at the top left of the blank prescription pad. Literally it means recipe, or "take thou."

Line 4. *Inscription.* This includes the name of the medication, the desired form (e.g., liquid, tablet, capsule), and the strength (e.g., 250 mg, 500 mL).

Line 5. *Subscription.* This states the amount to be dispensed (e.g., 60 tablets, 120 mL).

Line 6. *Signature.* This section notes any instructions for taking the medication (e.g., with meals, three times a day, four times a day).

Line 7. *Refills.* The number of times a prescription can be refilled should be indicated on the prescription and is generally no more than 5 times within 6 months. If no refills are indicated, the word none should be circled, or 0 should be written in.

Line 8. *Physician's signature.* The physician is responsible for prescriptions written in his or her office and should check and sign all prescriptions.

Line 9. *Generic.* Some physicians and insurance companies allow generic substitutes for some medications but not others. Note on the prescription whether generic substitutions can be made. If the physician does not want a specific medication substituted with a generic drug, "DAW" can be written on the prescription, which means "dispense as written."

All prescribed medications must be documented in full in the patient's record (Fig. 8-3). Prescriptions that are called or faxed to the pharmacist must also be

DATE	TIME	ORDERS
7/5/XX	1000	Prescription for ampicillin 250mg, p.o., qid X7 days as ordered by Dr. Smith.
		Sally Smith, CMA

Figure 8-3 Documentation of a prescribed medication in a patient record.

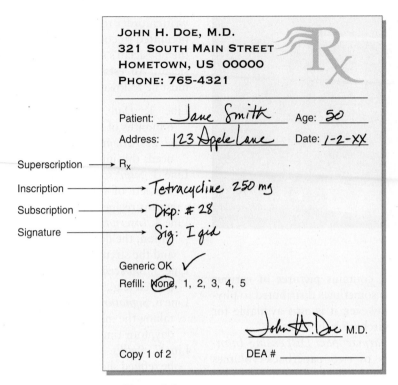

JOHN H. DOE, M.D.
321 SOUTH MAIN STREET
HOMETOWN, US 00000
PHONE: 765-4321

Patient: _Jane Smith_   Age: _50_
Address: _123 Apple Lane_   Date: _1-2-XX_

Superscription ──→ R~x~

Inscription ──────→ Tetracycline 250 mg

Subscription ─────→ Disp: # 28

Signature ────────→ Sig: I qid

Generic OK ✓
Refill: None, 1, 2, 3, 4, 5

John H. Doe M.D.

Copy 1 of 2   DEA # _____

Figure 8-4 Prescription form.

documented. The chart is a legal document and may be called into court in the event of legal action. If the medication order is not recorded, it will be presumed that the medication was never ordered. Figure 8-4 shows a sample prescription form.

Refilling Prescriptions

In most situations, a patient needing one or more prescriptions refilled will be required to make an appointment to see the physician, especially if the medications are controlled substances. Occasionally, a patient may phone the office requesting an emergency refill for a medication that is prescribed to be taken daily but has no additional refills noted on the bottle by the pharmacist. You should pull the patient's chart and check with the physician before calling any prescriptions into the pharmacy. This is also true if the pharmacist calls the medical office requesting the refill for the patient. Always check with the physician before authorizing the refill of any medication.

Some drugs, such as digoxin, have a cumulative effect and may become toxic if blood levels are not monitored closely. For this reason, it is important that you be familiar with the medications prescribed by the physician and promptly schedule any laboratory tests ordered by the physician. In addition, you should be vigilant about notifying the physician with the results of any patient laboratory blood tests that may be ordered to monitor the effects of medications. Patients who request phone refills for medications that need blood monitoring should be encouraged to comply with the physician's recommendations for such laboratory tests. It will be your responsibility to help patients understand the importance of maintaining therapeutic blood levels of these medications.

 CHECKPOINT QUESTION

5. What does the superscription on the prescription indicate, and how does it differ from the subscription?

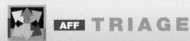 **TRIAGE**

Three patients have called the office asking you for prescription refills. It is 10 a.m. What is the correct priority order for looking at the patient's medical record and calling the pharmacy for a refill?

A. A 52-year-old patient says she went to take her methyldopa (Aldomet™) this morning but was out of it. She takes it every morning at 9:00 for her blood pressure.

B. A mother says her 3-year-old son spilled the bottle of ampicillin on the floor. The next dose is due at 2:00 this afternoon.

(continued)

C. A 66-year-old patient says she is out of her sleeping pills. She wants a refill for temazepam (Restoril™).

How do you sort these patients? Which prescription should be called in to the pharmacy first? Second? Third?

Important: Before calling any medication refill into the pharmacy, you must look at the patient's medical record and be sure there are refill orders on the chart. Also, you must follow your office's policy on prescription refills.

Patient A should be done first; it is important that blood pressure medications be taken at the same time every day. Patient B is next so that the 2:00 pm dose is not missed. Patient C's prescription should be handled last.

español SPANISH TERMINOLOGY

Tome este medicamento tres veces al día.
Take this medicine 3 times a day.

Debe ir a la farmacia para conseguir este medicamento.
Go to the pharmacy to get this medicine.

¿Ha tomado algun medicamento o remedio para aliviar su malestar?
Have you taken any medications or remedies for this (illness)?

Esta medicina puede provocarle cansancio.
This medicine may make you tired.

No maneje si está tomando este medicamento.
Do not drive while taking this medicine.

MEDIA MENU

- **Student Resources on thePoint**
  - **Animation: Drug Absorption**
  - **Animation: Drug Distribution**
  - **Animation: Drug Binding**
  - **Animation: Drug Excretion**
  - **CMA/RMA Certification Exam Review**
- **Internet Resources**

  The Food and Drug Administration
  http://www.fda.gov/medwatch

  The *Physician's Desk Reference*
  http://www.pdr.net

  MedlinePlus, National Institutes of Health
  http://www.nlm.nih.gov/medlineplus/druginformation.html

  National Center of Complementary and Alternative Medicine
  http://nccam.nih.gov

  MedicineNet
  http://www.MedicineNet.com

  American Society of Health-System Pharmacists
  http://www.ashp.org

- Medications are administered, dispensed, or prescribed to patients to produce therapeutic effects. They are available in many forms and can be administered in various ways.
- Some medications, called controlled substances, may result in dependency and abuse. These drugs are strictly regulated by the federal government.
- As a medical assistant, you will need to keep current on the legal regulations concerning the manufacture, sale, and prescribing of medications. You must also understand the actions, effects, and interactions of drugs to carry out a physician's medication orders.
- Whether administering medications in the office or refilling a prescription order to a pharmacy over the phone, you must always have a physician order. Never recommend any medication, even an over-the-counter remedy, to a patient.

Warm Ups for Critical Thinking

1. What type of information regarding medications do patients need to know? Is there anything they do not need to know?
2. Using a drug reference book such as the PDR, look up a medication that you have taken. What are the medication's trade and generic names? Are there any side effects or contraindications? Explain what you learned about this medication that you did not already know.
3. How would you interact with a patient who insists that he/she should leave immediately after receiving an injection when the office policy states that patients should remain in the office for 15 minutes after receiving an injection?
4. Describe how you could keep prescription pads secure during the typical day working in the medical office.

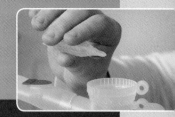

Outline

**Medication Administration
  Basics**
Safety Guidelines
Seven Rights for Correct
  Medication Administration
Systems of Measurement

**Routes of Medication
  Administration**
Oral, Sublingual, and Buccal
  Routes
Parenteral Administration
Other Medication Routes

**Principles of Intravenous
  Therapy**
Intravenous Equipment
Troubleshooting Problems

Learning Outcomes

Cognitive Domain

*Note: AAMA/CAAHEP 2008 Standards are
italicized.*

1. Spell and define the key terms
2. *Demonstrate knowledge of basic math computations*
3. *Apply mathematical computations to solve equations*
4. *Identify measurement systems*
5. *Define basic units of measurement in metric, apothecary, and household systems*
6. *Convert among measurement systems*
7. *Identify both abbreviations and symbols used in calculating medication dosages*
8. List the safety guidelines for medication administration
9. Explain the differences between various parenteral and nonparenteral routes of medication administration
10. Describe the parts of a syringe and needle and name those parts that must be kept sterile
11. List the various needle lengths, gauges, and preferred site for each type of injection

12. Compare the types of injections and locate the sites where each may be administered safely
13. Describe principles of intravenous therapy

Psychomotor Domain

*Note: AAMA/CAAHEP 2008 Standards are
italicized.*

1. Administer oral medications (Procedure 9-1)
2. Prepare injections (Procedure 9-2)
3. *Prepare proper dosages of medication for administration*
4. Administer an intradermal injection (Procedure 9-3)
5. Administer a subcutaneous injection (Procedure 9-4)
6. Administer an intramuscular injection (Procedure 9-5)
7. Administer an intramuscular injection using the Z-track method (Procedure 9-6)
8. *Administer parenteral medications (excluding IV)*
9. *Select proper sites for administering parenteral medication*

10. Apply transdermal medications (Procedure 9-7)
11. Obtain and prepare an intravenous site (Procedure 9-8)
12. *Practice standard precautions*
13. *Document accurately in the patient record*

Affective Domain

Note: AAMA/CAAHEP 2008 Standards are italicized.

1. *Apply critical thinking skills in performing patient assessment and care*
2. *Verify ordered doses/dosages prior to administration*
3. *Show awareness of patients' concerns regarding their perceptions related to the procedure being performed*
4. *Demonstrate empathy in communicating with patients, family, and staff*
5. *Apply active listening skills*
6. *Use appropriate body language and other nonverbal skills in communicating with patients, family, and staff*
7. *Demonstrate awareness of territorial boundaries of the person with whom you are communicating*

8. *Demonstrate sensitivity appropriate to the message being delivered*
9. *Demonstrate recognition of the patient's level of understanding in communications*
10. *Recognize and protect personal boundaries in communicating with others*
11. *Demonstrate respect for individual diversity, incorporating awareness of one's own biases in areas including gender, race, religion, age, and economic status*

ABHES Competencies

1. Demonstrate accurate occupational math and metric conversions for proper medication administration
2. Apply principles of aseptic techniques and infection control
3. Maintain medication and immunization records
4. Use standard precautions
5. Prepare and administer oral and parenteral medications as directed by physician
6. Document accurately
7. Dispose of biohazardous materials

Key Terms

ampule	induration	ophthalmic	vial
apothecary system	infiltration	otic	Z-track method
buccal	Mantoux test	parenteral	
diluent	metric system	sublingual	
gauge	nebulizer	topical	

Administering medications in most physician offices may be an important part of the clinical duties assigned to medical assistants. Become familiar with the laws in the state where you live—some states do not allow medical assistants to administer medications. However, there are many states that do permit medical assistants to administer medications. Medical assistants living in those states have a responsibility to perform these skills with accuracy and competence. This chapter gives detailed information about the preparation and administration of medications in the medical office.

COG Medication Administration Basics

Before administering any medications in the medical office, you should be familiar with the medication ordered by the physician and the procedures necessary to administer the drug accurately and safely. As a clinical medical assistant, you must look up any drugs you are not familiar with to determine the drug classification, the usual dosage, and the route of administration. In addition, you should be thoroughly familiar with the terminology, abbreviations, symbols, and signs used in prescribing, administering, and documenting medications. The abbreviations listed in Table 9-1 are most commonly used and should be memorized. The abbreviations listed in red have been identified as potentially dangerous to use by The Joint Commission and may result in medication errors.

Safety Guidelines

To ensure safety when administering medications, follow these guidelines:

1. Know the policies of your office regarding the administration of medications.
2. Give only the medications that the physician has ordered in writing. Do not accept verbal orders.
3. Check with the physician if you have any doubt about a medication or an order.
4. Avoid conversation and other distractions while preparing and administering medications. It is important to remain attentive during this task.
5. Work in a quiet, well-lighted area.
6. Check the label when taking the medication from the shelf, when preparing it, and when replacing it on the shelf or disposing of the empty container. This is known as the three checks for safe administration.
7. Place the order and the medication side by side to compare for accuracy.
8. Check the strength of the medication (e.g., 250 versus 500 mg) and the route of administration.
9. Read labels carefully. Do not scan labels or medication orders.
10. Check the patient's medical record for allergies to the actual medication or its components before administering.
11. Check the medication's expiration date. Outdated medications should be discarded according to office policy and should never be administered to a patient.
12. Be alert for color changes, precipitation, odor, or any indication that the medication's properties have changed. If the medication has changed in consistency, color, or odor, discard it appropriately.
13. Measure exactly. There should be no bubbles in liquid medication.
14. Have sharps containers as close to the area of use as possible.
15. Put on gloves for all procedures that might result in contact with blood or body fluids.
16. Stay with the patient while he or she takes oral medication. Watch for any reaction and record the patient's response.
17. Never return a medication to the container after it is poured or removed.
18. Never recap, bend, or break a used needle.
19. Never give a medication poured or drawn up by someone else.
20. Never leave the medication cabinet unlocked when not in use.
21. Never give keys for the medication cabinet to an unauthorized person. Limit access to the medication cabinet by limiting access to the cabinet keys.
22. Never document medication given by someone else, and do not ask someone else to document medication that you have administered.

When the physician writes a prescription for a medication, you will often be the health care provider who gives this prescription to the patient and records that this medication was ordered on the medication record in the patient health record (see Legal Tip box). In some cases, the physician may ask you to dispense a sample of the prescribed medication provided by the pharmaceutical representative to the patient until the prescription can be filled later at the pharmacy. Once the patient takes the prescription to the pharmacy, the pharmacy will fill the prescription according to the physician orders. In addition, the pharmacist will give the patient written information about taking the medication and any side effects that might be encountered. Also, the pharmacist will note any specific instructions and warnings on the medication container. Patients should always be encouraged to contact the office for any questions or problems concerning medications ordered by the physician.

 CHECKPOINT QUESTION

1. When are the "three checks" for safe medication administration performed?

Seven Rights for Correct Medication Administration

Medication errors should not occur during careful preparation or administration. By observing the seven rights during medication administration, you will eliminate the potential for many errors. The seven rights are as follows:

1. Right patient. Ask the patient to state his or her name. Some patients will answer to any name, so simply saying the name is not assurance that you have the correct patient.
2. Right time. Most medications ordered to be given in the office are to be given before the patient leaves. Some patients may have to be told when the next dose is due.
3. Right dose. Check doses carefully. Many medications come in various strengths.

TABLE 9-1   Abbreviations

The abbreviations in red have been identified as potentially dangerous to use by The Joint Commission and may result in medication errors. However, most physician offices are not accredited by The Joint Commission and may use these abbreviations.

Abbreviation	Meaning	Abbreviation	Meaning
ac	before meals	NS	normal saline
ad lib	as desired	OD	right eye
AM, am, A.M.	morning	OS	left eye
amp	ampule	OU	both eyes
amt	amount	oz	ounce
AD	**right ear**	p	after
AS	**left ear**	pc	after meals
AU	**both ears**	PM, pm, P.M.	afternoon or evening
aq	aqueous	po, PO	by mouth
bid	twice a day	prn, PRN	whenever necessary
c̄	with	q	every
cap	capsule	**qd**	**every day**
cc	**cubic centimeter**	qh	every hour
DC, disc, d/c	**discontinue**	q2h	every 2 hours
disp	dispense	q3h	every 3 hours
dl, dL	deciliter	qid	four times a day
elix	elixir	**qod**	**every other day**
et	and	qs	quantity sufficient
ext	extract	qt	quart
fl, fld	fluid	R	right, rectal
g, gm	gram	Rx	take, prescribe
gr	**grain**	s̄	without
gt(t)	drop(s)	SC, subcu, S/Q, SQ	subcutaneously
h, hr	hour	Sig	label
hs, HS	hour of sleep	SL	sublingual
Id, ID	intradermal	ss	one-half
IM	intramuscular	stat, STAT	immediately
IV	intravenous	supp	suppository
Kg	kilogram	syr	syrup
L, l	liter	tab	tablet
lb	pound	T, tb, tbs, tbsp	tablespoon
mcg, μg	**microgram**	t, tsp	teaspoon
mEq	milliequivalent	tid	three times a day
ml, mL	milliliter	tinc	tincture
NaCl	sodium chloride	**u**	**units**
NKA	no known allergies	ung	ointment
NPO	nothing by mouth		

4. Right route. Some medications are prepared for administration by a variety of routes. Is it oral, **parenteral, otic, ophthalmic,** or **topical**?
5. Right drug. Many medication names are very much alike; for instance Orinase™ and Ornade™ may be confused if you are not careful. Always look up unfamiliar medications in a drug reference book such as the *Physician's Desk Reference* (PDR).
6. Right technique. Check how the medication is to be given, such as orally and with or without food. Intramuscular, subcutaneous, and intradermal injections should be given only after carefully choosing a site and with the correct procedure.
7. Right documentation. The medical record is a legal document. Make sure that the medication is documented after it is administered (not before) and that you have documented it in the correct medical record. All medications given in the medical office must be documented immediately with the name of the medication, the dose, route, and site (if injected), and the documentation must be signed by the medical assistant. The patient's response should be charted as well, when appropriate.

 CHECKPOINT QUESTION

2. What information should be recorded in the patient's medical record after administering any medication?

 LEGAL TIP

MEDICATION ERRORS

Even if you are extremely careful, you may make an error when administering a medication. It is imperative that you report the error to the physician and that intervention measures start immediately. The error and all corrective actions must be documented thoroughly in the patient's medical record. An incident report should be completed for the error and filed in the medical office as verification that all possible precautions were taken for the patient.

Systems of Measurement

The most common system of measurement used in the medical office is the **metric system;** however, the **apothecary system** of measurement may still used by some physicians. The household system of measurement is most often used by patients (Box 9-1). Both the apothecary and the household systems of measurement should be avoided in the medical setting, since the measurements

---

BOX 9-1

HOUSEHOLD MEASURES

Household measurements include cups, medicine droppers, teaspoons, and tablespoons. Some of the approximate equivalents to household measurements are:

1 teaspoon = 1 fluid dram = 5 mL
1 tablespoon = 1/2 fluid ounce = 4 fluid drams = 15 mL
2 tablespoons = 1 fluid ounce = 30 mL

Caution patients who will be using household measurements to avoid using table flatware and regular cups. Standard measuring spoons and cups are more accurate.

---

are not as accurate as in the metric system. While working in the clinical setting, you may find it necessary to convert from one system to another. In addition, you may be required to calculate a dose in one system of measurement using mathematical equations. It is necessary to master the elements of the systems of measurement before attempting to calculate dosages.

Metric, Household, and Apothecary

The metric system is used in the United States and throughout the world. Because the metric system is based on multiples of 10, decimals, not fractions, are used in calculating and recording dosages. In the metric system, the base unit of *length* is the *meter* (m). The base unit of *weight* is the *gram* (g or gm), and the liter (L or l) is used to measure fluid and gas volume. Prefixes used in the metric system show a fraction or multiple of the base. The following prefixes are often used:

- Micro- (0.000001)
- Milli- (0.001)
- Centi- (0.01)
- Deci- (0.1)
- Kilo- (1,000.0)

For example, using the base unit of a gram, fractional measurements are as follows:

- Microgram (mcg, μg), one-millionth of a gram (×0.000001)
- Milligram (mg), one-thousandth of a gram (×0.001)
- Kilogram (kg), 1,000 grams (×1,000.0)

Decagrams and centigrams are not used in medication administration.

With the base unit of a liter (1 L = approximately 1.06 quarts), fractional measurements in milliliters (ml, mL) are commonly used in medication administration.

TABLE 9-2	Most Commonly Used Approximate Equivalents	
Metric	**Apothecary**	**Household**
60 mg	gr i	
0.06 mL	minim i	1 drop
1.0 g	gr xv	
1.0 mL	minim xv	1/5 tsp
5.0 mL	1 dram	1 tsp
15 mL	1/2 oz	1 tbsp
30 mL	1 oz	2 tbsp
500 mL	6 oz	1 pint
1,000 mL	2 oz	1 quart

There are many discrepancies among these approximate equivalents. For example, 30 mL is the accepted equivalent for 1 oz, but 29.57 mL is the exact equivalent. Such discrepancies are inevitable when equivalencies between the two systems are not exact. The discrepancies are within a 10% margin of error, which usually is acceptable in pharmacology.

Reprinted with permission from Taylor C, Lillis C, Le Mone P. Fundamentals of Nursing: The Art and Science of Nursing Care, ed 2. Philadelphia: Lippincott, 1993:1347.

Also, 1 cubic centimeter (cc) is equivalent to 1 mL, and therefore, the measures are used interchangeably at times.

The apothecary system is used less frequently now than in the past and is gradually being replaced by the metric system. In the apothecary system, liquid measurements include drop (gt) or drops (gtt), minim (min, m), fluid dram (fl dr), fluid ounce (fl oz), pint (pt), quart (qt), and gallon (gal). Measurements for solid weights include grain (gr), dram (dr), ounce (oz), and pound (lb). Roman numerals are used for smaller numbers, and fractions may be used when necessary. Decimals are never used in the apothecary system.

The household system of measurement includes measures such as the teaspoon (tsp), tablespoon (tbsp), ounce (oz), cup (c), pint (pt), quart (qt), and pound (lb). While this system is not used in the medical office for calculating doses, patients may need to be instructed on the proper household measurement for taking medications ordered in the metric system (e.g., 5 mL is equivalent to 1 tsp). Table 9-2 lists commonly used equivalents in the metric, apothecary, and household systems of measurement.

CHECKPOINT QUESTION

3. What are three systems of measurement? Which is the most commonly used in the medical office?

Converting Between Systems of Measurement

Apothecary or Household to Metric

To convert from one system to another system, use the following rules:

- To change grains (apothecary system) to grams (metric system), divide the number of grains ordered by 15. Example: gr 30 ÷ 15 = 2 g.
- To change grains (apothecary system) to milligrams (metric system), multiply the grains by 60. Use this rule with less than 1 grain. Example: gr 1/4 × 60 = 15 mg.
- To change ounces (household) to milliliters (metric system), multiply the ounces by 30. Example: 4 oz × 30 = 120 mL.
- To change milliliters (metric system) to fluid ounces (household system), divide the milliliters by 30. Example: 150 mL ÷ 30 = 50 oz.
- To change kilograms (metric system) to pounds (household system), multiply the kilograms by 2.2. Example: 50 kg × 2.2 = 110.0 lb.
- To change pounds to kilograms (metric system), divide the pounds (household system) by 2.2. Example: 44 lb ÷ 2.2 = 20 kg.

Metric to Metric

In the metric system, it is sometimes necessary to convert measurements using the same unit of measure. For example, the physician may order 0.5 grams of medication, and the medication label reads 500 mg. To convert within the metric system, use the following rules:

- To change grams to milligrams, multiply grams by 1,000 or move the decimal point three places to the right. Example: 0.5 g × 1,000 = 500 mg.
- To change milligrams to grams, divide the milligrams by 1,000 or move the decimal point three places to the left. Example: 500 mg ÷ 1,000 = 0.5 g.
- To change milligrams to micrograms, multiply the milligrams by 1,000 or move the decimal point three places to the right. Example: 5 mg × 1,000 = 5,000 μg.
- To change micrograms to milligrams, divide the micrograms by 1,000 or move the decimal point three places to the left. Example: 500 μg ÷ 1,000 = 0.5 mg.
- To change liters to milliliters, multiply the liters by 1,000 or move the decimal point three places to the right. Example: 0.01 L × 1,000 = 10 mL.
- To change milliliters to liters, divide the milliliters by 1,000 or move the decimal point three places to the left. Example: 100 mL ÷ 1,000 = 0.1 L.

There is no conversion necessary when changing cubic centimeters to milliliters; they are approximately the same.

Calculating Adult Dosages

Administration of medication is an exact science; errors in calculation can kill the patient. Although the physician will order the amount of medication to be administered to the patient, you may have to calculate the amount of medication to withdraw into a syringe or pour into a medicine cup. In addition to the physician's order, you must also be aware of the label on the medication container (Fig. 9-1) since both the physician's order and the information on the medication label are used to calculate the amount given. There are two methods by which doses are most frequently calculated for adults: the ratio method and the formula method. Measurements must be in the same system (preferably metric) and unit before a calculation can be made. For example, if the medication is ordered in the apothecary or household system but is packaged in the metric system, you must first convert the order (apothecary or household) to the metric system. If the medication is ordered in grams but is packaged in milligrams, the ordered dose must be converted to milligrams before any calculations can be made. When using the metric system, be careful to keep the decimal point in the correct place during calculations and be sure to convert fractions to decimals.

Ratio and Proportion

When using the ratio method to calculate doses, you must use the amount of medication ordered and the information on the medication label to create a ratio.

Once the ratio has been determined, the proportion, or relationship between the two ratios, can be calculated to give you the amount of medication to administer. To calculate a dose using the ratio and proportion method, set up the problem as follows:

Dose on hand: Known quantity = Dose desired: Unknown quantity

Example 1. The physician orders erythromycin 250 mg. The label on the package reads erythromycin 100 mg/mL. The equation can be written as:

$$100 \text{ mg}: 1 \text{ mL} = 250 \text{ mg}: X$$

Multiply the extremes (first and fourth terms) = 100X
Multiply the means (second and third terms) = 250

Write the proportion as follows: 100X = 250

Divide both sides of the equal sign by 100 to solve for X.

$$250 \div 100 = 2.5$$

Therefore, you administer 2.5 mL of erythromycin for the patient to receive the 250 mg ordered by the physician. *Note:* When you document the medication after administration, the amount given is the amount ordered by the physician in milligrams, not the amount in milliliters administered.

Example 2. The physician orders phenobarbital 25 mg. On hand are 12.5-mg tablets. State the equation:

$$12.5 \text{ mg}: 1 \text{ tablet} = 25 \text{ mg}: X$$

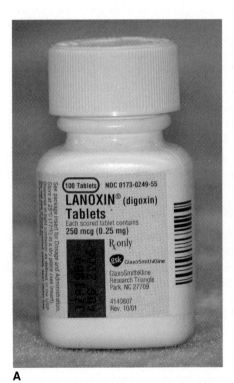

A

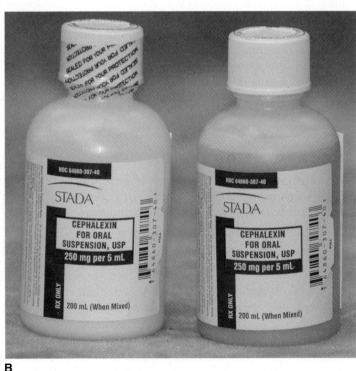

B

Figure 9-1 Medication labels include the name of the medication and the dose per unit such as (**A**) 0.25 mg per tablet or (**B**) 250 mg per 5 mL.

Multiply the extremes = 12.5X
Multiply the means = 25 mg

$$25 = 12.5X$$

Divide both sides by 12.5

$$25 \div 12.5 = 2 \text{ tablets}$$

In this example, you administer two tablets of phenobarbital to the patient and record that 25 mg was given.

The Formula Method

The formula method is written as follows:

$$(\text{Desired} \div \text{On hand}) \times \text{Quantity} = \text{Dose}$$

Example 1. The physician orders ampicillin 0.5 g. On hand, you have ampicillin 250-mg capsules. How much ampicillin should be administered? Remember, both doses must be in the same unit of measure. Convert grams in the physician's order to milligrams by multiplying the grams by 1,000 (or move the decimal point three places to the right). The answer is 0.5 g equals 500 mg. With this information, you may set up your problem:

500 mg (desired) ÷ 250 mg (on hand) × 1 (quantity) = 2 × 1 = 2

In this example, the quantity (one capsule) is how the medication (ampicillin 250 mg) comes supplied. You administer two capsules and chart that 0.5 g or 500 mg was given to the patient.

Example 2. The physician orders 0.35 g of a medication, and you have on hand a liquid form of the medication that is labeled 700 mg/mL. How many milliliters do you prepare to administer? Remember, measurements must be in equivalent units, so 0.35 g must be changed to 350 mg before setting up the formula.

$$(350 \text{ mg} \div 700 \text{ mg}) \times 1 \text{ mL} = 0.5 \text{ mL} = 0.5 \text{ mL}$$

 CHECKPOINT QUESTION

4. Before calculating a dose, what must be done with the measurements if the physician orders the medication in milligrams and the medication is supplied in grams?

Calculating Pediatric Dosages

Although several formulas may be used to calculate children's doses, one method uses the body surface area (BSA) and is considered to be the most accurate method for children up to 12 years of age or adults who are below normal percentiles for body weight. A scale known as a nomogram (Fig. 9-2) is used to estimate the BSA in square meters according to the patient's height and weight. A straight line is drawn from the

Height		Surface Area	Weight	
Feet	Centimeters	Square Meters	Pounds	Kilograms

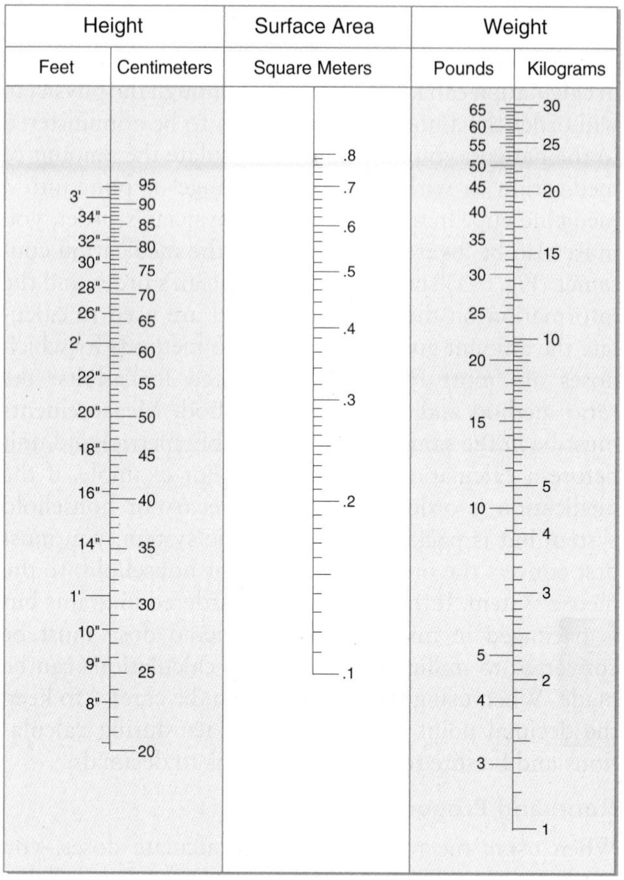

Figure 9-2 Nomogram for estimating surface area of infants and young children. To determine the surface area of the patient, draw a straight line between the point representing the height on the left vertical scale and the point representing the weight on the right vertical scale. The point at which this line intersects the middle vertical scale represents the patient's surface area in square meters.

patient's height in inches or centimeters in column 1 to the patient's weight in kilograms or pounds in column 3 (Fig. 9-3). The line intersects on the BSA column (column 2) to give the BSA of the child. Once the BSA is determined, the following formula is used to calculate the medication dosage:

$$(\text{BSA} \times \text{Adult dose}) \div 1.7 = \text{Child's dose}$$

Other rules for calculating pediatric doses include Young's rule, Clark's rule, and Fried's rule. Young's rule is used to calculate doses for children aged 12 months to 12 years. This method requires that you determine the age of the child in years and divide by the age of the child in years plus 12. This number is multiplied by the adult dose.

$$\text{Pediatric dose} = \times \text{Adult dose}$$

Clark's rule is more accurate than Young's rule because it allows for variations in body size and weight for different ages. Using Clark's rule, the weight of the child is divided by 150 (presumed weight of average

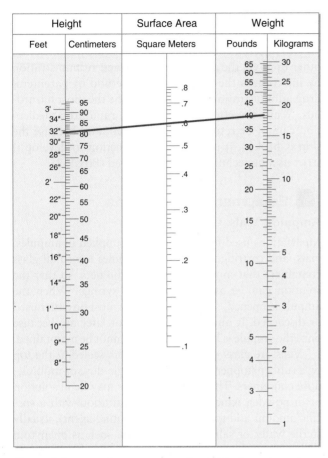

Height		Surface Area	Weight	
Feet	Centimeters	Square Meters	Pounds	Kilograms

Figure 9-3 Using the nomogram, the child who is 32 inches tall and weighs 40 pounds has a BSA of 0.6 m².

adult) and multiplied by the average adult dose to determine the pediatric dose.

$$\text{Pediatric dose} = \times \text{Adult dose}$$

Fried's rule, which is used for calculating doses for infants less than 2 years of age, bases the dose on the age of the child in months. In this case, 150 used in calculations is the age in months of a 12.5-year-old child, presuming that a child of that age would be eligible for an adult dose. Using Fried's rule, the child's age in months is divided by 150 and then multiplied by the average adult dose.

$$\text{Pediatric dose} = \times \text{Adult dose}$$

Some medications that require careful calibration are dosed per kilogram of body weight. Instructions for calculation are included in the package insert that comes with the medication or in the *Physician's Desk Reference*. For instance, the insert may state to give adults and children over 25 kg (55 lb) 500 mg of a particular medication and use the formula 25 mg/kg for children who weigh less than 25 kg. If the child weighs 20 lb, this weight must be converted to kilograms before any calculations are made. Since 1 kg is equal to 2.2 lb, the child

who weighs 20 lb also weighs 9 kg. The equation for calculating the child's dosage would be set up as follows:

$$25 \text{ mg} \times 9 \text{ kg} = 225 \text{ mg}$$

Therefore, the physician will use this calculation to determine how much medication (225 mg) is appropriate for the child who weighs 20 lb (9 kg).

CHECKPOINT QUESTION

5. When calculating how much medication to prescribe for an infant or child, which method for calculating pediatric dosages is most often used?

WHAT IF?

A child is brought to the medical office having difficulty breathing and needing emergency medications? How does the physician have time to calculate the dose for the child's body weight?

In such a situation, the physician does not have the time to perform the calculations and instead may rely on a printed graph that lists precalculated emergency drug doses or on medication reference books. There is also computer software that is available that will automatically calculate and print a list of pediatric emergency medications and their doses. In this situation, it is important to remain calm and notify emergency services as directed by the physician since these trained professionals will have the knowledge and equipment required to resuscitate a child should the emergency situation deteriorate.

Routes of Medication Administration

Medication can be administered in many ways and is chosen by the physician after considering many factors. Sometimes the route is chosen because of cost, safety, or the speed by which the drug will be absorbed into the body. Certain drugs may be administered by only one route, while others may be administered in a variety of ways. Some drugs may be toxic if given by a certain route, some may be effective only if given by a specific route, and sometimes absorption will occur only through one particular route.

Oral, Sublingual, and Buccal Routes

Of all of the medication routes, the oral route is most preferred by patients and is the easiest to administer. However, medications taken orally, or by mouth, are usually slow to take effect, and this route cannot be

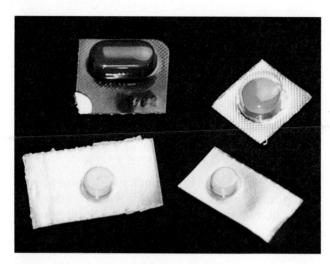

Figure 9-4 Unit dose packages.

used for unconscious patients, those with nausea and vomiting, or those who are ordered to take nothing by mouth. Drugs given orally may be administered as tablets, capsules, pills, or liquids (Procedure 9-1). Most are absorbed through the walls of the gastrointestinal tract. Drugs given orally in the medical office usually come in unit dose packs that contain the amount of the drug for a single dose (Fig. 9-4). These may be left by pharmaceutical sales representatives to be given as samples to patients. Unit dose packages are labeled with the trade name, generic name, precautions, instructions for storage, and an expiration date. Table 9-3 lists common solid and liquid forms of oral medications.

The physician may also order medications to be taken by either the **sublingual** or **buccal** routes. Medication taken sublingually is placed under the patient's tongue; it must not be swallowed. The drug is dissolved by the saliva in the mouth and is absorbed directly into the bloodstream through the oral mucosa covering the sublingual vessels. Caution the patient not to eat or drink until the medication has totally dissolved.

Medication given by the buccal route is placed in the pouch between the cheek and gum at the side of the mouth. Buccal absorption of medication occurs through the vascular oral mucosa. Although few medications are manufactured for this route, the patient must not eat or drink until the medication is completely absorbed if this method is used to administer medications.

 CHECKPOINT QUESTION

6. What are the disadvantages of the oral route for medication administration?

Parenteral Administration

If a patient cannot take medications orally, if the drug cannot be absorbed through the gastrointestinal system,

or if rapid absorption of the drug is desired, the parenteral route is used. Parenteral administration refers not only to injections but to all ways drugs are administered other than via the gastrointestinal tract. Administration by injection is the most efficient method of parenteral drug administration, but it can also be the most hazardous. While the effects may be quite rapid, the medication cannot be retrieved once injected, and because the skin is broken, it is possible for infection to develop if strict aseptic technique is not followed (Box 9-2).

 ### Equipment for Injections

Ampules, Vials, Cartridges

Medications used for injections are supplied in **ampules**, **vials**, and cartridges (Fig. 9-5). Ampules are small glass containers that must be broken at the neck so that the solution can be aspirated into the syringe. When the ampule is opened, all medication in it must be either used or discarded. It must not be saved for later use because once the ampule is broken, sterility cannot be maintained.

Vials are glass or plastic containers sealed at the top by a rubber stopper. They may be single-dose or multiple-dose containers. The contents of vials may be in solution or in powder, which requires reconstitution with a specific amount and type of **diluent** (diluting agent), usually sterile water or saline. Certain drugs, such as phenytoin (Dilantin), require a special diluent supplied by the manufacturer. When a powdered drug is reconstituted in a multiple-dose vial, the following must be written on the label:

1. Date of reconstitution
2. Initials of the person who reconstituted the drug
3. Diluent used

To reconstitute dry medication, withdraw the diluent using aseptic technique, add the diluent to the vial containing the powder, and roll the bottle between your palms to dissolve the medication completely. Shaking the vial may cause unnecessary bubbles. When the powder has completely dissolved, calculate the dose based on the amount of diluent added to the powder. The instructions from the manufacturer of the drug usually indicate how much diluent to add to the powder and the resulting concentration of the mixture necessary for calculating dosages. You should always check the vial label or manufacturer's instructions before adding the diluent to determine the resulting dosage.

Vials intended for multiple doses may hold up to 50 mL and may be used repeatedly by inserting a needle through the self-sealing rubber stopper to remove a portion of the solution. Unit dose vials usually contain 1 to 2 mL, and all of the solution is removed for a single injection.

Prefilled syringes contain a premeasured amount of medication in a disposable cartridge with a needle attached. The prefilled cartridge and needle are placed in a holder for administration (Fig. 9-6). Examples of

TABLE **9-3**	Forms of Oral Medications
Form	**Description**
Solids	
Buffered Caplet	Agents are added to decrease or counteract the medication's acidity to prevent gastric irritation.
Capsule	Powdered or granulated medication is enclosed in a gelatin capsule designed to dissolve in gastric enzymes or high in the small intestines.
Enteric Coated Tablet	A compressed dry form of a medication coated to withstand the gastric acidity and dissolve in the intestines. These may be medications that would be destroyed by the gastric enzymes or might be damaging to the gastric mucosa. Never crush or break enteric coated tablets.
Gelcap	An oil-based medication enclosed in a soft gelatin capsule.
Lozenge	A firm, compressed form of medication, usually for a local effect in the mouth or throat. Caution patients to let lozenges dissolve slowly and avoid drinking any fluids for a period of time after using the lozenge.
Powder	A finely ground form of medication; may be difficult for some patients to swallow.
Spansule or Time-Release Capsule	Gelatin capsules are filled with forms of the medication that will dissolve over a period of time rather than all at once. Never open spansules unless this is recommended by the manufacturer.
Tablet	Medication is formed into many shapes and colors for easy identification. Tablets usually dissolve high in the gastrointestinal tract. These may be broken into halves only if they have been scored for that purpose.
Liquids	
Elixir	Medication is dissolved in alcohol, and flavoring is added. These are less sweet than syrups and are usually preferred by adults. They should not be used with alcoholics or diabetics.
Emulsion	Medication is combined with water and oil. Emulsions must be thoroughly shaken to disperse the medication evenly.
Extract	This is a very concentrated form of medication made by evaporating volatile plant oils. Extracts may be administered as drops and are usually given in a liquid to disguise their strong taste.
Gel	Medication is suspended in a thin gelatin or paste base.
Suspension	Particles are dissolved in a liquid that must be shaken well before administered.
Syrup	This very sweet form of medication is used frequently for children's medications and is usually flavored in addition to having a high sugar content.

BOX 9-2

INJECTIONS: MAINTAINING STERILITY

The following parts of a hypodermic setup must be kept sterile:

- Syringe tip
- Inside of barrel
- Shaft of plunger
- Needle

prefilled cartridges and holders are the Tubex™ and the Carpuject™. After a prefilled cartridge and holder are used, only the used cartridge should be discarded in a sharps biohazard container. The holder is reusable.

Needles and Syringes

The choice of needle and syringe used for an injection depends on the type of injection and the size of the patient. The 1-mL and 3-mL hypodermic syringe are the sizes most commonly used for injections. In the medical office, syringes designed to hold 5 mL or more are

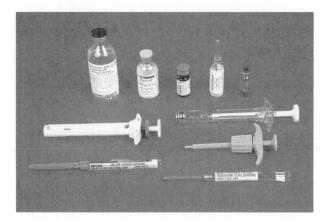

Figure 9-5 Ampules, vials, prefilled cartridges, and holders.

usually used for irrigation only, not for injections. All syringes consist of a plunger, body or barrel, flange, and tip (Fig. 9-7). Types of syringes used for parenteral administration include tuberculin, or 1-mL, syringes,

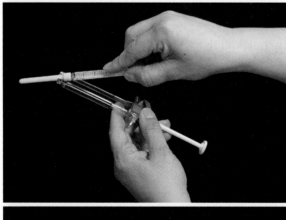

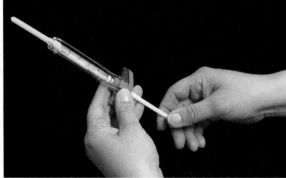

Figure 9-6 Prefilled syringes. (**A**) Prefilled medication cartridges and injector devices. (**B**) Inserting the cartridge into the injector device. (**C**) Ready for injection.

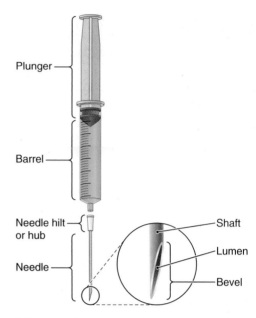

Figure 9-7 Parts of a syringe and needle. (Reprinted with permission from Cohen BJ. Medical Terminology: An Illustrated Guide, 6th Ed. Philadelphia: Lippincott Williams & Wilkins, 2011.)

3-mL syringes, and insulin syringes that are calibrated in units and are used for insulin only (Fig. 9-8).

Needle lengths vary from 3/8 inch to 1 1/2 inch for standard injections. **Gauge** refers to the diameter of the needle lumen. Needle gauge varies from 18 (large) to 30 (small); the higher the number, the smaller the gauge. Medical supply companies package hypodermic needles separately in color-coded packages (Fig. 9-9) or in color-coded envelopes with the syringe attached. The sizes are also written on the package. Choose the package with a needle length and gauge appropriate for the route of the injection. For example, an intramuscular injection for an adult requires a needle length of 1 to 1 1/2 inches, depending on the size of the patient and

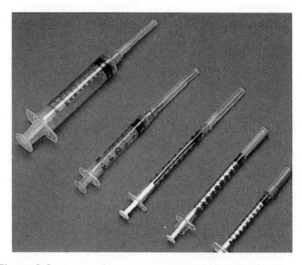

Figure 9-8 Syringes (*from top to bottom*): 10 mL, 3 mL, tuberculin or 1 mL, insulin, and low-dose insulin.

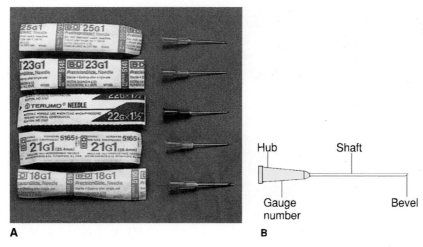

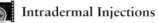

Figure 9-9 Needles. (**A**) Different gauges and lengths. (**B**) Parts of a needle.

the fat to muscle ratio. The needle gauge varies from 20 to 25 depending on the thickness of the medication to be administered. Thick medications, such as penicillin and hormones, are difficult to draw into a syringe using a small-gauge needle, such as a 25 or 27, and equally difficult to inject into the patient. Subcutaneous injections are generally given using a short, small-gauge needle: 23 to 25 gauge, 5/8 inch to 1/2 inch.

All hypodermic syringes are marked with 10 calibrations per milliliter on one side of the syringe. Each small line represents 0.1 mL. The other side of the syringe may be marked in minims (m), which are rarely used today. The tuberculin (TB) syringe is narrow and has a total capacity of 1 mL. There are 100 calibration lines marking the TB 1-mL syringe, with each line representing 0.01 mL. Every tenth line is longer than the others to indicate 0.1 mL. TB syringes are used for newborn and pediatric doses, for intradermal skin tests, and any time small amounts of medication (less than 1 mL) are to be given. The needle size for intradermal injections using a TB syringe is 25 to 27 gauge, 3/8 to 5/8 inch.

The insulin syringe is used strictly for administering insulin subcutaneously to diabetic patients and has an orange cap. It has a total capacity of 1 mL; however, the 1-mL volume is marked as 100 units (U) to represent the strength of 100 U insulin per milliliter when full. Each group of 10 U is divided by five small lines, and each line represents 2 U. Most of the insulin used today is U-100, which means that it has 100 U of insulin in each milliliter. The insulin syringe must be marked U-100 to match the insulin used.

Procedure 9-2 describes the steps required for preparing an injection.

CHECKPOINT QUESTION

7. What are ampules and vials, and how do they differ?

Types of Injections

Intradermal Injections

Intradermal medications are administered into the dermal layer of the skin by inserting the needle at a 10° to 15° angle, almost parallel to the skin surface (Fig. 9-10). When an intradermal injection is administered correctly, the needle tip and lumen are slightly visible under the skin, and a small bubble, known as a wheal, is raised in the skin. Recommended sites for intradermal injections include the anterior forearm

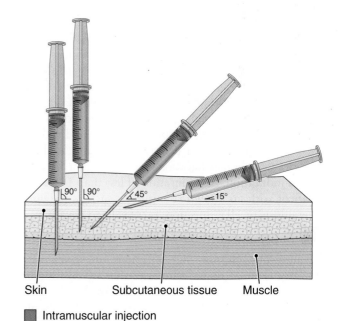

Figure 9-10 Comparison of the angles of insertion for intramuscular, subcutaneous, and intradermal injections. (Reprinted with permission from Cohen BJ. Medical Terminology: An Illustrated Guide, 6th Ed. Philadelphia: Lippincott Williams & Wilkins, 2011.)

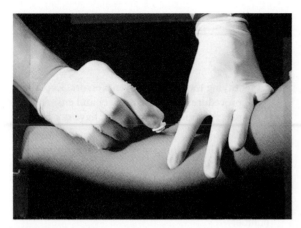

Figure 9-11 Administering the tine test for tuberculosis screening.

and the back. Intradermal injections are used exclusively to administer skin tests for tuberculosis screening, the **Mantoux test,** and allergy testing. Procedure 9-3 describes the steps for giving an intradermal injection.

The tine test is another skin test used for routine screening of tuberculosis, but it is not considered as diagnostic as the Mantoux test. Both methods use purified protein derivative (PPD) from a live tuberculin bacillus culture to test for the presence of tuberculin antibodies. The tine applicator contains small tines impregnated with PPD. After cleansing the forearm, press the tine applicator firmly into the intradermal layer of the skin (Fig. 9-11). A positive tine test is usually followed by a Mantoux test. Both the tine test and the Mantoux test must be read within 48 to 72 hours. A positive Mantoux reaction has **induration,** a hard raised area over the injection site, larger than 10 mm. This positive reaction indicates the possibility of exposure to tuberculosis; however, it does not indicate that the patient has active tuberculosis (see Chapter 15). A complete medical history and further testing by sputum culture and radiography are required for a definitive diagnosis. Redness over the intradermal injection site should not be considered induration. An induration of less than 10 mm in a patient with no known risk factors, such as previous tuberculosis or HIV infection, is considered negative.

Subcutaneous Injections

Subcutaneous (SQ or SC) injections are given into the fatty layer of tissue below the skin by positioning the needle and syringe at a 45° angle to the skin (see Fig. 9-10). The SQ route is chosen for drugs that should not be absorbed as rapidly as through the intramuscular (IM) or intravenous (IV) route. Common sites include the upper arm, thigh, back, and abdomen. Procedure 9-4 describes the steps for administering a SQ injection.

Intramuscular Injections

IM injections are given by positioning the needle and syringe at a 90° angle to the skin (see Fig. 9-10).

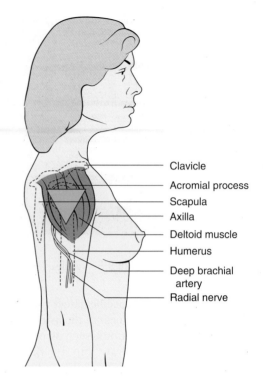

Figure 9-12 The deltoid muscle site for intramuscular injection is located by palpating the lower edge of the acromial process. At the midpoint, in line with the axilla on the lateral aspect of the upper arm, a triangle is formed. Medications are administered within this triangle.

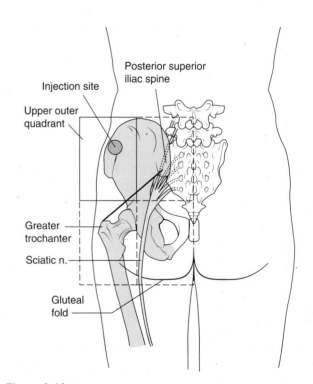

Figure 9-13 The dorsogluteal site for administering an IM injection is lateral and slightly superior to the midpoint of a line drawn from the trochanter to the posterior superior iliac spine. Correct identification of this site minimizes the possibility of accidentally damaging the sciatic nerve.

Absorption of IM medications is fairly rapid because of the rich vascularity of muscle. If slower absorption is desired, the medication is mixed with an oil base rather than saline or water to prolong absorption time. A 1-inch to 1 1/2–inch needle is required to administer an intramuscular injection to an adult. The length of the needle depends on the muscle chosen for injection and the size of the patient.

Recommended muscles used for IM injections include the deltoid (Fig. 9-12), dorsogluteal (Fig. 9-13), ventrogluteal (Fig. 9-14), and vastus lateralis (Fig. 9-15). The rectus femoris (Fig. 9-16) can also be used when the other sites are contraindicated. It is recommended that no more than 1 mL be injected into the deltoid muscle and no more than 3 mL be injected into the other muscles in an adult. Children younger than 2 years of age should never receive injections in the gluteal muscle, since this muscle is not well developed until the child is walking. The muscle chosen for the injection depends on the preference of the medical assistant, the patient, and the amount of medication to be administered. Also, some pharmaceutical companies recommend specific sites for medications to be injected intramuscularly, and the medical assistant should use these sites as indicated. Gold sodium thiomalate, a medication used to treat arthritis, and some vaccines are examples of medications that have specific guidelines for administration set forth by the manufacturer. Procedure 9-5 describes the steps for administering an intramuscular injection.

Z-Track Method of Intramuscular Injections

The **Z-track method** is used for IM administration of medications that may irritate or damage the tissues if

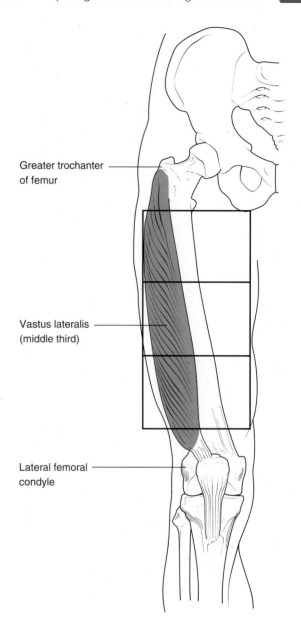

Figure 9-15 The vastus lateralis site for IM injections is identified by dividing the thigh into thirds horizontally and vertically. The injection is given in the outer middle third.

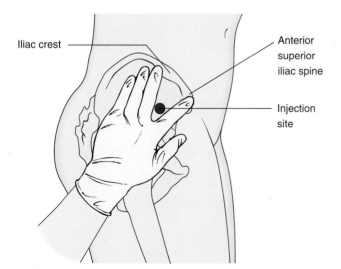

Figure 9-14 The ventrogluteal site is located by placing the palm on the greater trochanter and the index finger toward the anterior superior iliac spine. The middle finger is then spread posteriorly away from the index finger as far as possible. A "V" or triangle is formed by this maneuver. The injection is made in the middle of the triangle.

allowed to leak back along the line of injection. An example of a medication that should be administered using this technique is iron dextran, which is used to treat iron deficiency anemia. The Z-track method prevents leakage by sealing off the layers of skin along the route of the needle (Fig. 9-17). If the medication is extremely caustic, directions may include changing the needle after drawing up the solution. An additional precaution may include drawing up to 0.5 mL of air into the syringe after the medication has been aspirated into the syringe. When the medication is injected at a 90° angle, the additional air rises to the top of the syringe and is injected after the medication. This clears the needle

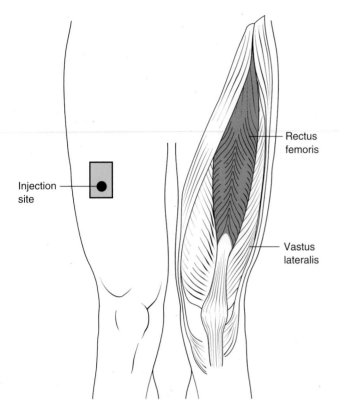

Figure 9-16 The rectus femoris site for IM injections is used only when other sites are contraindicated.

and the path of the injection (Fig. 9-18). Procedure 9-6 describes the steps for administering an intramuscular injection using the Z-track method.

 CHECKPOINT QUESTION

8. Name the types of injections and the possible sites for each type.

Other Medication Routes

Rectal Administration

Rectal medications are packaged in the form of suppositories or liquids administered as a retention enema (Fig. 9-19). They can provide a local effect or be absorbed through the rectal mucosa for a systemic effect. Rectal medications may be used for patients who are NPO (allowed nothing by mouth) or who have nausea and vomiting, but they are never used for patients who have diarrhea. Suppositories have a cocoa butter or glycerin base that melts at body temperature. They should be stored in the refrigerator to prevent melting. Rectal medications are rarely administered in the medical office, but you may be required to instruct the patient in the proper technique for administration at home. Both retention enemas and rectal suppositories should be retained by the patient for about 20 to 30 minutes before elimination.

PATIENT EDUCATION

ADMINISTERING RECTAL MEDICATIONS AT HOME

Some medications have to be administered rectally. You should teach the patient or family member to perform this procedure if the medication is to be taken at home. Here are some key points to discuss:

- Gloves should be worn.
- A small amount of a lubricant should be added to the suppository for easy insertion. The lubricant may be supplied with the suppository, or it can be purchased separately at the pharmacy.
- Advise the patient to remain lying on the bed for about 15 minutes after the suppository is inserted.
- The suppository should be inserted past the anal sphincter.

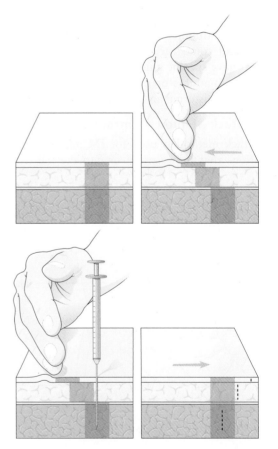

Figure 9-17 The Z-track technique is used to administer medications that are irritating to SQ tissue. The skin is pulled to one side, the needle is inserted, and the solution is injected after careful aspiration. When the needle is withdrawn and the displaced tissue is allowed to return to its normal position, the solution is prevented from escaping from the muscle tissue.

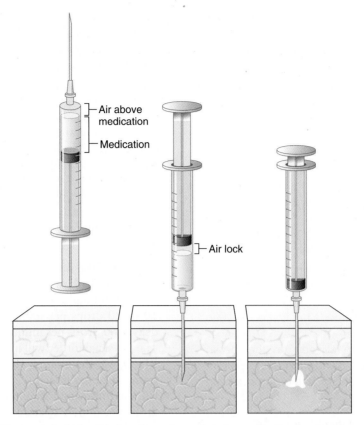

Figure 9-18 An air bubble added to the syringe after the medication has been accurately measured helps to expel solution that is trapped in the shaft of the needle when the injection is given. It also helps to trap the injected solution in the IM tissue.

Vaginal Administration

Vaginal medications include creams, tablets, cocoa butter–based suppositories, and solutions for douches. Examples include hormonal creams and antibiotic or antifungal preparations (Fig. 9-20). Very few medications other than those for local effects are prescribed for vaginal administration. Instruct the patient to remain lying for a while after the insertion of vaginal medications. For comfort, the patient may have to wear a light pad to absorb any drainage.

 ## Transdermal Administration

Dermal medications, which are applied to the skin, include topical creams, lotions, ointments, and transdermal medications. Topical medications (creams, ointments, sprays, and lotions) produce local effects, while transdermal medications produce systemic effects. Medication administered transdermally is delivered to the body by absorption through the skin. Delivery is slow and maintains a steady, stable level of medication. You should never cut a transdermal patch, since doing so alters the rate of absorption. Dermal patches are placed on the skin, usually on the chest or back, upper arm, or behind the ear (for medications that prevent motion sickness). Procedure 9-7 describes the steps for applying transdermal medications.

Inhalation

Inhalation is administration of medication, water vapor, or gas by inspiration of the substance into the lungs. Medication administered by inhalation is absorbed quickly through the alveolar walls into the capillaries, but a disease condition may make absorption difficult to predict. Patients with chronic pulmonary disease or disorder may self-administer certain medications with a handheld **nebulizer** or inhaler, both producing a fine spray of medicated mist that is inhaled directly into the lungs (see Chapter 15).

 ### CHECKPOINT QUESTION

9. How are medications given by the inhalation route absorbed?

Principles of Intravenous Therapy

With the IV route, a sterile solution of a drug is injected through a catheter or needle that has been inserted into a vein by a procedure known as *venipuncture* (refer to Chapter 26). IV medication has the quickest action because it enters the bloodstream immediately. In most cases, the physician administers IV medications, but some ambulatory care centers expect medical assistants to be proficient at setting up the equipment and fluids for an IV, performing the venipuncture, and regulating the IV fluids as directed by the physician. Some states may have laws that prohibit a medical assistant from starting an IV line or administering IV medications. Only drugs intended for IV administration should be given by this route.

 AFF **TRIAGE**

While you are working in a medical office setting, the following three situations arise:

A. A 50-year-old man is complaining of dyspnea, and the doctor has ordered a nebulizer treatment.

B. A 65-year-old woman needs her first dose of an antibiotic.

C. A 47-year-old woman slipped on the ice in the parking lot and is having moderate pain in the right ankle. The doctor has ordered a pain medication injection.

How do you sort these patients? Who do you see first? Second? Third?

Patient A should be treated first; any patient with chest pain or shortness of breath should be treated as a number 1 priority. Patient C should be medicated for pain control. Last, patient B should be given the antibiotic. Remember, you must closely monitor this patient for 30 minutes for signs of an allergic reaction. All three of these patients need to be closely evaluated after receiving their medications. Ask yourself, is the patient breathing better? Is the pain better? Communicate your findings with the physician.

Intravenous Equipment

The equipment necessary for starting an IV includes the fluids (determined by the physician), the IV catheter (angiocatheter), and the tubing and valve that connect the IV fluids to the catheter and regulate the flow of fluids into the patient (Fig. 9-21). Once the IV line is started, the fluids are administered through the vein either to replace fluids lost by the patient or to administer medications through special ports on the tubing.

Examples of fluids that come prepackaged for use in IV therapy are Ringer's lactate (RL), dextrose 5% and water (D_5W), 0.9% normal saline, 0.45% normal saline, or a combination (D_5NS, D_5RL). The physician

chooses the type and amount of fluid to be administered. An administration set (tubing) is used, with one end (the end with the drip chamber) inserted into the IV fluid bag and the other end inserted into the IV catheter after it is in the vein (Procedure 9-8). After securing the IV catheter and attaching the administration set tubing, adjust the flow of fluids by adjusting the roller clamp and carefully watching the fluids drip into the drip chamber. Carefully count the drops per minute so you can adjust the flow of fluids to the exact rate desired. The amount of fluid to be administered is ordered by the physician in terms of milliliters per hour (e.g., 125 mL/hour). Using this physician order, determine how fast to run the solution following this procedure:

- Determine the drop factor (number of drops needed to deliver 1 mL of fluid) as noted on the administration set tubing package (macrodrip systems deliver 10 or 20 drops per milliliter, and microdrip systems deliver 60 drops per milliliter.)
- The physician order will include the type of fluid (e.g., RL, D_5W), the amount (e.g., 125 mL), and the time frame (e.g., per hour).
- Use the following formula to calculate the number of drops per minute necessary to deliver the amount of fluid:

(Volume in milliliters ÷ Time in minutes) × Drop factor (gtt/min) = Drops per minute

For example, if the physician orders an IV of RL at 100 mL/hour and the administration set delivers 10 gtt/mL, the formula would be set up as follows:

$$(100 \text{ mL} \div 60 \text{ minutes}) = 1.67$$

1.67×10 gtt/mL = 17 gtt/min (16.7 rounded up to nearest tenth = 17)

In this situation, you would regulate the roller clamp so that 17 drops per minute flow into the drip chamber to deliver 100 mL/hour as ordered by the physician. If the physician would like the patient to have an IV line available, but not necessarily for administering fluids, a to-keep-open (TKO) or keep-vein-open (KVO) rate will be ordered. The flow of fluids into the vein to prevent clotting may be 15 to 30 mL/hour as determined by the physician. The same formula is used to calculate this rate: (rate = volume ÷ time × drop factor).

Troubleshooting Problems

The medical assistant must be vigilant about watching the IV fluids and the site of venipuncture. **Infiltration** occurs when IV fluid infuses into the tissues surrounding the vein, usually because the catheter has been dislodged. Carefully securing the IV catheter and the administration tubing usually prevents infiltration. In

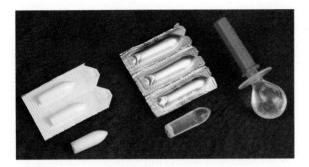

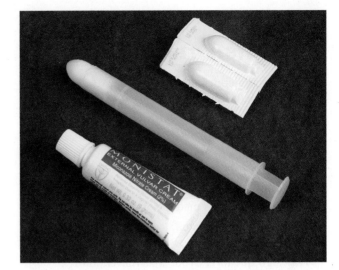

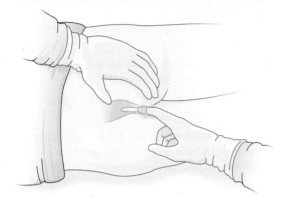

Figure 9-19 (**A**) These are examples of suppositories. (**B**) Rectal suppositories should be introduced into the anus well beyond the internal sphincter.

case of infiltration, stop the flow of fluids, remove the catheter, and notify the physician. Infiltration is characterized by the following:

- Swelling and pain at the IV site
- A slow or absent flow rate into the drip chamber of the administration set with the roller clamp open
- No blood return or backup into the tubing when the fluid bag is below the level of the heart

Phlebitis may occur when the IV catheter has caused inflammation in the vein or when there is an infection present. Often the irritation or infection occurs at the insertion site and is characterized by redness, swelling, and tenderness. There may also be a red streak starting at the insertion site and following the vein upwards on the extremity. Although the IV may be flowing without difficulty, signs of infection or inflammation indicate that the IV line should be removed and reinserted as ordered by the physician.

Regardless of the reason for reinserting an IV, you must use either the other arm or a site above the level of infiltration or infection. Procedure 9-8 outlines the steps for the initial insertion or reinsertion of an IV line.

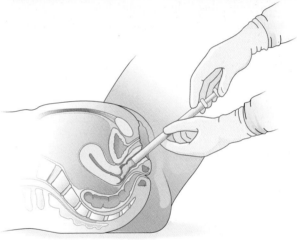

Figure 9-20 (**A**) Vaginal suppository and applicator. (**B**) Insertion of vaginal cream using applicator.

CHECKPOINT QUESTION

10. How would you explain an IV that is not flowing even with the roller clamp open?

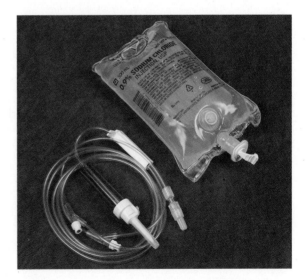

Figure 9-21 IV equipment including the fluid and tubing.

SPANISH TERMINOLOGY

español

¿Es alérgico/alérgica a algo?
Do you have allergies?

Tome tres cucharaditas cuatro veces al día.
Take three teaspoons 4 times a day.

Tengo que ponerle una inyección.
I need to give you an injection.

No mastique este medicamento.
Do not chew this medication.

¿Quiere un poco de agua?
Would you like some water?

¿Hay algo que lo/la ayude a aliviar el dolor?
Does anything help the pain?

MEDIA MENU

- **Student Resources on thePoint**
  - **Animation: Intramuscular Injection**
  - **Animation: Intravenous Injection**
  - **CMA/RMA Certification Exam Review**
  - **Video: Administering Oral Medications (Procedure 9-1)**
  - **Video: Preparing Injections (Procedure 9-2)**
  - **Video: Administering an Intradermal Injection (Procedure 9-3)**
  - **Video: Administering a Subcutaneous Injection (Procedure 9-4)**
  - **Video: Administering an Intramuscular Injection and the Z-Track Method (Procedures 9-5 and 9-6)**
  - **Video: Applying Transdermal Medications (Procedure 9-7)**
- **Internet Resources**

  Medwatch
  http://www.fda.gov/medwatch

  Physician's Desk Reference
  http://www.pdr.net/Default.aspx

  FDA Medication Guides
  http://www.fda.gov/Drugs/DrugSafety/ucm085729.htm

  National Center for Complimentary and Alternative Medicine
  http://nccam.nih.gov

  Institute for Healthcare Improvement
  http://www.ihi.org/IHI

  Patient Safety and Quality Healthcare
  http://www.psqh.com/index.html

PSY PROCEDURE 9-1: | **Administering Oral Medications**

Purpose: Accurately administer oral medications
Equipment: Physician's order, oral medication, disposable calibrated cup, glass of water, patient medical record

Steps	Reasons
1. Wash your hands.	Handwashing aids infection control.
2. Review the physician's medication order and select the correct medication. Compare the label to the physician's instructions. Note the expiration date. Check the label three times: when taking it from the shelf, while pouring, and when returning it to the shelf.	Carefully dispensing medications helps prevent errors. Outdated medication should not be administered but should be discarded appropriately.
3. Calculate the correct dosage to be given if necessary.	Some medications, such as vaccines, are given in specific milliliters and do not need to have a dosage calculated.
4. If using a multidose container, remove the cap from the container, touching only the outside of the lid. Single, or unit-dose, medications come individually wrapped in packages that may be opened by pushing the medication through the foil backing or peeling back a tab on one corner.	The inside of the lid of a multidose bottle will be contaminated if touched.
5. According to your calculations and the label, remove the correct dose of medication. A. For solid medications: (1) Pour the capsule or tablet into the bottle cap to prevent contamination.	The amount the physician orders is in milligrams. You will need to calculate the amount of milliliters to administer to deliver the milligrams ordered.

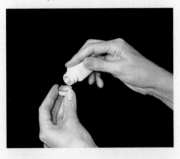

Step 5A (1). Pour the tablet into the bottle cap.

(2) Transfer the medication to a disposable cup.

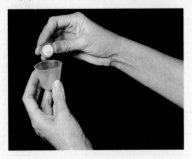

Step 5A (2). Transfer the medication into a disposable cup.

B. For liquid medications:

   (1) Open the bottle and place the lid on a flat surface with the open end up to prevent contamination of the inside of the cap.

(continued)

> **PSY** **PROCEDURE 9-1:** **Administering Oral Medications** *(continued)*

Steps	Reasons
(2) Palm the label to prevent liquids from dripping onto the label and possibly damaging it or making it illegible. 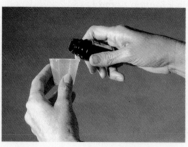 (3) With the opposite hand, place your thumbnail at the correct calibration on the cup. Holding the cup at eye level, pour the proper amount of medication into the cup, using your thumbnail as a guide.	**Step 5B (2).** Palm the label of the container when pouring liquids.
6. Greet and identify the patient. Explain the procedure. Ask the patient about medication allergies that might not be noted on the chart.	Identifying the patient prevents errors. Explaining the procedure helps ease anxiety and may improve compliance. The medical record should be checked for allergies, but the patient should also be asked, since allergies may not have been noted.
7. Give the patient a glass of water to wash down the medication unless contraindicated and administer the medication by handing the patient the disposable cup containing the medication.	Water helps the patient swallow the medication, but water is contraindicated for medications intended for a local effect (such as cough syrup or lozenges) and for buccal or sublingual medications.
8. Remain with the patient to be sure that all of the medication is swallowed. Observe any unusual reactions, report them to the physician, and enter them in the medical record.	You cannot assume that the patient swallowed the medication unless you observe it.
9. **AFF** Explain how to respond to a patient who is hearing impaired.	Make sure the patient can see your face as you are speaking. Speak clearly, not loudly.
10. Thank the patient and give any appropriate instructions.	
11. Wash your hands.	Always wash your hands after a patient encounter.
12. Record the procedure in the patient's medical record, noting the date, time, name of medication, dose administered, route of administration, and your name.	Procedures are considered not to have been done if they are not recorded.

Charting Example:

12/14/2012 8:45 am Ampicillin 125 mg PO given to pt. NKA ———————————————————— T. Jones, CMA

Note: The medical assistant may sign his or her name in the patient record using only the "CMA" credential if the office has a signature log denoting the entire credential as "CMA(AAMA)."

PSY PROCEDURE 9-2: **Preparing Injections**

Purpose: Accurately prepare a medication by injection
Equipment: Physician's order, medication for injection (ampule or vial), antiseptic wipes, needle and syringe of appropriate size, small gauze pad, biohazard sharps container, patient's medical record

Steps	Reasons
1. Wash your hands.	Handwashing aids infection control.
2. Review the medication order and select the correct medication. Compare the label to the physician's instructions. Note the expiration date. Check the label three times: when taking it from the shelf, while drawing it up into the syringe, and when returning it to the shelf.	Carefully dispensing medications helps prevent errors. Outdated medication should not be administered to a patient but should be discarded appropriately.
3. Calculate the correct dosage to be given if necessary.	
4. Choose the needle and syringe according to the route of administration, type of medication, and size of the patient.	A shorter needle is used for SQ medications, whereas a larger gauge may be necessary for thick medications.
5. Open the needle and syringe package. Assemble if necessary. Make sure the needle is firmly attached to the syringe by grasping the needle at the hub and turning it clockwise onto the syringe. **Step 5.** Grasp the needle at the hub and turn it clockwise.	Needles and syringes often are preassembled, or they may be purchased separately. A needle that is not firmly attached may be detached during the procedure.
6. Withdraw the correct amount of medication: A. From an ampule: (1) With the fingertips of one hand, tap the stem of the ampule lightly to remove any medication in or above the narrow neck. (2) Wrap a piece of gauze around the ampule neck to protect your fingers from broken glass. Grasp the gauze and ampule firmly with the fingers. Snap the stem off the ampule with a quick downward movement of the gauze. Be sure to aim the break away from your face. Dispose of the ampule top in a biohazard sharps container to prevent injury. 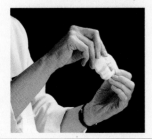 **Step 6A (2).** Grasp the gauze and ampule firmly.	Administering an incorrect amount of medication will result in the patient getting too little or too much of a medication.

(*continued*)

PSY PROCEDURE 9-2: Preparing Injections *(continued)*

Steps

Reasons

(3) After removing the needle guard, insert the needle lumen below the level of the medication. Withdraw the medication by pulling back on the plunger of the syringe without letting the needle touch the contaminated edge of the broken ampule. Withdraw the desired amount of medication and dispose of the ampule in a biohazard sharps container.

(4) Remove any air bubbles by holding the syringe with the needle up and gently tapping the barrel of the syringe until the air bubbles rise to the top. Draw back on the plunger to add a small amount of air, then gently push the plunger forward to eject the air out of the syringe. Be careful not to eject any medication if the required dosage has been drawn up.

B. From a vial:

(1) Using the antiseptic wipe, cleanse the rubber stopper of the vial to avoid introducing bacteria into the medication.

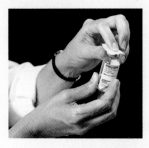

Step 6B (1). Clean the rubber stopper with an antiseptic wipe.

(2) Remove the needle guard and pull back on the plunger to fill the syringe with an amount of air equal to the amount of medication to be removed from the vial.

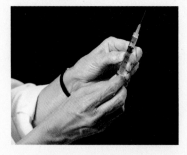

Step 6B (2). Pull back on the plunger, sucking air into the syringe.

(3) Insert the needle into the vial through the center of the cleansed vial top. Inject the air from the syringe into the vial above the level of the medication to avoid producing foam or bubbles in the medication.

PSY PROCEDURE 9-2:   **Preparing Injections** *(continued)*

Steps	**Reasons**

Injecting an equal amount of air into the vial will prevent a vacuum from forming in the vial, which would make withdrawal of the medication difficult.

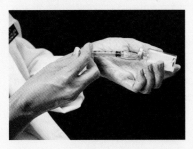

(4) With the needle inside the vial, invert the vial, holding the syringe at eye level. Aspirate, or withdraw, the desired amount of medication into the syringe.

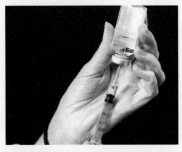

(5) Displace any air bubbles in the syringe by gently tapping the barrel of the syringe with the fingertips. Remove the air by pushing the plunger slowly and forcing the air into the vial.

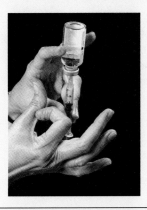

Step 6B (3). Insert the needle through the rubber stopper.

Step 6B (4). Invert the vial.

Step 6B (5). Tap the barrel gently to remove air bubbles from the medication.

---

7. Carefully recap the needle by placing the needle guard on a hard, flat surface, and without contaminating the needle, insert the needle into the cap and scoop up the cap with one hand.

Recapping the needle protects the sterility of the needle until the medication can be administered. Recapping with two hands should be avoided to prevent needle sticks, especially after giving an injection.

PSY PROCEDURE 9-3: **Administering an Intradermal Injection**

Purpose: Accurately prepare and administer a medication by intradermal injection
Equipment: Physician's order, medication for injection (ampule or vial), antiseptic wipes, needle and syringe of appropriate size, small gauze pad, biohazard sharps container, clean exam gloves, patient's medical record

Steps	Reasons
1. Wash your hands.	Handwashing aids infection control.
2. Review the order and select the correct medication. Compare the label to the physician's instructions. Note the expiration date. Check the label three times: when taking it from the shelf, while drawing it up into the syringe, and when returning it to the shelf or discarding the unit dose vial or ampule.	Carefully dispensing medications helps prevent errors. Outdated medication should not be administered to a patient but should be discarded appropriately.
3. Prepare the injection according to the steps in Procedure 9-2.	Regardless of the type of injection, the preparation is the same.
4. Greet and identify the patient. Explain the procedure and ask the patient about medication allergies that might not be noted on the medical record.	Correctly identifying the patient prevents errors.
5. Select the appropriate site for the injection. Recommended sites are the anterior forearm and the middle of the back.	The anterior forearm is used for tuberculosis testing, whereas the back is often used for allergy testing.
6. Prepare the site by cleansing with an antiseptic wipe using a circular motion starting at the anticipated injection site and working toward the outside. Do not touch the site after cleaning.	The site must be prepared by first removing microorganisms from the area. Wiping in a circular motion will carry the microorganisms away from the site.
7. Put on gloves.	Standard precautions must be followed for protection against potential exposure to blood.
8. Remove the needle guard. Using your nondominant hand, pull the patient's skin taut.	Stretching the skin allows the needle to enter the skin with less resistance and secures the patient against movement.
9. With the bevel of the needle facing upward, insert the needle at a 10° to 15° angle into the upper layer of the skin. When the bevel of the needle is under the skin, stop inserting the needle. The needle will be slightly visible below the surface of the skin. It is not necessary to aspirate when performing an intradermal injection.	The needle should be inserted almost parallel to the skin to ensure that penetration occurs within the dermal layer. The bevel of the needle facing up will allow the wheal to form. If the bevel faces downward, no wheal will be formed.

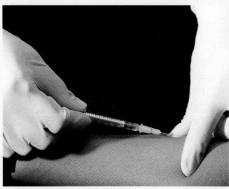

Step 9. Insert the needle at a 10° to 15° angle.

PSY **PROCEDURE 9-3:** | **Administering an Intradermal Injection (continued)**

Steps	Reasons
10. Inject the medication slowly by depressing the plunger. A wheal will form as the medication enters the dermal layer of the skin. Hold the syringe steady for proper administration. 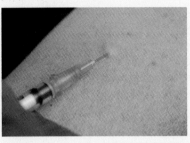	Moving the needle once it has penetrated the skin will cause discomfort to the patient.
	Step 10. A wheal is formed when the medication is injected under the skin in an intradermal injection.
11. Remove the needle from the skin at the angle of insertion. Do not use an antiseptic wipe or gauze pad when withdrawing the needle. Do not press or massage the site. Do not apply an adhesive bandage.	Pressure on the wheal may press the medication into the tissues or out of the injection site. Any redness or swelling produced by applying an adhesive bandage could result in an inaccurate reading of the test.
12. **AFF** Explain how to respond to a patient who has dementia.	Solicit assistance from a caregiver or other staff member to help during the procedure. Give simple directions to the patient about what he or she should do. Speak clearly, not loudly.
13. Do not recap the needle. Dispose of the needle and syringe in an approved biohazard sharps container. The sharps container should be placed where you have easy access to it after the injection is given.	Discarding the needle and syringe without recapping helps reduce the risk of an accidental needle stick.
14. Remove your gloves and wash your hands.	
15. Depending upon the type of skin test administered, the length of time required for the body tissues to react, and the policies of the medical office, perform one of the following: A. Read the test results. Inspect and palpate the site for the presence and amount of induration. B. Tell the patient when to return (date and time) to the office to have the results read. C. Instruct the patient to read the results at home. Make sure the patient understands the instructions. Have the patient repeat the instructions if necessary.	To make sure the results are accurate and that the patient does not have a serious reaction, you must be familiar with the skin test given and follow all procedures accordingly.
16. Document the procedure, site, results, and any instructions given to the patient.	Procedures are considered not to have been done if they are not recorded.

Charting Example:

05/04/2012 10:35 am Mantoux test, 0.1 mL PPD ID, (L) anterior forearm. Pt. given verbal and written instructions to
RTO in 48–72 hrs to have results read. Pt. verbalized understanding ———————————— P. King, CMA

Note: The medical assistant may sign his or her name in the patient record using only the "CMA" credential if the office has a signature log denoting the entire credential as "CMA(AAMA)."

PSY PROCEDURE 9-4:   **Administering a Subcutaneous Injection**

Purpose: Accurately prepare and administer a medication by SQ injection
Equipment: Physician's order, medication for injection (ampule or vial), antiseptic wipes, needle and syringe of appropriate size, small gauze pad, biohazard sharps container, clean exam gloves, adhesive bandage, patient's medical record

Steps	Reasons
1. Wash your hands.	Handwashing aids infection control.
2. Review the medication order and select the correct medication. Compare the label to the physician's instructions. Note the expiration date. Check the label three times: when taking it from the shelf, while drawing it up into the syringe, and when returning it to the shelf.	Carefully dispensing medications helps prevent errors. Outdated medication should not be administered to a patient but should be discarded appropriately.
3. Prepare the injection according to the steps in Procedure 9-2.	Regardless of the type of injection, the preparation is the same.
4. Greet and identify the patient. Explain the procedure and ask the patient about medication allergies that may not be noted on the medical record.	Correctly identifying the patient prevents errors.
5. Select the appropriate site for the injection. Recommended sites include the upper arm, thigh, back, and abdomen.	These areas of the body usually have additional adipose tissue.
6. Prepare the site by cleansing with an antiseptic wipe using a circular motion starting at the anticipated injection site and working toward the outside. Do not touch the site after cleaning.	The site must be prepared by first removing microorganisms from the area. Wiping in a circular motion will carry the microorganisms away from the site.
7. Put on gloves.	Standard precautions must be followed for protection against exposure to blood.
8. Remove the needle guard. Using your nondominant hand, hold the skin surrounding the injection site in a cushion fashion. **Step 8.** Cushion the tissue between your fingers for the SQ injection.	Holding the skin up and away from the underlying muscle will ensure entrance into the SQ tissues. Proper technique will help ensure that the SQ tissue, not the muscle, is entered.
9. With a firm motion, insert the needle into the tissue at a 45° angle to the skin surface. Hold the barrel between the thumb and the index finger of the dominant hand and insert the needle completely to the hub. **Step 9.** Insert the needle at a 45° angle for a SQ injection.	A quick, firm motion is less painful to the patient. Full insertion ensures that the medication is inserted into the proper tissue.

PSY PROCEDURE 9-4:   **Administering a Subcutaneous Injection** *(continued)*

Steps	Reasons
10. Remove your nondominant hand from the skin.	Your nondominant hand will be used to pull back on the plunger in the next step.
11. Holding the syringe steady, pull back on the syringe gently. If blood appears in the hub or the syringe, a blood vessel has been entered. If this occurs, do not inject the medication. Remove the needle and prepare a new injection.	If medication intended for SQ administration is administered into a blood vessel, the medication can be absorbed too quickly, producing undesirable results.
12. Inject the medication slowly by depressing the plunger.	If medication is injected too rapidly, pressure is created, which will cause patient discomfort and may cause tissue damage.
13. Place a gauze pad over the injection site and remove the needle at the angle at which it was inserted. Gently massage the injection site with the gauze pad with one hand while discarding the needle and syringe into the sharps container with the other hand. Do not recap the used needle. Apply an adhesive bandage if needed.	Discarding the needle and syringe without recapping helps reduce the risk of an accidental stick. Massaging helps to distribute the medication so that it can be more completely absorbed.
14. **AFF** Explain how to respond to a patient who is deaf, hearing impaired, visually impaired, or does not speak English.	Solicit assistance from anyone who may be with the patient or a staff member who speaks his or her native language to interpret if available. If no interpreter is available, use hand gestures or pictures to explain procedure to the patient.
15. Remove your gloves and wash your hands.	
16. An injection given for allergy desensitization requires that the patient remain in the office for at least 30 minutes for observation of any reaction. If the patient experiences any unusual reaction after any injection, notify the physician immediately.	An unusual reaction after an allergy injection could be fatal.
17. Document the procedure, site, results, and instructions if given.	Procedures are considered not to have been done if they are not recorded.

Charting Example:

03/04/2012 9:30 am Regular insulin 5 units SQ (R) posterior upper arm ———————————— M. Collins, CMA

Note: The medical assistant may sign his or her name in the patient record using only the "CMA" credential if the office has a signature log denoting the entire credential as "CMA(AAMA)."

PSY PROCEDURE 9-5: **Administering an Intramuscular Injection**

Purpose: Accurately prepare and administer a medication by IM injection

Equipment: Physician's order, medication for injection (ampule or vial), antiseptic wipes, needle and syringe of appropriate size, small gauze pad, biohazard sharps container, clean exam gloves, adhesive bandage, patient's medical record

Steps	Reasons
1. Wash your hands.	Handwashing aids infection control.
2. Review the order and select the correct medication. Compare the label to the physician's instructions. Check the label three times: when taking it from the shelf, while drawing it up into the syringe, and when returning it to the shelf.	Carefully dispensing medications helps prevent errors. Outdated medication should not be administered to a patient but should be discarded appropriately.
3. Prepare the injection according to the steps in Procedure 9-2.	Regardless of the type of injection, the preparation is the same.
4. Greet and identify the patient. Explain the procedure and ask the patient about medication allergies that might not be noted on the medical record.	Correctly identifying the patient prevents errors.
5. Select the appropriate site for the injection. Recommended sites include the deltoid, vastus lateralis, dorsogluteal, and ventrogluteal areas; however, the site should be chosen based on the medication and age and size of the patient.	Skill and accuracy are crucial when locating IM injection sites since major blood vessels and nerves may lie near the muscles.
6. Prepare the site by cleansing with an antiseptic wipe using a circular motion starting at the anticipated injection site and working toward the outside. Do not touch the site after cleaning.	The site must be prepared by first removing microorganisms from the area. Wiping in a circular motion will carry the microorganisms away from the site.
7. Put on gloves.	Standard precautions must be followed for protection against potential exposure to blood.
8. Remove the needle guard. Using your nondominant hand, hold the skin surrounding the injection site taut with the thumb and index fingers or grasp the muscle in a small person with little body fat.	Holding the skin taut in an average or overweight person will allow for easier insertion of the needle. Bunching the muscle produces a deeper muscle mass in a very thin person.

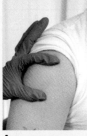

A

Step 8 (A). Hold the skin taut for an average size person.

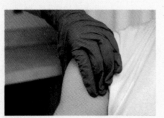

B

Step 8 (B). Bunch the muscle in a thin person.

PSY PROCEDURE 9-5: | **Administering an Intramuscular Injection (continued)**

Steps	Reasons
9. While holding the syringe like a dart, use a quick, firm motion to insert the needle into the tissue at a 90° angle to the surface. Hold the barrel between the thumb and the index finger of the dominant hand and insert the needle completely to the hub. 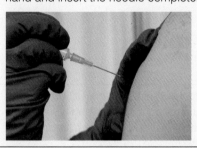	A quick, firm motion is less painful to the patient. Full insertion at 90° ensures that the medication is inserted into the proper muscle tissue. **Step 9.** Insert the needle at a 90° angle to the hub.
10. Remove your nondominant hand from the skin and gently pull back on the plunger while holding the syringe steady. If blood appears in the hub or the syringe, a blood vessel has been entered. If this occurs, do not inject the medication. Remove the needle and prepare a new injection.	If medication intended for IM administration is administered into a blood vessel, the medication can be absorbed too quickly, producing undesirable results.
11. Inject the medication slowly by depressing the plunger.	If medication is injected too rapidly, pressure is created, which will cause patient discomfort and may cause tissue damage.
12. Place a gauze pad over the injection site and remove the needle at the same angle at which it was inserted. Gently massage the injection site with the gauze pad with one hand while discarding the needle and syringe into the sharps container with the other hand. Do not recap the used needle. Apply an adhesive bandage if needed.	Discarding the needle and syringe without recapping helps reduce the risk of an accidental needle stick. Massaging helps to distribute the medication into the tissues so that it can be more completely absorbed.
13. **AFF** Explain how to respond to a patient who is visually impaired.	Face the patient when speaking and always let him or her know what you are going to do before touching him or her.
14. Remove your gloves and wash your hands.	
15. Observe the patient for any unusual reactions. If the patient experiences any unusual reaction after any injection, notify the physician immediately.	Unusual reactions after administering injections may be the beginning of a life-threatening emergency.
16. Document the procedure, the site, results, and instructions if given.	Procedures are considered not to have been done if they are not recorded.

Charting Example:

05/06/2012 2:00 pm Solu-Medrol 20 mg IM (L) DG ——————————————— O. Campbell,.CMA

Note: The medical assistant may sign his or her name in the patient record using only the "CMA" credential if the office has a signature log denoting the entire credential as "CMA(AAMA)."

PSY **PROCEDURE 9-6:**   **Administering an Intramuscular Injection Using the Z-Track Method**

Purpose: Accurately prepare and administer a medication by Z-track IM injection
Equipment: Physician's order, medication for injection (ampule or vial), antiseptic wipes, needle and syringe of appropriate size, small gauze pad, biohazard sharps container, clean exam gloves, adhesive bandage, patient's medical record

Steps	Reasons
1. Follow Steps 1 through 7 as described in Procedure 9-5 (Administering an Intramuscular Injection). *Note:* The ventrogluteal, vastus lateralis, and dorsogluteal sites work well for the Z-track method; the deltoid does not.	
2. Remove the needle guard. Rather than pulling the skin taut or grasping the tissue as you would for an IM injection, pull the top layer of skin to the side and hold it with the nondominant hand throughout the injection.	The skin pulled to the side will eventually be released after the medication is administered and will act as a barrier to prevent the medication from leaving the injection site in the muscle.
A **B**	**Step 2.** Pull the top layer of skin to one side using the edge of your nondominant hand.
3. While holding the syringe like a dart, use a quick, firm motion to insert the needle into the tissue at a 90° angle to the skin surface. Hold the barrel between the thumb and the index finger of the dominant hand and insert the needle completely to the hub. Continue to hold the skin to one side with the nondominant hand.	A quick, firm motion is less painful to the patient. Full insertion at 90° ensures that the medication is inserted into the proper muscle tissue.
4. Aspirate by withdrawing the plunger slightly. If no blood appears, push the plunger in slowly and steadily. Count to 10 before withdrawing the needle.	If medication intended for IM administration is administered into a blood vessel, the medication can be absorbed too quickly, producing undesirable results. Counting to 10 before removing the needle allows time for the tissues to begin absorbing the medication.
5. Remove the needle at the same angle at which it was inserted while releasing the skin. Do not massage the area. Discard the needle and syringe into the sharps container. Apply an adhesive bandage if needed.	Discarding the needle and syringe without recapping helps reduce the risk of an accidental needle stick.
6. Remove your gloves and wash your hands.	

PSY PROCEDURE 9-6: **Administering an Intramuscular Injection Using the Z-Track Method** *(continued)*

Steps	Reasons
7. Observe the patient for any unusual reactions. If the patient experiences any unusual reaction after any injection, notify the physician immediately.	An unusual reaction may be the start of a life-threatening emergency.
8. Document the procedure, the site, the results, and the instructions if given.	Procedures are considered not to have been done if they are not recorded.

Charting Example:

07/11/2012 3:30 pm Imferon 25mg IM Z-track (R) DG ———————————————— E. Edwards, CMA

Note: The medical assistant may sign his or her name in the patient record using only the "CMA" credential if the office has a signature log denoting the entire credential as "CMA(AAMA)."

PSY PROCEDURE 9-7: **Applying Transdermal Medications**

Purpose: Accurately prepare and administer a transdermal medication
Equipment: Physician's order, medication, clean exam gloves, patient's medical record

Steps	Reasons
1. Wash your hands.	Handwashing aids infection control.
2. Review the order and select the correct medication. Compare the label to the physician's instructions. Note the expiration date. Check the label three times: when taking it from the shelf, before taking it into the patient exam room, and before applying it to the patient's skin.	Carefully dispensing medications helps prevents errors. Outdated medications should not be administered to a patient but should be discarded appropriately.
3. Greet and identify the patient. Explain the procedure and ask the patient about medication allergies that might not be noted on the medical record.	Correctly identifying the patient prevents errors.
4. Select the appropriate site and perform any necessary skin preparation. The sites are usually the upper arm, the chest or back surface, or behind the ear. These sites should be rotated. Ensure that the skin is clean, dry, and free from any irritation. Do not shave areas with excessive hair; trim the hair closely with scissors	Shaving may abrade the skin and cause the medication to be absorbed too rapidly.
5. If there is a transdermal patch already in place, remove it carefully while wearing gloves. Discard the patch in the trash container. Inspect the site for irritation.	Touching the medication with bare hands may cause it to be absorbed into your skin, causing undesirable reactions.

(continued)

PSY PROCEDURE 9-7: Applying Transdermal Medications (continued)

Steps	Reasons
6. Open the medication package by pulling the two sides apart. Do not touch the area of medication.	Touching the area of medication will remove some and prevent the patient from getting the prescribed amount.
	Step 6. Open the transdermal medication by pulling the wrapper apart.
7. Apply the medicated patch to the patient's skin following the manufacturer's directions. Press the adhesive edges down firmly all around, starting at the center and pressing outward. If the edges do not stick, fasten with tape.	Starting at the center eliminates air spaces that may prevent contact with the skin.
8. **AFF** Explain how to respond to a patient who is uncomfortable exposing skin on areas such as the chest or arms due to cultural or religious beliefs.	Be respectful of cultural differences by explaining why procedures are important. Provide additional privacy measures if necessary.
9. Wash your hands.	Always wash your hands after a patient encounter.
10. Document the procedure and the site of the new patch in the medical record.	Procedures are considered not to have been done if they are not recorded.

Charting Example:

09/06/2012 8:30 am Transdermal nitroglycerin 0.2mg/hr patch to (L) anterior chest ————————— R. Evans, RMA

Note: The medical assistant may sign his or her name in the patient record using only the "CMA" credential if the office has a signature log denoting the entire credential as "CMA(AAMA)."

PSY PROCEDURE 9-8: **Obtaining and Preparing an Intravenous Site**

Purpose: Accurately start a peripheral IV line
Equipment: Physician's order including the type of fluid to be used and the rate, IV solution, infusion administration set, IV pole, blank labels, IV catheter (Angiocath), antiseptic wipes, tourniquet, small gauze pad, biohazard sharps container, clean exam gloves, bandage tape, adhesive bandage, patient medical record

Steps	Reasons
1. Wash your hands.	Handwashing aids infection control.
2. Review the physician's order and select the correct catheter, solution, and administration set. Compare the label on the infusion solution to the physician's order. Note the expiration dates on the infusion solution and the administration set.	Carefully checking the order and the solution helps prevent errors. Outdated solutions should not be used but should be discarded appropriately.
3. Prepare the solution by attaching a label to the solution indicating the date, time, and name of the patient, and hang the solution on an IV pole. Remove the administration set from the package and close the roller clamp.	Although there may be other clamps on the administration set, close only the roller clamp, since this is the primary clamp that will be used to adjust the flow rate.
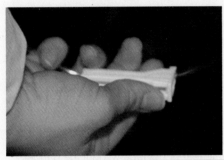	
	Step 3. Close the roller clamp on the administration set.
4. Remove the end of the administration set by removing the cover on the spike (above the drip chamber). Remove the cover from the infusion port (on the bottom of the bag) and insert the spike end of the administration set into the IV fluid.	Maintain sterility of the end of administration set and the port on the infusion solution bag at all times.
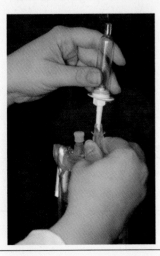	
	Step 4. The spike on the administration set tubing will be inserted completely into the port on the IV solution bag.

(continued)

PSY PROCEDURE 9-8: **Obtaining and Preparing an Intravenous Site** *(continued)*

Steps	Reasons
5. Fill the drip chamber on the administration set by squeezing the drip chamber until it is about half full. 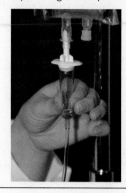	Do not fill the drip chamber completely. You must observe the flow of drops into this chamber to determine the rate.
	Step 5. Fill the drip chamber about half full.
6. Open the roller clamp and allow fluid to flow from the drip chamber through the length of the tubing, displacing any air. Do not remove the cover protecting the end of the tubing. Close the roller clamp when the fluid has filled the tubing and no air is noted. Drape the filled tubing over the IV pole and perform a venipuncture.	The air should be displaced out of the tubing before the IV is started.
7. Greet and identify the patient. Explain the procedure and ask the patient about medication allergies that might not be noted on the medical record.	Correctly identifying the patient prevents errors.
8. Prepare the IV start equipment by tearing or cutting two to three strips of tape that will be used to secure the IV catheter after insertion. Also, inspect each arm for the best available vein.	After inserting the IV, you will not be able to let go of the catheter to tear or cut tape without the danger of the catheter falling out or being pulled out by the weight of the tubing.
9. Wearing gloves, apply the tourniquet 1 to 2 inches above the intended venipuncture site. The tourniquet should be snug but not too tight. Ask the patient to open and close the fist of the selected arm to distend the veins. 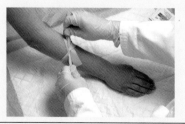	Standard precautions must be followed for protection against potential exposure to blood. Making a fist raises the vessels out of the underlying tissues and muscles.
	Step 9. Pull tourniquet snugly around the arm.
10. Secure the tourniquet by using the half-bow. Make sure the ends of the tourniquet extend upward to avoid contaminating the venipuncture site.	
11. Select a vein by palpating using your gloved index finger to trace the path of the vein and judge its depth. Release the tourniquet after palpating the vein if it has been left on for more than 1 minute.	

PSY PROCEDURE 9-8: **Obtaining and Preparing an Intravenous Site *(continued)***

Steps	Reasons
12. Prepare the site by cleansing with an antiseptic wipe using a circular motion starting at the anticipated venipuncture site and working outward. Do not touch the site after cleaning. 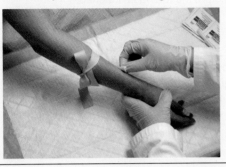 **Step 12.** Prepare the venipuncture site by working outward from the center.	Sterile technique must be used for the venipuncture.
13. Place the end of the administration set tubing on the exam table for easy access after venipuncture. Anchor the vein to be punctured by placing the thumb of the nondominant hand below the intended site and holding the skin taut.	Holding the vein in place will prevent it from rolling once the needle is inserted.
14. Remove the needle cover from the IV catheter. Using the dominant hand, insert the needle and catheter unit directly into the top of the vein with the bevel of the needle up at a 15° to 20° angle for superficial veins and while holding the catheter by the flash chamber, not the hub of the needle. Watch for blood in the flash chamber located next to the catheter hub during insertion of the catheter into the vein.	Holding the catheter by the hub may prevent you from seeing problems during insertion of the catheter. A blood flashback indicates that the needle, not necessarily the catheter, has been correctly inserted into the vein. A "pop" may be felt when the vein has been entered.
15. When the blood flashback is observed, lower the angle of the needle until flush with the skin and slowly advance the needle and catheter unit about 1/4 inch. 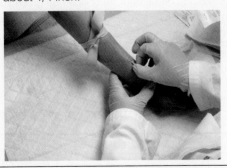 **Step 15.** After needle and catheter unit has been inserted into the vein, slowly advance the unit about 1/4 inch and then stop.	When blood is seen, the needle is in the vein and should only be inserted enough to make sure the bevel is completely in the vein.
16. Once the needle and catheter unit have been inserted slightly into the lumen of the vein, hold the flash chamber of the needle steady with the nondominant hand and slide the catheter (using the catheter hub) off of the needle and into the vein with the dominant hand. The catheter should be advanced into the vein up to the hub.	The needle will not be advanced into the vein; however, the catheter will be inserted up to the hub.

(continued)

PSY PROCEDURE 9-8: **Obtaining and Preparing an Intravenous Site (continued)**

Steps	Reasons
17. With the needle partly occluding the catheter, release the tourniquet. Remove the needle and discard into a biohazard sharps container. Connect the end of the administration tubing to the end of the IV catheter that has been inserted into the vein. Open the roller clamp and adjust the flow according to the physician's order.	A sterile 2 × 2 gauze pad may be placed under the catheter hub to absorb blood that will flow back out of the catheter after the needle has been completely removed before the tubing is attached.
18. Secure the hub of the IV catheter with tape by placing one small strip, sticky side up, under the catheter and crossing one end over the hub and adhering onto the skin on the opposite side of the catheter. Cross the other end of the tape in the same fashion and adhere to the skin on the opposite side of the hub. A transparent membrane adhesive dressing can then be applied over the entire hub and insertion site.	Avoid placing tape directly over the insertion site so that signs of infection or other problems can be observed readily.

Step 18. Tape the catheter in place carefully and apply an adhesive dressing over the entire hub and insertion site.

Steps	Reasons
19. Make a small loop with the administration set tubing near the IV insertion site and secure with tape.	This will prevent the catheter from being pulled if the tubing should be pulled or tugged.
20. **AFF** Explain how to respond to a patient who is from a older generation than yourself.	Refer to an elderly patient by his or her correct title (Mr., Mrs., Miss, etc.). Be respectful to the patient by only using his or her first name after he or she has given you permission to do so. Do not assume the patient is hearing or cognitively impaired because of his or her age.
21. Remove your gloves, wash your hands, and document the procedure in the medical record indicating the size of the IV catheter and the location, type of infusion solution, and rate.	Procedures are considered not to have been done if they are not recorded.

Charting Example:

05/11/2012 11:45 am IV started with #22 Angiocath, (L) anterior forearm, 1,000 mL RL solution
at TKO rate ———————————————————————————————————— J. Partin, CMA

Note: The medical assistant may sign his or her name in the patient record using only the "CMA" credential if the office has a signature log denoting the entire credential as "CMA(AAMA)."

- The administration of medication is one of the most challenging and exacting procedures performed in the medical office.
- Few other procedures require such intense concentration and attention to detail or include such potential for danger to the patient.
- You will be asked to practice interpersonal skills, such as tact and diplomacy, to make these procedures acceptable to the patient and to allay the anxiety felt by almost all patients during the administration of medications.
- It is also your responsibility to be familiar with and follow the laws in your state regarding the administration of medications.

Warm Ups for Critical Thinking

1. Design a patient education brochure that will teach patients about administering rectal medications at home.
2. After inserting the needle while giving an IM injection, you aspirate by pulling back slightly on the plunger. As you do this, blood appears in the syringe. What has happened? What should you do?
3. Another coworker has just given an oral medication to a patient in the office. She asks you to document the procedure. How would you handle this situation?
4. When preparing a medication for injection, you become distracted and forget how much medication you need to draw up into the syringe. What should you do?

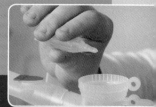

CHAPTER

10 Diagnostic Imaging

Outline

Principles of Radiology
X-Rays and X-Ray Machines
Outpatient X-Rays
Patient Positioning
Examination Sequencing
Radiation Safety
Diagnostic Procedures
Mammography
Contrast Medium Examinations
Fluoroscopy

Computed Tomography
Sonography
Magnetic Resonance Imaging
Nuclear Medicine
Interventional Radiologic
Procedures
Radiation Therapy
The Medical Assistant's Role
in Radiologic Procedures
Calming the Patient's Fears

Assisting with Examinations
Handling and Storing
Radiographic Films
Transfer of Radiographic
Information
Teleradiology

Learning Outcomes

Cognitive Domain

Note: AAMA/CAAHEP 2008 Standards are
italicized.

1. Spell and define the key terms
2. Explain the theory and function of x-rays and x-ray machines
3. State the principles of radiology
4. Describe routine and contrast media, fluoroscopy, computed tomography, sonography, magnetic resonance imaging, nuclear medicine, and mammographic examinations
5. Explain the role of the medical assistant in radiologic procedures
6. *Describe body planes, directional terms, quadrants, and cavities*
7. *Describe implications for treatment related to pathology*
8. *Identify critical information required for scheduling patient admissions and/or procedures*

Psychomotor Domain

Note: AAMA/CAAHEP 2008 Standards are
italicized.

1. Assist with x-ray procedures (Procedure 10-1)
2. *Instruct patients according to their needs to promote health maintenance and disease prevention*
3. *Prepare a patient for procedures and/or treatments*
4. *Document patient education*
5. *Schedule patient admissions and/or procedures*
6. *Perform within scope of practice*
7. *Apply local, state, and federal health care legislation and regulation appropriate to the medical assisting practice setting*

Affective Domain

Note: AAMA/CAAHEP 2008 Standards are italicized.

1. *Apply critical thinking skills in performing patient assessment and care*
2. *Use language/verbal skills that enable a patient's understanding*
3. *Demonstrate respect for diversity in approaching patients and families*
4. *Explain the rationale for performance of a procedure to the patient*
5. *Demonstrate empathy in communicating with patients, family, and staff*
6. *Apply active listening skills*
7. *Use appropriate body language and other nonverbal skills in communicating with patients, family, and staff*
8. *Demonstrate awareness of the territorial boundaries of the person with whom you are communicating*
9. *Demonstrate sensitivity appropriate to the message being delivered*
10. *Demonstrate recognition of the patient's level of understanding in communications*
11. *Recognize and protect personal boundaries in communicating with others*
12. *Demonstrate respect for individual diversity, incorporating awareness of one's own biases in areas including gender, race, religion, age, and economic status*

ABHES Competencies

1. Assist the physician with the regimen of diagnostic and treatment modalities as they relate to each body system
2. Comply with federal, state, and local health laws and regulations
3. Communicate on the recipient's level of comprehension
4. Serve as a liaison between the physician and others
5. Show empathy and impartiality when dealing with patients

Key Terms

cassette	fluoroscopy	radiography	radiopaque
computed tomography (CT)	magnetic resonance imaging (MRI)	radiologist	teleradiology
		radiology	ultrasound
contrast medium	nuclear medicine	radiolucent	x-rays
film	radiograph	radionuclides	

The discovery of **x-rays** in the late 19th century forever changed the practice of medicine. Routine x-ray imaging, **computed tomography (CT)**, sonography, **magnetic resonance imaging (MRI)**, and **nuclear medicine** are now commonly used diagnostic and therapeutic procedures. Advances in radiation therapy continue to be at the forefront of the treatment for cancer.

COG Principles of Radiology

Radiology continues to evolve through technologic changes that provide ever-increasing diagnostic information to physicians. As the technology advances, the need to teach patients becomes even more important. Medical assistants are often directly involved in preparing patients for outpatient radiographic procedures, performing basic radiographic procedures in the medical office, and assisting in the general educational process.

X-Rays and X-Ray Machines

X-rays are high-energy waves that cannot be seen, heard, felt, tasted, or smelled and that can penetrate fairly dense objects, such as the human body. This penetrating ability is what allows x-rays to be powerful diagnostic and therapeutic tools. Diagnostically, these penetrating waves create two-dimensional shadowlike images on **film** that is similar to photographic film. Unprocessed film must be protected from light and kept in a special holder called a **cassette** before use. Once the film inside

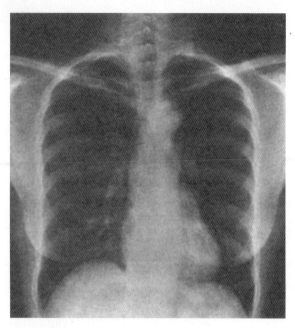

Figure 10-1 Radiograph of chest.

the cassette has been exposed to x-rays, the cassette is placed in a special machine that removes the film and processes it. The processed film containing a visible image is called a **radiograph** (Fig. 10-1). The process by which these films are produced is called **radiography**.

Electricity of extremely high voltage in the x-ray tube produces x-rays. The x-rays leave the tube in one primary direction as a beam, through a device used to control the size of the beam. The light that shines on the patient is not part of the beam but is a positioning aid that illuminates the area covered by the beam. A patient may hear noises coming from the tube area during an exposure, but these are made by the equipment, not the x-rays.

Today, x-ray machines are sophisticated and technologically advanced. Many are designed to work with computers to produce digital images of the body. Fluoroscopic units can reveal motion within the body. Most permanently installed radiographic units include a special table, some of which can be electronically rotated from the horizontal to the vertical. In this situation, the radiographic film is placed in a cassette that slides into a slot or opening on the table.

Images are formed on the x-ray film as the rays either pass through or are absorbed by the tissues of the body. **Radiolucent** tissues, such as air in the lungs, permit the passage of x-rays, while **radiopaque** tissues, such as bone, do not permit the passage of x-rays. Because bone is dense and absorbs much of the radiation beam, these structures appear white on a radiograph. Air is not dense and does not absorb much radiation. Therefore, air in a structure shows up dark on a radiograph. Other body tissues, such as muscle, fat, and fluid, show as varying shades of gray because of the way each tissue absorbs

the x-rays. Physicians who specialize in interpreting the images on the processed film are **radiologists**.

Outpatient X-Rays

The medical community is making a conscious effort to have as much treatment as possible done on an outpatient basis, and thus, some medical offices have on-site x-ray equipment. Outpatient diagnostic imaging centers have also been created to offer these services. Some companies specialize in providing minimal x-ray services to patients in long-term care facilities or the patients' homes.

In some states, you may be permitted to take and process simple images such as bone or chest radiographs as permitted by state law. The training for medical assistants varies, but some programs include a formal course in the theory of radiography and a written examination offered by the state radiographic association for the general operator. In other states, only licensed radiographers may take and process radiographs. You should be familiar with your state laws and comply with any regulations.

 CHECKPOINT QUESTION

1. How would you describe x-rays to a patient?

Patient Positioning

The x-ray exposure on film is a two-dimensional image. Because the human body is a three-dimensional structure, x-ray examinations usually require a minimum of two exposures taken at 90° to each other. For instance, a chest radiographic examination requires one exposure from the back and another from the side (Fig. 10-2). Other examinations necessitate three or more exposures at different angles. These different angles of exposure are the basis for standard positioning for x-ray examinations (Box 10-1).

Examination Sequencing

Most radiographic procedures can be performed in any order of convenience, but certain procedures must follow certain sequences in specific situations. For example, patients with gallbladder symptoms may go through a series of procedures, progressing from the simple noninvasive oral cholecystogram (an x-ray of the gallbladder after the ingestion of a **contrast medium** orally) to the more complex operative cholangiogram (x-ray of the bile ducts after injection with a contrast medium during a surgical procedure).

Another example is barium studies, the name given to examinations performed after administration of barium sulfate. A patient with gastrointestinal (GI) symptoms

Anteroposterior projection

Posteroanterior projection

Right lateral projection

Left lateral projection

Left posterior oblique projection

Right posterior oblique projection

Left anterior oblique projection

Right anterior oblique projection

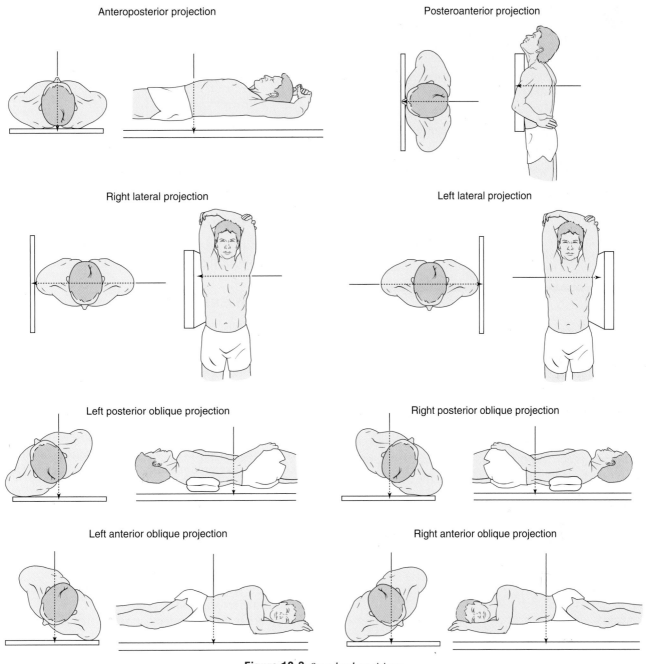

Figure 10-2 Standard positions.

may undergo a series of barium studies to assist the physician in diagnosis. Because of the nature of the barium studies and the length of time required to eliminate the barium from the digestive tract, barium enemas are usually scheduled before upper GI examinations. If an endoscopic study, such as an esophagogastroscopy, is ordered, it is imperative that these be scheduled before other procedures involving barium to avoid having the barium obstruct or interfere with the visualization of internal structures.

The barium study that requires filling only the large intestine with barium is the barium enema. Because this procedure involves the last part of the GI tract, this barium can be eliminated fairly quickly so that other examinations can be performed. If an upper GI examination, commonly referred to as an upper GI or barium swallow, is performed first, it may be several days before all of the barium is out of the patient's system. Any residual barium in the GI tract can obscure vital structures in subsequent procedures, preventing them from contributing diagnostic information. The proper sequencing of scheduling the barium enema first and the upper GI last will usually provide diagnostic information in a shorter time.

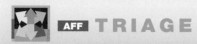 **AFF TRIAGE**

While working in a medical office setting, the physician has asked you to call the hospital and schedule Mrs. Roberts for the following three tests:

A. An esophagogastroduodenoscopy (EGD)
B. Barium enema
C. Barium swallow

What is the correct order for scheduling these tests to be performed?

The correct order is the EGD, the barium enema, and finally the upper GI series or barium swallow. It is important that these procedures be scheduled in this order to ensure optimal results.

BOX 10-1

STANDARD TERMINOLOGY FOR POSITIONING AND PROJECTION

Radiographic View
Describes the body part as seen by an x-ray film or other recording medium, such as a fluoroscopic screen. Restricted to the discussion of a *radiograph* or *image*.

Radiographic Position
Refers to a specific body position, such as supine, prone, recumbent, erect, or Trendelenburg. Restricted to the discussion of the *patient's physical position.*

Radiographic Projection
Restricted to the discussion of the *path of the central ray.*

Positioning Terminology
Lying Down
1. *Supine*, lying on the back
2. *Prone*, lying face downward
3. *Decubitus*, lying down with a horizontal x-ray beam
4. *Recumbent*, lying down in any position

Erect or Upright
1. *Anterior position*, facing the film
2. *Posterior position*, facing the radiographic tube
3. *Oblique position*, (erect or lying down)
   A. Anterior, facing the film
      i. *Left anterior oblique*, body rotated with the left anterior portion closest to the film
      ii. *Right anterior oblique*, body rotated with the right anterior portion closest to the film

B. *Posterior*, facing the radiographic tube
   i. *Left posterior oblique*, body rotated with the left posterior portion closest to the film
   ii. *Right posterior oblique*, body rotated with the right posterior portion closest to the film

From The American Registry of Radiologic Technologists ® "Content Specifications for The Examination in Radiography." Publication date: July 2004.

 CHECKPOINT QUESTION

2. Why is it important to schedule a barium enema before an upper GI or barium swallow?

Radiation Safety

Of primary concern to all radiation workers and patients is the proper and safe use of radiant energy. The hazards of radiation have been known for many decades, and warnings about x-ray radiation are usually posted in appropriate areas (Fig. 10-3). X-rays have the potential to cause cellular or genetic damage to the body, and the results of this damage may not manifest for several years after exposure. The adverse effects are most extreme for rapidly reproducing cells. Pregnant women, children, and reproductive organs of adults are at the highest risk because of their rapid cell division and growth.

Radiation safety procedures for patients include the following:

1. Minimizing exposure amounts.
2. Avoiding unnecessary examinations.
3. Limiting the area of the body exposed.
4. Shielding sensitive body parts, such as the gonads and the thyroid gland.
5. Evaluating the pregnancy status of female patients before performing examinations.

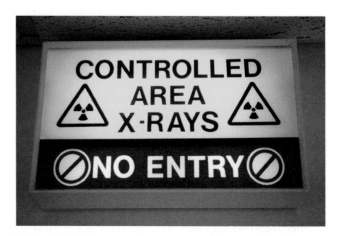

Figure 10-3 X-ray warning sign.

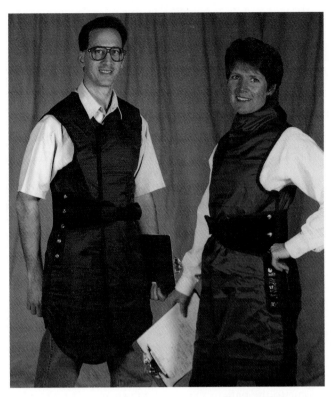

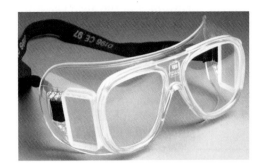

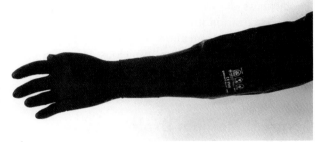

Figure 10-4 X-ray protection equipment.

Safety procedures for clinical staff working around x-ray equipment include the following:

1. Limiting the amount of time exposed to x-rays.
2. Staying as far away from the x-rays as possible during exposure, preferably standing behind a barrier such as a wall lined with lead.
3. Using available shielding for protection, such as lead aprons and gloves (Fig. 10-4).
4. Avoiding holding patients during exposures. For children requiring assistance, a parent wearing a lead apron may be recruited during the procedure.
5. Wearing individual dosimeters, which are small devices that contain radiographic film clipped to the outside of the uniform, to record the amount of radiation, if any, to which the worker has been exposed (Fig. 10-5). These badges are provided by the employer and are obtained from companies that specifically monitor any radiation exposure of individual health care providers.
6. Ensuring proper working condition of the equipment by scheduling routine maintenance.

For both patients and medical assistants working around radiation, these concerns can be summed up in what is called the *ALARA concept*: doing whatever is necessary to keep radiation exposure as low as reasonably achievable.

COG Diagnostic Procedures

Routine radiographic examinations require little or no preparation of the patient and are the most commonly performed examinations. These procedures are most readily accepted by the patient and are named for the part of the body involved in the radiographic procedure (Table 10-1). These studies are performed for viewing primarily bone structure or abnormalities.

CHECKPOINT QUESTION

3. How does the dosimeter protect you from radiation?

Mammography

Mammography, an x-ray examination of the breast, is used as a screening tool for breast cancer (Box 10-2). Each breast is compressed in a specialized device to even

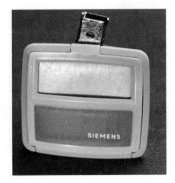

Figure 10-5 Dosimeter badge.

TABLE 10-1	Routine Radiographic Examinations by Body Region
Region	**Patient Preparation**
Trunk	Disrobing of the area: chest, ribs, sternum, shoulder, scapula, clavicle, abdomen, hip, pelvis, sternoclavicular, acromioclavicular, sacroiliac joints
Extremities	Removing jewelry or clothing that might obscure parts of interest: fingers, thumb, hand, wrist, forearm, elbow, humerus, toes, foot, os calcis, ankle, lower leg, knee, patella, femur
Spine	Disrobing of the appropriate area: cervical, thoracic, or lumbar spine; sacrum; coccyx
Head	Removing eyewear, false eyes, false teeth, earrings, hairpins, and hairpieces: skull, sinuses, nasal bones, facial bones and orbits, optic foramen, mandible, temporomandibular joints, mastoid and petrous portion, zygomatic arch

the thickness, allowing for an optimal diagnostic image. Needle localization studies using the information gained from the mammogram allow the physician to withdraw small amounts of cells from suspicious areas in a minimally invasive procedure. Mammography has become a vital adjunct to biopsy (Fig. 10-6).

Contrast Medium Examinations

Within the abdomen, many structures having similar radiation absorption rates are superimposed on each other. This makes differentiating structures difficult. The use of a radiopaque contrast medium helps differentiate between body structures by artificially changing the absorption rate of a particular structure. For example, barium sulfate absorbs radiation and shows white on a radiograph (Fig. 10-7). There are many contrast media for various applications. Iodinated compounds are used in many areas of the body, including the kidneys and blood vessels, and in some CT scans. Patients who may have an intestinal perforation may be given an iodinated contrast medium instead of barium because that material spilling into the peritoneum is much less troublesome to the patient than barium.

Radiographic examinations using contrast media are performed to evaluate not only a structure, but also its function. For example, patients having excretory urography have a contrast medium injected, and the anatomic structure of each kidney is evaluated as the medium passes through the urinary tract. Contrast media may be introduced into the body in several ways, including by mouth, intravenously, or through a catheter, depending on the material and area of the body being examined. It is important that you ask the patient about allergies, especially shellfish allergies. Usually, patients allergic to

---

BOX 10-2

AMERICAN CANCER SOCIETY (ACS) GUIDELINES FOR BREAST CANCER SCREENING

The American Cancer Society recommends mammography for women yearly starting at the age of 40. However, women with known risk factors such as a family history of breast cancer may have mammography screenings earlier than the age of 40 years. The following breast cancer screenings are recommended:

- Mammography over the age of 40 every year.
- Clinical breast exam, or breast exam by a physician or nurse, yearly to palpate the presence of lumps or other changes.
- Breast self-exam monthly to check for the presence of lumps, changes in the size or shape of the breast, or any other changes in the breasts or underarm.
- A mammography and MRI of the breast yearly for women at high risk for developing breast cancer.

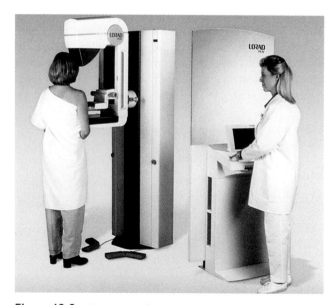

Figure 10-6 Mammography machine.

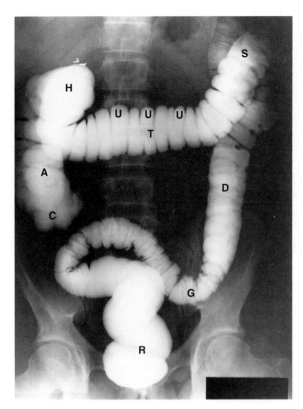

Figure 10-7 Barium-filled large intestine.

shellfish are actually allergic to the high iodine content of the shellfish, and because injectable contrast media are iodine based, this information needs to be relayed to the radiology center before the patient is scheduled. Another concern for patients undergoing radiographic procedures requiring contrast media is the preparation they must undergo before some of these procedures, especially barium studies. Preparation of the patient for a barium study might include the following:

- Liquid diet only for the evening meal on the day before the examination.
- Laxatives the day preceding the examination to help clean the intestinal tract.
- Nothing by mouth (NPO) after midnight the day before the examination. This usually includes no gum chewing or cigarette smoking because both activities increase gastric secretions that may interfere with the ability of the contrast medium to coat the wall of the intestine.

This general preparation applies to any contrast examination of the abdominal structures. Although this type of radiographic procedure is not performed in the medical office, you must ensure that the patient has proper instructions for preparing for the procedure and is notified of the scheduled time and facility. If patients are not properly prepared for contrast studies, they may have to be rescheduled for another time and day and must undertake the preparations again. Explaining the importance of the preparation can be one of the most important contributions you can make to the patient's care in contrast examinations.

 CHECKPOINT QUESTION

4. How does contrast media aid in differentiating between body structures?

Fluoroscopy

Fluoroscopy, or fluoro studies, use x-rays to observe movement within the body. The movement of a contrast medium in the body could include barium sulfate through the digestive tract or iodinated compounds in the blood as it flows through the heart or blood vessels. Fluoroscopy is also used as an aid to other types of treatments, such as reducing fractures and implanting devices such as pacemakers.

Computed Tomography

CT is a procedure in which the x-ray tube and film move in relation to one another during the exposure, blurring out all structures except those in the focal plane. CT uses a combination of x-rays from a tube circling the patient and computers that analyze the x-rays to create cross-sectional images of the body. CT may be done with or without contrast medium. In addition, some CT units can create three-dimensional images so that organs can be viewed from all angles (Fig. 10-8).

 CHECKPOINT QUESTION

5. What procedures would require the use of fluoroscopy?

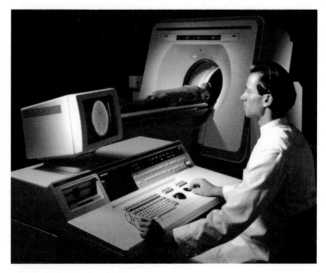

Figure 10-8 A CT scanner.

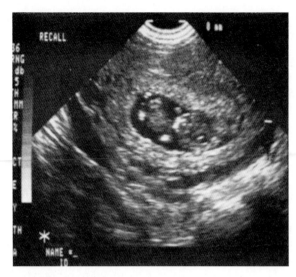

Figure 10-9 A sonogram.

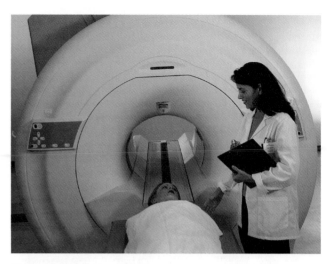

Figure 10-10 An open MRI.

Sonography

Ultrasound, or sonography, uses high-frequency sound waves, not x-rays, to create cross-sectional still or real-time (motion) images of the body, usually with the help of a computer. This application is often used to demonstrate heart function or abdominal or pelvic structures. It is commonly used in prenatal testing to visualize the developing fetus. Many obstetricians routinely schedule at least one sonogram before the fourth month of pregnancy (Fig. 10-9).

Magnetic Resonance Imaging

MRI uses a combination of high-intensity magnetic fields, radio waves, and computer analysis to create cross-sectional images of the body. MRI does not use x-rays. The image depends on the chemical makeup of the body. MRI is commonly used for a variety of studies, including the central nervous system and joint structure. Some MRI studies are performed with contrast. Typically, the patient must be prepared for a long procedure snugly enclosed in a machine that makes numerous knocking and whirring noises. Some facilities use open MRI, which does not make a patient feel as claustrophobic as the closed MRI (Fig. 10-10). Patients with a fear of enclosed places may require a mild sedative before closed MRI.

Nuclear Medicine

Nuclear medicine entails the injection of small amounts of **radionuclides,** which are radioactive materials with short life spans, designed to concentrate in specific areas of the body. Sophisticated computer cameras detect the radiation and create an image. This technique is commonly used to study the thyroid, brain, lungs, liver, spleen, kidney, bone, and breast. These examinations are commonly called scans.

A sophisticated nuclear medicine study, *positron emission tomography* (*PET*), uses specialized equipment to produce detailed sectional images of the body's physiologic processes. Another procedure, *single photon emission computed tomography* (*SPECT*), is a nuclear study that produces sectional images of the body as detectors move around the patient. Both of these procedures are useful in the early diagnosis of physiologic and cellular abnormalities, such as those associated with cancerous tumors.

 CHECKPOINT QUESTION

6. Which diagnostic imaging technique would most likely be ordered for diagnosing cancer in the early stages?

COG Interventional Radiologic Procedures

Interventional radiologic techniques are designed to treat specific disease conditions. For some patients, these therapeutic techniques are so effective that there is no need for surgery. Some interventional procedures may be lifesaving. The following are some types of techniques:

• *Percutaneous transluminal coronary angioplasty* (*PTCA*), also known as *balloon angioplasty*, is used to enlarge the lumen of a coronary artery with a balloon-tipped catheter. Using fluoroscopy, the catheter is placed at a point of partial occlusion or stenosis. The balloon is then briefly inflated, compressing the plaque against the sides of the vessel. After the balloon is deflated, the catheter is removed, and the lumen of the vessel remains larger, allowing for improved blood flow through the blood vessel. Balloon angioplasties may be performed in almost any blood vessel.

- *Laser angioplasties* use laser beams to remove deposits in vessels using fluoroscopy.
- *Vascular stents* (plastic or wire tubes) may be inserted into the stenosed, or constricted, area of a vessel to maintain its patency. Fluoroscopy is used to guide placement of the stent.
- *Embolizations* artificially stop active bleeding from a blood vessel or reduce blood flow to a diseased area of an organ.

COG Radiation Therapy

A major force in the fight against cancer for many years has been radiation therapy. The use of high-energy radiation to destroy cancer cells may not only prolong the lives of many patients but also saves lives. Used in conjunction with surgery, chemotherapy, or both, radiation is possibly the best-known treatment for cancer. Because the radiation is intense enough to destroy cancer cells, it may also damage adjacent normal cells. Therefore, treatments must be planned carefully and precisely by a radiologist, a physician who specializes in radiology.

Treatment consists of a precise, carefully planned regimen of therapy, including the frequency and amount of radiation to be used and the number of exposures during a given period. The area of the body to be exposed must be defined exactly so that each treatment is identical. The therapy consists of placing the patient in a position described by the treatment plan and having the exact amount of radiation administered by a radiology technician. Usually the patient has little to do but lie still.

The patient's prognosis varies with the situation. Most patients have some side effects, which may include hair loss, weight loss, loss of appetite, skin changes, and digestive system disturbances. Once the treatment plan is carried out, most of the side effects disappear.

CHECKPOINT QUESTION

7. What type of health care practitioner is responsible for prescribing and monitoring the effects of radiation therapy for the treatment of cancer?

COG The Medical Assistant's Role in Radiologic Procedures

Because professional medical assistants have a variety of responsibilities in patient care, they often are in an ideal position to help alleviate patients' anxiety regarding radiology. Patient anxiety may be relieved by giving patients information about examinations they do not understand, by making patients feel comfortable enough to ask questions, and by answering questions in terms the patient can understand.

Calming the Patient's Fears

Some patients who have experience with the medical system have learned to overcome their anxieties and to find answers to their questions. No matter how much they have been through before, however, there is always something new or something they do not understand that may make them feel as if they have lost control of their situation. Being sensitive to patients' feelings is one of the greatest talents anyone in medicine can possess and should be an important part of your training and personality.

Unfortunately, many patients must undergo procedures they do not understand and do not know enough about to be able to ask relevant questions. Many feel like spectators rather than participants in their own care. Medical assistants can affect a patient's emotional response to a radiologic procedure by explaining what to expect in simple, everyday language, not technical medical terms. The technical aspects of radiology make it difficult for patients to understand. The key to success in explaining radiology procedures to patients is simplicity, leaving the details to the physician.

As noted earlier, explaining the preparations for examinations and their importance is vital to the success of many procedures. Equally important may be an explanation of what to do after the procedure. A barium enema, for instance, can lead to constipation if the patient does not drink enough fluids after the examination. This simple direction can save the patient much distress.

AFF WHAT IF?

A patient has been scheduled for a barium study at a local outpatient facility but calls your office to ask what to do if he ate breakfast this morning. What should you do?

As a medical assistant, you must understand the reason for fasting before certain diagnostic procedures. In this situation, the patient should be instructed to call the diagnostic facility for further instructions, which will include rescheduling the procedure. Emphasize to the patient the importance of following all instructions carefully since not doing so will interfere with the procedure and/or the results. Not following instructions will result in further inconvenience of the patient and delay of a possible diagnose, further delaying treatment and outcomes for the patient.

Assisting with Examinations

As a medical assistant, you may be expected to assist with radiologic examinations in the following ways:

• Tell the patient what clothing to remove or assist with clothing removal as needed.
• Help the patient take the position for the procedure, emphasizing the importance of remaining still and following breathing directions.
• Perform specific radiologic procedures, such as bone or chest radiography, as permitted by your state's laws and your education and training.
• Place film in an automatic processor and reload new film into the cassette.
• Distribute or file radiographs and reports appropriately.

Procedure 10-1 details the procedure for assisting with x-ray procedures.

Handling and Storing Radiographic Films

Advancing technology and the need for quality control have led to automated processing and developing of film to eliminate human error. Automated processing machines produce a film usually in less than 2 minutes. Because processors vary by manufacturer, you need to be proficient in the operation of your particular facility's equipment.

Unexposed film must be protected from moisture, heat, and light by storage in a cool, dry place, preferably in a lead-lined box. Film packets, exposed or unexposed, must be opened in a darkroom using only the darkroom light for illumination. The film is placed in a cassette for use in any area outside the darkroom. Intensifying screens in the cassette are used to reduce the amount of exposure required. Special sleeves or envelopes of various sizes are available for storing the film that has been labeled with the name of the patient (Fig. 10-11). Film must be protected and stored in a cool, dry area.

 CHECKPOINT QUESTION

8. How can the medical assistant help with radiologic examinations?

COG Transfer of Radiographic Information

Radiographic images obtained on site for use by the physician remain part of the patient's permanent record. Digital images can be saved on a computer diskette or compact disk. In many cases, however, radiographic studies are performed at one site for consultation or

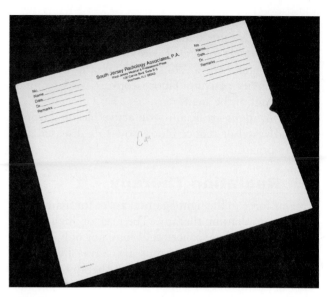

Figure 10-11 An x-ray envelope.

referral at another site. X-ray films belong to the site where the study was performed. The examining physician or radiologist generally writes a summary of the examination to the referring physician. You may need the patient's permission to have the summary of findings sent to the office physician.

With a short-term referral, the examining physician usually returns the films to the referring physician. Patients who have ongoing concerns or who change physicians may request the information contained in their records after submitting written consent. In addition, the patient may obtain copies of the original radiographs if necessary.

 AFF WHAT IF?

What if your patient asks you to give him the results of a recently taken chest x-ray?

Many patients are anxious to find out test results including the results of radiology procedures. Often, these patients will ask you for the results before the physician has had an opportunity to read any radiology reports or to look at the actual radiograph. You should tell this patient that the physician would prefer to talk to him about the results and any questions can be answered at that time by the physician. Although you may have access to radiology reports, it is not appropriate to discuss the results with the patient unless the physician has given you permission to do so.

Teleradiology

The use of computed imaging and information systems, **teleradiology**, is providing new benefits in medicine. Many institutions use a picture archiving and communication system (PACS) in which computers store and transmit images. Digital images from CT, for instance, can be transmitted via telephone lines to distant locations. This allows consultation with experts on a difficult case within a matter of minutes. Previously unavailable expertise can be brought to rural areas for greatly improved patient care. The result is improved patient care over large geographic areas, not just in specific locations. The term *teleradiology* is often used to describe this radiology over a great distance.

 CHECKPOINT QUESTION

9. If digital images are taken, how are these records stored?

 PATIENT EDUCATION

ADVANCES IN SURGICAL PROCEDURES

Today, many surgeries that once required large abdominal incisions and extended hospital stays are performed in outpatient ambulatory surgical centers through small incisions and a laparoscope. For example, gallstones are removed with a laparoscope guided by an interventional radiologist, and the patient returns home the same day of surgery. Abdominal aortic aneurysms are treated with a similar procedure, resulting in shorter hospital admissions and less pain. You need to stay current regarding new procedures and surgical techniques so that you can be informed and reassure patients and their families who may not be as aware of the advances made in health care.

SPANISH TERMINOLOGY

Tiene que estar en ayunas antes de la prueba.
You must not eat or drink anything before the test.

Puede tomar una comida ligera la noche antes de la prueba.
You may eat a light supper the night before the test.

Debe seguir estas instrucciónes al pie de la letra.
You must follow these directions exactly.

Tengo que hacerle una radiografía una placa.
I have to take an x-ray.

MEDIA MENU

• **Student Resources on thePoint**
  • **CMA/RMA Certification Exam Review**

• **Internet Resources**

  Radiology Info
  http://www.radiologyinfo.org

  Virtual Hospital
  http://www.vh.org

  American Society of Radiologic Technologists
  http://www.asrt.org

  Access Excellence Resource Center: The Living Skeleton
  http://www.accessexcellence.org/RC/VL/xrays/index.php

  Medline Plus: X-Rays
  http://www.nlm.nih.gov/medlineplus/xrays.html

  The Registry of Radiologic Technologists
  http://www.arrt.org

PSY PROCEDURE 10-1: **Assist with X-Ray Procedures**

Purpose: Prepare the patient for general x-ray procedure
Equipment: Patient gown and drape
Standard: This procedure should take 5 minutes.

Steps	Reasons
1. Wash your hands.	Handwashing aids infection control.
2. Greet the patient by name, introduce yourself, and escort him or her to the room where the x-ray equipment is maintained.	Identifying the patient by name prevents errors.
3. **AFF** Explain how to respond to a patient who speaks English as a second language (ESL).	With the patient's permission, have an interpreter in the room to assist with translation. Arrange this before the patient comes into the office if possible. If one is not available, utilize a picture chart or nonverbal gestures to help the patient understand.
4. Ask female patients about the possibility of pregnancy. If the patient is unsure or indicates pregnancy in any trimester, consult with the physician before proceeding with the x-ray procedure.	Fetal exposure to x-rays may be damaging to developing organs and tissues.
5. After explaining what clothing should be removed, if any, give the patient a gown and provide privacy.	For a chest x-ray, you will have the patient remove all clothing from the waist up. Jewelry such as necklaces may also have to be removed since these will show up on the x-ray and may obscure the images the physician needs to view for diagnosis.
6. Notify the x-ray technician or physician that the patient is ready for the x-ray procedure. Stay behind the lead-lined wall during the x-ray procedure to avoid exposure to x-rays during the procedure.	Depending on state law, you may or may not be permitted to be trained to perform x-ray procedures.
7. After the x-ray, ask the patient to remain in the room until the film has been developed and checked for accuracy and readability.	On occasion, the x-ray will need to be repeated for clarity or adjusted patient position.
8. Once you have determined that the exposed film is adequate for the physician to view for diagnosis, have the patient get dressed and escort him or her to the front desk.	At that time, you can explain any further physician instructions or billing procedures.
9. Document the procedure in the medical record.	Procedures are considered not to have been done if they are not recorded.

Charting Example:

10/19/2012 AP Chest x-ray obtained per x-ray tech. Radiograph placed on viewbox—Dr. Jones notified ————
———————————————————————————————— S. Smith, CMA

Medical assistant may sign his or her name in the patient record using only the "CMA" credential if the office has a signature log denoting the entire credential as "CMA(AAMA)."

- Radiology is continually evolving as a tool to diagnose and treat disease. As a medical assistant:
- You must understand the common types of diagnostic and therapeutic radiologic procedures that may be ordered by the physician.
- You may also be responsible for teaching patients about these procedures in general and about any particular preparations required.
- When assisting the physician, you must always follow radiation safety precautions carefully for the protection of yourself and your patient.

Warm Ups for Critical Thinking

1. While preparing a female patient for an x-ray procedure, she explains to you that she might be pregnant. How would you handle this situation?
2. Create a poster for your office summarizing the key points of radiation safety.
3. Constipation is a common problem among patients who have barium studies. How can patient education diminish this problem?
4. An elderly woman is concerned about having an ultrasound of her gallbladder and states that she does not want to have any more x-rays. Based on what you know about sonography, how would you respond to this patient?
5. Explain the importance of patient privacy laws (Health Insurance Portability and Accountability Act of 1996 [HIPAA]) and teleradiology. What is your role in maintaining privacy in using teleradiology?

Medical Office Emergencies

Outline

Medical Office Emergency Procedures

Preparation for an Emergency

Patient Assessment

Types of Emergencies

Learning Outcomes

Cognitive Domain

Note: AAMA/CAAHEP 2008 Standards are italicized.

1. Spell and define key terms
2. *State principles and steps of professional/provider CPR*
3. *Describe basic principles of first aid*
4. Identify the five types of shock and the management of each
5. Describe how burns are classified and managed
6. Explain the management of allergic reactions
7. Describe the management of poisoning and the role of the poison control center
8. List the three types of hyperthermic emergencies and the treatment for each type
9. Discuss the treatment of hypothermia
10. Describe the role of the medical assistant in managing psychiatric emergencies

Psychomotor Domain

Note: AAMA/CAAHEP 2008 Standards are italicized.

1. Administer oxygen (Procedure 11-1)
2. Perform cardiopulmonary resuscitation (Procedure 11-2)
3. Use an automatic external defibrillator (Procedure 11-3)
4. Manage a foreign body airway obstruction (Procedure 11-4)
5. Control bleeding (Procedure 11-5)
6. Respond to medical emergencies other than bleeding, cardiac/respiratory arrest, or foreign body airway obstruction (Procedure 11-6)
7. *Perform first aid procedures*
8. *Practice standard precautions*
9. *Document accurately in the patient record*
10. *Perform within scope of practice*
11. *Select appropriate barrier/personal protective equipment for potentially infectious situations*

Affective Domain

Note: AAMA/CAAHEP 2008 Standards are italicized.

1. *Apply critical thinking skills in performing patient assessment and care*
2. *Show awareness of patients' concerns regarding their perceptions related to the procedure being performed*
3. *Demonstrate empathy in communicating with patients, family, and staff*
4. *Apply active listening skills*
5. *Use appropriate body language and other nonverbal skills in communicating with patients, family, and staff*

6. *Demonstrate awareness of territorial boundaries of the person with whom you are communicating*
7. *Demonstrate sensitivity appropriate to the message being delivered*
8. *Demonstrate recognition of the patient's level of understanding in communications*
9. *Recognize and protect personal boundaries in communicating with others*
10. *Demonstrate respect for individual diversity, incorporating awareness of one's own biases in areas including gender, race, religion, age, and economic status*

ABHES Competencies

1. Document accurately
2. Recognize and respond to verbal and nonverbal communication
3. Adapt to individualized needs
4. Apply principles of aseptic techniques and infection control
5. Recognize emergencies and treatments and minor office surgical procedures
6. Use standard precautions
7. Perform first aid and CPR
8. Demonstrate professionalism by exhibiting a positive attitude and sense of responsibility

Key Terms

allergen	frostbite	hypothermia	partial-thickness burn
anaphylactic shock	heat cramps	hypovolemic shock	seizures
cardiogenic shock	heat exhaustion	infarction	septic shock
contusions	heat stroke	ischemia	shock
ecchymosis	hematomas	melena	splint
full-thickness burn	hyperthermia	neurogenic shock	superficial burn

Emergency medical care is the immediate care given to sick or injured persons. When properly performed, it can mean the difference between life or death, rapid recovery or long hospitalization, and temporary or permanent disability. Emergency care in the medical office entails identifying the emergency, delivering basic first aid, and furnishing temporary assistance or basic life support until a rescue squad and advanced life support can be obtained.

COG Medical Office Emergency Procedures

An emergency can occur anywhere, to anyone, at any time. For example, a patient who is being seen for a routine examination may have a heart attack, collapse, and require immediate cardiopulmonary resuscitation (CPR). A diabetic patient or co-worker may lapse into a diabetic coma (see Chapter 21 for diabetic emergency procedures). A patient may fall down a flight of stairs and receive trauma to the head or limbs. In a life-threatening situation, the well-prepared medical assistant can obtain important information and perform lifesaving procedures before the ambulance or rescue squad arrives, increasing the patient's chance for survival. Medical assistants should be certified in CPR, using the automatic external defibrillator (AED), and removing foreign body airway obstructions. Currently, the American Association of Medical Assistants (AAMA) requires certified medical assistants (CMAs) to demonstrate proof of current CPR certification to recertify their credential. This training may be provided by the American Red Cross, American Heart Association, American Safety and Health Institute, or National Safety Council. You should contact one of these agencies for specific information regarding training and certification. This chapter is not meant to provide a comprehensive study of all aspects of emergency care; instead, it briefly reviews the information in such a training course.

Preparation for an Emergency

Every medical office should have an emergency action plan, including the following:

- The local emergency rescue service telephone number (usually 911)
- Location of the nearest hospital emergency department

- Telephone number of the local or regional poison control center
- Procedures for various emergencies
- List of office personnel who are trained in CPR
- Location and list of contents of the emergency medical kit or crash cart

Whether confronted with a cardiac emergency or psychiatric crisis, medical assistants must be able to coordinate multiple ongoing events while rendering patient care. Contributing to the complexity of a medical emergency are such factors as panicky family members, the arrival of emergency personnel, and possibly language barriers. You must be able to remain calm in these situations while reacting competently and professionally.

Emergency Medical Kit

Proper equipment and supplies should be readily available in a medical emergency. Although the office's equipment and supplies vary with the medical specialty, emergency equipment and supplies are fairly standard. This equipment should be kept in a designated location that is accessible to all staff. Standard supplies for a medical emergency kit are listed in Box 11-1. Although items used during an emergency should be replaced as soon as possible, a medical assistant or other staff member should check the contents of the emergency kit or crash cart regularly, perhaps weekly, to verify that contents are available and that no item has gone beyond the expiration date. If so, the expired items should be replaced immediately.

The Emergency Medical Services System

The initial element of any emergency medical services (EMS) system is citizen access. The availability of rapid, systematic intervention by personnel specifically trained in providing emergency care is an integral part of the EMS system. Most communities have a 911 system to report emergencies and summon help by telephone. The communications operator at the local EMS station will answer the call, take the information, and alert the EMS, fire, or police department as needed. In communities without a 911 system, emergency calls are usually made directly to the local ambulance, fire, or police department. You should know the emergency system used in your community. Emergency phone numbers should be prominently displayed by all telephones in the medical office.

Some communities have an enhanced 911 system that automatically identifies the caller's telephone number and location. If the telephone is disconnected or the caller loses consciousness, the communications operator can still send emergency personnel to the scene. In the medical office, an emergency requiring notification of the EMS includes situations that are life threatening or

---

BOX 11-1

EMERGENCY MEDICAL KIT AND EQUIPMENT

The following are standard supplies that can be used to make up an emergency medical kit:

- Acetic acid solution (4%–6%) or vinegar
- Activated charcoal
- Adhesive strip bandages, assorted sizes
- Adhesive tape, 1- and 2-inch rolls
- Alcohol (70%)
- Alcohol wipes
- Antimicrobial skin ointment
- Chemical ice pack
- Cotton balls
- Cotton swabs
- Disposable gloves
- Elastic bandages, 2- and 3-inch widths
- Gauze pads, 2 × 2– and 4 × 4–inch widths
- Roller, self-adhesive gauze, 2- and 4-inch widths
- Safety pins, various sizes
- Scissors
- Spray bottle for cool water
- Syrup of ipecac
- Thermometer
- Tweezers

In addition to these contents, the following equipment should be available:

- Blood pressure cuff (pediatric and adult)
- Stethoscope
- Bag-valve mask device with assorted size masks
- Flashlight or penlight
- Portable oxygen tank with regulator
- Oxygen masks
- Suction unit and catheters

Additional equipment that may be available includes:

- Various sizes of endotracheal tubes
- Laryngoscope handle and various sizes of blades
- AED
- IV supplies (catheters, administration set tubing, assorted solutions)
- Emergency drugs including atropine, epinephrine, and sodium bicarbonate

---

have the potential to become life threatening, such as the symptoms of a heart attack, shock, or severe breathing difficulties. In each of these cases, the medical assistant provides immediate care to the patient, including CPR if necessary, while directing another staff member to notify the physician. During assessment of the emergency by the physician, the medical assistant should continue to provide first aid or be prepared to assist the physician in administering first aid while another staff member notifies the EMS. The staff member who calls EMS should be able to describe the emergency to the communications operator. The operator will then know what level of emergency personnel and rescue equipment to send. Excellent communication skills and cooperation between health care team members is essential during a medical office emergency.

Documentation in the medical record is an important responsibility in all patient care, including emergency care. EMS personnel depend on accurate and complete information regarding the patient's symptoms, the nature of the emergency, and any treatment performed prior to their arrival. This information should be placed in the patient's record in chronological order as events occurred or treatments were performed. Any vital signs taken during the emergency should also be recorded. Emergencies that involve visitors or staff must also be documented, and in this case, a blank paper or progress note page will be sufficient to record the details and outline the care provided. Information should include but not be limited to the following:

1. Basic identification, including name, age, address, and location of the patient's emergency contact if known
2. The chief complaint if known
3. Times of events, beginning with recognition of the emergency, management techniques, and changes in patient's condition
4. The patient's vital signs
5. Specific emergency management rendered in the office, such as CPR, bandaging, splinting, and medications administered before and after the emergency
6. Observations of the patient's condition, including any slurred speech, lethargy, confusion, and so on
7. Any medical history, allergies, or current medications if known

When the EMS personnel arrive, assist them as necessary. Let them examine the patient and take over the emergency care. You can also help by removing any obstacles to removal of the patient by stretcher and keeping family members in the reception area or a private room.

 CHECKPOINT QUESTION

1. What should you document before the ambulance arrives in an emergency?

Patient Assessment

The two primary objectives in assessment of the patient are to identify and correct any life-threatening problems and provide necessary care. Each step of the assessment must be managed effectively before proceeding to the next. For example, airway, breathing, and circulation must be intact before you take a history. In addition, survey the scene quickly to identify hazards or clues to the patient's condition. For example, an elderly person found at the bottom of a stairway will likely have head or neck injuries and should be treated in such a way as to avoid moving the head, neck, or spinal column. Emesis found near a person that resembles coffee grounds may be a clue to bleeding in the gastrointestinal system that may result from peptic ulcer disease and hemorrhage.

Recognizing the Emergency

When providing emergency care, do not assume that the obvious injuries are the only ones. Less noticeable or internal injuries may also have occurred during an accident. You should look for the causes of the injury, which may provide a clue to the extent of physical damage. For example, the elderly patient who fell down the stairs may have a noticeable bump on the forehead; this is obvious, but perhaps the patient has an injury in the cervical spine that is not as readily noticeable. In the case of an injury to the head or back when spinal fracture is possible, be especially careful not to move the victim any more than necessary and avoid rough handling.

The Primary Assessment

Once you are at the victim's side, an initial survey of the patient is the first step in emergency care. This is a rapid evaluation, usually done in less than 45 seconds. The purpose of the primary assessment is to identify and correct any life-threatening problems. Quickly assess the following aspects of the patient:

- Responsiveness
- Circulation
- Airway
- Breathing

Checking for responsiveness means noting whether the patient is conscious or unconscious. If the patient is unconscious, attempt to awaken the patient by speaking and touching the shoulder. If no response occurs, check for circulation. Evaluate circulation in adults and children by checking the carotid pulse (Fig. 11-1). The brachial pulse is used to evaluate circulation in infants. If no pulse is found, begin CPR chest compressions immediately (Fig. 11-2). Some medical offices may have an AED as part of the emergency medical kit (Fig. 11-3). Training to use the AED is included in most CPR classes. Many public places such as airports and shopping malls have AED units available for use by those individuals trained appropriately. If no pulse present, begin chest compressions.

After 30 compressions, assess the patient's airway by using the head tilt–chin lift method (Fig. 11-4). Patients

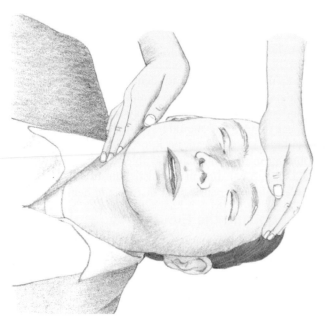

Figure 11-1 Check for circulation by palpating the carotid pulse. (From Nursing Procedures, 4th Edition. Ambler: Lippincott Williams & Wilkins, 2004.)

who may have neck injuries should have the airway opened using the jaw thrust method to avoid further injury to the spinal cord (Fig. 11-5). An unconscious patient who is supine is likely to have a partial or total airway obstruction caused by the tongue falling back into the oropharynx, producing snoring respirations or total airway obstruction. Opening the patient's airway may be necessary to allow adequate respirations. In the event of a foreign body airway obstruction, it will be necessary to clear the airway to perform effective rescue breathing.

Once the airway is open, evaluate the patient's breathing by watching for movement of the chest up or down while listening and feeling over the mouth and nose for signs of adequate ventilation. If the patient

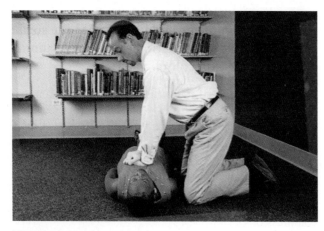

Figure 11-2 Chest compressions should be started if no signs of circulation, including a pulse, are present.

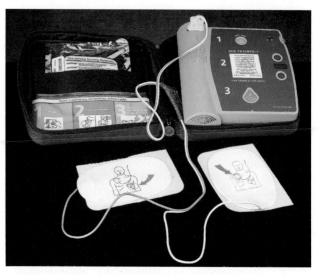

Figure 11-3 The AED can be used to defibrillate a life-threatening heart rhythm.

is not breathing, rescue breathing must be started immediately. A face mask with a one-way valve or a bag–valve–mask device is required when performing rescue breathing (Fig. 11-6). Respirations that are too fast, too slow, or irregular also require medical intervention. Immediate intervention for these conditions may include breathing into a mask or paper bag for respirations that are too fast (hyperventilation) or administering oxygen as directed by the physician. Any obvious noises, such as stridor or wheezes, are

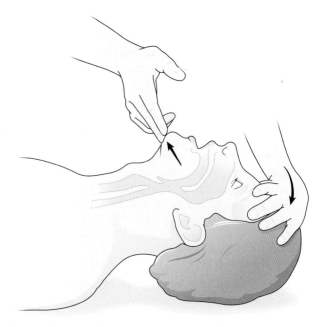

Figure 11-4 The head tilt–chin lift technique for opening the airway. The head is tilted backward with one hand (*down arrow*) while the fingers of the other hand lift the chin forward (*up arrow*).

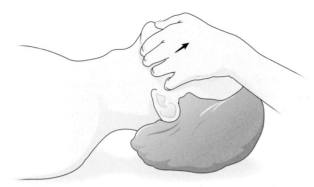

Figure 11-5 The jaw thrust technique for opening the airway. The hands are placed on either side of the head. The fingers of both hands grasp behind the angle of the jaw, bringing it up (*arrow*).

noted and reported to the physician (see Chapter 15). Continue cardiopulmonary procedures until relieved by another healthcare staff member or EMS personnel arrive and take over. Procedure 11-1 describes the procedure for administering oxygen in the medical office, while Procedures 11-2, 11-3, and 11-4 explain CPR, the use of the AED, and managing a patient with a foreign body airway obstruction.

During the primary assessment, also check for any hemorrhage, and if found, control the bleeding quickly (Procedure 11-5). Evaluate perfusion, or blood flow through the tissues, by checking the temperature and moisture of the skin.

✓ CHECKPOINT QUESTION

2. What is the purpose of the primary assessment?

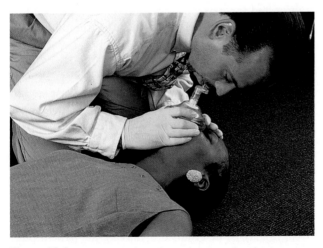

Figure 11-6 Using a mask with a one-way valve, begin rescue breathing if no breathing is noted in the primary survey.

PATIENT EDUCATION

CHOKING

Although the danger of choking is always present with small children, many adults choke to death each year. Here are some important tips to prevent choking in adults:

- Always chew food carefully before swallowing. Focus on eating by avoiding eating and driving a car at the same time.
- Avoid excessive alcohol consumption, especially while eating.
- Laughter and talking increase your chance of choking. Do not talk with food in your mouth.
- Older adults who wear dentures should go for an annual dental evaluation to make sure dentures fit snugly.
- With age, saliva production decreases, making it more difficult to swallow. Encourage older patients to take smaller bites and chew food longer, sipping liquids as needed.

The Secondary Assessment

After conducting a primary assessment and assessing that the patient's airway, breathing, and circulation are adequate, a secondary assessment can be performed. The secondary assessment includes asking the patient questions to obtain additional information and performing a more thorough physical evaluation to find less obvious problems than those noted in the primary assessment. To gain an accurate impression during the secondary assessment, the following four areas are assessed:

1. *General appearance.* The patient's skin color and moisture, facial expression, posture, motor activity, speech, and state of alertness provide important clues about the mental and physical condition. Check for a medical bracelet or necklace. Medicine bottles in a pocket or purse can also be helpful.
2. *Level of consciousness.* By the time you have completed the primary survey and noted the patient's general appearance, the level of consciousness may be apparent. A decrease in oxygen to the cells of the brain, neurologic damage from a cerebrovascular accident (stroke), and intracranial swelling are just some of the conditions that may alter a patient's level of consciousness. The AVPU system uses a common language to describe the patient's level of consciousness:

- A, **A**wake and alert
- V, responds to **V**oice
- P, responds only to **P**ain
- U, **U**nresponsive or unconscious

3. *Vital signs.* After noting the general appearance and determining the level of consciousness, assess the vital signs, including the pulse and respiratory rates and blood pressure. Assessment of temperature is important for patients who have altered skin temperature or have been exposed to environmental temperature extremes. Patients with a history of infection, chills, or fever and children with **seizures** should always have their temperature taken.

4. *Skin.* An initial evaluation of the temperature and moisture of skin should have been noted during the primary survey. A more thorough look should now be taken. Skin is normally dry and somewhat warm. Moist, cool skin may indicate poor blood flow to the tissues and possibly shock. The color of the skin should be noted as an indication of the circulation near the surface of the body and oxygenation of the tissues.

WHAT IF?

What if your patient has a cervical fracture?

Fractures to the cervical spine can be life threatening or seriously disabling. There are seven cervical vertebrae in the neck, and fractures to the first cervical vertebra (C1), the most superior vertebra, tend to be fatal unless immediately and aggressively treated by emergency services personnel before transport to a trauma center. Fractures to the second and third cervical vertebrae (C2 and C3) often result in permanent or long-term respiratory dependency on a mechanical ventilator since the involuntary respiratory center of the brain is affected. Vertebrae fractures of the fourth to seventh cervical vertebrae (C4 to C7) will result in various levels of paralysis and motor impairment. If you suspect a patient has a cervical fracture or other vertebral fracture, keep the head and neck of the patient still and call for emergency personnel. Never move the patient unless the patient is in immediate danger. The emergency medical technicians will properly immobilize the head and neck of the patient for transport to the hospital, where radiographic tests will diagnose the extent of the injury.

The Physical Examination

A head-to-toe survey that includes examination of the head and neck, chest and back, abdomen, and extremities in this sequence should be done only after completing the primary and secondary surveys. Although the physician usually performs this examination, you must be prepared to assist as needed while continuing to reassure the patient.

Head and Neck

If a cervical spine injury is suspected, immediately immobilize the spine and avoid manipulating the neck during examination of the head. Inspect the face for edema, bruising, bleeding, and drainage from the nose or ears. Examine the mouth for loose teeth and dentures. The condition and severity of a neurologic injury or patient with altered consciousness can be assessed by checking the pupils with a flashlight or penlight. The pupils should be checked for several characteristics:

- Equality in size
- Dilation bilaterally in darkness or dim light
- Rapid constriction to light in both eyes
- Equal reaction to light

To evaluate the pupils for these qualities, shade both eyes from the light and use a flashlight or small penlight at an angle 6 to 8 inches from each eye. The conscious patient should not look directly into the light. Report the findings to the physician.

Chest and Back

The anterior chest is evaluated to some degree when the patient's respiratory status is evaluated. A further inspection of the chest should be done after removing clothing from a patient with trauma or abnormal vital signs. Patients with cardiac or respiratory complaints should also have their chest more thoroughly evaluated. Palpation of the chest and back may reveal the possibility of rib fractures.

Abdomen

The abdomen of all patients is evaluated, but it is particularly important for those with GI symptoms or suspicion of blood or fluid loss as seen in vaginal bleeding, vomiting, or **melena** (blood in the stool). The abdomen is inspected for scars, bruises, and masses. A distended abdomen may indicate hemorrhage in the abdominal cavity.

Arms and Legs

An examination of the arms and legs is the last step of the head-to-toe survey. Inspect the arms and legs for swelling, deformity, and tenderness. Also note any tremors in the hands. To determine the neurologic status of the arms and legs, assess strength, movement, range of motion, and sensation, including comparing one side of the body with the other. Muscle strength in the upper extremities is checked by having the patient squeeze both of your hands at the same time. Leg strength may be determined by having the patient push each foot against your hand, again at the same time, while noting any weakness in one side or the other.

Assess sensation by using a safety pin or other tool to determine the patient's response to pain. Throughout the examination, you must note the comparison of both sides, including any weakness or decreased sensation in one side or the other. Again, the physician will most likely be performing this examination, but you must be prepared to assist as needed.

 CHECKPOINT QUESTION

3. What diagnostic signs are evaluated in the secondary assessment?

Types of Emergencies

Shock

Shock is lack of oxygen to the individual cells of the body, including the brain, as a result of a decrease in blood pressure. Although the cause of the low blood pressure varies, the body initially adjusts for any type of shock by increasing the strength of the heart contractions and the heart rate while constricting the blood vessels throughout the body. As shock progresses, the body has more difficulty trying to adjust, and eventually tissues and body organs have such severe damage that the shock becomes irreversible and death ensues. The signs and symptoms of shock include:

- Low blood pressure
- Restlessness or signs of fear
- Thirst
- Nausea
- Cool, clammy skin
- Pale skin with cyanosis (bluish color) at the lips and earlobes
- Rapid and weak pulse

Types of Shock

Hypovolemic shock is caused by loss of blood or other body fluids. If the cause is blood loss, it is hemorrhagic shock. Dehydration caused by diarrhea, vomiting, or profuse sweating can also lead to hypovolemic shock. **Cardiogenic shock** is an extreme form of heart failure that occurs when the function of the left ventricle is so compromised that the heart can no longer adequately pump blood to body tissues. This type of shock may follow death of cardiac tissue during a myocardial infarction (heart attack). **Neurogenic shock** is caused by a dysfunction of the nervous system following a spinal cord injury. Normally, the diameter of all blood vessels is controlled by the involuntary nervous system and smooth muscles surrounding the vessels. After a spinal cord injury, the nervous system loses control of the diameter of the blood vessels, and vasodilation ensues. Once the blood vessels are dilated, there is not enough blood in the general circulation, so that blood pressure

falls and shock ensues. **Anaphylactic shock** is an acute general allergic reaction within minutes to hours after the body has been exposed to an offending foreign substance. You must carefully observe patients for this type of shock after giving medications and during allergy testing (see later section on anaphylaxis). **Septic shock** is caused by a general infection of the bloodstream in which the patient appears seriously ill. It may be associated with an infection such as pneumonia or meningitis, or it may occur without an apparent source of infection, especially in infants and children. Initially, a fever is present, but the body temperature falls, a clinical sign suggestive of sepsis.

Management of the Patient in Shock

Because shock can result from many types of medical situations or trauma, you should always be prepared to treat the patient for shock in any emergency situation that occurs in the medical office. After performing the primary and secondary assessments, the following list of general guidelines for managing a patient in shock should be observed:

1. Observe the patient for and maintain an open airway and adequate breathing.
2. Control bleeding.
3. Administer oxygen as directed by the physician.
4. Immobilize the patient if spinal injuries may be present.
5. Splint fractures.
6. Prevent loss of body heat by covering the patient with a blanket, especially if the patient is cold.
7. Assist the physician with starting an intravenous (IV) line as ordered (see Chapter 9).
8. Elevate the feet and legs of a patient with low systemic blood pressure.
9. Transport the patient to the closest hospital as soon as possible by notifying the EMS as directed by the physician.

 CHECKPOINT QUESTION

4. What does it mean when a patient is in shock?

Bleeding

Soft tissue injuries involve damage to the skin and/or underlying musculature. When a blunt object strikes the body, it may crush the tissue beneath the skin. Although the skin does not always break, severe damage to tissue and blood vessels may cause bleeding within a confined area. This is called a closed wound. Types of closed wounds include **contusions, hematomas,** and crush injuries. A contusion is a bruise or collection of blood under the skin or in damaged tissue (Fig. 11-7). The site may swell immediately or 24 to 48 hours later. As blood accumulates in the area, a characteristic black and blue mark, called **ecchymosis,** is seen.

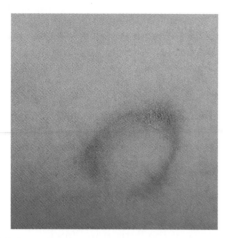

Figure 11-7 A closed wound; contusion.

A blood clot that forms at the injury site, generally when large areas of tissue are damaged, is a hematoma. As much as a liter of blood can be lost in the soft tissue when a large bone is fractured. Crush injuries are usually caused by extreme external forces that crush both tissue and bone. Even though the skin remains intact, underlying organs may be severely damaged. Regardless of the type of swelling in a closed wound, the treatment includes the application of ice to reduce and prevent additional swelling to the area (see Procedure 13-2 in Chapter 13).

In an open wound, the skin is broken, and the patient is susceptible to external hemorrhage and wound contamination. An open wound may be the only surface evidence of a more serious injury, such as a fracture. Open wounds include abrasions, lacerations, major arterial lacerations, puncture wounds, avulsions, amputations, and impalements (Fig. 11-8). When managing any patient with an open wound, follow standard precautions to protect yourself against disease transmission and to protect the patient from further contamination. An open injury to these tissues is a wound. Box 11-2 describes common soft tissue injuries and wounds.

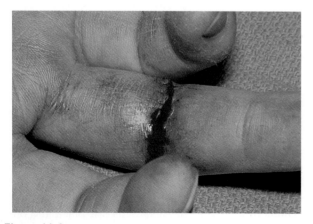

Figure 11-8 An open wound; laceration.

BOX 11-2

TYPES OF SOFT TISSUE INJURIES

- *Abrasion*, the least serious type of open wound, is little more than a scratch on the surface of the skin. All abrasions, regardless of size, are painful because of the nerve endings involved.
- *Laceration* results from snagging or tearing of tissues that leaves a freely bleeding jagged wound. Skin may be partly or completely torn away, and the laceration may contain foreign matter that can lead to infection. A wound caused by a broken bottle or a piece of jagged metal is a laceration.
- *Major arterial laceration* can cause significant bleeding if the sharp or jagged instrument cuts the wall of a blood vessel, especially an artery. Uncontrolled major arterial bleeding can result in shock and death.
- *Puncture wounds* can result from sharp, narrow objects like knives, nails, and ice picks. Punctures also can be caused by high-velocity penetrating objects, such as bullets. A special case of the puncture wound is the *impaled object wound*, in which the instrument that caused the injury remains in the wound. The object can be anything—a stick, arrow, piece of glass, knife, steel rod—that penetrates any part of the body.
- *Avulsion* is a flap of skin torn loose; it may either remain hanging or tear off altogether. Avulsions usually bleed profusely. Most patients who present with an avulsion work with machinery. Home accidents with lawn mowers and power tools are common causes of avulsion.
- *Amputation* is caused by the ripping, tearing force of industrial and automobile accidents, often great enough to tear away or crush limbs from the body.

Management of Bleeding and Soft Tissue Injuries

Management of open soft tissue injuries includes controlling bleeding by applying direct pressure (Procedure 11-5). Sterile gauze should be used to cover the wound if possible to avoid introducing microorganisms into the wound. Management of an amputated body part includes controlling the bleeding but also preserving the severed part for possible reattachment later. To preserve the severed body part:

- Place the severed part in a plastic bag.
- Place this bag in a second plastic bag. This second bag will provide added protection against moisture loss.
- Place both sealed bags in a container of ice or ice water, but do not use dry ice.

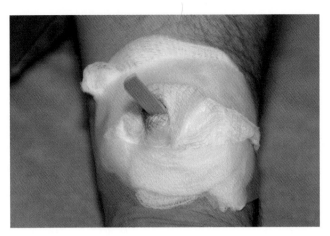

Figure 11-9 An impaled object.

An impaled object should not be removed but requires careful immobilization of the patient and the injured area of the body (Fig. 11-9). Because any motion of the impaled object can cause additional damage to the surface wound and underlying tissue, you must stabilize the object without removing it by placing gauze pads around the object and securing with tape. The immobilized impaled object can be carefully removed after transportation to the hospital.

 CHECKPOINT QUESTION

5. How should an open wound that is bleeding be treated?

Burns

The four major sources of burn injury are thermal, electrical, chemical, and radiation. *Thermal burns*, also called heat burns, result from contact with hot liquids, solids, superheated gases, or flame. *Electrical burns* are caused by contact with low- or high-voltage electricity. Lightning injuries are also considered electrical burns. *Chemical burns* result when wet or dry corrosive substances come into contact with the skin or mucous membranes. The amount of injury with a chemical burn depends on the concentration and quantity of the chemical agent and the length of time it is in contact with the skin. *Radiation burns* are similar to thermal burns and can occur from overexposure to ultraviolet light or from any extreme exposure to radiation.

Classification of Burn Injuries

Classification of burn injuries depends on the depth, or tissue layers involved. Factors that determine the depth of the burn include the agent causing the burn, the temperature, and the length of time exposed. Burns are classified according to the depth of injury: **superficial** (first-degree), **partial-thickness** (second-degree), or **full-thickness** (third-degree) **burns** (Fig. 11-10).

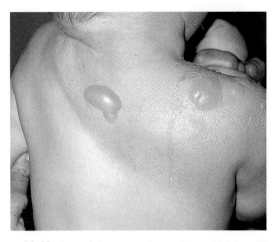

Figure 11-10 Second-degree sunburn. (From Fleisher GR, MD, Ludwig S, MD, Baskin MN, MD. Atlas of Pediatric Emergency Medicine. Philadelphia: Lippincott Williams & Wilkins, 2004.)

Calculation of Body Surface Area Burned

The extent of body surface area (BSA) injured by the burn is most commonly estimated by a method called the rule of nines. This method calculates the percentage of total body surface of individual sections of the body. With the rule of nines for an adult, 9% of the skin is estimated to cover the head and another 9% for each arm, including front and back (Fig. 11-11). Twice as much, or 18%, of the total skin area covers the front of the trunk, another 18% covers the back of the trunk, and

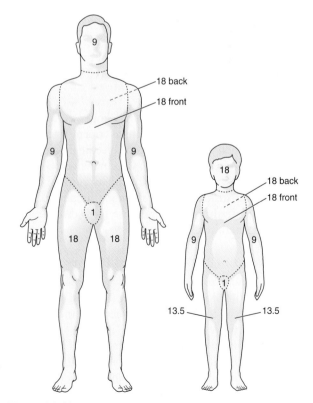

Figure 11-11 The rule of nines.

18% covers each lower extremity. The area around the genitals is the additional 1% of the BSA. In infants and children, the percentages are the same except that the head is 18% and each lower extremity is 13.5% of the total BSA. Usually, the emergency room physician determines the percentage of body burned using this rule, not the medical assistant.

Management of the Burn Victim

Follow these guidelines for managing burn patients in the medical office:

1. Eliminate the source of the burn, if necessary, by washing the area with cool water.
2. Have someone notify the physician, and take the patient immediately to an examination or treatment room.
3. Continually assess the patient's airway, breathing, and circulation. Begin CPR if necessary.
4. Remove all jewelry and clothing as necessary to evaluate the extent of the burn.
5. Administer oxygen as instructed by the physician.
6. Treat the patient for shock and accompanying low blood pressure.
7. Notify the EMS as directed by the physician.
8. Document the time and type of treatments given.
9. Assist with the necessary procedures for transporting the patient to the hospital.

 CHECKPOINT QUESTION

6. What are the four major sources of burn injuries?

Musculoskeletal Injuries

Injuries to muscles, bones, and joints are some of the most common problems encountered in providing emergency care. The seriousness varies widely, from simple injuries, such as a fractured finger, to major or life-threatening conditions, such as open fracture to the femur, which can cause severe bleeding. Injuries to muscles, tendons, and ligaments occur when a joint or muscle is torn or stretched beyond its normal limits. Fractures and dislocations are usually associated with external forces, although some arise from disease, such as bone degeneration.

Management of Musculoskeletal Injuries

It is often difficult to distinguish between strains, sprains, fractures, and dislocations in an emergency. Therefore, in most cases, assume the area is fractured and immobilize it accordingly. Proper splinting includes immobilizing the joint above and below the fracture site. Splinting helps prevent further injury to soft tissues, blood vessels, and nerves from sharp bone fragments and relieves pain by stopping motion at the fracture site. As soon as possible, apply ice to the injured area to reduce the swelling

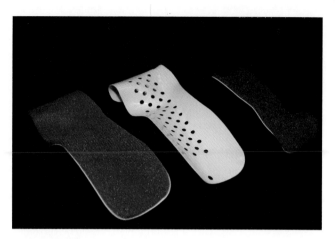

Figure 11-12 Types of splints.

that commonly occurs with this type of injury, but never attempt to reduce, or put back into place, a dislocated area. For injuries to the upper extremities, an arm sling may be ordered (Procedure 13-1 in Chapter 13 describes how to apply an arm sling).

Types of Splints

Any device used to immobilize a sprain, strain, fracture, or dislocated limb is a **splint**. Splinting material may be soft or rigid and can be improvised from almost any object that can provide stability. Commercial types include traction, air, wire ladder, and padded board splints (Fig. 11-12). Regardless of the type of splint, once applied, you must examine the extremity for signs of impaired circulation. To check the circulation of an extremity:

- Observe the skin color and nail beds of the affected extremity. A pale or cyanotic color indicates that the circulation is impeded.
- Locate a pulse in the artery distal to the affected extremity. A weak or absent pulse also indicates that circulation is decreased to the area.
- Watch for increased swelling of the extremity. Although this may not indicate that the circulation is impaired, the swelling itself can reduce circulation.

If the circulation is impaired with the splint in place, it must be removed or loosened immediately to provide for adequate blood flow, or tissue **ischemia** (decrease in oxygen) and **infarction** (death) may occur.

 CHECKPOINT QUESTION

7. What is the purpose of applying a splint?

Cardiovascular Emergencies

According to the American Heart Asociation, cardiovascular disease is the leading cause of death in adults age 75 and older and second for adults 45 to 74 years of age. The most common problem is coronary artery disease. Approximately two thirds of sudden deaths from coronary artery disease occur out of the hospital, and most occur within 2 hours of the onset of symptoms. As coronary artery disease progresses, less and less oxygen can get to the cardiac muscle, which leads to tissue ischemia and eventual infarction of the cardiac tissue. The early symptoms of a myocardial infarction (heart attack) include the following:

- Chest pain not relieved by rest
- A complaint of pressure in the chest or upper back
- Nausea or indigestion
- Chest pain that radiates up into the neck and jaw or down one arm
- Anxiety

Early treatment, including basic life support, early defibrillation, and advanced life support can prevent many of these deaths. If CPR is initiated promptly and the patient is rapidly and successfully defibrillated, the patient's survival chances improve. As noted earlier, an AED may be available in your medical office and should be used as soon as possible after it is determined that the victim does not have a pulse. When applied to the patient's chest, the AED will analyze the rhythm and advise the operator to shock, or defibrillate, the patient by simply pressing a button.

Neurologic Emergencies

A seizure is caused by an abnormal discharge of electrical activity in the brain. During a seizure, erratic muscle movements, strange sensations, and a complete loss of consciousness can occur. A seizure is not a disease but a manifestation or symptom of an underlying disorder. Epilepsy, head injury, and drug toxicity can cause seizures in adults. Children may also have seizures due to an elevated body temperature. A thorough patient history is important when assessing these patients. It should include the following:

- Information about previous seizure disorders
- Frequency of seizures if recurrent
- Prescribed medications
- Any history of head trauma
- Alcohol or drug abuse
- Recent fever
- Stiff neck (as seen in meningitis)
- A history of heart disease, diabetes, or stroke.

In managing a patient having a seizure, you must give priority to assessing the patient's responsiveness, airway, breathing, and circulation. In certain types of seizures, the patient loses consciousness and, therefore, cannot protect the airway. During the seizure, the muscles of the body, including those of the face, will contract tightly. If you attempt to force an object between the teeth to prevent the patient from biting the tongue,

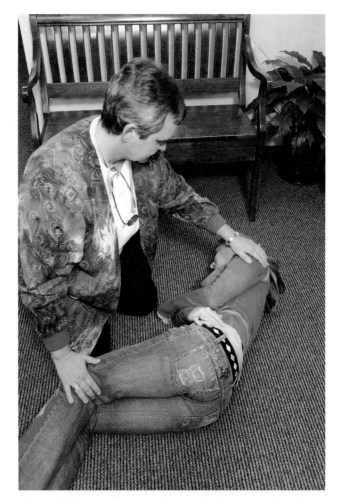

Figure 11-13 Patient in recovery position.

the result will most likely be injury to you or the patient. Frequently, a patient may vomit during the seizure and lose bowel or bladder control. Particular attention and care are necessary to clear and maintain the airway without causing injury to yourself or the patient. Assisting the patient into the recovery position (on one side) will help secretions such as blood or vomit drain from the mouth (Fig. 11-13). Secretions may be removed from the mouth using a suction machine if available. It is helpful to also note how long the seizure lasted including the time between seizures if the patient experiences multiple seizures. Be sure to report this information to the physician and the emergency services personnel.

The most important thing you can do for a patient during a seizure is protect the patient from injury. If the patient lost consciousness and fell at the beginning of the seizure, care will be necessary to protect the neck and cervical spine until immobilization can occur.

 CHECKPOINT QUESTION

8. What are some causes of seizure activity in a patient?

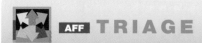

AFF TRIAGE

While working in a busy medical urgent care center, the following three patients arrive at the same time:

A. A 4-year-old child arrives, carried in by his mother who states that he has had vomiting and diarrhea for approximately 2 days but has recently become "sleepy and hard to arouse."

B. A 36-year-old female comes in complaining of pain in her hand after spilling a cup of hot coffee on it. You notice that the palm of her left hand is red and has several small blisters on it.

C. A 40-year-old man had cut his thumb while using a box cutter at work. He has a towel on it and notes that the bleeding has "stopped," but he still would like to have it evaluated by the physician.

How do you sort these patients? Who do you see first? Second? Third?

Anytime there is change in anyone's mental status, it should be treated as a priority. See patient A first since he may be dehydrated and headed for hypovolemic shock. Patient B should be seen next. She has a first- and second-degree burn, and although these may be painful, she is not in immediate danger of shock. Patient C should be seen last. The patient is capable of holding pressure to the site to control bleeding, but he may need sutures to close the wound as well as a tetanus injection.

Allergic and Anaphylactic Reactions

A severe allergic reaction called anaphylaxis causes most emergency department visits related to allergies. An allergic reaction is a generalized reaction that can occur within minutes to hours after the body has been exposed to a substance recognized by the immune system as foreign and to which it is oversensitive. The systemic signs and symptoms of anaphylaxis are more severe compared to a simple allergic reaction, but repeated exposure to a substance that produces allergic reactions may ultimately lead to an anaphylactic reaction and should be avoided.

Common Allergens

An **allergen** is a substance that gives rise to hypersensitivity or allergy. The allergen may be a drug, insect venom, food, or pollen and may be injected, ingested, inhaled, or absorbed through the skin or mucous membranes. A person may have symptoms within seconds after exposure to an allergen, or the reaction may be delayed for several hours. You must ask every patient about allergies at every visit and note these on the front of the patient's chart and the medication record. Check the patient's medical record and ask about allergies *before* administering any medications in the office; this is essential to prevent allergic reactions or anaphylaxis in patients with known hypersensitivity.

Although the exact incidence of anaphylactic reactions is difficult to pinpoint, it is estimated that 1% to 2% of patients who receive penicillin in the United States have some form of allergy to the drug and that one in 50,000 injections of penicillin results in death from anaphylaxis. However, you must be alert to the signs and symptoms of allergic reactions after administering any medication, not just penicillin. Patients with moderate to severe allergy symptoms often receive frequent injections of specific allergens to reduce the symptoms associated with allergies. These patients should be monitored closely for anaphylaxis and they should not be permitted to leave the office for a prescribed amount of time, often 20 to 30 minutes after the injection. When documenting that an injection was given, you should also note the condition of the patient upon discharge.

Signs and Symptoms

The initial signs and symptoms of an allergic reaction may include severe itching, a feeling of warmth, tightness in the throat or chest, or a rash. The primary rule for any exposure is that the sooner the symptoms occur after the exposure, the more severe the reaction is likely to be. Be observant and ready to treat any patient who has these symptoms. Airway obstruction, cardiovascular collapse, and shock can occur if the situation worsens. Because the primary cause of death in an anaphylactic reaction is swelling of the tissues in the airway causing airway obstruction, observe the patient closely for signs of airway involvement, including wheezing, shortness of breath, and coughing. Choking or tightness in the neck and throat may signal this danger. Tachycardia, hypotension, pale skin, dryness of the mouth, diaphoresis (profuse sweating), and other signs of shock may also be present.

Management of Allergic and Anaphylactic Reactions

The patient having a severe allergic reaction will often be anxious. Some allergic reactions are mild, without respiratory problems or signs of shock. These simple reactions can be managed by administering oxygen or medications such as antihistamines to relieve symptoms as directed by the physician. If respiratory involvement occurs without signs of shock, the physician may order that epinephrine (1:1,000) be given subcutaneously. The patient with a severe anaphylactic reaction who is in shock needs more aggressive therapy, including additional medications, an IV line, and monitoring of the cardiac rhythm.

The primary goal when treating a patient having an anaphylactic reaction is restoring respiratory and circulatory function. The following steps are required for managing allergic reactions, including anaphylaxis:

- Do not leave the patient, but have another staff member request that the physician immediately evaluate the patient and bring the emergency kit or cart, including oxygen.
- Assist the patient to a supine position.
- Assess the patient's respiratory and circulatory status by obtaining the blood pressure, pulse, and respiratory rates.
- Observe the skin color and warmth.
- If the patient complains of being cold or is shivering, cover him or her with a blanket.
- Upon the direction of the physician, start an IV line (see Chapter 9) and administer oxygen.
- As ordered by the physician, administer medications such as epinephrine as ordered.
- Document vital signs and any medications and treatments given, noting the time each set of vital signs is taken or medications are administered.
- Communicate relevant information to the EMS personnel, including copies of the progress notes or medication record as needed.

 CHECKPOINT QUESTION

9. What is the primary cause of death in anaphylaxis?

Poisoning

The likelihood that one will be exposed to toxins in the home or workplace is increasing. In addition to over-the-counter and prescription medications often found in the home, household chemicals are an additional hazard and are often designed to have a pleasant odor and color. Industrial chemicals offer another possibility of poisoning. These chemicals may affect a single victim or many victims in the event of a hazardous materials incident. Most toxic exposures occur in the home, and almost 50% occur in children aged 1 to 3 years (Fig. 11-14). Although about 90% of reported poisonings are accidental, intentional exposures usually affect adolescents and adults, and they tend to have a higher death rate. Fortunately, deaths from drug overdoses and poisoning are rare, but you must know how to respond if a patient comes to the office or telephones with a possible poisoning.

Poison Control Center

The American Association of Poison Control Centers (AAPCC) has established standards and regional poison control centers throughout the country. These centers are staffed by physicians, nurses, and pharmacists.

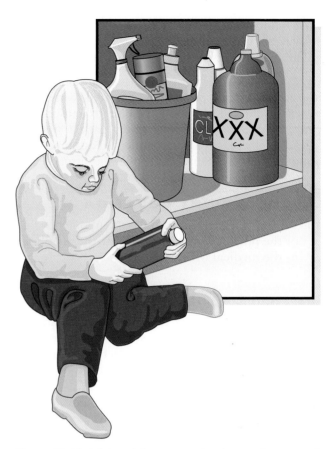

Figure 11-14 Advise adults to store cleaning products out of the reach of small children.

When information about a poisoning or drug overdose is not readily available, the poison control center is a valuable resource, and the phone number should be posted near all phones in the medical office. The professionals at the poison control center can usually evaluate a potential or known toxic exposure, instruct the caller in the use of syrup of ipecac to induce vomiting if indicated, and check on the patient's progress by follow-up telephone calls.

Management of Poisoning Emergencies

Exactly how and when a poison control center is consulted should be part of the medical office's protocol. Few toxic substances have specific antidotes, so the management of the poisoning is aimed at treating the signs and symptoms and assessing the involved organ systems. The patient may go to the medical office after the poisoning, or more commonly, the patient or caregiver telephones the office requesting information. In either situation, you must obtain the following information *before* making the call to poison control:

- The nature of the poisoning (ingested, inhaled, skin exposure)
- The age and weight of the victim
- The name of the substance

- An estimate of the amount of poison
- When the exposure occurred
- The patient's present signs and symptoms

Once the poison control center has been notified and instructions given, you must be prepared to treat the patient as directed and notify the EMS to transport the patient to the hospital. Never give a patient syrup of ipecac or otherwise induce vomiting unless directed to do so by the professionals at the poison control center.

 CHECKPOINT QUESTION

10. Why is it important to have the phone number of the poison control center near the telephone in the medical office?

Heat- and Cold-Related Emergencies

Environmental temperature is one of the many variables to which the body normally adjusts, maintaining equilibrium. Human beings depend on the ability to control core body temperature within a range of several degrees. Measured rectally, this core temperature is 37.6°C (99.6°F). The peripheral temperature is usually lower (98.6°F orally). Several conditions can disrupt the normal heat-regulating mechanisms of the body. These are divided into two main categories: **hyperthermia** and **hypothermia**.

Hyperthermia

Hyperthermia is the general condition of excessive body heat. Correct management depends on assessment of the underlying cause. The first type of hyperthermia and the least severe includes **heat cramps**, which is muscle cramping that follows a period of heavy exertion and profuse sweating in a hot environment. While sweat is primarily water, it also contains the electrolyte sodium, which is needed for muscle function. Heavy sweating, which is a normal compensatory mechanism to cool the body, will result in a sodium deficit, which compromises muscle function and produces muscle cramps. A patient with heat cramps often complains of cramping in the calves of the legs and in the abdomen. Cramping may also occur in the hands, arms, and feet. Mental status and blood pressure usually remain normal, although an increased pulse rate is common.

Heat cramps signal the need for cooling and rest. In uncomplicated cases, the patient is encouraged to take fluids by mouth, but nausea may make IV infusion necessary. If the patient is able to take fluids by mouth, give a commercial electrolyte solution or salt can be added to water or fruit juice at 1 teaspoon per pint. Cramps can sometimes be prevented entirely with similar oral intake before physical exertion and every 20 minutes during exercise. Salt tablets are not recommended because they may cause nausea.

Heat exhaustion results most often from physical exertion in a hot environment without adequate fluid replacement and may follow heat cramps that are not treated. Body temperature usually remains normal or slightly above normal. Patients have central nervous system symptoms such as headache, fatigue, dizziness, or syncope (fainting). Although the skin is typically moist and the pulse rate is high, skin color, blood pressure, and respiratory rate vary with the degree to which the body is able to hold off the distress. Patients in late stages of heat exhaustion have pale skin, low blood pressure, and rapid respiration. Treatment includes having the patient lie down in a cool room, remove clothing, and spraying the patient a cool water spray. The patient should also be encouraged to drink cool fluids including water or a commercial electrolyte solution as with heat cramps.

Heat stroke is a true emergency and is the most serious of the heat related emergencies. The body is no longer able to compensate for the rapid rise in body temperature (past 105°F) and the patient may undergo brain damage or death. Heat stroke victims can deteriorate quickly to coma, and many patients have seizures. The skin is classically hot, flushed, and dry. Vital signs are elevated initially but may drop, with ensuing cardiopulmonary arrest. Heat stroke demands rapid cooling of the body by immersing the patient in cold water up to the chin or wrapping the body in sheets or towels that have been soaked in cold water. This patient will need transported to the hospital immediately and you may be required to activate the EMS and communicate appropriately and clerarly.

For any heat related emergency, you should alert the physician and follow office policy for the management of hyperthermia including these basic steps:

- Move the patient to a cool area.
- Remove clothing that may be holding in the heat.
- Place cool, wet cloths or a wet sheet on the core surface areas of the body where the ability to cool the central blood is the greatest: the scalp, neck, axilla, and groin.
- Administer oxygen as directed by the physician and apply a cardiac monitor.
- Notify the EMS for transportation to the hospital as directed by the physician.

Hypothermia

The body's core temperature can drop several degrees without loss of normal body function. The body usually tolerates a 3° to 4°F drop in temperature without symptoms; hypothermia is an abnormally low body temperature, below 35°C (95°F). Internal metabolic factors and significant heat loss to the external environment can lead to hypothermia. Very cold air and immersion in cold water can cause a rapid drop in core temperature. The following are the signs and symptoms of hypothermia:

- Cool, pale skin
- Lethargy and mental confusion
- Shallow, slow respirations
- Slow, faint pulse rate

Basic management of hypothermia includes handling the patient gently, removing wet clothing, and covering the patient to prevent further cooling. If there is evidence of rewarming (skin warm, respirations approaching normal, no shivering) and the patient is alert and able to swallow, give warm fluids by mouth. Avoid drinks that constrict peripheral blood vessels, such as those that contain caffeine (coffee and tea). Fluids that cause dilation of the blood vessels, such as alcohol, should also be avoided. Warm beverages with sugar, such as hot chocolate, can be given to begin replacement of the fuel that the body needs to restore normal heat production. No fluids should be given by mouth to patients who have a diminished or changing level of consciousness.

Frostbite

Windy subfreezing weather creates the greatest risk for **frostbite**. Small body parts with a high ratio of surface area to tissue mass (fingers, toes, ears, and nose) are most vulnerable to frostbite, although larger areas of the extremities are also vulnerable during profound cooling. Exposure to cold can cause tissues to freeze, and the frozen cells will die.

The type and duration of contact are the two most important factors in determining the extent of frostbite injury. Touching cold fabric, for example, is not nearly as dangerous as coming into direct contact with cold metal, particularly if the skin is wet or even damp. The combination of wind and cold is dangerous. *Superficial frostbite* appears as firm and waxy gray or yellow skin in an area that loses sensation after hurting or tingling. Prolonged exposure can lead to blistering and eventually *deep frostbite*, which most often affects the hands and feet. No warning symptoms appear after the initial loss of feeling. Freezing progresses painlessly once the nerve endings are numb. Skin becomes inelastic and the entire area feels hard to the touch. Deep frostbite results in tissue death, and the affected tissue must be removed surgically or amputated.

Superficial frostbite can be managed by warming the affected part with another body surface, for example placing an ungloved hand over the nose or ears. Management for more than superficial frostbite is rapid rewarming after any system-wide hypothermia has been corrected. Deep frostbite should be managed only in the hospital to prevent further damage to the tissue. You

may be asked to do the following as directed by the physician:

- Immerse the frozen tissue in lukewarm water (41°C, 105°F) until the area becomes pliable and the color and sensation return.
- Do not apply dry heat.
- Do not massage the area; massage may cause further tissue damage.
- Avoid breaking any blisters that may form.
- Upon the direction of the physician, notify the EMS for transportation to a hospital.

If rewarming is not attempted, bandage the frostbitten part with dry sterile dressings. Frostbitten tissue is similar to burned tissue in that it is vulnerable to infection. Take care to keep the affected part as clean as possible. All frostbite victims should be assessed for hypothermia. Clothing offers good protection against weather only if it is loose enough to avoid restricting circulation. Tight gloves, cuffs, boots, and straps add to the danger.

CHECKPOINT QUESTION

11. What is the difference between heat exhaustion and heat stroke?

Behavioral and Psychiatric Emergencies

Psychological distress may be mild, moderate, or severe. The degree of intensity determines the type and amount of intervention necessary. A psychiatric emergency is different from an emotional crisis, and you must know how to differentiate between the two. A psychiatric emergency is any situation in which the patient's moods, thoughts, or actions are so disordered or disturbed that harm or death may result for the patient or others if no intervention occurs. An emotional crisis, on the other hand, is a situation with much less intensity. While it may be distressing to the patient, in most cases, it is not likely to end in danger, harm, or death without immediate intervention. However, if neglected entirely, an emotional crisis may escalate to a full psychiatric emergency.

A true behavioral emergency, like a medical emergency, carries a serious threat. Urgent behavioral situations usually require some form of professional psychological evaluation and intervention and require transportation to the hospital. The following guidelines are useful for handling a psychiatric emergency:

- Notify the physician and EMS as directed
- Offer reassurance and general support to the patient and any caregivers or family members who may be present
- Accurately document information including vital signs and the patient's behavior

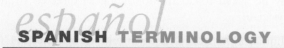

SPANISH TERMINOLOGY

¿Le duele algo?
  Dop you have pain?

¿Tiene dificultad para respirar?
  Are you having any problem breathing?

¿Cuándo ocurrió el accidente?
  When did the accident happen?

Calmese, por favor. La ambulancia está de camino.
  Calm down, please. The ambulance is on the way.

MEDIA MENU

- **Student Resources on thePoint**
  - **CMA/RMA Certification Exam Review**
  - **Video: Administering Oxygen (Procedure 11-1)**

- **Internet Resources**

  American Association of Poison Control Centers
  http://www.aapcc.org

  American Heart Association
  http://www.heart.org

  American Red Cross
  http://www.redcross.org

  Safety and Health Institute
  http://www.hsi.com

  National Safety Council
  http://www.nsc.org /Pages/Home.aspx

  Occupational Health and Safety Administration
  http://www.osha.gov

PSY PROCEDURE 11-1: **Administer Oxygen**

Purpose: Administer oxygen according to the physician's order
Equipment: Oxygen tank with regulator, oxygen delivery system (nasal cannula, mask)

Steps	Reasons
1. Wash your hands.	Handwashing aids infection control.
2. Check the physician order for the amount of oxygen and the delivery method (nasal cannula, mask).	
3. Assemble the equipment.	
4. Greet and identify the patient. Explain the procedure.	Identifying the patient prevents errors. Explaining the procedure helps ease anxiety and may improve compliance.
5. **AFF** Explain how to respond to a patient who has dementia.	Solicit assistance from caregiver or other staff member to help during the procedure. Give simple directions to the patient about what he/she should do. Speak clearly, not loudly.
6. Connect the distal end of the tubing on the oxygen delivery method (nasal cannula or mask) to the adapter on the regulator, which is connected to the oxygen tank. 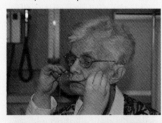	The oxygen tank must have a regulator attached that allows the nasal cannula or mask tubing to be connected. The tubing cannot be connected with a regulator on the oxygen tank.
	Step 6. Connect the distal end of the oxygen tubing to the regulator on the oxygen tank.
7. Place the oxygen delivery system (nasal cannula or mask) on the patient. 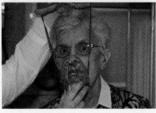	
	Step 7. Step 7A: Place the nasal cannula into the patient's nares, or Step 7B: Secure the mask over the nose and mouth.

(continued)

PSY PROCEDURE 11-1: | **Administer Oxygen (continued)**

Steps	Reasons
8. Turn the regulator dial to the appropriate number of liters per minute as ordered by the physician. 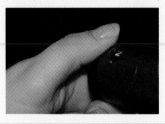	Oxygen is considered a medication and must be ordered by a physician.

Step 8. Turn on the oxygen by rotating the dial on the oxygen tank regulator. |
| 9. Record the procedure in the patient's medical record. | Procedures are considered not to have been done if they are not recorded. |

Charting Example:

12/23/2012 2:15 p.m. Oxygen applied per nasal cannula at 4 L/min as ordered ———————— J. Leigh, CMA

Note: The medical assistant may sign his or her name in the patient record using only the "CMA" credential if the office has a signature log denoting the entire credential as "CMA(AAMA)."

PSY PROCEDURE 11-2: | **Perform CPR (Adult)**

Purpose: Perform rescue breathing and chest compressions (cardiopulmonary resuscitation) on an adult
Equipment: CPR mannequin for practice, mouth-to-mask barrier device, gloves
Note: Demonstration of competency depends upon the individual student and the most current structured educational protocol by certified trainers for the American Heart Association, American Red Cross, or the National Safety Council.

Steps	Reasons
1. Determine unresponsiveness by shaking the patient and shouting "Are you okay?" Instruct another staff member to get the physician, emergency cart/supplies, and AED. If gloves are easily accessible, put clean gloves on both hands. Otherwise, put them on when the emergency medical cart arrives.	Establishing unresponsiveness prevents rescue measures being taken for a patient who does not need them. High quality CPR and early defibrillation will improve survival from sudden cardiac arrest.
2. If the patient does not respond, assess for cardiac function by feeling for a pulse using the carotid artery on the side of the patient's neck.	The most current guidelines require rescuers to check for a pulse *before* checking the airway or breathing.
3. If no pulse is present, follow the protocol for chest compressions according to the standards of the training provided by the American Heart Association, the American Red Cross, or the National Safety Council.	Instead of using the acronym "ABC," use "CAB" (Circulation, Airway, Breathing). The physician will probably want EMS notified at this point since quick access to advanced care will increase the patient's chance for survival.

PSY PROCEDURE 11-2: Perform CPR (Adult) (continued)

Steps	Reasons
4. After 30 compressions, check for airway patency and respiratory effort using the head tilt–chin lift maneuver with the patient in a supine position.	If you suspect a neck injury, use the jaw thrust maneuver to open the airway after rolling the patient carefully to his/her back without twisting or moving the neck.
5. After opening the airway, begin rescue breathing by placing a mask over the patient's mouth and nose and giving two slow breaths, causing the chest to rise without overfilling the lungs.	Giving slow breaths will provide oxygen without overfilling the lungs. Overfilling the lungs with air may cause gastric distention and vomiting.
6. Continue chest compressions and rescue breathing at a ratio of 30:1 until relieved by another health care provider or EMS arrives.	If an AED is available, follow the recommended guidelines for using this device.
7. Utilize the recovery position if the patient regains consciousness or a pulse and adequate breathing.	The recovery position includes the patient lying on his/her side, which facilitates respirations and prevents aspiration of emesis in the event that the patient vomits.

Note: In the clinical situation, respiratory barrier devices and gloves will be available to protect you from the patient's oral secretions and should be used appropriately.

All health care professionals should receive training for proficiency in CPR in an approved program. The procedure described here is not intended to substitute for proficiency training with a mannequin and a structured protocol.

Charting Example:

10/14/ 2012 10:30 am Pt c/o chest pain. Skin diaphoretic, color pale. Pulse 125 and regular, BP
88/54 (L). Collapsed in exam room, Dr. Barton notified. Pulse and respirations absent, CPR started. EMS notified per
Dr. Barton ———————————————————————————————————— S. Pencil, CMA
10/14/2012 10:40 am CPR continued per EMS, pt. unresponsive. Transported to General Hospital.
Patient's wife, Helen, notified of transport ——————————————————— S. Pencil, CMA

Note: The medical assistant may sign his or her name in the patient record using only the "CMA" credential if the office has a signature log denoting the entire credential as "CMA(AAMA)."

PSY PROCEDURE 11-3: Use an AED (Adult)

Purpose: Correctly apply and use an AED on an adult patient
Equipment: Practice AED, chest pads with connection cables appropriate for the AED machine, scissors, dry gauze pads, gloves, and mannequin

Steps	Reasons
1. Determine unresponsiveness by shaking the patient and shouting, "Are you okay?"	Establishing unresponsiveness prevents rescue measures being being taken for a patient who does not need them.
2. Have another staff member get the physician, medical emergency cart or bag, and AED. Follow the procedure for CPR procedures according the most recent guidelines (see Procedure 11-2).	High quality CPR and early defibrillation will improve survival from sudden cardiac arrest.

(continued)

PSY PROCEDURE 11-3: **Use an AED (Adult)** *(continued)*

Steps	Reasons
3. When the AED is available, continue CPR while a second rescuer removes the patient's shirt and prepares the chest for the AED electrodes. This second rescuer will be in control of operating the AED. 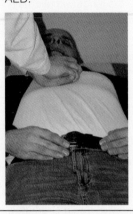	If the patient's skin is wet, use a dry towel or cloth to dry the chest. If the patient is wearing a transdermal medication patch on the chest, remove the patch and wipe any excess medication off of the chest. If there is excessive hair on the patient's chest, use a disposable razor to remove any hair over where the chest electrode pads will be placed. **Step 3.** The first rescuer continues CPR while the second rescuer prepares the AED.
4. After removing the sticky paper backing on the AED electrode pads, apply the chest electrodes onto the patient's chest, one on the upper right chest and the other on the lower left chest. 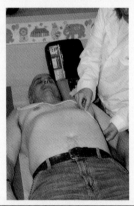	Placing the electrodes on the chest as directed will allow the best conduction of electricity to the heart muscle. **Step 4.** Place the AED pads on the upper right chest and the lower right chest.
5. Once the electrodes are in place, connect the wire from the electrodes to the AED unit and turn the AED on. 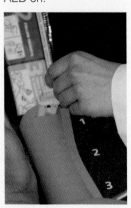	Although AED machines vary, most ask you to place the electrodes on the patient *before* connecting the wires to the AED machine. **Step 5.** Connect the AED electrode wires to the AED machine.

PSY PROCEDURE 11-3:   Use an AED (Adult) (continued)

Steps	Reasons
6. Follow the instructions given by the AED as the heart rhythm is being analyzed. Do not touch the patient during the analysis, including doing CPR. If no shock is necessary, the AED will indicate this and instruct you to resume CPR.	The AED will verbally tell you what to do. Listen to all instructions and follow the directions given by the machine.
7. If the AED instructs you that an electrical shock is necessary, the second rescuer will operate the machine, making sure that no person is touching the patient or the exam table (if the patient is on a table) before pressing the appropriate button on the AED to deliver the electrical shock. 	If another person is touching the patient or the exam table when an electrical shock is delivered, the shock will be given to that person as well as the patient. **Step 7.** The second rescuer delivers the electrical shock if indicated.
8. After delivering the shock, the AED will again analyze the patient's heart rhythm. The patient must not be touched during this process.	If a shock is not advised and CPR is resumed, the AED will ask you to stop CPR periodically to reanalyze the rhythm. Do not touch the patient while the AED is analyzing the heart rhythm.
9. Continue to follow the instructions given by the AED, which will include either reshocking the patient or resuming CPR.	Continue this pattern until EMS arrives and takes over the emergency procedures.

Note: All health care professionals should take an approved training course in CPR and use of an AED. This procedure is not intended to substitute for proficiency training with a mannequin in a structured educational protocol.

Charting Example:

11/15/2012 3:15 pm Pt. became unresponsive while waiting in reception area; no pulse or respiratory effort.
Dr. Barton notified, CPR started ——————————————————————— J. Crete, CMA

11/15/2012 3:18 pm AED applied, 2 electrical shocks delivered, pulse returned, no respiratory effort.
Rescue breathing resumed ——————————————————————— J. Crete, CMA

11/15/2012 3:25 pm EMS here. Pt. transported to General Hospital ——————————— J. Crete, CMA

Note: The medical assistant may sign his or her name in the patient record using only the "CMA" credential if the office has a signature log denoting the entire credential as "CMA(AAMA)."

PSY PROCEDURE 11-4: **Manage a Foreign Body Airway Obstruction (Adult)**

Purpose: Respond appropriately to an adult (conscious and unconscious) with a foreign body airway obstruction

Equipment: Mouth to Mask with barrier device, gloves, CPR mannequin

Steps	Reasons
1. For a conscious patient, ask, "Are you choking?" If the patient can speak or cough, the obstruction is not complete. Observe the patient for increased distress and assist as needed, but do not perform abdominal thrusts.	The patient who is coughing or speaking can breathe and may be able to remove the obstruction without assistance. Performing abdominal thrusts on a patient who is not in need of assistance may cause injury.
2. If the patient cannot speak or cough and is displaying the universal sign of distress (grasping the throat with both hands), follow these steps to perform abdominal thrusts and have a co-worker notify the physician: A. Stand behind the patient and wrap your arms around his or her waist. B. Make a fist with your nondominant hand, with the thumb side against the patient's abdomen between the navel and the xiphoid process.	Excess pressure on the xiphoid process may cause it to break off. Applying pressure at or below the navel may not produce enough force on the diaphragm to expel the foreign object.

Step 2B. Make a fist, with the thumb side against the abdomen.

C. Grasp your fist with your dominant hand and give quick upward thrusts. Completely relax your arms between each thrust and make each thrust forceful enough to dislodge the obstruction in the airway.	
3. Repeat the thrusts until the object is expelled and the patient can breathe or the patient becomes unconscious.	Several thrusts may be necessary to expel the object.
4. If the patient is unconscious OR becomes unconscious, perform a tongue-jaw lift followed by a finger sweep to remove the object if possible.	Before performing the tongue-jaw lift and finger sweep, apply clean examination gloves to avoid contact with the patient's oral secretions.
5. Open the airway and try to give the patient two rescue breaths.	Repositioning the patient's head ensures that the airway obstruction is not caused by improper head position.
6. If rescue breaths are obstructed, begin abdominal thrusts: A. Straddle the patient's hips. B. Place the palm of one hand between the patient's navel and the xiphoid process. C. Lace your fingers with the other hand against the back of the properly positioned hand.	

PSY PROCEDURE 11-4:   Manage a Foreign Body Airway Obstruction (Adult) *(continued)*

Steps	Reasons
7. Give five abdominal thrusts, and then repeat the tongue-jaw lift and finger sweep maneuver. Attempt to give rescue breaths. If rescue breaths adequately ventilate the patient, continue rescue breaths until the patient resumes breathing *or* EMS arrives, as indicated by the physician. While you are performing rescue breathing, periodically check for a carotid pulse and be prepared to start chest compressions if necessary.	A patient with a foreign object may not be able to breathe; however, cardiac function may continue.
8. If no object is removed after the finger sweep or the lungs cannot be inflated during the attempted rescue breaths, continue the cycle of abdominal thrusts, tongue-jaw lift, finger sweep, and rescue breaths until EMS arrives.	

Note: Obese or pregnant patients require chest thrusts rather than abdominal thrusts. Children over the age of 8 years are considered to be adults for the purpose of foreign body airway obstruction.

All health care professionals should take an approved training course in CPR, use of an AED, and managing a foreign body airway obstruction in an approved program. This procedure is not intended to substitute for proficiency training with a mannequin in a structured educational protocol.

Charting Example:

07/09/2012 2:15 pm Pt. choked on a throat lozenge in the examination room. Abdominal thrusts x6 administered;

lozenge removed. Dr. Kramer notified. Pulse 104, respirations 26, BP 160/98 (R) ———————————— R. Lent, CMA

Note: The medical assistant may sign his or her name in the patient record using only the "CMA" credential if the office has a signature log denoting the entire credential as "CMA(AAMA)."

Purpose: Adequately control external bleeding to prevent further hemorrhage and shock
Equipment: Gloves, sterile gauze pads

Steps	Reasons
1. Identify the patient and determine, if possible, what type of accident caused the external bleeding. Immediately escort the patient to an examination room and have someone notify the physician.	Injuries that are due to the use of a weapon will require reporting to the local law enforcement authorities.
2. Obtain clean examination gloves and an adequate supply of sterile gauze pads, preferably 4 × 4–size pads.	The gloves will protect you from the patient's blood, whereas the sterile gauze pads will prevent micro-organisms from entering the open wound. If sterile gauze pads are not immediately available, the use of nonsterile gauze pads to control bleedings is appropriate until sterile pads can be obtained.
3. Apply the exam gloves and quickly open two to three packages of gauze pads. Instruct the patient to lie down on the exam table if he or she has not already done so.	Having the patient lie down reduces the risk of fainting and falling.
4. Using the sterile gauze pads, apply direct pressure to the wound. Maintain pressure until the bleeding stops. Hold pressure for at least 20 minutes without removing the gauze to check for bleeding.	Lifting the gauze to check for continued bleeding may remove any clots that are beginning to form, causing the bleeding to resume or worsen.
	Step 4. Apply direct pressure to the wound.
5. If the bleeding continues or seeps through the gauze, do not remove it. Apply additional gauze on top of the saturated gauze while continuing to apply direct pressure.	Removing the saturated gauze may dislodge a blood clot that is trying to form, causing an increase in bleeding.
6. As directed by the physician, apply direct pressure to the artery delivering blood to the area while continuing to apply direct pressure to the wound.	Pressure points include the brachial artery, the radial artery, the femoral artery, and the popliteal artery.
7. Once the bleeding is controlled, be prepared to assist the physician with a minor office surgical procedure to close the wound *or* notify EMS for transport to the hospital as directed by the physician.	Always monitor the patient for signs of shock and treat the patient appropriately.

Charting Example:

01/20/2012 1:45 pm Pt. presented with laceration to left hand due to hand saw accident at home. Wound
approximately 4 inches across palm of hand and bleeding profusely. Direct pressure applied. Dr. Smith notified ————
——— *S. Jones, CMA*

01/20/2012 1:50 pm Bleeding controlled after direct pressure to brachial artery per Dr. Smith. Wound bandaged, pt.
transported to General Hospital emergency room per EMS ———————————————— *S. Jones, CMA*

Note: The medical assistant may sign his or her name in the patient record using only the "CMA" credential if the office has a signature log denoting the entire credential as "CMA(AAMA)."

PSY PROCEDURE 11-6: **Respond to Medical Emergencies Other than Bleeding, Cardiac/Respiratory Arrest, or Foreign Body Airway Obstruction**

Purpose: Adequately respond to a variety of medical emergencies.
Equipment: A medical emergency kit that contains a minimum of personal protective equipment including gloves, low-dose aspirin tablets, 2×2 and 4×4 sterile gauze pads, vinegar or acetic acid solution, blood pressure cuff and stethoscope, sterile water or saline for irrigation, ice bags, towel or rolled gauze bandage material

Steps	Reasons
1. Identify the patient and determine, if possible, what type of medical emergency is involved. Immediately escort the patient to an examination room.	Injuries that are due to the use of a weapon will require reporting to the local law enforement authorities.
2. Have another staff member get the physician, medical emergency cart or bag, and AED.	High quality CPR and early defibrillation will improve survival from sudden cardiac arrest should the medical emergency progress to cardiac or respiratory arrest.
3. Apply clean examination gloves and other personal protective equipment as appropriate.	The gloves will protect you from the patient's blood or body fluids.
4. Assist the patient to the exam table and have him or her lie down if he/she has not already done so.	Having the patient lie down reduces the risk of fainting and falling.
5. Treat the patient according to the physician instructions and the most current guidelines for first aid procedures:	
A. Chest pain: Activate EMS and have patient chew one (1) adult non–enteric-coated aspirin or two (2) low-dose aspirin tablets unless contraindicated.	Patients who have a history of aspirin allergy or recent gastrointestinal bleeding should not be give aspirin.
B. Snakebite: Apply pressure bandage to *all* venomous snakebites. A blood pressure cuff may be used to apply pressure.	Applying pressure will slow the lymph flow and reduce the absorption of the venom. Use the following mmHg guidelines if a blood pressure cuff is used to apply pressure: Upper extremity: >40 mm Hg and <70 mm Hg. Lower extremity: >55 mm Hg and <70 mm Hg
	Step 5B. Teeth marks of a poisonous snake **(A)** as compared with that of **(B)** a nonpoisonous snake. (From Neil O. Hardy, Westpoint, CT.)
C. Jellyfish sting: Wash the area for at least 30 seconds with acetic solution, such as vinegar or a 4%–6% acetic acid solution.	Washing with acetic solution will deactivate the venom.
Remove nematocysts and apply or immerse the area in hot water for 20 minutes.	Removing the nematocysts and applying hot water will reduce the pain.
	Step 5C. Jellyfish sting. Note the whiplike shape of the lesions. (From Goodheart HP, MD. Goodheart's Photoguide of Common Skin Disorders, 2nd Edition. Philadelphia: Lippincott Williams & Wilkins, 2003.)

(continued)

PSY PROCEDURE 11-6: **Respond to Medical Emergencies Other than Bleeding, Cardiac/Respiratory Arrest, or Foreign Body Airway Obstruction (continued)**

Steps	Reasons
D. Dental Injuries:	
Chipped tooth: Patient should follow up with a dentist.	A chipped tooth may not be painful but may require repair to prevent further problems or for cosmetic reasons.
Cracked or broken tooth: Patient should follow up with a dentist as soon as possible to prevent further damage.	A root canal or tooth extraction may be necessary. Patient may experience pain and sensitivity to hot/cold and air.
Tooth removed: Rinse tooth with water but do not do not scrub the tooth or remove any attached tissue. Do not allow the tooth to dry. Attempt to reinsert the tooth into the socket or store it in a container of milk. The patient should see a dentist immediately.	Rinsing removes any debris. The tooth should be reimplanted by a dentist within 30 minutes for the best success with reimplantation; however, there may be success for up to 2 hours.
Broken jaw: Secure the jaw with a towel tied around the jaw over the top of the head. Depending on the assessment of the physician, the patient may need to be transported to the hospital emergency room or a dentist or oral surgeon may be consulted.	The physician will determine the extent of the injury and if additional treatment is warranted.

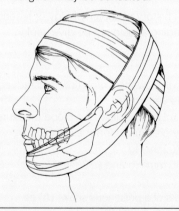

Step 5D. Barton's bandage used to support a fractured mandible. (From Harwood-Nuss A, MD, FACEP, Wolfson AB, MD, FACEP, FACP, et al. The Clinical Practice of Emergency Medicine, 3rd Edition. Philadelphia: Lippincott Williams & Wilkins, 2001.)

6. If the patient develops cardiac or respiratory arrest, follow the procedure for CPR according to the most recent guidelines (see Procedures 11-2 and 11-3).	High quality CPR and early defibrillation will improve survival from sudden cardiac arrest.

Charting Example:

01/20/2012 1:45 pm Pt. presented with complaint of snakebite to right anterior forearm. No identification of snake
determined, forearm shows 2 small pinpoint wounds with increased redness and swelling. Dr. Jones notified.
Sterile gauze placed over wound and pressure applied via a blood pressure cuff at 50 mmHg. EMS notified as
ordered. Pt. anxious, pulse 122, respirations 32, nonlabored. ——————————— B. Reynolds, CMA

Note: The medical assistant may sign his or her name in the patient record using only the "CMA" credential if the office has a signature log denoting the entire credential as "CMA(AAMA)."

Chapter Summary

Dealing with a medical emergency will require you to:

- Communicate clearly and calmly.
- Recognize the need for immediate medical intervention.
- Perform emergency procedures immediately and competently.
- Provide first aid and life support measures that can mean the difference between life and death.
- Reassure the patient and family members.
- Work with the physician and other health care team members efficiently and with confidence.

Warm Ups   for Critical Thinking

1. When an emergency occurs, the patient's family members may become anxious and emotionally distraught. How can you help to calm an anxious family member?

2. Investigate the Good Samaritan law in your state. Prepare a poster describing the laws in your state.

3. While obtaining a chief complaint, your patient complains of shortness of breath. His respiratory rate is 36, and his skin is cool and clammy. What should be your next steps? Why?

4. The mother of a 15-year-old boy calls the office and tells you that her son has just been stung by a bee. She says he has never been stung before, and she is concerned about the amount of swelling around the site of the sting on his arm. However, you hear him coughing in the background. Are there any questions that you might want to ask the mother? How would you handle this call?

5. On a hot summer day, the mail carrier comes into your office to deliver the mail and collapses on the floor in the reception area. You notice that his skin is flushed and hot to touch. Should you move this person to an exam room? What could be the possible cause for his symptoms? How would you treat this patient?

TWO

Clinical Duties Related to Medical Specialties

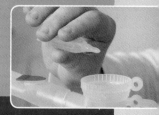

12 Dermatology

Outline

Common Disorders of the Integumentary System
Skin Infections
Inflammatory Reactions
Disorders of Wound Healing
Disorders Caused by Pressure
Alopecia

Disorders of Pigmentation
Skin Cancers
Diagnostic Procedures
Physical Examination of the Skin
Wound Cultures
Skin Biopsy

Urine Melanin
Wood's Light Analysis
Bandaging
Types of Bandages
Bandage Application Guidelines

Learning Outcomes

Cognitive Domain

Note: AAMA/CAAHEP 2008 Standards are italicized.

1. Spell and define key terms
2. Describe common skin disorders
3. *Describe implications for treatment related to pathology*
4. Explain common diagnostic procedures
5. Prepare the patient for examination of the integument
6. Assist the physician with examination of the integument
7. Explain the difference between bandages and dressings and give the purpose of each
8. Identify the guidelines for applying bandages

Psychomotor Domain

Note: AAMA/CAAHEP 2008 Standards are italicized.

1. Apply a warm or cold compress (Procedure 12-1)
2. Assist with therapeutic soaks (Procedure 12-2)
3. Apply a tubular gauze bandage (Procedure 12-3)

4. *Assist physician with patient care*
5. *Practice standard precautions*
6. *Document patient care*
7. *Document patient education*
8. *Practice within the standard of care for a medical assistant*

Affective Domain

Note: AAMA/CAAHEP 2008 Standards are italicized.

1. *Apply critical thinking skills in performing patient assessment and care*
2. *Use language/verbal skills that enable patients' understanding*
3. *Demonstrate empathy in communicating with patients, family, and staff*
4. *Use appropriate body language and other nonverbal skills in communicating with patients, family, and staff*
5. *Demonstrate awareness of the territorial boundaries of the person with whom you are communicating*
6. *Demonstrate sensitivity appropriate to the message being delivered*

7. *Demonstrate recognition of the patient's level of understanding in communications*
8. *Recognize and protect personal boundaries in communicating with others*
9. *Demonstrate respect for individual diversity, incorporating awareness of one's own biases in areas including gender, race, religion, age, and economic status*
10. *Apply active listening skills*
11. *Apply local, state, and federal health care legislation and regulation appropriate to the medical assisting practice setting*

ABHES Competencies

1. Assist the physician with the regimen of diagnostic and treatment modalities as they relate to each body system
2. Comply with federal, state, and local health laws and regulations
3. Communicate on the recipient's level of comprehension
4. Serve as a liaison between the physician and others
5. Show empathy and impartiality when dealing with patients

Key Terms

alopecia	erythema	intertrigo	pustule
bulla	folliculitis	macule	seborrhea
carbuncle	furuncle	neoplasm	urticaria
cellulitis	herpes simplex	pediculosis	verruca
dermatophytosis	herpes zoster	pruritus	vesicle
eczema	impetigo	psoriasis	vitiligo

The skin, or integument, is the largest organ of the body. Clear skin glowing with health indicates a good general state of wellness; pallor, cyanosis, or dry, scaly skin indicates poor general health. Although it has many functions, including maintaining homeostasis, one of the most important functions of the integumentary system is to protect the underlying tissues and organs from the external environment. Figure 12-1 shows a cross section of the normal anatomy of the skin and accessory structures. Unbroken skin provides a protective barrier that prevents the entrance of microorganisms and is the body's first line of defense against infection. In addition, the skin protects the body from mechanical injury, damaging substances, and the ultraviolet rays of the sun. The study of the skin is dermatology, and a physician who specializes in disorders of the skin is a dermatologist. The general practice physician may diagnose diseases of the integumentary system or may refer patients to the dermatologist.

CHECKPOINT QUESTION

1. How does the skin help to prevent infectious microorganisms from entering the body?

COG Common Disorders of the Integumentary System

Skin Infections

Many integumentary disorders are manifested by lesions or abnormalities in skin tissue (Fig. 12-2A–P). These lesions may be primary or secondary to primary lesions. When working with a patient who may have a skin infection, you should always wear protective equipment, such as examination gloves, since the drainage from any lesions may be infective.

Bacterial Infections

Impetigo

Impetigo is a contagious bacterial infection of the skin that is common in young children. It may be caused by *Staphylococcus* or *Streptococcus* microorganisms. Lesions appear on exposed areas, such as the face and neck. Terms used to describe many skin lesions, not just those seen in a patient with impetigo, include the following:

Macule: small, flat skin discoloration (see Fig. 12-2A).
Vesicle: small fluid-filled sac (see Fig. 12-2D).

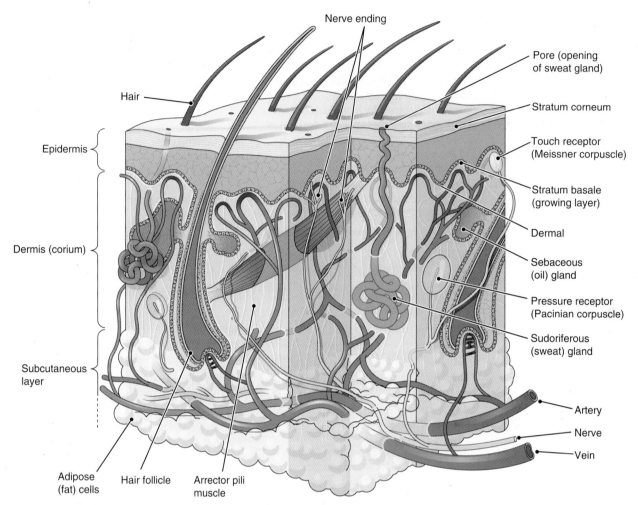

Figure 12-1 Cross section of the skin. (Reprinted with permission from Cohen BJ. Memmler's The Human Body in Health and Disease, 11th ed. Philadelphia: Lippincott Williams & Wilkins, 2009.)

Bulla: large fluid-filled sac (see Fig. 12-2E).
Pustule: pus-filled sac (see Fig. 12-2F).

Initially, impetigo may appear as an area of **erythema;** however, patches of vesicles that produce honey-colored drainage and crusts follow the redness (see Fig. 12-2K). These vesicles leave red areas when the crusts are removed. Treatment is washing the area two or three times a day and applying a topical antibiotic as ordered by the physician. Oral antibiotics may also be prescribed for severe cases. Scratching must be discouraged to prevent the spread of the infection, and patients must be instructed to wash towels, washcloths, and bed linens daily. Individuals at risk for developing impetigo are those in poor health, those with conditions such as anemia or malnutrition, and those with poor hygiene; however, any person handling contaminated laundry or otherwise exposed to the infectious material should be encouraged to practice frequent medical asepsis such as handwashing.

Folliculitis

Folliculitis is a superficial infection of a hair follicle (see Fig. 12-2N). It is characterized by itching, burning, and the formation of a pustule. Treatment is aimed at promoting drainage and healing. Saline soaks or compresses (Procedures 12-1 and 12-2) may be ordered for 15 minutes twice a day followed by application of an anti-infective ointment or cream and a dressing to absorb any drainage. If folliculitis is left untreated, it may lead to the formation of an abscess. An abscess is formed when a small sac of pus, or purulent material, accumulates at the site of inflammation. The causative agent of these infections is often *Staphylococcus.*

Furuncle

A **furuncle,** more commonly known as a *boil,* is a deep-seated infection of a hair follicle or gland (see Fig. 12-2O). Friction and pressure at the site may contribute to its formation. A hard, painful nodule forms

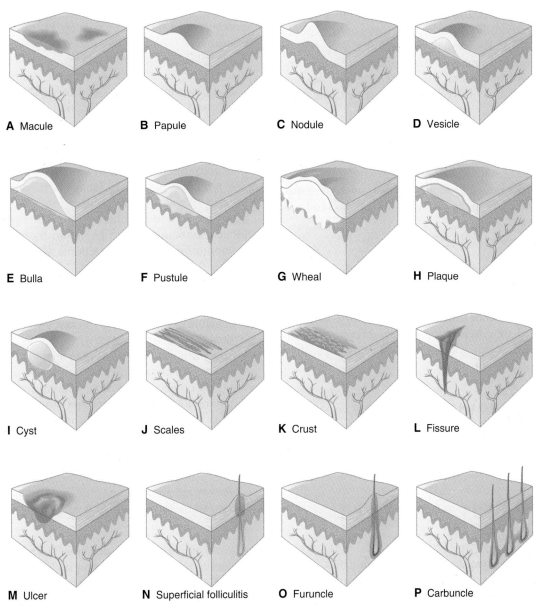

Figure 12-2 Skin lesions. Primary lesions: (**A**) Macule. Flat, circumscribed discoloration. (**B**) Papule. Palpable elevated solid lesion smaller than 1 cm; colors vary. (**C**) Nodule. Raised solid lesion larger than 1 cm. (**D**) Vesicle. Small elevation filled with clear fluid. (**E**) Bulla. Vesicle or blister larger than 1 cm. (**F**) Pustule. Lesion containing pus. (**G**) Wheal. Transient elevation of the skin caused by edema of the dermis and surrounding capillary dilation. (**H**) Plaque. Elevated solid lesion on skin or mucosa; larger than 1 cm. (**I**) Cyst. Tumor that contains semisolid or liquid material. Secondary lesions: (**J**) Scales. Heaped-up horny layer of dead epidermis. (**K**) Crust. Covering formed from serum, blood, or pus drying on the skin. (**L**) Fissures. Cracks in the skin. (**M**) Ulcer. Lesion formed by local destruction of the epidermis and part of the underlying dermis. Other lesions: (**N**) Superficial folliculitis. Local infection of a hair follicle. (**O**) Furuncle. Acute inflammation deep within hair follicle. (**P**) Carbuncle. Infection involving subcutaneous tissues around several hair follicles.

(see Fig. 12-2C), enlarges for several days, and then erupts, with pus oozing from the site. The cause of the infection is often *Staphylococcus*. Treatment of a furuncle includes application of moist heat to assist in ripening it, or bringing it to a head, and antibiotic therapy. Often a minor surgical procedure known as *incision and drainage (I & D)* is performed to remove the purulent material and facilitate healing. (Chapter 7 discusses incision and drainage in detail.)

Carbuncle

A **carbuncle** consists of infection in an interconnected group of hair follicles or several furuncles joined together in a mass (see Fig. 12-2P). The subcutaneous tissue in the surrounding area is also involved, and *Staphylococcus* is often responsible. Carbuncles are hard, round, extremely painful swellings that enlarge over several days to a week. Eventually they soften and erupt, discharging pus from several sites. When the skin sloughs away, a scarred cavity remains. The patient often has a fever.

Treatment of a carbuncle is with systemic antibiotics, moist heat (Procedures 12-1 and 12-2), and incision and drainage once the lesion has matured. A topical anti-infective agent and loose bandages are also applied to the area. The site may require a wick, or sterile gauze packing, to remain in the cavity for several days to facilitate healing.

Cellulitis

When an existing wound is infected and the infection spreads to the surrounding connective tissue, **cellulitis** results. The skin becomes hot, red, and edematous (Fig. 12-3). If it is not treated, the underlying tissue may be destroyed or develop an abscess. A systemic anti-infective, such as an antibiotic, usually provides rapid and successful treatment.

 CHECKPOINT QUESTION

2. Which of the listed bacterial infections develop in the hair follicles?

 PATIENT EDUCATION

MRSA

A strain of *Staphylococcus areus* bacteria that must be considered as the cause of some skin infections is **methicillin resistant Staphylococcus aureus** or MRSA (pronounced "mersa"). This microorganism is resistant to many antibiotics used to treat common staphylococcus skin infections. Patients who become infected with MRSA in a health care setting such as a hospital or long-term care facility have HA-MRSA (health-care associated MRSA) while those who become infected in the community have CA-MRSA (community-associated MRSA). In a health care facility, MRSA may be contracted as a result of invasive procedures such as surgeries and intravenous or urinary catheters. In the community, MRSA is contracted through direct contact (skin-to-skin) with the microorganism. The microorganism may be present on objects or the skin of people who are not infected. Symptoms of CA-MRSA include one or more painful skin boils that eventually drain purulent material. Diagnosis is made by obtaining a culture of the exudates and

sending to a lab for evaluation of the causative microbe.

People at risk include those who live in crowded living spaces, child care workers, students who participate in contact sports such as wrestling, and anyone who is immunosuppressed. Treatment includes incision and drainage (I & D) of the abscessed area and the administration of specific antibiotics that are effective at killing the microorganism. Although hospitalized patients are typically placed in isolation to prevent the spread of this microorganism, patients may be seen in the medical office. The following preventative measures should be taken by health care personnel working with patients with skin infections:

- Frequent handwashing. Hand sanitizer may be used when access to soap and water are not possible, however, the product should be at least 60 percent alcohol.
- Cover wounds. Infected areas should be covered with sterile dressings and bandages until completely healed to prevent infected exudate from coming into contact with other areas of the body, other people, or objects in the environment.
- After each patient encounter, sanitize and disinfect items in the exam room, such as the exam table, that come into contact with patients.

Patient education must include the preventative measures noted above and should also include these:

- Avoid sharing personal items such as towels, sheets, razors, clothing, and athletic equipment. MRSA spreads on contaminated objects as well as through direct contact.
- Personal hygiene should include frequent showers, especially for student athletes after athletic games or practices. Showering should include the use of soap and water.
- Towels and bed linens should be washed frequently in hot water using an appropriate laundry detergent and the addition of bleach if possible. Washed items should be dried in a hot dryer.

Your role may also include educating family and the general community about MRSA including preventative measures. Because of the negative stigma that some patients and their families have about MRSA, education and a nonjudgmental attitude will go a long way towards reducing fear and preventing the spread of this microbe!

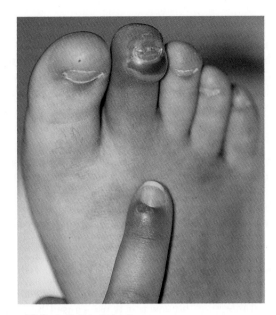

Figure 12-3 Cellulitis infection.

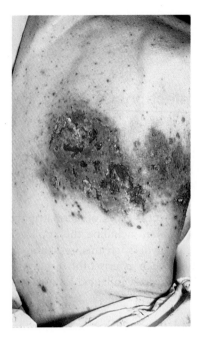

Figure 12-4 Herpes zoster (shingles).

Viral Infections

Herpes Simplex

Herpes simplex infections produce lesions commonly known as *cold sores* or *fever blisters*. The lesions, which appear on the lips, mouth, face, and nose, are small vesicles grouped on a red base. They eventually erupt, leaving a painful ulcer and then a crust. The infection may be precipitated by other infections, such as upper respiratory infections, or by menstruation, fatigue, trauma, stress, or exposure to the sun.

The causative agent is herpes simplex virus I (HSVI). Herpes simplex II is responsible for the sexually transmitted disease known as *genital herpes*. Typically, HSVI infections are recurrent, and no effective treatment eliminates or controls the disease. During an outbreak, the lesions appear and demonstrate the characteristics noted earlier and should be considered infectious. Antiviral drugs, such as valacyclovir or acyclovir, have been shown to decrease the severity of the outbreaks in some people, but they do not offer a cure. Treatment is aimed at relieving discomfort with topical anesthetic ointment to relieve the pain until the lesions heal, usually in 5 to 7 days.

Herpes Zoster

Herpes zoster, or shingles, is caused by the same virus that causes chicken pox. It is believed that, after an initial infection with the varicella virus, the virus lies dormant in the nervous system for years. Herpes zoster usually occurs in adults and may become active in times of physical or emotional stress or immunosuppression. When reactivated, the virus spreads down a nerve to the skin, causing redness, swelling, and pain. After about 48 hours, a band of lesions develops (Fig. 12-4). They begin as papules, which are small, red solid elevations on the skin (see Fig. 12-2B). Shingles commonly appear on the face, back, and chest and are frequently unilateral. These lesions progress to vesicles and pustules and then dry crusts and may last for 2 to 5 weeks. Scarring and alterations in pigmentation are common. Pain often remains after the lesions have disappeared, in some cases for several months.

The treatment of a herpes zoster breakout includes an opioid analgesic for the discomfort or nerve block for severe pain. Locally, calamine lotion may be used for itching. The area must be protected from air and the irritation of clothing. Antiviral medications such as acyclovir or Valtrex™ may be prescribed to alleviate the severity of the disease. A vaccine for shingles is available, and, although it may not prevent an outbreak, it may decrease the course and duration of the disease.

Verruca

A **verruca** is a wart, or squamous cell papilloma (benign skin tumor), that appears as a rough, raised lesion with a pitted surface. Verruca may occur singly or in groups and may be found anywhere on the skin or mucous membranes. They commonly appear on the fingers, hands, or feet and may vary in size, shape, and appearance. The causative agents include papilloma viruses, and the treatment is removal. Removing a wart may be achieved with keratolytic agents, which cause softening and shedding of the skin; liquid nitrogen, which freezes and destroys the affected tissue; podophyllum resin, a caustic agent found in many over-the-counter wart medications; laser therapy, which removes the affected tissue using radiation of the visible infrared spectrum of light; or surgical excision. They may also disappear spontaneously.

CHECKPOINT QUESTION

3. How can viral skin infections be prevented?

Fungal Infections

Fungal infection of the skin (**dermatophytosis**) is caused by a group of molds called *dermatophytes*. The group of fungal diseases called *tinea* is collectively known as *ringworm*; its members are named according to the area of the body infected. All tinea infections are considered contagious.

There are several types of dermatophytes, but the treatment is similar, including the application of topical antifungal powders, creams, or shampoos. Antifungal medications such as griseofulvin may be prescribed orally for severe cases. Inflamed lesions may be treated with wet compresses or soaks.

Tinea Capitis

Tinea capitis affects the scalp. It is contagious and appears most frequently in children. It is characterized by round gray scaly patches (dried skin flakes) and areas of **alopecia** (baldness). There are usually no symptoms except light itching.

Tinea Corporis

Tinea corporis (also known as *tinea circinata*) manifests on hairless portions of the body. It is characterized by itchy red rings that are clear in the center with a scaly border (see Fig. 12-2J). It is frequently found on the face and arms but may also be found on the trunk (Fig. 12-5).

Tinea Cruris

Tinea cruris, known in lay terms as jock itch, is found on the skin in the groin area and the gluteal folds. The lesions, which cause marked itching, are red macules with clear centers and scaly borders.

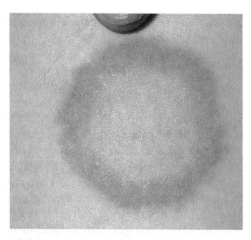

Figure 12-5 Tinea corporis (ringworm) fungal infection.

Tinea Pedis

Tinea pedis, or athlete's foot, is characterized by itching, burning, and stinging between the toes and on the soles of the feet. The lesions may appear as red, weepy vesicles, as chronic dry scales, or as fissures (crack-like lesions) between the toes (see Fig. 12-2L).

Tinea Unguium

Also known as *onychomycosis*, tinea unguium causes thickening, discoloration, and crumbling of the nails, most often the toenails. It is difficult to cure and often requires months of local antifungal preparations. In severe cases, an oral antifungal medication, griseofulvin, is prescribed.

Tinea Versicolor

Tinea versicolor, also known as *pityriasis versicolor*, is a fungal infection; however, it is not caused by dermatophytes. It is not known exactly what sort of fungus is the causative agent. The disease causes a multicolor rash, generally over the upper trunk. It is most common in young people during warm weather, and it is chronic. Its lesions vary from macular to raised, round, or oval; vary from darkly pigmented to depigmented; and are slightly scaly. There are usually no symptoms. Diagnosis of tinea versicolor is determined with a Wood's light, an ultraviolet light used in a darkened room to show abnormalities in the skin as fluorescent. Treatment includes the use of selenium sulfide for 7 days along with topical antifungal cream or lotion.

CHECKPOINT QUESTION

4. Why should you avoid direct contact with skin lesions?

PATIENT EDUCATION

PREVENTING FUNGAL INFECTIONS

Because fungi thrive in moist conditions, a general measure for treating fungal infections and preventing the spread of infection is to keep the infected area clean and dry. Instruct patients diagnosed with fungal infections to wear loose-fitting clothing and launder clothing daily. Socks and underclothing should be changed frequently, and clothing should not be shared with others. Shower shoes should be worn in public showers and pools since these areas are usually wet, providing an optimum environment for the fungus to grow on floors and be transmitted directly to the feet.

Parasitic Infections

Scabies

Scabies is a contagious skin disorder caused by the itch mite *Sarcoptes scabiei*. It is spread by direct contact and produces small vesicles or pustules between the fingers and at the inner wrist, elbows, axillae, waist, and groin. The itching caused by the mite is worst at night, when the female burrows under the epidermis to lay her eggs.

Treatment for scabies is aimed at disinfestation. For adults, an antiparasitic such as 1% lindane cream is applied from the neck down at bedtime. One application of 5% permethrin, or Elimite, cream is effective and is the drug of choice for children. All bedding and clothing for the entire family should be laundered daily until the infestation is resolved.

Pediculosis

Pediculosis is an infestation of the skin with a parasite known commonly as *lice*. Three types of the louse *Pediculus humanus* infest the body: *P. humanis* var. *capitis* infests the scalp (pediculosis capitis) and the eyelashes or eyelids (pediculosis palpebrarum); and *P. humanis* var. *corporis* or *var. vestimenti* is found on the body (pediculosis corporis) and the pubic hairs (pediculosis pubis). Wherever they are found, itching is intense, and the skin often becomes secondarily infected from scratching. Lice feed on human blood and lay eggs (nits) on body hair or clothing fibers. Nits may be seen on hair shafts close to the skin or in seams of clothing.

Pediculosis is common among populations with overcrowding, such as head lice in schools, and poor hygiene. The infestation is transmitted through physical contact with an infested person, by sitting on an infested toilet seat, or by sharing a comb, brush, clothing, or bedding that is infested. Benzene hexachloride creams, lotions, or shampoos are used for all types of pediculosis. All clothing and linen must be dry cleaned or washed in hot water and ironed. Sealing items in plastic bags for 30 days or heating them to 140°F will kill lice on items that cannot be laundered.

 CHECKPOINT QUESTION

5. How are parasitic skin infections spread?

Inflammatory Reactions

Eczema

Eczema is an inflammatory skin disorder usually involving only the epidermal layer of the skin. It is more common in children than adults and is characterized by itching and lesions that generally begin as red patches, proceed to weepy vesicles, and end up as dry scaly

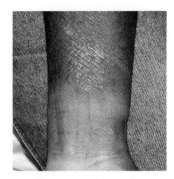

Figure 12-6 Eczema.

crusts (Fig. 12-6). They appear on the face, neck, bends of the knees and elbows, and the upper trunk. It is not clear why some patients develop this disorder, which is chronic and may have periods of remission and exacerbation. Possible causes of eczema depend on the individual and may include the following:

- Food allergies to fish, eggs, and milk products
- Medication or chemical allergies
- Sensitivity to irritating soaps, household cleaning products, deodorants, and perfumes
- Inhalants such as pollen, dust, or animal dander
- Poor circulation to a body part
- Ultraviolet rays

Treatment is removing the cause and promoting healing of the lesions. The causative agent should be avoided if it is known. The patient should maintain good hydration and keep the skin well moistened with emollients. A humid environment is recommended. Warm, not hot, baths should be taken daily with a nondrying soap. The skin should be dried immediately, and scratchy clothing should be avoided.

Exudative lesions are treated with soaks, baths, or wet dressings for 10 to 30 minutes three or four times daily. Domeboro™, Aveeno™, or bicarbonate is good for these purposes. In addition, the physician may order the following treatments:

- Topical corticosteroid lotion, cream, or ointment to be used twice a day
- Bandages at night to protect against scratching
- Antihistamines for severe **pruritus** (itching)
- For scales, a topical steroid ointment. Systemic corticosteroids, such as prednisone, may be ordered in severe cases.

Seborrheic Dermatitis

Seborrheic dermatitis (skin inflammation), also known as **seborrhea**, is an overproduction of sebum. It is a chronic disorder resulting in greasy yellow scales primarily on the scalp, where it is called *seborrheic dandruff*. Underlying redness and pruritus may be present. The eyelids, face, chest, back, umbilicus, and body folds may also be affected. It is thought that seborrhea is caused by a genetic predisposition and a combination of hormones, nutrition, infection, or stress. It is treated with shampoo and topical corticosteroid lotion.

Urticaria

Urticaria, or hives, is an acute inflammatory reaction of the dermis. It begins with itching, followed by erythema and swelling. The wheals (see Fig. 12-2G) have a pale center with a red edge. They resemble a mosquito bite and appear in clusters anywhere on the body. Hives are self-limiting, lasting from a few days to a few weeks. The most common causes include contact with these substances:

- Foods, including shellfish, strawberries, tomatoes, citrus fruits, eggs, and chocolate
- Inhalants, including feathers or animal dander
- Chemicals, cosmetics, and medications
- Sunlight
- Insect bites or stings
- Heat, cold, or pressure on the skin
- Infection
- Stress

Treatment of urticaria is reduction of the inflammatory response. The cause should be avoided if known. Antihistamines are usually given to reduce itching and swelling, and a short course of prednisone is sometimes ordered. Starch or Aveeno baths twice a day may be ordered to make the patient more comfortable. Epinephrine is given if the symptoms of urticaria develop rapidly and are associated with dyspnea. These symptoms are indicative of anaphylaxis, a severe life-threatening emergency (see Chapter 11).

Acne Vulgaris

Acne vulgaris is an inflammatory disease of the sebaceous glands. Its cause is not known in all cases, and, although it may occur in any adult, it more commonly occurs during adolescence as a result of the increase in hormone production. It is characterized by pimples, comedones (blackheads), cysts (fluid-filled sacs beneath the skin) (see Fig. 12-2I), and scarring. The lesions may occur on the face, neck, upper chest, back, and shoulders. Overactive sebaceous glands produce excessive sebum that gets trapped in a follicle, producing a dark substance that results in a blackhead. Leukocytes accumulate, producing pus.

Treatment for acne includes a regimen of tretinoin (Retin-A™), benzoyl peroxide, and tetracycline. Sunlamp treatments are sometimes used to dry the lesions.

Psoriasis

Psoriasis is a chronic inflammatory skin disorder characterized by bright red plaques (see Fig. 12-2H) covered

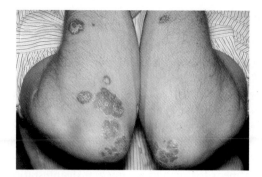

Figure 12-7 Psoriasis.

with dry, silvery scales. Although the cause is unknown, it is a chronic disorder and often difficult to treat. Psoriasis is usually found on the scalp, elbows, knees, base of the spine, palms, soles, and around the nails (Fig. 12-7). There are usually no vesicles, and itching varies from mild to severe. Exacerbations are common during cold weather, stress, and pregnancy. Treatment includes tar preparations and topical steroid cream or ointment. Exposure to ultraviolet light three times a week may also be prescribed.

 CHECKPOINT QUESTION

6. How are eczema and psoriasis different?

Disorders of Wound Healing

Keloids

Keloids, an overproduction of scar tissue, occur as a complication of wound healing. The scar tissue forms as a result of excessive collagen accumulation. A raised nodule forms and does not resolve with time. The cause is unknown. It occurs most frequently in young women, especially during pregnancy, and is particularly common in African Americans. The most common sites are the neck and shoulders. Injections of cortisone are sometimes effective in treating keloids.

Disorders Caused by Pressure

Callus and Corn

A callus, sometimes called a *callosity*, is a raised painless thickening of the epidermis. It is caused by pressure or friction on the hands and feet. A corn is a hard, raised thickening of the stratum corneum on the toes. It results from chronic friction and pressure, especially from poorly fitting shoes. The pressure compresses the dermis, making it thin and tender and causing pain and inflammation. Soft corns can form between the toes.

The treatment for calluses and corns begins with relieving the pressure. Shoes should be made of soft leather and fit properly. Liners may be inserted in shoes to relieve pressure. Bandages and corn pads also help correct the problem. In some cases, the physician recommends surgical intervention or use of a keratolytic agent to cause chemical peeling.

Decubitus Ulcers

Decubitus ulcers are also called *pressure sores* and are caused by prolonged pressure to an area of the body, usually over a bony prominence (see Fig. 12-2M). The pressure impairs blood supply, oxygen, and nutrition to the area, which results in an ulcerative lesion and eventual tissue death. The most common sites are over the sacrum and hips, but these ulcers may also occur on the back of the head, ears, elbows, heels, and ankles (Fig 12-8). They are most common in aged, debilitated, and immobilized patients. Bedridden and wheelchair-bound patients are at risk for developing decubiti unless they are repositioned frequently, every 2 hours, to relieve pressure. Special mattresses, pads, and pillows are useful in preventing pressure sores.

Decubitus ulcers are graded, or staged, according to the degree of tissue involvement (Table 12-1). Treatment consists of topical antibiotic powder and adhesive absorbent bandages and dressings. Deep infections may require systemic antibiotics and possibly surgical débridement.

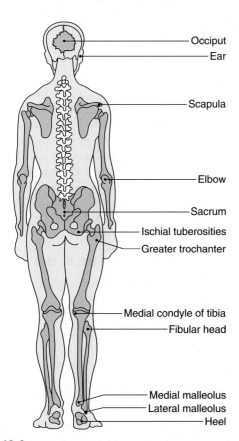

Figure 12-8 Areas susceptible to pressure sores. (From Nettina, Sandra M., MSN, RN, CS, ANP. The Lippincott Manual of Nursing Practice, 7th ed. Lippincott, Williams & Wilkins, 2001.)

Labels: Occiput, Ear, Scapula, Elbow, Sacrum, Ischial tuberosities, Greater trochanter, Medial condyle of tibia, Fibular head, Medial malleolus, Lateral malleolus, Heel

WHAT IF?

An elderly patient comes into the office with multiple decubitus ulcers. What should you do?

Older adults are always at risk for developing skin ulcerations; however, the physician must assess the situation to determine whether the patient is receiving adequate care at home. Patients who arrive in the medical office with multiple ulcers in different stages of healing may be abused or neglected. Elder abuse is less often identified, but some experts believe it is as common as child abuse. If you suspect elder abuse, contact your local department of social services. The investigation may substantiate the abuse (requiring referral to law enforcement) or may identify ways to alleviate the situation (caregiver education, respite care) without removing the patient from home. In some states, the law requires reporting elder abuse. The physician who fails to do so can be fined or be subject to other penalties.

Intertrigo

Intertrigo is a disorder of skin breakdown that occurs in the body folds of obese persons. The combination of heat, moisture, and friction of the skin against itself in these areas causes the skin to break down. Humid climates and poor hygiene often aggravate the condition. Erythema and skin fissures result, and the affected area itches, stings, and burns.

Treatment for intertrigo is proper hygiene and an attempt to keep the area clean and dry. Talcum powder or cornstarch is often recommended. Antibacterial or antifungal lotion or powder is necessary if secondary infection is present.

CHECKPOINT QUESTION

7. What patients are most at risk for developing decubitus ulcers?

Alopecia

Alopecia, or baldness, may be the result of physical trauma, systemic disease, bacteria or fungal infection, chemotherapy, excessive radiation, hormonal imbalance, or genetic predisposition. Baldness caused by scarring and inherited male pattern baldness are permanent and cannot be reversed; however, the drug minoxidil may be recommended by the physician to stimulate hair growth in male pattern baldness. For other causes of baldness, treatment of the underlying disorder often results in new hair growth.

TABLE 12-1	Staging or Grading for Decubitus Ulcers
Stage	**Description**
I	Red skin does not return to normal when massaged or when pressure is relieved.
II	Skin is blistered, peeling, or cracked superficially.
III	Skin is broken, with loss of full thickness; subcutaneous tissue may be damaged; serous or bloody drainage may be present.
IV	Deep, crater-like ulcer shows destruction of subcutaneous tissue; fascia, connective tissue, bone, or muscle may be exposed and may be damaged.

Disorders of Pigmentation

Albinism

Albinism is a genetically determined condition of partial or total absence of the pigment melanin in the skin, hair, and eyes. The skin is pale, the hair is white, and the irises of the eyes appear pink (Fig. 12-9). The skin will not tan and is prone to sunburn. Because no pigment is present to protect the underlying eye structures from the ultraviolet rays of the sun, eye problems may develop as a result of this disorder. Albinism has no treatment.

Vitiligo

Vitiligo is a progressive chronic destruction of melanocytes, which are cells in the epidermis that produce melanin, a skin pigment. This disorder is thought to be an autoimmune disorder in patients with an inherited predisposition. The depigmented areas occur as white patches that sometimes have a hyperpigmented border. It usually occurs in exposed areas of the skin.

There is no effective treatment for vitiligo. Patients are advised to protect the areas from the sun because they are prone to sunburn in the absence of melanin. Waterproof cosmetics may be used to cover the area.

Leukoderma

Leukoderma is a permanent local loss of skin pigment that results from damage caused by skin trauma. It is particularly common in African Americans. Causes of leukoderma include contact with caustic chemicals and the sequela of burns or infection.

Nevus

A nevus, also known as a *birthmark* or *mole*, is a congenital pigmented skin blemish. It is usually circumscribed and may involve the epidermis, connective tissue, nerves, or blood vessels. Nevi are usually benign, not cancerous, but may become malignant (cancerous). Patients should be cautioned to watch for changes in the color, size, and texture of any nevus. Bleeding and itching should also be reported (Box 12-1).

 CHECKPOINT QUESTION

8. Which of the disorders of pigmentation are inherited?

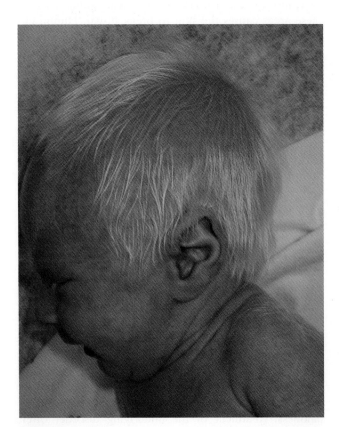

Figure 12-9 Albinism.

Skin Cancers

Basal Cell Carcinoma

Basal cell carcinoma is a slow-growing cancer that appears most commonly on exposed areas of the body, usually the face, but may also occur on the shoulders or chest. The lesion has a waxy appearance with a depressed center and a rolled edge where blood vessels may be apparent. Metastasis (spreading to other areas of the body) almost never occurs, but if left untreated,

WHEN IS A SKIN LESION ABNORMAL?

Most melanomas, a type of skin cancer, are pigmented, elevated skin lesions that frequently develop from a new or existing mole. The key to treatment of this potentially deadly cancer is early detection of changes in size, color, shape, elevation, texture, or consistency of any pigmented area, old or new, or of any spot or bump. Being familiar with what is normal for you will help you notice what is abnormal.

The eventual outcome of melanoma is governed by how deeply it has invaded the skin, which also determines how aggressively the cancer will be treated. Because many skin cancers develop from overexposure to the sun, a cancer prevention message first used in Australia and currently being promoted in the United States is, "Slip! Slop! Slap! Wrap!" This may help individuals to remember how to protect the skin: slip on a shirt, slop on sunscreen, slap on a hat, and put on wrap-around sunglasses to protect your eyes and the skin around them.

the lesions will grow locally and may ulcerate and damage surrounding tissues (Fig. 12-10). The most common treatment for basal cell carcinoma is surgical removal, and this may be done in the physician's or dermatologist's office. Radiation therapy and cryosurgery, or removal using a cold agent such as liquid nitrogen, are alternative treatments.

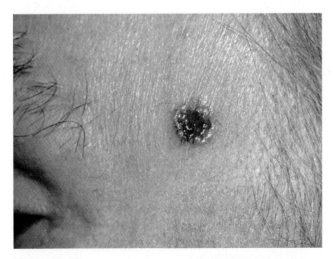

Figure 12-10 Basal cell carcinoma. (Reprinted with permission from Goodheart HP. Goodheart's Photoguide of Common Skin Disorders. Philadelphia: Lippincott Williams & Wilkins, 2003.)

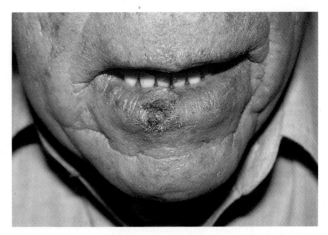

Figure 12-11 Squamous cell carcinoma. (Reprinted with permission from Goodheart HP. Goodheart's Photoguide of Common Skin Disorders. Philadelphia: Lippincott Williams & Wilkins, 2003.)

Squamous Cell Carcinoma

Squamous cell carcinoma is slightly less common than basal cell carcinoma and occurs in any squamous (scaly) epithelial area of the body, such as the lungs, cervix, or anus, but is most frequently found on the skin (Fig. 12-11). This type of skin cancer is a slow-growing, malignant **neoplasm** (tumor). The lesions are firm, red, horny or prickly, and painless, and they range widely in size. Those on exposed areas are thought to result from exposure to the sun. Other areas not normally exposed, such as mucous membranes, are thought to be affected as the result of frequent irritation. Treatment is the same as for basal cell carcinoma. Although basal cell carcinoma is not generally metastatic, squamous cell carcinoma will spread readily through underlying and surrounding tissues.

Malignant Melanoma

Malignant melanoma is a cancer of the skin that forms from melanocytes. Lesions vary from macules to nodules and often have an irregular border and a variety of colors (Fig. 12-12). Mixtures of white, blue, purple, and red are the most common. The tumor grows both in radius and in depth into the dermis. The American Cancer Society notes that melanoma is primarily a disease of whites, who are 10 times more likely to have a melanoma compared to African Americans. The rates for men getting this type of cancer are 50% higher than for women.

Risk factors for developing malignant melanoma include a personal or family history of melanoma and the presence of multiple moles. In some cases, skin cancer grows in a preexisting nevus, so patients should be encouraged to have new, unusual, or changing skin lesions evaluated by the physician. Other risk factors include those for all types of skin cancer: sensitivity to

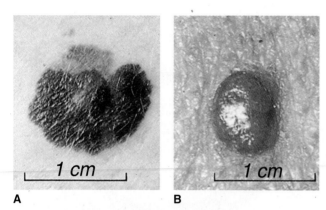

A   **B**

Figure 12-12 Malignant melanoma. (**A**) Left: Superficial melanoma. (**B**) Right: Nodular melanoma.

the sun (e.g., fair skin, blond or red hair) and a history of sunburns, tanning, preexisting immunosuppressive diseases, and a past history of basal or squamous cell skin cancers (Box 12-2).

Treatment of malignant melanoma is surgical removal after a biopsy, possibly including removal of lymph tissue. The patient's prognosis depends on the depth of the tumor. Tumors over 1.5 mm often metastasize to the lymph nodes, liver, lungs, and brain and are often fatal.

 CHECKPOINT QUESTION

9. Which is more likely to metastasize, basal cell or squamous cell carcinoma?

BOX 12-2

EFFECTS OF SUNLIGHT ON THE SKIN

In addition to sunburn and premature aging, exposure to the sun's ultraviolet rays is the major cause of skin cancers. Primary prevention of skin cancer consists of limiting exposure to ultraviolet light by wearing proper clothing and using sunscreen. Exposure to the sun is not recommended during the 5 peak hours of the day: 10:00 a.m. to 3:00 p.m. A sunscreen with at least a 15 SPF (sun protective factor) is considered good protection in blocking ultraviolet rays. Although many sunscreens contain PABA (aminobenzoic acid), which may cause allergy in some people, a number of PABA-free sunscreens are available. Exposure to ultraviolet rays through the use of sunlamps and tanning beds should also be discouraged.

 PATIENT EDUCATION

PLAYING IT SAFE IN THE SUN

During the summertime, many teenagers enjoy lying on the beach and acquiring a tan, while others are exposed to the sun by working outdoors in jobs such as lifeguarding. These two habits can lead to long-term skin problems. As a medical assistant, you can help educate teenagers about these risks. The following patient education tips are useful reminders for any patient who is exposed to excessive sunlight:

- The powerful rays of the sun can injure your eyes. Always wear sunglasses.
- Even one sunburn can increase your potential for developing skin cancer.
- A hat can prevent sunburn on the scalp. Also, a hat can help keep the sun away from the face.
- Use the highest level of sun block that is available. Apply it frequently.
- Do not apply oil to the skin to tan faster.
- Avoid lying on the beach during peak sun hours. Enjoy beach activities during the early morning or late afternoon.

COG Diagnostic Procedures

Physical Examination of the Skin

Examination of the skin is performed primarily by inspection. Many lesions can be diagnosed by the characteristic size, shape, and distribution on the skin; however, laboratory studies may be necessary to confirm a diagnosis. As the medical assistant, you may assemble the equipment as directed by the physician, verify that an informed consent has been obtained for surgical procedures, and properly direct specimens to the appropriate laboratories. Observe standard precautions when handling any specimens, including those obtained from the skin.

Before the examination, prepare the examination room and the patient. Use a gown and draping appropriate to the patient's symptoms and area to be examined. During the examination, aid the physician by ensuring that the lighting is adequate and directed properly, assisting in obtaining wound cultures, maintaining asepsis, and applying topical medications, sterile dressings, and bandages. Protect skin lesions from further infection by using medical or surgical asepsis as indicated.

After the dermatologic examination, reinforce the physician instructions about caring for the skin condition at home, including:

- Keeping bandages clean and dry
- Returning to the office to have sutures or staples removed

- How long to avoid getting the area wet
- Applying topical medications

When the patient has left the office, clean and disinfect the examination room according to the office policy.

Wound Cultures

Obtain a wound culture by getting a sample of wound exudate (drainage) using a sterile swab, applying the specimen to a growth medium, and allowing the microorganisms to grow. A sample of the culture is typically collected by the medical assistant and sent to an outside laboratory. At the laboratory, the specimen is placed on a slide and observed under a microscope to diagnose the type of the bacterial or fungal infection. Chapter 29 describes the specific procedure for collecting a wound specimen and preparing the specimen for transport to an outside laboratory.

 CHECKPOINT QUESTION

10. What are the responsibilities of the medical assistant regarding diagnosing skin lesions?

Skin Biopsy

The purpose of a skin biopsy is to remove a small piece of tissue from a lesion so that it may be examined under a microscope to determine whether it is a benign or malignant growth. A local anesthetic is injected by the physician, and sterile asepsis is used throughout the procedure (see Chapter 7). The three types of skin biopsy performed by the physician are excision, punch, and shave. In an excision biopsy, the entire lesion is removed for evaluation. When a punch biopsy is done, a small section is removed from the center of the lesion. A shave biopsy cuts the lesion off just above the skin line. Regardless of the method used to obtain the skin biopsy, samples of tissue are sent to the laboratory for analysis.

 LEGAL TIP

INFORMED CONSENT

Some dermatology procedures, such as biopsies, are invasive and require a sample of tissue for analysis. Although some office procedures may be considered "minor," patients must always be informed of the actual procedure and the potential risks involved. It is in the best interest of the medical office to have consent forms signed no matter how minor the surgical procedure.

Although the physician is responsible for informing the patient about the procedure, including the benefits and risks, it is the responsibility of the medical assistant to make sure the consent form is signed and in the medical record before the procedure is started. In some cases, you may be asked to obtain the signature of the patient on the consent form. This is acceptable; however, if the patient has specific questions about the procedure or feels unsure if this is the right decision, always let the physician know before the patient signs the form so that questions and concerns can be addressed. It is always better to err on the side of caution than proceed without a signed consent form or with a signed form when the patient was not truly informed.

Urine Melanin

Melanin is not normally present in the urine unless the patient has malignant melanoma. A urine test to detect the presence of melanin is done with a random sample of urine from the patient. The specimen is sent to the laboratory, allowed to sit for 24 hours, and then examined under a microscope for the presence of melanin. Chapter 28 describes the procedure for instructing a patient on collecting a urine sample and transporting the sample to the laboratory.

Wood's Light Analysis

Wood's light is a dark, ultraviolet light that is used to primarily detect a fungal infection. However, alterations in pigment, scabies, and other types of infections may also be detected with a Wood's light. Normally, the skin does not appear fluorescent when exposed to this type of ultraviolet light. Any areas that appear fluorescent when exposed to a Wood's light are considered abnormal and can be diagnosed by the physician and treated accordingly. This procedure is not invasive and requires no preparation by the patient or the medical assistant; however, any creams or ointments may need to be removed before using the Wood's light on the skin.

 CHECKPOINT QUESTION

11. Why are skin biopsies performed?

COG Bandaging

Bandages are strips of woven materials, typically absorbent, that are used for many purposes, such as:

1. Applying pressure to control bleeding
2. Holding a dressing in place
3. Protecting dressings and wounds from contamination
4. Immobilizing an injured part of the body
5. Supporting an injured part of the body

Types of Bandages

* *Roller bandages* are soft woven materials packaged in a roll. Roller bandages are available in various lengths and widths from 1 inch to 6 or more inches (Fig. 12-13). The bandage size used depends on the part being bandaged and the desired thickness of the completed bandage. Most bandages are made of a porous, lightweight material and may be either sterile or clean. Gauze bandages conform easily to angular surfaces of the body. A crepe-like stretchy gauze is made to adjust to various body contours and resists unrolling much better than plain roller gauze. Kling™ and Conform™ are two frequently used brands.

* *Elastic bandages*, such as the Ace brand, are special bandage rolls with elastic woven throughout the fabric (Fig. 12-14). They are generally brownish tan. Unlike other types of roller gauze, elastic bandages can be given to the patient to take home to be washed and reused many times. Because of the elastic fibers, great care must be exercised when applying the bandage to prevent compromising circulation and still provide support to the injured part. Elastic bandages should be applied without wrinkling in concentric or overlapping layers. Bandages should fit snugly but not too tightly. Adjust the bandage if it seems too loose or if the patient says it is uncomfortable or tight. Some elastic bandages have an adhesive backing, which helps keep the layers in place and provides a secure, snug, and comfortable fit. To avoid applying it too tightly, never stretch or pull on the elastic bandage during application. Ask the patient how tight the bandage feels as it is being applied, and instruct the patient on signs of impaired circulation by checking the extremity distal to the bandage for the following indications:
  * Increased swelling or pain
  * Pale skin
  * Cool skin compared to the other extremity

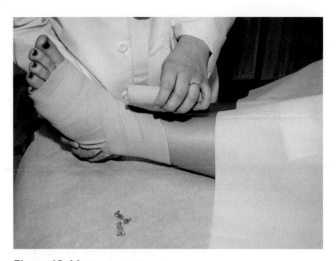

Figure 12-14 An elastic bandage.

* *Tubular gauze bandages* are used to enclose rounded body parts. The bandage resembles a hollow tube and is very stretchy (Fig. 12-15). It is used to enclose fingers, toes, arms, and legs and even the head and trunk. Tubular gauze bandages are available in various widths to fit any part of the body from 1/2 inch to 7 inches. Tubular gauze is applied using a metal or plastic tubular frame-like applicator. The applicator is available in various sizes and should be slightly larger than the body part to be covered. This enables the gauze to slide easily over the body part. Applicators are marked according to a size number that corresponds to different sizes of tubular gauze. Procedure 12-3 describes the specific steps for applying a tubular gauze bandage.

Bandage Application Guidelines

When properly applied, bandages should feel comfortably snug and should be fastened securely enough to remain in place until removed. Bandages can be fastened

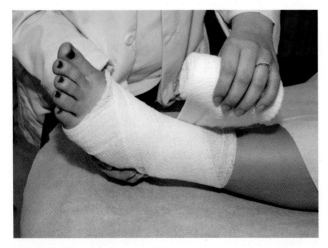

Figure 12-13 Gauze roller bandage.

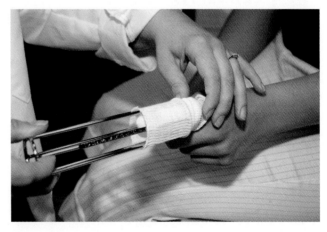

Figure 12-15 A tubular bandage.

with safety pins, adhesive tape, or clips. You gain the patient's confidence when you apply a bandage that is comfortable and neat looking and that stays in place. Patients become understandably upset when bandages fall off during normal activities. The following are general guidelines for applying bandages:

1. Observe the principles of medical asepsis, including handwashing, to prevent the transfer of pathogens. Surgical asepsis is not necessary. The bandage may be used to cover a sterile dressing or may be used alone if there is no open wound.

2. Keep the area to be bandaged and the bandage itself dry and clean because moisture may wick bacteria into the wound. A moist bandage encourages the growth of pathogens and is uncomfortable for the patient.

3. Never place a bandage directly over an open wound. Apply a sterile dressing first, and cover it with a bandage for protection. The bandage should extend approximately 1 to 2 inches beyond the edge of the dressing.

4. Never allow skin surfaces of two body parts to touch each other under a bandage. Wound healing may cause opposing surfaces to adhere and result in scar tissue formation. For example, burned fingers must be dressed separately but may be bandaged together.

5. Pad joints and any bony prominence to help prevent skin irritation caused by the bandage rubbing against the skin over a bony area.

6. Bandage the affected part in the normal position: joints should be slightly flexed to avoid muscle strain, discomfort, and pain. Muscle spasms may occur if the part is made to assume an unnatural position.

7. Apply bandages beginning at the distal part and extending to the proximal part of the body. Bandage turns that extend distal to proximal aid in return of venous blood to the heart and help make the bandage more secure.

8. Always talk with the patient during the bandaging. If the patient complains that it is too tight or too loose, adjust the bandage. Instruct the patient to do the same at home. The bandage should fit snugly, but if it is too tight, it may impair circulation. If it is too loose, it may fall off.

9. When bandaging hands and feet, leave the fingers and toes exposed whenever possible to make it easier to check for circulatory impairment. If the skin feels cold or looks pale, the nail beds look cyanotic, or the patient complains of swelling, numbness, or tingling of the toes or fingers, remove the bandage immediately and reapply it correctly.

Figure 12-16A–F illustrates various techniques for wrapping bandages.

 AFF TRIAGE

While working in a medical office setting, the following three situations occur:

A. The physician has asked you to apply a new dressing to a 24-year-old man who lacerated his finger today and just had four sutures inserted by the physician.

B. The receptionist informs you that a patient has arrived and signed in but is complaining of a rash that is "itching." The receptionist is concerned that the scratching patient may be contagious, and she would like him put into an examination room right away.

C. A 32-year-old woman is waiting in the procedure room to have a suspicious mole removed from her back. You need to set up the sterile tray for this minor office surgical procedure.

How do you sort these patients? Who do you see first? Second? Third?

Patient B should be taken directly to an examination room since the cause for the patient's symptom (itching) is not known. If you will be expected to assist the physician with the minor surgical procedure, it would be best to take care of patient A because applying a dressing should take only a few minutes. After applying the dressing and discharging the patient, then you can set up for the surgical procedure and assist the physician. However, if your physician does not usually require you to assist during minor procedures, it might be more logical to set up for the procedure then apply the dressing to patient A, allowing plenty of time for wound care instructions if necessary.

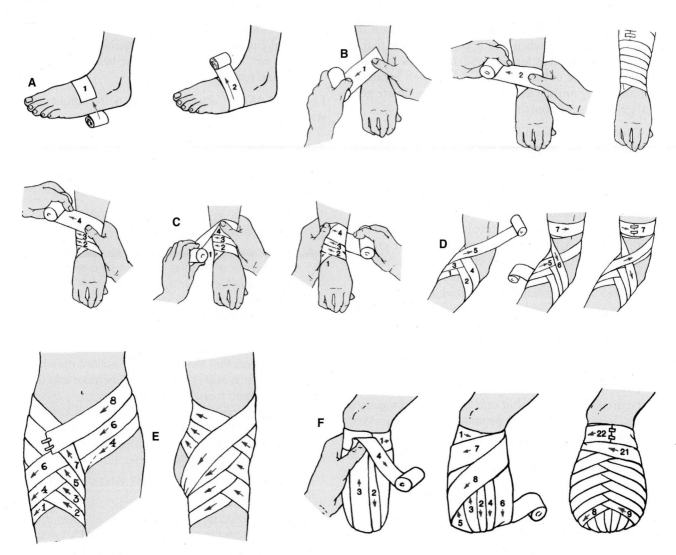

Figure 12-16 The six basic techniques for wrapping a roller bandage. (**A**) A *circular turn* is used to anchor and secure a bandage when it is started and ended. Hold the free end of the rolled material in one hand and wrap it about the area and back to the starting point. (**B**) A *spiral turn* partly overlaps a previous turn. The overlapping varies from half to three-fourths of the width of the bandage. Spiral turns are used to wrap a cylindrical part of the body like the arms and legs. (**C**) A *spiral reverse turn* is a modification of a spiral turn. The roll is reversed halfway through the turn. This works well on tapered body parts, such as the forearm and wrist. (**D**) A *figure-of-eight turn* is best used when an area spanning a joint, like the elbow or knee, requires bandaging. It is made by making oblique turns that alternately ascend and descend, simulating the number 8. (**E**) A *spica turn* is a variation of the figure-of-eight turn. It differs in that the wrap includes a portion of the trunk or chest. (**F**) The *recurrent turn* is made by passing the roll back and forth over the tip of a body part. Once several recurrent turns have been made, the bandage is anchored by completing the application with another basic turn like the figure-of-eight. A recurrent turn is especially beneficial when wrapping the stump of an amputated limb.

Medication Box

Commonly Prescribed Dermatology Medications

Note: The generic name of the drug is listed first and is written in all lower case letters. Brand names are in parentheses and the first letter is capitalized.

acyclovir (Zovirax)	Capsules: 200 mg Injection: 500 mg/vial, 1 g/vial Suspension: 200 mg/5 mL Tablets: 400 mg, 800 mg	Antiviral
crotamiton (Eurax)	Cream: 10% Lotion: 10%	Scabicide
diphenhydramine hydrochloride (Benadryl)	Capsules: 25 mg, 50 mg Injection: 50 mg/mL (IM) Tablets: 25 mg, 50 mg	Antihistamine
epinephrine (adrenaline) (Epi-Pen)	Injection (IM or SC): 0.1 mg/mL (1:10,000); 0.5 mg/mL (1:2,000); 1 mg/mL (1:1,000)	Bronchodilator
famciclovir (Famvir)	Tablets: 125 mg, 250 mg, 500 mg	Antiviral
hydrocortisone (Cortizone 5, 10; Scalpicin; Dermolate)	Cream: 0.5%, 1%, 2.5% Topical solution: 1%, 2.5%	
isotretinoin (Accutane)	Capsules: 10 mg, 20 mg, 30 mg, 40 mg	Retinoic acid derivative
itraconazole (Sporanox)	Capsules: 100 mg Oral solution: 10 mg/mL	Antifungal
ketoconazole (Nizoral)	Tablets: 200 mg	Antifungal
lindane (Hexit)	Cream: 1% Lotion: 1% Shampoo: 1%	Pediculicide; Scabicide
linezolid (Zyvox)	Tablets: 600 mg	Antibiotic
minoxidil (Rogaine)	Topical foam: 5% Topical solution: 2%, 5%	Vasodilator
permethrin (Acticin, Elimite, Nix)	Cream: 5% Lotion: 1% Topical liquid (cream rinse): 1%	Pediculicide
Pyrethrins and piperonyl butoxide (RID, A-200, Pronto)	Lotion: 0.3% and 2% Mousse: 0.33% and 4% Shampoo: 0.33% and 4% Topical gel: 0.3% and 3%	Pediculicide
terbinafine hydrochloride (Lamisil)	Oral granules (packets): 125 mg, 187.5 mg Tablets: 250 mg	Antifungal
tetracycline hydrochloride (Sumycin)	Capsules: 250 mg, 500 mg Oral suspension: 125 mg/5mL	Antibiotic
tretinoin (Retin-A; Atralin)	Cream: 0.02%, 0.025%, 0.05% 0.1% Gel: 0.05%, 0.01%, 0.025% Microsphere gel: 0.04%, 0.1%	Retinoid
triamcinolone acetonide (Kenalog, Triderm)	Cream: 0.025%. 0.1%, 0.5% Lotion: 0.025%, 0.1% Ointment: 0.025%, 0.1%, 0.5%	Corticosteroid
vancomycin hydrochloride (Vancocin)	Capsules: 125 mg, 250 mg Powder for Injection (IV): 500 mg vial, 1 g vial	Antibiotic
zoster vaccine, live (Zostavax)	Injection: single dose (SC)	Vaccine

español SPANISH TERMINOLOGY

¿Desde hace cuánto tiene usted ese lunar?
  How long have you had that mole?

He tenido este lunar desde hace cinco 5 años.
  I have had this mole for 5 years.

Esta ampolla es dolorosa.
  This blister is painful.

MEDIA MENU

- **Student Resources on thePoint**
  - **Animation: Acute Inflammation**
  - **Animation: Wound Healing**
  - **Video: Applying A Tubular Gauze Bandage (Procedure 12-3)**
  - **CMA/RMA Certification Exam Review**
- **Internet Resources**

  American Cancer Society
  http://www.cancer.org

  American Academy of Dermatology
  http://www.aad.org

  American Board of Dermatology
  http://www.abderm.org

  American Society of Dermatology
  http://www.asd.org

  Dermatology Image Atlas, Johns Hopkins University
  http://dermatlas.med.jhmi.edu

PSY PROCEDURE 12-1: **Applying a Warm or Cold Compress**

Purpose: Apply warm or cold compresses according to a physician's order
Equipment: Warm compresses: appropriate solution (water with possible antiseptic if ordered) warmed to 110°F or recommended temperature, bath thermometer, absorbent material (cloth, gauze), waterproof barriers, hot water bottle (optional), clean or sterile basin, gloves; Cold compresses: appropriate solution, ice bag or cold pack, absorbent material (cloth, gauze), waterproof barriers, gloves

Steps	Reasons
1. Wash your hands.	Handwashing aids in infection control.
2. Check the physician's order and assemble the equipment and supplies.	Hot and cold compresses must be ordered by the physician.
3. Pour the appropriate solution into the basin. For hot compresses, check the temperature of the warmed solution.	The solution must not be hot enough to injure the patient.

Step 3. Check hot solution with a bath thermometer.

4. Greet and identify the patient. Explain the procedure.	Identifying the patient prevents errors in treatment. Explaining the procedure helps ease anxiety and ensure compliance
5. Ask patient to remove clothing as appropriate and to put on a gown. Drape as appropriate.	Privacy must always be provided.
6. **AFF** Explain how to respond to a patient who is hearing impaired.	Solicit assistance from anyone who may be with the patient or a staff member who knows sign language to interpret if available. If no interpreter is available, use hand gestures or pictures to explain the procedure to the patient.
7. Protect the examination table with a waterproof barrier.	Wet surfaces are uncomfortable for the patient and may cause chilling.
8. Place absorbent material or gauze in the prepared solution. Wring out excess moisture.	Compresses should be moist but not dripping; avoid wetting the patient.
9. Lightly place the compress on the patient's skin and ask about the temperature for comfort. Observe the skin for changes in color.	Always ask the patient whether the temperature of the compress is causing pain or discomfort.

(continued)

Steps	Reasons
10. Gently arrange the compress over the area and contour the material to the area. Insulate the compress with plastic or other waterproof barrier. 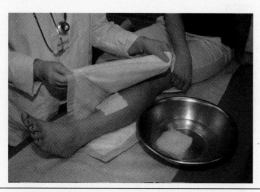	Unless the material is against the skin, temperature will not be transferred to the area of concern. Insulating the area with the waterproof barrier will retard temperature loss and avoid getting the rest of the patient wet.
	Step 10. Place a waterproof barrier over the compress material.
11. Check the compress frequently for moisture and temperature. Hot water bottles or ice packs may be used to maintain the temperature. Rewet absorbent material as needed.	The temperature should stay fairly constant. If the material dries, benefits will be lost.
12. After the prescribed amount of time, usually 20 to 30 minutes, remove the compress, discard disposable materials, and disinfect reusable equipment.	Equipment should be available for the next use. Cross-contamination must be avoided.
13. Remove your gloves and wash your hands.	
14. Document the procedure, including duration the treatment, type of solution, temperature of solution if a warm compress was used, skin color after treatment, assessment of the area, and the patient's response.	Procedures are considered not to have been done if they are not recorded

Note: If the compress is being applied to an area with an open lesion, sterile technique is required.

Warm compresses will speed suppuration to increase healing. Cold compresses will slow bleeding and decrease inflammation.

Charting Example:

10/16/2013 10:45 AM Hot compress applied to the left ankle ×20 min. Skin pink after treatment; no broken areas or blisters noted on the skin ———————————————————————————— B. Barth, CMA

Note: The medical assistant may sign his or her name in the patient record using only the "CMA" credential if the office has a signature log denoting the entire credential as "CMA(AAMA)."

PSY PROCEDURE 12-2: Assisting with Therapeutic Soaks

Purpose: Perform a therapeutic soak as directed by the physician
Equipment: Clean or sterile basin or container in which to place the body part comfortably, solution and/or medication, dry towels, bath thermometer, gloves

Steps	Reasons
1. Wash your hands.	Handwashing aids in infection control.
2. Assemble the equipment and supplies, including a basin or container of the appropriate size.	If the container is uncomfortably small, soaking the body area will be difficult and may cause muscle spasms. Surfaces should be padded for comfort.
3. Fill the container with solution and check the temperature with a bath thermometer. The temperature should be below 110°F to avoid blood pressure changes caused by vasodilation.	Assessing the temperature will prevent burning or injuring tissues.
4. Greet and identify the patient. Explain the procedure.	Identifying the patient prevents errors in treatment. Explaining the procedure helps ease anxiety and ensure compliance.
5. Slowly lower the area to be soaked into the container and check the patient's reaction. Arrange the part comfortably. Check for pressure areas and pad the edges as needed for comfort.	Immersing the part too quickly can shock the patient. If the patient is not comfortable, muscle spasms or strain may result

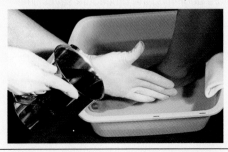

Step 5. The basin should be large enough to immerse the entire body area.

Steps	Reasons
6. **AFF** Explain how to respond to a patient who has dementia.	Solicit assistance from a caregiver who may have accompanied patient to the office visit or ask another staff member to help during the procedure if necessary. Give simple directions to the patient about what he or she should do. Speak clearly, not loudly.
7. While soaking, check the temperature of the solution every 5 to 10 minutes. If additional water or solution must be added to maintain the temperature, remove some of the solution and then add warmed solution while holding your hand between the patient and the stream of the solution being poured. Mix or swirl the soak to ensure constant, even temperature.	The proper temperature must be maintained for maximum benefit. Avoid pouring the solution or water directly against the patient's skin.

Step 7. Shield the patient's skin when adding warm solution to the soak.

(continued)

PSY PROCEDURE 12-2: **Assisting with Therapeutic Soaks (continued)**

Steps	Reasons
8. Soak for the prescribed amount of time, usually 15 to 20 minutes. Remove the part from the solution and carefully dry the area with a towel.	The area may be sensitive to brisk rubbing but must be dried to prevent chilling the patient or causing discomfort.
9. Properly care for the equipment; appropriately dispose of single-use supplies.	
10. Document the procedure, including duration of treatment, type and temperature of solution, skin color after treatment, assessment of the area, including the condition of any lesions, and the patient's response.	Procedures are considered not to have been done if they are not recorded.

Charting Example:

4/19/2013 12:20 PM Left great toe soaked in Betadine solution × 15 min. Mod. amount of tan drainage from edges of toenail noted after soak ———————————————————————————————————— J. Brighton, RMA

Note: The medical assistant may sign his or her name in the patient record using only the "CMA" credential if the office has a signature log denoting the entire credential as "CMA(AAMA)."

PSY PROCEDURE 12-3: **Applying A Tubular Gauze Bandage**

Purpose: Apply tubular gauze bandage to a digit or extremity
Equipment: Tubular gauze, applicator, tape, scissors

Steps	Reasons
1. Wash your hands.	Handwashing aids in infection control.
2. Greet and identify the patient. Explain the procedure.	This prevents error in treatment, helps gain the patient's compliance, and eases anxiety.
3. **AFF** Explain how to respond to a patient who is visually impaired.	Face the patient when speaking and always let him or her know what you are going to do before touching him or her.
4. Choose the appropriate size tubular gauze applicator and gauze width according to the size of the area to be covered. Manufacturers of tubular gauze supply charts with suggestions for the appropriate size for various body parts.	The applicator and gauze should slip easily over the body part. Choose an applicator slightly larger than the part to be covered. The gauze designed to fit the chosen applicator will provide a secure fit.
5. Select and cut or tear adhesive tape in lengths to secure the gauze ends.	Tape ensures that the gauze will not slip off. Having it at hand before beginning the procedure saves time and effort.
6. Place the gauze bandage on the applicator in the following manner: A. Be sure the applicator is upright (open end up) and placed on a flat surface. B. Pull a sufficient length of gauze from the stock box; do not cut it yet.	The gauze bandage and applicator are clean and will protect the sterile dressing on the wound.

PSY PROCEDURE 12-3: **Applying A Tubular Gauze Bandage** *(continued)*

Steps	Reasons

C. Open the end of the length of gauze and slide it over the upper end of the applicator; estimate and push the amount of gauze that will be needed for this procedure onto the applicator.

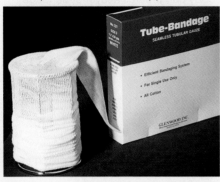

Step 6 C. Place the applicator upright and slide the end of the gauze over the applicator.

D. Cut the gauze when the required amount of gauze has been transferred to the applicator.

7. Place the applicator over the distal end of the affected part (finger, hand, toe, leg) and begin to apply the gauze by pulling it over the applicator onto the skin. Hold it in place as you move to Step 8.

The applicator should begin distally and work proximally.

8. Slide the applicator up to the proximal end of the affected part. Holding the gauze at the proximal end of the affected part, pull the applicator and gauze toward the distal end.

This keeps the bandage from slipping. If the bandage is not held in place at the early stages of application, it may not completely cover the part

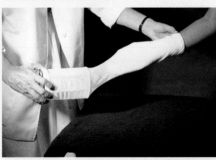

Step 8. Hold the gauze at the proximal end of the affected part and pull the applicator toward the distal end.

9. Continue to hold the gauze in place at the proximal end. Pull the applicator 1 to 2 inches past the end of the affected part if the part is to be completely covered. Sometimes the gauze need not extend beyond a limb but covers only the area the wound.

The bandage will be secured at the distal end if the part is to be completely covered. If the distal portion of the limb is not to be covered, the bandage must extend at least 1 inch beyond the wound site to ensure adequate coverage.

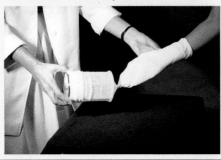

Step 9. Pull the applicator 1 to 2 inches past the affected area.

(continued)

PSY PROCEDURE 12-3: **Applying A Tubular Gauze Bandage** *(continued)*

Steps	Reasons
10. Turn the applicator one full turn to anchor the bandage.	The bandage will be securely held in place by the twist.
11. Move the applicator toward the proximal part as before.	Moving the applicator and gauze up and down over the affected body part creates a layer of bandage material, adding additional protection to the wound.

Step 11. Move the applicator toward the proximal part.

12. Move the applicator forward about 1 inch beyond the original point. Anchor the bandage again by turning it as before.	Anchoring provides a secure fit.

Step 12. Move the applicator forward about 1 inch beyond the starting point.

13. Repeat the procedure until the desired coverage is obtained. The final layer should end at the proximal part of the affected area. Any extra length of gauze can be cut from the applicator. Remove the applicator.	The part should be adequately covered to protect the wound.
14. Secure the bandage in place with adhesive tape, or cut the gauze into two tails and tie them at the base of the tear. Tie the two tails around the closest proximal joint. Use the adhesive tape sparingly to secure the end if not using a tie.	The bandage must be securely fastened to keep it in place until it is changed.

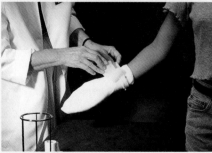

Step 14. Secure the bandage with adhesive tape.

PSY **PROCEDURE 12-3:** **Applying A Tubular Gauze Bandage** *(continued)*

Steps	Reasons
15. Properly care for or dispose of equipment and supplies. Clean the work area. Wash your hands.	Standard precautions must be followed.
16. Record the procedure.	Procedures are considered not to have been done if they are not recorded.

Charting Example:

02/08/2013 9:15 am Sterile dressing change to right index finger, tubular bandage applied and secured over dressing
———————————————————————————————————— T. Matthews, CMA

Note: The medical assistant may sign his or her name in the patient record using only the "CMA" credential if the office has a signature log denoting the entire credential as "CMA(AAMA)."

- The skin and its accessories make up the largest and most visible organ of the body.
- Assessment of the integument offers the first glimpse into a person's total state of health.
- The medical physician who treats disorders of the skin is called a *dermatologist*; however, the medical assistant working in other offices will also be exposed to various types of integumentary system disorders.
- A responsibility of the medical assistant includes assisting the physician in correctly identifying and treating various forms of skin lesions.

- Typically, the medical assistant will be responsible for applying sterile dressings directly over a skin lesion or wound and should always remember to follow sterile technique.
- Always provide patient instruction during and after bandaging, alerting the patient to the signs and symptoms of impaired circulation.
- Bacterial skin infections may be contagious, and you should follow standard precautions, including good handwashing, after being with any patient with a skin disorder that may be infectious.

Warm Ups for Critical Thinking

1. Sunlight or ultraviolet rays are needed to convert vitamin D, which is necessary for calcium and phosphorous absorption. Why is it important that children be exposed to sunlight regularly during their growing years?
2. After considering the factors needed for any microorganism to thrive, explain why molds and fungi thrive in a public shower or pool.
3. Create a patient information sheet describing the difference between eczema and psoriasis.

4. Using a drug reference book, research the usual dosage, side effects, and contraindications of the drug minoxidil, which is used to treat alopecia.
5. How would you respond to a patient who complains that his friend has recently been diagnosed with vitiligo and he is worried that he might also get this disease?

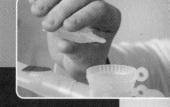

CHAPTER 13

Orthopedics

Outline

The Musculoskeletal System and Common Disorders
Sprains and Strains
Dislocations
Fractures
Bursitis
Arthritis
Tendonitis
Fibromyalgia
Gout
Muscular Dystrophy
Osteoporosis
Bone Tumors

Spine Disorders
Abnormal Spine Curvatures
Herniated Intervertebral Disc
Disorders of the Upper Extremities
Rotator Cuff Injury
Adhesive Capsulitis, or Frozen Shoulder
Lateral Epicondylitis, or Tennis Elbow
Carpal Tunnel Syndrome
Dupuytren Contracture

Disorders of the Lower Extremities
Chondromalacia Patellae
Plantar Fasciitis
Common Diagnostic Procedures
Physical Examination
Diagnostic Studies
The Role of the Medical Assistant
Warm and Cold Applications
Ambulatory Assist Devices

Learning Outcomes

Cognitive Domain

Note: AAMA/CAAHEP 2008 Standards are italicized.

1. Spell and define the key terms
2. List and describe disorders of the musculo-skeletal system
3. Compare the different types of fractures
4. Identify and explain diagnostic procedures of the musculoskeletal system
5. Discuss the role of the medical assistant in caring for the patient with a musculoskeletal system disorder
6. Describe the various types of ambulatory aids
7. *Identify common pathologies related to each body system*
8. *Describe implications for treatment related to pathology*

Psychomotor Domain

Note: AAMA/CAAHEP 2008 Standards are italicized.

1. Apply an arm sling (Procedure 13-1)
2. Apply cold packs (Procedure 13-2)
3. Use a hot water bottle or commercial hot pack (Procedure 13-3)
4. Measure a patient for axillary crutches (Procedure 13-4)
5. Instruct a patient in various crutch gaits (Procedure 13-5)
6. *Assist physician with patient care*
7. *Prepare a patient for procedures and/or treatments*
8. *Practice standard precautions*
9. *Document patient care*
10. *Document patient education*
11. *Practice within the standard of care for a medical assistant*

Affective Domain

Note: AAMA/CAAHEP 2008 Standards are italicized.

1. *Apply critical thinking skills in performing patient assessment and care*
2. *Use language/verbal skills that enable patients' understanding*
3. *Demonstrate empathy in communicating with patients, family, and staff*
4. *Use appropriate body language and other nonverbal skills in communicating with patients, family, and staff*
5. *Demonstrate awareness of the territorial boundaries of the person with whom you are communicating*
6. *Demonstrate sensitivity appropriate to the messeage being delivered*
7. *Demonstrate recognition of the patient's level of understanding in communications*
8. *Recognize and protect personal boundaries in communicating with others*
9. *Demonstrate respect for individual diversity, incorporating awareness of one's own biases*

in areas including gender, race, religion, age, and economic status
10. *Apply active listening skills*
11. *Apply local, state, and federal health care legislation and regulation appropriate to the medical assisting practice setting*

ABHES Competencies

1. Assist the physician with the regimen of diagnostic and treatment modalities as they relate to each body system
2. Comply with federal, state, and local health laws and regulations
3. Communicate on the recipient's level of comprehension
4. Serve as a liaison between the physician and others
5. Show empathy and impartiality when dealing with patients
6. Document accurately

Key Terms

ankylosing spondylitis	callus	goniometer	phonophoresis
arthrograms	contracture	iontophoresis	prosthesis
arthroplasty	contusions	kyphosis	reduction
arthroscopy	electromyography	lordosis	scoliosis
bursae	embolus	Paget disease	

Muscles allow movement of the body through contraction and relaxation. Bones support the body and respond to the contractions and relaxations (Fig. 13-1). Because the two systems depend on each other to function, they are often referred to as a single system—the musculoskeletal system. Within this system are joints, areas where two or more bones are held together by connective tissue and cartilage. The integrity of the entire system is required for normal body support and movement (Fig. 13-2).

COG The Musculoskeletal System and Common Disorders

When there is a problem with the musculoskeletal system, orthopedists and physical therapists often provide appropriate treatment and rehabilitation. However,

medical assistants working in other specialties, such as family practice or urgent care centers, also care for patients with musculoskeletal disorders. The most common disorders of the musculoskeletal system are sprains, dislocations, fractures, joint disruptions, and degeneration. The musculoskeletal system reacts to injury or disease with pain, swelling, inflammation, deformity, and/or limitation of range and function (Box 13-1).

Sprains and Strains

Injury to a joint capsule and its supporting ligaments is called a *sprain*, and injury to a muscle and its supporting tendons is called a *strain*. Damage to a muscle, ligament, or tendon may result in joint instability. If the ligament is completely torn, it cannot efficiently stabilize the joint.

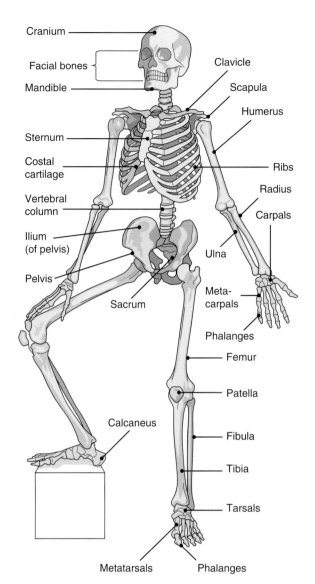

Cranium

Facial bones

Mandible

Clavicle

Scapula

Humerus

Sternum

Costal cartilage

Vertebral column

Ilium (of pelvis)

Pelvis

Sacrum

Ribs

Radius

Carpals

Ulna

Meta-carpals

Phalanges

Femur

Patella

Calcaneus

Fibula

Tibia

Tarsals

Metatarsals

Phalanges

Figure 13-1 The axial skeleton is shown in yellow; the appendicular skeleton is shown in blue. (Reprinted with permission from Cohen BJ. Memmler's The Human Body in Health and Disease, 11th ed. Philadelphia: Lippincott Williams & Wilkins, 2009.)

Common symptoms are inflammation and pain. Applying ice at the time of injury helps reduce swelling and pain. For mild sprains, treatment includes exercise to prevent joint stiffness and muscle atrophy. Therapeutic devices and compression wraps reduce swelling. Moderate sprains must be treated with care to prevent further injury because the ligaments are weakened and healing may take 6 to 8 weeks. Severe sprains often require surgery, and the recovery may take longer than 8 weeks.

In the spine, a sprain to the facet joint (the area between vertebrae) can cause pain not only at the point of difficulty, but also radiating into an extremity (radicular pain) as a result of impingement on the nerve root that passes close to the joint. For example, an injury to the facet joint between vertebrae of the lower back often causes pain in the back that radiates down one leg or the other. An injury to the anterior cruciate ligament in the knee greatly compromises the joint's stability. The knee becomes swollen, painful, and unstable and has limited motion. Complete tears in the ligaments of the knee require surgery and extensive rehabilitation. An injury to the Achilles tendon in the lower posterior leg is extremely painful and limits the ability to walk. A tear in this tendon requires surgery followed by immobilization.

Dislocations

Dislocation of a joint, also called a *luxation*, occurs when the end of the bone is displaced from its articular surface. It can be caused by trauma or disease, or it may be congenital. Common sites of dislocations include the shoulders, elbows, fingers, hips, and ankles. A *subluxation* is a partial dislocation in which the bone is pulled out of the socket but all joint structures maintain their proper relationships. Partial dislocations can result from weakness, decreased muscle tone, gravity, or neurologic deficit. The muscles bear most of the responsibility for preventing subluxation. Common symptoms of dislocations include pain, pressure, limited movement, and deformity. Numbness and loss of a pulse in the affected extremity can also occur. Treatment includes realigning the bones and immobilization of the joint. The patient may have to do exercises to strengthen supporting muscles to avoid recurrences.

 CHECKPOINT QUESTION

1. How does a luxation differ from a subluxation?

Fractures

A fracture is a break or disruption in a bone caused by falls, other trauma, disease, tumors, or unusual stress. There are many types of fractures, each with its own set of problems (Table 13-1). However, all fractures have one symptom in common: pain. Other manifestations may include swelling, hemorrhage, lack of movement or unusual movement, **contusions**, and deformity of the body part involved.

Treatment of a fracture is known as a **reduction** (realigning the bones) by placing the broken ends into proper alignment. Casting, splinting, wrapping, and taping are means of maintaining and immobilizing a closed reduction while the bone heals. If it is not possible to obtain proper alignment by a closed reduction, surgery is required; this open reduction may require the insertion of pins, a plate, or other hardware to maintain alignment of the bones. Fractures in the shoulder are serious because the immobilization necessary for

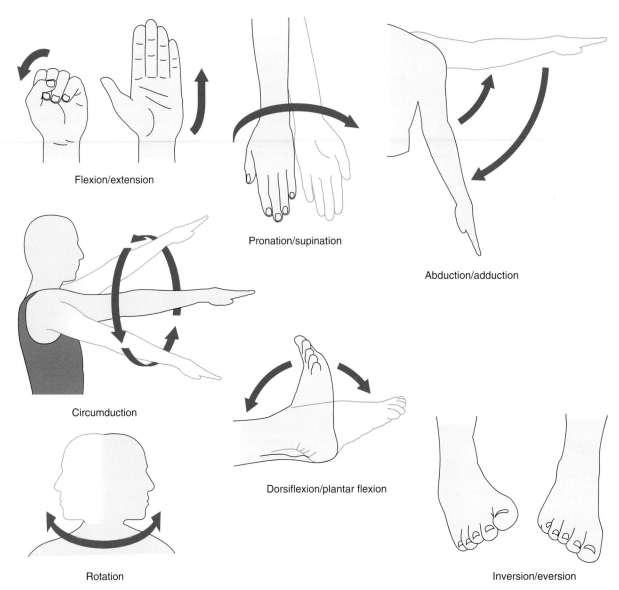

Figure 13-2 Normal range of motion of selected joints: flexion/extension; pronation/supination; abduction/adduction; circumduction; dorsiflexion/plantar flexion; inversion/eversion; and rotation. (Reprinted with permission from Cohen BJ. Memmler's The Human Body in Health and Disease, 11th ed. Philadelphia: Lippincott Williams & Wilkins, 2009.)

healing may cause scar tissue (adhesions) to form in the capsule, resulting in a severe loss of motion and function. These patients require extensive physical therapy to regain complete use of the involved arm.

Casts

Fractures must be immobilized to facilitate healing of the bone in the proper alignment. In most instances, both proximal and distal joints are included in the cast to ensure that movement is restricted. Box 13-2 describes various types of casts. The casting material is either plaster or fiberglass. Traditional plaster casts are bandages impregnated with calcium sulfate crystals and are supplied as rolls of material in widths appropriate to a variety of sites. After water is added to the dry

rolls of bandage and the wet material is applied to the extremity, a chemical reaction generates heat that may be uncomfortable to the patient for a short time, usually less than 30 minutes. This chemical reaction is necessary to produce a rigid dressing when dry. The bandage will mold smoothly to the casting site as it is applied.

A plaster cast is rather soft until it is fully dry, which can take as long as 72 hours. Patients must be cautioned not to exert pressure on the drying cast so as to avoid pressure sores from indentations. Plaster casts must be kept dry at all times.

Because of its lighter weight, water resistance, and durability, fiberglass is often used for casting. While the application is similar to the plaster cast, the polyurethane additives harden in minutes, eliminating the

MUSCULOSKELETAL PAIN

Rest, immobilization, or both may be needed to relieve pain in acute soft tissue strains, sprains, and inflammations. Because painful movement may cause further damage to the injured tissue, restriction of movement may also be required. This can be accomplished by rest and by the use of a cast, brace, sling, splint, collar, elastic wrap, or corset. If weight bearing is painful or inadvisable because of fracture or musculoskeletal pathology, an ambulatory aid (e.g., cane, walker, or crutches) may be used.

The use of hot moist packs, a heating pad, or warm baths can help increase circulation, relax spasms, and ease sore muscles. Ice packs help prevent swelling, decrease inflammation, and reduce contusions, which may follow a direct blow on a muscle.

With contusions, the capillaries (small blood vessels) rupture and bleed into the tissue. Swelling and inflammation may result. Reduction of the bleeding is crucial; it is accomplished by applying cold packs and a pressure bandage. Immobilization to prevent further injury is also important. Within a few days, pain-free exercises and heat applications should be introduced to begin healing.

Generally, movement should begin as soon as possible after a soft tissue injury to maintain a healthy joint and resilient muscles. Gentle active or passive movement in the pain-free range, mild joint immobilization, traction, or exercise can be effective in maintaining normal range, function, and strength.

extended drying time. After the cast has set, the material will not soften when wet but must be dried to prevent skin lesions. The fabric has a more open weave than plaster, which helps maintain skin integrity.

Assisting with Plaster or Fiberglass Cast Application

After positioning the patient comfortably before the procedure begins, drape the patient to expose only the part to be casted, avoiding unnecessary exposure and protecting other skin areas from the casting material. The part to be casted should be clean and dry; apply a bandage or dressing to any lesions before casting. Assemble the following items:

- Tubular soft fabric stocking material large enough to encircle the limb
- Roller padding, also called *sheet wadding*
- Casting material
- Bucket of cool or tepid water
- Plaster or cast knife
- Utility gloves

The limb is covered first with the soft knitted tubular material with extra fabric above and below the projected casting length to allow for a padded fold at each end. The soft roller padding is applied in fairly thick layers over bony prominences (Fig. 13-3). The limb is wrapped from the distal end to the proximal end with the soaked casting material. You may be responsible for soaking the material until bubbles no longer form around the rolls. The rolls should be pressed, not wrung, until they are wet through but not dripping. Wear utility gloves to protect your hands from the material. When the site is adequately covered, rough edges are trimmed with the plaster knife, and the knitted fabric is folded back to form cuffs at each end. The skin outside the cast is cleansed of casting material to avoid discomfort and skin breakdown.

Because of the unsupported weight an arm cast may put on the shoulder muscles, a sling is ordered to relieve and redistribute the weight. Slings are also used when casting is not necessary but the arm must be immobilized to facilitate healing. Procedure 13-1 describes the steps for applying a sling; however, many commercially made slings are now available that adjust easily depending on the size of the patient.

PATIENT EDUCATION

CAST CARE

Instruct patients with casts to do the following:

- Be aware of the initial warmth of the drying cast; this will diminish in 20 to 30 minutes.
- Keep a plaster cast dry.
- Avoid indentations by allowing the cast to dry completely before handling or propping it on a hard surface.
- Note that the fingers and toes are left uncovered to check for color, swelling, numbness, and temperature; report any impairment to the physician immediately.
- Report odors, staining, or undue warmth of the cast.
- Prevent swelling by elevating the limb for at least 24 hours after casting and as often as possible after that time.
- Never insert any object under the cast to scratch beneath it. Breaks in the skin may become infected and require that the cast be removed prematurely.

TABLE **13-1**   Types of Fractures

Type	Description
Simple or closed	Does not protrude through the skin; usually treated with a closed reduction
Compound or open	Broken end protrudes through the skin; infection a major concern; surgery often required
Spiral	Occurs with torsion or twisting injuries; appears to be S-shaped on radiographs
Impacted	One bone segment driven into another
Greenstick	Common injury in children; partial or incomplete break in which only one side of a bone is broken, like a green stick
Transverse	At right angles to axis of bone; generally caused by excessive bending force or direct hit on bone
Oblique	Slanted across axis of bone
Comminuted	Bone is fragmented, usually by much direct force; difficult to reduce because many pieces of bone must be held in proper alignment; more complicated to treat if articular surface if involved, so surgery usually required; severe soft tissue damage common because of the force necessary to cause the fracture
Compression	Damage from application of strong force against both ends, such as a fall; vertebrae susceptible to compression fractures, especially in older adults
Depressed	Fracture of flat bones (usually skull), causing fragment to be driven below surface of bone
Avulsion	Caused by strong force applied to bone by sharp twisting, pulling motion of attached ligaments or tendons resulting in a tearing away of bone fragments
Pathologic	Usually result of disease process such as osteoporosis (brittle bones), **Paget disease** (a chronic skeletal disease in older adults with bowing of the long bones), bone cysts, tumors, or cancers

Closed   Open   Greenstick   Comminuted

A

(**A**) Types of fractures: closed, open, greenstick, comminuted.

TABLE **13-1**   Types of Fractures *(continued)*

Type	Description

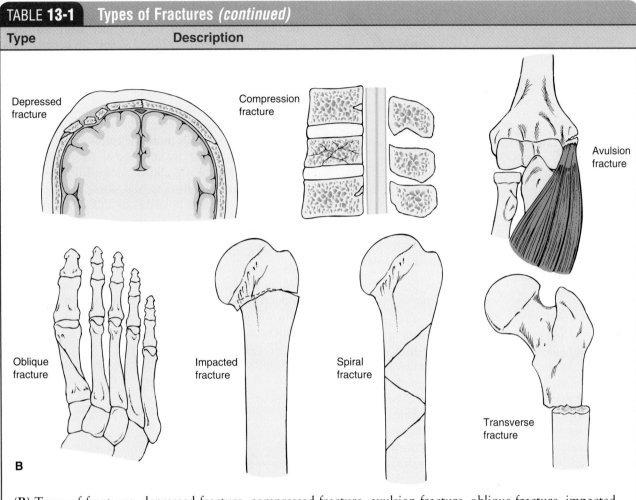

(B) Types of fractures: depressed fracture, compressed fracture, avulsion fracture, oblique fracture, impacted fracture, spiral fracture, transverse fracture.

BOX 13-2

TYPES OF CASTS

- *Short arm cast* extends from below the elbow to mid palm.
- *Long arm cast* extends from the axilla to mid palm. The elbow is usually at a 90° angle.
- *Short leg cast* extends from below the knee to the toes; the foot is in a natural position.
- *Long leg cast* extends from the upper thigh to the toes; the knee is slightly flexed, and the foot is in a natural position.
- *Walking cast* may be either short leg or long leg; the cast is extra strong to bear weight and may include a walking heel.
- *Body cast* encircles the trunk, usually from the axilla to the hip.
- *Spica cast* encircles part of the trunk and one or two extremities.

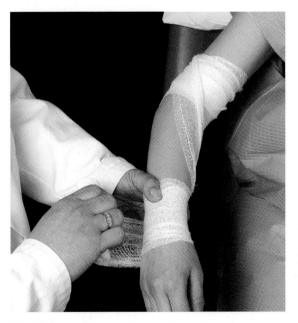

Figure 13-3 Applying a roller bandage before the casting material.

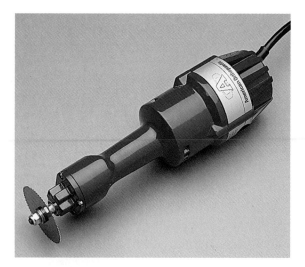

Figure 13-4 A cast cutter and saw. (Courtesy of M-PACT Worldwide, Eudora, KS.)

Plaster or Fiberglass Cast Removal

To remove a plaster or fiberglass cast, cuts are made in the cast through its length on opposite sides, dividing it into halves. An electric oscillating circular saw known as a *cast cutter* is used (Fig. 13-4). Assure the patient that this will not cut the skin. Wear safety goggles to protect your eyes from flying particles and caution the patient also. The cast will be split apart with a cast spreader, and the padding will be cut with utility scissors. The patient should be warned that the skin will be pale and dry and the muscle will be weak and shrunken from disuse. Also explain that the skin may be sensitive to touch and temperature. Creams and lotions help alleviate the dryness, and physical therapy and exercise will restore the muscle tone.

 CHECKPOINT QUESTION

2. Why is it important to not touch plaster casts until completely dry?

 LEGAL TIP

ASSESSING CIRCULATION AFTER A CAST APPLICATION

A cast that is applied improperly can lead to nerve and vascular damage, resulting in permanent loss of function to the extremity. In extreme situations, a surgical amputation may be required. To ensure proper care and to avoid lawsuits, it is essential that distal extremity circulation be assessed and documented before and after reductions and casting. Also, the patient should be taught to watch for and report signs of impaired circulation.

Healing of Fractures

The most important criterion for successful healing of a fracture is an adequate blood supply. In dermatology, the term "callus" describes a raised painless thickening of the epidermis. However, the blood secretes an important glue-like substance also known as **callus**, which is deposited around a break in any bone. Callus holds the ends of the bones together; with time, the callus turns to bone. The bone cells mold the callus and smooth the fracture site to close to its original size. Immobilization of the fracture site allows successful molding and reshaping. Older adults may heal slowly, and prosthetic joint replacement may be necessary if bone restructuring is inadequate (Box 13-3).

If the blood supply is inadequate to the healing bone or tissue, union may be delayed or absent. If damage is sufficient or if severe trauma, disease, tumor, or complications are involved, amputation may be necessary. Amputation is a drastic measure that is performed only when all other avenues are exhausted. A **prosthesis** enables the amputee to resume functional activities such as walking, grasping, and holding.

A potentially life-threatening complication of a fracture is a fat **embolus**. This type of embolus results from

BOX 13-3

BONE HEALING IN OLDER ADULTS

A fractured femur in older adults raises special concerns. Bone-repairing osteoblasts are less able to use calcium to restructure bone tissue at any site in older adults, but the neck of the femur, the most common fracture site, is especially vulnerable to delayed or imperfect healing because the blood supply is poor. Fractures through this area, involving the femoral head or neck or just inferior to the greater trochanter, may require hip arthroplasty or total hip replacement.

Most hip joint replacement prostheses are metal or polyethylene molded to conform to the joints they are designed to replace. Total hip replacement, usually used for degenerative joint disease or rheumatoid arthritis, replaces the head and neck of the femur and the acetabular surface. Knee replacement replaces both the head of the tibia and the distal epiphysis of the femur.

Early repair and return to mobility prevent contractures and atrophy of the supporting muscles. Postoperative walking prevents many of the complications associated with prolonged confinement in older adults, such as pathologic fractures, static pneumonia, and renal calculi.

BOX 13-3 *(continued)*

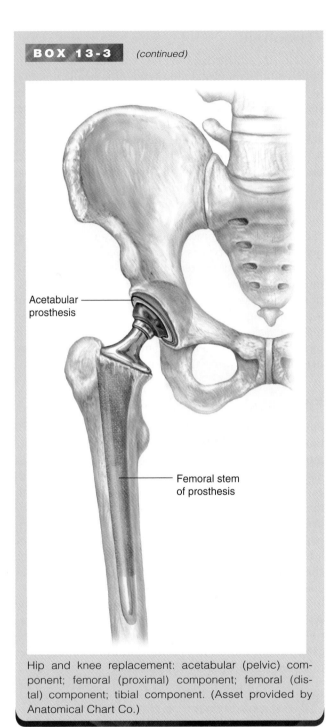

Acetabular prosthesis

Femoral stem of prosthesis

Hip and knee replacement: acetabular (pelvic) component; femoral (proximal) component; femoral (distal) component; tibial component. (Asset provided by Anatomical Chart Co.)

PATIENT EDUCATION

HELPING ELDERLY PATIENTS AVOID HIP FRACTURES

Older patients are particularly likely to fall and fracture bones, and when this happens, one of the most common bones broken is the head of the femur. These fractures take a long time to heal and often result in the patient being admitted to a skilled nursing facility for rehabilitation. Therefore, it is important for you to teach older patients fall prevention techniques. Here are some important tips:

- Always wear shoes with good, solid tie strings.
- Be sure that lighting is adequate, both inside and outside the home.
- Remove scatter rugs inside the home.
- Place grab bars throughout the home where extra assistance may be needed in getting out of chairs or off of the toilet.

Advise the patient that one-floor living is best, and teach the patient ways to reorganize the home to avoid climbing stairs.

Bursitis

Bursae, small pad-like sacs filled with a clear synovial fluid, surround some joints in areas of excessive friction, such as under tendons and over bony prominences. Their primary purposes are to reduce friction between moving parts and to prevent damage. The subdeltoid bursa in the shoulder between the deltoid muscle and the joint capsule is the most common site of bursitis, an inflammation of the bursa. Other frequent sites include the olecranon process at the elbow, the trochanter at the hip, the prepatellar bursae at the knee, and the heel.

The most common symptom of bursitis is pain during range-of-motion movement (see Fig. 13-2). In subdeltoid bursitis, pain occurs in the midrange of abduction but not at the beginning or end of the range. Pain occurs in the shoulder and arm when the inflamed bursa is pinched between the head of the humerus and the clavicle during abduction.

Treatment for bursitis usually consists of anti-inflammatory medications, rest, heat or cold applications, ultrasound to promote healing, and activities within the pain-free range. Physical therapy for range-of-motion exercises may also be ordered by the physician.

the release of fat droplets from the yellow marrow of the long bones. If the embolus lodges in the coronary or pulmonary vessels or in a large vessel in the brain, it can block the vessel, causing an infarction and death.

 CHECKPOINT QUESTION

3. What is the difference between an open and closed reduction of a fracture?

 CHECKPOINT QUESTION

4. What is the most common site of bursitis?

Arthritis

Osteoarthritis, or degenerative joint disease, is caused by wear and tear on the weight-bearing joints. As the articular cartilage degenerates, the ends of the bones enlarge, causing an intrusion of bone into the joint cavity. The patient has pain and restricted movement in the affected joint. Treatment of osteoarthritis includes administration of anti-inflammatory medications and intra-articular corticosteroid injections to control the pain and inflammation. Patients may also require the use of an ambulatory aid such as a cane, walker, or crutches to decrease joint stress.

Rheumatoid arthritis is a systemic autoimmune disease that attacks the synovial membrane lining of the joint. Ultimately it leads to inflammation, pain, stiffness, and crippling deformities (Fig. 13-5). It usually begins in non–weight-bearing joints such as the fingers but eventually may affect many joints, including the hands, wrists, elbows, feet, ankles, knees, and neck.

Marie-Strumpell disease, or **ankylosing spondylitis**, is rheumatoid arthritis of the spine. It is characterized by extreme forward flexion of the spine and tightness in the hip flexors. Rheumatoid arthritis in children is known as *Still disease*.

The treatment for rheumatoid arthritis is similar to the treatment for osteoarthritis: anti-inflammatory medications orally and corticosteroid or gold injections into the affected joint, heat and cold applications, and protection of painful joints with splints or braces. In severe cases, the joint may be surgically replaced with an artificial one.

CHECKPOINT QUESTION

5. How does osteoarthritis differ from rheumatoid arthritis?

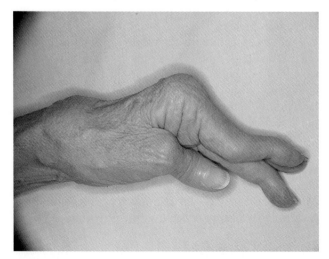

Figure 13-5 Hand of a patient with rheumatoid arthritis. (From Strickland JW, Graham TJ. Master Techniques in Orthopeadic Surgery: The Hand, 2nd Edition. Philadelphia: Lippincott Williams & Wilkins, 2005.)

Tendonitis

Muscles are attached to bones by tendons, which aid the body's mobility and stability. Tendonitis is inflammation of these structures. This disorder usually occurs after strains, sprains, overuse, or overstretching of the tissue. Although pain does not occur with passive movement, active movement is painful, and resistance to movement is intensely painful because the tissue must contract during active and resisted movement. Local tenderness is usual. The most common site of tendonitis is at the supraspinatus tendon in the shoulder, one of the rotator cuff muscles. Palpation over the tendon will elicit extreme pain. Sometimes tendonitis is caused by calcium deposits, and this type is called *calcific tendonitis*.

The treatment for tendonitis consists of oral anti-inflammatory medications, rest, heat or cold applications, ultrasound, **iontophoresis** (electrical transfer of ions), massage, and transverse friction massage (deep massage across the fibers of the tendons). Usually the patient is referred to a licensed massage therapist for the massage or transverse friction massage.

Fibromyalgia

Fibromyalgia causes multiple and often nonspecific symptoms including widespread pain in specific body areas, muscular stiffness, fatigue, and difficulty sleeping. This disorder varies from person to person, and the symptoms can be intermittent, making diagnosis difficult. Although the exact cause of this disorder is not known, some evidence suggests abnormalities in the immune system, perhaps resulting from a viral infection. Although it does not lead to other serious diseases, fibromyalgia tends to be chronic and is diagnosed by ruling out all other diseases and disorders with similar symptoms.

Treatment for fibromyalgia is based on relieving the symptoms with nonsteroidal anti-inflammatory medications, exercise, rest, and personal counseling, as indicated for the clinical depression that often accompanies this disorder because it is chronic.

CHECKPOINT QUESTION

6. What is the usual cause of tendonitis?

Gout

Gout, a metabolic disease of overproduction of uric acid, is a form of arthritis caused by the deposit of uric acid crystals into a joint, usually in the great toe. Although the cause of gout is unknown, the patient may have a history of injury to the joint, obesity, and a high-protein diet, especially a diet high in purines (alcoholic beverages, turkey, sardines, trout, bacon, and organ meats). The patient with gout complains of a painful, hot, inflamed joint; symptoms worsen unless treated (Fig. 13-6). Periods of

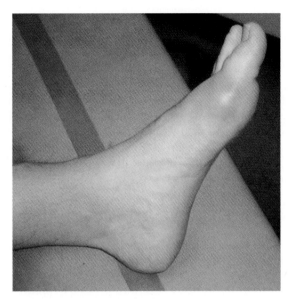

Figure 13-6 Tenderness and erythema on the medial aspect of the first metatarsophalangeal joint caused by gout. (From Dale Berg and Katherine Worzala, Atlas of Adult Physical Diagnosis. Philadelphia: Lippincott Williams & Wilkins, 2006.)

remission and exacerbation may occur. Gout may become chronic and can lead to multiple joint involvement with chronic pain, degeneration, and deformity. Symptoms are relieved by taking nonsteroidal anti-inflammatory medications and by avoidance of purine-rich foods and alcohol. Medication to prevent uric acid formation or foster its excretion from the body may also be prescribed.

 CHECKPOINT QUESTION

7. What foods should be avoided in the patient with gout?

Muscular Dystrophy

The congenital disorders collectively known as *muscular dystrophy* are characterized by varying degrees of progressive wasting of skeletal muscles. There is no neurologic involvement, but the skeletal muscles waste and weaken. Some forms of the disease affect the heart and other organs. The most common type of muscular dystrophy, Duchenne, is apparent in males in early childhood and is usually fatal by young adulthood as respiratory and cardiac muscles fail. Several forms, such as facioscapulohumeral and limb girdle dystrophy, progress slowly from a childhood onset and result in varying degrees of disability. Duchenne, facioscapulohumeral, and limb girdle dystrophies are genetically transmitted.

Diagnosis of muscular dystrophy is based on family and patient history. The characteristic signs are frequently the most obvious diagnostic indicators of the disease. They include muscle weakness, clumsiness, frequent falling, and muscle spasms. **Electromyography**

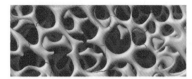
Healthy bone

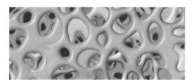
Bone with osteoporosis

Figure 13-7 Healthy bone versus bone with osteoporosis.

and muscle biopsy are used to rule out nervous system involvement. There is no known cure for any form of muscular dystrophy; however, exercise, physical therapy, and the use of splints or braces can relieve the symptoms. As mobility decreases, the use of a cane, walker, or wheelchair may be useful in maintaining independence.

Osteoporosis

Porous bones, or osteoporosis, is a condition in which the bones are deficient in calcium and phosphorus, making them brittle and vulnerable to fractures (Fig. 13-7). The cause may be dietary, with general deficiencies in calcium, vitamin D, or phosphorus, or it may be primary progressive inability to metabolize calcium brought on by estrogen deficiency in elderly women or sedentary lifestyle, alcoholism, liver disorder, or rheumatoid arthritis.

There are few signs of osteoporosis other than a gradual loss of stature or height, progressive kyphosis (or dowager's hump), and spontaneous, nontraumatic fractures (Fig. 13-8). Diagnosis includes bone scan, densitometry (a test that measures the density of the bones), thyroid and parathyroid studies, and serum calcium and phosphorus determinations. Treatment is preventing

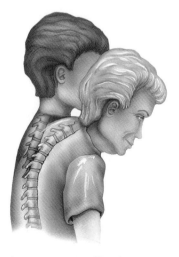

Figure 13-8 The progression of kyphosis in osteoporosis.

fractures by increasing appropriate levels of exercise to strengthen the bones. Hormone therapy with estrogen or a combination of estrogen and progesterone may be prescribed for postmenopausal women to prevent loss of minerals from the bones that occurs with the natural decrease in these hormones during menopause. Calcium and vitamin D supplements are beneficial to arrest the progression but will not cure the underlying degenerative factors once osteoporosis has begun.

Bone Tumors

Bone tissue is rarely the primary site for malignancies but is frequently a site of metastasis. Primary osteosarcomas occur most often in young men, although they may occur at any age in either sex. Osteogenic sarcomas originate in the bony tissue, while nonosseous tumors seed to the bones from other sites. Ewing sarcoma, originating in the marrow and invading the shaft of the long bones, is common in young adults, especially adolescent boys.

There is no known cause of malignant skeletal tumors, but one hypothesis is that rapid development of

bone tissue during growth spurts is a predisposing factor. Bone pain is the most common early sign. The pain is most intense at night, is usually dull and centered at the site, and is not relieved by resting the body part. Depending on the site, the mass may be palpable through the skin and muscles. Biopsy is the definitive diagnostic test after a bone scan suggests the need. Surgical treatment includes excision of the tumor, including a large margin of surrounding bone structure and nearby lymph nodes, or amputation if the tumor is in an extremity. Chemotherapy and radiation are usually indicated also.

CHECKPOINT QUESTION

8. Why is exercise used to treat or prevent osteoporosis?

Spine Disorders

The vertebral column (Fig. 13-9) is made up of 33 vertebrae and numerous joints. The cervical, thoracic, and lumbar

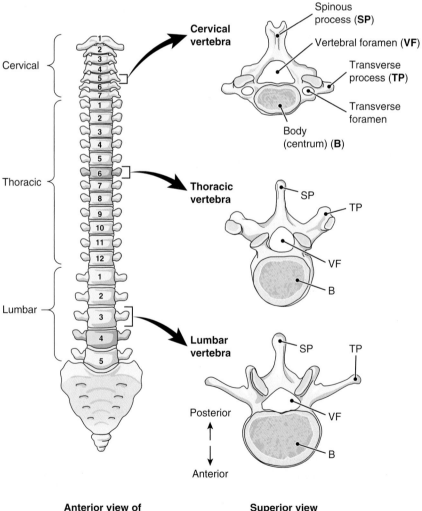

Figure 13-9 (Left) Front view of the vertebral column. (Right) Vertebrae from above. (Reprinted with permission from Cohen BJ. Memmler's The Human Body in Health and Disease, 11th ed. Philadelphia: Lippincott Williams & Wilkins, 2009.)

BOX 13-4

AVOIDING BACK STRAIN

You can prevent back strain by using good body mechanics:

- When lifting a heavy object, keep the object close to your body. Never lift an object with extended arms.
- Never lift and twist at the same time. Lift the object, and then reposition your feet by pivoting or taking two steps to turn.
- Bend your knees, not your back, when lifting.
- Ask for assistance from co-workers when you must lift or move obese patients or heavy objects.
- Maintain proper posture at all times; slouching causes muscle strain.
- If you do sustain an injury at work, inform your supervisor immediately and document what happened. Complete an incident report in accordance with the facility's policy.

---

vertebrae are separated from each other by 23 intervertebral discs; the vertebrae of the sacrum and coccyx are fused, with no discs separating the bones. These vertebrae and their discs absorb and transmit the shock of running, walking, and jumping and keep the spine flexible for a high degree of mobility. Many strong ligaments and structures support and protect the spine, including the anterior and posterior longitudinal ligaments and the four natural curves in the spine. However, back injuries are common and are a leading cause of work-related injury among health care professionals. Box 13-4 offers some suggestions for avoiding back strain, and patients can use these general guidelines as well.

 PATIENT EDUCATION

POSTURE AND BACK PAIN

Although there are many reasons for poor posture including the aging process, the result of poor posture includes back pain, which often results in more pain and poor posture. In patients with poor posture, the bones are not aligned properly, and the muscles, joints, and ligaments become strained and stressed. As the discs between the vertebra become less resilient, there is increased pressure from forces such as gravity and body weight, which results in the loss of flexibility in the muscles of the back and spine and spine degeneration. Weak, tight, and inflexible muscles cannot support the back's natural curves.

The most common posture faults are the forward head posture and rounded shoulders. Maintaining good posture—or correcting poor posture—can help reduce a bulging disc or relieve the biomechanical stress caused by poor skeletal alignment, greatly aiding musculoskeletal system functioning.

Abnormal Spine Curvatures

Exaggerated or abnormal curvatures of the spine affect the posture and the alignment of the shoulders and hips. An abnormally deep lumbar curve is **lordosis**, or swayback. Abnormal thoracic curvature, particularly of the upper portion, is called **kyphosis**, or hunchback. A side-to-side or lateral curvature is called **scoliosis**; it is commonly screened for in school children, especially girls, and if severe enough, it is surgically corrected during adolescence (Fig. 13-10).

Treatment of abnormal spinal curvatures entails the use of bracing to straighten the curve to a normal position. Transcutaneous muscle stimulation devices cause the muscles on one side to contract and draw the spine into its proper position. When necessary, orthopedic surgery is performed to straighten the spinal column.

Herniated Intervertebral Disc

The lumbar spine is one of the most frequently injured parts of the body because it absorbs the body's full weight and the weight of anything that is carried. Because most of the movement in the lumbar spine occurs at the L4 to L5 and L5 to S1 segments, most herniated discs are seen

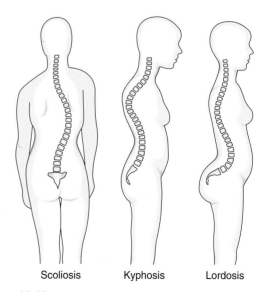

Scoliosis   Kyphosis   Lordosis

Figure 13-10 Abnormalities of the spinal curves. (Reprinted with permission from Cohen BJ. Memmler's The Human Body in Health and Disease, 11th ed. Philadelphia: Lippincott Williams & Wilkins, 2009.)

SAGITTAL VIEW OF LOWER SPINE

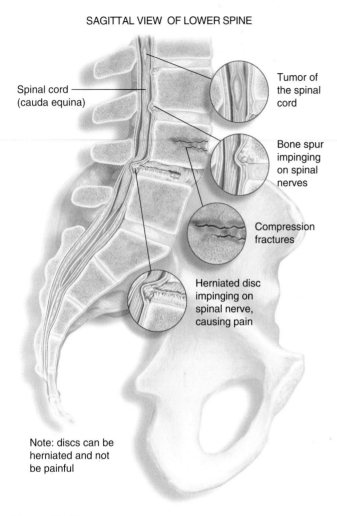

Spinal cord (cauda equina)

Tumor of the spinal cord

Bone spur impinging on spinal nerves

Compression fractures

Herniated disc impinging on spinal nerve, causing pain

Note: discs can be herniated and not be painful

Figure 13-11 Causes of low back pain.

at these levels, but injury can occur in any disc in the spine (Fig. 13-11).

A disc herniates when its soft center, known as the *nucleus*, ruptures through its tough outer layer to protrude into the spinal canal, sometimes pressing on the spinal cord. It is usually caused by severe trauma, degenerative change, or strenuous strain. Common symptoms include severe back pain, numbness in one or both extremities, spasms, weakness, and limitation of movement. Flexion radiates pain into the extremities, and extension is restricted and causes pain at the spinal segment. Having the patient raise one leg from the supine position (known as the *straight leg raise test*) indicates whether the back pain is from a disc. A positive sign includes back pain with the leg at 45° to 60°. A flattened lumbar curve and a lateral shift of the spine are fairly common. Radiography may show a narrowed disc space.

Because bone strength throughout the body is diminished during confinement or inactivity, total bed rest is no longer a common treatment for most musculoskeletal disorders, including herniated discs, although pain

limits activity. The treatment for herniated discs may include physical therapy for traction, massage, and mild extension exercises. While most disc herniations and bulges can be treated successfully without surgery, severe, unremitting pain, numbness, and progressive weakness of an extremity are indications for surgery to remove the injured disc.

 CHECKPOINT QUESTION

9. What are the three abnormal curvatures of the spine? Briefly describe each.

COG **Disorders of the Upper Extremities**

The structures of the upper extremity include the shoulder, elbow, wrist, and hand. Movement of the shoulder occurs in a ball-and-socket joint, which is the most mobile joint in the body. The elbow, a hinge joint, is made up of the articulation of the humerus with the radius (lateral) and the ulna (medial) and allows movement in one direction only.

The complex structure of the wrist allows for a variety of movements, including flexion, extension, ulnar deviation, radial deviation, and circumduction. However, the most intricate and specialized movements of the musculoskeletal system occur in the hand. The thumb, the first digit, accounts for 50% of hand function. The muscles that control the precision movements and fine motor activities of the hand are known as *intrinsic muscles* because they have both of their attachments, origin (the end of the muscle that stays relatively stationary or fixed) and insertion (the more movable end of the muscle), in the hand.

Rotator Cuff Injury

The rotator cuff is formed by the tendons of four muscles that hold the joint surfaces together during joint motion. Injury to the rotator cuff muscles in the shoulder can cause severe pain, weakness, and loss of function (Fig. 13-12). Surgical intervention for rotator cuff injury is often necessary because the tendons do not heal quickly on their own. An extended period of postoperative rehabilitation and physical therapy is usually needed to increase range of motion and strength and to regain the use of the shoulder. Professional athletes, particularly baseball pitchers, are prone to rotator cuff injuries.

Adhesive Capsulitis, or Frozen Shoulder

Frozen shoulder, a shortening of the muscles and joint structures known as a **contracture**, affects the entire

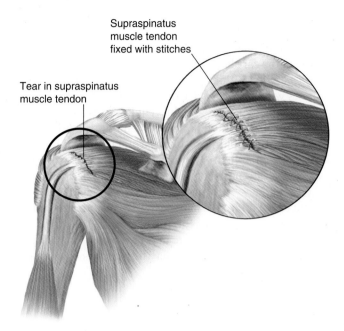

Supraspinatus muscle tendon fixed with stitches

Tear in supraspinatus muscle tendon

Figure 13-12 Rotator cuff tear.

shoulder joint and its capsule. It usually results from a fracture or disease process that prevents movement; however, anything that causes pain or restricts motion (e.g., tendonitis, bursitis, nerve damage, stroke, sprain, or strain) can lead to a frozen shoulder.

Contractures develop when the joint is immobilized, allowing the collagen fibers to stick to each other and thereby limit the movement in the joint. Adhesions and additional collagen are produced in response to injury, which results in a painful, tight, and constricted capsule. The shoulder movements most restricted are abduction and external rotation. Because full active range of motion is not possible, weakness and atrophy ensue.

Treatment consists of administration of anti-inflammatory medications and heat or cold applications. The physician may also prescribe physical therapy to include ultrasound, mobilization or manipulation, and stretching exercises. Recovery is slow and typically painful. Contractures in the joints are often preventable with proper management and by moving the joint through a full range of motion each day.

Lateral Epicondylitis, or Tennis Elbow

Lateral epicondylitis, often called *tennis elbow*, is a common elbow injury involving a sprain or strain of the tendons of origin of the wrist and finger extensor muscles. Symptoms include extreme pain with extension of the wrist, such as when trying to lift a cup or glass. Resistance to wrist extension and supination are the diagnostic tests for tennis elbow because both movements greatly increase the pain.

Treatment consists of ice applications, **phonophoresis** (ultrasound with cortisone) or iontophoresis, avoiding

movements that cause the pain, use of a forearm strap just distal to the elbow to take the pressure off the tendon, transverse friction massage, and gentle passive exercise to maintain mobility. In prolonged, extreme cases, surgery may be indicated.

 CHECKPOINT QUESTION

10. Which of the disorders of the upper extremities may result from decreasing movement of the arm and shoulder?

Carpal Tunnel Syndrome

A repetitive motion injury, carpal tunnel syndrome occurs when the carpal bones and transverse carpal ligaments compress the median nerve at the wrist. Symptoms include numbness in the thumb and index and middle fingers and pain and weakness in the affected hand and wrist. Often pain awakens the patient at night.

Diagnostic tests for carpal tunnel syndrome include the Phalen test, in which holding the wrist in flexion reproduces the symptoms; Tinel's test, in which the wrist is held in hyperextension and the transverse carpal ligament is thumped, causing tingling in the hand and fingers; and nerve conduction tests.

Treatment of carpal tunnel syndrome can be conservative, with anti-inflammatory medications and immobilization of the wrist with a brace or splint. If surgical intervention is necessary, it consists of release of the transverse carpal ligament.

PATIENT EDUCATION

LIVING WITH CARPAL TUNNEL SYNDROME

Patients with carpal tunnel syndrome should be questioned regarding their work environment. This syndrome is common among typists, computer operators, assembly line workers, and other professions that demand frequent grasping, twisting, and flexion of the wrist. Caution a patient who does a lot of word processing or typing to maintain good body alignment at all times in a properly proportioned and well-constructed chair. Palm supports for computer keyboards decrease the degree of wrist flexion. Advise the patient to take breaks and, if possible, to alternate computer work with other tasks. A physical therapist may offer range-of-motion exercises that the patient can do throughout the day to alleviate wrist tension. An occupational therapist can evaluate the work area and make suggestions for changes. Always consult the physician before making referrals.

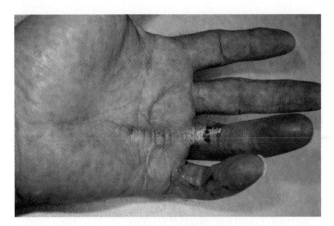

Figure 13-13 A Dupuytren contracture.

Dupuytren Contracture

Dupuytren contracture results in flexion deformities of the fingers, most often the ring and little fingers. It is caused by contractures of the fascia in the palm of the hand due to the proliferation or overgrowth of fibrous tissue (Fig. 13-13). As the fibrous tissue grows thicker, function is lost because the fingers cannot be straightened. Dupuytren contracture is easily diagnosed by inspection and palpation. Surgery is often required to release the contractures. Although no medications are available to treat this disorder, corticosteroid injections may temporarily improve function in the hand. Stretching of the tight structures in the early stages may slow the progression.

 CHECKPOINT QUESTION

11. What is the treatment for carpal tunnel syndrome?

COG **Disorders of the Lower Extremities**

The musculoskeletal structures of the lower extremities include the hip, knee, ankle, and feet. The hip, a ball-and-socket joint, is important for weight bearing and walking. The acetabulum, the socket of the hip joint, is deep enough to hold most of the femoral head and is surrounded by three strong ligaments.

The largest joint in the body, however, is the knee. Locking the knee into extension allows one to stand for long periods without using the muscles. An integral part of the knee is the patella, which lies inside the quadriceps tendon and protects the hinge joint. Two important sets of ligaments, the collateral and cruciate ligaments, stabilize the knee. The knee is often injured because it is supported entirely by muscles and ligaments and because it is one of the most stressed joints, lying as it does between the two longest bones in the body.

Chondromalacia Patellae

Chondromalacia patellae is a degenerative disorder affecting the cartilage that covers the back of the patella, or kneecap. It usually occurs in young women and in athletes who perform activities that stress the knee, such as running, jumping, and bicycling. A common complaint is pain when walking down stairs or getting out of a chair. Rest, physical therapy, bracing or taping the knee, anti-inflammatory medications, ice therapy, and exercises to strengthen the quadriceps muscles can help to relieve the symptoms. If these treatments are not effective, an endoscope may be used to examine the joint and surrounding tissue for further problems (**arthroscopy**) (Fig. 13-14). In severe and chronic cases, a surgical procedure, **arthroplasty**, may be performed to repair or remove damaged cartilage.

Plantar Fasciitis

Plantar fasciitis, inflammation of the plantar fascia ligament that stretches across the bottom of the foot, is the most frequent cause of pain in the bottom of the foot. Although the cause of plantar fasciitis is not always known, repetitive activities that stress the plantar fascia ligament, such as running and walking for extended periods on hard surfaces, may cause it. Factors that may aggravate it include wearing improperly fitted shoes and being overweight. Diagnosis includes a history of pain in the foot and heel when getting out of bed or after sitting for long periods. Deep palpation over the plantar (sole) surface of the heel bone will elicit pain. Radiography of the foot may be ordered to identify stress fractures, bone cysts, or heel spurs; however, ligaments do not show up clearly on radiographs, which are not routinely ordered to diagnose plantar fasciitis.

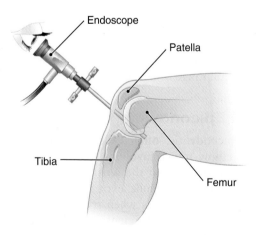

Figure 13-14 An arthroscopic examination of the knee. (Reprinted with permission from Cohen BJ. Medical Terminology: An Illustrated Guide, 6th ed. Philadelphia: Lippincott Williams & Wilkins, 2011.)

The treatment of choice for plantar fasciitis is a foot orthotic device (splint or heel pad) to support the arch and distribute the weight evenly. Physical therapy to stretch the ligament, ice therapy, massage, ultrasound, and nonsteroidal anti-inflammatory medications may also relieve the pain. Chronic planter fasciitis may necessitate wearing a night splint, which holds the affected foot at a 90° angle, preventing shortening and tightening of the plantar fascia during the night. Surgery is rarely done because of the high incidence of recurrence.

COG Common Diagnostic Procedures

Physical Examination

The physician's evaluation of the musculoskeletal system usually includes an assessment of structure and function, movement, and pain. An important part of the evaluation is the history, which includes the patient's description of the events and circumstances that led to the decision to seek medical help.

The physician observes the patient's overall physical state by noting how the patient walks, sits, stands, and moves. Concentrating on the area of concern, the physician evaluates the problem by visual inspection, palpation, and diagnostic tests. Pain and limited or compromised functions are warning signals. Strength also affects function and is a part of any musculoskeletal evaluation. Other important considerations are skin color, temperature, tone, and tenderness; abnormal findings may indicate underlying disease.

Diagnostic Studies

The most frequently used tools for detecting disorders of the musculoskeletal system are radiology and diagnostic imaging, which are used to diagnose fractures, dislocations, and degeneration or diseases of the bones and joints. Other radiographic studies include **arthrograms**, x-ray studies of the joints that may show joint disease, and myelograms, which help detect intervertebral disc conditions. A bone scan analyzes bone growth, density, tumors, and other pathology.

Computed tomography (CT) and magnetic resonance imaging (MRI) may reveal soft tissue disease, such as tumor, metastatic lesions, and ruptured or bulging discs. Electromyography and nerve conduction velocity tests measure the health and fitness of the nerves as they relate to conduction of nerve impulses and muscle function.

Goniometry is measurement of the amount of movement available in a joint by a protractor-like device called a **goniometer** (Fig. 13-15). A bone or muscle biopsy is also a valuable diagnostic tool. It allows intense examination of the tissue under a microscope to determine cell damage, neoplasms (tumor or growth), or other types of diseases.

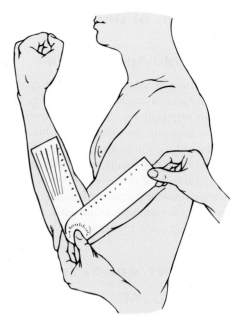

Figure 13-15 A goniometer. (Reprinted with permission from Weber J, Kelley J. Health Assessment in Nursing. Philadelphia: Lippincott Williams & Wilkins, 2003.)

 CHECKPOINT QUESTION

12. What procedures can be used to diagnose musculoskeletal disorders?

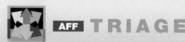 **AFF TRIAGE**

While working in a medical office setting, the following three situations occur:

A. You need to teach a 78-year-old patient how to use a walker.

B. A 47-year-old woman just arrived in the office complaining of pain in her left wrist. She fell in the parking lot. You have been instructed to apply a cold pack to her wrist.

C. A 12-year-old patient needs a sling applied to her right arm.

How do you sort these patients? Who do you see first? Second? Third?

Patient B should be attended first. A cold pack should be applied to the injured wrist as soon as possible to help control the swelling and decrease the pain. Patient C should be seen next. Applying a sling will take less time than teaching patient A how to use the walker. Teaching an older patient may take extra time, skill demonstration, and return demonstration. In addition, a detailed patient education instruction pamphlet about the use of the walker should be given to the patient and explained in detail.

COG The Role of the Medical Assistant

Warm and Cold Applications

Because of the time necessary for warm or cold applications, these procedures are not often done in the office. However, your responsibility may include instructing the patient in administering the treatments at home. Patients should understand the purpose of the procedure, how to perform it, the expected results, and any precautions or danger signs. Table 13-2 discusses the types of heat and cold applications and the purposes of each. Procedure 13-2 describes the steps for applying a cold pack, and Procedure 13-3 describes a hot pack application.

 PATIENT EDUCATION

HEATING PADS

Heating pads are not often used in the office, but a heating pad may be ordered by the physician for the patient to use at home. The patient must be aware of the potential for injury if strict guidelines are not followed. Share these safety tips with your patient:

1. Most heating pads are equipped with a cover to ensure comfort and safety. If one is not provided, wrap the pad in a soft cover before applying to the skin.
2. Do not fold or bend the pad; wires may break and form an electrical short if not kept in alignment.
3. Do not use safety pins on the heating pad. Pins may cause malfunction if they come into contact with the wiring inside the pad.

4. Never place heating pads under the body; heat may build up as it is reflected from the surface below and cause burns.
5. Set the temperature to be comfortably warm at first touch (usually the low or medium setting); do not turn the temperature up to high as the body adjusts to the temperature.
6. Keep to the recommended time for heat treatments and allow circulation to return to normal at intervals.

Precautions

When exposed to cool or warm temperatures, the body quickly adapts. For example, the water in a swimming pool feels cool at first, but after a short while, the body becomes used to the temperature, and it no longer feels cool. The body has adapted. Using this reasoning, patients should be instructed that the benefits of heat or cold therapy are continuing even though they may not be able to feel the initial temperature change.

The body responds to extremes of temperature for extended periods by exerting an opposite effect called the *rebound phenomenon*. For example, heat applied to an area will cause dilation of the blood vessels, or vasodilation. However, if heat is applied beyond 30 minutes, vasoconstriction will occur as the body attempts to compensate for the heat. Therefore, applications left on longer than recommended by the physician will have an opposite effect to the one intended.

Some areas of the body with thin skin and few nerve receptors, such as the abdomen, are more sensitive to heat than areas such as the palms of the hands. When applying heat, remember that the very young, older adults, the confused or disoriented patient, and patients with circulatory disorders or diabetes are particularly subject to burns.

TABLE **13-2**	Heat and Cold Treatments: Types and Purposes	
Dry Heat	**Moist Heat**	**Purposes**
Hot water bottle	Compresses	Relieve muscle spasms or tension; relieve pain; hasten healing by increasing blood flow to an area; provide local or systemic warming
Heating pad	Warm soaks	
Thermal pad		
Disposable heat pack		
Heat lamp		
Dry Cold	**Moist Cold**	**Purposes**
Ice bag	Compresses	Limit initial edema by decreasing capillary permeability (caution: cold retards edema by decreasing blood flow to the area); decrease bleeding or hemorrhage; decrease inflammation; relieve pain by numbing nerve pathways; provide local or systemic cooling
Ice collar	Cold soaks	
Disposable ice pack		

Generally, the temperature of heat and cold therapy should be kept within the following guidelines:

- Warm: tepid, 95° to 98°F, to very warm, 115°F
- Cold: neutral, 93° to 95°F, to very cold, 50°F

After checking with the physician, you should caution patients as follows:

Do not use heat:

- Within 24 hours after an injury, because it may increase bleeding
- For noninflammatory edema, because increased capillary permeability will allow additional tissue fluid to build up
- In cases of acute inflammation, because increased blood supply will increase the inflammatory process
- In the presence of malignancies, because cell metabolism will be enhanced
- Over the pregnant uterus
- On areas of erythema or vesicles, because it will compound the existing problem
- Over metallic implants, because it will cause discomfort

Do not use cold:

- On open wounds, because decreased blood supply will delay healing
- In the presence of already impaired circulation, because it will further impair circulation

 CHECKPOINT QUESTION

13. How does the body respond to prolonged exposure to temperature extremes?

Ambulatory Assist Devices

Patients may lose their ability to move normally because of an accident or injury, disease process, neurologic or muscular defect, or degeneration. Patients who require assistance to maintain mobility may use crutches, a cane, a walker, or a wheelchair. Medical assistants often are responsible for teaching patients how to use these ambulatory aids safely. Remind the patient to:

- Check the rubber tips frequently and replace worn tips immediately. (Most ambulatory aids require rubber tips, although some walkers have rollers.)
- Check screws and bolts frequently; tighten as needed.
- Remove scatter rugs and small pieces of furniture that may cause falls.
- Use caution on wet surfaces to avoid falling.
- To avoid damage to the axillary nerve, do not place the axillary bars against the axilla.
- Avoid back and neck strain by standing straight and looking ahead.

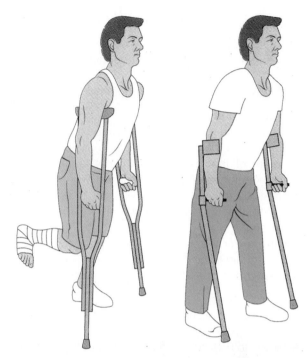

Figure 13-16 Types of crutches. **(A)** Axillary crutches. **(B)** Lofstrand crutches (also known as *Canadian* or *forearm crutches*).

 Crutches

Crutches may be made of wood or tubular aluminum and may be ordered for short-term use or when the patient will need assistance long term for several months or years. Axillary crutches are the most common form and extend from just under the patient's axillae to the floor with hand grips to distribute weight to the palms. These crutches are typically prescribed for short-term conditions when the patient cannot bear weight on one extremity. The Lofstrand, or Canadian, crutch is usually aluminum and reaches just to the forearms, with a metal cuff to maintain its position on the arms and a covered hand grip to distribute the weight (Fig. 13-16A,B). Lofstrand crutches allow the patient to release and use the hands without losing the crutches. These work well for patients who will need crutches for a long period or for those who have poor coordination. Procedure 13-4 explains the steps necessary for measuring and fitting a patient with axillary crutches, and Procedure 13-5 explains how to teach a patient the proper gait techniques.

 PATIENT EDUCATION
TIPS FOR CRUTCH WALKING

To go up stairs:
- Stand close to the bottom step.
- With the body's weight supported on the hands, step up on the first step with the unaffected leg.

(continued)

- Bring the affected side and the crutches up to the step at the same time.
- Resume balance before proceeding to the next step.
- *Remember:* The good side goes up first!

To go down stairs:
- Stand close to the edge of the top step.
- Bend from the hips and knees to adjust to the height of the lower step. Do not lean forward (leaning forward may cause a fall).
- Carefully lower the crutches and the affected leg to the next step before moving the other extremity.
- Next, lower the unaffected leg to the lower step and regain balance.
- *Remember:* The affected foot goes down first!

To sit:
- Back up to the chair until you feel its edge on the back of your legs.
- Move both crutches to the hand on the affected side and reach back for the chair with the hand on the unaffected side.
- Lower yourself slowly into the chair.

Canes

A cane is used when the patient needs extra support and stability but requires only a small measure of assistance with weight bearing. The standard cane may be used when the patient needs very slight assistance. The tripod (three legs) or quad cane (four legs) is useful when the patient needs greater stability (Fig. 13-17A–C). Tripod and quad canes can stand alone when patients need to use their hands or have other support. They tend to be bulkier and heavier than standard canes, but because they offer greater stability and safety, they are good for patients who need more support than the standard cane affords.

To measure for proper cane length, have the patient stand erect. The cane should be level with the patient's greater trochanter, and the patient's elbow should be bent at a 30° angle. To walk with a cane, the patient should:

1. Position the cane on the unaffected side about 4 to 6 inches to the side and about 2 inches ahead of the foot.
2. Advance the cane and the affected leg together.
3. Bring the unaffected leg forward to a position just ahead of the cane.
4. Repeat the steps.

Walkers

A walker is a comfortable aid for older adults and others with conditions that cause weakness or poor

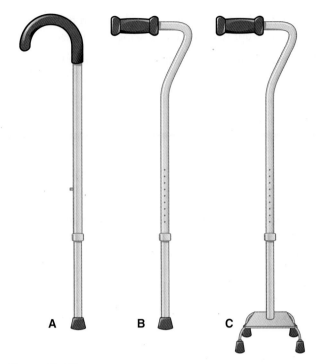

Figure 13-17 Three types of canes. (**A**) Single-ended canes with half-circle handles are recommended for patients requiring minimal support. (**B**) Single-ended canes with straight handles are recommended for patients with hand weakness. (**C**) Three- or four-prong canes are recommended for patients with poor balance.

coordination. A walker is a lightweight aluminum frame shaped like three sides of a rectangle; however, because walkers are somewhat bulky, maneuvering in close quarters can be difficult. The walker frame should

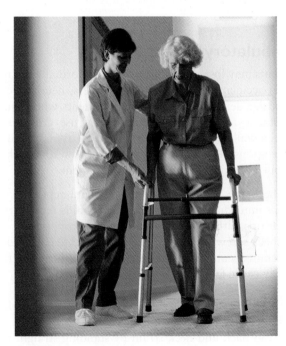

Figure 13-18 A properly adjusted walker.

be level with the patient's hip, and the patient's elbow should be bent at about a 30° angle (Fig. 13-18). To use a walker:

1. Stand erect and move the walker ahead about 6 inches.
2. Using an easy walking gait with hands on the walker grips, step into the walker.

3. Move the walker ahead again.
4. Repeat the steps.

 CHECKPOINT QUESTION

14. On which side of the body is the cane positioned?

Medication Box

Commonly Prescribed Orthopedic Medications

Note: The generic name of the drug is listed first and is written in all lower case letters. Brand names are in parentheses and the first letter is capitalized.

acetylsalicylic acid (aspirin) (Bayer, Ecotrin)	Tablets: 325 mg, 500 mg	Analgesic
acetaminophen and codeine (Tylenol #3)	Tablets: 300 mg acetaminophen and codeine 30 mg	Analgesic
adalimumab (Humira)	Injection: 40 mg/0.8 mL prefilled syringe	Antirheumatic
alendronate sodium (Fosamax)	Tablets: 5 mg, 10 mg, 35 mg, 40 mg, 70 mg	Antiresorptive
allopurinol (Lopurin, Zyloprim)	Tablets: 100 mg, 300 mg	Antigout
calcium citrate (Citracal)	Tablets: 250 mg, 950 mg	Calcium
carisoprodol (Soma)	Tablets: 250 mg, 350 mg	Muscle Relaxant
celecoxib (Celebrex)	Capsules: 50 mg, 100 mg, 200 mg, 400 mg	NSAID
colchicines (Colcrys)	Tablets: 0.6 mg	Antigout
cyclobenzaprine (Flexeril, Amrix)	Capsules: 15 mg, 30 mg	Muscle Relaxant
gold sodium thiomalate (Aurolate, Myochrysine)	Injection: 50 mg/mL (IM)	Antirheumatic
hydrocodone and acetaminophen (Vicodin, Lortab)	Tablets: 500 mg acetaminophen and 5 mg hydrocodone	Analgesic
ibandronate sodium (Boniva)	Tablets: 2.5 mg, 150 mg Injection: 3 mg/3 mL prefilled syringe (IV)	Antiresorptive
ibuprofen (Motrin, Advil)	Capsules: 200 mg Tablets: 100 mg, 200 mg, 400 mg, 800 mg	NSAID
indomethacin (Indocin)	Capsules: 25 mg, 50 mg Oral suspension: 25 mg/5 mL	NSAID
meperidine hydrochloride (Demerol)	Tablets: 50 mg, 100 mg Injection (IM): 25 mg/mL, 50 mg/mL, 75 mg/mL	Analgesic
morphine sulfate (Duramorph, Kadian, Roxanol)	Tablets: 15 mg, 30 mg Capsules: 30 mg to 120 mg Oral solution: 10 mg/5 mL	Analgesic

(continued)

Medication Box *(continued)*

Commonly Prescribed Orthopedic Medications

naproxen (Naprosyn)	Tablets: 200 mg, 250 mg, 375 mg, 500 mg	NSAID
oxycodone (OxyContin, Roxicodone)	Capsules: 5 mg Oral solution: 5 mg/5 mL Tablets: 5 mg, 10 mg, 15 mg, 20 mg, 30 mg	Analgesic
tramadol hydrochloride (Ultram)	Tablets: 50 mg	Analgesic

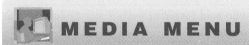

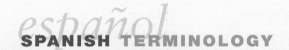

SPANISH TERMINOLOGY

Voy a ponerle una tabilla en la pierna.
I am going to put a splint on the leg.

Voy a examinarle la pierna.
I am going to examine your leg.

Doble las rodillas, no la espalda.
Bend your knees, not your back.

¿Le duelen las conyonturas?
Do you have pain in your joints?

MEDIA MENU

- **Student Resources on thePoint**
  - **Animation: Muscle Contraction**
  - **Video: Measure a Patient for Axillary Crutches and Instruct in Various Gaits (Procedures 13-4 and 13-5)**
  - **CMA/RMA Certification Exam Review**
- **Internet Resources**

  Arthritis Foundation
  http://www.arthritis.org

  Muscular Dystrophy Association
  http://www.mdausa.org

  About.com: What you need to know about orthopedics
  http://orthopedics.about.com

  American Association of Neurological Surgeons
  http://www.aans.org/Patient%20Information.aspx

PSY PROCEDURE 13-1: **Apply an Arm Sling**

Purpose: Correctly apply an arm sling
Equipment: A canvas arm sling with adjustable straps

Steps	Purpose
1. Wash your hands.	Handwashing aids infection control.
2. Assemble the equipment and supplies.	Be prepared before beginning any procedure.
3. Greet and identify the patient and explain the procedure.	Identifying the patient prevents errors in treatment. Explaining the procedure helps ease anxiety and ensure compliance.
4. **AFF** Explain how to respond to a patient who does not speak English or speaks English as a second language (ESL).	Solicit assistance from anyone who may be with the patient or get another staff member who speaks his or her native language to interpret if available. If no interpreter is available, use hand gestures or pictures to explain the procedure to the patient.
5. Position the affected limb with the hand at slightly less than a 90° angle so that the fingers are a bit higher than the elbow.	This position helps reduce swelling of the hand and fingers.
6. Insert the arm into the pouch end of the sling with the elbow fitting into the pocket corner.	The elbow should fit snugly into the sling.

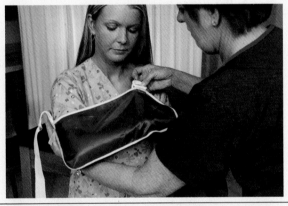

Step 6. Insert elbow into pocket of sling.

7. Bring the strap across the back and over the opposite shoulder to the front of the patient.	The back and unaffected shoulder will support the weight of the affected arm.

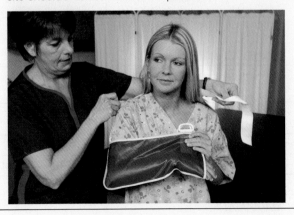

Step 7. Bring strap across back and to front of patient.

(continued)

PSY **PROCEDURE 13-1:** **Apply an Arm Sling** *(continued)*

Steps	Purpose
8. Secure the velcro end of the strap by inserting the end of it under the loop on the sling. Pull the strap through the loop an adequate amount so that the arm and hand inside the sling continue to be slightly elevated at a 90° angle.	The arm and hand should be at 90° to prevent swelling of the hand and fingers.

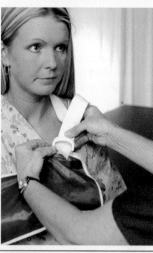

Step 8. Bring strap through loop.

Steps	Purpose
9. Press the velcro ends together and check the patient's comfort and distal extremity circulation.	Check circulation by palpating a radial pulse.

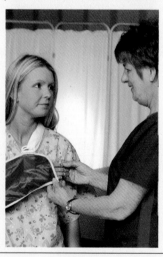

Step 9. Check circulation.

Steps	Purpose
10. Document the application in the patient's chart.	Procedures are considered not to have been done if they are not recorded.

Charting Example:

10/28/2014 11:15 AM Arm sling applied to (R) arm as ordered. Fingers to (R) hand warm and pink, no swelling.

To RTO in 4 days ————————————————————————————— T. Burton, RMA

Note: The medical assistant may sign his or her name in the patient record using only the "CMA" credential if the office has a signature log denoting the entire credential as "CMA(AAMA)."

PSY PROCEDURE 13-2: ██ **Apply Cold Packs**

Purpose: Apply a cold pack appropriately according to the physician's order
Equipment: Ice bag and ice chips or small cubes or a disposable cold pack, small towel or cover for the ice pack, gauze or tape

Steps	Purpose
1. Wash your hands.	Handwashing aids infection control.
2. Assemble the equipment and supplies, checking the ice bag for leaks. If using a commercial cold pack, read the manufacturer's directions.	Avoid wetting and chilling the patient. Small bits of ice help the bag to conform to the patient's contours better than large pieces.
3. Fill a reusable ice bag about two-thirds full. Press it flat on a surface to express air from the bag. Seal the container.	If the bag is too full of ice or air, it will not conform easily to the patient's contours.
4. If using a commercial chemical ice pack, activate it according to the manufacturer's instructions.	Commercially prepared chemical ice packs contain chemicals that must be mixed before the pack will become cold.
5. Cover the bag in a towel or other suitable cover.	The cover will absorb condensation and make the procedure more comfortable for the patient.

Step 5. Place the ice pack in a protective cover.

Steps	Purpose
6. Greet and identify the patient. Explain the procedure.	Identifying the patient prevents errors in treatment. Explaining the procedure helps ease anxiety and ensures compliance.
7. **AFF** Explain how to respond to a patient who has cultural or religious beliefs that prohibit disrobing.	Be respectful of the cultural differences by explaining why procedures are important. Provide additional privacy if necessary.
8. After assessing the skin for color and warmth, place the covered ice pack on the area.	The area must be assessed for the documentation before treatment begins. The cold pack should not come into direct contact with the skin.
9. Secure the ice pack with gauze or tape.	The ice pack should lie securely against the patient's skin for the greatest benefit. Pins may puncture the ice bag.

Step 9. Secure the ice pack with gauze or tape.

(continued)

PSY PROCEDURE 13-2:   Apply Cold Packs *(continued)*

Steps	Purpose
10. Apply the treatment for the prescribed amount of time and no longer than 30 minutes.	Longer than the prescribed time or 30 minutes may cause an adverse rebound effect, causing increased blood flow and swelling.
11. During the treatment, assess the skin under the pack frequently for mottling, pallor, or redness. Remove the ice pack at once if these appear.	These signs indicate an adverse reaction and should be reported to the physician immediately after removing the ice pack.
12. Properly care for or dispose of equipment and supplies. Wash your hands.	If the equipment is reusable, it should be prepared for the next patient by disinfecting according to office policy. If it is disposable, discard it appropriately.
13. Document the procedure, site of the application, results including the condition of the skin after the treatment, and the patient's response.	Procedures are considered not to have been done if they are not recorded.

Charting Example:

> 11/22/2014 10:45 AM Ice bag applied to (L) anterior thigh as ordered ×20 minutes. Skin before treatment swollen, with large contusion noted, no break in skin. After treatment, area pale and cool to touch, swelling decreased. Verbal and written instructions given for application qid at home; pt. verbalized understanding —————————B. Barry, CMA

Note: The medical assistant may sign his or her name in the patient record using only the "CMA" credential if the office has a signature log denoting the entire credential as "CMA(AAMA)."

PSY PROCEDURE 13-3:   Apply a Hot Water Bottle or Commercial Hot Pack

Purpose: Apply a hot pack appropriately according to the physician's order
Equipment: A hot water bottle or commercial hot pack, towel or other suitable covering for the hot pack

Steps	Purpose
1. Wash your hands.	Handwashing aids infection control.
2. Assemble equipment and supplies, checking the hot water bottle for leaks.	Checking for leaks avoids wetting the patient.
3. Fill the hot water bottle about two-thirds full with warm (110°F) water; place the bottle on a flat surface with the opening up and press out the excess air.	Excess air will prevent the bottle from conforming to the patient's contours.

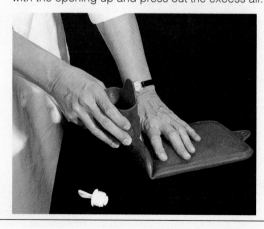

Step 3. Express air from the bottle before capping.

PSY PROCEDURE 13-3: **Apply a Hot Water Bottle or Commercial Hot Pack** *(continued)*

Steps	Purpose
4. If using a commercial hot pack, follow the manufacturer's directions for activating it.	Commercially prepared chemical hot packs contain chemicals that must be mixed before the pack will become hot.
5. Wrap and secure the pack or bottle before placing it on the patient's skin. **Step 5.** Wrap and secure the bag before placing on the patient's skin.	Covering the bag will increase the patient's comfort and prevent burning the skin.
6. Greet and identify the patient. Explain the procedure.	Identifying the patient prevents errors in treatment.
7. After assessing the color of the skin where the treatment is to be applied, place the covered hot pack on the area.	The area must be assessed for documentation before the treatment begins. The hot pack should not touch the skin. Heat therapy should be used cautiously in patients with circulatory disorders, diabetics, and older adults.
8. **AFF** Explain how to respond to a patient is from a different (older) generation than you.	Refer to an elderly patient by his or her correct title (Mr., Mrs., Miss, etc.). Be respectful to the patient by only using his or her first name after they have given you permission to do so. Do not assume the patient is hearing or cognitively impaired because of his or her age.
9. Secure the hot pack with gauze or tape.	It should be securely against the patient's skin for the greatest benefit. Pins may puncture the hot pack.
10. Apply the treatment for the prescribed amount of time but for no longer than 30 minutes.	Longer than the prescribed time or 30 minutes may cause an adverse rebound effect and decreased blood flow to the area.
11. During the treatment, assess the skin every 10 minutes for pallor (rebound), excessive redness (pack too hot), and swelling (tissue damage). If you see any of these signs, immediately remove the hot pack.	These signs indicate an adverse reaction and should be reported to the physician immediately after you remove the hot pack.
12. Properly care for or dispose of equipment and supplies. Wash your hands.	Reusable equipment should be disinfected for the next patient. Disposables should be discarded appropriately.

(continued)

PSY PROCEDURE 13-3: **Apply a Hot Water Bottle or Commercial Hot Pack** *(continued)*

Steps	Purpose
13. Document the procedure, site of the application, results including condition of the skin after treatment, and the patient's response.	Procedures are considered not to have been done if they are not recorded.

Charting Example:

7/11/2014 3:00 PM Hot pack to (L) shoulder × 30 minutes as ordered. Skin pink before treatment, slightly reddened
after treatment. Pt. stated pain in upper back and shoulder relieved. Oral and written instructions given for
applications at home qid, Pt. verbalized understanding —————————————————————— S. Rose, CMA

Note: The medical assistant may sign his or her name in the patient record using only the "CMA" credential if the office has a signature log denoting the entire credential as "CMA(AAMA)."

PSY PROCEDURE 13-4: **Measure a Patient for Axillary Crutches**

Purpose: Accurately measure a patient for axillary crutches
Equipment: Axillary crutches with tips, pads for the axilla, and hand rests as needed

Steps	Purpose
1. Wash your hands.	Handwashing aids infection control.
2. Assemble the equipment, including crutches correct size.	Axillary crutches must always be fitted to the of the height of the patient.
3. Greet and identify the patient.	This helps avoid errors in treatment.
4. Ensure that the patient is wearing low-heeled shoes with safety soles.	Low-heeled shoes with good soles assist with adjusting the crutches to the patient's height and help prevent falls. While using the crutches, patients should wear shoes with the same heel height to avoid an improper crutch fit.
5. Have the patient stand erect. Support the patient as needed.	Standing will allow you to adjust the crutches to the correct height.
6. **AFF** Explain how to respond to a patient who is hearing impaired.	Make sure the patient can see your face as you are speaking. Speak clearly, not loudly.
7. While standing erect, have the patient hold the crutches naturally with the tips about 2 inches in front of and 4 to 6 inches to the sides of the feet. This is called the *tripod position*, and all crutch gaits start from this position.	This is the *tripod position*, and all crutch gaits start from this position.

PSY **PROCEDURE 13-4:** **Measure a Patient for Axillary Crutches** *(continued)*

Steps	Purpose
8. Adjust the central support in the base so that the axillary bar is about two finger-breadths below the patient's axillae. Tighten the bolts for safety at the proper height.	If the axillary bar presses on the axillae, nerve damage may occur. If it is too low, the crutches will be difficult to manage and will cause poor posture and back strain.

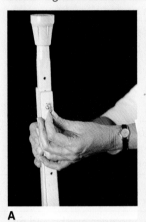 A 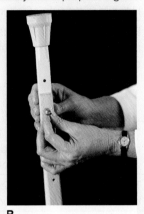 B

Step 8. (A) Adjust the crutches to the patient's height by removing the wing nut and bolt and moving the extension. **(B)** Tighten the bolt securely.

Steps	Purpose
9. Adjust the hand grips by raising or lowering the bar so that the patient's elbow is at a 30° angle when the bar is gripped. Tighten bolts for safety.	Hand grips that are too high or too low will compromise safety and may cause nerve pressure.

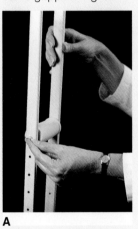 A 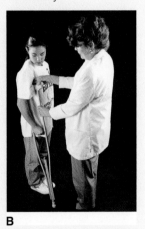 B

Step 9. (A) Adjust the hand grips by raising or lowering along the shaft of the crutch. **(B)** Crutches are properly adjusted when the patient's elbow is at a 30° angle and two fingers can be inserted under the axilla on top of the crutch axillary bar.

Steps	Purpose
10. If needed, pad axillary bars and hand grips with soft material, such as large gauze pads or small towels and secure with tape to prevent friction.	If padding is used on the axillary bars, make sure the padding is not touching the axilla; this is to avoid pressure and damage to the axillary nerve.
11. Wash your hands and record the procedure.	Procedures are considered not to have been done if they are not recorded.

Charting Example:

3/17/2014 4:40 PM Pt. measured for axillary crutches as ordered; no pressure to axilla, elbows at a 30° angle. Given

oral and written instructions for crutch safety and the 3-point and swing-through gaits. Demonstrated both gaits

without difficulty. Verbalized understanding of instructions. Reinforced physician order for no weight bearing on

(L) leg × 3 days, to return to office in 4 days —————————————————— *B. Daye, RMA*

Note: The medical assistant may sign his or her name in the patient record using only the "CMA" credential if the office has a signature log denoting the entire credential as "CMA(AAMA)."

PSY PROCEDURE 13-5: **Instruct a Patient in Various Crutch Gaits**

Purpose: Properly instruct a patient in various gaits using axillary crutches
Equipment: Axillary crutches measured appropriately for a patient

Steps	Purpose
1. Wash your hands.	Handwashing aids infection control.
2. Have the patient stand up from a chair, holding both crutches on the affected side, then sliding to the edge of the chair. The patient pushes down on the chair arm on the unaffected side, then pushes to stand. With one crutch in each hand, he or she rests on the crutches until balance is restored.	Encourage the patient to use the large leg and arm muscles to stand instead of back muscles to avoid straining the back.
3. **AFF** Explain how to respond to a patient who is visually impaired.	Observe patients carefully to prevent injury. Face the patient when speaking and always let him or her know what you are going to do before touching him or her.
4. Assist the patient to the tripod position.	To ensure safety and proper balance, crutches should be in this position before proceeding with any gait.
5. Depending on the patient's weight-bearing ability, coordination, and general state of health, instruct the patient in one or more of the following gaits: A. Three-point gait, most commonly used for crutch training. For use when only one leg can bear weight or only partial weight bearing is allowed on the affected leg. Used by amputees, those with injury to one leg, and leg or foot surgery patients. Requires coordination and upper body strength. (1) Move both crutches forward with the unaffected leg bearing weight. (2) Supporting weight on hand grips, bring unaffected leg past crutches. (3) Repeat. B. Two-point gait, requires partial weight bearing and good coordination. Two points are raised, and two points are always on the floor. (1) Move right crutch and left foot forward. (2) As these points rest, move right foot and left crutch forward. (3) Repeat. C. Four-point gait, slowest and safest of the gaits. At least three points are on the ground at all times. The affected leg must bear partial weight. Used by patients with degenerative diseases, spasticity, or poor coordination. (1) Move right crutch forward. (2) Move left foot just ahead of left crutch. (3) Move left crutch forward. (4) Move right foot just ahead of right crutch. (5) Repeat. D. Swing-through gait. (1) Move both crutches forward. (2) With weight on hands, swing body ahead of crutches, with both legs leaving the floor together.	Most patients will use one or two gaits and should be taught how to use those gaits safely.

PSY PROCEDURE 13-5: | **Instruct a Patient in Various Crutch Gaits** *(continued)*

Steps	Purpose

(3) Move crutches ahead.
(4) Repeat.
  E. Swing-to gait.
    (1) Move both crutches forward.
    (2) With weight on hands, swing body even with crutches, with both legs leaving the floor.
    (3) Move crutches ahead.
    (4) Repeat.

4 POINT GAIT	2 POINT GAIT	3 POINT GAIT	SWING TO	SWING THROUGH
• Partial weight bearing both feet • Maximal support provided • Requires constant shift of weight	• Partial weight bearing both feet • Provides less support than 4 point gait • Faster than a 4 point gait	• Non weight bearing • Requires good balance • Requires arm strength • Faster gait • Can use with walker	• Weight bearing both feet • Provides stability • Requires arm strength • Can use with walker	• Weight bearing • Requires arm strength • Requires coordination/balance • Most advanced gait
4. Advance right foot	4. Advance right foot and left crutch	4. Advance right foot	4. Lift both feet/swing forward/land feet next to crutches	4. Lift both feet/swing forward/land feet in front of crutches
3. Advance left crutch	3. Advance left foot and right crutch	3. Advance left foot and both crutches	3. Advance both crutches	3. Advance both crutches
2. Advance left foot	2. Advance right foot and left crutch	2. Advance right foot	2. Lift both feet/swing forward/land feet next to crutches	2. Lift both feet/swing forward/land feet in front of crutches
1. Advance right crutch	1. Advance left foot and right crutch	1. Advance left foot and both crutches	1. Advance both crutches	1. Advance both crutches
Beginning stance	Beginning stance	Beginning stance	Beginning stance	Beginning stance

Step 4: Crutch gaits.

(continued)

PSY PROCEDURE 13-5: **Instruct a Patient in Various Crutch Gaits** *(continued)*

Steps	Purpose
6. Wash your hands and record the procedure.	Procedures are considered not to have been done if they are not recorded.

Charting Example:

See Charting Example for Procedure 13-4.

- The musculoskeletal system has many functions including:
  - Providing support and protection for vital organs
  - Allowing movement and mobility
  - Providing a frame (the skeleton) on which muscles are attached and the bones are held together at the joints
  - Providing stability and flexibility of the body
- Although the orthopedic physician specializes in the diagnosis and treatment of these conditions, you should expect to see patients with disorders of the musculoskeletal system in various medical offices, including pediatrics and family practice. In this chapter, you learned:

- Common disorders of the musculoskeletal system including the upper and lower extremities.
- Diagnostic procedures including x-ray procedures that may be ordered by the physician to assist in diagnosing disorders of the musculoskeletal system.
- Various types of ambulatory assist devices that may be necessary for patients who have mobility problems related to disorders of the musculoskeletal system including canes and crutches.
- Your role in working with patients in the medical office who may have disorders of the musculoskeletal system.

Warm Ups for Critical Thinking

1. Create a patient education brochure for the use of ambulatory aids. Be sure to include a brief description of the purpose of each aid along with the procedure steps.
2. The youth baseball league playoffs are coming to your town, and you are asked to staff the first aid station. What kinds of orthopedic injuries do you expect to see, and why? Develop a list of the first aid supplies that you want to have available and explain the reasons for your selections.
3. How would you respond to a patient with impaired circulation who tells you that he often uses a heating pad to relieve the pain in his legs although the physician has warned him not to do so?

4. Your patient with plantar fasciitis asks you why the pain is worse in the morning when first getting out of bed. Describe how you could explain this condition to a patient with limited understanding of human anatomy.
5. Using a drug reference book, look up several anti-inflammatory medications (naproxen sodium, ibuprofen). What gastrointestinal disorders may result from taking these medications, and how can these side effects be avoided?

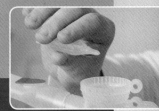

Ophthalmology and Otolaryngology

Learning Outcomes

Cognitive Domain

Note: AAMA/CAAHEP 2008 Standards are italicized.

1. Spell and define the key terms
2. List and define disorders associated with the eye and identify commonly performed diagnostic procedures
3. List and define disorders associated with the ear and identify commonly performed diagnostic procedures
4. List and define disorders associated with the nose and throat and identify commonly performed diagnostic procedures
5. Describe patient education procedures associated with the eye, ear, nose, and throat

6. *Identify common pathologies related to each body system*
7. *Describe implications for treatment related to pathology*

Psychomotor Domain

Note: AAMA/CAAHEP 2008 Standards are italicized.

1. Measure distance visual acuity with a Snellen chart (Procedure 14-1)
2. Measure color perception with an Ishihara color plate book (Procedure 14-2)
3. Instill eye medication (Procedure 14-3)
4. Irrigate the eye (Procedure 14-4)
5. Irrigate the ear (Procedure 14-5)

6. Administer an audiometric hearing test (Procedure 14-6)
7. Instill ear medication (Procedure 14-7)
8. Instill nasal medication (Procedure 14-8)
9. *Assist physician with patient care*
10. *Prepare a patient for procedures and/or treatments*
11. *Practice standard precautions*
12. *Document patient care*
13. *Perform patient screening using established protocols*
14. *Practice within standard of care for a medical assistant*

Affective Domain

Note: AAMA/CAAHEP 2008 Standards are italicized.

1. *Apply critical thinking skills in performing patient assessment and care*
2. *Use language/verbal skills that enable patients' understanding*
3. *Demonstrate empathy in communicating with patients, family, and staff*
4. *Use appropriate body language and other nonverbal skills in communicating with patients, family, and staff*
5. *Demonstrate awareness of the territorial boundaries of the person with whom you are communicating*

6. *Demonstrate sensitivity appropriate to the message being delivered*
7. *Demonstrate recognition of the patient's level of understanding in communications*
8. *Recognize and protect personal boundaries in communicating with others*
9. *Demonstrate respect for individual diversity, incorporating awareness of one's own biases in areas including gender, race, religion, age, and economic status*
10. *Apply active listening skills*
11. *Apply local, state, and federal health care legislation and regulation appropriate to the medical assisting practice setting*

ABHES Competencies

1. Assist the physician with the regimen of diagnostic and treatment modalities as they relate to each body system
2. Comply with federal, state, and local health laws and regulations
3. Communicate on the recipient's level of comprehension
4. Serve as a liaison between the physician and others
5. Show empathy and impartiality when dealing with patients
6. Document accurately

Key Terms

astigmatism	hyperopia	optician	refraction
cerumen	intraocular pressure	optometrist	retinal degeneration
decibel (db)	myopia	otolaryngologist	strabismus
fluorescein angiography	myringotomy	otoscope	tinnitus
hordeolum	ophthalmologist	presbycusis	tonometry
	ophthalmoscope	presbyopia	

Medical assistants working for **ophthalmologists**, who specialize in disorders of the eyes, or **otolaryngologists**, who specialize in disorders of the ears, nose, and throat (also known as *ENT physicians*), are expected to perform basic procedures associated with these body systems. Medical assistants working in general family practice and pediatric offices also encounter patients with eye or ear disorders and are expected to perform basic procedures associated with the eyes, ears, nose, and throat in

these settings as well. This chapter describes the various disorders, diagnostic tests, and treatment modalities that are included in the eye, ear, nose, or throat examination.

COG Common Disorders of the Eye

Light waves are reflected off of all objects and are transmitted through various structures of the eye including the cornea, lens, and retina (Fig. 14-1). These impulses

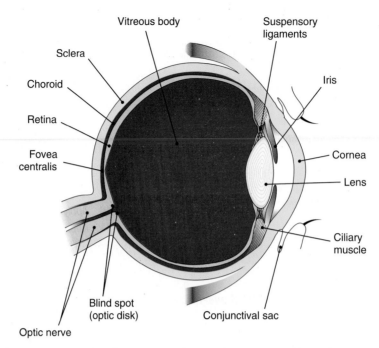

Figure 14-1 The eye. (Reprinted with permission from Cohen BJ. Memmler's The Human Body in Health and Disease, 11th ed. Philadelphia: Lippincott Williams & Wilkins, 2009.)

are transmitted via the optic nerve to the occipital lobe of the cerebral cortex in the brain. When the rays of light are bent, or refracted, by the curvature of the cornea and lens, the occiput recognizes whether the objects are in or out of focus. If the objects are out of focus to the occiput, impulses are sent to change the shape of the lens or the position of the extrinsic muscles to sharpen the image.

While the eye is a complex, highly developed organ, any of its many components may malfunction or become infected or diseased. The most common eye disorders that you may encounter in a medical office are described in the following sections. In addition, Box 14-1 describes guidelines for assisting sight-impaired patients in a medical office.

Cataract

A cataract is an opacity, or clouding, of the lens that leads to decreased visual acuity. Most commonly, cataracts are bilateral and seen in older adults. A rare condition in infancy can result from maternal exposure to the rubella virus. This condition is known as *congenital cataracts*. Occasionally, trauma to the lens or chemical toxicity causes clouding of the lens.

The symptoms include gradual blurring and loss of vision over months as the clouding of the lens slowly progresses. The observer may see a milky opacity at the pupil rather than the normal black opening (Fig. 14-2). An examination with an **ophthalmoscope** reveals the white area behind the pupil if the cataract has not advanced to the point where it can be seen unassisted.

The treatment for cataracts is surgical removal of the opaque lens. This surgery is beneficial in 95% of patients and is usually an outpatient procedure. After the cloudy lens has been removed, an intraocular lens is implanted, or the patient's vision is corrected by contact lenses or special glasses.

BOX 14-1

ASSISTING SIGHT-IMPAIRED PATIENTS

Follow these tips to assist a sight-impaired patient:

- Ask patients how you can help, and follow their requests and suggestions. Many sight-impaired patients know best what they need.
- When escorting the patient, offer your arm. Tell the patient the approximate length of the hallway and advise the patient of any turns, such as, "It should be about 20 steps and then we'll take a right." Avoid stairs if possible, but if you must assist a sight-impaired patient up or down stairs, advise the person of the number of steps. Many patients prefer to hold the railings for balance.
- If the patient has a guide dog, do not approach the dog without first speaking to the patient and receiving approval.
- If the patient needs extensive teaching on a particular subject, suggest using a tape recorder to record the instructions.

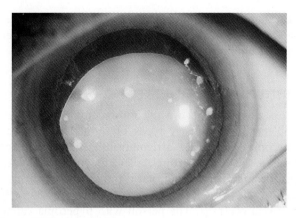

Figure 14-2 An eye with a cataract.

Sty or Hordeolum

A sty, or **hordeolum,** is an infection of any of the lacrimal glands of the eyelids, causing redness, swelling, and pain. The causative infectious organism is often *Staphylococcus aureus,* a microorganism commonly found on the skin. Warm compresses will hasten suppuration of the infection, and topical antibiotic drops or ointments attack the microorganism. You may be responsible for teaching the patient the procedure for applying warm compresses and instilling ophthalmic drops or ointment.

 CHECKPOINT QUESTION

1. What are the symptoms of a cataract?

Conjunctivitis

Conjunctivitis, an infection of the mucous membrane covering the sclera and cornea (conjunctiva) of the eye, is caused by several species of bacteria or viruses. Additional causes of conjunctivitis include allergens or irritants without an infectious process. Many pathogens cause unilateral conjunctivitis, but allergic conjunctivitis is almost always bilateral.

Signs and symptoms of conjunctivitis include tearing and occasionally exudates and pain (Fig. 14-3).

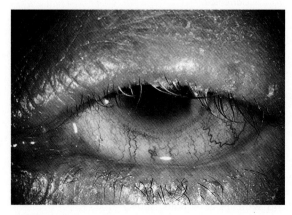

Figure 14-3 Conjunctivitis.

Bacterial and viral conjunctivitis, or pink eye, is highly contagious and can rapidly spread through schools and day care centers. It is spread by contact; for example, an infectious child rubs the eyes, handles objects such as toys or books, and spreads the infection to the next child who comes into contact with the contaminated object. The infected child should not go to school or day care until the infection is treated and has been resolved. Good hygiene, including handwashing, helps prevent the spread of infectious conjunctivitis. Antibiotic ophthalmic drops or ointment are prescribed by the physician if the cause of the conjunctivitis is bacterial. To prevent the spread of conjunctivitis, you should instruct the patient to do the following:

- Avoid rubbing the eyes to prevent spreading the infection to the other eye or to other people.
- Discard all eye makeup that may be infectious.
- Wash all towels, washcloths, and pillowcases after use.

Corneal Ulcer

A corneal ulcer is erosion of the surface of the cornea, leaving scar tissue that may lead to visual disturbances or blindness. Corneal ulcers are caused by several types of bacteria, fungi, viruses, and protozoa or by trauma, allergen, or toxin. Signs and symptoms include tearing, pain on blinking, and sensitivity to light. A visual examination with a penlight shows an irregular corneal surface. A fluorescein dye is administered by placing a strip gently in the sulcus of the eye; this stains the perimeter of the ulcer to confirm the diagnosis. Treatment includes rest and antibiotic therapy.

 CHECKPOINT QUESTION

2. Explain the difference between a sty and conjunctivitis.

Retinopathy

Retinopathy is a general term for disease or disorder affecting the retina. A decrease in the blood supply to the highly vascular retina will cause **retinal degeneration,** pathologic changes in cell structure that impair or destroy the retina's function. The causes include atherosclerosis that impedes blood flow to the retina, the microcirculatory changes associated with diabetes (diabetic retinopathy), and vascular changes resulting from long-term hypertension. Depending on the cause, the patient's loss of vision may be sudden or gradual. Loss of vision may be preceded by small intraocular hemorrhages, night blindness, or loss of the central visual field. If small vessels rupture and scar, they may pull against the retina and cause retinal detachment that results in blindness.

Diagnosis of retinopathy is made by a thorough eye examination and **fluorescein angiography**. This procedure involves injection of fluorescent dye into one of the veins of the arms and photographing the blood vessels of the eye as the dye moves through it. The treatment of retinopathy is based on treating the underlying cause. Although some forms of retinopathy respond well to treatment, others progress to full blindness.

Glaucoma

Glaucoma describes a group of disorders that result in increased **intraocular pressure**, or pressure within the eye. As aqueous humor is formed in the posterior chamber just in front of the lens, it flows through the pupil to the anterior chamber just behind the cornea. It eventually filters into the canal of Schlemm. Any pathology that impedes the outflow of aqueous humor (genetics, vasoconstriction) will increase the pressure, either very gradually or quite suddenly. The gradual form of glaucoma (open-angle glaucoma) may present with mild or no pain, visualizing halos around lights, and loss of peripheral vision. Most adult glaucoma patients have this type of glaucoma. Angle-closure glaucoma, an acute and sudden blockage, is characterized by severe eye pain, blurred vision, headache, nausea, and vomiting. Blindness may result within days of the onset of acute glaucoma unless the condition is diagnosed and treated quickly.

Treatment for chronic glaucoma includes medication, often a diuretic, to decrease intraocular pressure by slowing the formation of aqueous humor within the eyes or by improving the flow. Acute glaucoma may necessitate an iridectomy, or removal of part of the iris, to increase the outflow of the humor. Frequent eye examinations, including **tonometry**, may detect glaucoma and facilitate treatment before visual deficiencies and blindness result.

Refractive Errors

Errors of **refraction** are the most common of all eye problems. The primary types of refractive errors are **hyperopia, myopia, astigmatism,** and **presbyopia** (Fig. 14-4A,B). Hyperopia, also known as *farsightedness*, occurs in an eyeball that is too short from front to back to allow the lines of vision to reflect distinctly on the fovea centralis. The person with hyperopia cannot focus on objects near the face.

Myopia, also known as *nearsightedness*, results when the eyeball is too long. The lines of vision converge before they reach the fovea centralis and begin to diverge again at the fovea. Objects must be near the face for the image to be focused far back on the retina.

Astigmatism is unfocused refraction of light rays on the retina resulting from lens or corneal irregularities. If the cornea is not smooth, images refracted through it will not project sharply onto the retina; the effect is much like peering through wavy glass.

Presbyopia is vision change resulting from loss of lens elasticity with age. The lens normally adjusts to refract light from near or far. As a person ages, the ciliary bodies that hold and adjust the lens and the lens itself lose elasticity and no longer accommodate near vision; far vision may be unaffected. Symptoms usually begin gradually around age 40 years. Most adults are affected to some degree by age 50 years.

All refractive errors are treated with either corrective lenses or reshaping the lens with laser surgery

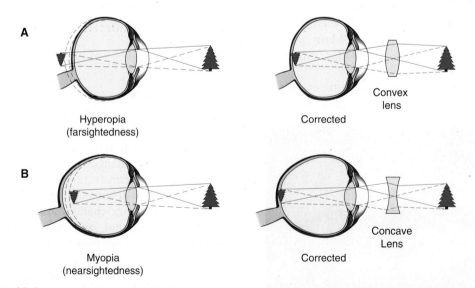

Hyperopia
(farsightedness)

Convex
lens

Corrected

Myopia
(nearsightedness)

Concave
Lens

Corrected

Figure 14-4 Errors of refraction. (**A**) The hypertrophic eye with convex corrective lens. (**B**) The myopic eye with concave corrective lens. (Reprinted with permission from Cohen BJ. Memmler's The Human Body in Health and Disease, 11th ed. Philadelphia: Lippincott Williams & Wilkins, 2009.)

LASER SURGERY TO CORRECT ERRORS OF REFRACTION

A procedure that is popular among patients to correct myopia, hyperopia, and astigmatism is a surgical procedure called *LASIK*, which stands for laser in situ keratomileusis. An ophthalmologist uses a laser to reshape the cornea, allowing the light to properly focus on the retina and correcting these errors of refraction. Advantages of this procedure include:

- It is an outpatient procedure that takes very little time to perform.
- The vision of most people is corrected within 24 hours.
- There is a quick recovery time with very little pain.
- There is no need for glasses or contacts in most patients after the procedure.

Disadvantages include:

- The procedure is expensive.
- Changes made to the cornea cannot be reversed.
- Some side effects, such as dry eyes, may be experienced by some patients.

Patients wanting to know more about this procedure should be referred to an ophthalmologist.

(Box 14-2). An **optometrist** is a trained specialist who measures errors of refraction and prescribes lenses. An **optician** is a trained specialist who grinds lenses to fulfill corrective prescriptions written by either an optometrist or an ophthalmologist, a medical doctor who treats eye disorders or performs surgical corrections.

 CHECKPOINT QUESTION

3. What are the four common refractive errors? Briefly explain each.

Strabismus

Strabismus is a misalignment of eye movements, usually caused by muscle incoordination. Although most newborns are born with some degree of strabismus, coordination improves as the infant grows and the eye muscles strengthen. However, the strabismus does not resolve in some cases and requires medical intervention. Strabismus may take any of the following forms (Fig. 14-5A–C):

- Esotropic, also known as *cross eyes* or *convergent eyes*
- Exotropic, also known as *wall eyes* or *divergent eyes*
- Hypotropic, deviation downward
- Hypertropic, deviation upward
- Concomitant, with both eyes moving together
- Nonconcomitant, with the two eyes moving independently

Treatment may require only patching, or covering, the unaffected eye to force the affected eye's muscles to strengthen. In some cases, surgery is required to correct the deviant muscle or muscles.

Color Deficit

Color deficit is an absence of or a defect in color perception. Red, green, or blue perception may be impaired or absent. The term "color deficient" or "color deficit" is commonly used rather than referring to the disorder as *color blindness*.

This disorder is usually inherited on the X chromosome and affects more men than women. Occasionally, color deficit results from damage to the cones by medications or other substances that are toxic to the color-receptive nerve cells. Color deficit has no cure or correction.

 CHECKPOINT QUESTION

4. How is strabismus corrected?

COG **Diagnostic Studies of the Eye**

In most medical offices, the basic examination equipment includes the ophthalmoscope, the lighted instrument used to examine the inner surfaces of the eye (Fig. 14-6). In many instances, visually examining the interior structures of the eyes can alert the physician to a number of vascular and hypertensive conditions because the blood vessels of the eye and the inner structures, such as the retina, are easily viewed.

Visual Acuity Testing

Visual acuity, or clearness, is commonly assessed in the medical office using the Snellen eye chart. These charts are hung 20 feet from the patient at eye level in an area with good lighting and few distractions (Procedure 14-1). Normal vision (20/20) means the patient can see at 20 feet what the normal eye sees at 20 feet. The figures on the charts—letters, numbers, a series of E's, or common symbols—become progressively smaller to test levels of perception (Fig. 14-7). For patients who cannot read

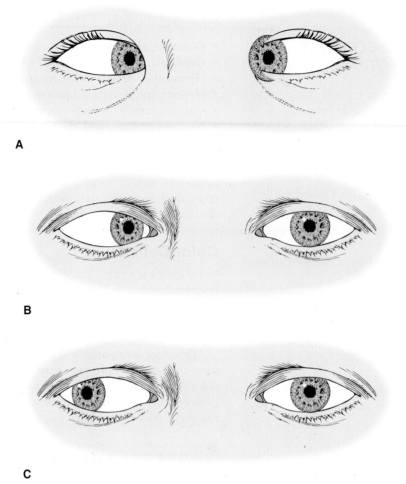

A

B

C

Figure 14-5 Forms of strabismus. (**A**) Esotropic. (**B**) Exotropic. (**C**) Hypotropic. (From Weber J, Kelley J. Health Assessment in Nursing. 2nd ed. Philadelphia: Lippincott Williams & Wilkins, 2003.)

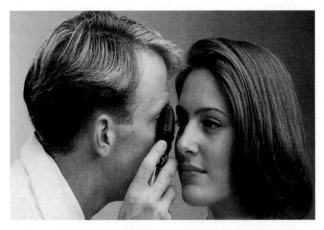

Figure 14-6 Examination of the eye with an ophthalmoscope. (Reprinted with permission from Willis MC. Medical Terminology: A Programmed Learning Approach to the Language of Health Care. Baltimore: Lippincott Williams & Wilkins, 2002.)

or who do not speak English, the E chart may be used. A patient who can see only the line (letters or E's) on the chart at the 20/40 level has visual acuity at 20 feet equivalent to what a person with normal vision can see at 40 feet. The patient should wear any corrective lenses for the test unless the physician requests that the examination be done without them. Each eye is tested separately, with the opposite eye covered but not closed.

The picture chart is used for children. If a child is to be tested, first spend a few moments familiarizing the child with the objects on the chart. For example, if the picture is of a dog and the child has never seen one, the illustration may not be recognized as a dog. If necessary, enlist a parent or coworker to help with the eye cover.

 CHECKPOINT QUESTION

5. When is the E chart used to test visual acuity?

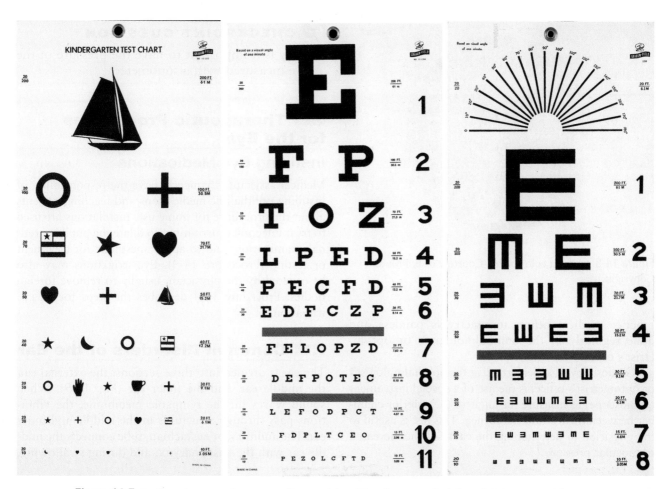

Figure 14-7 Snellen charts used to assess distant vision. The charts on the left and right are used for young children and illiterate adults.

PATIENT EDUCATION

PREVENTATIVE EYE CARE

Preventive care of the eye is a vital component of patient education. Regular eye checkups, proper care of contact lenses, control of diabetes and hypertension, annual tonometer checks for glaucoma yearly after age 40 years, and proper attention to eye injuries are important aspects of eye health maintenance.

Advise patients to wear sunglasses with ultraviolet protection during any sun exposure to avoid damage to the eyes. Children should also be fitted for sunglasses to protect their eyes against sun damage.

Advise patients not to rub their eyes. This can spread infection from person to person and can damage the cornea if a small foreign object is in the eye. Wearing goggles or safety glasses at appropriate times can prevent disease transmission and injury caused by foreign bodies.

Color Deficit Testing

The Ishihara method is used to test for color deficits (Procedure 14-2). It consists of 14 color plates with many four-colored dots forming a number, a letter, or a pattern of contrasting color in arrangement of dots (Fig. 14-8). Patients with deficient color perception are unable to see the design, numbers, or letters on plates 1 to 11, depending on the color deficiency. Although there is no cure or treatment for color deficits, knowledge of the deficit may help the patient with regard to coordinating clothing or choosing colors for decorating.

Tonometry and Gonioscopy

Using a tonometer, the physician measures the intraocular pressure or tension in the eye. The anterior eye is anesthetized with eye drops, and the instrument is moved against the cornea to measure the pressure required to produce an indentation or to flatten a small area of the cornea. This test is an important part of the eye examination to diagnose glaucoma. Although it is not routinely performed at the general

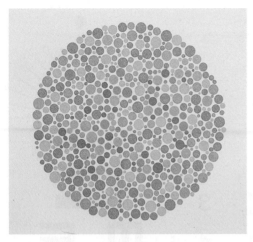

Figure 14-8 Ishihara color plate. (Courtesy of B. Proud. Copyright.)

practice medical office, tonometry is painless and done regularly at the ophthalmologist's or optometrist's office.

Gonioscopy, also performed at the ophthalmologist's or optometrist's office, is the use of a special instrument (gonioscope) to measure the angle of the anterior chamber between the iris and the cornea. This test is useful to the physician in determining the cause of the increased intraocular pressure.

 CHECKPOINT QUESTION

6. Why is it important to have the pressure of the eye measured with a tonometer?

COG **Therapeutic Procedures for the Eye**

Instilling Eye Medications

Medical assistants frequently have the responsibility of instilling ophthalmic medications and teaching patients about the procedure for home use. Instillations are used to treat infection or irritation, to dilate the pupil for retinal examination, and to apply anesthetic for treatment or testing (Procedure 14-3). Eye irrigations may also be ordered by the physician, usually to remove foreign bodies. Procedure 14-4 describes the steps for an eye irrigation.

COG **Common Disorders of the Ear**

The ear is divided into three sections: the external ear, the middle ear, and the inner ear (Fig. 14-9). When sound waves hit the tympanic membrane, the vibrations pass through structures in the middle and inner ear. The auditory, or eustachian, tube connects the middle ear with the nasopharynx, and during swallowing,

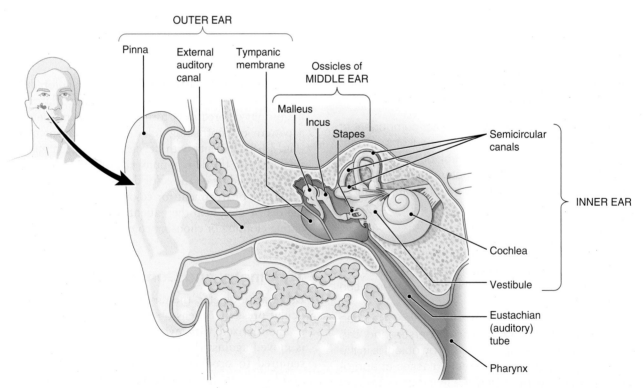

Figure 14-9 The ear, showing the outer, middle, and inner subdivisions. (Reprinted with permission from Cohen BJ. Memmler's The Human Body in Health and Disease, 11th ed. Philadelphia: Lippincott Williams & Wilkins, 2009.)

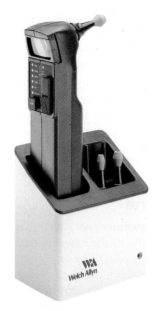

Figure 14-10 The audiometer.

pressure is equalized in the middle ear. This equalization through the eustachian tube prevents pressure from building up in the middle ear and rupturing the tympanic membrane.

Patients who have problems with the ear or hearing are often referred to an otolaryngologist. Medical assistants in general practices also encounter patients with various disorders of the ears because pain and hearing loss are a frequent outcome of certain diseases and can occur at any age. Box 14-3 describes guidelines for assisting hearing-impaired patients in a medical office.

Ceruminosis

Ceruminosis, or impacted earwax, is a frequent reason for diminished hearing. **Cerumen** is usually soft and moist and leaks out in such small amounts that it is unnoticed. Occasionally, the cerumen becomes hard and dry or excessive hair in the ear holds the wax in the ear canal, causing it to build up against the tympanic membrane.

The presenting symptoms may be a gradual hearing loss or **tinnitus,** an extraneous noise heard in one or both ears. An examination of the ear canal with an **otoscope** shows the obvious reason. The wax may be softened by warm ear drops or hydrogen peroxide and removed by an ear curet or by gently washing with an irrigating device using water at room temperature (Procedure 14-5).

Conductive and Perceptual Hearing Loss

Conductive and perceptual hearing loss are the two categories of hearing impairment. In conductive loss, sound waves are not appropriately transmitted to the level of the cochlea. In perceptual, or sensorineural, loss, transmission from the oval window to the receptors in the brain is impaired. Many patients present with both, a condition called *mixed deafness.*

Causes of hearing loss include heredity, infection, trauma, ototoxic drugs, some neurologic diseases, exposure to loud noises, and **presbycusis.** Presbycusis usually results from a hardening of the joints between the ossicles (three small bones in the middle ear), which occurs with aging.

Diagnosis of hearing loss of any type is done by testing the hearing using an audiometer (Fig. 14-10) in the medical office. Procedure 14-6 describes the steps for performing a hearing test using the audiometer. Treatment is aimed at addressing the underlying cause of the hearing loss if possible. A stapedectomy may be performed for otosclerosis, with a replacement for the impaired joint. Cochlear implants are gaining favor for those whose hearing loss is caused by impairment in the cochlear receptors. Conductive hearing loss can be treated successfully in most instances with hearing aids; perceptual loss is far more difficult to correct.

 CHECKPOINT QUESTION

7. What is the difference between conductive and perceptual hearing loss?

Ménière Disease

Ménière disease, a degenerative condition of unknown cause, affects the inner ear and upsets the body's ability to maintain equilibrium in addition to causing loss of hearing. The symptoms include vertigo, sensorineural hearing loss, and tinnitus. Severe symptoms may lead to nausea and vomiting. Periods of remission are followed by exacerbation. Although there is no cure, many of the symptoms can be treated with palliative medication. If the symptoms persist or increase and become incapacitating, it may be necessary to destroy the organs of the inner ear. The result of this drastic measure is immediate relief of symptoms, but the patient is irreversibly deaf.

Otitis Externa

Also known as *swimmer's ear*, otitis externa is an inflammation or infection of the external ear. It is common in the summer and is caused by any number of pathogens that grow in the warm, moist ear canal. The presenting symptoms include pain on movement of any adjoining structures around the ear, jaw, and auricle. Otoscopy reveals a red, swollen ear canal (Fig. 14-11). Although the physician may order that debris (pus or excessive cerumen) be gently washed from the area, otitis externa is best treated by an antibiotic, either topical (Procedure 14-7) or systemic, warm compresses, and medication to relieve pain.

Applying an alcohol solution after swimming can help prevent this problem. Encourage patients who are prone to otitis externa to wear earplugs while swimming and to avoid using objects such as swabs or hairpins to clean inside the ear canal.

Otitis Media

Otitis media, an inflammation or infection of the middle ear, is frequently caused by an upper respiratory infection. Pathogens responsible for pharyngitis, nasopharyngitis, and the common cold frequently travel through the warm, moist eustachian tube to the middle ear. As the infection increases, the mucous membranes of the eustachian tubes swell, closing off the opening to the middle ear. With no way to drain, fluid builds up as a response to the infection and causes pain and pressure on the flexible tympanic membrane. If pressure is sufficient, the membrane may tear or perforate spontaneously to relieve the pressure.

This disorder is common in infants and children because of the relatively horizontal position of the eustachian tube between the nasopharynx and middle ear. Children have very short, almost horizontal eustachian tubes, which can be problematic if microorganisms from the nasopharynx are forced into the middle ear by coughing. The problem is compounded for children who are put to bed with a bottle of milk or formula. The milk acts as a hospitable medium for bacteria.

Symptoms include severe pain, fever of varying degrees, and mild to moderate hearing loss. Infants may be fussy and tug at their ears. Any elevation in a child's temperature should be a warning to check for otitis media. Diagnosis is usually made by otoscopy, which may reveal a reddened, bulging tympanic membrane (Fig. 14-12). Bubbles can sometimes be seen behind the thin membrane. Treatment is an antibiotic for bacterial infection and an analgesic for pain relief. A decongestant may reduce some of the swelling. In severe chronic cases, a **myringotomy** (surgical incision into the tympanic membrane) may be performed to relieve pressure. Tubes may be inserted through the tympanic membrane and remain for several months to equalize the pressure if the problem persists.

 CHECKPOINT QUESTION

8. What are the symptoms of otitis media in an infant?

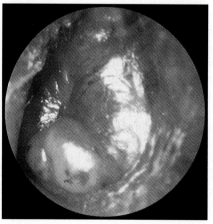

Otitis media

Figure 14-12 A bulging tympanic membrane of a patient with otitis media. (From Moore KL, Dalley AF II. Clinical Oriented Anatomy. 4th ed. Baltimore: Lippincott Williams & Wilkins, 1999.)

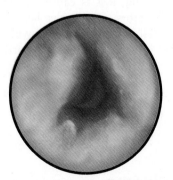

Figure 14-11 The red, swollen ear canal of a patient with otitis externa. (From Bickley LS, Szilagyi P. Bates' Guide to Physical Examination and History Taking. 8th ed. Philadelphia: Lippincott Williams & Wilkins, 2003.)

PATIENT EDUCATION

OTOLOGIC DISORDERS

Teach patients to recognize symptoms of oto-logic disorders (hearing loss, pain, drainage) and to report them promptly to the physician. Proper attention at the early stage of an infection or injury can often prevent serious or irreversible damage.

Instruct patients that it is acceptable to clean the external ear with a cotton-tipped applicator but that they should not put the applicator inside the ear canal. This drives cerumen deeper into the ear and creates more impaction than may already be present.

Tell children not to put small objects such as beans, peas, or small parts of toys in their ears because they may become lodged and removal may require surgery. Caution parents to complete all antibiotic treatment for children's ear infections even though the symptoms subside. The infection may linger after the patient is asymptomatic. Ear recheck appointments should be kept as scheduled to ensure that the child is free of infection.

Otosclerosis

Otosclerosis is a disorder of the ossicles of the middle ear, especially the stapes bone. This disorder, thought to be hereditary, results from ossification or hardening of the bones causing loss of hearing of low tones. The treatment for otosclerosis is hearing aids or microsurgical implantation of a stapedial prosthesis to replace the sclerotic joint and allow movement of the bones.

COG Diagnostic Studies of the Ear

Visual Examination

Using an otoscope, the physician can view the auditory canal and eardrum (Fig. 14-13). Disposable otoscopes are available; reusable otoscopes use disposable speculum covers that are changed between patients. Some reusable otoscopes use the same base as an ophthalmoscope.

Audiometry and Tympanometry

An audiometer can be used to detect hearing loss (Procedure 14-6). Audiometers produce pure tones of various **decibel (dB)** levels and frequencies heard through earphones or an instrument that resembles an otoscope. The decibel is a unit for measuring the intensity of sound. Speech audiometry uses voice tones rather than pure tones to assess hearing.

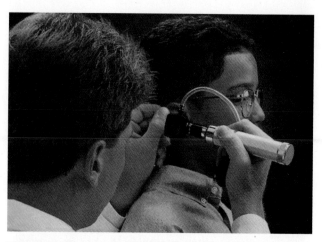

Figure 14-13 Examination of the ear with an otoscope. (Reprinted with permission from Willis MC. Medical Terminology: A Programmed Learning Approach to the Language of Health Care. Baltimore: Lippincott Williams & Wilkins, 2002.)

Impedance audiometry evaluates tympanic membrane and ossicle mobility. A probe is inserted into the auditory meatus and emits tones of various intensity levels that bounce back to the probe receiver. If the tympanic membrane and ossicles are normal, the movement is transmitted and rebound is picked up by the receiver to produce a curve on the graph. If the tympanic membrane and ossicles are less mobile than normal, much of the sound transmitted bounces back and is reflected to the instrument to produce a distinct curve on the graph. Tympanometry works like the audiometer but uses air pressure rather than tones to produce the graph.

CHECKPOINT QUESTION

9. Which of the tests described allows the physician to visualize the ear canal and tympanic membrane?

Tuning Fork Tests

Two tests that may be performed using the tuning fork are the Rinne test and the Weber test. The Rinne test entails lightly tapping the tuning fork, placing the end of it on the mastoid bone, and then moving it to the external auditory meatus to determine conductive hearing loss. In normal hearing, the sound is louder through the external auditory meatus than the bone. The Weber test entails gently tapping the tuning fork and placing it on the midline of the forehead to differentiate between conductive and sensorineural hearing loss. In conductive loss, the sound is louder in the affected ear; in sensorineural loss, the sound is louder in the unaffected ear. Although the physician most likely is the one who performs the tuning fork tests, you should ensure that the tuning fork is available and assist as needed.

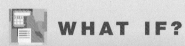

WHAT IF?

What if your patient asks you if a hearing aid could help her?

Hearing aids help many people, but they do not fully restore the ability to hear. The purpose of the aid is to amplify sound waves. Not all patients with hearing loss are good candidates for hearing aids. For example, patients who have permanent nerve damage generally do not have significant improvement with standard hearing aids.

The two basic types of aids are bone conduction receivers, which sit behind the ear and press against the skull, and air conduction receivers, which fit into the auditory canal. The size and type of hearing aid depends on the patient's specific condition and need. Binaural (both ears) aids are available and often can be fitted into eyeglasses for inconspicuous appearance.

Patients must understand that a hearing aid will improve their hearing, not correct it. Teach patients about maintenance requirements so they can keep the device in good working condition, and explain how to adjust the volume control. Have the patient speak to the physician regarding any concerns about purchasing and using a hearing aid.

COG Therapeutic Procedures for the Ear

Irrigations and Instillations

Ear irrigations are performed to relieve pain, to remove debris or foreign objects, or to apply medication solutions. Ear instillations may include a local anesthetic for the relief of pain associated with otitis externa or otitis media or a topical antibiotic for otitis externa. These medications include the words "for otic use" on the label. For medication irrigations and instillations, observe the principles of medication administration, including checking the medication label for the expiration date.

COG Common Disorders of the Nose and Throat

Allergic Rhinitis

Allergic rhinitis is inflammation of the mucous membranes of the nasal passages usually resulting from exposure to an allergen. Symptomatic treatment with antihistamine medication is usually offered to relieve the symptoms. It is also known as *hay fever* or *seasonal allergic rhinitis* when it appears in response to seasonal plant pollens. If the symptoms are present year round, it is perennial allergic rhinitis and is usually a reaction to household irritants, such as dust mites and pet dander. The signs are obvious, with paroxysmal sneezing, intense rhinorrhea (nasal drainage), congestion, and watery reddened eyes.

Diagnosis usually entails history and differential diagnosis. Mucous secretions may reveal an increase in immunoglobulin E in response to the allergens. An allergist may isolate the offending protein by skin testing. Allergy treatment entails exposure to the allergen in minute doses to desensitize the immune reaction.

Epistaxis

Commonly known as *nosebleed*, epistaxis generally occurs from trauma to the nasal membranes, but it may be secondary to another disorder, such as hypertension, malignancy, polyps, or the fragile capillaries associated with pregnancy. Diagnosis necessitates a history and inspection of the nasal mucosa with a nasal speculum (Fig. 14-14). The initial therapy for simple epistaxis is having the patient sit upright with the head slightly forward to avoid postnasal drainage that may lead to nausea. Compress the nares against the septum for 5 to 10 minutes with either ice or a cold, wet compress. Advise the patient to remain still and not to blow the nose until the physician concludes that all danger is past.

Bleeding that continues more than 10 minutes after treatment begins is considered severe. For severe epistaxis, the physician may insert nasal packing or a balloon catheter that may remain in place several hours to several days. For secondary bleeding, treatment of the underlying cause may be indicated. Cautery to an exposed blood vessel helps if that is the only cause.

CHECKPOINT QUESTION

10. What factors may contribute to epistaxis?

Nasal Polyps

Nasal polyps are small pendulous tissues that obstruct breathing. Polyps usually occur in the mucous membranes

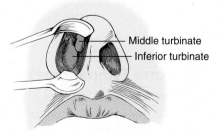

Middle turbinate
Inferior turbinate

Figure 14-14 Physical examination of the nose with a nasal speculum. (Reprinted with permission from Nettina SM. The Lippincott Manual of Nursing Practice. Philadelphia: Lippincott Williams & Wilkins, 2001.)

of the nasal passages as a response to long-term allergies. Symptoms include a feeling of fullness or congestion and occasionally a nasal discharge. Diagnosis requires direct examination with a nasal speculum or radiography of the nasal structures. Treatment may be corticosteroids applied either topically or by injection directly into the polyps. The underlying allergy must be treated to prevent recurrence of polyps. If conservative treatment is not effective, conventional or laser surgery is required.

Sinusitis

Sinusitis, or inflammation of one or more of the sinus cavities, can be either acute or chronic. Acute sinusitis is usually the result of an upper respiratory infection and is fairly easily resolved. Chronic sinusitis is more persistent and more difficult to control. Either form is particularly common when microorganisms are forced into the moist sinus cavities during hard nose blowing.

Symptoms of sinusitis include the obvious signs of an upper respiratory infection, with the addition of a purulent nasal discharge and facial pain over the sinus areas. Diagnosis requires direct visualization using a nasal speculum, radiography of the sinuses, needle puncture of the sinuses to withdraw a specimen for culture, and ultrasound.

Serious complications in the brain and middle ear may occur if sinusitis is not treated promptly with antihistamines or ephedrine nose drops to shrink mucosal tissue and relieve pressure. Steroidal nasal sprays may also be prescribed. Procedure 14-8 describes the steps for instilling nasal medication. If the cause of the sinusitis is a bacterial infection, antibiotics are prescribed by the physician and effectively relieve symptoms within 7 to 10 days. Chronic sinusitis may require treatment for 4 to 6 weeks. Total blockage of the sinus cavity may result if the disorder is not treated; this may require surgery to puncture the wall between the nose and the involved sinus cavity to allow drainage.

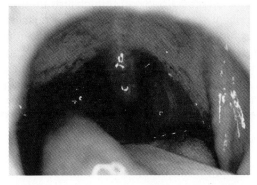

Figure 14-15 Pharyngitis with swollen tonsils. (From The Wellcome Trust, National Medical Slide Bank, London, United Kingdom.)

CHECKPOINT QUESTION

11. What is the usual cause of a sinus infection?

PATIENT EDUCATION
NASAL DISORDERS

Patients need to be alert for any changes in their breathing pattern. The early symptoms of any nasal disorder must be treated as soon as possible to prevent complications. Instruct children not to put small pieces of food or toys in the nose.

Instruct patients about the rebound phenomena of nasal sprays and drops. If used without the advice of a physician, these medications may become addictive. After frequent use, the nasal mucosa responds to withdrawal of the medication with congestion. Nasal preparations should never be used more than four times a day for 3 days unless specified by the physician.

Pharyngitis and Tonsillitis

Inflammation of the epithelial tissues of the throat and of the tonsils produces similar symptoms of sore throat and difficulty swallowing. Examination of the throat reveals red, swollen tissues and possibly pustules on the tonsils or in the throat (Fig. 14-15). You may be asked to obtain a throat specimen from these patients for transportation to an outside laboratory for a culture, or you may be required to perform a rapid strep test on the specimen in the office. (Chapter 29 describes the steps for collecting throat specimens.) Treatment of a sore throat may include gargles, an analgesic, and an antibiotic, especially if the throat culture reveals a bacterial infection. Tonsillitis may be treated with an antibiotic, or if the problem is chronic, the tonsils may be surgically removed—a tonsillectomy. This procedure usually includes removal of both pharyngeal tonsils (adenoids) and palatine tonsils.

LEGAL TIP

A patient calls the office at 4:45 p.m. complaining of a sore throat. Scheduled appointments are running 1 to 2 hours behind. Because it is the middle of flu season, you think it is safe to tell the patient that he has a virus and can be seen in the morning. During the night, the patient's throat closes because of the infection and obstructs his airway. The patient dies, and the autopsy report shows a tonsillar abscess. Could the patient's family sue

(continued)

you? Yes! As a medical assistant, you cannot presume to diagnose medical conditions. You made a medical decision and diagnosed the patient when you decided that the symptoms indicated a virus. Only the physician can make a diagnosis. Always follow office policy regarding telephone advice, and document all phone conversations after bringing them to the physician's attention.

Laryngitis

Inflammation of the larynx can result from an infection, irritation, or overuse of the voice. The result is hoarseness, cough, and difficulty speaking. Diagnosis is made after a thorough history and visual inspection of the pharynx for redness and signs of infection. Laryngitis may be treated with an antibiotic if it is thought to be caused by a bacterial infection, but more often, it is left to resolve on its own. The patient is told to rest the voice and speak as little as possible. A cool-mist humidifier may be helpful in soothing the throat.

 CHECKPOINT QUESTION

12. Describe the symptoms of a patient with laryngitis.

COG Diagnostic Studies of the Nose and Throat

Visual Inspection

Examination of the nose and throat entails visually inspecting the nose using a nasal speculum or viewing the throat using a penlight and tongue depressor. The physician may order radiography and culture to identify infectious microorganisms. The physician may also palpate the lymph nodes in the neck and other neck structures related to the upper airway. You may be responsible for preparing the patient and assisting during the examination.

COG Therapeutic Procedures for the Nose and Throat

Throat Culture

A throat culture in cases of suspected pharyngitis or tonsillitis can help determine what microorganism is causing the problem. The patient's throat is gently swabbed with a sterile culture swab to obtain the specimen. A sterile swab is necessary to avoid culturing microorganisms not in the throat. After the specimen is obtained, it is either processed in the office with a commercially prepared test kit such as those that check for streptococcal bacteria or sent to a laboratory for analysis. If the specimen is sent to the laboratory, it must be placed in a culture medium, labeled, and sent in a biohazard bag with the appropriate laboratory request. (Chapter 29 describes the steps for collecting throat specimens.)

 CHECKPOINT QUESTION

13. Why is it necessary to use a sterile swab to obtain the throat culture specimen?

 AFF **TRIAGE**

You have the following three tasks:

A. Patient A is on the phone asking for advice on pain and blurred vision in his left eye after wearing his contact lens through the night.

B. Patient B is waiting in an examination room for you to complete a visual acuity and Ishihara test required for a pre-employment physical exam.

C. A pharmacist telephones with a question about a patient's prescription for glaucoma medication.

How do you sort these tasks? What do you do first? Second? Third?

After asking the receptionist to take a message from the pharmacist calling regarding patient C, address patient A since he will need an appointment to be seen right away. Wearing contact lenses longer than prescribed can scratch the cornea, and the patient should be seen as soon as possible to avoid further damage. Next, complete and record the eye examinations for patient B's physical examination. Once these situations are resolved, call the pharmacist and answer any questions, clarify concerns, or refer the matter to the physician.

Medication Box

Commonly Prescribed Otic and Ophthalmic Medications

Note: The generic name of the drug is listed first and is written in all lower case letters. Brand names are in parentheses and the first letter is capitalized.

amoxicillin and clavulanate (Augmentin)	Tablets: 250 mg, 500 mg Oral Suspension: 125 mg/5 mL	Antibiotic
amoxicillin trihydrate (Amoxil)	Capsules: 250 mg, 500 mg Tablets: 500 mg, 875 mg Oral suspension: 50 mg/mL	Antibiotic
atropine sulfate (Isopto Atropine)	Ophthalmic solution: 0.5%, 1%, 2%	Antimuscarinic
azithromycin (Zithromax)	Tablets: 250 mg, 500 mg, 600 mg	Antibiotic
betaxolol hydrochloride (Betoptic)	Ophthalmic solution: 0.5% Ophthalmic suspension: 0.25%	Antiglaucoma
bimatoprost (Latisse)	Ophthalmic solution: 0.03%	Antiglaucoma
brimonidine tartrate (Alphagan P)	Ophthalmic solution: 0.1%, 0.15%, 0.2%	Antiglaucoma
ceftriaxone sodium (Rocephin)	Injection (IM): 250 mg, 500 mg, 1 g, 2 g	Antibiotic
dexamethasone (Maxidex)	Ophthalmic solution: 0.1% Ophthalmic suspension: 0.1%	Corticosteroid
gentamicin sulfate (Genoptic)	Ophthalmic ointment: 0.3% Ophthalmic solution: 0.3%	Anti-infective
latanoprost (Xalatan)	Ophthalmic solution: 0.005%	Antiglaucoma
loratadine (Claritin, Alavert)	Capsules: 10 mg Syrup: 1 mg/mL Tablets: 10 mg	Antihistamine
tobramycin (Tobrex)	Ophthalmic ointment: 0.3% Ophthalmic solution: 0.3%	Anti-infective

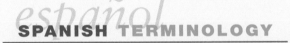

español SPANISH TERMINOLOGY

El ojo
The eye

Los oídos
(inner) ears

Las orejas
(outer) ears

La nariz
The nose

La garganta
The throat

¿Cuándo fue la ultima vez que se hizo un examen de la vista?
When was the last time you had a vision test?

¿Padece de dolor de oído?
Do you have earaches?

MEDIA MENU

- **Student Resources on thePoint**
  - **CMA/RMA Certification Exam Review**
- **Internet Resources**

  American Academy of Otolaryngology, Head and Neck Surgery
  http://www.entnet.org

  Journal of Pediatric Ophthalmology and Strabismus
  http://www.slackjournals.com/jpos

  American Foundation for the Blind
  http://www.afb.org

  Foundation Fighting Blindness
  http://www.blindness.org

  Prevent Blindness America
  http://www.preventblindness.org

  American Optometric Association
  http://www.aoa.org

  Hearing Loss Association of America
  http://www.shhh.org

PSY PROCEDURE 14-1:   Measuring Distance Visual Acuity

Purpose: To assess and document the distance visual acuity of a patient in both eyes, with or without corrective lenses
Equipment: Snellen eye chart, paper cup or eye paddle

Steps	Purpose
1. Wash your hands.	Handwashing aids infection control.
2. Prepare the examination area. Make sure the area is well lighted, a distance marker is placed exactly 20 feet from the chart, and the chart is at eye level.	All distance visual acuity testing is done at 20 feet for consistency of results.
3. Greet and identify the patient. Explain the procedure.	Patients who understand the procedure are likely to be compliant and produce an accurate test result.
4. **AFF** Explain how to respond to a patient who is hearing impaired.	Speak clearly, not loudly, and face the patient.
5. Position the patient at the 20-foot marker.	The patient may stand or sit as long as the chart is at eye level and the patient is 20 feet from it.
6. Observe whether the patient is wearing glasses. If not, ask the patient about contact lenses and mark the results of the test accordingly.	The visual acuity examination is usually performed with patients wearing their corrective lenses, if they have them. If the patient wears his or her corrective lenses, then the record must indicate that the lenses were worn for the test.
7. Have the patient cover the right eye with the cup or the eye paddle. Instruct the patient to keep both eyes open. Also tell him or her to not lean forward and to avoid squinting during the test.	The test starts with the right eye covered for paper consistency. The hand should not be used to cover the eye, since pressure against the eye or peeking through the fingers affects the results. Closing one eye will cause squinting of the other, which changes the vision and skews the findings.

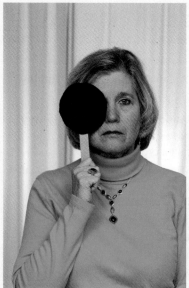

Step 7. Have the patient cover the right eye.

8. Stand beside the chart and point to each row as the patient reads aloud the indicated lines, starting with the 20/200 line. This number is on the right side of the chart next to each line.	It is generally best to start at about the second or third row to judge the patient's response. If these lines are read easily, move down to smaller figures. If the patient has difficulty reading the larger lines, notify the physician.

PSY PROCEDURE 14-1: **Measuring Distance Visual Acuity** *(continued)*

Steps	Purpose
9. Record the smallest line that the patient can read with two errors or less according to office policy. If the patient reads line 5 with one error with the left eye, it will be recorded as OS (ocularis sinistra) 20/40–1. If that same line is read with two mistakes, it is recorded as OS 20/40–2. If no errors are read at the 20/40 line, it is recorded as OS 20/40. Your physician may prefer that only lines read without any error be counted as correct.	Many offices will consider up to two mistakes acceptable when recording visual acuity.
10. Repeat the procedure with the left eye covered and record as in Step 9, using OD (ocularis dexter).	
11. Wash your hands and document the procedure.	Procedures are considered not to have been done if they are not recorded.

Charting Example:

01/16/2013 4:30 PM Visual acuity OD 20/40–1 OS 20/20 with correction. Dr. Smart aware. ————— C. Mayers, CMA

PSY PROCEDURE 14-2: **Measuring Color Perception**

Purpose: To assess and document color perception
Equipment: Ishihara color plates, gloves

Steps	Purpose
1. Wash your hands, put on gloves, and get the Ishihara color plate book.	Handwashing aids infection control. Gloves in this case are to protect the plates, not the patient or health care worker. Oils from the hands can alter the colors and interfere with the test results.
2. Greet and identify the patient and explain the procedure.	Greeting the patient establishes rapport and identifying the patient ensures you have the correct patient.
3. Ensure that the patient is seated comfortably in a quiet, well-lighted room. Indirect sunlight is best. (Sunlight should not shine directly on the plates; the colors fade with exposure to bright lights.) Patients who wear glasses or contact lenses should keep them on.	The Ishihara tests color perception, not visual acuity. Corrective lenses do not interfere with accurate test results.
4. **AFF** Explain how to respond to a patient who is developmentally challenged.	Depending on the level of impairment, speak to the patient accordingly. Explain the procedure using words the patient can understand. Solicit assistance from the caregiver who may be with the patient.

(continued)

PSY PROCEDURE 14-2: Measuring Color Perception *(continued)*

Steps	Purpose
5. After opening the book, hold the first plate in the book about 30 inches from the patient and ask if he or she can see the number in the dots on the plate. 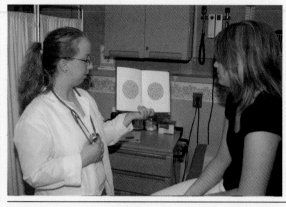	The first plate should be obvious to all patients and serves as an example.
	Step 5. Hold the first plate about 30 inches from the patient.
6. Record the results of the test by noting the number or figure the patient reports on each plate, using the plate number followed by the response. If the patient cannot distinguish the pattern, record as the plate number followed by the letter X. The patient should not take more than 3 seconds to read the plates and should not squint or guess. These indicate that the patient was unsure and are recorded as X.	Procedures not recorded in the medical record are considered not to have been done.
7. Record the results for plates 1 to 10. Plate 11 requires the patient to trace the winding bluish-green line between the two x's. Patients with a color deficit will not be able to trace the line.	If 10 or more of the first 11 plates are read correctly without difficulty, the patient does not have a color deficit. Plates 12, 13, and 14 are usually used to detect the degree of deficiency in patients with red–green color deficiencies. Procedures are considered not to have been done if they are not recorded.
8. Store the book in a closed, protected area away from light.	Storing the book in a dark cabinet will safeguard the integrity of the colors.
9. Remove your gloves and wash your hands.	Wash your hands after any patient contact.

Charting Example:

12/22/2013 10:30 AM Ishihara color deficit testing performed:

Plate 1	*12*	*Plate 7*	*X (normal 45)*
Plate 2	*8*	*Plate 8*	*X (normal 2)*
Plate 3	*5 (normal 2)*	*Plate 9*	*2 (normal X)*
Plate 4	*X*	*Plate 10*	*X (normal 16)*
Plate 5	*21 (normal 74)*	*Plate 11*	*X (traceable)*
Plate 6	*X (normal 7)*		

—*B. Cotton, CMA*

PSY PROCEDURE 14-3: Instilling Eye Medications

Purpose: Instill and document ophthalmic medications as ordered by the physician
Equipment: Physician's order and patient record, ophthalmic medication, sterile gauze, tissues, gloves

Steps	Purpose
1. Wash your hands.	Handwashing aids infection control.
2. Obtain the patient's medical record, including the physician's order, correct medication, sterile gauze, and tissues.	The medication must specify ophthalmic use. Check the label three times before administering the ophthalmic solution or ointment. Medications formulated for other uses may be harmful if used in the eyes.
3. Greet and identify the patient. Explain the procedure. Ask the patient about any allergies not recorded in the chart.	Identifying the patient prevents errors in treatment.
4. **AFF** Explain how to respond to a patient who does not speak English or who speaks English as a second language (ESL).	Solicit assistance from anyone who may be with the patient or a staff member who speaks the patient's native language to interpret if available. If no interpreter is available, use hand gestures or pictures to explain the procedure to the patient.
5. Position the patient comfortably.	The patient may lie or sit with the head tilted slightly back and the affected eye slightly lower to avoid the medication running into the unaffected eye.
6. Put on gloves and pull down the lower eyelid with sterile gauze while asking the patient to look up.	Since there is potential for contact with secretions from the eye, you must wear gloves. Pulling down the lower lid exposes the conjunctival sac to receive the medication. If the patient is looking up and away from the medication, the blink reflex may not be triggered.

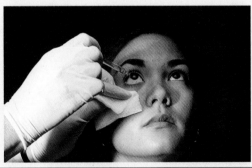

Step 6. Pull the lower eyelid down and ask the patient to look up.

Steps	Purpose
7. Instill the medication: A. Ointment: Discard the first bead of ointment from the container onto a tissue without touching the end of the medication tube to the tissue. Place a thin line of ointment across the inside of the lower eyelid, moving from the inner canthus outward. Release the ointment by twisting the tube slightly. Do not touch the tube to the eye. B. Drops: Hold the dropper close to the conjunctival sac (about half an inch away) but do not touch the patient. Release the proper number of drops into the sac. Discard any medication left in the dropper.	The first bead of ointment is considered contaminated. Placing the ointment in the sac avoids touching the eye with the tip of the ointment tube. Twisting the tube releases the ointment. Discarding the remaining medication prevents contaminating the remainder of a multiple dose container.
8. Release the lower lid and have the patient gently close the eye and roll it to disperse the medication.	Closing the eye will prevent the medication from leaking out. Rolling the eye around will distribute the medication.

(continued)

PSY PROCEDURE 14-3: **Instilling Eye Medications (continued)**

Steps	Purpose
9. Wipe off any excess medication with the tissue. Instruct the patient to apply light pressure to the puncta lacrimalis for several minutes.	Pressing the puncta prevents the medication from running into the nasolacrimal sac and duct.
10. Properly care for or dispose of equipment and supplies. Clean the work area and wash your hands.	Always clean up after procedures as soon as possible. Wash your hands after any patient contact.
11. Record the procedure.	Procedures are considered not to have been done if they are not recorded.

Charting Example:

10/14/2013 8:45 AM Garamycin ophthalmologic ointment applied to OS ———————————— B. Marker, CMA

PSY PROCEDURE 14-4: **Irrigating the Eye**

Purpose: Irrigate the eye as ordered by the physician and document the procedure
Equipment: Physician's order and patient record, small sterile basin if sterile solution is used, irrigating solution (water) and medication (if ordered), protective barrier or towels, emesis basin, sterile bulb syringe, tissues, gloves

Steps	Purpose
1. Wash your hands and put on gloves.	Handwashing aids infection control. You must wear gloves when you may be exposed to body fluids
2. Assemble the equipment, supplies, and medication if ordered. Check the label three times as recommended for medication administration, and make sure the label indicates ophthalmic use. Note: If both eyes are to be treated, use separate equipment (solution and bulb syringe) to avoid cross-contamination.	Unless water is ordered for the eye irrigation, solutions for the eye must be sterile and must be formulated for ophthalmic use.
3. Greet and identify the patient. Explain the procedure.	Identifying the patient prevents errors in treatment. Patients who understand the procedure are generally cooperative and compliant.
4. **AFF** Explain how to respond to a patient who is hard of hearing.	Make sure the patient can see your face as you speak. Speak clearly, not loudly.
5. Position the patient comfortably, either with the head tilted and the affected eye lower or lying with the affected eye down.	With the affected eye down, there is little chance of contamination running into the unaffected eye.
6. Drape the patient with the protective barrier or towel.	A protective barrier will prevent wetting the patient's clothing.
7. Place the emesis basin against the upper cheek near the eye with the towel under the basin. With clean gauze, wipe the eye from the inner canthus outward to remove debris from the lashes.	Debris from the lashes may be washed into the eye.

PSY PROCEDURE 14-4: **Irrigating the Eye** *(continued)*

Steps	Purpose
8. Separate the lids with the thumb and forefinger of your nondominant hand. To steady your hand, you may lightly support your dominant hand, holding the syringe with solution on the bridge of the patient's nose parallel to the eye.	Because of the natural reflex to close the eye, you must use your nondominant hand to physically separate the eyelids.

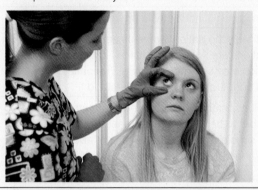

Step 8. Separate the eyelids with the thumb and forefinger.

Steps	Purpose
9. Gently irrigate from the inner to the outer canthus, holding the syringe 1 inch above the eye. Use gentle pressure and do not touch the eye. The physician will order the time or amount of solution to be used. Debris from the lashes may be washed into the eye.	The solution must flow from the inner to the outer canthus to avoid washing pathogens into the punctum. With the syringe 1 inch above the eye, there is little chance of touching the eye and causing discomfort

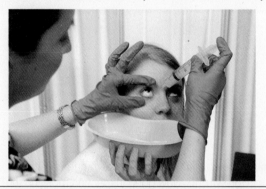

Step 9. Hold the syringe 1 inch above the eye.

Steps	Purpose
10. Use tissues to wipe any excess solution from the patient's face.	This prevents the spread of microorganisms.
11. Properly dispose of equipment or sanitize as recommended and remove your gloves. Wash your hands.	Always clean up as soon as possible after completing procedures. Hands should be washed after patient contact to prevent the spread of disease.
12. Record the procedure in the patient's record, including the amount, type, and strength of the solution; which eye was irrigated; and any observations.	Procedures are considered not to have been done if they are not recorded.

Charting Example:

04/16/2013 11:30 AM OD irrigated with 500 mL sterile NS, return clear ———————————— J. Penta, CMA

PSY PROCEDURE 14-5:   Irrigating the Ear

Purpose: Irrigate the ear as ordered and document the procedure
Equipment: Physician's order and patient's record, emesis or ear basin, waterproof barrier or towels, otoscope, irrigating solution (water), bowl for solution, gauze

Steps	Purpose
1. Wash your hands.	Handwashing aids infection control.
2. Assemble the equipment and supplies.	Ear irrigation is not a sterile procedure.
3. Greet and identify the patient. Explain the procedure.	Identifying the patient prevents errors in treatment. Ear irrigations are not usually painful, but the flow of the solution may be uncomfortable. The patient may be more cooperative if this is understood.
4. **AFF** Explain how to respond to a patient who has dementia.	Solicit assistance from a caregiver or other staff member to help during the procedure as needed. Give simple directions to the patient about what he or she should do. Speak clearly, not loudly.
5. Position the patient comfortably erect.	The patient who is comfortably seated may be more cooperative during the procedure.
6. View the affected ear with an otoscope to locate the foreign matter or cerumen.	The area of treatment must be visualized before irrigation begins. If debris from the external auricle is not removed, it may be washed into the canal.

A. Adults: Gently pull ear up and back to straighten the auditory canal.
B. Children: Gently pull ear slightly down and back to straighten the auditory canal.

Step 6. The shape of the ear canal changes with growth. To allow good inspection, position the ear as illustrated.

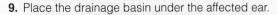

7. Drape the patient with a waterproof barrier or towel.	Wet clothing would be uncomfortable for the patient.
8. Tilt the patient's head toward the affected side.	Tilting the head will facilitate the flow of solution.
9. Place the drainage basin under the affected ear.	

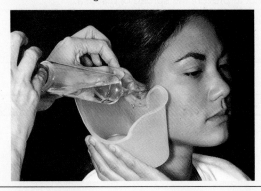

Step 9. Place the basin under the ear.

PSY PROCEDURE 14-5:   Irrigating the Ear *(continued)*

Steps	Purpose
10. Fill the irrigating syringe or turn on the irrigating device.	Some offices have special systems for irrigating ears, whereas others may have you use a 20 cc or bulb syringe.
11. Gently position the auricle as described, using your nondominant hand.	The canal must be straight for visualization and treatment.
12. With your dominant hand, place the tip of the syringe in the auditory meatus and direct the flow of the solution gently up toward the roof of the canal.	Directing the flow against the upper surface prevents pressure against the tympanic membrane and facilitates the outflow of solution.
13. Continue irrigating for the prescribed period or until the desired result (cerumen removal) is obtained.	If the patient complains of pain or discomfort, stop the irrigation and notify the physician.
14. Dry the patient's external ear with gauze. Have the patient sit for awhile with the affected ear down to drain the solution.	Solution left in the ear is uncomfortable.
15. Inspect the ear with the otoscope to determine the results.	It may be necessary to repeat the procedure, and it is always necessary to inspect the area to record the results.
16. Properly care for or dispose of equipment and supplies. Clean the work area. Wash your hands.	This prevents the spread of microorganisms.
17. Record the procedure in the patient's chart.	Procedures are considered not to have been done if they are not recorded.

Note: If the tympanic membrane appears to be perforated, do not irrigate without checking with the physician; solution may be forced into the middle ear through the perforation. Remove any obvious debris at the entrance of the canal before beginning the irrigation.

Charting Example:

03/17/2013 3:30 PM AD irrigated with 500 mL sterile water; return clear with 2 large pieces of yellow-brown
cerumen noted ———————————————————————————————— S. Stark, CMA

PSY PROCEDURE 14-6:   Perform Audiometric Hearing Test

Purpose: To accurately assess and document a hearing test using audiometry
Equipment: Audiometer, otoscope

Steps	Purpose
1. Wash your hands.	Handwashing aids infection control.
2. Greet and identify the patient. Explain the procedure. Take the patient to a quiet area or room for testing.	Patients who understand the procedure are likely to be compliant, producing accurate results. A quiet room allows for accurate results without distraction. Determine the signal (raising the hand, saying yes) to indicate that the tones are heard.
3. **AFF** Explain how to respond to a patient who is visually impaired.	Face the patient when speaking and always let him or her know what you are going to do before touching him or her.

(continued)

PSY PROCEDURE 14-6:   Perform Audiometric Hearing Test (continued)

Steps	Purpose
4. Using an otoscope or audioscope with a light source, visually inspect the ear canal and tympanic membrane before the examination.	Looking into the ear canal verifies that there are no obstructions, such as cerumen, to interfere with the test. If you see an obstruction, notify the physician.
5. Choose the correct size tip for the end of the audiometer. Attach a speculum to fit the patient's external auditory meatus, making sure the ear canal is occluded with the speculum in place.	The design of the tip or speculum obviates bulky ear phones. The tip should block any environmental noise during the test.
6. With the speculum in the ear canal, retract the pinna: up and back for adults; down and back for children.	Pulling the pinna up and back for adults and down and back for children straightens the ear canal.

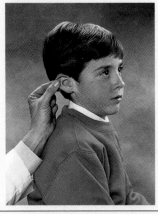

Step 6. Pull the pinna down and back for children. (Courtesy of Welch-Allyn.)

Steps	Purpose
7. Turn the instrument on and select the screening level. There is a pretest tone for practice if necessary. Press the start button and observe the tone indicators and the patient's responses.	The signal (raising the hand, saying yes) was determined before you began the test. The audiometer will proceed down each tone with a light indicator.

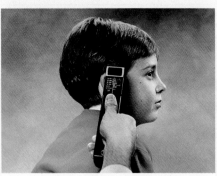

A

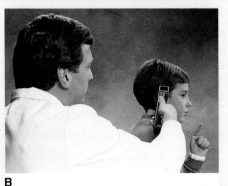

B

Step 7. **(A)** Place the audiometer tip in the patient's ear. **(B)** The patient should give a signal when each tone is heard. (Courtesy of Welch-Allyn.)

PSY PROCEDURE 14-6: **Perform Audiometric Hearing Test (continued)**

Steps	Purpose
8. Screen the other ear.	Each ear is screened separately.
9. If the patient fails to respond at any frequency, rescreening is required.	If the patient does not hear a specific tone, a second opportunity should be given.
10. If the patient fails rescreening, notify the physician.	A patient who fails to hear one or more tones may be referred to an audiologist.
11. Record the results in the medical record.	Procedures are considered not to have been done if they are not recorded.

Charting Example:

02/14/2013 9:00 AM Audiometry testing performed AU, results in chart _____ *S. Smythe, RMA*

PSY PROCEDURE 14-7: **Instilling Ear Medication**

Purpose: Instill otic medication as ordered and document the instillation
Equipment: Physician's order and patient's record, otic medication with dropper, cotton balls
Standard: This procedure should take 5 minutes.

Steps	Purpose
1. Wash your hands.	Handwashing aids infection control.
2. Check the medication label three times as specified for medication administration. The label should specify otic preparation.	Medication for otic instillation is formulated for that purpose.
3. Greet and identify the patient. Explain the procedure.	Identifying the patient prevents errors in treatment. Patients who understand the procedure are generally compliant.
4. Ask the patient about any allergies not documented in the medical record.	The patient may have developed allergies since the medical record was last updated.
5. **AFF** Explain how to respond to a patient who does not speak English or who speaks English as a second language (ESL).	Solicit assistance from anyone who may be with the patient or a staff member who speaks the patient's native language to interpret if available. If no interpreter is available, use hand gestures or pictures to explain the procedure.
6. Have the patient seated with the affected ear tilted upward.	The medication must be allowed to flow through the canal to the tympanic membrane.
7. Draw up the ordered amount of medication.	Only administer the amount prescribed.
8. Straighten the canal. A. Adults: Pull the auricle slightly up and back. B. Children: Pull the auricle slightly down and back.	Straightening the ear canal will prevent the medication from pooling in the ear canal.

(continued)

PSY PROCEDURE 14-7: Instilling Ear Medication (continued)

Steps	Purpose
9. Insert the tip of the dropper without touching the patient's skin and let the medication flow along the side of the canal.	Touching the patient will contaminate the dropper. The medication should flow gently to avoid discomfort.

Step 9. Insert the tip of the dropper without touching the ear.

Steps	Purpose
10. Have the patient sit or lie with the affected ear up for about 5 minutes after the instillation.	The medication should rest against the tympanic membrane for as long as possible.
11. If the medication is to be retained in the ear canal, insert a moist cotton ball into the external auditory meatus without force.	A slightly moist cotton ball will keep the medication in the canal and not wick it out. Forcing the cotton ball into the ear canal could be painful to the patient.
12. Properly care for or dispose of equipment and supplies. Clean the work area. Wash your hands.	This prevents the spread of microorganisms.
13. Record the procedure in the patient record.	Procedures are considered not to have been done if they are not recorded.

Charting Example:

06/15/2013 12:30 PM Neosporin otic solution, 2 gtt instilled into AS as ordered —————————— D. Barth, CMA

PSY PROCEDURE 14-8: Instilling Nasal Medication

Purpose: Instill nasal medication as ordered and document the instillation
Equipment: Physician's order and patient's record, nasal medication, drops or spray, tissues, gloves

Steps	Purpose
1. Wash your hands.	Handwashing aids infection control.
2. Assemble the equipment and supplies. Check the medication label three times.	Medications for use in the nasal passages must be formulated for these surfaces.
3. Greet and identify the patient. Explain the procedure and ask the patient about any allergies not documented.	Identifying the patient prevents errors in treatment. Nasal instillations are uncomfortable but should not be painful; patients will be more cooperative if they understand the procedure.
4. **AFF** Explain how to respond to a patient who has dementia.	Solicit assistance from the caregiver or another staff member to help during the procedure. Give simple directions to the patient about what he or she should do. Speak clearly, not loudly.

PSY PROCEDURE 14-8:   Instilling Nasal Medication (continued)

Steps	Purpose
5. Position the patient comfortably recumbent. Extend the patient's head beyond the edge of the examination table or place a pillow under the shoulders. Support the patient's neck to avoid strain as the head tilts back.	The patient must be properly positioned if the medication is to reach the upper nasal passages.

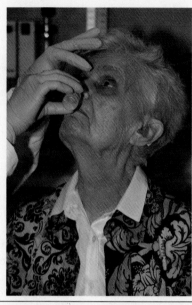

Step 5. Tilt the patient's head back.

Steps	Purpose
6. Administer the medication. A. Hold the dropper upright just above each nostril and dispense one drop at a time without touching the nares. Keep the patient recumbent for 5 minutes. B. Place the tip of the bottle at the naris opening without touching the patient's skin or nasal tissues and spray as the patient takes a deep breath.	Touching the dropper to the nostril would contaminate the dropper. For effective treatment, the patient must allow the medication to reach the upper nasal passages. The medication must reach the upper passages; if the patient breathes out while the medication is being sprayed, the medication is exhaled and does not reach the nasal passages.
7. Wipe any excess medication from the patient's skin with tissues.	Excess medication around the nares is uncomfortable.
8. Properly care for or dispose of equipment and supplies. Clean the work area. Remove your gloves and wash your hands.	This prevents the spread of microorganisms.
9. Record the procedure in the patient's chart.	Procedures are considered not to have been done if they are not recorded.

Charting Example:

06/15/2013 12:00 PM Oxymetazoline hydrochloride 0.05% nasal spray, 2 sprays to each nostril as ordered

per Dr. Greene ——————————————————————————————— D. Pratt, CMA

Although not all patients who have disorders of the eyes or ears need a referral to an ophthalmologist or otolaryngologist, you will routinely encounter patients who need to have these conditions properly diagnosed and treated. Keep in mind that:

- Disorders of the eyes, ears, nose, and throat may affect any patient at any age.

- Severe complications, such as an infection of the brain or hearing loss, can result in patients who are not receiving adequate attention or not following the physician's instructions for treatment.
- You will play a vital role by assisting with ear, nose, and throat examinations and educating patients regarding their treatment.

Warm Ups for Critical Thinking

1. The mother of a 10-month-old boy explains to you that the baby has had a runny nose and has been fussy for the past 2 days. You notice that he is pulling at his right ear. What equipment do you anticipate that the physician will need for examining the child?

2. A 16-year-old girl complains of a sore throat. Her vital signs are T 102.8 (O), P 112, R 24, and BP 112/84. The physician examines her and tells you to obtain a throat specimen for a rapid strep test to determine whether the pharyngitis is due to an infection with streptococcal bacteria. The patient is reluctant to let you obtain a throat culture, saying it will make her gag and vomit. How do you handle this situation?

3. The school nurse at the local high school phones your office asking for information about a student who has been out of school the past 3 days with conjunctivitis. Specifically, she wants to know whether this student has been diagnosed with this condition or is simply truant. How do you handle this phone call?

4. An elderly patient is having difficulty hearing and would like you to explain why the physician wants you to irrigate his ears for ceruminosis. He is concerned that the procedure will be uncomfortable. What could you say to the patient to ease his anxiety?

5. You notice that another medical assistant working in the office is getting frustrated with an adult male during a visual acuity test using the Snellen eye chart. The patient doesn't seem to know the letters of the alphabet and you suspect that he is illiterate, but may have been embarrassed to tell the other MA before the examination started. Would you intervene? What would you say?

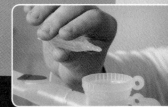

CHAPTER

15 Pulmonary Medicine

Learning Outcomes

Cognitive Domain

Note: AAMA/CAAHEP 2008 Standards are italicized.

1. Spell and define the key terms
2. Identify the primary defense mechanisms of the respiratory system
3. *Identify common pathologies related to each body system*
4. Explain various diagnostic procedures of the respiratory system
5. *Describe implications for treatment related to pathology*
6. Describe the physician's examination of the respiratory system
7. Discuss the role of the medical assistant with regard to various diagnostic and therapeutic procedures

Psychomotor Domain

Note: AAMA/CAAHEP 2008 Standards are italicized.

1. Instruct a patient in the use of the peak flowmeter (Procedure 15-1)
2. Administer a nebulized breathing treatment (Procedure 15-2)
3. Perform a pulmonary function test (Procedure 15-3)

4. *Assist physician with patient care*
5. *Prepare a patient for procedures and/or treatments*
6. *Practice standard precautions*
7. *Perform patient screening using established protocols*
8. *Document patient care*
9. *Document patient education*
10. *Practice within the standard of care for a medical assistant*

Affective Domain

Note: AAMA/CAAHEP 2008 Standards are italicized.

1. *Apply critical thinking skills in performing patient assessment and care*
2. *Use language/verbal skills that enable patients' understanding*
3. *Demonstrate empathy in communicating with patients, family, and staff*
4. *Use appropriate body language and other nonverbal skills in communicating with patients, family, and staff*
5. *Demonstrate awareness of the territorial boundaries of the person with whom you are communicating*

6. *Demonstrate sensitivity appropriate to the messeage being delivered*
7. *Demonstrate recognition of the patient's level of understanding in communications*
8. *Recognize and protect personal boundaries in communicating with others*
9. *Demonstrate respect for individual diversity, incorporating awareness of one's own biases in areas including gender, race, religion, age, and economic status*
10. *Apply active listening skills*
11. *Apply local, state, and federal health care legislation and regulation appropriate to the medical assisting practice setting*

ABHES Competencies

1. Assist the physician with the regimen of diagnostic and treatment modalities as they relate to each body system
2. Comply with federal, state, and local health laws and regulations
3. Communicate on the recipient's level of comprehension
4. Serve as a liaison between the physician and others
5. Show empathy and impartiality when dealing with patients
6. Document accurately

Key Terms

atelectasis	dyspnea	laryngectomy	tidal volume
chronic obstructive pulmonary disease (COPD)	forced expiratory volume	palliative	tracheostomy
	hemoptysis	status asthmaticus	
		thoracentesis	

The respiratory system provides the body with the oxygen that all cells need to perform their functions (Fig. 15-1). It also eliminates carbon dioxide, a waste product, and water from the body. The respiratory system works closely with the cardiovascular system to deliver oxygen to every cell in the body. When a cell is too long deprived of oxygen, the cell dies, and when many cells die, so does the tissue.

The upper airways, tracheobronchial tree, and alveoli come into contact with air from the atmosphere or environment, which can contain dust, pathogenic microorganisms, and other irritants. In healthy individuals, defense mechanisms in the respiratory system help to protect the body from disease and illness caused by these environmental contaminants. Table 15-1 summarizes the major defense mechanisms of the respiratory system. Disease can occur, however, when these defenses are overwhelmed by cigarette smoke, air pollution, infectious organisms, or other irritants.

COG Common Respiratory Disorders

Upper Respiratory Disorders

The most common problems of the upper respiratory tract are caused by infectious microorganisms and by allergic reactions that produce inflammation.

Acute rhinitis, sinusitis, pharyngitis, tonsillitis, and laryngitis are described in Chapter 14; these are also considered upper respiratory disorders.

Lower Respiratory Disorders

Diseases of the lower respiratory tract may be acute (sudden in onset with relatively short duration) or chronic (progressing over time or recurring frequently). Acute diseases of the lower respiratory tract include bronchitis and pneumonia. Chronic diseases include asthma, chronic bronchitis, and emphysema. The last two diseases are usually grouped as chronic obstructive pulmonary disease because most patients have elements of both emphysema and chronic bronchitis.

 PATIENT EDUCATION

EFFECTS OF SMOKING ON THE AIRWAYS

Cigarette smoking has many harmful effects on the body. Smoke from a cigarette irritates the airways and causes the membrane to produce more mucus. This increased production of mucus, along

(box continued on page 364)

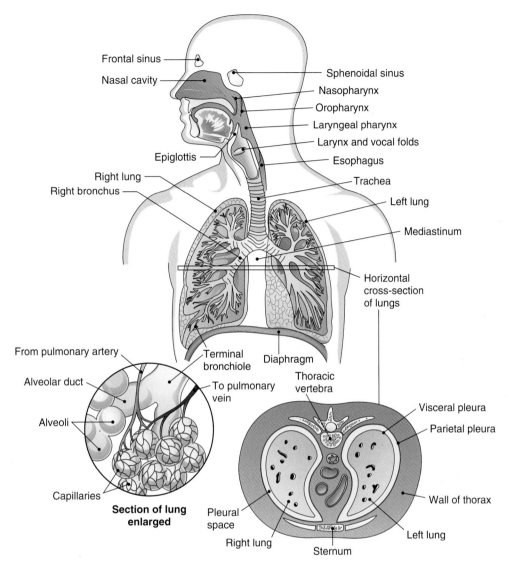

Figure 15-1 The respiratory system. (Reprinted with permission from Cohen BJ. Memmler's The Human Body in Health and Disease, 11th ed. Philadelphia: Lippincott Williams & Wilkins, 2009.)

TABLE **15-1**	Defenses of the Respiratory System
Defense	**Function**
Nasal hairs	Filter large dust particles from the air
Mucous membranes	Trap dust and other particles, add moisture
Turbinates in nose	Whirl air around to increase warming, humidifying, filtering
Epiglottis	Closes over trachea to prevent aspiration during swallowing
Airway reflexes	Trigger cough to clear irritants in pharynx, larynx, trachea
Airway smooth muscles	Constrict when irritation occurs to prevent entry of foreign substances
Macrophage in alveoli	Phagocytize ("eat") bacteria, other foreign cells, debris
Tonsils	Filter air moving through passageways to protect against bacterial invasion; aid in formation of white blood cells

with the increase in dust and debris that collects in the mucus, slows down the body's normal clearing processes. The smoke anesthetizes the cilia lining the respiratory tract so they stop waving the debris away. Over time, large amounts of thick, sticky mucus are retained in the lungs, blackening the lung tissue and sealing the alveolar sacs. This thick, tarry mucus causes the patient to cough frequently, especially in the mornings, and to be prone to bronchitis, both acute and chronic, as a result of the destruction of the protective mechanisms of the airway from the heat and tar inhaled in the smoke.

Bronchitis

Bronchitis is an inflammation of the mucous membranes of the bronchi caused by infection or irritation that induces increased production of mucus in the trachea, bronchi, and bronchioles. The most prominent symptom of bronchitis is a productive cough. If a bacterial or viral infection is present, the sputum may change color from the normal white or clear to yellow, green, gray, or tan. If an infection is suspected, you may be asked to obtain a sputum specimen for culture and sensitivity to determine the causative microorganism and appropriate antibiotic therapy. (Chapter 29 outlines the procedure for collecting a sputum specimen.) In many cases, the physician bases a diagnosis of bronchitis on the history and symptoms of the patient without ordering a sputum culture.

The treatment of bronchitis generally includes an antibiotic for bacterial infection, smoking cessation, rest, and increased fluid intake. A cough suppressant may be prescribed, especially for use at night, but this is controversial because of the body's need to clear secretions from the airways. Retained secretions can become infected and lead to pneumonia.

Pneumonia

Pneumonia is a bacterial or viral infection in the alveoli, or tiny air sacs that are the site of gas exchange in the lungs. The buildup of fluid and congestion in the alveoli prevents effective gas exchange. Diagnostic testing usually includes analysis of a sputum specimen and chest radiography. Bacterial pneumonias tend to be sudden and severe in onset, causing a fever, cough, chills, and **dyspnea**. Infections caused by bacteria also tend to be local to one lobe or area of the lung. Treatment of bacterial pneumonia primarily includes an appropriate antibiotic, bed rest, and medication to relieve symptoms. Pneumonia caused by bacteria often requires hospitalization for administration of intravenous antibiotics and oxygen, especially in the elderly or debilitated patients.

Viral pneumonia is usually more gradual in onset but can be just as serious. Antibiotics are ineffective in

PATIENT EDUCATION

PULMONARY FIBROSIS

Pulmonary fibrosis is a lung disease that occurs due to damage and scarring of the lung tissue. As more scarring develops, the lungs become stiff and the ability of the alveoli to exchange oxygen and carbon dioxide is decreased. Symptoms of pulmonary fibrosis include dyspnea, a dry cough, fatigue, and weight loss. In some patients, the disease may develop quickly and be severe while other patients are diagnosed and the disease progresses more slowly, perhaps over months or years. As the disease progresses, the patient will become more short of breath with exertion.

The cause of this disease is often unknown (idiopathic pulmonary fibrosis); however, some patients have developed this disease due to the following:

- Long-term exposure to occupational or environmental pollutants such as asbestos, grain dust, or bird droppings.
- Medications such as those used for chemotherapy, cardiac arrhythmias, and some antibiotics may damage the lungs and result in pulmonary fibrosis months or years after taking the drug.
- Underlying medical conditions including tuberculosis, pneumonia, rheumatoid arthritis, and systemic lupus erythematosus may cause lung damage that results in pulmonary fibrosis.

Although there is no cure for pulmonary fibrosis, some patients may have significant lung damage and may receive a lung transplant. Most patient care is aimed at education and support including:

- Corticosteroids such as prednisone and/or drugs that suppress the immune system.
- Oxygen therapy may be ordered by the physician to decrease symptoms associated with decreased blood-oxygen levels.
- A referral for pulmonary rehabilitation may be prescribed by the physician to provide patients with exercises to improve endurance, breathing techniques to improve lung efficiency, emotional support, and nutritional counseling.

Encourage patients who are diagnosed with this disease to:

- Participate in treatment as much as possible.
- Stop smoking and avoid environments where cigarette or cigar smoke is in the air.
- Maintain nutritional status by increasing calories and frequency of meals.

• Receive vaccines as ordered by the physician to avoid respiratory infections.

As the patient's disease progresses, support to both the family and the caregivers will be essential. Discussions for end-of-life care should be directed to the physician and any decisions made respected by the health care team working with the patient and family.

treating viral pneumonia; however, the physician may order an antibiotic to prevent a secondary bacterial infection. Viral pneumonia tends to spread throughout the lung fields and often is marked by a fever and productive cough. Treatment may include bed rest or hospitalization.

 CHECKPOINT QUESTION

1. What are the characteristics of bacterial and viral pneumonia?

 Asthma

Asthma is a reversible inflammatory process involving primarily the small airways such as the bronchi and bronchioles. Asthma manifests as constriction of the smooth muscle lining the airways, spasms of the bronchi and bronchioles (bronchospasm), swelling of the mucous membranes of the airways, and increased mucus production with productive coughing. All three of these manifestations narrow the airways, making it difficult for the patient to move air into and out of the lungs.

The patient having an asthma attack may have dyspnea, coughing, wheezing, and, in severe cases, cyanosis. Patients with asthma usually have exacerbations, which are periods of frequent attacks, and remissions, which are periods when they are relatively symptom free. Attacks may be triggered by exposure to allergens, such as mold or dust; inhaled irritants, such as cigarette smoke; upper respiratory infections; psychological stress; cold air; or exercise. In some instances, the immediate cause of the asthma attack is unknown. While asthma is considered a chronic disorder that occurs in children or adults, many children with asthma outgrow it by adulthood.

Many medications are available to prevent or control the symptoms of asthma, but it is important that they be used properly. On days that the patient has no symptoms of asthma, he or she should use a device called a peak flowmeter (Fig. 15-2) to determine the amount of air moving into and out of the lungs (Procedure 15-1). Instruct the patient to use the peak flowmeter correctly and record the results on a chart or diary provided by the medical office. This record, known as the patient's personal best, assists the physician in establishing and maintaining a medication protocol.

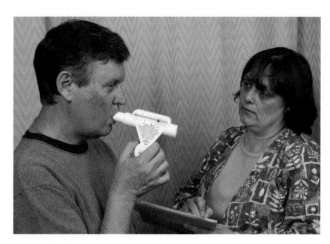

Figure 15-2 The peak flowmeter.

Patients with symptoms of asthma, including wheezing and difficulty breathing, may be prescribed a nebulized breathing treatment with a bronchodilator, a medication to dilate the bronchi, such as albuterol (Procedure 15-2). After the bronchodilator is in the nebulizer administration setup, the machine is turned on and causes the liquid medication to break apart into a fine spray that is inhaled by the patient through a mouthpiece or mask. Since bronchodilator medications cause an increase in the heart rate, you should monitor the patient's pulse before, during, and after the treatment. If the patient becomes lightheaded, discontinue the treatment, have the patient lie down, obtain the vital signs, and notify the physician.

An asthma attack that does not respond to medication is an emergency known as **status asthmaticus**. Because such attacks can be fatal, the patient needs immediate emergency medical services and hospitalization.

 CHECKPOINT QUESTION

2. What factors may trigger an asthma attack?

 PATIENT EDUCATION

USING MORE THAN ONE INHALER FOR ASTHMA

Asthmatics may use more than one inhaler. One medication is usually a bronchodilator to open the bronchioles and control bronchospasms. Another type of inhaler is a corticosteroid. Steroids help to control inflammation in the bronchioles and generally are prescribed only during a respiratory illness. Teach the patient to use the bronchodilator first, wait 5 minutes, and then use the steroid. Using the steroid inhaler after the bronchodilator allows for more steroid medication to enter the lung tissue, making it more effective.

(continued)

Some patients are prescribed two inhaled bronchodilators. One type is used daily to prevent asthma attacks, and the other is used as a rescue inhaler. The rescue inhaler should be used only when the asthma cannot be controlled with the daily regimen. Before teaching a patient about the correct pattern for using the inhalers, clarify the information with the physician. Each asthmatic responds differently and requires an individualized approach to care.

Chronic Obstructive Pulmonary Disease

Chronic bronchitis and emphysema are most commonly caused by cigarette smoking. As a result, patients who have smoked over a long period often exhibit signs and symptoms of both of these disorders. Chronic bronchitis is a chronic inflammation and swelling of the airways with excessive mucus production, obstruction of the bronchi, and trapping of air behind mucus plugs. The trapping of this air overinflates the alveoli. Chronic bronchitis is not usually an infectious process but, instead, is produced by chronic irritation of the airways by cigarette smoke or other pollutants. However, because of the increase in sputum and the difficulty these patients have in clearing their sputum, they are prone to develop respiratory infections.

Emphysema is a disease process in which the walls of the damaged alveoli stretch and break down after repeated exposure to irritants such as cigarette smoke and air pollution. The pulmonary capillaries also break down, and the tiny airways leading to each alveolus weaken and collapse. The end result is a sharp reduction in surface area for gas exchange, and once again, air is trapped in the enlarged air sacs that were once clusters of tiny alveoli.

The combination of these diseases, together called **chronic obstructive pulmonary disease (COPD)**, produces characteristic symptoms. COPD is a likely cause of shortness of breath, chronic cough, sputum production, and wheezing in the patient with a history of smoking. The onset of these symptoms is usually slow and gradual over years, and the patient may go a long time without realizing that he or she has signs and symptoms of a disease. Many people with COPD have some of the signs and symptoms of asthma, and many of these patients take asthma medications.

Once a patient is diagnosed with COPD, the disease process is not usually reversible. Many patients have a hard time accepting that fact and insist that their physician provide a cure or restore the lungs to normal function. Although the disease is not curable, the progression of COPD can be slowed and the quality of life improved significantly through education about the disease, a prescribed exercise regimen, proper use of medications, good nutrition, and home oxygen therapy.

PATIENT EDUCATION

LIVING WITH COPD

To improve the quality of life, encourage a patient diagnosed with COPD to follow these suggestions:

1. Quit smoking if you haven't already done so! Even though the lungs have been permanently damaged, further deterioration will be reduced if you stop smoking now.
2. Get a flu vaccination each fall and make sure you have had the pneumonia vaccine.
3. Avoid crowds, especially in the winter, when the viruses that cause colds and influenza are prevalent.
4. If pollution is high, stay indoors with the air conditioning on if possible.
5. Use your abdominal muscles instead of your shoulder and neck muscles to avoid strain and fatigue in these muscles.
6. Drink lots of fluids unless the physician has limited your fluid intake. Water is the best fluid. Good fluid intake is the best way to keep the mucus in your airways thin so that it is easy to cough up.
7. Follow a healthy, balanced diet.
8. Avoid doing difficult physical tasks (e.g., vacuuming or mowing the lawn) all in one day. If you must do these chores, do them in short periods spaced throughout the day with frequent rest periods.
9. Organize your home to minimize standing, reaching, and lifting.

WHAT IF?

What if a patient requires home oxygen therapy?

Many patients with severe COPD or end-stage lung cancer are discharged from the hospital with oxygen to use at home. Most surgical supply companies and pharmacies can arrange to have oxygen therapy equipment delivered to the home. The oxygen is usually supplied by a machine called a concentrator that runs on electricity. The concentrator separates oxygen out of room air and concentrates it for delivery to the patient. Attached to the cylinder is a flowmeter, or regulator, that indicates the amount of oxygen being delivered. The patient should be instructed to leave the oxygen at the setting prescribed by the physician. Too much oxygen can be toxic for some patients, such as those with emphysema. A cannula (plastic tube with pronged openings that fit into the nares) is attached to the flowmeter and delivers oxygen to the patient's airways. The company supplying the oxygen should instruct the patient regarding safe home oxygen administration. Since oxygen is highly flammable, you should reinforce safety precautions during oxygen use, including avoiding open flames and sparks. In addition, the supplier should be available 24 hours a day for emergency oxygen maintenance.

Tuberculosis

Tuberculosis is an infectious disease spread by respiratory droplets from a person infected with *Mycobacterium tuberculosis*. The patient with active tuberculosis has signs and symptoms such as a productive cough, night sweats, and malaise. Although no tuberculosis vaccine is available, a screening test can be administered to detect a previous infection. However, a patient with a positive screening test for tuberculosis does not necessarily have active disease and therefore may not be contagious. The procedure for administering and reading the results of the screening tests (Mantoux and tine tests) for tuberculosis is described in Chapter 9. Patients with symptoms of tuberculosis should be treated as contagious and encouraged to wear a protective mask over the nose and mouth to prevent spreading the disease through infected droplets released into the air during speaking and coughing. In addition, you are required to report any diagnosis of tuberculosis to the local public health department. The treatment for tuberculosis includes a regimen of antibiotic therapy that lasts for months. You should provide emotional support for these patients, since the treatment lasts up to a year, and encourage compliance with the prescribed regimen at each office visit.

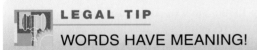

LEGAL TIP

WORDS HAVE MEANING!

Patients with chronic and irreversible diseases, such as COPD, must never be led to believe that the doctor can cure the disease. Avoid making statements such as, "Everything will be okay" or "The doctor can help you," and also be careful not to indicate that the patient will return to normal function. Legally, the doctor is responsible for your actions, including promises, even if they are innocent and were said only to make the patient feel better. These statements may be taken as a guarantee, and if the results are not achieved, the patient may file a lawsuit on the grounds that a contract was broken and the promised results were not delivered.

 CHECKPOINT QUESTION

3. What two disease processes are present in a patient with COPD?

Common Cancers of the Respiratory System

Laryngeal Cancer

Cancer of the larynx is seen most commonly in heavy smokers and alcoholics. The presenting symptoms are usually hoarseness that lasts longer than 3 weeks, a feeling of a lump in the throat, or pain and burning in the throat when drinking citrus juice or hot liquids. A patient with laryngeal cancer may be treated with radiation, surgery, or both. Surgery usually is a **laryngectomy**, or removal of the larynx, and formation of a permanent **tracheostomy** stoma (Fig. 15-3). Patients who have had a laryngectomy are unable to speak normally but can be trained to use esophageal speech or a prosthetic speech device.

Lung Cancer

Lung cancer is one of the most common causes of death in both men and women. Cigarette smoking is believed to be the most common cause; 80% of lung cancer patients are smokers. Prognosis is generally poor for patients with lung cancer, with only 8% of men and 12% of women surviving for 5 years. One of the reasons is that symptoms tend to present rather late in the disease, when it has already had a chance to metastasize, or spread to other organs. Also, many of the symptoms are nonspecific and are seen in most heavy smokers. These symptoms include chronic cough, wheezing, dyspnea, **hemoptysis**, and chest pain.

Diagnosis of lung cancer is made by chest radiography, sputum cytology, bronchoscopy, biopsy, or **thoracentesis**. Treatment is generally **palliative**, giving relief but not a cure, and usually includes surgery, radiation, and chemotherapy. These treatments may improve the patient's prognosis and prolong survival.

 CHECKPOINT QUESTION

4. What factor appears to contribute to both laryngeal cancer and lung cancer?

Common Diagnostic and Therapeutic Procedures

Physical Examination of the Respiratory System

The traditional examination of the chest consists of four parts: inspection, palpation, percussion, and auscultation. Each is briefly described in the following

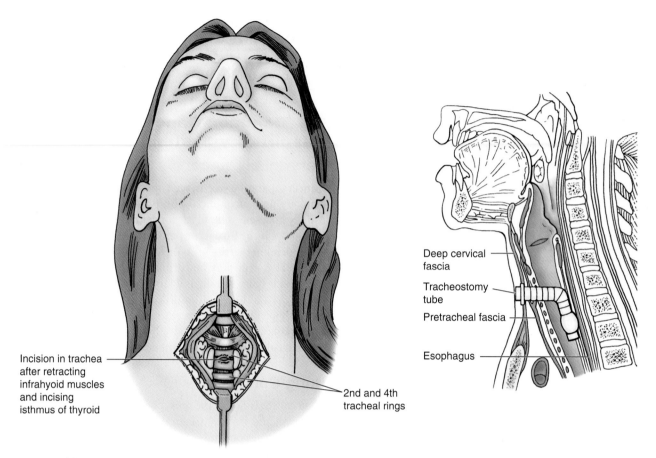

Incision in trachea
after retracting
infrahyoid muscles
and incising
isthmus of thyroid

2nd and 4th
tracheal rings

Deep cervical
fascia

Tracheostomy
tube

Pretracheal fascia

Esophagus

Figure 15-3 The patient with a tracheostomy. (From Moore KL, Dalley AF II. Clinical Oriented Anatomy. 4th ed. Baltimore: Lippincott Williams & Wilkins, 1999.)

sections. For the physician to perform this examination efficiently, the patient should be sitting up, and all clothing should be removed from the waist up. The patient should be given a gown and draped appropriately (see Chapter 5).

Inspection

Inspection consists of a visual examination of the chest and the patient's respiratory pattern (Table 15-2). During inspection, the physician looks for abnormal shape of the thorax, use of accessory muscles to breathe, surgical scars, cyanosis, and any other visible signs of previous or current respiratory disease.

Palpation

In palpation, the physician uses his or her hands to feel the patient's throat for lumps, areas of tenderness, and location of the trachea, which may be displaced by a tumor. The patient may be asked to say "99" while the physician feels the chest wall in different places to assess the vibrations produced. Solid masses (such as tumors) or fluids (as in pneumonia) increase vibrations, whereas increased air (as seen in emphysema) reduces the vibrations.

Percussion

Percussion is placing a finger (or fingers) on the chest and striking it with the fingers of the other hand. The physician listens for the sound to determine whether it is normal (resonant), like the sound produced by a drum. Dull or flat sounds are heard in patients with consolidation of pulmonary tissue, such as **atelectasis**, pneumonia, or a tumor. A hyperresonant sound is hollow and is heard in patients with emphysema. Children with cystic fibrosis (see Chapter 22) often require chest percussion to loosen the thick respiratory secretions throughout the day.

Auscultation

Auscultation is listening to the patient's lungs and airway passages with a stethoscope. The physician systematically listens to each side of the chest in each area to compare the sounds bilaterally. The patient should breathe deeply, with an open mouth and the head turned away from the physician's face. The patient is encouraged not to breathe too rapidly to avoid hyperventilation, which can cause dizziness. During auscultation, the physician listens for abnormal or adventitious sounds, such as crackles and wheezes, which may also indicate a disease process (Table 15-3).

TABLE **15-2**	Abnormal Respiratory Patterns
Pattern	**Description**
Apnea	No respirations
Bradypnea	Slow respirations
Cheyne-Stokes	Rhythmic cycles of dyspnea or hyperpnea subsiding gradually into brief apnea
Dyspnea	Difficult or labored respirations
Hypopnea	Shallow respirations
Hyperpnea	Deep respirations
Kussmaul	Fast and deep respirations
Orthopnea	Inability to breathe except while sitting or standing
Tachypnea	Fast respirations

CHECKPOINT QUESTION

5. What are the four methods used to examine the respiratory system?

Sputum Culture and Cytology

Sputum cultures are obtained to aid with diagnosis and treatment decisions in patients with suspected pneumonia, tuberculosis, or other infectious diseases of the lower airway. A microbiology laboratory will culture and incubate the specimen to identify any pathogenic microorganisms. Sputum specimens obtained for cytology are analyzed in the laboratory for abnormal cells that may indicate precancerous or cancerous conditions of the lung or airway. In all cases, it is important to obtain a specimen that the patient has coughed up and expectorated from the lower airways, with minimal contamination by oral and pharyngeal secretions. The patient is asked to cough deeply and collect the specimen in a sterile container (see Chapter 29). After instructing the patient on coughing and collecting the specimen, you process the specimen and prepare the laboratory request for transportation to the laboratory for analysis.

Sputum collection for suspected cancer or for tuberculosis may be required over three consecutive mornings. The specimens should be brought into the office as soon as possible to avoid deterioration of the specimen. Most diagnostic specimens are obtained early in the morning, when the greatest volume of secretion has accumulated. If this is not possible, a specimen may also be collected after a nebulized breathing treatment with a bronchodilator. The patient may be weak from illness, thick mucus may be difficult to bring up, and coughing may exhaust the patient. A cool-mist humidifier may be ordered for use at home to help loosen thick secretions. It is vitally important that the patient understand that the specimen must be collected from the lung fields and not from the mouth. The difference between saliva and sputum should be explained to the patient at his or her level of understanding.

TABLE **15-3**	Abnormal Breath Sounds
Breath Sound	**Description**
Bubbling	Gurgling sounds as air passes through moist secretions in airways
Crackles (rales)	Crackling sound, usually inspiratory, as air passes through moist secretions in airways. Fine to medium crackles indicate secretions in small airways and alveoli. Medium to coarse crackles indicate secretions in larger airways.
Friction rub	Dry, rubbing or grating sound
Rhonchi	Low-pitched, continuous sound as air moves past thick mucus or narrowed air passages
Stertor	Snoring sound on inspiration or expiration; indicates a partial airway obstruction
Stridor	Shrill, harsh inspiratory sound; indicates laryngeal obstruction
Wheeze	High-pitched musical sound, either inspiratory or expiratory; indicates partial airway obstruction

Chest Radiography

Chest radiography can help in the diagnosis of a large variety of pulmonary problems, including pneumonia, lung cancer, emphysema, tuberculosis, and pulmonary edema. Often the physician orders two views: a posteroanterior (PA) view and a lateral view. This gives the physician a three-dimensional view. If the procedure is performed at the hospital or other outpatient facility, you may have to schedule it and request the results after the radiographs are interpreted by the radiologist.

 CHECKPOINT QUESTION

6. What is being analyzed in a sputum specimen?

Bronchoscopy

Bronchoscopy is an endoscopic procedure in which a lighted scope is inserted into the trachea and bronchi for direct visualization. This procedure is considered invasive and requires the patient's written consent. It is usually performed in an outpatient surgical setting, and you may have to schedule it. Bronchoscopy can be used for many diagnostic purposes, such as obtaining sputum specimens, obtaining tissue for biopsy, and visually assessing airway changes caused by chronic pulmonary diseases such as COPD or asthma. It can also be used therapeutically, for example to clear out mucus plugs or to remove a foreign body.

 Pulmonary Function Tests

Pulmonary function tests are performed with a spirometer that measures the amount of air a patient can move in and out of the lungs (Fig. 15-4). The patient breathes into a mouthpiece and performs several breathing maneuvers that you explain during the test. By measuring the patient's airflow and comparing the results with

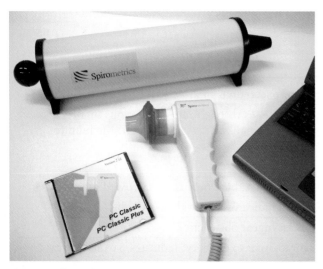

Figure 15-4 A pulmonary function testing machine. (Courtesy of Spirometrics.)

predicted values for the patient's height, weight, gender, age, and race, the physician gains valuable information concerning whether the patient has mild, moderate, or severe obstructive or restrictive disease. The patient's **tidal volume** and **forced expiratory volume** are two measurements that can be obtained during the pulmonary function test. Procedure 15-3 describes the steps for performing the pulmonary function test.

 AFF **TRIAGE**

While working in a medical office, the following three situations occur this afternoon:

A. Patient A is an elderly male with emphysema who is wheezing. The doctor has ordered a nebulized treatment with a bronchodilator.

B. Patient B is a 34-year-old woman who is scheduled to have a pulmonary function test today as part of a pre-employment physical. She is anxious about getting the test "over with" so that she can pick up her children from school.

C. Patient C has been seen and discharged by the doctor but is waiting for you to schedule a bronchoscopy that the physician has ordered to be done later this week.

How do you sort these patients? Who do you see first? Second? Third?

Patient A should be seen first. Anyone who has trouble breathing or a respiratory problem must be treated as a priority. It is important to monitor this patient closely for any changes in condition before, during, and after treatment. Place patient B in an examination room and tell her that you will start the test within 10 minutes or advise her that she can reschedule the test for later this week. Inform patient C that you will schedule her procedure and notify her by phone of the exact date and time. Patients often become anxious about impending tests and can easily become upset with delays. Offer reassurance to the patient as needed.

Arterial Blood Gases

Arterial blood gas (ABG) determinations measure the pH and pressures of oxygen and carbon dioxide in arterial blood. The results can indicate whether the patient's lungs are adequately exchanging gases. ABGs can also give information about metabolic acid–base problems, such as diabetic ketoacidosis. Drawing blood from an artery takes special training and is not routinely done in the medical office. However, you may be required to schedule a patient for an arterial puncture at a laboratory or hospital and record the results, which are usually phoned to the office.

Pulse Oximetry

Many medical offices have a pulse oximeter, which quickly and painlessly determines the percentage of oxygen saturation on a patient's capillary blood cells (Fig. 15-5). The pulse oximeter is small, fitting into the palm of the hand, and includes a digital display that notes the patient's pulse rate and oxygen saturation when a sensor cable is attached to the nail bed of the patient's index finger. Pulse oximeter readings should be obtained as a baseline for patients with chronic respiratory conditions and for patients with respiratory signs and symptoms, such as complaints of dyspnea or wheezing. The results should be recorded as a percentage; readings above 95% are considered normal. Although patients with chronic conditions such as emphysema may have readings of 90% or higher, readings below 90% should be reported to the physician immediately.

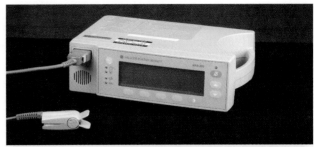
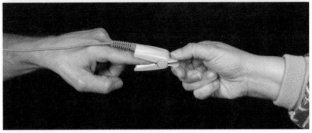

Figure 15-5 Pulse oximetry is used to measure oxygen saturation of arterial blood. (Reprinted with permission from Cohen BJ. Medical Terminology: An Illustrated Guide. Philadelphia: Lippincott Williams & Wilkins, 2003.)

 CHECKPOINT QUESTION

7. What are the ways the physician can obtain information to help diagnose respiratory disorders?

Medication Box

Commonly Prescribed Respiratory System Medications

Note: The generic name of the drug is listed first and is written in all lower case letters. Brand names are in parentheses and the first letter is capitalized.

albuterol sulfate (Proventil, Ventolin)	Inhalation aerosol: 90 mcg/metered spray Solution for inhalation: 0.083%, 0.5%, 0.42% Tablets: 2 mg, 4 mg	Bronchodilator
benzonatate (Tessalon)	Capsules: 100 mg, 200 mg	Local anesthetic
budesonide (Pulmicort Respules)	Powder: 90 mcg/dose Inhalation suspension: 0.25 mg, 0.5 mg, 1 mg	Corticosteroid
cefdinir (Omnicef)	Capsules: 300 mg Suspension: 125 mg/5 mL, 250 mg/5 mL	Antibiotic
cephalexin (Keflex)	Capsules: 250 mg, 333 mg, 500 mg, 750 mg Oral suspension: 125 mg/5 mL	Antibiotic
cetirizine hydrochloride (Zyrtec)	Tablets: 5 mg, 10 mg Oral solution: 5 mg/5 mL	Antihistamine
dextromethorphan hydrobromide (Delsym, Robitussin, Triaminic)	Gelcaps: 15 mg, 30 mg Solution: 3.5 mg/5 mL, 5 mg/5 mL	Cough suppresant
fexofenadine hydrochloride (Allegra)	Tablets: 30 mg, 60 mg, 180 mg Oral suspension: 30 mg/5 mL	Antihistamine
fluticasone propionate (Flonase)	Nasal spray: 50 mcg/metered spray	Corticosteroid
guaifenesin (Mucinex, Robitussin)	Syrup: 100 mg/5 mL Capsules: 200 mg Tablets: 100 mg, 200 mg, 400 mg	Mucolytic (expectorant)

(continued)

Medication Box *(continued)*

Commonly Prescribed Respiratory System Medications

influenza virus vaccine, live intranasal (FluMist)	Intranasal spray: 0.2 mL	Vaccine
ipratropium bromide (Atrovent)	Inhaler: 17 mcg/metered dose	Bronchodilator
ipatropium bromide and albuterol (Combivent)	Inhaler: 18 mcg ipatropium and 90 mcg albuterol/metered dose	Bronchodilator
isoniazid (INH)	Injection: 100 mg/mL (IM) Tablets: 100 mg, 300 mg Oral solution: 50 mg/5 mL	Antibiotic
levalbuterol (Xopenex)	Inhalation aerosol: 3 mL vials: 45 mcg Solution for inhalation: 0.31 mg, 0.63%, 1.25 mg; 5 mL vials: 1.25 mg	
levofloxacin (Levaquin)	Tablets: 250 mg, 500 mg, 750 mg Oral solution: 25 mg/mL	Antibiotic
loratadine (Claritin, Alavert)	Capsules: 10 mg Syrup: 1 mg/mL Tablets: 10 mg	Antihistamine
oseltamivir phosphate (Tamiflu)	Capsules: 30 mg, 45 mg, 75 mg Oral suspension: 12 mg/mL	Antiviral
pirbuterol acetate (Maxair)	Inhaler: 0.2 mg/metered dose	Bronchodilator
rifampin (Rifadin, Rimactane)	Capsules: 150 mg, 300 mg	Antibiotic
theophylline (Theochron, Theo-24)	Tablets (Theochron): 100 mg to 600 mg; Capsules (Theo-24): 100 mg to 400 mg	Bronchodilator
zanamivir (Relenza)	Powder for inhalation: 5 mg/blister	Antiviral

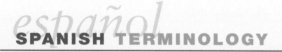

SPANISH TERMINOLOGY

¿Tose con flema?
　Do you cough up any phlegm?

¿De qué color es la flema?
　What color is it?

Transparente
　Clear

Blanca
　White

Amarilla
　Yellow

Verde
　Green

Oscura
　Dark

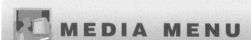

MEDIA MENU

- **Student Resources on thePoint**
  - **Animation: Asthma**
  - **Animation: Breathing Sounds**
  - **Animation: Oxygen Transport**
  - **Video: Administering a Nebulized Breathing Treatment (Procedure 15-2)**
  - **Video: Perform a Pulmonary Function Test (Procedure 15-3)**
  - **CMA/RMA Certification Exam Review**
- **Internet Resources**
  - **Centers for Disease Control and Prevention**
    http://www.cdc.gov
  - **American Lung Association**
    http://www.lungusa.org
  - **American Association of Respiratory Care**
    http://www.acr.org
  - **American Thoracic Society**
    http://www.thoracic.org
  - **American Cancer Society**
    http://www.cancer.org

PSY PROCEDURE 15-1: **Instructing a Patient on Using the Peak Flowmeter**

Purpose: Instruct the patient on the correct procedure for using and recording measurements using the peak flowmeter.
Equipment: Peak flowmeter, recording documentation form

Steps	Reasons
1. Wash your hands.	Handwashing aids infection control.
2. Assemble the peak flowmeter, disposable mouthpiece, and patient documentation form.	The flowmeter is used to instruct patients in performing a peak flow reading. A disposable mouthpiece should be used. In some offices, the patient is instructed in using a peak flowmeter that is given to him or her to take home and use. In this case, no disposable mouthpiece is necessary.
3. Greet and identify the patient and explain the procedure.	Identifying the patient prevents errors.
4. **AFF** Explain how to respond to a patient who is developmentally challenged.	Always explain procedures to the caregiver who accompanies the patient.
5. Holding the peak flowmeter upright, explain how to read and reset the gauge after each reading.	In the upright position, the meter is calibrated with numbers and contains a sliding gauge that should move freely up and down the meter next to the numbers.

Step 5. The peak flowmeter and sliding gauge.

6. Instruct the patient to put the peak flowmeter mouthpiece in the mouth, forming a tight seal with the lips. After taking a deep breath, the patient should blow hard into the mouthpiece without blocking the back of the flowmeter.	The patient should close the lips around the mouthpiece without biting down. Blocking the back of the flowmeter will interfere with the movement of the gauge.
7. Note the number on the flowmeter corresponding to the level at which the sliding gauge stopped after the patient blew hard into the mouthpiece. Reset the gauge to zero.	A normal range provided with the flowmeter is based on the patient's age, height, and weight. Ideally, the patient's readings should be within this range.

(continued)

PROCEDURE 15-1: **Instructing a Patient on Using the Peak Flowmeter** *(continued)*

Steps	Purpose
8. Instruct the patient to perform this procedure three times consecutively, in the morning and at night, and to record the highest reading on form.	The highest reading is the patient's best reading. Recording the readings on the form allows the patient to follow his or her progress based on the medication therapy or exposure to allergens.

Peakflow Meter Daily Record

Name: Jane Doe

Date:	3/05	3/06	3/07							
Time:	8am	8:30	8:15							
750										
650										
550		•								
450	•									
350		•								
250										
150										

Step 8. A peak flowmeter documentation form.

9. Explain to the patient the procedure for cleaning the mouthpiece by washing with soapy water and rinsing without immersing the flowmeter in water.	Cleaning the mouthpiece is sanitary and prevents the spread of microorganisms.
10. Document the procedure.	Procedures are considered not to have been done if they are not recorded.

Charting Example:

12/11/2013 3:30 PM Pt. instructed on using a flowmeter—return demonstration without difficulty, verbalized
understanding. Given patient documentation form, instructed to record readings in morning and evening. Today's
reading 400 LPM. No dyspnea, c/o wheezing or SOB ————————————————————E. Michael, CMA

Note: The medical assistant may sign his or her name in the patient record using only the "CMA" credential if the office has a signature log denoting the entire credential as "CMA(AAMA)."

PSY PROCEDURE 15-2: **Performing a Nebulized Breathing Treatment**

Purpose: Set up and administer a nebulized breathing treatment in the medical office
Equipment: Physician order, patient's medical record, inhalation medication, nebulizer disposable setup, nebulizer

Steps	Reasons
1. Wash your hands.	Handwashing aids infection control.
2. Assemble the equipment and medication; check the medication label three times, as when administering any medications.	Checking the medication label three times prevents errors.

PSY PROCEDURE 15-2: **Performing a Nebulized Breathing Treatment (continued)**

Steps	Purpose
3. Greet and identify the patient and explain the procedure.	Properly identifying the patient will avoid errors. Explaining the procedure promotes understanding and compliance.
4. **AFF** Explain how to respond to a patient who does not speak English or who speaks English as a second language (ESL).	Solicit assistance from anyone who may be with the patient or a staff member if available who speaks the patient's language. If no interpreter is available, use hand gestures or pictures to explain the procedure to the patient.
5. Remove the nebulizer treatment cup from the setup and add the exact amount of medication ordered by the physician. 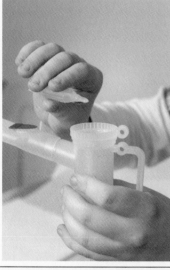 **Step 5.** The nebulizer medication cup.	The physician bases the amount of bronchodilator on the age and weight of the patient.
6. Place the top on the cup securely, attach the T piece to the top of the cup, and position the mouthpiece firmly on one end of the T piece. 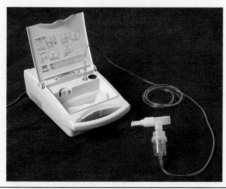 **Step 6.** A nebulizer machine and disposable setup with mouthpiece.	The top of the mouthpiece usually screws onto the bottom of the cup, providing a reservoir for the medication and saline.
7. Attach one end of the tubing securely to the connector on the cup and the other end to the connector on the nebulizer machine.	

(continued)

PSY **PROCEDURE 15-2:** **Performing a Nebulized Breathing Treatment (continued)**

Steps	Purpose
8. Ask the patient to put the mouthpiece in the mouth and make a seal with the lips without biting the mouthpiece. Instruct the patient to breathe normally during the treatment, occasionally taking a deep breath.	The patient may have difficulty breathing or be wheezing but should be encouraged to breathe as normally as possible. Breathing too rapidly may cause hyperventilation. Occasionally taking a deep breath will allow medication to be administered to deeper lung tissues.

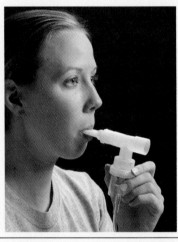

Step 8. The T piece and medication cup.

Steps	Purpose
9. Turn the machine on. The medication in the reservoir cup will become a fine mist to be inhaled by the patient.	A fine mist will come from the opposite end of the T piece when the patient exhales.
10. Before, during, and after the breathing treatment, take and record the patient's pulse.	Most bronchodilators cause a slight increase in the heart rate. Notify the physician if the increase is significant or if the patient has symptoms such as dizziness.
11. When the treatment is over and the medication cup is empty, turn the machine off and have the patient remove the mouthpiece.	The treatment typically takes about 15 minutes.
12. Disconnect the disposable treatment setup and dispose of all parts in a biohazard container. Properly put away the machine.	The setup equipment, including the mouthpiece, may be contaminated with hazardous microorganisms and should be handled and disposed of properly.
13. Wash your hands and document the procedure, including the patient's pulse before, during, and after the treatment.	Procedures are considered not to have been done if they are not recorded. Again, the bronchodilator used for nebulized treatments may cause the heart rate to increase, and the pulse should be noted and recorded during and after the treatment.

Charting Example:

11/26/2013 9:15 AM Pt. given nebulized breathing treatment with albuterol 2 mg for inhalation—pulse before
treatment 88, during treatment 100, and after treatment 110. Pt. states she is "breathing easier" after treatment, skin
warm and dry, color pink ———————————————————————————————— J. Barker, CMA

Note: The medical assistant may sign his or her name in the patient record using only the "CMA" credential if the office has a signature log denoting the entire credential as "CMA(AAMA)."

PSY **PROCEDURE 15-3:** | **Perform a Pulmonary Function Test**

Purpose: Perform a pulmonary function test and record the procedure
Equipment: Physician order, patient's medical record, spirometer and appropriate cables, calibration syringe and log book, disposable mouthpiece, printer, nose clip

Steps	Reasons
1. Wash your hands.	Handwashing aids infection control.
2. Assemble the equipment.	Having all the necessary equipment and supplies saves time when the patient is ready to undergo the procedures.
3. Greet and identify the patient and explain the procedure.	Identifying the patient prevents errors, and explaining the procedure promotes compliance.
4. **AFF** Explain how to respond to a patient who is visually impaired.	Observe patients carefully to prevent injury and ask before offering assistance or taking hold of their arms to guide. Face the patient when speaking and always let him or her know what you are going to do before touching him or her.
5. Turn the spirometer on, and, if it has not been been calibrated according to office policy, calibrate it using the calibration syringe according to the manufacturer's instructions. Record the calibration in the appropriate log book.	The spirometer must be calibrated daily to ensure accurate results.

Step 5. The calibration syringe used for checking the spirometer.

6. With the machine on and calibrated, attach the appropriate cable, tubing, and mouthpiece according to the type of machine being used.	One cable is plugged into an electrical outlet, and another cable or tube is connected to the spirometer and the patient's mouthpiece.
7. Using the keyboard on the machine, enter the patient's name or identification number, age, weight, height, sex, race, and smoking history.	The spirometer automatically takes these parameters into consideration when providing the results.
8. Ask the patient to remove any restrictive clothing, such as a necktie, and show the patient how to apply the nose clip.	Restrictive clothing can stop the chest from fully expanding, causing an inaccurate result. The nose clip stops air from being expelled from the nose during the test.

(continued)

PSY PROCEDURE 15-3: **Perform a Pulmonary Function Test (continued)**

Steps	Purpose
9. Ask the patient to stand, breathe in deeply, and blow into the mouthpiece as hard as possible. The patient should continue to blow into the mouthpiece until the machine indicates that it is appropriate to stop blowing. A chair should available in case the patient becomes dizzy or lightheaded.	Some machines signal to stop blowing with a buzz or beep; however, you may have to instruct the patient if the machine gives only a visual signal. Some patients become lightheaded during this procedure and should be observed closely for be signs of difficulty or imbalance.

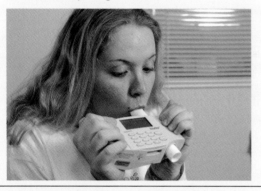

Step 9. The patient should blow into the mouthpiece as instructed.

Steps	Purpose
10. During the procedure, coach the patient as necessary to obtain an adequate reading.	Many patients feel that they have exhaled all air from the lungs when the machine is instructing them to continue. All air must be exhaled to obtain accurate results. The machine will indicate whether the reading or maneuver is adequate.
11. Continue the procedure until three adequate readings, or maneuvers, are performed.	Three maneuvers are usually required to obtain the patient's best result. The patient may rest between readings if necessary.
12. After printing the results, properly care for the equipment and dispose of the mouthpiece into the biohazard container. Wash your hands.	The mouthpiece may be contaminated and must be handled and discarded properly.
13. Document the procedure and place the printed results in the patient's medical record.	The three maneuvers will be recorded on one printout. Procedures are not considered to have been done if not properly recorded.

Charting Example:

06/12/2013 3:00 pm PFT performed for employment physical as ordered by Dr. John. ×3 maneuvers obtained without difficulty. Dr. John notified of results in chart——————————————————— J. Barker, CMA

Note: The medical assistant may sign his or her name in the patient record using only the "CMA" credential if the office has a signature log denoting the entire credential as "CMA(AAMA)."

You can play an important role in helping the patient to maintain healthy lungs and in assisting the physician to diagnose and treat respiratory disease. It is important that you remember that:

- Because the air that we breathe is open to the atmosphere, the respiratory system is susceptible to infection and irritant injury.
- Disorders of the respiratory system can affect either the upper respiratory system or the lower respiratory system.

- Chronic disorders of the respiratory system include emphysema and asthma, while acute disorders include sinusitis and the common cold.
- The peak flowmeter is used by patients at home to assess breathing, while a pulmonary function test is done in the office and gives the physician more information about the health of the lungs.
- Diagnosis of infectious respiratory infections can be done through the sputum culture.

Warm Ups   for Critical Thinking

1. Why do you think it is better to inhale through the nose than through the mouth?
2. Mr. Gardner, age 55 years, has been diagnosed with COPD and has many questions about his condition. Identify the characteristics of COPD. How do you explain this disease to Mr. Gardner?
3. Your patient has recently had an upper respiratory infection and was seen today for bronchitis. Why would the physician tell the patient to take the cough suppressant only at night? Use a drug reference book and look up some possible cough suppressants that might be ordered by the physician. Are there any precautions that the patient

should be made aware of before taking these medications?
4. The mother of an 8-year-old child with asthma tells you that the child has tested positive for an allergy to cats. Unfortunately, their family owns two cats. The mother tells you that she is reluctant to give the cats away since her son will "probably outgrow his asthma" according to a family friend whose daughter also has asthma. How would you respond? Could the allergy to cats trigger an asthma attack?
5. Develop a patient brochure on the effects of smoking. Investigate the products available for smoking cessation and include these in your brochure.

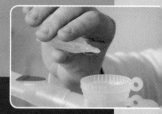

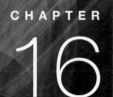

Outline

Common Disorders of the Cardiovascular System
Disorders of the Heart
Disorders of the Blood Vessels

Common Diagnostic and Therapeutic Procedures
Physical Examination of the Cardiovascular System
Electrocardiogram
Holter Monitor

Chest Radiography
Cardiac Stress Test
Echocardiography
Cardiac Catheterization and Coronary Arteriography

Learning Outcomes

Cognitive Domain

Note: AAMA/CAAHEP 2008 Standards are italicized.

1. Spell and define key terms
2. List and describe common cardiovascular disorders
3. Identify and explain common cardiovascular procedures and tests
4. Describe the roles and responsibilities of the medical assistant during cardiovascular examinations and procedures
5. Discuss the information recorded on a basic 12-lead electrocardiogram
6. Explain the purpose of a Holter monitor
7. *Identify common pathologies related to each body system*
8. *Describe implications for treatment related to pathology*

Psychomotor Domain

Note: AAMA/CAAHEP 2008 Standards are italicized.

1. *Perform electrocardiography (Procedure 16-1)*
2. Apply a Holter monitor for a 24-hour test (Procedure 16-2)
3. *Assist physician with patient care*
4. *Prepare a patient for procedures and/or treatments*
5. *Practice standard precautions*

6. *Document patient care*
7. *Document patient education*
8. *Practice within the standard of care for a medical assistant*

Affective Domain

Note: AAMA/CAAHEP 2008 Standards are italicized.

1. *Apply critical thinking skills in performing patient assessment and care*
2. *Use language/verbal skills that enable patients' understanding*
3. *Demonstrate empathy in communicating with patients, family, and staff*
4. *Use appropriate body language and other nonverbal skills in communicating with patients, family, and staff*
5. *Demonstrate awareness of the territorial boundaries of the person with whom you are communicating*
6. *Demonstrate sensitivity appropriate to the message being delivered*
7. *Demonstrate recognition of the patient's level of understanding in communications*
8. *Recognize and protect personal boundaries in communicating with others*
9. *Demonstrate respect for individual diversity, incorporating awareness of one's own biases in areas including gender, race, religion, age, and economic status*

10. *Apply active listening skills*
11. *Apply local, state, and federal health care legislation and regulation appropriate to the medical assisting practice setting*

ABHES Competencies

1. Assist the physician with the regimen of diagnostic and treatment modalities as they relate to each body system
2. Perform electrocardiograms
3. Comply with federal, state, and local health laws and regulations
4. Communicate on the recipient's level of comprehension
5. Serve as a liaison between the physician and others
6. Show empathy and impartiality when dealing with patients
7. Document accurately

Key Terms

aneurysm
angina pectoris
artifacts
atherosclerosis
bradycardia
cardiomegaly
cardiomyopathy
cerebrovascular

accident (CVA)
congestive heart failure
coronary artery bypass graft (CABG)
electrocardiography (ECG)
endocarditis

lead
myocardial infarction (MI)
myocarditis
palpitations
percutaneous transluminal coronary angioplasty (PTCA)

pericarditis
tachycardia
transient ischemic attack (TIA)

Cardiovascular disease is a major cause of illness and death. The cardiologist is a physician who specializes in disorders of the heart, and many patients with chronic cardiac conditions are referred to the cardiology office for treatment and follow-up. However, many of these patients are seen in internal medicine or family practice medical offices also. Because medical assistants see patients who have cardiovascular disorders regardless of the medical specialty, you must understand the cardiovascular system, associated disorders, and common tests and procedures that are ordered for diagnosis and treatment.

COG Common Disorders of the Cardiovascular System

The cardiovascular system consists of the heart (Fig. 16-1) and blood vessels, including the arteries, capillaries, and veins. The rhythmic contractions of the heart pump oxygen-rich blood from the lungs throughout the body to oxygenate and nourish the tissues and remove wastes for elimination. Although the heart and blood vessels are a closed system for the flow of blood (Fig. 16-2), disorders anywhere in this system may adversely affect other body systems that depend on the cardiovascular system for delivery of oxygen and nutrients. Depending on the body system affected by the lack of oxygen and nutrients being delivered, the following can be symptoms of various heart disorders:

- Chest pain
- Dyspnea
- Fatigue
- Diaphoresis
- Nausea and vomiting
- Irregular heartbeat
- Changes in peripheral circulation
- Edema
- Skin ulcers that do not heal
- Pain that increases with walking and decreases with rest
- Changes in skin color

Although some of these symptoms can indicate disorders not related to the heart or blood vessels, you should obtain an accurate history and chief complaint and communicate any finding to the physician through complete documentation.

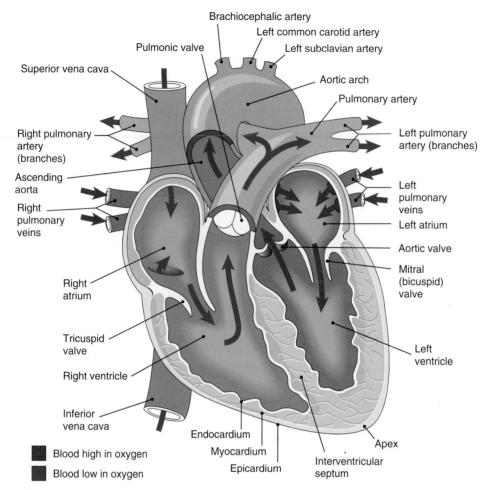

Figure 16-1 The heart and great vessels. (Reprinted with permission from Cohen BJ. Memmler's The Human Body in Health and Disease, 11th ed. Philadelphia: Lippincott Williams & Wilkins, 2009.)

Disorders of the Heart

Carditis

Cardiac inflammation, or carditis, may affect any of the layers of the heart muscle, and, although other factors may be involved, it is usually the result of a systemic infection. **Pericarditis**, an inflammation of the sac that covers the outside of the heart, may be acute or chronic. It is caused by a pathogen, neoplasm, or autoimmune disorder, such as systemic lupus erythematosus or rheumatoid arthritis. Other causes of pericarditis include certain chemicals, radiation, and uremia in patients with kidney failure. Signs and symptoms include a sharp pain in the same locations as with a **myocardial infarction (MI)**, except that pain increases on inspiration and on lying down but decreases on sitting up and leaning forward. Dyspnea, tachycardia, neck venous distention, pallor, and hypertension are warning signs that serous fluid is compressing the heart and interfering with cardiac function. Treatment is relieving the symptoms and, if possible, correcting the underlying cause, including administering an antibiotic for bacterial infection.

Myocarditis may be diffused through the heart muscle or may be local to a focal point. Causes include radiation, chemicals, and bacterial, viral, or parasitic infection. Signs and symptoms of early acute episodes are usually nonspecific, such as fatigue, fever, and mild chest pain. Chronic cases may lead to heart failure with **cardiomegaly** (an enlarged heart muscle), arrhythmias, and valvulitis. Treatment is supportive care and medication as ordered by the physician to kill the responsible pathogen.

Chronic or acute **endocarditis** is infection or inflammation of the inner lining of the heart, the endocardium. The lining of the heart and its valves may gather clusters of platelets, fibrin, and white blood cells to trap the pathogens. These clusters, called *vegetations*, may break away to become emboli that travel to the spleen, kidneys, lungs, or nervous system. These formations may also scar the valves and erode the chordae tendinea, small tendons that attach the heart valves to the ventricles. The destruction of these structures may result in reflux, or backflow, of the valves or blood. Diagnosis of endocarditis requires a blood culture to identify the

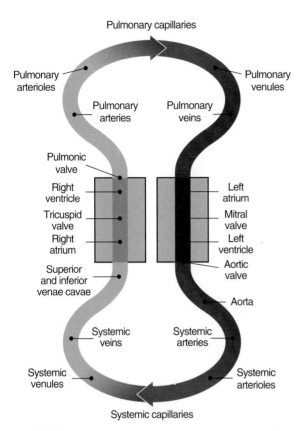

Pulmonary capillaries

Pulmonary
arterioles

Pulmonary
arteries

Pulmonary
venules

Pulmonary
veins

Pulmonic
valve

Right
ventricle

Tricuspid
valve

Right
atrium

Superior
and inferior
venae cavae

Left
atrium

Mitral
valve

Left
ventricle

Aortic
valve

Aorta

Systemic
veins

Systemic
arteries

Systemic
venules

Systemic
arterioles

Systemic capillaries

Figure 16-2 Blood vessels form a closed system for the flow of blood. Blood high in oxygen (oxygenated) is shown in red; blood low in oxygen (deoxygenated) is shown in blue. Changes in oxygen content occur as blood flows through capillaries. (Reprinted with permission from Cohen BJ. Memmler's The Human Body in Health and Disease, 11th ed. Philadelphia: Lippincott Williams & Wilkins, 2009.)

causative agent. Treatment is directed at eliminating the infecting organism.

 CHECKPOINT QUESTION

1. How does the pain in pericarditis differ from pain of myocardial infarction?

Congestive Heart Failure

Congestive heart failure (CHF) is a condition in which the heart cannot pump effectively. Failure of the right ventricle causes congestion of the peripheral extremities, while failure of the left ventricle leads to pulmonary congestion. Many patients have failure of both sides of the heart; their signs and symptoms include edema of the lower extremities and dyspnea. As blood flow to organs such as the brain and kidneys decreases, patients may also have complaints related to the organs

involved. Progressive heart failure results in damage to vital organs and death.

The causes of CHF include coronary artery disease, myocardial disease, valvular heart disease, and hypertension. While there is no cure for it, treatment is aimed at relieving symptoms and preventing permanent damage to vital organs. Medications given to CHF patients include drugs to increase cardiac function and decrease edema.

Myocardial Infarction

Death of any part of the heart muscle, called *myocardial infarction*, occurs when one or more of the coronary arteries becomes totally occluded, usually by atherosclerotic plaques or by an embolism. An MI may occur suddenly without prior symptoms or in patients with diagnosed atherosclerotic coronary artery disease. Symptoms of myocardial infarction may be similar to those felt during **angina pectoris** in patients with ischemic heart disease, but this disorder is distinguished by pain that lasts longer than 20 to 30 minutes and is unrelieved by rest. Box 16-1 describes criteria that the physician will use to distinguish the chest pain of angina pectoris from the chest pain of MI. Other symptoms include nausea, diaphoresis, weakness, vomiting, and abdominal cramps. The patient may complain of feeling a viselike grip around the chest cavity. The skin may become cool, clammy, and pale, and the patient may feel anxiety or impending doom. Some patients have nonspecific symptoms such as indigestion and therefore do not seek medical attention. In 20% of patients, the MI may be silent, diagnosed only by routine **electrocardiography (ECG)**. It is imperative not to ignore or dismiss complaints by patients with symptoms of MI or to accept the patient's own diagnosis that "It's only indigestion." Although the death of myocardial tissue that occurs during an MI cannot be reversed, early medical intervention may reduce the amount of tissue that dies and increase the patient's chances of survival. Procedures such as **percutaneous transluminal coronary angioplasty (PTCA)** and **coronary artery bypass graft (CABG)** are performed to increase blood flow to the cardiac muscle (Box 16-2).

 CHECKPOINT QUESTION

2. Why is it important to treat a patient with myocardial infarction as early as possible?

Cardiac Arrhythmia

When the electrical conduction system of the heart is not functioning normally, cardiac arrhythmias may develop and can be detected on the electrocardiography. Cardiac arrhythmia or dysrhythmia is an abnormal

---

BOX 16-1

IS IT ANGINA OR MYOCARDIAL INFARCTION?

The pain felt with angina and MI is brought about by myocardial anoxia, or an increased need for oxygen to the heart muscle because of exertion, stress, or extremes of heat or cold. Typically, angina is relieved by rest or nitroglycerin, a vasodilator. However, pain from an MI is not relieved by these measures. The following is a brief comparison of these two disorders:

	Angina	Myocardial Infarction
Description	Moderate pressure deep in the chest; squeezing, suffocating feeling	Severe deep pressure not relieved by reducing stressors; crushing pressure
Onset	Pain gradual or sudden; subsides quickly, usually in less than 30 minutes; can be relieved by nitroglycerin, rest, or reducing stressors	Pain sudden; remains after stressors reduced or relieved; not relieved by nitroglycerin
Location	Mid-anterior chest, usually diffuse, radiates to back, neck, arms, jaw, and epigastric area	Mid-anterior chest with same radiating patterns
Signs and symptoms	Dyspnea, nausea, signs of indigestion, profuse sweating	Nausea, vomiting, fear, diaphoresis, pounding heart, palpitations

Any patient who calls the medical office complaining of chest pain must be examined immediately. The office should have an established protocol for handling these calls. The physician must be consulted to decide whether the patient should be directed to the nearest emergency department or come directly to the office.

---

heart rhythm that may occur as a primary disorder or as a response to a systemic problem. Arrhythmia may also be a reaction to a drug toxicity or an electrolyte imbalance. Normally, the sinoatrial (SA) node is the pacemaker of the heart (Fig. 16-3), initiating an electrical impulse in the adult at rest 60 to 100 times a minute. This is sinus rhythm. Arrhythmia may occur if the SA node initiates electrical impulses too fast or too slowly. If the SA node is damaged or the conduction pathway is blocked, the heart will beat too slowly to meet the body's demands. This type of arrhythmia, called **bradycardia**, is characterized by a heart rate less than 60 beats per minute. If the SA node initiates an electrical impulse faster than 100 times per minute, the arrhythmia is called **tachycardia**.

More serious arrhythmias occur when the ventricles beat too fast, a condition known as *ventricular tachycardia (VT)*. This condition occurs when some of the electrical signals originate in the ventricles rather than in the SA node. Once the ventricles begin to beat at a very rapid rate, less blood is pumped out of the heart with each contraction, since the heart's chambers do not have time to fill with blood before the next contraction begins. As less blood is pumped into circulation, less oxygen is carried to the tissues. This lack of adequate blood and oxygen may cause dizziness, unconsciousness, or cardiac arrest.

Another arrhythmia is ventricular fibrillation. Ventricular fibrillation is a medical emergency that occurs when the heart is quivering rather than contracting in an organized fashion. In this condition, very little blood is pumped out of the heart, and the patient will fall unconscious and die very quickly unless a shock with a cardiac defibrillator is administered immediately to restore normal cardiac electrical activity. Automatic external defibrillators (AED) are now available in many medical offices and public places, such as airports and shopping malls. All professional medical assistants should receive certification in cardiopulmonary resuscitation (CPR) and use of the AED, which is relatively easy to operate (Box 16-3). Patients who require frequent defibrillation may benefit from the insertion of an implantable cardiac defibrillator that will automatically deliver an electrical shock to restore normal cardiac conduction. These devices should not be confused with cardiac pacemakers, which help to regulate the normal rhythm of the heart.

Artifical Pacemakers

When a patient's heart conduction system cannot maintain normal sinus rhythm without assistance, an electrical source can be implanted to assist or replace the sinoatrial node. The permanent or temporary artificial pacemaker is surgically implanted either between the chest wall and the rib cage or within the chest cavity (Fig. 16-4). The pacemaker may be programmed to fire, or initiate an electrical charge, continuously at a predetermined rate or on demand,

BOX 16-2

CORRECTIVE CARDIAC SURGERY

The least traumatic form of cardiac surgery is the *PTCA*. A double-lumen catheter with a balloon surrounding the upper portion is inserted into a vessel in the groin or axilla. This catheter is threaded into the coronary vessels, with the surgeon watching a fluoroscopic screen while performing the procedure. When the occlusion is found, the balloon is inflated to press the atherosclerotic plaque against the arterial walls and relieve the occlusion. A laser may be used to remove the plaque. A spring or mesh (called a *stent*) may be inserted and left in place within the vessel to maintain patency. This procedure is less invasive than bypass surgery, but occasionally the artery rebuilds plaque at the site, or the stent may fill with plaque and the artery may occlude again.

CABG is performed by grafting a piece of vessel from another part of the body to the area beyond the occlusion and to the ascending aorta, providing a patent passage for the blood. The surgery requires a still field of surgery, so the heart must be stopped and the patient supported by a cardiopulmonary bypass machine for the length of the operation. The saphenous vein may be used for multiple bypasses; the internal mammary artery is used if the surgery is not extensive. Hospitalization may be as long as 5 to 7 days, and 20% of patients develop a repeat thrombus within 1 year.

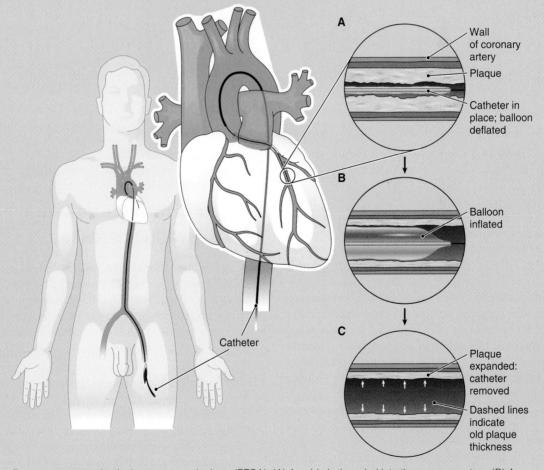

Percutaneous transluminal coronary angioplasty (PTCA). (A) A guide is threaded into the coronary artery. (B) A balloon catheter is inserted through the occlusion. (C) The balloon is inflated and deflated until plaque is flattened and the vessel is opened.

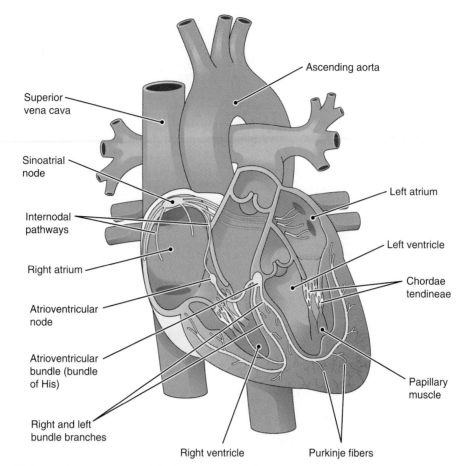

Figure 16-3 Conduction system of the heart. (Reprinted with permission from Cohen BJ. Memmler's The Human Body in Health and Disease, 11th ed. Philadelphia: Lippincott Williams & Wilkins, 2009.)

only when the patient's normal heart rate falls below a preset number.

Pacemaker programming initially occurs when the pacemaker is inserted in an outpatient or inpatient surgical facility. If additional programming or assessment is necessary, the pacemaker may be evaluated by telephone monitoring: the patient uses the telephone receiver to transmit the rate and function of the pacemaker to a physician at the receiving site. If battery function is failing and replacement is not possible or advisable, batteries can be recharged transdermally. A charging unit is placed over the implantation site and plugged into an ordinary electrical outlet. The power cell is recharged through the skin with no discomfort to the patient. Pacemakers are battery operated and usually are manufactured to retain their charge for up to 20 years. Recharging or changing the battery in an implanted pacemaker usually requires an outpatient surgical procedure under a local anesthetic.

 CHECKPOINT QUESTION

3. Which two cardiac arrhythmias are emergencies requiring immediate intervention by the medical assistant?

 PATIENT EDUCATION

NITROGLYCERIN

A medication commonly prescribed to increase blood flow to the cardiac muscle is nitroglycerin, a vasodilator. Vasodilators open the lumen of vessels, increasing blood supply to the heart muscle. Patient education should include the following instructions:

- Keep the medication in the dark bottle supplied by the pharmacy because nitroglycerin can be deactivated if exposed to light.
- Be alert for any side effects, such as lightheadedness, syncope, and hypotension. Caution patients not to drive or operate other machinery until these symptoms have passed.
- Be aware that nitroglycerin may be prescribed and dispensed as either tablets or a spray to be used as needed, or it may be ordered as a transdermal patch worn constantly to maintain vasodilation. The usual administration guidelines are for three doses at 5-minute intervals. If pain persists, the patient should be advised to call for emergency medical services.

- Patients with arthritis or visual impairment should use nitroglycerin spray. These patients may find the spray easier to use than tablets, since the tablets are very small.
- Check the expiration date of the medication frequently, and always have an adequate supply available at home and when traveling.
- Encourage patients prescribed nitroglycerin to obtain and wear a Medic Alert bracelet or necklace. In the event of an emergency, first responders can assist with administering this medication if necessary.
- Ensure that the medication is kept out of the reach of children.

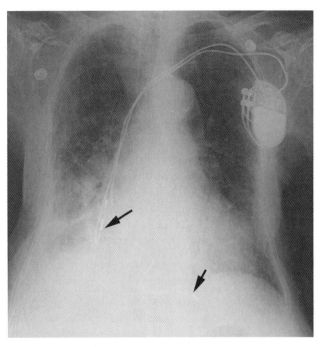

Figure 16-4 Chest x-ray of an intracardiac pacemaker showing the leads (*arrows*) in the right atrium and right ventricle. (From Richard H. Daffner, Clinical Radiology The Essentials, 3rd Edition. Philadelphia: Lippincott Williams & Wilkins, 2007.)

BOX 16-3

THE AUTOMATIC EXTERNAL DEFIBRILLATOR

The automatic external defibrillator (AED) is becoming more widely supplied in public places and medical offices because of the minimal training required and potential to save the life of a patient with sudden cardiac arrest without waiting for emergency medical services or transportation to a hospital.

The device is a small defibrillator in a zippered bag that is usually orange or red with the acronym *AED* written clearly on the front. Inside the bag are also disposable chest pads connected to a cord that is inserted into the connection on the AED. A small washcloth for drying the skin before placing the chest pads if necessary, disposable razor to shave excess chest hair, and examination gloves in the event of possible exposure to blood or other body fluids during the procedure may be added to the AED bag because these items may be necessary to ensure adequate contact between the patient's skin and the chest pads.

In the event that an unconscious patient or victim is found with no pulse (refer to cardiopulmonary resuscitation criteria), the rescuer should apply the chest pads as trained, and using the pictures provided on the pads as a guide, connect the cable to the machine and turn the machine on. The machine has verbal commands to guide the user through the steps necessary to provide an electrical shock if necessary. Do not touch or move the patient while the machine is analyzing the patient's cardiac rhythm or when the machine determines that an electrical shock is necessary.

Congenital and Valvular Heart Disease

Valvular disease is an acquired or congenital abnormality of any of the four cardiac valves. Valvular heart disease is characterized by stenosis and obstructed blood flow or by valvular degeneration and backflow of the blood against the course of the circulatory pathway. The valves in the left side of the heart are most often affected. The most common congenital valve diseases include atrial septal defect (ASD), ventricular septal defect (VSD), patent ductus arteriosus (PDA), coarctation of the aorta, aortic or pulmonic stenosis, bicuspid aortic valve, mitral valve prolapse, and tetralogy of Fallot (Table 16-1).

Rheumatic heart disease, an acquired valvular disease, presents clinically as a generalized inflammatory disease occurring 10 to 21 days after an upper respiratory infection caused by group A beta-hemolytic streptococci. It is characterized by inflammatory lesions of the connective tissues, particularly in the heart, joints, and subcutaneous tissues. The heart valves are damaged by an abnormal response of the immune system caused by the turbulence of the infected blood. This damage results in a systolic murmur. Although it usually attacks children aged 5 to 15, rheumatic heart disease has declined significantly since the 1940s.

Mitral valve stenosis, a condition that occurs when the leaflet cusps of the mitral valve fuse and thicken, may result from rheumatic heart disease. When the valve cusps thicken and fuse, the result is an abnormally

TABLE 16-1	Diseases of the Cardiac Valves and Congenital Cardiac Defects	
Disorder	Description	Treatment
ASD	Abnormal opening between atria, allowing unoxygenated blood in right atrium to mix with oxygenated blood in left atrium; congenital	Surgery to close
VSD	Abnormal opening between ventricles, allowing unoxygenated blood in right ventricle to mix with oxygenated blood in left ventricle; congenital	Surgery to close
PDA	Abnormal opening between pulmonary artery and aorta; congenital	Surgery to close
Coarctation of the aorta	Narrowing of the aorta resulting in high blood pressure in upper extremities and low blood pressure in lower extremities; congenital	Surgery to increase diameter of aorta
Bicuspid aortic valve	Aortic valve having two cusps instead of three, resulting in incomplete closure between aorta and left ventricle during systole and diastole; congenital	Surgical replacement of aortic valve
Aortic or pulmonic stenosis	Narrowing of aortic or pulmonary artery valve leaflets, causing overwork of cardiac muscle and hypertrophy of ventricles; as stenosis increases, valve becomes less flexible	Dilation of stenosed area or surgical replacement of valve
MVP	Drooping of one or both cusps of mitral (bicuspid) valve into left ventricle during systole, resulting in incomplete closure of valve and backflow of blood from left ventricle into left atrium	Usually benign; treatment is alleviating any symptoms (palpations, chest pain); prophylactic antibiotic may be ordered before dental procedures
Tetralogy of Fallot	Four defects: pulmonary stenosis, dextraposition of aorta, ventricular septal defect, and hypertrophy of right ventricle; congenital	Surgery to correct

narrow valve; hence mitral regurgitation, or backflow, of blood from the left ventricle into the left atrium occurs. Patients with mitral stenosis often have dyspnea, or shortness of breath, and their ability to exert themselves physically may be limited. Pulmonary edema may also develop and cause symptoms such as dyspnea and a productive cough.

Treatment of valvular disease depends on the type and severity of the abnormality. Severe cases may require medication, low-sodium diet, and prophylactic antibiotic before surgery or dental work. If medication is not successful, surgical replacement of the involved valves may be necessary.

 CHECKPOINT QUESTION

4. What microorganism may be responsible for rheumatic heart disease and cardiac valvular damage?

Disorders of the Blood Vessels

Atherosclerosis

Diseases of blood vessels—arteries or veins—often begin with collection of fatty plaques made of calcium and cholesterol inside the walls of the vessels. These plaques narrow the lumen, or opening, of the blood vessels and impede blood flow. This condition, which is known as **atherosclerosis**, is problematic in arteries because oxygen and nutrients are prevented from reaching various tissues of the body. In addition to the occlusion that occurs with atherosclerosis, the plaques are rougher than the walls of a normal artery and may remain stationary as a thrombus or break away from the wall of the artery as an embolus (Fig. 16-5). Signs and symptoms of atherosclerosis usually result from ischemia to a body part and may include pain or numbness, loss of normal blood flow, or loss of a palpable pulse to the affected body area.

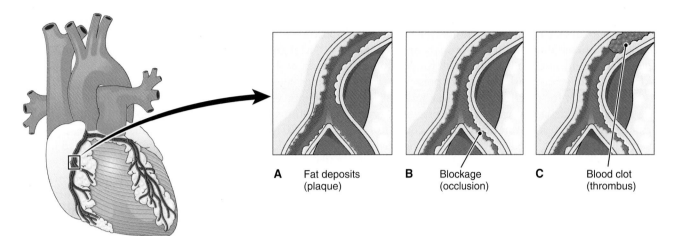

Figure 16-5 Coronary atherosclerosis. (**A**) Fat deposits narrow an artery, leading to ischemia. (**B**) Blockage of the coronary artery. (**C**) Formation of a blood clot (thrombus), leading to MI. (Reprinted with permission from Cohen BJ. Memmler's The Human Body in Health and Disease, 11th ed. Philadelphia: Lippincott Williams & Wilkins, 2009.)

If the coronary arteries are involved, the condition is coronary artery disease (CAD), the most common type of heart disease and the leading cause of death in men and women in the United States. Patients with CAD may have the following symptoms:

- Angina pectoris (pain radiating to the arm, jaw, shoulder, back, or neck, usually felt on exertion and relieved by rest)
- Pressure or fullness in the chest, felt most severely during exertion and relieved by rest
- Syncope (fainting)
- Edema of the extremities, especially the legs
- Unexplained cough, generally without respiratory symptoms
- Excessive fatigue
- Dyspnea

Predisposing conditions for atherosclerosis and coronary artery disease (CAD) include a diet high in saturated fats and a family history of hypercholesterolemia. Other risk factors include cigarette smoking, diabetes mellitus, and hypertension. Consuming a diet low in cholesterol and saturated fats, participating in a moderate exercise program, maintaining normal body weight and blood pressure, and not smoking may minimize the chances for developing atherosclerosis and CAD or reduce the progression if a diagnosis has been made. If necessary, the physician may order lipid-lowering medication for patients whose blood cholesterol and triglyceride levels are not affected by dietary or other behavioral changes.

Diagnosis of atherosclerosis is often made by angiography to locate the occlusion and evaluate the degree of obstruction (Fig. 16-6). In this procedure, a catheter is inserted into the blood vessel, and radiographic images are taken as a contrast medium is injected into the vessel. The radiographs are evaluated for the presence and amount of plaque buildup or the presence of a thrombus. Doppler ultrasonography, a test that uses sound waves to produce an image of the blood vessel, may also be ordered to detect atherosclerosis. Doppler ultrasonography, or echocardiography, can be used to determine the ability of the heart to fill and pump blood. This noninvasive test uses sound waves to produce a picture of the heart on a video monitor to detect areas of poor blood flow or damaged muscle.

A relatively new noninvasive test for CAD is cardiac calcium scoring using electron beam computed

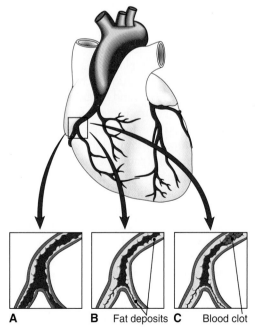

Figure 16-6 Atherosclerotic coronary occlusion. (Reprinted with permission from Rubin E, Farber JL. Pathology. Philadelphia: Lippincott Williams & Wilkins, 2005.)

tomography (CT). In this procedure, CT of the coronary arteries using an electron beam identifies the amount of fat and calcium buildup within the coronary arteries. An elevated score indicates an increased risk for developing CAD, especially if other risk factors are present.

The treatment for atherosclerosis often includes lifestyle changes, as described earlier, to reverse or prevent further atherosclerotic formations. If the condition is severe, lipid-lowering medication may be prescribed. Surgery to remove the plaque or improve blood flow through an artery may also be indicated for some patients. Your responsibilities will include coordinating diagnostic procedures based on the physician's orders and insurance requirements and teaching patients about behaviors that can prevent atherosclerosis and CAD. Patients diagnosed with atherosclerosis and CAD require emotional support to encourage compliance with medication and lifestyle changes, such as diet and exercise.

 CHECKPOINT QUESTION

5. What are four predisposing factors for heart disease?

Hypertension

Patients with a resting systolic blood pressure above 140 mm Hg and a diastolic pressure above 90 mm Hg are said to be hypertensive. Hypertension cannot be diagnosed on the basis of one blood pressure measurement, since other factors, such as emotional upset or anxiety, may cause a temporary increase in blood pressure. Since many factors may affect the blood pressure, the physician often requires several blood pressure readings before making the diagnosis of hypertension. Once a diagnosis of hypertension is made, you may play a major role in assisting with the control of this condition by regularly monitoring the patient's blood pressure and medication prescriptions; teaching the patient about dietary and lifestyle changes, such as smoking cessation and weight loss; and recording complete and accurate information regarding the medical history each time the patient visits the office. Refer to Table 4-6 in Chapter 4 for more information regarding blood pressure readings and what constitutes normal, prehypertension, and hypertension I and II.

One type of hypertension, essential hypertension, is a major cause of stroke and renal failure and is a major consequence of atherosclerosis anywhere in the circulatory system. The long-term effects of essential hypertension may include weakening of the arteries throughout the body and enlargement of the left ventricle of the heart. Left ventricular hypertrophy, or enlargement, occurs gradually as the heart works harder to overcome the higher pressure in the arteries. Essential hypertension is often called a "silent killer" because the disease is gradual and

frequently produces no symptoms in the patient, striking anyone regardless of age, race, sex, or ethnic origin.

Malignant hypertension is severe and sudden in onset and is most common in African-American men under age 40 years regardless of other risk factors. Patients with malignant hypertension have signs and symptoms including diastolic blood pressure greater than 120 mm Hg and blurred vision, headache, and possibly confusion. The physician should be notified immediately if these symptoms are present.

While the cause of essential hypertension may be unknown, its correlation with an elevated serum cholesterol level has been shown. After diagnosis, some patients can control the high blood pressure with a low-sodium, low-fat diet, an exercise program, weight reduction if needed, and antihypertensive and lipid-reducing medications. Diuretic medication may be prescribed to reduce the amount of sodium in the body, which in turn reduces the total fluid volume. The decrease in fluid volume reduces strain on the heart and blood vessels. Patients should also be informed of methods to reduce the cholesterol and triglycerides in their diet.

Patients who have been prescribed antihypertensive medications should be instructed to take that medication as prescribed. Many patients feel that because their blood pressure has reached a manageable level, they do not need to continue the prescribed medication. Explain that the medication is the cause of the lowered blood pressure and that discontinuing the treatment without consulting the physician may jeopardize their recovery.

 CHECKPOINT QUESTION

6. What two disorders may result from untreated hypertension?

Varicose Veins

Varicosities, the most common circulatory disease of the lower extremities, occur when the superficial veins of the legs swell and distend (Fig. 16-7). Eventually the valves in the veins fail to close properly, allowing blood to pool and stretch the walls of the veins. People who sit or stand for long periods without moving or contracting their leg muscles are predisposed to varicose veins. A hereditary weakness in the vein walls is also a predisposing factor. Varicosities may also be secondary to deep vein thrombosis. Signs and symptoms of varicose veins are swelling, aching, and a feeling of heaviness in the legs. Varicosities may also be asymptomatic. Many patients consider varicose veins unattractive and seek treatment even without symptoms.

Treatment of varicose veins is usually conservative, with instructions to avoid standing or sitting for long periods to reduce symptoms and prevent the development of further varicosities. Other helpful measures that may be

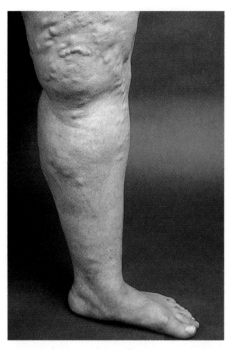

Figure 16-7 Varicose veins of the lower extremities. (Reprinted with permission from Bickley LS, Szilagy PG. Bates' Guide to Physical Examination and History Taking. Philadelphia: Lippincott Williams & Wilkins, 2003.)

ordered by the physician include wearing elastic support stockings or wrapping the legs with elastic bandages and elevating the legs for specified periods. Surgery to remove the veins is usually the last approach. Another treatment technique is injection of a sclerosing agent into small varicose vein segments, but this is not suggested for large areas.

Venous Thrombosis and Pulmonary Embolism

Thrombi, or blood clots, in the peripheral or pulmonary veins commonly affect patients with underlying cardiovascular disease. Risk factors for developing thrombi may be either primary (inherited) or secondary (acquired). Primary causes include hemolytic anemia and sickle cell disease, and secondary factors include long-term immobility, chronic pulmonary disease, thrombophlebitis, varicosities, and defibrillation after cardiac arrest. Chemical contraceptives for women have also been implicated in a higher risk of developing thrombi in young women who have none of the usual predisposing factors. The risk increases in women who smoke. A thrombus in the peripheral venous circulatory system may dislodge and become an embolus. This embolus is dangerous to the patient, since the blood clot can lodge in the pulmonary circulation (causing a pulmonary embolism), the cardiac circulation (causing MI), or the cerebral circulation (causing a **cerebrovascular accident [CVA]**).

Peripheral vascular occlusion may also lead to stasis ulcers, which are caused by breakdown of the skin and

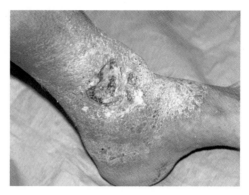

Figure 16-8 Stasis dermatitis with venous stasis ulcer. (From Goodheart HP, MD. Goodheart's Photoguide of Common Skin Disorders, 2nd Edition. Philadelphia: Lippincott Williams & Wilkins, 2003.)

underlying tissue due to inadequate circulation to the area. These ulcers develop as deep red discolorations, itching, edema, and large areas of scaling skin leading to fissures and ulcers (Fig. 16-8). Increasing circulation to the lower extremities with use of support stockings, weight reduction, and elevating the limbs may prevent formation of these ulcers.

A blood clot lodged in the pulmonary circulation is a pulmonary embolism. Signs and symptoms of a pulmonary embolism include dyspnea, syncope, and severe pleuritic chest pain with respiration. Diagnosis may include chest radiography, an electrocardiogram, a lung scan, or a pulmonary arteriogram. Doppler studies are used to diagnose deep vein thrombosis. Depending on the severity, treatment may include bed rest with elevation of the affected extremity, anticoagulant medication such as coumadin, or surgery.

 CHECKPOINT QUESTION

7. What disease occurs when the superficial veins in the legs become swollen and distended?

 PATIENT EDUCATION

ANTICOAGULANT THERAPY

Patients with certain types of cardiac problems are prescribed anticoagulant medications, commonly called *blood thinners*, which are used to decrease the risk of a thrombus or embolus developing. Coumadin is a common oral anticoagulant. Lovenox™, another anticoagulant, is given as an injection. Teach patients who are prescribed anticoagulants as follows:

• Monitor the mouth, urine, and stool for any signs of bleeding.

(continued)

- Use a soft-bristle toothbrush.
- Call the office if any signs of bleeding occur.
- Avoid injuries and falls while taking anticoagulant medications.
- Be aware that needlesticks from injections or venipuncture require prolonged application of pressure afterward to control bleeding and bruising.
- Comply with orders for blood work. Anticoagulant medications necessitate frequent tests for blood counts and bleeding times.
- Limit the intake of foods high in vitamin K (asparagus, cabbage, fish, broccoli, cheese, pork, spinach, cauliflower, and rice). These patients should be given a printed flyer on dietary restrictions.
- Avoid taking over-the-counter (OTC) medications containing aspirin or ibuprofen without consulting the physician. These drugs may cause an increase in bleeding times, interfering with the actions of the anticoagulant.
- Take the medication at the same time every day. If a dose is missed, take it as soon as it is remembered that day, but do not take a double dose.

Cerebrovascular Accident

CVA, sometimes called *stroke*, results suddenly when damage to the blood vessels in the brain occurs. The damage blocks the circulation, resulting in ischemia, or lack of oxygen, to that part of the brain. Brain tissue dies without adequate oxygen. A common cause of CVA is blockage of the cerebral artery by thrombus or embolus. Hemorrhage, atherosclerotic heart disease, and hypertension are additional causes of CVAs. Unfortunately, CVAs are the most common nervous system disorder in the elderly and one of the leading causes of death in the United States.

Patients who have CVAs usually have varying degrees of weakness or paralysis of one side of the body, with possible involvement of language and comprehension. Symptoms vary according to which artery and which part of the brain is affected. CVAs are fatal when vital centers of the brain are damaged. Once the brain tissue is damaged by a CVA, treatment is aimed at reducing further death of cerebrovascular tissue and assisting the patient to regain any affected function. Patients who have CVAs need many months of rehabilitation, including physical therapy, occupational therapy, and speech therapy. You must remember that, although these patients may not be able to communicate effectively with you, they are capable of understanding and should be treated with respect, dignity, and compassion.

Ischemia to small areas of the brain over short periods is known as **transient ischemic attack (TIA)**. TIA, or mini-stroke, should be considered a warning sign for a possible impending cerebrovascular accident. TIAs may be caused by atherosclerotic plaques narrowing the arteries supplying blood to the brain, a small embolus that reduces the flow of blood to an area, or spasms of the blood vessels. The symptoms vary according to the arteries affected but usually include the following:

- Mild numbness or tingling in the face or a limb
- Difficulty swallowing
- Coughing and choking
- Slurred speech
- Unilateral visual disturbance
- Dizziness

As many as 50% to 80% of patients who exhibit symptoms of TIAs progress to a stroke. The signs of a major stroke may begin as a TIA and progress to loss of consciousness, hyperpnea (deep, gasping breaths), anisocoria (unequal pupils), and hemiplegia (unilateral paralysis). Any patient who has the signs and symptoms of a TIA or a CVA should be sent to the emergency room following all physician instructions and office policies.

Aneurysm

Weakened blood vessel walls are predisposed to abnormal dilation. Dilation in the form of an **aneurysm** may occur in any vessel, but arteries are most often affected (Fig. 16-9A–C). Because of the high pressure so close to the heart, the aorta is the most common site. The normally elastic vessel wall develops a ballooning effect in one or many forms, all of them dangerous:

- A *dissecting aneurysm* tears the inner walls of the artery and allows blood to leak into the lining of the vessel; the wall will eventually die and tear open.
- A *sacculated aneurysm* balloons from the arterial wall into a sac, which may burst.
- A *berry aneurysm* is usually a congenital defect in a cerebral artery.

Causes of aneurysms include trauma, hypertension, atherosclerosis, certain fungal infections, syphilis, and congenital defects. Symptoms include pain or pressure at the site. Death may occur quickly if the tear is not repaired. Diagnosis is based on a thorough history and examination, an arteriogram or aortogram, computed tomography, or magnetic resonance imaging. Surgical resection is the only option.

 CHECKPOINT QUESTION

8. What is the physiologic reason for a stroke?

Anemia

Deficiencies in hemoglobin or in the numbers of red blood cells result in anemia. Anemia is not considered

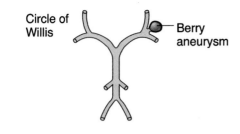

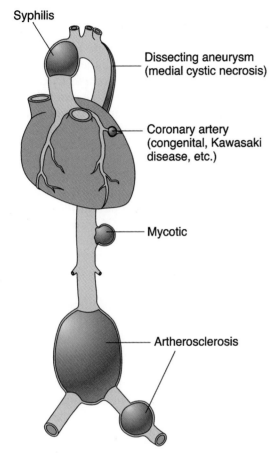

Figure 16-9 The locations of aneurysms. (Reprinted with permission from Rubin's Pathology: Clinicopathologic Foundations of Medicine. Philadelphia: Lippincott Williams & Wilkins, 2005.)

a disease but is a symptom of an underlying disorder. Anemia can result from any of the following:

- Blood loss due to hemorrhage or slow internal bleeding
- A diet low in iron or a malabsorption condition (nutritional anemia)
- Suppressed (by chemotherapeutic medication) or diseased bone marrow, resulting in decreased blood cell formation (aplastic anemia)
- Vitamin B12 deficiency due to a lack of intrinsic factor (pernicious anemia)
- Genetic abnormality (sickle cell anemia, thalassemia)
- Destruction of functioning red blood cells by various means, such as liver or spleen dysfunction or toxins (hemolytic anemia)

Symptoms of anemia may include cardiovascular alterations such as tachycardia and pallor, anorexia and weight loss, dyspnea on exertion, and fatigue. Treatment of anemia must address the cause; it can include increasing dietary iron, blood transfusions, and injection of vitamin B12 (cyanocobalamin) on a regular basis. Aplastic anemia may require a bone marrow transplantation. Unfortunately, genetic abnormalities, such as sickle cell anemia and thalassemia, cannot be corrected at this time.

COG Common Diagnostic and Therapeutic Procedures

Testing for cardiovascular disorders may be either invasive or noninvasive. Invasive techniques require entering the body by the use of a tube, needle, or other device. Noninvasive techniques do not require entering the body or puncturing the skin. Depending on the patient's symptoms, testing may be basic and can be done easily during the general physical examination by auscultating the heart and chest cavity. Additional tests the physician may order that you perform in the medical office can include chest radiography or 12-lead ECG. Sometimes initial findings indicate the need for a more sophisticated procedure, such as cardiac catheterization, which is performed at an outpatient surgical center or hospital.

Physical Examination of the Cardiovascular System

The cardiovascular examination is the most basic noninvasive procedure used to assess the heart and blood vessels. When preparing a patient for a cardiovascular examination, you will obtain vital information, including accurate determination of weight, blood pressure, heart and respiratory rates, body temperature, and cardiovascular history. It is also important to obtain a complete list of the patient's medications and current dosages, including any herbal and vitamin supplements and OTC medications. A brief social and family history should include lifestyle and familial risk factors for cardiovascular disorders. The patient should be questioned regarding a history of smoking tobacco, alcohol intake, family history of heart disease, hypercholesterolemia, diet, and exercise. Specifically, you should ask the following questions to elicit important information from a patient with cardiovascular problems:

- Why are you seeing the cardiologist or physician today?
- What symptoms have you been having?
- How long have you had the pain, discomfort, distress, or unusual sensations? (Patients may not think of chest discomfort as a cardiac symptom.)
- Where is the pain or discomfort? Does it stay in one place or radiate in any direction?

- Is the pain associated with any other symptoms, such as shortness of breath, nausea, weakness, sweating, or dizziness?
- If you have been short of breath, does it restrict any of your activities or require you to sleep on additional pillows at night?
- Are you a smoker?
- Do you drink alcoholic beverages?

As you proceed with the interview, keep in mind that patients with cardiovascular problems are usually understandably anxious and concerned. They may bring with them family members who are also concerned or anxious. It is your responsibility to help ease apprehension and to offer reassurance and support when appropriate.

The physician or cardiologist usually begins the examination with a review of the patient's history and reason for the office visit. The physician also reviews the patient's vital signs and medications, noting any allergies to medications and other substances. The physician inspects the patient to evaluate the general appearance, noting the circulation and any swelling of the extremities, color of the skin, and jugular vein distention. Palpation is used to evaluate the efficiency of the circulatory pathways and peripheral pulses. Using auscultation with a stethoscope, the physician can evaluate the sounds made as blood flows through the heart and the valves open and close. Abnormal heart sounds, such as bruits and murmurs, may be detected (Box 16-4).

In addition to obtaining important information and data before the physician examines the patient, you must also provide instructions and materials for proper

gown wearing and draping. After the examination, the physician may order an ECG, which you will perform and give to the physician for diagnosis.

CHECKPOINT QUESTION

9. What is a heart murmur?

 ## Electrocardiogram

One of the most valuable diagnostic tools for evaluating the electrical pathway through the heart is the electrocardiogram, known by the acronym ECG or EKG. The ECG is the graphic record of the electrical current as it progresses through the heart. It can be performed as part of a routine physical examination or as needed for a patient with chest pain, discomfort, or other signs and symptoms of possible cardiac problems. During the ECG, you are responsible for explaining the procedure to the patient and applying combinations of electrodes, called **leads**, on the patient's limbs and precordial area (anterior chest). ECGs are used to assist in diagnosing ischemia, delays in impulse conduction, hypertrophy of the cardiac chambers, and arrhythmias. They are not used to detect anatomic disorders, such as heart murmurs.

The ECG tracing is printed on graph paper that is either blue or black with a heat-labile white coating. Graph lines are printed over the white coating, appearing as small blocks with thicker lines outlining every five small blocks. On standard ECG paper, each small block is 1 mm^2. The large blocks are 5 mm^2 (Fig. 16-10A). Some older ECG machines contain a stylus that heats and melts the white coating, exposing the dark background beneath to record the movement of the stylus as the electrical impulses are detected. Newer ECG machines dispense ink from a cartridge into the stylus to mark the ECG tracing paper. The ECG paper may be affected by pressure as well as heat and should be handled carefully to prevent extraneous markings. Each small horizontal block represents time (0.04 seconds), and the vertical small blocks represent voltage (0.1 millivolts). After the heart's electrical markings are traced on the paper, the heart rate and time required for the electrical impulses to spread through the heart can be determined (Fig. 16-10B).

ECG Leads

Over the years, a standard system of electrode placement has evolved, and nomenclature has been developed for the recordings from different electrode combinations. Each lead records the electrical impulse through the heart from a different angle. Viewing the conduction of the electrical impulses in these various angles gives the physician a fairly complete view of the entire heart.

BOX 16-4

ABNORMAL HEART SOUNDS

Abnormal heart sounds, called *murmurs*, are sounds the blood makes as it courses through the heart valves. The sounds vary with the severity and location of the abnormality. For instance, they may blow, rasp, rub, bubble, whistle, whoosh, and/or click. A murmur is not a disease, but it may indicate organic heart disease.

Functional murmurs may only occur during elevations in body temperature or during times of physical stress and are not usually a cause for concern. *Organic murmurs* indicate structural abnormalities of varying degrees and are always present. A cardiologist evaluates the murmur by noting its location in the heart, when it occurs in the cardiac cycle, how long it lasts, and its characteristic sound.

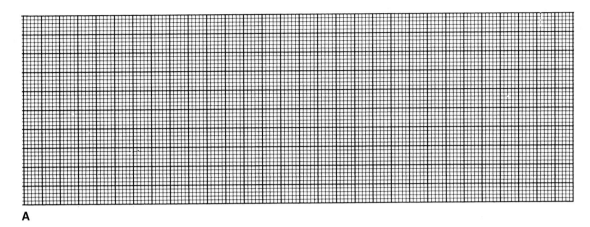

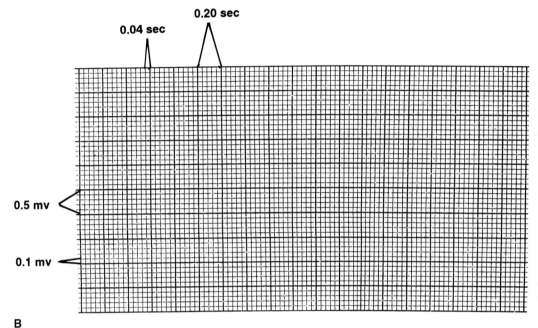

Figure 16-10 ECG graph paper. (**A**) Each small square is 1 mm × 1 mm. Each fifth line is marked darker to make a cube of 5 mm × 5 mm (actual size). (**B**) Horizontally, the graph paper represents time in seconds. Each small square represents 0.04 seconds, and each large square represents 0.2 seconds. Five large squares = 1 second (5 × 0.2).

The standard ECG has 12 leads that produce a three-dimensional record of the impulse wave. Four wires are labeled and color coded for the limb that the wire should be connected to, and six wires are labeled for connection to electrodes placed on the anterior chest (Box 16-5). The four limb electrodes should be positioned away from bony areas and on muscular areas, such as the calves, outer thighs, and above the elbow. Adjustments may be necessary for patients with amputations, surgery to the extremity, or trauma to the arms or legs.

The right leg (RL) electrode, the grounding lead, helps reduce alternating current (AC) interference and keeps the average voltage of the patient the same as that of the recording instrument. The other three limb leads

BOX 16-5

ABBREVIATIONS USED IN PERFORMING ECGS

RA	right arm
LA	left arm
LL	left leg
RL	right leg
V_1-V_6	chest leads
aVR	augmented voltage right arm
aVL	augmented voltage left arm
aVF	augmented voltage left foot or leg

attached to electrodes on the patient's left leg and arms make up the combinations necessary for the first six views of the heart in the 12-lead ECG. The first three combinations, which are standard bipolar leads also known as *Einthoven leads*, allow frontal visualization of the heart's electrical activity from side to side. Each lead provides specific measurements:

- Lead I measures the difference in electrical potential between the right arm (RA) and the left arm (LA).
- Lead II measures the difference in electrical potential between the right arm (RA) and the left leg (LL).
- Lead III measures the difference in electrical potential between the left arm (LA) and the left leg (LL).

The same limb electrodes provide measurement of the signal between one electrode and the average of the remaining two. These second three combinations, the augmented unipolar limb leads, allow visualization from a frontal view top to bottom:

- Lead aVR (LL 1 LA) to RA measures the potential at the right arm.
- Lead aVL (LL 1 RA) to LA measures the potential at the left arm.
- Lead aVF (RA 1 LA) to LL measures the potential at the left foot.

For a closer look at the electrical conduction through the heart, electrodes are placed directly on the anterior chest wall, but the limb electrodes must remain attached to the patient. The positioning of the chest electrodes must be precise for accuracy. These leads, the unipolar precordial (chest) leads, show the comparison of the chest electrode potential to the average of the three limb electrodes (Box 16-6). All electrodes must connect to the wires of the ECG machine. Each lead is clearly marked on the ECG paper as it

TABLE **16-2**	Coding ECG Leads		
Lead	Code	Lead	Code
I	.	V1	-.
II	..	V2	-..
III	...	V3	-...
aVR	-	V4	-....
aVL	—	V5	-.....
aVF	—-	V6	-......

is printed, or specific codes may be printed on the paper to denote each lead (Table 16-2). The recording of the ECG on paper varies from one machine to another, but the principles and techniques are universal (Procedure 16-1).

ECG Interpretation

The physician's interpretation of the standard 12-lead ECG includes an examination of various waveforms associated with the cardiac cycle (Fig. 16-11). Commonly measured components of an ECG tracing are discussed in the following sections.

PR Interval

The time from the beginning of the P wave to the beginning of the QRS complex is called the *PR interval*. This time interval represents depolarization of the atria

---

BOX 16-6

POSITIONING OF UNIPOLAR PRECORDIAL (CHEST) LEADS

- LV_1 = (RA + LA + LL) to V_1: Fourth intercostal space at right margin of sternum
- LV_2 = (RA + LA + LL) to V_2: Fourth intercostal space at left margin of sternum
- LV_3 = (RA + LA + LL) to V_3: Midway between V_2 and V_4
- LV_4 = (RA + LA + LL) to V_4: Fifth intercostal space at junction of midclavicular line
- LV_5 = (RA + LA + LL) to V_5: Horizontal level of V_4 at left anterior axillary line
- LV_6 = (RA + LA + LL) to V_6: Horizontal level of V_4 and V_5 at midaxillary line

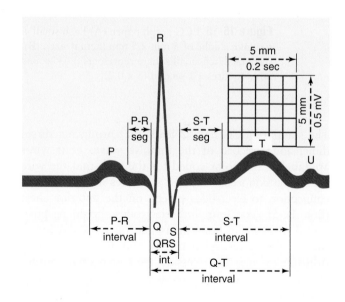

Figure 16-11 The cardiac cycle waves, segments, and intervals. (Reprinted with permission from Cohen BJ. Medical Terminology: An Illustrated Guide. Philadelphia: Lippincott Williams & Wilkins, 2003.)

and the spread of the depolarization wave up to and including the atrioventricular node.

PR Segment

The PR segment represents the period between the P wave and QRS complex.

ST Segment

The distance between the QRS complex and the T wave from the point where the QRS complex ends (J-point) to the onset of the ascending limb of the T wave is called the *ST segment*. On the ECG, this segment is a sensitive indicator of myocardial ischemia or injury.

Ventricular Activation Time

The time from the beginning of the QRS complex to the peak of the R wave, the *ventricular activation time*, represents the time necessary for the depolarization wave to travel from the inner surface of the heart (endocardium) to the outer surface of the heart (epicardium).

During the ECG, the paper speed on the machine should be set at 25 mm per second, which allows the electrical impulses (seen as waves) on the ECG to be measured using the blocks on the ECG paper as a reference (each small horizontal block is 0.04 seconds). Movement of the electricity through the atria is noted and measured on the ECG tracing as the PR interval (the normal PR interval is 0.12 to 0.20 seconds). Electrical movement through the ventricles is measured and noted on the ECG as the QRS complex, which is normally less than 0.12 seconds. The following elements are taken into consideration:

- Rate: how fast the heart is beating
- Rhythm: regularity of cardiac cycles and intervals
- Axis: position of the heart and direction of depolarization, or electrical movement, through the heart
- Hypertrophy: size of the heart
- Ischemia: decrease in blood supply to an area of the heart
- Infarction: death of heart muscle resulting in loss of function

Under usual diagnostic conditions, the 12-lead ECG provides sufficient data. As the medical assistant, you are responsible for obtaining a good-quality ECG without avoidable **artifacts**. An artifact is an abnormal signal that does not reflect electrical activity of the heart during the cardiac cycle. Artifacts can be due to movement by the patient, mechanical problems with the ECG machine, or improper technique. Table 16-3 describes three types of artifacts and how to prevent them.

Sometimes the physician requests a rhythm strip along with the ECG. A rhythm strip is a long strip of a certain lead or a combination of leads. It may be used to define certain cardiac arrhythmias. While most ECG machines have a button that automatically records the 12 views in the 12-lead ECG, a rhythm strip must be obtained using the manual mode on the ECG machine.

CHECKPOINT QUESTION

10. Which three waves represent a cardiac cycle on an ECG?

WHAT IF?

What if the physician asks you to perform an ECG on a child?

Although pediatric cardiac problems may not be encountered daily in the medical office, obesity, elevated cholesterol and triglyceride blood levels, and type 2 diabetes are conditions that are seen increasingly frequently in pediatric and family practice offices, and these conditions may require intervention, including electrocardiography. Although the placement of the electrodes is similar to that for an adult, smaller electrodes for use on the smaller patient allow for easier placement. A standard ECG can be done on children over 8 or 9 years of age; however, for younger children, the sensitivity, or gain, on the machine should be changed according to the physician's orders or office policy and procedure manual. If the sensitivity or gain is changed, this must be noted on the ECG before it goes into the medical record.

Holter Monitor

In many instances, an ECG that records the electrical activity of the heart for a brief moment in the medical office does not reveal cardiac problems. For diagnosis of intermittent cardiac arrhythmias and dysfunctions, a monitor that records for at least 24 hours is used. The Holter monitor is small and portable and can be worn comfortably for long periods without interfering with daily activities (Fig. 16-12). It may be set to record continuously or only when the patient presses a record button when feeling symptoms. This record button is also known as an "incident" or "event" button. When applying the Holter monitor, you must instruct the patient to keep a diary of daily activities. The physician will interpret the ECG tracing recorded by the Holter monitor and compare these findings with activities recorded in the diary to get an accurate view of what activities, if any, precipitate cardiac arrhythmias. Procedure 16-2 describes the steps for applying a Holter monitor.

TABLE 16-3 Types of Artifacts

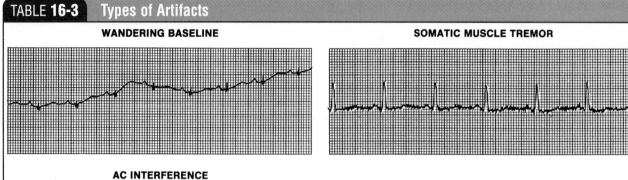

WANDERING BASELINE

SOMATIC MUSCLE TREMOR

AC INTERFERENCE

Wandering baseline, somatic muscle temor, and alternating current (AC) interference.

Artifact	Possible Cause	How to Prevent Problems
Wandering baseline	Electrodes too tight or too loose; electrolyte gel dried out; skin has oil, lotion, or excessive hair	Apply electrodes properly; apply new electrodes; prepare skin before applying electrodes
Muscle or somatic artifact	Patient cannot remain still because of tremors or fear	Reassure patient; explain procedure and stress the need to keep still; patients with disease may be unable to stay motionless
Alternating artifact	Improperly grounded ECG machine	Check cables to ensure properly current grounded machine before beginning test
	Electrical interference in room in immediate area	Move patient or unplug appliances
	Dangling lead wires	Arrange wires along contours of patient's body

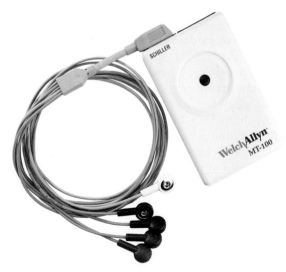

Figure 16-12 A Holter Monitor. (Courtesy of Welch Allyn.)

PATIENT EDUCATION

THE HOLTER MONITOR PATIENT DIARY

A patient with a Holter monitor must keep a diary of daily activities. When the patient has symptoms, he or she depresses an incident (or event) button on the machine and then records in the diary the activity that caused the incident, including the symptoms. At intervals, the patient also records daily activities such as working quietly at a desk, driving a car, eating a meal, watching television, and sleeping. All activities must be noted, including elimination, sexual intercourse, anger, laughter, and so on. Some monitors are equipped with small tape recorders so the patient can keep an audio diary instead of a written one.

Chest Radiography

Chest radiography provides valuable basic information about the anatomic location and gross structures of the heart, great vessels, and lungs. It also aids in the evaluation of such disorders as CHF and pericardial effusions. Many patients with CHF have an enlarged heart, especially the ventricles, and pericardial effusions appear as white markings around the heart on the film. Many patients with chronic cardiac conditions also have pulmonary problems, and the chest film can be used to assess the lungs. Any abnormal swelling or growth of the heart or great vessels (aorta, inferior vena cava, superior vena cava, pulmonary arteries) can also be assessed.

Cardiac Stress Test

To measure the response of the cardiac muscle to increased demands of oxygen, the physician may request a cardiac stress test. The heart is usually tested with the patient walking on a treadmill (Fig. 16-13) with periodic increases in the rate or angle of the walk or run, but it may also be done on a stationary bicycle. The patient is attached to an ECG monitor for constant tracing during the test, and the blood pressure is monitored

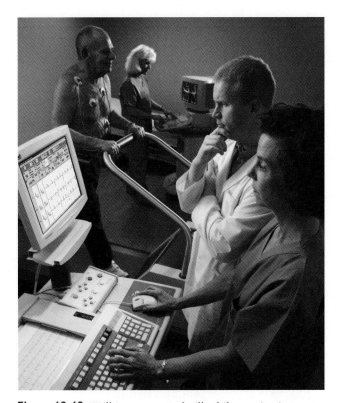

Figure 16-13 Walking on a treadmill while monitoring the heart's activity with an ECG machine is one way to determine the ability of the heart to adapt to increased work during exercise. (Courtesy of Borgess Medical Center, Kalamazoo, MI.)

before, during, and after the test. The test is performed according to the physician's orders, and the ECG is interpreted by the physician, but you may be responsible for attaching the electrodes, monitoring and recording the blood pressure, and assisting the physician in watching the patient for signs of light-headedness. Emergency resuscitation equipment should be available in case of cardiac or respiratory difficulties. This test may indicate the need for further cardiac testing. The cardiac stress test may be done as part of a routine physical examination in adults without symptoms or as a diagnostic tool for patients who have intermittent periods of angina pectoris or **palpitations**.

CHECKPOINT QUESTION

11. What is the purpose of a cardiac stress test?

Echocardiography

An echocardiogram, or echo, uses sound waves generated by a small device called a *transducer*. These waves travel through the cardiac chambers, walls, and valves and are transmitted back to a screen, where they can be viewed and interpreted. Echocardiograms help the physician to diagnose suspected or known valvular disease in adults and children. Echocardiograms also aid in diagnosing the severity of heart failure and **cardiomyopathy**. In addition, this test can be used to detect injuries to the heart in patients with trauma. Only the most specialized cardiac medical offices have the equipment and personnel (ultrasonographers) to obtain echocardiographs. In most instances, your role is to schedule the outpatient procedure and give the patient any instructions required by the facility. Usually no patient preparations are required for echocardiography.

 AFF **T R I A G E**

While working in a medical office, the following three situations occur:

A. A 29-year-old woman has been seen by the physician, who orders application of a Holter monitor. She also needs instruction on the importance of completing the diary.

B. A 62-year-old woman needs an ECG. She is complaining of heaviness in her chest.

C. A 17-year-old patient and his mother have just arrived in the office with written orders from an orthopedic surgeon that he needs a "stat preop" ECG. The patient is scheduled for knee surgery in the morning.

(continued)

How do you sort these patients? Who do you see first? Second? Third?

Do the ECG for patient B first. Her chest heaviness may be due to a cardiac problem, and the physician should assess this ECG immediately. See patient A next, since she has been waiting. After applying the Holter monitor and explaining the diary, do the ECG for patient C. Every surgeon has standard orders for various tests he or she wants completed before doing surgery. ECGs are commonly ordered and read by a cardiologist or internist before a surgical procedure. Although the written order is written as stat, the test can be done as soon as possible and convenient.

Cardiac Catheterization and Coronary Arteriography

Cardiac catheterization is a common invasive procedure used to help diagnose or treat conditions affecting the coronary arterial circulation. It may be performed on patients with shortness of breath, angina, dizziness, palpitations, fluttering in the chest, rapid heartbeat, and other cardiovascular symptoms to determine the severity or cause of the problem. It is often indicated after a cardiac stress test or echocardiogram reveals an abnormality. This procedure is not done in the medical office, but the medical assistant may be responsible for scheduling diagnostic cardiac catheterizations at a local outpatient facility or hospital and giving the patient any instructions required by the outpatient facility. If the procedure is for treatment, it must be done at an inpatient facility that has immediate access to open heart surgical equipment and personnel in the event of an emergency.

During the catheterization, the physician, usually a cardiologist, inserts a flexible tube into a blood vessel in either the arm or the groin and gently guides it toward the heart. When the catheter is in place, coronary arteriography is performed by injecting contrast medium, revealing the heart's chambers, valves, great vessels, and coronary arteries on a monitor. If atherosclerotic plaques are found, an angioplasty may be performed or scheduled for later (see Box 16-2).

 CHECKPOINT QUESTION

12. How is the echocardiography obtained?

Medication Box

Commonly Prescribed Cardiovascular System Medications

Note: The generic name of the drug is listed first and is written in all lowercase letters. Brand names are in parentheses, and the first letter is capitalized.

amlodipine (Novasc)	Tablets: 2.5 mg, 5 mg, 10 mg	Antianginal; antihypertensive
atenolol (Tenormin)	Tablets: 25 mg to 100 mg	Antihypertensive
carvedilol (Coreg)	Tablets: 3.125 mg to 25 mg	Antihypertensive
digoxin (Lanoxin)	Tablets: 0.125 mg, 0.25 mg	Inotropic
diltiazem hydrochloride (Cardizem)	Capsules (extended release): 60 mg to 420 mg Tablets: 30 mg to 120 mg	Antianginal; antihypertensive
enalapril (Vasotec)	Tablets: 2.5 mg to 20 mg	Antihypertensive
ezetimibe (Zetia)	Tablets: 10 mg	Antilipemic
furosemide (Lasix)	Tablets: 20 mg to 80 mg	Diuretic; antihypertensive
gemfibrozil (Lopid)	Tablets: 600 mg	Antilipemic
hydrochlorothiazide (Microzide)	Tablets: 12.5 mg to 100 mg Capsules: 12.5 mg	Diuretic
lisinopril (Prinivil; Zestril)	Tablets: 2.5 mg to 40 mg	Antihypertensive
metoprolol succinate (Toprol XL)	Tablets: 25 mg to 200 mg	Antihypertensive
metoprolol tartrate (Lopressor)	Tablets: 25 mg to 100 mg	Antihypertensive
nadolol (Corgard)	Tablets: 20 mg to 160 mg	Antianginal; antihypertensive

Commonly Prescribed Cardiovascular System Medications *(Continued)*		
nitroglycerin (Nitrostat; Nitro-dur; Nitrolingual)	Capsules: 2.5 mg, 6.5 mg, 9 mg	Antianginal
	Tablets (sublingual): 0.3 mg, 0.4 mg, 0.6 mg	
	Transdermal: 0.1 mg/hr to 0.8 mg/hr	
pravastatin sodium (Pravachol)	Tablets: 10 mg to 80 mg	Antilipemic
propranolol (Inderal)	Tablets: 10 mg to 80 mg,	Antianginal; antihypertensive
	Capsules (extended release): 60 mg to 160 mg	
ramipril (Altace)	Capsules: 1.25 mg to 10 mg	Antihypertensive
simvastatin (Zocor)	Tablets: 1.25 mg to 10 mg	Antilipemic
	Tablets: 5 mg to 80 mg	
verapamil hydrochloride (Calan; IsoptinSR)	Capsules (extended release): 100 mg to 300 mg	Antianginal; antihypertensive
	Tablets: 40 mg to 120 mg	

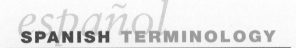

SPANISH TERMINOLOGY

¿Padece de presion alta?
  Do you have high blood pressure?

¿Tiene dolor de pecho?
  Do you have chest pain?

¿Ha sentido dolor en el brazo izquierdo?
  Have you ever had pain in the left arm?

¿Se marea?
  Do you have dizzy spells?

MEDIA MENU

- **Student Resources on thePoint**
  - **Animation: Cardiac Cycle**
  - **Animation: Congestive Heart Failure**
  - **Animation: Hypertension**
  - **Animation: Myocardial Blood Flow**
  - **Animation: Stroke**
  - **Video: Perform a Basic 12-Lead Electrocardiogram (Procedure 16-1)**
  - **Video: Applying a Holter Monitor (Procedure 16-2)**
  - **CMA/RMA Certification Exam Review**
- **Internet Resources**
  American Heart Association
  http://www.heart.org
  American Red Cross
  http://www.redcross.org
  National Safety Council
  http://www.nsc.org
  American College of Cardiology
  http://www.cardiosource.org/acc
  American Society of Hypertension, Inc.
  http://www.ash-us.org
  American Medical Association
  http://www.ama-assn.org

Performing a 12-Lead Electrocardiogram

Purpose: Prepare a patient and obtain a 12-lead ECG that is free from artifacts
Equipment: Physician's order, patient record, ECG machine with cable and lead wires, ECG paper, disposable electrodes that contain coupling gel, gown and drape, skin preparation materials including a razor and antiseptic wipes

Steps	Reasons
1. Wash your hands.	Handwashing aids infection control.
2. Assemble the equipment.	Obtain all necessary equipment and supplies before beginning the procedure.
Step 2. The ECG machine.	
3. Greet and identify the patient. Explain the procedure.	This avoids errors in treatment and helps gain compliance.
4. Turn the machine on and enter appropriate data, including the patient's name and/or identification number, age, sex, height, weight, blood pressure, and medications.	This information will assist the physician in determining a proper diagnosis.
5. Instruct the patient to disrobe above the waist, and provide a gown for privacy. Female patients should also be instructed to remove any nylons or tights.	Clothing may interfere with proper placement of the leads. Patients wearing pants do not have to remove them if they can be pulled up to expose the lower legs.
6. Position the patient comfortably supine with pillows as needed for comfort. Drape the patient for warmth and privacy.	If the patient is uncomfortable, too cool, or improperly draped, movement is likely, which will result in artifacts on the ECG tracing.
7. Prepare the skin as needed by wiping away skin oil and lotions with the antiseptic wipes or shaving any hair that will interfere with good contact between the skin and the electrodes.	Skin preparation ensures properly attached leads and helps avoid improper readings and lost time repeating the test.
8. Apply the electrodes snugly against the fleshy, muscular parts of the upper arms and lower legs according to the manufacturer's directions. Apply chest electrodes, V_1–V_6.	Electrodes that are not snug against the skin or are on bony prominences may cause improper reading and artifact. In case of an amputation or the otherwise inaccessible limb, place the electrode on the uppermost part of the existing extremity or on the anterior shoulder (upper extremity) and groin (lower extremity).

PSY **PROCEDURE 16-1:** **Performing a 12-Lead Electrocardiogram** *(continued)*

Steps	Reasons

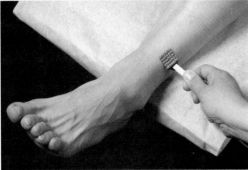

A

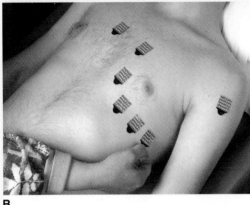

B

Step 8. **(A)** Applying limb electrodes. **(B)** Applying chest electrodes.

9. Connect the lead wires securely according to the color-coded notations on the connectors (RA, LA, RL, LL, V_1–V_6). Untangle the wires before applying them to prevent electrical artifacts. Each lead must lie unencumbered along the contours of the patient's body to decrease the likelihood of artifacts. Double-check the placement.

Improperly placed leads will result in both time lost to an inaccurate reading and retesting.

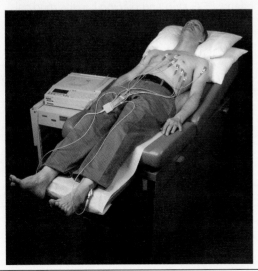

Step 9. The wires should lie along the contours of the patient's body.

(continued)

PSY PROCEDURE 16-1:   **Performing a 12-Lead Electrocardiogram (continued)**

Steps	Reasons
10. Determine the sensitivity, or gain, and paper speed settings on the ECG machine before running the test. Set sensitivity or gain on 1 and paper speed on 25 mm/second.	A sensitivity setting of 1 and a paper speed of 25 mm/second are necessary to obtain an accurate ECG. These settings should not be changed without a direct order from the physician and the changes noted on the final ECG tracing.
11. Depress the automatic button on the ECG machine to obtain the 12-lead tracing. The machine will automatically move from one lead to the next without your intervention.	If the physician wants only a rhythm strip tracing, use the manual mode of operation and select the lead manually.
12. When the tracing is complete and printed, check the ECG for artifacts and a standardization mark. Normal Standard Standardization mark is 10 mm high **A** One-Half Standard Standardization mark is 5 mm high **B** Double Standard Standardization mark is 20 mm high **C**	With sensitivity set on 1, the standardization mark should be 2 small squares wide and 10 small squares high. The standardization mark documents accuracy of operation and provides a reference point. **Step 12. (A)** Normal standardization mark is 10 mm high. **(B)** One-half standardization mark is 5 mm high. **(C)** Double standardization mark is 20 mm high.
13. If the tracing is adequate, turn off the machine and remove and discard the electrodes. Assist the patient to a sitting position and help with dressing if needed.	Some patients become dizzy while lying supine.
14. **AFF** Explain how to respond to a patient with dementia.	Solicit assistance from a caregiver or other staff member to help during the procedure. Give simple directions to the patient about what he or she should do. Speak clearly, not loudly.
15. If a single-channel machine was used (each lead produced on a roll of paper, one lead at a time), carefully roll the ECG strip without using clips to secure the roll. This ECG must be mounted on 8 × 11–inch paper or a form before going into the medical record according to the office policy and procedure.	Folding the ECG tracing or applying clips may make marks on the surface, obscuring the reading. Special forms may be purchased specifically for mounting a single-channel ECG strip and placing it in the medical record.
16. Record the procedure in the patient's medical record.	Procedures are considered not to have been done if they are not recorded.
17. Either place the ECG tracing and the patient's medical record on the physician's desk or give it directly to the physician, as instructed.	

Charting Example:

12/02/2014 9:45 AM Pre-employment 12-lead ECG obtained and placed in chart——————————— A. Perez, CMA

Note: The medical assistant may sign his or her name in the patient record using only the "CMA" credential if the office has a signature log denoting the entire credential as "CMA(AAMA)."

PSY PROCEDURE 16-2: **Applying a Holter Monitor**

Purpose: Prepare and instruct a patient on wearing a Holter monitor for continuous cardiac monitoring
Equipment: Physician's order, patient record, Holter monitor with appropriate lead wires, fresh batteries, carrying case with strap, disposable electrodes with coupling gel, adhesive tape, gown and drape, skin preparation materials including a razor and antiseptic wipes, diary
Standard: This procedure should take 10 minutes.

Steps	Reasons
1. Wash your hands.	Handwashing aids infection control.
2. Assemble the equipment.	Obtain all necessary equipment and supplies before beginning the procedure.
3. Greet and identify the patient. Explain the procedure, reminding the patient that it is important to carry out all normal activities for the duration of the test.	Identifying the patient and explaining the procedure avoids errors in treatment and helps gain compliance. A normal routine is essential to allow the physician to identify areas of concern.
4. Explain the purpose of the incident diary, emphasizing the need to carry it at all times during the test. Ask the patient to remove all clothing from the waist up and put on the gown, and drape appropriately for privacy.	The chest must be exposed for proper placement of the electrodes.
5. With the patient seated, prepare the skin for electrode attachment. Provide privacy. Shave the skin if necessary and cleanse with antiseptic wipes.	Shaving and cleansing the skin will improve adherence of the adhesive on the electrodes.
6. Expose the adhesive backing of the electrodes and follow the manufacturer's instructions to attach each firmly. Apply the electrodes at the specified sites: **A.** Right manubrium border **B.** Left manubrium border **C.** Right sternal border at the fifth rib **D.** Fifth rib at the anterior axillary line **E.** Right lower rib cage over the cartilage as a ground lead.	The electrodes will be worn by the patient for up to 24 hours and must be secure.

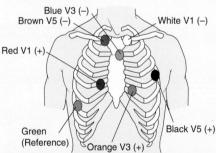

A

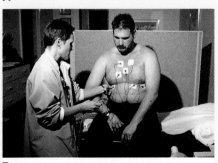

B

Step 6. (A) Sites for Holter electrodes. **(B)** Place the Holter electrodes as directed by the manufacturer.

(continued)

PSY PROCEDURE 16-2: **Applying a Holter Monitor** *(continued)*

Steps	Reasons
7. Check the security of the attachments.	Electrodes that are not securely attached will result in poor tracings.
8. Position electrode connectors down toward the patient's feet. Attach the lead wires and secure with adhesive tape.	Application of adhesive tape over the connections will help ensure that the leads do not work loose during the day.

Step 8. Securely tape each electrode. Tape the lead wires to the patient's body.

Steps	Reasons
9. Connect the cable and run a baseline ECG by hooking the Holter to the ECG machine with the cable hookup.	Check for accurate function of the Holter before the patient leaves.
10. Assist the patient to dress carefully with the cable extending through the garment opening. Clothing that buttons down the front is convenient.	This prevents pulling and strain on the leads.
11. Plug the cable into the recorder and mark the diary. If needed, explain the purpose of the diary to the patient again. Give instructions for a return appointment to evaluate the recording and the diary.	Keeping the diary is an important part of wearing the Holter monitor and will assist the physician in an accurate diagnosis.
12. Record the procedure in the patient's medical record.	Procedures are considered not to have been done if they are not recorded.

Charting Example:

11/28/2014 1:00 PM Holter monitor ordered and applied; baseline ECG done. Oral and written instructions given
regarding care and use of monitor. Instructions for completion of diary also given. Pt. verbalized understanding of use
of monitor and completion of diary. To RTO tomorrow pm for removal of the monitor————————— R. Steele, CMA

Note: The medical assistant may sign his or her name in the patient record using only the "CMA" credential if the office has a signature log denoting the entire credential as "CMA(AAMA)."

- The circulatory system is a closed transport system kept in motion by the force of the beating heart.
- Nutrients are delivered to cells, cellular wastes are picked up, hormones are directed to target cells, and disease-fighting mechanisms are transported to areas of concern.
- The patient with undiagnosed cardiac disease may complain of lethargy, shortness or breath, or swelling of the extremities.
- Your responsibility includes:
  - Obtaining a complete cardiac history from all patients.
- Assisting with the physical examination.
- Performing or assisting with diagnostic testing.
- Scheduling any cardiac procedures that are not performed in your medical office.
- Obtaining necessary referrals from third-party payers when the physician concludes that the patient should be evaluated by a cardiologist.
- Educating patients at every opportunity to prevent cardiac disease and offering support once a cardiac diagnosis has been made by the physician.

Warm Ups | for Critical Thinking

1. Draw a diagram of the heart and a cardiac cycle as seen on the ECG. How would you explain an ECG to a patient? How would you assist the patient in relaxing for this procedure?

2. Compare and contrast the signs and symptoms of a CVA and a TIA. What kind of help does a patient need at home after a stroke? What language barriers might you encounter with the patient who has had a stroke, and how could you overcome these barriers?

3. Explain anemia and identify its symptoms. Why does anemia cause these symptoms? What dietary instructions should be given to a patient with iron deficiency anemia?

4. Prepare a patient education brochure that describes hypertension and its causes, symptoms, and possible treatments. In this brochure, explain why hypertension is often referred to as the silent killer.

5. Using a drug reference book, look up nitroglycerin. What is the usual dosage? How often can this drug be taken for the pain of angina?

6. Research the reason for why many patients with mitral valve disease are prescribed prophylactic anitbiotics before dental procedures. What would you say to a patient who does not want to take these antibiotics before a dental procedure?

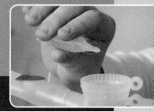

Gastroenterology

Outline

Common Gastrointestinal Disorders
Mouth Disorders
Esophageal Disorders
Stomach Disorders
Intestinal Disorders
Liver Disorders

Gallbladder Disorders
Pancreatic Disorders
Common Diagnostic and Therapeutic Procedures
History and Physical Examination of the GI System

Blood Tests
Radiology Studies
Nuclear Imaging
Ultrasonography
Endoscopic Studies
Fecal Tests

Learning Outcomes

Cognitive Domain

Note: AAMA/CAAHEP 2008 Standards are italicized.

1. Spell and define key terms
2. List and describe common disorders of the alimentary canal and accessory organs
3. Identify and explain the purpose of common procedures and tests associated with the gastrointestinal system
4. Describe the roles and responsibilities of the medical assistant in diagnosing and treating disorders of the gastrointestinal system
5. *Identify common pathologies related to each body system*
6. *Describe implications for treatment related to pathology*

Psychomotor Domain

Note: AAMA/CAAHEP 2008 Standards are italicized.

1. Assist with colon procedures (Procedure 17-1)
2. *Assist physician with patient care*
3. *Prepare a patient for procedures and/or treatments*
4. *Practice standard precautions*
5. *Document patient care*

6. *Document patient education*
7. *Practice within the standard of care for a medical assistant*

Affective Domain

Note: AAMA/CAAHEP 2008 Standards are italicized.

1. *Apply critical thinking skills in performing patient assessment and care*
2. *Use language/verbal skills that enable patients' understanding*
3. *Demonstrate empathy in communicating with patients, family, and staff*
4. *Use appropriate body language and other nonverbal skills in communicating with patients, family, and staff*
5. *Demonstrate awareness of the territorial boundaries of the person with whom you are communicating*
6. *Demonstrate sensitivity appropriate to the message being delivered*
7. *Demonstrate recognition of the patient's level of understanding in communications*
8. *Recognize and protect personal boundaries in communicating with others*
9. *Demonstrate respect for individual diversity, incorporating awareness of one's own biases in areas including gender, race, religion, age, and economic status*

10. *Apply active listening skills*
11. *Apply local, state, and federal health care legislation and regulation appropriate to the medical assisting practice setting*

ABHES Competencies

1. Assist the physician with the regimen of diagnostic and treatment modalities as they relate to each body system
2. Prepare patient for examinations and treatments

3. Recognize and understand various treatment protocols
4. Comply with federal, state, and local health laws and regulations
5. Communicate on the recipient's level of comprehension
6. Serve as a liaison between the physician and others
7. Show empathy and impartiality when dealing with patients
8. Document accurately

Key Terms

anorexia	hepatomegaly	melena	stomatitis
ascites	hepatotoxins	metabolism	turgor
dysphagia	insufflator	obturator	
guaiac	leukoplakia	peristalsis	
hematemesis	malocclusion	sclerotherapy	

The gastrointestinal (GI) system, or tract, is responsible for the ingestion, digestion, transportation, and elimination of the food we eat (Fig. 17-1). Nutrients are broken down by the action of digestive enzymes into units that can be absorbed through the walls of the GI system into the circulatory and lymphatic systems. This process starts when something is put into the mouth, chewed, and mixed with the enzymes in saliva. Through **peristalsis**, food is pushed along the GI tract, further breaking it down into segments and mixing it with enzymes to hasten the breakdown into nutrients. **Metabolism** is the breakdown of food into usable units through these physical and chemical changes. Any unused food material is eliminated as waste from the GI system as feces.

Disorders of the GI system may affect the alimentary canal, also called the *GI tract*, or accessory organs such as the liver, gallbladder, and pancreas. This chapter describes common disorders of the GI system and the accessory organs, diagnostic procedures, and your role as a medical assistant working with patients with GI disorders. Although the physician who specializes in disorders of the GI system is the gastroenterologist, medical assistants working in other offices, such as family practice and internal medicine, often encounter patients with disorders of this body system.

Common Gastrointestinal Disorders

Mouth Disorders

Although disorders of the teeth, gums, and oral cavity are typically diagnosed and treated by the dentist, patients requiring a referral to a dentist or oral surgeon may be seen first in the medical office. Physicians and other health care professionals should be aware of these disorders and their importance to the nutrition, digestion, and overall health status of the patient. Your role includes taking an accurate medical history, including inquiring about the condition of the oral cavity and teeth, making referrals as ordered by the physician, and educating patients about the care of the gums and teeth to prevent health problems and loss of teeth.

Caries

Dental caries (tooth decay) is the most widespread disease of the oral cavity. Bacteria allowed to remain on the teeth erode the enamel and allow infection to reach the inner portions of the tooth. Factors that may contribute to the development of dental caries include a poor diet, inadequate dental hygiene, and **malocclusion**, which is

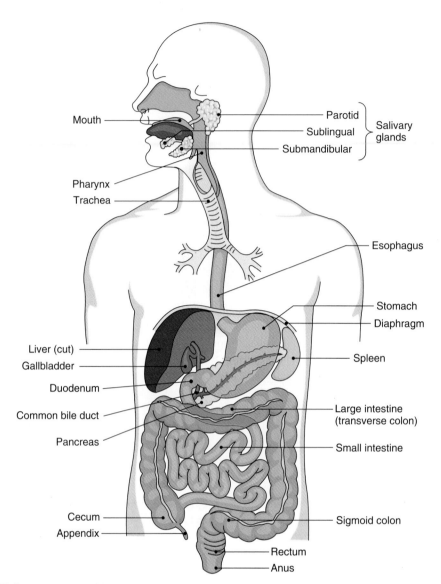

Figure 17-1 The digestive system. (Reprinted with permission from Cohen BJ. Memmler's The Human Body in Health and Disease, 11th ed. Philadelphia: Lippincott Williams & Wilkins, 2009.)

abnormal contact between the upper teeth and the lower teeth. Prevention of dental caries includes consuming a balanced diet low in sugars, good oral hygiene as prescribed by the dentist, and frequent professional dental care. Treatment may include drilling the dental caries and replacing the space with a filling or extraction of the affected teeth. Because dental caries can cause discomfort with chewing or biting, they may affect nutrition and ultimately digestion and the overall health of the patient.

Stomatitis

Stomatitis, an inflammation of the oral mucosa, may be caused by a virus, bacteria, or fungus. The two most common forms are herpetic stomatitis, caused by the herpes simplex virus, and candidiasis, caused by the fungus *Candida albicans.*

Herpes simplex is usually self-limiting after the initial exposure to the virus. The virus is usually transmitted hand to mouth, mouth to mouth, or by vector (e.g., shared drinking glasses or eating utensils). The infection presents as a painful sore on the mucosa of the mouth (commonly called a *canker sore*) or on the lips (commonly called a *fever blister* or *cold sore*). After the initial infection, the virus lies dormant for long periods, with exacerbations during illness, stress, overexposure to the sun, or other trigger. Although there is no cure for herpes simplex, palliative measures such as ointments or creams may be purchased over the counter to relieve the discomfort.

C. albicans, formerly called *Monilia albicans,* is an opportunistic yeast or fungus. This organism is always present in the mouth but is kept in check by other normal microorganisms found in the mouth including bacteria. When the normal bacterial balance in the mouth is altered,

C. albicans microorganisms multiply, causing an infection that appears as a white substance covering the oral cavity and tongue. Factors that can upset the balance of these microorganisms in the mouth include the use of broad-spectrum antibiotics that kill many bacteria throughout the body, including the mouth, allowing the opportunistic organisms to grow without control. In babies, the disease is called *thrush* and commonly is caused by a favorable environment for the growth of *C. albicans*, as milk changes the pH of the mouth. In adults or infants, treatment with an antifungal agent usually cures the disorder and restores the balance of microbes in the mouth.

CHECKPOINT QUESTION

1. What are the two most common causes of stomatitis?

Gingivitis

Gingivitis is an inflammation of the gingiva, or gums. It may lead to periodontitis, or inflammation, and possible destruction of the supporting structures of the teeth, including the gingiva, periodontal ligament, and mandibular or maxillary bone. In Americans, more teeth are lost to gum disease than to tooth decay. Good oral hygiene and frequent dental care help prevent premature loss of teeth. Once diagnosed, gingivitis is usually treated with an antibiotic.

Oral Cancers

Cancers of the oral cavity are common, especially among individuals who use tobacco products. The constant irritation of the tobacco causes white spots or patches, called **leukoplakia**, to form on the oral mucosa, particularly the lips and tongue. These lesions have clearly defined borders and frequently become malignant. Treatment includes surgery or chemical agents such as radiation or chemotherapy. Although cancer of the lips usually responds well to radiation or surgery, cancers of the margins of the tongue metastasize quickly and are commonly difficult to treat effectively.

CHECKPOINT QUESTION

2. How can gingivitis be prevented?

Esophageal Disorders

Hiatal Hernia

Hiatal hernia, or diaphragmatic hernia, occurs when the stomach protrudes up into the diaphragm through a weakened or enlarged cardiac sphincter at the bottom of the esophagus, allowing a portion of the stomach to slide up into the chest cavity. This type of hernia is a common condition that frequently affects people over age 40 years. Weight gain, either recent or prolonged, can be a contributing factor. Normally, the cardiac sphincter, a muscle that separates the end of the esophagus from the beginning of the stomach, prevents gastroesophageal reflux, or backflow of gastric acids from the stomach into the esophagus. The presence of a hiatal hernia enables the stomach acid to backflow into the esophagus, causing considerable discomfort, including indigestion and epigastric pain in the upper abdomen (Fig. 17-2).

The symptoms of a hiatal hernia include abdominal pain and indigestion, especially after eating. Diagnosis

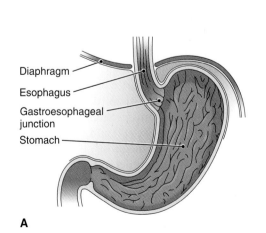

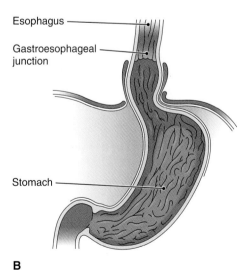

A   **B**

Figure 17-2 **(A)** Normal. **(B)** Hiatal hernia. The stomach protrudes through the diaphragm into the thoracic cavity, raising the level of the junction between the esophagus and the stomach. (Reprinted with permission from Cohen BJ, Wood DL. Memmler's The Human Body in Health and Disease, 11th ed. Philadelphia: Lippincott Williams & Wilkins, 2009.)

is made by taking a careful medical history, chest radiographs, barium swallow, or endoscopy. Medical treatment is usually preferred to surgical intervention because surgically corrected hiatal hernias frequently recur. Medical interventions include diet modifications such as small, frequent meals with no food for at least 2 hours before bedtime. In addition, the physician may order antacids, weight loss, elevating the head of the bed when sleeping, and drug therapy to increase the tone of the cardiac sphincter.

Constant exposure to gastric acid from gastroesophageal reflux can lead to esophagitis, a condition that resembles abraded tissue along the lining of the esophagus. Constant irritation of the lining of the esophagus, also known as *Barrett esophagus*, may lead to malignancy. Patients with Barrett esophagus have a 30% to 40% chance of developing adenocarcinoma. If the source of irritation is gastroesophageal reflux, it will be diagnosed and treated much the same as a hiatal hernia.

Gastroesophageal Reflux Disease (GERD)

Patients who complain of any type of chest pain, including heartburn, should be assessed immediately because the chest pain of gastroesophageal reflux disease (GERD) may be similar to the chest pain of a patient having cardiac problems. In addition to the chest pain, signs and symptoms of myocardial involvement can include:

• Shortness of breath
• Nausea or vomiting
• Pain that spreads from the chest to the jaw, back, or arms

Chest pain that is not cardiac may be diagnosed by the physician as GERD, a chronic disorder characterized by discomfort in the chest (heartburn) due to the backflow of gastric contents into the esophagus. This disorder is caused by a weak lower esophageal sphincter that normally closes after food is swallowed, keeping the material in the stomach. The symptoms of GERD include:

• Frequent heartburn or indigestion relieved by antacids
• Hoarseness or laryngitis
• Sore throat
• A feeling of a lump in the throat
• Chronic cough

A thorough examination by the physician plus endoscopic and radiologic procedures are usually necessary to diagnose GERD. Once diagnosed, this disorder can be treated with appropriate medications. Untreated, GERD can lead to erosion of the esophagus and complications such as esophageal bleeding. GERD may also be the cause of esophageal cancers in some patients.

PATIENT EDUCATION

PREVENTING GASTRIC REFLUX

• Avoid spicy foods and chocolate, especially in the evening.
• Limit caffeine.
• Maintain optimum weight.
• Avoid overeating.
• Wait 1 hour after eating before exercising.
• Do not eat just before going to bed.
• Do not lie down just after eating.
• Stop smoking.
• Place blocks, bricks, or a stack of books under the legs of the bed to elevate the head, chest, and abdomen approximately 12 inches.
• See the physician if symptoms persist.

Esophageal Varices

Varicose veins (varices) of the esophagus result from pressure within the esophageal veins. This condition is commonly seen in patients diagnosed with cirrhosis of the liver. Since drainage from the portal vein is impaired by the liver damage, the veins of the esophagus become distended, resulting in varices. The most common and dangerous problem that results from esophageal varices is hemorrhaging if the distended veins rupture. Before a rupture occurs, the treatment of choice is **sclerotherapy**, which uses a chemical agent to cause fibrosing (hardening) of the area around the varices, preventing hemorrhaging. In the event of esophageal hemorrhage, the patient should be transported immediately to the emergency room, where pressure tubes can be applied directly to the varices to control the bleeding.

Esophageal Cancer

Cancer of the esophagus is most common among older men and is usually fatal. Predisposing factors for this type of cancer include chronic gastroesophageal reflux, smoking, and drinking alcohol. The malignancy narrows the lumen of the esophagus and causes **dysphagia** (difficulty swallowing). As the mass enlarges, swallowing solid food may become extremely painful. Vomiting and weight loss occur as the symptoms progress. A barium swallow with fluoroscopy outlines the lesion, and esophagoscopy with biopsy confirms the diagnosis. If the disease is local, surgical resection, chemotherapy, and radiation are the therapies of choice. No treatment has proven satisfactory, however, and the survival rates are very low.

 CHECKPOINT QUESTION

3. What is a hiatal hernia, and how can it affect the esophagus?

Stomach Disorders

Gastritis

Gastritis, an inflammation of the lining of the stomach, can be acute or chronic. The most common causes include irritants such as alcohol and certain drugs, including aspirin and nonsteroidal anti-inflammatory medications (NSAIDs). The bacterium *Helicobacter pylori*, also often implicated, is presumed to enter the body through food contaminated with infected fecal material (fecal–oral route) or from eating or drinking from a utensil also used by someone who is infected with the bacteria (oral–oral route). It resides in the mucous lining of the stomach and secretes enzymes that attack the mucous membrane.

Gastritis can cause significant oozing of blood and may result in a positive test for occult (hidden) blood in the stool. In elderly patients, sufficient blood loss can result in anemia. Signs and symptoms of gastritis include evidence of GI bleeding, epigastric discomfort, nausea, and vomiting. Diagnosis is usually made by obtaining a careful and complete history and direct visualization of the gastric mucosa through an endoscopic procedure known as a gastroscopy. Treatment usually involves eliminating the irritant, restoring the proper gastric acidity, and administering antibiotics as prescribed by the physician.

Peptic Ulcers

Ulcers in the GI tract are erosions or sores left by sloughed tissues. These erosions can expose small blood vessels and produce bleeding and pain. Peptic ulcers occur from the exposure of the lining of the stomach and first part of the small intestine (duodenum) to hydrochloric acid (HCl), a caustic chemical produced and secreted by the lining of the stomach that may cause erosion if too much is excreted. As the mucosa erodes, the patient has abdominal pain that intensifies during peristalsis, especially after eating. As the erosions and mucosa become more irritated, the ulcers bleed. The bleeding may range from slight oozing to life-threatening hemorrhage. Heavy bleeding will lead to **melena** (black tarry stools) or **hematemesis** (vomiting blood). Ulcers in the upper GI tract may perforate into the abdominal cavity with life-threatening consequences such as hypovolemic shock and peritonitis (Box 17-1). Chronic ulcerative conditions may also progress to malignancies.

The causes of peptic or gastric ulcers may include the use of chemicals that irritate the gastric mucosa, including aspirin, NSAIDs, and alcohol. Many gastric ulcers are also caused by an infection with *H. pylori*, which can be treated effectively with an antibiotic. Overproduction of gastric HCl also irritates the gastric mucosa and may produce erosions. Gastric acid production is under nerve and hormonal control and increases during times of emotional stress. Diagnosis of an ulcer is similar to the diagnosis of gastritis, including a thorough

---

> ### BOX 17-1
>
> ## PERITONITIS
>
> Peritonitis, an infection of the lining of the abdominal cavity, is a serious complication of several GI disorders that may occur if contents of the intestines or other organs leak into the abdominal cavity. The patient will be acutely ill and will have a fever and elevated white blood cell count. In addition, the patient will be complaining of severe abdominal pain. Treatment of peritonitis requires hospitalization with intravenous antibiotics and continuous monitoring of the patient for signs of septic shock. This condition can quickly become fatal if not treated appropriately and aggressively.

---

history and possibly endoscopic examination. The prescribed treatment for ulcers is avoiding the irritants causing the erosion, limiting the production of hydrogen by the gastric cells to neutralize the acid in the stomach, and an antibiotic as prescribed. Surgery to cut or disconnect the vagus nerve (vagotomy), which also reduces the secretion of HCl, may be performed if methods to decrease production of gastric acid are ineffective in treating the ulcer.

Gastric Cancer

Gastric cancer has no known cause, although smoking, excessive alcohol intake, ingesting foods high in preservatives, and genetic predisposition may contribute. Gastric cancer spreads rapidly to adjacent organs (the liver and pancreas) and throughout the peritoneal cavity. Signs and symptoms include chronic indigestion, weight loss, **anorexia**, anemia, and fatigue. The patient may have hematemesis with bright blood or coffee ground vomitus with dark blood. There may also be dark, bloody stools.

Diagnosis of gastric cancer requires an upper GI series with fluoroscopy, fiberoptic gastroscopy, and biopsy of the lesion or tumor. The extent of the disease can be determined by computed tomography (CT) and biopsy of the suspected metastatic sites, including adjacent organs. Surgery to remove the lesion may range from a subtotal gastric resection (removal of part of the stomach) to a total gastrectomy (removal of the entire stomach). If the cancer has metastasized, other organs may be removed, and radiation and chemotherapy may be necessary.

 CHECKPOINT QUESTION

4. What microorganism is found to be the cause of peptic ulcers in some patients?

Intestinal Disorders

Gastroenteritis

Gastroenteritis is general inflammation of the stomach, small intestine, and/or colon. This condition is caused by ingesting food or water that contains bacteria, viruses, parasites, or irritating agents such as spices. Food allergies and reactions to certain medications, such as antibiotics, may also inflame these organs. Symptoms include abdominal pain and cramping, nausea, vomiting, diarrhea, and fever.

The symptoms of gastroenteritis are self-limiting in most adults, usually lasting a few hours to a couple of days. However, because of the dehydration that can accompany the diarrhea and vomiting, gastroenteritis may be life threatening in the elderly, young children, and persons with diabetes mellitus. Treatment is palliative; it includes reducing the work of the GI tract by limiting food intake; treating the nausea, vomiting, and diarrhea; and maintaining the fluid balance by hydrating the body as needed. In severe cases, intravenous fluids must be administered to prevent dehydration and death, especially in the young and the elderly. If the cause of the inflammation is a bacterial or parasitic infection, an antibiotic or antiparasitic medication may be prescribed once the causative microorganism has been identified through a stool culture and analysis.

Duodenal Ulcers

Ulcerative lesions in the duodenum are often caused by exposure to highly corrosive gastric acid that is secreted by the stomach or other irritants that pass through the pylorus to the small intestine. Unlike the stomach, the duodenum has a normally alkaline pH, and the mucosa is not as well protected as the gastric mucosa. When food material passes through the pylorus and brings excessive acid or other irritants with it, an ulcer may form in the duodenum. As with the peptic ulcer, an overproduction of gastric acid may arise from ingestion of highly spicy foods or from overproduction of stress hormones, which also increases production of gastric acid. Treatment for duodenal ulcers is limiting or avoiding the irritating factors and reducing gastric acidity. If these measures are not successful, surgery may be an option. Ulcers in the duodenum left untreated may perforate the lining of the small intestine or may progress to cancerous lesions.

Malabsorption Syndromes

Malabsorption syndromes prevent the normal absorption of certain nutrients through the walls of the small intestines. Commonly, fat is not absorbed. A sign that a patient has a problem with malabsorption of fats includes stools that are frothy and pale. Because fat is necessary for the metabolism of vitamins A, D, E, and K, patients with this disorder require supplemental vitamin therapy.

Celiac sprue is a malabsorption syndrome marked by intolerance to gluten, a protein found in wheat and wheat byproducts. Celiac sprue can develop at any stage of life and often causes diarrhea high in fat. The cause of celiac sprue is not known, but it runs in families, suggesting a genetic factor.

Regardless of the nutrient involved in a patient with malabsorption syndrome, the patient is typically treated by addressing the suspected causes and avoiding or replacing the malabsorbed substances.

 CHECKPOINT QUESTION

5. How are peptic and duodenal ulcers different?

 PATIENT EDUCATION

BARIATRIC SURGERY TO TREAT OBESITY

Bariatrics is the study of morbid obesity. A popular surgical procedure to treat obesity is gastric bypass. Here are a few facts about this procedure:

- According to the American Society for Metabolic and Bariatric Surgery (http://www.asmbs.org), candidates for the surgery must be severely obese and have failed to lose weight with other methods.
- Candidates for gastric bypass surgery must have either a body mass index greater than 40 (approximately 80–100 pounds over the ideal weight for height) or significant medical problems associated with being overweight.
- The abdomen is incised, and the stomach is reduced to about the size of a thumb. The large remainder of the stomach is bypassed, and the new, smaller stomach is attached directly to the small intestine.
- The surgery comes with risks and requires lifestyle changes. Anemia and nutritional deficiencies are long-term risks that must be monitored and prevented or corrected.
- Since weight reduction after this procedure is often quick and dramatic, patients should be encouraged to begin an exercise program following the surgery as indicated by the surgeon.

Crohn Disease

Crohn disease, also known as *regional enteritis*, is an inflammation of the deep lining of the bowel ranging from very mild to severe and debilitating. The cause of Crohn disease is unclear, but it is thought to be an autoimmune disorder with a possible genetic link. Crohn disease can affect the small bowel and the colon but is more common in the area of the ileocecal valve.

The bowel walls become inflamed, and the lymph nodes enlarge, leading to edema of the bowel wall. When the lining of the bowel is swollen, the fluid from the intestinal contents cannot be absorbed, causing diarrhea and cramping, which may lead to more irritation and bleeding. Patients may also have periods of constipation, anorexia, and fever.

Although Crohn disease is a chronic disorder, each episode of inflammation causes scarring. The scarring may lead to narrowing of the colon, obstructing the bowel. Bowel obstruction can be life threatening and is a medical emergency. Diagnosis of Crohn disease necessitates a thorough history and analysis of the blood, which shows an increase in white blood cells and the erythrocyte sedimentation rate. A barium enema, or lower GI radiographic examination, if ordered by the physician, shows strictures alternating with normal bowel. Sigmoidoscopy and colonoscopy show patchy areas of inflammation within the bowel.

The treatment of Crohn disease is symptomatic; it includes restoration of fluids and electrolytes, administering corticosteroids to reduce inflammation, rest, and a low-fiber diet. Surgery is performed in cases of perforation or hemorrhage. If the situation is severe, a colectomy with an ileostomy may be performed (Fig. 17-3).

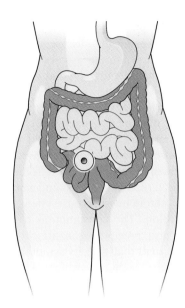

Figure 17-3 An ileostomy. The shaded portion indicates the section of the bowel that has been removed or is inactive. (Modified with permission from Cohen BJ. Medical Terminology: An Illustrated Guide. Philadelphia: Lippincott Williams & Wilkins, 2003.)

is thought to be an abnormal GI immune reaction to foods or microorganisms. Ulcerative colitis is a chronic condition, and the symptoms can be mild or severe with periods of remission.

The tissue that lines the colon becomes congested and edematous, eventually sloughing off and leading to ulcers and bloody diarrhea. Sometimes pus and mucus are present in the stool. Malabsorption of fluids causes weakness, anorexia, nausea, and vomiting. Scarring can occur as the ulcers heal. The colon may produce pseudopolyps, which can be precancerous. Diagnosis may be determined by endoscopic examination or by a barium enema, and biopsy confirms the diagnosis. Colonoscopy is used to evaluate strictures caused by scarring and to assess the risk of cancer.

Treatment of ulcerative colitis requires controlling the inflammation and preventing the loss of fluids and nutrients during periods of exacerbation. If the disease is severe, a corticosteroid is prescribed to relieve the inflammation. Surgery is a last resort and usually involves a proctocolectomy with an ileostomy.

LEGAL TIP

REMINDER: CONFIDENTIALITY AND PRIVACY

Patients with any chronic disease process, such as Crohn disease, often have concerned family members who may call or contact the office for information regarding the health of the patient. It is important to include family members in the care of the patient with a disorder such as this; however, information about the patient or their condition cannot be released without written permission of the patient no matter how well-meaning the requests or questions appear. Many offices have all patients sign a statement annually giving permission as to what family members, if any, can get information about the patient including leaving messages on answering machines about lab or test results. Always check the medical record for signed consents regarding private information and if no consent is available, do not share any information about the patient.

CHECKPOINT QUESTION

6. Which of the inflammatory bowel diseases can lead to life-threatening bowel obstruction? How?

Ulcerative Colitis

Like Crohn disease, ulcerative colitis is an inflammatory bowel disease affecting the lining of the colon. It occurs most often in young women but may occur at any age and may affect men also. The cause is not known but

Irritable Bowel Syndrome

Patients with irritable bowel syndrome frequently complain of bouts of constipation alternating with diarrhea.

Although the patient may have signs and symptoms resembling those of Crohn disease or ulcerative colitis, irritable bowel syndrome usually does not result in weight loss, and the prognosis is good. However, this disorder can be debilitating because there is no warning for the bouts of diarrhea caused by the spastic colon. Women are more likely than men to have this chronic disorder, whose symptoms may range from mild to severe even though endoscopic examination shows no signs of disease. The origin of irritable bowel syndrome is thought to be psychogenic, a reaction to stress and emotions and the actions of the autonomic nervous system, which partly controls the colon. The consumption of specific food irritants may also precipitate an attack; however, the particular food item that triggers symptoms varies from person to person. Diagnosis requires a careful history, both physical and emotional. Other diseases are ruled out by testing. Treatment is stress management and identifying the offending food irritants. For severe flare-ups, the physician may order corticosteroids and antibiotics.

Diverticulosis

Diverticulosis is a chronic condition of thinning of the bowel wall, causing small out-pouches in the lining of the intestinal wall (Fig. 17-4). This disorder usually occurs in the sigmoid colon but may occur anywhere in the GI tract. The cause has been attributed to a diet deficient in roughage. While many people have diverticulosis without symptoms, the condition becomes more serious when the bowel wall becomes so thin that veins and arteries are exposed. Bleeding can occur when the wall is nicked by a piece of stool and may be severe enough to require surgery to stop the hemorrhage. A diet high in fiber and use of stool softeners may be ordered by the physician to prevent the signs and symptoms of this disorder.

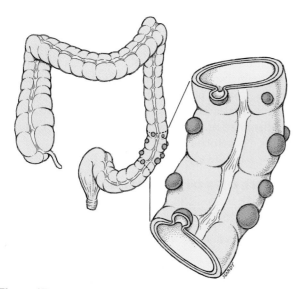

Figure 17-4 Diverticulosis of the sigmoid colon. (Reprinted with permission from Neil Hardy, Westpoint, CT.)

Diverticulosis may progress to diverticulitis, or inflammation of these areas of weakness in the bowel wall. The inflammation is usually caused by fecal material becoming lodged in the thin pockets. The symptoms are fever and abdominal pain. As the bowel becomes swollen and distended, the diseased areas may rupture, exposing the peritoneum to fecal material and resulting in peritonitis. The pouches are visualized on films produced from a barium enema or directly through endoscopic studies. During the acute phase, treatment includes a bland diet and stool softeners until the inflammation has subsided.

 PATIENT EDUCATION

MAINTAINING GOOD BOWEL HABITS

By following these guidelines, patients can prevent common problems of elimination:

- Eat a variety of foods, especially fresh fruits, vegetables, and whole grains. Limit the intake of highly processed foods.
- Drink eight glasses of water a day to keep the stools moist and easy to pass and to hydrate the tissues.
- Get some form of exercise daily. Even a walk around the block will aid muscle tone and help prevent sluggish metabolism.
- Make time for bowel movements when the stimulus is felt. Avoiding or delaying defecation results in loss of moisture from the stool and may make the bowel insensitive to the stimulus.
- Do not use laxatives or enemas. Frequent use may result in a lazy bowel that responds only to these chemical and physical stimuli.

The frequency of bowel elimination is an individual characteristic. If stools are passed only several times a week but are soft, formed, and passed with little effort, there should be no concern about constipation. However, constipation may be a problem if stools are passed daily but are hard, dry, and difficult to pass.

Polyps

Colon polyps are masses of benign mucous membrane lining the large intestine that are usually slow growing but may become cancerous. Polyps are usually discovered by a barium enema or during a colonoscopy. If the polyps are discovered at an early stage and removed, cancer of the colon may be prevented. Cancer of the colon may invade the muscle of the bowel and metastasize through the lymph system to other organs.

Hernias

The anterior abdominal wall is covered with various muscles that assist with movement and support and protect the internal structures of the abdomen. When these muscles weaken, the underlying organs or intestines may protrude through the weakened muscle wall, resulting in a hernia. Factors that may increase the risk for developing a hernia include a genetic predisposition to muscular weakness, lifting heavy objects, obesity, and pregnancy. The signs and symptoms of abdominal hernia include a protrusion or bulge over the area of the hernia. Specific types of abdominal hernias are named according to the area of the abdomen: the inguinal hernia occurs in right or left inguinal (groin) areas; the ventral hernia occurs in the front of the abdomen; and the umbilical hernia occurs over the umbilicus. The treatment for abdominal hernias includes surgically repairing the weakened muscle (herniorrhaphy) using grafting material as necessary. To prevent abdominal hernias, encourage the use of abdominal support and good body mechanics when lifting and weight reduction as prescribed by the physician.

 CHECKPOINT QUESTION

7. What has generally been noted as the cause of diverticulosis?

Appendicitis

The vermiform appendix, a small pouch of tissue protruding from the cecum or first part of the large intestine, is approximately 4 inches long. Although the function of this tissue is not clear, there is no direct involvement with the process of digestion. Appendicitis occurs when the vermiform appendix becomes infected and fills with bacteria, pus, and blood. Adolescents and young adult men are most commonly affected by this condition, but women and young children can also develop appendicitis. The symptoms include severe abdominal pain with tenderness over the right lower quadrant, vomiting, a fever, and an elevated white blood count. A thorough history should be obtained from any patient with these symptoms, and once the physician determines the diagnosis of appendicitis, it is necessary to make arrangements for immediate surgical removal of the infected appendix. If a diagnosis is not made quickly or the appendectomy is delayed, perforation of the appendix and peritonitis can result and make recovery more difficult for the patient (see Box 17-1).

Hemorrhoids

Hemorrhoids are external or internal dilated veins (varicosities) in the rectum. Internal hemorrhoids may enlarge and may bleed during defecation. A patient with external hemorrhoids may complain of rectal pain and itching and bleeding with bowel movements. Poor abdominal and pelvic floor muscle tone, poor dietary habits including a diet low in fiber, and chronic constipation may cause hemorrhoids. The diagnosis of external hemorrhoids is made by visual inspection, while internal hemorrhoids are diagnosed by anoscopy or proctoscopy. Treatment involves regulating the diet to control constipation, providing local pain relief, using a stool softener, and surgical ligation (hemorrhoidectomy) using standard surgical techniques, laser, or cryosurgery (freezing).

Colorectal Cancers

Cancer of the colon and rectum is often fatal, but the patient's chances for survival are better with early diagnosis and treatment. Although the cause of colorectal cancer is unknown, it has been linked to diets high in animal fats and low in fiber. It is commonly seen in patients with a history of ulcerative colitis or colorectal polyps and affects the first and last parts of the colon more often than other areas (Fig. 17-5). Early signs of colorectal cancer are vague abdominal pains with occasional bloody stools. Later signs depend on the section and amount of the colon involved and the degree of metastasis to other organs and tissues.

Many rectal cancers are discovered by a digital examination or an anoscopy, but sigmoidoscopy or colonoscopy is used to determine the extent of involvement. A barium enema with contrast air aids in the diagnosis. Laboratory tests include **guaiac** tests, such as the Hemoccult™, which test for occult (hidden) blood in the stool. Surgical removal of the affected area, usually

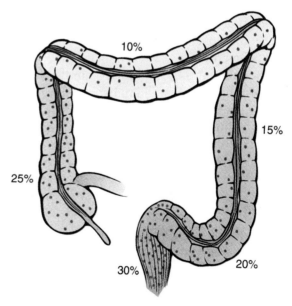

Figure 17-5 Percent distribution of cancer sites in the colon and rectum.

followed by chemotherapy and radiation, is the treatment of choice.

Functional Disorders

Functional disorders of the GI tract include the common disorders of constipation, diarrhea, and intestinal gas. Normally, peristalsis causes the products of digestion to move at a constant rate, not too slowly and not too quickly. Constipation occurs when the lower colon retains fecal material too long so that too much moisture is absorbed, making the stool hard and dry. Most constipation is caused by poor bowel habits (avoiding defecation and overusing laxatives), low-fiber diet, and inadequate fluid intake. The quality of the stool is more important than the quantity. To avoid constipation, patients should be encouraged to increase oral fluid intake, eat foods high in fiber, such as raw vegetables and fruit, and maintain regular bowel habits. The physician may also prescribe a stool softener and an over-the-counter fiber product as needed.

When the fluid contents of the bowel are rushed through, as in diarrhea, the water and minerals are not reabsorbed into the system, and the stool is loose and watery. Bacterial or viral infection or a GI irritant causes the smooth muscles and mucous membranes to work to flush out the bowel as quickly as possible. The treatment for diarrhea includes medication to slow peristalsis, a bland diet, and increasing oral fluids to replace fluids and electrolytes lost in the stool.

Intestinal gas, produced by bacterial decomposition of proteins in the digestive tract, can lead to abdominal discomfort. Gas in the intestinal tract causes a feeling of fullness. The gas may be expelled from the stomach through the mouth (eructation, or belching) or from the intestines through the rectum (flatulence). The production of intestinal gas is due to intolerance of milk products, swallowing air through excessive talking or gum chewing, consuming gas-producing spicy or fatty foods, or slow emptying of the stomach and bowels. The problem can usually be relieved by avoiding the offending foods or behaviors. Various over-the-counter preparations and prescription medications can be used if the problem persists.

 CHECKPOINT QUESTION

8. What causes hemorrhoids?

Liver Disorders

Liver disorders are assessed by observing the cardinal signs of liver dysfunction: jaundice, **ascites** (fluid accumulation in the peritoneal cavity), and **hepatomegaly** (enlargement of the liver). It is vital to obtain a complete medical history from patients with a suspected liver disorder. Particular concern focuses on jaundice, anemia, splenectomy, alcohol use, travel to developing countries, blood transfusions, use of **hepatotoxins** (drugs that are damaging to the liver), and abuse of controlled substances. Diagnostic tests for liver disorders include the following:

- Liver function tests, including prothrombin time and levels of bilirubin, alkaline phosphatase, albumin, and cholesterol
- Radiography and barium study
- Radioisotope liver scan
- Percutaneous peritoneoscopy and biopsy
- Surgical laparotomy and liver biopsy

Hepatitis

Hepatitis is an inflammation or infection of the liver that may lead to liver destruction and necrosis of hepatic cells. The five types of viral hepatitis are summarized in Table 17-1 and listed here:

- *Hepatitis A (HAV)*, the most common type of viral hepatitis, is also known as infectious hepatitis. HAV spreads in food and water contaminated with fecal material or seafood high in coliform bacteria. It is highly contagious, but the prognosis for recovery after an infection with hepatitis A is good.
- *Hepatitis B (HBV)*, also known as *serum hepatitis*, can be transmitted by contaminated blood and other body fluids. HBV may be so severe that death results, but the use of standard precautions will prevent spread. Fortunately, there is a vaccine to protect

TABLE **17-1**	Types of Viral Hepatitis	
Virus	**Transmission**	**Precautions**
HAV	Fecal–oral route	Handwashing; HAV vaccine
HBV	Sera and body fluids	Standard precautions; HBV vaccine
HCV	Blood transfusions Percutaneous contamination	Standard precautions
HDV	Coinfection with HBV	Standard precautions; HBV vaccine
HEV	Fecal–oral route	Handwashing; standard precautions

against HBV, and it is recommended for all health care workers.

- *Hepatitis C (HCV)*, also known as *non-A, non-B hepatitis*, can be transmitted via blood transfusion or percutaneous contamination. After the initial infection, HCV frequently progresses to chronic hepatitis that may be asymptomatic but is communicable. As with HBV, the use of standard precautions prevents spread.
- *Hepatitis D (HDV)* occurs only in patients who have had HBV; it cannot survive without HBV.
- *Hepatitis E (HEV)* spreads in food or water contaminated with fecal material and ingested by the unsuspecting individual.

While the viruses responsible for the individual types of viral hepatitis are physically different, the symptoms of all types are similar. They may include fatigue, joint pain, flulike symptoms with fever, jaundice, dark urine, and light stools. Complications of hepatitis include long-term impaired liver function, chronic hepatitis, liver cancer, and death.

Diagnosis of the various types of viral hepatitis is made by obtaining a complete medical history, blood analysis for hepatitis antibodies, and liver function studies. There is no cure once infection occurs, but the patient is encouraged to rest and take in a supportive diet. Interferon-α is given to some patients to assist the immune system in responding to viral hepatitis. Standard precautions must be observed to protect caregivers and health care workers from contracting hepatitis.

Another cause of hepatitis, toxic hepatitis, is exposure to chemical toxicants or hepatotoxic substances, including certain medications and alcohol. If the offending toxicant is eliminated early enough, the prognosis for recovery is good. The symptoms of toxic hepatitis resemble viral hepatitis, and the diagnosis is similar. A liver biopsy may identify the underlying pathology.

Cirrhosis or Fibrosis

Cirrhosis is a chronic disease characterized by destruction of liver cells and the formation of scar tissue or fibers throughout the liver, altering its function and efficiency. The causes of cirrhosis include a history of exposure to hepatotoxins, alcoholism, prolonged biliary obstruction, and a history of hepatitis. In the early stages, symptoms include vague GI discomfort. In the late stages, respiratory efficiency decreases because of ascites that forces the abdominal contents against the diaphragm. Bleeding tendencies result from the loss of clotting factors formed in the liver. Dermal pruritus (itching), jaundice, and hepatomegaly are usually present. Diagnosis is made by liver biopsy, liver scan, and blood work. Treatment includes avoiding the hepatotoxins or abstinence from alcohol to prevent further death of hepatic cells, a good diet, vitamin supplements, and supportive care. In cases of liver failure that

accompanies increased destruction of liver tissue, the physician may recommend a liver transplantation.

CHECKPOINT QUESTION

9. How does the cause of viral hepatitis differ from that of toxic hepatitis?

Liver Cancer

The liver is rarely a primary site for cancer but is frequently a target site of metastasis. This type of cancer is more common in men than in women and is rapidly fatal. There is no known cause, but primary liver cancers are thought to be due to exposure to carcinogenic chemicals, including hepatotoxins. Patients who have cirrhosis or hepatitis B are more likely than the general population to develop liver cancer.

In the early stages of the disease, patients usually complain of weight loss, weakness, and right upper quadrant pain. Jaundice may be present and will definitely develop as the disease progresses (Fig. 17-6). Diagnosis is confirmed by biopsy, liver function tests, and computed tomography (CT) or magnetic resonance imaging (MRI). If the lesion is small and local, resection is possible. Chemotherapy may be used in some instances. If there is no metastasis, a liver transplantation may be possible.

Gallbladder Disorders

Cholelithiasis and Cholecystitis

Cholelithiasis is the formation of gallstones made of cholesterol and bilirubin (Fig. 17-7). When the peristaltic action of the gallbladder is sluggish and bile pools in

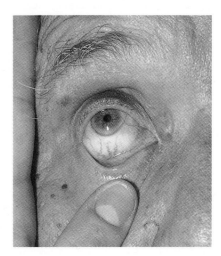

Figure 17-6 A patient with jaundice. (From Bickley LS, Szilagyi P. Bates' Guide to Physical Examination and History Taking. 8th ed. Philadelphia: Lippincott Williams & Wilkins, 2003.)

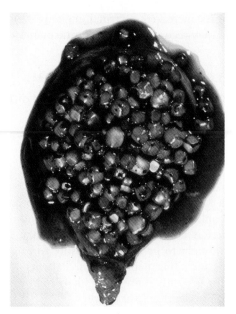

Figure 17-7 Cholelithiasis. The gallbladder has been opened to reveal numerous yellow cholesterol gallstones. (Reprinted with permission from Rubin E, Gorstein F, Rubin R, Schwarting R, Strayer D. Rubin's Pathology: Clinicopathologic Foundations of Medicine. Philadelphia: Lippincott Williams & Wilkins, 2005.)

the sac, fluid is absorbed, leaving the solids to concentrate and solidify into stones. Cholecystitis is an acute or chronic inflammation of the gallbladder, usually resulting from an impacted stone in the duct. Cholecystitis or cholelithiasis usually causes pain as peristalsis presses bile against the blockage, especially after a fatty meal.

Signs and symptoms of any gallbladder disorder include acute right upper abdominal quadrant pain that may radiate to the shoulders, back, or chest; indigestion; nausea; and intolerance of fatty foods. Later in the illness, jaundice may appear as the ducts to the liver become blocked. Tests to determine the cause of the symptoms include cholecystography after the ingestion of a radiopaque dye, percutaneous transhepatic cholangiography, endoscopic retrograde cholangiopancreatography (ECRP), and duodenal endoscopy. Noninvasive procedures include ultrasound and CT. Flat plate radiographs are not especially accurate for evaluating gallbladder disorders. The treatment may be supportive or palliative, including pain medication and avoiding fatty foods; however, surgical removal of the stones (cholecystectomy) may be necessary, usually through endoscopic laparotomy. Lithotripsy (crushing the gallstones using sound waves) may also be used to break the stones into small pieces that can pass easily through the bile ducts and into the digestive system for elimination.

Gallbladder Cancer

Cancer of the gallbladder is rare and difficult to diagnose. Since the symptoms are similar to those of cholecystitis, this cancer is usually discovered during routine gallbladder tests performed to diagnose general gallbladder disease. The signs and symptoms include right upper quadrant pain, nausea and vomiting, weight loss, and anorexia. However, cholecystitis pain is usually sporadic, whereas pain due to malignancy is usually chronic and severe. The gallbladder may be palpable, and jaundice may be present. It is most common in older women and is rapidly fatal. The cause is not known, but theory suggests that cholelithiasis is a predisposing factor. Diagnosis includes liver function tests, CT, MRI, and cholecystography. Surgical cholecystectomy is the primary treatment, but survival rates are low.

 CHECKPOINT QUESTION

10. How are cholelithiasis and cholecystitis different?

Pancreatic Disorders

Pancreatitis

Pancreatitis is an inflammation of the pancreas that may be related to alcoholism, trauma, gastric ulcer, or biliary tract disease. Signs and symptoms include vomiting and steady epigastric pain radiating to the spine. Signs of progressive disease include abdominal rigidity and decreased bowel activity. Complications include diabetes mellitus, hemorrhage, shock, coma, and death as the digestive enzymes cause the organ to digest itself. Diagnostic blood tests show an increase in serum amylase and glucose levels. Ultrasound and CT are useful for diagnosis. Treatment includes pain relief and medication to reduce pancreatic secretions while the organ recovers. Prognosis depends on the extent and severity of damage to the pancreas.

Pancreatic Cancer

One of the deadliest malignancies is pancreatic cancer, which kills most patients within a year of diagnosis. There is no definitive cause of pancreatic cancer, but it occurs most often in middle-aged African American men who smoke, who have a diet high in fats and proteins, or who are exposed to industrial chemicals for long periods. Patients complain of weight loss, back and abdominal pain, and diarrhea. Commonly they are jaundiced. Diagnosis is made by laparoscopic biopsy, CT, MRI, endoscopic retrograde cholangiopancreatography (ERCP), and pancreatic enzyme studies. Surgical removal of the pancreas (pancreatotomy), chemotherapy, and radiation therapy are used to treat pancreatic cancer, but the survival rate is very low.

 CHECKPOINT QUESTION

11. What are some complications of pancreatitis?

Common Diagnostic and Therapeutic Procedures

History and Physical Examination of the GI System

Before beginning any patient's care, an adequate history must be obtained. The patient presenting with GI concerns will be assessed for signs (e.g., vomiting) and symptoms (e.g., nausea). From that base, the physician will determine the direction of the diagnostic testing to rule out or to confirm possible diagnosis. The history must include occupation, family history, recent travel to developing countries, and current medications. Patients should also be required to complete a checklist of concerns, which may include heartburn, GI bleeding, weight gain or loss, history of alcohol use, and laxative and enema use.

The physician will assess skin **turgor** (elasticity), jaundice, edema, bruising, breath odor, size and shape of the abdomen, and presence and quality of bowel sounds. The physician will also palpate abdominal contents.

Blood Tests

Blood work ordered by the physician may include white and red blood cell counts. The red blood cells, hemoglobin, and hematocrit are used to assess possible anemia as the result of GI bleeding. White blood cell counts can help to detect infection, while the erythrocyte sedimentation rate is used to assess inflammatory processes, including inflammation of the GI system.

Blood may also be drawn and sent to the laboratory to determine liver function. Specifically, alkaline phosphatase, serum bilirubin, prothrombin time, and SGPT (serum glutamic pyruvic transaminase) levels are determined in a test collectively known as a *liver panel*. Pancreatic enzyme studies include evaluation of blood for levels of enzymes normally released by the pancreas, including trypsin, chymotrypsin, steapsin, and amylopsin. Results that fall outside of the normal ranges for these substances indicate pathology and necessitate further testing as determined by the physician.

Radiology Studies

Flat plate radiographs of the abdomen may be ordered for diagnosing GI problems, but without contrast medium, these radiographs are not so useful as contrast radiographs. Radiology studies of the stomach and intestines consist of instilling barium, a radiopaque liquid, into the GI tract orally or rectally to outline the organs and identify abnormalities. The radiographs include standard pictures taken at various intervals after the barium is administered by mouth or by enema. If a fluoroscope (special type of radiographic equipment) is used, movement of the chalky liquid barium is viewed while it fills the esophagus or colon, giving additional diagnostic information.

The barium swallow (also called an *upper GI* or *UGI*) series can reveal abnormal constrictions, masses, and obstruction in the esophagus, stomach, and duodenum. This examination requires that the patient have nothing by mouth (NPO) after midnight the night before the test. A small bowel series is an extension of the UGI that visualizes the barium flowing through the small intestine to diagnose abnormalities of the first part of the small intestine.

A barium enema, or lower GI study, provides an outline of the colon. It can reveal a blockage, cancerous growths, polyps, and diverticula. Since the lower GI study requires that the colon be empty of stool, the patient must be given specific instructions to follow before the examination. Box 17-2 outlines the standard preparation for a barium enema, which should be orally explained to the patient and given in written form.

Cholecystography is radiography of the gallbladder after the patient takes oral tablets containing a contrast material 12 hours prior to the procedure. The contrast medium is excreted from the liver into the gallbladder, and any abnormalities are viewed on the radiogram. After the initial films are taken, the patient is given a fatty meal that stimulates the contraction of the gallbladder to release bile and contrast medium into the bile ducts. Additional films may be taken to view any obstruction of these ducts by stones. The bile ducts may also be examined using

---

BOX 17-2

PATIENT PREPARATION FOR BOWEL STUDIES

Many bowel studies, such as barium enema and flexible sigmoidoscopy, require that the bowel be completely clear of fecal matter. With minor variations as directed by the physician, the bowel preparation usually includes the following:

- Liquid diet without dairy products for the full day before the procedure or a clear liquid evening meal
- A laxative or enema the evening preceding the procedure
- Nothing by mouth after midnight except water
- Rectal suppository, Fleet's enema, or cleansing enema the morning of the procedure

If inflammatory processes or ulcerations are suspected inside the bowel, only gentle cleansing will be used to avoid undue discomfort or possible perforation of lesions.

percutaneous transhepatic cholangiography, a test that entails injection of contrast material through a needle inserted through the skin into the hepatic duct. Once the dye is injected, radiography is performed for diagnosis by the physician.

The role of the medical assistant in radiographic procedures includes determining third-party payer (insurance) requirements for referrals or preauthorization, scheduling the procedure in an outpatient facility, and explaining to the patient the preparations for the examination as necessary. When the test is complete, the radiologist will submit a written report to the referring physician. Follow office policy and procedure for routing the report to the physician for review and advising the patient of the examination results.

 CHECKPOINT QUESTION

12. Why are contrast media used in radiography of the GI organs?

Nuclear Imaging

Radionuclides, or radioactive elements, are often used in the diagnosis of disorders of the liver. After the elements are injected into the body, images are taken using a nuclear scanning device, and abnormalities can be detected and evaluated by the radiologist. The injected radionuclide remains radioactive for a short specific period, and there is usually very little, if any, patient preparation required for this test. The role of the medical assistant includes coordinating any third-party payer requirements such as preauthorization, scheduling the test at a nuclear imaging center or hospital, and following up with the patient when the results are returned to the medical office as indicated in the policy and procedure manual. Test results indicating abnormalities necessitate additional evaluation and testing as determined by the physician.

Ultrasonography

The use of high-frequency sound waves to diagnose disorders of internal structures is used in many specialties, including gastroenterology. Abnormalities in the structure of various digestive accessory organs, such as the liver and gallbladder, can be easily viewed using ultrasonography and require very little if any preparation by the patient. As with other diagnostic tests ordered by the physician, your role includes verifying third-party payer guidelines and obtaining preauthorization if needed. Although ultrasound does not use radiation or radiography, ultrasounds are scheduled in the imaging department of many outpatient or inpatient facilities. Your role includes scheduling the test, advising the

patient of the date and time, following up after the test to obtain results if necessary, ensuring that the physician is aware of the results, and notifying the patient with any findings or additional instructions as ordered by the physician.

Endoscopic Studies

Fiberoptic technology has enabled physicians to pass soft, flexible tubes down the esophagus into the stomach and small intestine or up into the colon for direct visualization of these organs. Supplemental laboratory specimens, including tissue biopsy samples; samples of secretions for gastric analysis, including pH; culture sample to check for bacteria; bile for crystals that may lead to the formation of stones; and cells for cytology, including cancerous or otherwise abnormal cells, can be obtained. Endoscopic examinations are also used to diagnose biliary disorders.

ERCP (endoscopic retrograde cholangiopancreatography) is used to visualize the esophagus, stomach, proximal duodenum, and pancreas with a flexible endoscope. When the endoscope is in place, dye is injected directly into the ducts of the gallbladder and pancreas, and radiographs are taken to determine patency and function of these structures and the biliary ducts (Fig. 17-8). This procedure is usually performed in an outpatient surgical center under anesthesia. Your role includes scheduling the procedure, advising the patient on any instructions prior to the test, and follow-up when the written report is sent by the gastroenterologist or radiologist.

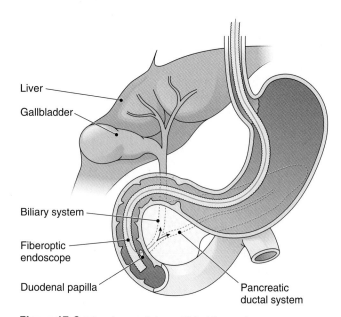

Figure 17-8 The ducts of the gallbladder and pancreas can be easily visualized during an ERCP. (From Cohen BJ. Medical Terminology. 4th ed. Philadelphia: Lippincott Williams & Wilkins, 2003.)

Anoscopy, which may be performed in the medical office, is insertion of a metal or plastic anoscope into the rectal canal for visual inspection of the anus and rectum and to swab for cultures. The sigmoidoscopy examination provides a visual examination of the sigmoid colon using either a rigid sigmoidoscope or the more widely accepted flexible fiberoptic sigmoidoscope. The rigid sigmoidoscope is about 25 cm (10 inches) long. This instrument is supplied as reusable metal or disposable plastic and is calibrated in centimeters. An **obturator** in the lumen allows the instrument to be inserted with minimal discomfort and can be removed after insertion allowing for better visualization and obtaining specimens. The lens at the end magnifies the view for closer observation of the intestinal mucosa and can be moved aside to allow the physician to swab, suction, or sample the mucosa for biopsy. The handle contains the light source. The scope may be equipped with a hand bulb **insufflator**, a device for blowing air into the colon to expand the walls for easier visualization.

The flexible fiberoptic sigmoidoscope is more popular because it offers better visualization and is less uncomfortable for the patient (Fig. 17-9). The scope is very thin, can bend and maneuver curves, and can be inserted much farther than the rigid scope (Fig. 17-10). The instrument is 35 cm (about 14 inches) or 65 cm (about 26 inches). It usually includes an insufflator and suction in addition to the light source. Although smaller in diameter than the rigid scope, it can also be used to obtain samples and cultures.

Some physicians prefer that the bowel be as free of feces as possible and may order a light, low-residue meal the evening before the endoscopic examination. An evening laxative may also be ordered to be followed by a cleansing enema on the morning of the procedure. A light breakfast may be allowed but only if ordered by the physician. Other physicians prefer to view the mucosa as it normally appears, without

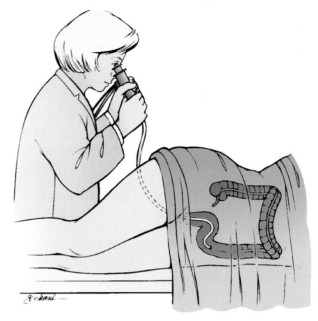

Figure 17-10 Sigmoidoscopy. The flexible scope is advanced past the proximal sigmoid colon and into the descending colon. (Reprinted with permission from Cohen BJ. Medical Terminology: An Illustrated Guide. Philadelphia: Lippincott Williams & Wilkins, 2003.)

preparation. Most medical offices note the preferred preparation in the policy and procedure manual. Your role includes informing the patient of the preferred preparation for the procedure, assisting the physician during the procedure, and offering reassurance and support to the patient. Procedure 17-1 describes the steps for assisting with colon procedures in the medical office.

CHECKPOINT QUESTION

13. What does anoscopy involve, and how does it differ from sigmoidoscopy?

Fecal Tests

As part of the routine examination for adult patients, many physicians recommend testing a stool specimen for the presence of occult, or hidden, blood. A stool specimen may also be ordered to test for ova (eggs) and parasites if the physician suspects the patient has a parasite infection. You may be responsible for instructing the patient in the procedure for collecting these specimens, and in some cases, such as in testing the stool for occult blood, you may be responsible for testing the stool specimen after the patient returns it to the office. Chapter 29 discusses the procedure for instructing a patient to collect a stool specimen and for processing the specimens for occult blood.

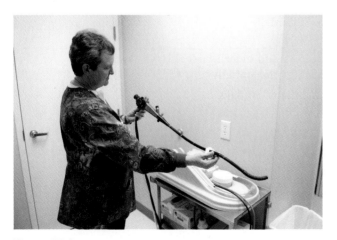

Figure 17-9 A flexible sigmoidoscope.

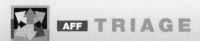

TRIAGE

While you are working in a medical office, the following three situations occur:

A. A 44-year-old man is scheduled for a routine physical. However, he arrives in the office complaining of "heartburn" and is taken to an exam room where the physician has ordered an ECG.

B. An 18-year-old boy comes into the office with lower right abdominal pain. The physician wants blood drawn immediately to determine a white blood cell count and rule out appendicitis.

C. A 52-year-old woman has just seen the physician and needs to be scheduled for a colonoscopy at the local outpatient ambulatory surgical center.

How do you sort these patients? Who do you see first? Second? Third?

First, you should do the ECG on patient A. A feeling of indigestion or epigastric discomfort can be a sign of cardiac disease. Next draw patient B's blood, since an elevation in the white blood cell count indicates the need for additional tests and/or surgery for appendicitis. Finally, schedule the outpatient procedure for patient C after checking for appropriate insurance referrals.

Note: This sequence is the accepted triage standard; however, the physician may opt for the blood work to be done first if he or she considers that patient A's discomfort is probably due to gastric difficulties and has ordered the ECG as a prophylactic measure. This decision is based on the physical examinations of both patients. You and the physician must work as a team to achieve the best outcomes.

Medication Box

Commonly Prescribed GI System Medications

Note: The generic name of the drug is listed first and is written in all lowercase letters. Brand names are in parentheses, and the first letter is capitalized.

bisacodyl (Dulcolax)	Tablets: 10 mg	Laxative
cimetidine (Tagamet)	Oral liquid: 300 mg/5 mL	Antiulcerative
	Tablets: 200 mg, to 800 mg	
dicyclomine (Bentyl)	Capsules: 10 mg, 20 mg	Anticholinergic
diphenoxylate (Lomotil)	Tablets: 2.5 mg	Antidiarrheal
	Liquid: 2.5 mg/5 mL	
esomeprazole (Nexium)	Capsules: 20 mg to 40 mg	Antiulcerative
famotidine (Pepcid)	Gelcaps: 10 mg	Antiulcerative
	Tablets: 10 mg to 40 mg	
hepatitis A vaccine, inactivated (Havrix, Vaqta)	Injection: 25 units/0.5 mL (intramuscular)	Vaccine
hepatitis B vaccine, recombinant (Engerix-B, Recombivax HB)	Injection: Adults (20 yr and older): First dose: 20 mcg intramuscular initially	Vaccine
	Second dose: 20 mcg after 30 days	
	Third dose: 20 mcg 6 months after second dose	
infliximab (Remicade)	100-mg vial (intravenous)	Immunosuppressant
lansoprazole (Prevacid)	Capsules: 15 mg and 30 mg	Antiulcerative
	Oral suspension: 15 or 30 mg/packet	

Commonly Prescribed GI System Medications *(continued)*		
metoclopramide (Reglan)	Tablets: 5 mg, 10 mg Intramuscular injection: 5 mg/mL	Antiemetic
omeprazole (Prilosec)	Capsules: 10 mg to 40 mg	Antiulcerative
ondansetron (Zofran)	Tablets: 4 mg, 8 mg, 24 mg	Antiemetic
pantoprazole (Protonix)	Tablet: 20 mg, 40 mg	Antiulcerative
phentermine (Adipex-P)	Capsules: 18.75 mg, 30 mg, 37.5 mg Tablets: 37.5 mg	Appetite suppressant
polyethylene glycol (MiraLax)	Powder: single-dose (17 g) 16 oz, 24 oz	Laxative
rabeprazole (Aciphex)	Tablets: 20 mg	Antiulcerative
rantidine (Zantac)	Tablets: 75 mg	Antiulcerative
scopolamine (Scopace; Transderm-Scop)	Tablets: 0.4 mg Transdermal patch: 1.5 mg/2.5 cm^2	Antiemetic
sibutramine (Meridia)	Capsules: 5 mg, 10 mg, 15 mg	Appetite suppressant

español SPANISH TERMINOLOGY

¿Tiene indigestion?
  Do you have indigestion?

¿Esta estreñido?
  Are you constipated?

¿Tiene diarreas?
  Do you have diarrhea?

¿Ha notado sangre o mucosidad en la escreta?
  Have you noticed any blood or mucus in the stools?

MEDIA MENU

- **Student Resources on thePoint**
  - **Animation: Cirrhosis**
  - **Animation: General Digestion**
  - **CMA/RMA Certification Exam Review**
- **Internet Resources**

  The American College of Gastroenterology
  http://www.acg.gi.org

  Centers for Disease Control and Prevention
  http://www.cdc.gov/hepatitis

  National Digestive Diseases Information Clearinghouse
  http://digestive.niddk.nih.gov/ddiseases/pubs/cirrhosis

PSY PROCEDURE 17-1:   Assisting with Colon Procedures

Purpose: Prepare the patient and assist with endoscopic colon procedures
Equipment: Appropriate instrument (flexible or rigid sigmoidoscope, anoscope, or proctoscope), water-soluble lubricant, gown and drape, cotton swabs, suction (if not part of the scope), biopsy forceps, specimen container with preservative, completed laboratory requisition form, personal wipes or tissues, equipment for assessing vital signs, examination gloves

Steps	Reasons
1. Wash your hands.	Handwashing aids infection control.
2. Assemble the equipment and supplies. Write the name of the patient on the label of the specimen container and complete the laboratory requisition.	The name of the patient must be clearly marked on the container and the laboratory requisition form must be complete for accurate identification and processing of any specimens taken.
3. Check the light source if a flexible sigmoidoscope is being used. Turn off the power after checking for working order to avoid a buildup of heat in the instrument.	If heat is permitted to build up in the scope, the patient may be burned. If the rigid sigmoidoscope, anoscope, or proctoscope is being used, check the examination light for working order.

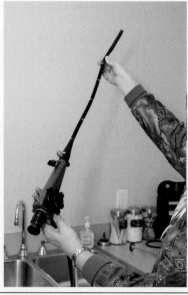

Step 3. Make sure the equipment, such as the sigmoidoscope, is in good working order.

4. Greet and identify the patient and explain the procedure. Inform the patient that a sensation of pressure or the need to defecate may be felt during the procedure and that the pressure is from the instrument and will ease. The patient may also feel gas pressure when air is insufflated during sigmoidoscopy. *Note:* The patient may have been ordered to take a mild sedative before the procedure.	Identifying the patient prevents errors in treatment. Explaining the procedure helps ease anxiety and ensure compliance.
5. Instruct the patient to empty the urinary bladder.	Pressure from the instrument may injure a full bladder. Urine in the bladder may increase discomfort.
6. Assess the vital signs and record them in the medical record.	Colon examination procedures may cause cardiac arrhythmias and a change in blood pressure in some patients. Baseline vital signs will allow you to detect variations from the patient's normal vital signs.
7. Have the patient undress completely from the waist down and put on a gown. Drape appropriately.	Drapes will provide privacy and warmth.

PSY PROCEDURE 17-1: Assisting with Colon Procedures (continued)

Steps	Reasons
8. Assist the patient onto the examination table. If the instrument is an anoscope or a fiberoptic device, Sims position or a side-lying position is most comfortable. If a rigid instrument is used, the patient will assume a knee-chest position or be placed on a proctology table that supports the patient in a knee-chest position. *Note:* Do not ask the patient to assume the knee-chest position until the physician is ready to begin. The position is difficult to maintain. Drape the patient appropriately. 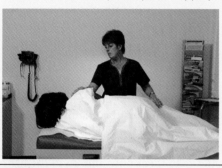	These positions facilitate the procedure by moving the abdominal organs up into the abdominal cavity rather than the pelvis.
	Step 8. This patient is in the Sims position.
9. **AFF** Explain how to respond to a patient who is visually impaired.	Observe patients carefully to prevent injury and always ask before offering assistance. Face the patient when speaking and always let him or her know what you are going to do before touching him or her.
10. Assist the physician as needed with lubricant, instruments, power, swabs, suction, and specimen containers.	Anticipating what the physician needs and being ready to hand items to the the physician will provide for a smooth and quick procedure.
11. During the procedure, monitor the patient's response and offer reassurance. Instruct the patient to breathe slowly through pursed lips.	Reminding the patient how to breathe will aid in relaxation during the procedure.
12. When the physician is finished, assist the patient into a comfortable position and allow a rest period. Offer personal cleaning wipes or tissues. Take the vital signs before allowing the patient to stand, and assist the patient from the table and with dressing as needed. Give the patient any instructions regarding care after the procedure and follow-up ordered by the physician.	A drop in blood pressure on standing is common after lying in any of these positions for an extended period. If the patient complains of dizziness or lightheadedness after sitting up, have him or her lie down. If any biopsy samples were taken, the patient may have slight rectal bleeding.
13. Clean the room and route the specimen to the laboratory with the requisition. Disinfect or dispose of the supplies and equipment as appropriate and wash your hands.	Follow standard precautions throughout the procedure.
14. Document the procedure.	Procedures are considered not to have been done if they are not recorded.

Charting Example:

> 05/31/2013 12:45 PM T 98.6 (O), P 100, R 20, BP 144/86 (L). Sigmoidoscopy performed by Dr. Jacobs and specimen obtained—pt. tolerated well. Specimen to Acme Lab, VS after procedure P 112, R 24, BP 146/86 (L). Pt. denied dizziness after procedure. Discharged per Dr. Jacobs. ————————————————————— S. Clay, CMA

Note: The medical assistant may sign his or her name in the patient record using only the "CMA" credential if the office has a signature log denoting the entire credential as "CMA(AAMA)."

Information regarding the care of a patient with GI disorders requires knowledge of the following:

- Any disruption of the processes of ingestion, absorption, or elimination is pathologic not only to the gastric system, but to other body systems and cells as well.
- Although the medical assistant working in the office of the gastroenterologist encounters many patients with disorders of the GI system, patients with gastric disorders are commonly seen in other offices, including family practice, internal medicine, and pediatrics.

- A thorough history is essential for an accurate diagnosis of any GI disorder.
- Assisting with various diagnostic procedures, such as colon examinations and stool testing, can also help the physician detect abnormalities in GI function.
- Patient education regarding diet and prevention of various gastric disorders is a critical aspect of the professional medical assistant's role and should be considered an ongoing process.

Warm Ups | for Critical Thinking

1. Review the preparation of the patient for an upper GI series and a barium enema. Create two handouts that include the following:
   - A description of each procedure
   - A list of reasons for the procedure
   - Preparations required to ensure reliable test results
2. Many endoscopic examinations require the patient to be in an uncomfortable and embarrassing position. How can you help alleviate the stress and anxiety?
3. Mrs. Barnes, a 43-year-old patient, was scheduled for a cholecystography at 11:00 a.m. today and was given all instructions and the oral contrast medium to take the morning of the examination. She calls the office at 10:30 a.m. and tells you that she forgot to take the dye tablets and wants to know whether she should take them now and go in for her test at the appointed time. What do you tell Mrs. Barnes?
4. Research the various surgeries used to treat obesity. In addition to the risks involved with having abdominal surgery, are there any side effects or risks with each procedure that may further affect the GI system or other body systems?
5. Explain how a patient with gallstones can develop pancreatitis.

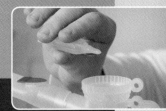

18 Neurology

Outline

Common Nervous System Disorders
  Infectious Disorders
  Degenerative Disorders
  Seizure Disorders
  Developmental Disorders
  Trauma

Brain Tumors
Headaches
Common Diagnostic Tests for Disorders of the Nervous System
  Physical Examination
  Radiologic Tests

Electrical Tests
Lumbar Puncture

Learning Outcomes

Cognitive Domain

Note: AAMA/CAAHEP 2008 Standards are italicized.

1. Spell and define key terms
2. Identify common diseases of the nervous system
3. Describe the physical and emotional effects of degenerative nervous system disorders
4. List potential complications of a spinal cord injury
5. Name and describe the common procedures for diagnosing nervous system disorders
6. *Identify common pathologies related to each body system*
7. *Describe implications for treatment related to pathology*

Psychomotor Domain

Note: AAMA/CAAHEP 2008 Standards are italicized.

1. Assist with a lumbar puncture (Procedure 18-1)
2. *Assist physician with patient care*
3. *Prepare a patient for procedures and/or treatments*
4. *Practice standard precautions*
5. *Document patient care*
6. *Document patient education*

7. *Practice within the standard of care for a medical assistant*

Affective Domain

Note: AAMA/CAAHEP 2008 Standards are italicized.

1. *Apply critical thinking skills in performing patient assessment and care*
2. *Use language/verbal skills that enable patients' understanding*
3. *Demonstrate empathy in communicating with patients, family, and staff*
4. *Use appropriate body language and other nonverbal skills in communicating with patients, family, and staff*
5. *Demonstrate awareness of the territorial boundaries of the person with whom you are communicating*
6. *Demonstrate sensitivity appropriate to the message being delivered*
7. *Demonstrate recognition of the patient's level of understanding in communications*
8. *Recognize and protect personal boundaries in communicating with others*
9. *Demonstrate respect for individual diversity, incorporating awareness of one's own biases in areas including gender, race, religion, age, and economic status*
10. *Apply active listening skills*

11. *Apply local, state, and federal health care legislation and regulation appropriate to the medical assisting practice setting*

ABHES Competencies

1. Assist the physician with the regimen of diagnostic and treatment modalities as they relate to each body system

2. Comply with federal, state, and local health laws and regulations
3. Communicate on the recipient's level of comprehension
4. Serve as a liaison between the physician and others
5. Show empathy and impartiality when dealing with patients
6. Document accurately

Key Terms

aura	dysphagia	meningocele	Romberg test
cephalalgia	dysphasia	migraine	seizures
concussion	electroencephalogram	myelogram	spina bifida occulta
contusion	(EEG)	myelomeningocele	
convulsion	herpes zoster	Queckenstedt test	

The nervous system is the chief communication and command center for all parts of the body. The nervous system has two divisions: the central nervous system (CNS) and the peripheral nervous system (PNS). The CNS includes the brain and spinal cord (Fig. 18-1), and the PNS contains the nerves that transmit impulses. Nerves are found throughout the body and in the brain. The autonomic nervous system (ANS), a division of the PNS, functions without voluntary action. Together these divisions of the nervous system allow skeletal movement, maintain vital homeostatic functions such as breathing and heart rate, and promote thought processes including memory and logic. The complexity of the nervous system and its connections with the muscular system make it subject to many disorders that can be difficult to diagnose and treat effectively.

Neurology deals with study of the nervous system and its disorders, and the physician who specializes in this area is a neurologist. The medical assistant who works in a neurology office has many interesting and challenging patients. Also, the medical assistant who works in other medical specialties may also have patients with diseases or disorders of the nervous system. This chapter focuses on some of the common disorders of the nervous system and the role of the medical assistant who works with these patients.

Common Nervous System Disorders

Infectious Disorders

Disorders of the nervous system range from minor inconveniences to lethal diseases. The following sections discuss the disorders in groups: infectious, degenerative, convulsive (**seizures**), developmental, traumatic, neoplastic (tumors), and headache.

Meningitis

Meningitis is characterized by inflammation of the meninges covering the spinal cord and the brain. The inflammation can result from either bacterial or viral infection. Viral meningitis is usually not life threatening and is often short lived, but bacterial meningitis is often severe and may be fatal. The infection is usually precipitated by an upper respiratory, sinus, or ear infection. Children are the age group most likely to develop meningitis. Meningitis can also result from head trauma when an open wound allows organisms to enter the cranium and nervous system.

Patients with meningitis have a variety of signs and symptoms, including nausea, vomiting, fever, headache, and a stiff neck. Patients may also complain of photophobia, or intolerance to light. A rash with small, reddish purple dots may appear on the body,

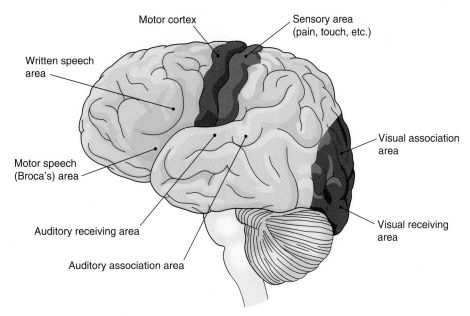

Motor cortex

Sensory area
(pain, touch, etc.)

Written speech
area

Visual association
area

Motor speech
(Broca's) area

Visual receiving
area

Auditory receiving area

Auditory association area

Figure 18-1 Functional areas of the cerebral cortex. (Reprinted with permission from Cohen BJ. Memmler's The Human Body in Health and Disease, 11th ed. Philadelphia: Lippincott Williams & Wilkins, 2009.)

and as patients become sicker, they may slip into a coma and have seizures.

To diagnose meningitis, the physician usually orders a complete blood count. If the white blood cell count is high, a lumbar puncture is performed, and cerebrospinal fluid (CSF) is sent to the laboratory for analysis to determine the infectious organism. The treatment of meningitis depends on the organism causing the infection. The treatment for viral meningitis includes fluids and bed rest, and bacterial meningitis is treated with antibiotics and generally requires hospitalization. The local health department must be notified of the diagnosis, and some states require that an infectious disease form be filed. Check your office policy and procedure manual to determine who is responsible for obtaining, completing, and submitting these reports, keeping in mind that, in many offices, it is the medical assistant's responsibility. Depending on the type of meningitis, individuals (family, friends, coworkers, classmates) who have had contact with the patient may require prophylactic treatment.

Encephalitis

Encephalitis is an inflammation of the brain that frequently results from a viral infection following a varicella (chicken pox), measles, or mumps infection. A strain of the virus is transmitted by mosquitoes. This type is primarily seen on the East and Gulf coasts. Symptoms of all forms include drowsiness, headache, and fever. Seizures and coma may occur in later stages. Diagnosis is made via lumbar puncture and analysis of CSF.

Treatment of encephalitis requires hospitalization for intravenous fluid therapy and supportive care.

The prognosis is usually good if the diagnosis is made early and treatment begins quickly. As with meningitis, the local health department should be notified to identify those who may have been exposed to the disease.

CHECKPOINT QUESTION

1. How does the treatment of viral meningitis differ from that of bacterial meningitis?

Herpes Zoster

Herpes zoster, or *shingles*, is caused by the virus that causes chicken pox and occurs only in those who have had a varicella infection (see Chapter 12). Herpes zoster usually occurs in adults, often in times of physical or emotional stress. The virus, which lies dormant after the initial infection, becomes reactivated and spreads down the length of a nerve, causing redness, swelling, and pain (Fig. 18-2). After about 48 hours, a band of papules develops on the skin following the nerve pathway. These lesions commonly appear on the face, back, and chest and progress to vesicles, pustules, and then dry crusts similar to chickenpox lesions. The lesions may last for 2 to 5 weeks, and the patient may have pain after the lesions disappear.

The treatment of a herpes zoster breakout includes an analgesic or nerve block for pain. Calamine lotion may be applied to the skin to reduce itching. Antiviral medication, such as acyclovir, may be prescribed to alleviate the severity of the disease.

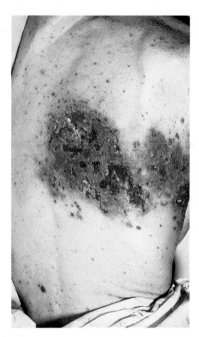

Figure 18-2 Primary skin lesions. Herpes zoster (shingles) is an acute, inflammatory, infectious skin disease caused by a herpes virus. (From Weber J RN, EdD and Kelley J RN, PhD. Health Assessment in Nursing, 2nd edition. Philadelphia: Lippincott Williams & Wilkins, 2003.)

Poliomyelitis

Commonly called *polio*, this highly contagious and resistant virus affects the brain and spinal cord. The virus can live outside the body for several months, making it almost impossible to eliminate once it has appeared in a community. It is transmitted by direct contact, usually through the mouth. In the United States, its incidence has been greatly reduced by aggressive immunization programs. However, because not all children have received the proper schedule of immunizations and because some adults have not been immunized at all, concern about the disease still exists.

In the acute phase, the patient may complain of a stiff neck, fever, headaches, and a sore throat. Nausea, vomiting, and diarrhea may also occur. As the disease progresses, paralysis may develop. Muscle atrophy leads to eventual deformities (Fig. 18-3). If the respiratory muscles are affected, the patient cannot breathe without artificial assistance.

A new dimension of the disease, postpoliomyelitis muscular atrophy (PPMA) syndrome, has been documented in some individuals who had polio as children. Many of these patients have signs and symptoms similar to those that signaled the onset of the original disease. They usually complain of muscle weakness and a lack of coordination. Typically, patients with PPMA are treated on an outpatient basis with supportive care. No cure is available.

During the acute stage of polio, treatment is palliative and supportive. After this acute stage has

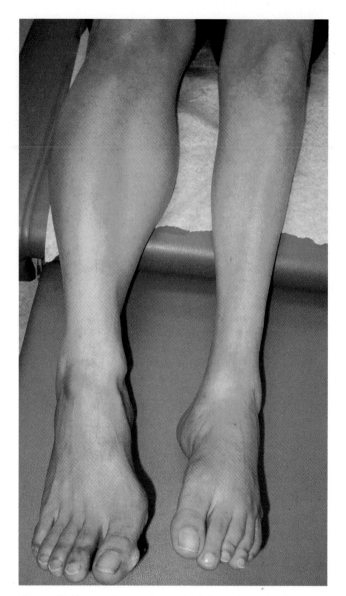

Figure 18-3 Muscle atrophy in the left leg due to polio. (Image provided by Stedman's.)

resolved, treatment of the patient is rehabilitation of the weakened extremities with a strong emphasis on physical and occupational therapy. To increase mobility, patients are fitted with mechanical supports such as braces and splints. Some patients must wear these devices indefinitely. Emotional support is important for these patients, particularly those with PPMA. Many need counseling to reconcile themselves to body image changes caused by the deformities and to allay fear of dependency.

Activities aimed at preventing polio are essential. You may be responsible for patient education regarding immunizations. The previously used oral polio vaccine contained a weakened form of the polio virus, but today's newer injectable form does not contain a live or weakened form of the virus. In the oral form, the virus could be shed in the stool of the immunized child, and caretakers who were not immunized could contract the disease. This is not possible with the newer form of the vaccine.

Tetanus

Tetanus, commonly called *lockjaw*, is an infection of nervous tissue caused by the tetanus bacillus, *Clostridium tetani*, which lives in the intestinal tract of animals and is excreted in their feces. The microorganism is also found in almost all soil. An infection occurs after the microbe enters the body through an open wound in the skin, often a puncture wound. Wounds caused by farm equipment involving manure are especially susceptible to a tetanus infection. All deep, dirty wounds should be treated as high risk for tetanus.

Tetanus has a slow incubation period. It may inhabit the body for up to 14 weeks before signs and symptoms appear. Initial symptoms include spasms of the voluntary muscles, restlessness, and stiff neck. As the disease progresses, seizures and **dysphagia** (difficulty swallowing) develop. The facial and oral muscles contract, leaving the mouth sealed with the teeth clenched tightly. Untreated, the respiratory muscles become paralyzed, and the disease is typically fatal.

Prevention is the best defense against tetanus. Wounds should be properly cleaned immediately. Dead tissue around the wound must be removed, and an antibiotic should be given if the wound appears infected. To obtain immunity early in life, immunizations are administered to infants and children on a schedule determined by the American Academy of Pediatrics and the Centers for Disease Control and Prevention. After the initial immunization schedule is complete, the vaccine must be given every 10 years for life. Patients who develop an infection with the tetanus microbe require immediate hospitalization and aggressive antibiotic therapy. The prognosis is guarded when tetanus has fully developed.

 CHECKPOINT QUESTION

2. What are the initial signs of a tetanus infection?

Rabies

Rabies is caused by a virus that is commonly transmitted by animal saliva through a bite wound from an infected animal and spreads to the organs of the central nervous system. Animals that commonly transmit rabies are skunks, squirrels, raccoons, bats, dogs, cats, coyotes, and foxes. Children are at highest risk for rabies because they are most likely to be bitten by such animals.

The incubation period for rabies ranges from 10 days to many months, depending on the location of the bite. Initial symptoms include fever, general malaise,

and body aches. As the disease progresses, mental derangement, paralysis, and photophobia develop. The patient's saliva becomes extremely profuse and sticky, and the throat muscles begin to spasm, making swallowing difficult or impossible, which causes profuse drooling. Muscle spasms of the throat occur at the sight of water or when attempting to drink water, resulting in hydrophobia. The progressive involvement of the tissues of the brain is often fatal.

Immediate treatment of a wound caused by an animal must be the first priority. After the wound is cleansed, the patient should receive an antibiotic and prophylactic vaccine therapy consisting of the human diploid cell vaccine and a rabies immune globulin vaccine. All animal bites must be reported to the city or county animal control center, and you may be responsible for completing and submitting the report. If possible, the animal should be quarantined and evaluated for behavioral changes. If the animal is domestic, a complete veterinary history must be obtained. A copy of the animal's rabies tag and certificate, if available, should be placed in the patient's chart.

Reye Syndrome

Reye syndrome, a devastating nervous system illness, typically occurs in children after a viral illness, commonly varicella (chicken pox). Studies have found that the use of aspirin in the presence of a viral illness increases the risk of developing Reye syndrome. No other antipyretic agents have been implicated in this disorder. Reye syndrome is not contagious.

While this disorder can affect all organs of the body, it most often affects the liver and the brain. Initial symptoms include vomiting and lethargy, and as the brain swelling continues, confusion, seizures, and coma may develop quickly. The signs and symptoms of Reye syndrome should be treated as a medical emergency because early diagnosis and treatment increase the chances of recovering. The prognosis depends on the amount and severity of cerebral edema. Diagnosis is made by obtaining blood samples to determine liver function, including ammonia, aspartate aminotransferase, and alanine aminotransferase levels. Patients with Reye syndrome require rapid hospitalization, aggressive antibiotic therapy to prevent secondary bacterial infection, and supportive care.

Degenerative Disorders
Multiple Sclerosis

The cause of multiple sclerosis (MS) is unknown, but possible origins include a viral infection, autoimmunity, immunologic response, and genetic predisposition. In MS, the myelin sheaths covering many neurons in the body degenerate and are replaced with plaque, which

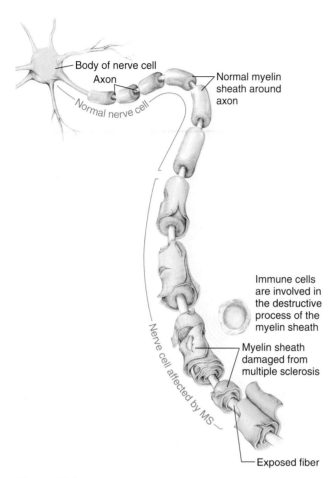

Body of nerve cell
Axon
Normal myelin sheath around axon
Normal nerve cell

Immune cells are involved in the destructive process of the myelin sheath

Nerve cell affected by MS

Myelin sheath damaged from multiple sclerosis

Exposed fiber

Figure 18-4 Nerve cell in multiple sclerosis.

impairs nerve impulse conduction (Fig. 18-4). Multiple sclerosis most commonly occurs in women aged 20 to 40 years and is characterized by remissions and exacerbations. Although there is no cure, the rate and severity of progression vary greatly among patients.

Typically, patients complain initially of progressive loss of muscle control. They may also complain of loss of balance, shaking tremors, and poor muscle coordination. Tingling and numbness can also be first signs of the disease. **Dysphasia** (difficulty speaking) may be another sign. As the disease progresses, bladder dysfunction and complaints of visual disturbances are common. Patients may also develop nystagmus (involuntary rapid movement of the eyeball in all directions).

Treatment of MS is palliative. Physical therapy is critical to limit the extent of muscle deterioration and to maintain existing muscle strength. As the disease progresses, the patient is often fitted for prosthetic appliances such as crutches to assist with mobility. Drug therapy includes muscle relaxants and steroids. Because this disease affects persons in the prime of life, patients with MS and their families require psychological support from all of their regular health care providers. Many support groups and counselors specialize in providing

therapy for persons with debilitating diseases, including MS, and this information should be shared with patients and families as appropriate.

Amyotrophic Lateral Sclerosis

Commonly known as *Lou Gehrig disease*, amyotrophic lateral sclerosis (ALS) causes a progressive loss of motor neurons. ALS is a terminal disease with no known cause, but a strong familial connection has been observed. It occurs most often in middle-aged men. It begins with loss of muscle mobility in the forearms, hands, and legs and then progresses to the facial muscles, causing dysphasia and dysphagia that worsen over time. Death usually occurs 3 to 5 years after the onset of symptoms.

Treatment of ALS consists of keeping the patient comfortable and educating the family. As the disease progresses, it becomes increasingly difficult for the patient to maintain an unobstructed airway. The family must be taught to prevent and manage choking. Often, the physician discusses advance directives, or end-of-life requests, with the family and the patient. Ideally, the medical assistant will be present for these discussions to provide emotional support.

Parkinson Disease

This disease is most often seen in older adults; however, it may begin in middle adulthood. Because the disease is a neurologic disorder affecting specific neurotransmitters, or chemicals, in the brain, the symptoms appear gradually and cause a decrease in muscle control. Common symptoms of this disease include rigid muscles, involuntary tremors, and difficulty walking. For more information about Parkinson disease, refer to Chapter 23.

CHECKPOINT QUESTION

3. Should health care professionals worry that multiple sclerosis is contagious?

Seizure Disorders

Seizures, commonly called **convulsions**, are involuntary contractions of voluntary muscles caused by a rapid succession of electrical impulses through the brain. Seizures have many causes, including chemical imbalance, trauma, pregnancy-induced hypertension, tumor, and withdrawal from drugs or alcohol. However, many seizures are idiopathic (have no known cause).

Epilepsy is the most common form of seizure disorder. Epilepsy may appear in early childhood or at any life stage. Diagnosis is made through **electroencephalogram (EEG)** studies, blood tests, and radiologic tests. Epileptic seizures are characterized as either petit mal or grand mal. Petit mal seizures, also called *absence seizures* or *partial seizures*, are briefer than grand mal seizures and usually occur only in childhood. The child may appear to fall asleep or drift away momentarily. Some muscle twitching may occur. Then the child awakes and continues the interrupted activity. Petit mal seizures may go undetected for many years.

Grand mal seizures, also called *tonic-clonic seizures*, are more involved than petit mal seizures. Generally, the patient will go through three phases:

1. The first phase is an **aura**, or warning that a seizure is impending. The aura may include tingling in the extremities, visual signs (such as flashing lights), or perception of a particular taste or odor. Not all patients have auras, but those who do usually perceive the same aural phenomena each time.
2. The second phase is complete loss of consciousness with extensive muscle twitching or contractions, which may be violent. The patient falls and usually loses control of bladder and bowel functions.
3. The third phase is the postictal phase. The patient slowly regains consciousness but remains drowsy for an extended time.

The primary treatment during the actual seizure is preventing injury to the patient (see Chapter 11). Epilepsy is treated with various pharmacologic agents that must be taken by the patient regularly to prevent seizure activity. Instruct patients to take their medication every day as prescribed by the physician, never missing a dose. Many epileptic patients who become stabilized and seizure free on medication decide they no longer need the medication. Remind these patients that stopping the medication may lead to the recurrence of seizures.

A patient who has seizures is usually permitted to have a driver's license, but each state has specific regulations requiring that patients be seizure free for a particular length of time. The patient may ask the physician to complete paperwork from the state issuing the driver's license, and you may be asked to assist with completion of these forms.

Febrile Seizures

Febrile (fever) seizures occur in a small number of children, most commonly aged 6 months to 3 years, with an elevated body temperature. Children with febrile seizures must have a complete physical and neurologic examination to rule out the possibility of organic origin of the seizures. Typically, children generally outgrow febrile seizures by age 6 or 7 years and have no further seizure activity.

Treatment is gently returning the child's body temperature to a more manageable level. Cool compresses are preferable to ice baths or alcohol sponge baths, which may cause hypothermia. Because of the danger of Reye syndrome, these children should not be given salicylates, or products containing aspirin, to reduce the temperature.

Focal Seizures

A focal, or *Jacksonian*, seizure begins as a small local seizure that spreads to adjacent areas. For instance, the small seizure may begin in the fingers and spread to the hand and arm. The cause of focal seizures must be researched to prevent the progression to general seizures.

 CHECKPOINT QUESTION

4. How do petit mal seizures differ from grand mal seizures?

 WHAT IF?

What if the mother of a 2-year-old child who recently had a febrile seizure tells you that she is scared that the child will have another seizure and that it will cause brain damage?

Because febrile seizures can be very scary for parents of small children, you can help them cope with these measures by doing the following:

- Reassure the parents that febrile seizures are common in young children and that they generally are not chronic.
- Allow the parents to be involved in the care of the child. If a seizure occurs in the medical office, urge the parents to hold and comfort the child after the seizure has subsided and the physician has evaluated the child.
- Provide easy-to-understand explanations for all procedures.
- Encourage parents to talk about their fears.
- Remain calm and demonstrate confidence in handling the situation.

Developmental Disorders

Neural Tube Defects

Many abnormalities may occur during the embryonic and fetal stages of development. As the embryo develops, the tissue over the neural tube (a tubelike section of the developing embryo) closes and evolves into the components of the CNS. If a developmental failure occurs on the proximal (upper) portion, anencephaly, or the absence of a brain, may result. An abnormality in development in the distal, or caudal, end of the neural tube results in spina bifida. **Spina bifida occulta** is the most benign form. In this condition, the posterior laminae of the vertebrae fail to close, typically at L5 or S1. There are usually no external signs of deformity, although there may be a skin dimple or dark tufts of

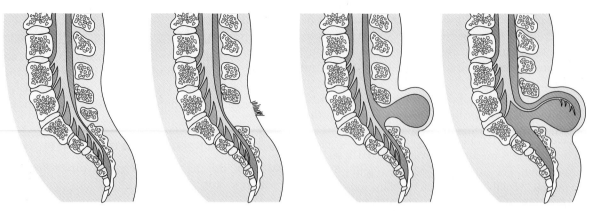

Figure 18-5 Spinal defects. (**A**) Normal spinal cord. (**B**) Spina bifida occulta. (**C**) Meningocele. (**D**) Meningomyelocele. (Reprinted with permission from Pillitteri A. Maternal and Child Health Nursing: Care of the Childbearing and Childrearing Family. 5th ed. Philadelphia: Lippincott Williams & Wilkins, 2007.)

hair over this area on the lower back. A **meningocele** occurs when the meninges protrude through the spina bifida. In spina bifida with **myelomeningocele**, the most severe form, the spinal cord and meninges protrude externally (Fig. 18-5A–D). The main treatment is surgical intervention; prognosis is based on the extent of spinal cord involvement.

PATIENT EDUCATION

ALPHA-FETOPROTEIN

This blood test is routinely performed during the second trimester (weeks 16 to 18) of pregnancy to check for maternal serum levels of alpha-fetoprotein and screen the fetus for defects in the neural tube. If this protein is found to be high, there may be nervous system disorders in the fetus, such as spina bifida, whereas low levels may indicate trisomy 13 or Down syndrome. Because abnormal results may occur due to more than one fetus or incorrect due dates, high or low results indicate the need for further studies such as sonography or amniocentesis before a definitive diagnosis is made.

Hydrocephalus

Hydrocephalus occurs when the arachnoid and ventricular spaces of the brain contain excessive CSF. Although it occurs most commonly in infants and children as the result of a defect in CSF production or absorption, hydrocephalus sometimes occurs in adults as a result of tumor or trauma. Treatment is surgical insertion of a shunt, which reroutes the excessive CSF from the brain to the right atrium of the heart or the peritoneal cavity. The prognosis is usually good if hydrocephalus is treated aggressively in the early stages, before CNS damage.

Cerebral Palsy

Cerebral palsy describes a group of neuromuscular disorders that result from CNS damage during the prenatal, neonatal, or postnatal period. Although cerebral palsy is not progressive, the damage may become more obvious as developmental delays are discovered. Impairment may range from slight motor dysfunction to catastrophic physical and mental disabilities. Prognosis varies with the site of the damage and its severity. Treatment is supportive and rehabilitative. No cure exists.

 CHECKPOINT QUESTION

5. What is spina bifida, and how does it develop?

Trauma

Traumatic injuries are the most common causes of neurologic disorders and the leading killer of individuals ages 1 to 24 years. The trauma often is a preventable injury to the head that causes edema in the brain tissue or blows to the posterior neck and back, injuring the spinal cord. You can help prevent these types of injuries and the lifelong impairments that accompany permanent damage to the CNS by encouraging parents to require their children to wear a helmet when bicycle riding, skating, skateboarding, and riding in a motor vehicle. Head trauma sustained in a motor vehicle accident often results from the passengers being tossed around the interior of the car or worse yet, ejected from the vehicle. Inexperienced teenage drivers should also be asked about the use of seat belts not just for themselves, but for their passengers as well.

Traumatic Brain Injuries

Children are at particularly high risk for head trauma. A child's head is large in proportion to the rest of the body; therefore, when children fall (as they frequently

TABLE 18-1	Spinal Cord Injuries
Level of Injury	**Resulting Disabilities**
C1, C2	Unable to breathe independently; no neck muscle control
C3, C4	May manipulate electric wheelchair with mouthpiece; some neck control possible
C5	Uses wheelchair with hand controls; eats with hand splints; good elbow flexion
C6	Transfers to wheelchair and bed with little or no assistance; good shoulder control
C7	Transfers independently to wheelchair and bed; eats with no special devices
T1, T4	Moves from wheelchair to floor with little or no assistance; normal upper extremity function
T5, L2	Limited walking with bilateral leg braces and crutches
L3, L4	Walks with short leg braces with or without crutches
L5, S3	Walks independently with no equipment if foot strength is good

C = cervical; L = lumbar; S = sacral; T = thoracic.

do), they often fall head first. Children are also prone to traumatic injuries because their reflex systems are immature. Traumatic injuries to the brain include **concussion**, **contusion**, and intracranial hemorrhage. A concussion is a nonlethal brain injury that results from blunt trauma. The patient may momentarily lose consciousness but promptly return to an awake and alert state. The treatment for concussion is rest and observation for signs of a more serious injury, contusion. A contusion is a focal alteration of cerebral circulation. Hemorrhages and extravasation, or pooling, of blood and fluid can result. Loss of consciousness results, and brain damage may occur. The patient may become confused and lethargic and have nausea and vomiting as the intracranial bleeding increases, causing pressure on the brain. Intracranial hemorrhage is bleeding of a vessel inside the skull due to trauma, congenital abnormality, or aneurysm.

Traumatic brain injuries are diagnosed with radiographic studies. Treatment for contusions and hemorrhages can be surgery, drug therapy, and supportive care. The prognosis for all brain injuries depends on the extent of damage and the location of the injury.

Spinal Cord Injuries

Spinal cord injuries are most common among individuals ages 15 to 35 years. Most spinal cord injuries are due to trauma from a motor vehicle accident, diving accident, or fall. A complete spinal cord injury is one in which the cord is transected and no neurologic abilities remain below the point of injury. An incomplete spinal cord injury is one in which the cord is injured or partially severed, causing minor to severe disability below the point of injury (Table 18-1). The higher in the spinal cord the injury is, the more serious the complications and paralysis for the patient. Table 18-2 describes the types of paralysis that a patient may have and the typical causes of each type.

In caring for patients who may have a spinal cord injury, the initial consideration is to prevent further damage. Accident victims with suspected spinal cord injuries must be kept immobile until proper emergency medical service personnel are present. Treatment in the emergency department is focused on stabilization, and patients usually require an extended hospitalization and rehabilitation, depending on the extent of the damage to the spinal cord.

In the physician's office, recovering trauma patients may receive follow-up treatment and evaluation. These patients are monitored for changes in their reflexes and evaluated for physical therapy and occupational therapy. The goal of long-term care is to prevent complications, which can include skin ulcerations (pressure

TABLE 18-2	Types of Paralysis	
Type	**Causes**	**Result**
Hemiplegia	Cerebrovascular accident; trauma to one side of brain; tumors	Paralysis on one side of body, opposite the side of involvement
Paraplegia	Spinal cord trauma; spinal tumors	Paralysis of any part of the body below the point of involvement
Quadriplegia	Spinal cord trauma; spinal tumors	Paralysis of all limbs (usually cervical or high thoracic vertebra involvement)

ulcers), hypostatic pneumonia, bladder infection, muscle contractures, and psychological depression. Most of the physical complications are treated with physical therapy and good care either in the home or in the long-term rehabilitation facility. The mental and emotional complications require intensive therapy by counselors who specialize in treating patients with debilitating disorders.

 CHECKPOINT QUESTION

6. How does a complete spinal cord injury differ from an incomplete one?

 PATIENT EDUCATION

SPINAL CORD AND TRAUMATIC BRAIN INJURIES

Spinal cord and traumatic brain injuries are common in young people. Both types of injuries can produce serious, and even fatal, results. As a medical assistant, you must take an active role in educating your community, patients, and friends about prevention of these injuries:

- Use seat belts in automobiles for all passengers.
- Secure infants and young children in approved car seats.
- Avoid alcohol when participating in sporting activities and driving.
- Obey traffic signs and speed limits.
- Avoid illicit drug use and any medication that impairs awareness.
- Wear a helmet while bicycling and riding a motorcycle.
- Never dive head first into water that is shallow or not clear.

Brain Tumors

A brain tumor may be either malignant or benign and may be a secondary or metastatic site. If the brain tumor is the primary site, it is named for the site of origin (e.g., glioma, meningioma, medulloblastoma). Both malignant and benign tumors can produce serious complications for the patient because of the limited space inside the cranium. Generally, the patient has vague complaints of headaches, blurred vision, personality changes, or memory loss. In more advanced cases, seizures, blindness, and dysphagia may be evident. The type of tumor and its location affect the presenting symptoms, their severity and onset, and the prognosis.

Diagnosis is made primarily with radiologic studies. The treatment can include surgery, radiation therapy, chemotherapy, or a combination of radiation and chemotherapy.

Headaches

It is estimated that 70% of the population has **cephalalgia**, or headaches. Headaches have a variety of origins, including stress, trauma, bone pathology, infection (e.g., sinus), or vascular disturbance. In many instances, the cause is never known.

Migraine headaches are one of the most common types. Migraines can be triggered by stress, high altitude, smoking, certain smells, or ingested chemicals (e.g., caffeine, alcohol, and certain food additives), but in many situations, the cause is unknown. Many patients who have migraines have an aura, or sensory perception such as flashing lights or wavy lines, before onset. Once the migraine headache begins, the symptoms usually include a unilateral temporal headache, photophobia, diplopia (double vision), and nausea. Generally these headaches are treated with an analgesic, and the patient may be instructed to rest in a dark, quiet room. The physician may also prescribe medication to arrest the headache and symptoms when the migraine begins. These medications, sometimes called *abortive headache medications*, include the triptans (sumatriptan succinate [Imitrex™], naratriptan hydrochloride [Amerge™], and eletriptan hydrobromide [Relpax™]).

Other common types of headaches include:

- *Tension headaches* are associated with contraction of the muscles of the neck and scalp due to stress. The treatment is a muscle relaxant, analgesic, and reversing the precipitating factors. Biofeedback techniques may also be useful to assist with coping with stress that cannot be avoided.
- *Cluster headaches* are similar to migraine headaches but typically occur at night. They are usually short lasting but may recur as often as 4 or 5 times a night for several weeks and then not again for weeks or months. Treatment is a muscle relaxant, analgesic, and stress relief techniques.

 CHECKPOINT QUESTION

7. What are some triggers for migraine headaches?

 LEGAL TIP

RISK MANAGEMENT

Risk management includes those activities performed in the medical office that may help reduce or eliminate litigation or lawsuits. A professional medical assistant can practice risk management by:

- Documenting concisely and accurately immediately following any patient encounter, either in person or on the telephone.

- Being familiar with the office policy and procedure manual and following the guidelines as written.
- Communicating clearly with patients and other health care providers while observing the laws regarding confidentiality.
- Maintaining compliance with state and federal laws with regard to filing insurance claims and billing procedures.
- Practicing within your scope of education and training.

Common Diagnostic Tests for Disorders of the Nervous System

The physician may perform a variety of tests to evaluate a patient's neurologic status. These tests may be invasive or noninvasive and may include radiologic and electrical tests along with physical examination.

Physical Examination

The physical examination, a key component of diagnosis of nervous system disorders, includes the following evaluations:

- Mental status and orientation
- Cranial nerve assessment
- Sensory and motor functions
- Reflex assessment

The patient's mental status is evaluated by routine questioning to establish mental alertness and orientation. For example, the examiner may ask the patient to count to 10 and to state the president's name and the year.

Cranial nerves are assessed according to the methods described in Table 18-3. Visual acuity may be tested on a chart such as the Snellen eye chart, and the results can indicate a refractive error or a more serious neurologic disorder. Sensory function is tested with the pin versus soft brush method for spinal nerves and cranial nerves. The instrument commonly used is the Buck neurologic

TABLE 18-3	Cranial Nerves and Assessment		
Nerve (Number)	**Type**	**Functions**	**Examination Methods**
Olfactory (I)	Sensory	Smell	Test each nostril for smell reception, interpretation
Optic (II)	Sensory	Vision	Test vision for acuity, visual fields
Oculomotor (III)	Motor	Pupil constriction, raise eyelids	Test papillary reaction to light, ability to open and close eyes
Trochlear (IV)	Motor	Downward, inward eye movement	Test for downward, inward eye movement
Trigeminal (V)	Motor	Jaw movements, chewing, mastication	Ask patient to open and clench jaws while palpating the jaw muscles
	Sensory	Sensation on face, neck	Test face and neck for pain sensations, light touch, temperature
Abducens (VI)	Motor	Lateral movement of eyes	Test ocular movement in all directions
Facial (VII)	Motor	Muscles of face	Ask patient to raise eyebrows, smile, show teeth, puff out cheeks
	Sensory	Sense of taste on anterior two thirds of tongue	Test for taste sensation with various agents
Acoustic (VIII)	Sensory	Hearing	Test hearing ability
Glossopharyngeal (IX)	Motor	Pharyngeal movement and swallowing	Ask patient to say "ah," yawn to observe upward movement of soft palate; elicit gag response; note ability to swallow
	Sensory	Taste on lower third of tongue	Test for taste with various agents
Vagus (X)	Motor	Swallowing, speaking	Ask patient to swallow, speak; note hoarseness
Accessory (XI)	Motor	Movement of shoulder muscles	Ask patient to shrug against resistance
Hypoglossal (XII)	Motor	Movement, strength of tongue against cheek	Ask patient to protrude tongue, push tongue

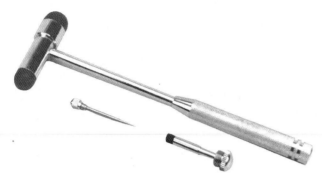

Figure 18-6 The Buck neurologic hammer.

hammer (Fig. 18-6). With the patient's eyes closed, the physician uses the pin and brush to determine the patient's ability to distinguish between sensations. The physician evaluates sensory reception and determines whether there is a reception difference on either side of the body.

Motor functioning is tested by watching the patient walk. Many disorders can be detected by observing a patient's gait. Part of this assessment includes the **Romberg test**. The patient is asked to stand with feet together and with the eyes closed. A positive Romberg sign is noted if the patient sways or is unsteady.

The last part of the examination is reflex testing (Table 18-4). Figure 18-7A–D depicts the correct method for tendon reflex testing. Reflexes are scored on the following scale:

0 = No response
1+ = Diminished response
2+ = Normal
3+ = Brisker than normal
4+ = Hyperactive with clonus, which is the repetitive jerking of a muscle and indicates a neurologic disorder

Patients with weak or slow responses to stimuli applied during reflex testing may require additional testing to determine the source of the problem. Since the muscles require electrical impulses from the nervous system to contract, the physician must determine whether the problem is with the muscles or if there is a disorder of the nervous system.

Radiologic Tests

The most common noninvasive radiologic tests include computed tomography (CT) and magnetic resonance imaging (MRI). These tests may be done with a contrast medium or dye. The contrast medium helps differentiate between the soft tissue areas of the nervous system and the tumors, lesions, or hemorrhages that may blend in with their supporting tissues.

A **myelogram** is an invasive radiologic test in which dye is injected into the CSF. After the dye is injected, the spinal cord is filmed, and any abnormalities, such as tumors or damage from injury, can be detected. The blood vessels of the brain can be visualized on radiographic film by injecting dye through a femoral artery catheter threaded up to the carotid artery in a test called *cerebral angiogram*.

Radiography of the skull may be used to rule out many possible disorders and is diagnostic for fractures.

Electrical Tests

Electroencephalography (EEG) is a noninvasive test that records electrical impulses in the brain. A variety of electrodes are placed on the patient's scalp, and tracings of brain wave activity are recorded. Typically, the patient is given a mild sedative to induce a quiet state. This test is used to assess hyperactive electrical responses in the brain as seen in patients with seizure disorders. In the inpatient acute care setting, EEG is used to determine brain activity in patients who are on life support but who may be brain dead and have no chance for recovery.

 CHECKPOINT QUESTION

8. What are the differences between a myelogram and an EEG?

TABLE **18-4**	Reflex Testing		
Reflex	**Method of Testing**	**Expected Response**	**Location**
Brachioradialis	Tap styloid process of radius	Flexion of elbow	C5, C6
Biceps	Tap biceps tendon	Flexion of elbow	C5, C6
Triceps	Tap triceps	Extension of elbow	C7
Patellar	Tap patellar tendon	Extension of leg	L2, L4
Achilles	Tap Achilles tendon	Plantarflexion of foot	S1
Corneal	Light touch on corneoscleral corner	Closure of eyelid	CN V, VII

C = cervical; L = lumbar; S = sacral; CN = cranial nerve.

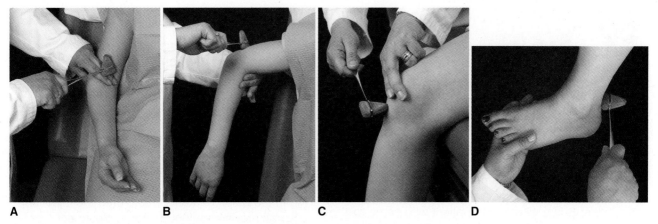

A   B   C   D

Figure 18-7 Techniques for eliciting major tendon reflexes. (**A**) Biceps reflex. (**B**) Triceps reflex. (**C**) Patellar reflex. (**D**) Ankle or Achilles reflex.

Lumbar Puncture

A lumbar puncture is used to diagnose infectious inflammatory or bleeding disorders affecting the brain and spinal cord or as a means of injecting pain control medication into the spinal column near the nerves producing the pain. A needle is inserted into the subarachnoid space at L4 to L5, below the level of the spinal cord (Fig. 18-8). If CSF is removed and sent to the laboratory, it may be tested for glucose, protein, bacteria, cell counts, and red blood cells, which indicate intracranial bleeding. It may also be performed to evaluate intracranial pressure. An obstruction to CSF flow can be determined with the **Queckenstedt test.** For this test, you will be directed to press against the patient's jugular veins in the neck (right, left, or both) while the physician monitors the pressure of CSF. If CSF pressure increases when the jugular vein is compressed, the finding is normal. If no increase in pressure occurs, the flow of CSF is blocked.

If a lumbar puncture is performed in the medical office, your responsibility includes assisting the patient into a side-lying curled position or a supported forward-bending sitting position and maintaining sterility of the items used during the puncture (see Chapter 7). The physical position is uncomfortable and difficult to maintain, and you should help the patient to relax as much as possible by encouraging slow, deep breathing during the procedure. The steps for assisting the physician with a lumbar puncture are described in Procedure 18-1.

If CSF has been removed, the physician may require that the patient lie flat for 6 to 12 hours to prevent a spinal headache. In addition, the patient may require intravenous fluid and pain medication. For these reasons, the lumbar puncture may be performed in outpatient clinics than in the medical office.

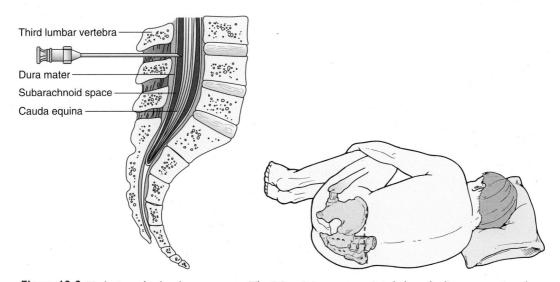

Third lumbar vertebra

Dura mater

Subarachnoid space

Cauda equina

Figure 18-8 Technique for lumbar puncture. The L3 to L5 spaces are just below the line connecting the anterior and superior iliac spines. (Taylor C, Lillis CA, LeMone P. Fundamentals of Nursing. 2nd ed. Philadelphia: Lippincott, 1993:543.)

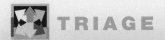 **TRIAGE**

While you are working in a medical office, the following three situations occur at the same time:

A. Patient A is a 35-year-old woman who came to the office with a severe migraine. She is sitting in the darkened examination room with an emesis basin because she has been nauseated and vomiting this morning. The physician has ordered an injection of Imitrex™.

B. Patient B is a 46-year-old patient who came to the office for an injection of anesthetic into the spinal column to relieve chronic pain caused by an injury that occurred on the job 2 years ago.

C. Patient C is phoning about a bill received after an office visit last month. The patient is angry and demanding to speak to the physician immediately.

How do you sort these patients? Who do you see first? Second? Third?

Patient C should quickly be referred to the office manager or billing supervisor in a calm and professional manner. In most offices, the clinical medical assistant does not have enough information about the patient's account to determine the nature of the problem. Next, patient A should be given the injection and allowed to remain in the examination room until the medication has taken effect or she feels able to leave. While she is resting in the quiet, darkened room after the injection, you can prepare patient B and the treatment room.

Medication Box

Commonly Prescribed Neurology System Medications

Note: The generic name of the drug is listed first and is written in all lowercase letters. Brand names are in parentheses, and the first letter is capitalized.

acetaminophen (Tylenol)	Tablets: 160 mg to 650 mg	Analgesic; antipyretic
	Caplets: 160 mg, 500 mg	
	Gelcaps: 500 mg	
	Oral suspension: 80 mg/0.8 mL	
	Suppositories: 80 mg, 120 mg	
acyclovir (Zovirax)	Capsules: 200 mg	Antiviral
	Injection: 500 mg/vial, 1 g/vial (*do not give intramuscularly or subcutaneously*)	
	Tablets: 400 mg, 800 mg	
carbamazepine (Tegretol)	Capsules: 100 mg, 200 mg, 300 mg	Anticonvulsant
	Tablets: 200 mg	
	Tablets (chewable): 100 mg	
cefadroxil (Duricef)	Capsules: 500 mg	Antibiotic
	Oral suspension: 125 mg/5 mL to 500 mg/mL	
	Tablets: 1 g	
clonazepam (Klonopin)	Tablets: 0.5 mg, 1 mg, 2 mg	Anticonvulsant
	Tablets (orally disintegrating): 0.125 mg, 0.25 mg, 0.5 mg, 1 mg, 2 mg	

Commonly Prescribed Neurology System Medications *(Continued)*		
elitriptan hydrobromide (Relpax)	Tablets: 20 mg, 40 mg	Antimigraine
fentanyl transdermal system (Duragesic)	Transdermal: Patches release 12.5 mcg, 25 mcg, 50 mcg, 75 mcg, or 100 mcg per hour	Opioid analgesic
gabapentin (Neurontin, Gabarone)	Capsules: 100 mg to 400 mg Oral solution: 250 mg/5 mL Tablets: 100 mg to 800 mg	Anticonvulsant
ibuprofen (Motrin, Advil, Excedrin IB)	Capsules: 200 mg Oral drops: 40 mg/mL Oral suspension: 100 mg/5 mL Tablets: 100 mg to 800 mg	Analgesic; antipyretic
meclizine hydrochloride (Antivert, Dramamine)	Tablets: 12.5 mg, 25 mg, 50 mg	Antiemetic
naratriptan (Amerge)	Tablets: 1 mg, 2.5 mg	Antimigraine
oxycodone hydrochloride (OxyContin)	Capsules: 5 mg Tablets: 5 mg, 10 mg, 15 mg, 20 mg 30 mg	Opioid analgesic
penicillin G sodium	Injection: (intramuscular or intravenous) 5-million-unit vial	Antibiotic
penicillin V potassium (Penicillin VK, Veetids)	Oral suspension: 125 mg/5 mL to 250 mg/mL (after reconstitution) Tablets: 250 mg, 500 mg	Antibiotic
phenobarbital (Solfoton)	Elixer: 15 mg/5 mL, 20 mg/5 mL Tablets: 15 mg to 100 mg	Anticonvulsant
phenytoin (Dilantin)	Tablets (chewable): 50 mg Oral suspension: 125 mg/5 mL	Anticonvulsant
sumatriptan succinate (Imitrex)	Injection: 4 mg/0.5 mL, 6 mg/0.5 mL Tablets: 25 mg, 50 mg Nasal solution: 5 mg/0.1 mL, 20 mg/0.1 mL	Antimigraine
tramadol hydrochloride (Ultram)	Tablets: 50 mg	Opioid analgesic
valacyclovir (Valtrex)	Tablets: 500 mg, 1,000 mg	Antiviral

español SPANISH TERMINOLOGY

¿Tiene una buena memoria?
   Is your memory good?

¿Le duele la cabeza?
   Have you any pain in the head?

¿Siente vértigo?
   Do you feel dizzy?

Voltése para el lado izquierdo (derecho).
   Turn on your left (or right) side.

MEDIA MENU

- **Student Resources on thePoint**
  - **Animation: Nerve Synapse**
  - **CMA/RMA Certification Exam Review**
- **Internet Resources**

  Centers for Disease Control and Prevention
  http://www.cdc.gov/rabies

  National Reye's Syndrome Foundation
  http://www.reyessyndrome.org

  National Institutes of Health
  http://www.nlm.nih.gov/medlineplus/seizures.html
  http://www.nlm.nih.gov/medlineplus/cerebralpalsy.html

  Association for Spina Bifida and Hydrocephalus
  http://www.asbah.org

  Spina Bifida Association of America
  http://www.spinabifidaassociation.org

  National Multiple Sclerosis Society
  http://www.nationalmssociety.org/index.aspx

  Amyotrophic Lateral Sclerosis Association
  http://www.alsa.org

  American Spinal Injury Association
  http://www.asia-spinalinjury.org

PSY PROCEDURE 18-1: Assisting with a Lumbar Puncture

Purpose: To prepare and assist the physician during a lumbar puncture
Equipment: Sterile and clean exam gloves, 3- to 5-inch lumbar needle with stylet (physician will specify gauge and length), sterile gauze sponges, sterile specimen container, local anesthetic and syringe, needle, adhesive bandages, fenestrated drape, sterile drape, antiseptic, skin preparation supplies (razor), biohazard sharps container, biohazard waste container

Steps	Purpose
1. Wash your hands.	Handwashing aids infection control.
2. Assemble the equipment, identify the patient, and explain the procedure.	Identifying the patient helps prevent errors in treatment. Explaining the procedure helps ease anxiety.
3. Check that the consent form is signed and in the chart. Warn the patient not to move during procedure. Tell the patient that the area will be numb but pressure may still be felt after the local anesthetic is administered.	Because this is an invasive procedure, informed consent should be obtained and the form kept in the the chart. Although there is little chance of damage to the spinal cord, movement may injure the patient and will probably contaminate the field.
4. **AFF** Explain how to respond to a patient who has dementia.	Solicit assistance from the caregiver or other staff member to help during the procedure. Give simple directions to the patient about what he or she should do. Speak clearly, not loudly.
5. Have the patient void. Direct the patient to disrobe and put on a gown with the opening the back.	Emptying the bladder will decrease discomfort during the procedure. The back must be exposed in for the procedure.
6. Prepare the skin unless this is to be done with sterile preparation. If the physician prefers to prepare the skin using sterile forceps after gloving, you may have to add sterile solution the field. Assist as needed with administration of the anesthetic.	Before beginning, assess the lumbar region. If the site is hairy, it may be necessary to shave the skin before the procedure. Strict medical and surgical asepsis must be observed to reduce the risk of to introducing microorganisms into the nervous system.
7. When the physician is ready, prepare the sterile field and assist with the initial preparations. Assist the patient into the appropriate position. A. For the side-lying position, stand in front of the patient and help by holding the patient's knees and top shoulder. Ask the patient to move so the back is close to the edge of the table.	These positions widen the space between the vertebrae to allow entrance of the needle. Your presence will help ensure that the patient does not move.

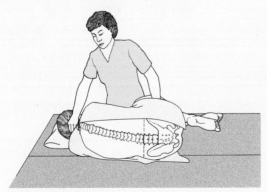

Step 7. The patient should be lying on the side with the knees drawn up, the head and neck down, and the back curled as much as possible.

B. For the forward-leaning, supported position, stand in front of the patient and rest your hands on the shoulders as a reminder to remain still. Ask the patient to breathe slowly and deeply.

(continued)

PSY PROCEDURE 18-1: Assisting with a Lumbar Puncture (continued)

Steps	Reasons
8. Throughout the procedure, observe the patient closely for signs such as dyspnea or cyanosis. Monitor the pulse at intervals and record the vital signs after the procedure. Note the patient's mental alertness and any leakage at the site, nausea, or vomiting. Assess lower limb mobility. Assist the physician as necessary.	When the physician has the needle securely in place, the physician may ask you to help the patient to straighten slightly to ease tension and to allow a normal CSF flow.
9. If specimens are to be taken, put on gloves to receive the potentially hazardous body fluid. Label the tubes in sequence as you receive them. Label them also with the patient's identification and place them in biohazard bags.	Standard precautions must be followed.
10. If the Queckenstedt test is to be performed, you may be required to press against the patient's jugular veins in the neck (right, left, or both) while the physician monitors the pressure of CSF.	Normally, the pressure of CSF will rise and drop rapidly as the veins in the neck are compressed. If an obstruction is present, the rise and return to normal may be slow, or there may be no response to the external application of pressure.
11. At the completion of the procedure, cover the site with an adhesive bandage and assist the patient to a flat position. The physician will determine when the patient is ready to leave the examining room and the office.	Some patients have headache after the procedure and must be monitored carefully during the recovery period.
12. Route the specimens as required. Clean the examination room and care for or dispose of the equiment as needed. Wash your hands.	Standard precautions must be followed throughout the procedure.
13. Chart all observations and record the procedure.	Procedures are considered not to have been done if they are not recorded.

Charting Example:

02/12/13 8:30 AM Pt. positioned and draped for lumbar puncture. VS 120/80 (R), 86, 18. LP per formed by

Dr. Alexander —————————————————————————————— B. Ryan, CMA

9:00 AM LP complete. Pt. tolerated procedure well. CSF specimen to lab. Post LP VS 114/74 (R) 76, 16 ————

—————————————————————————————————————— B. Ryan, CMA

9:30 AM Pt. denies discomfort. No n/v. No leakage at LP site. Bandage clean and dry. Pt and wife given discharge

instructions. Verbalized understanding. Pt. d/c per Dr. Alexander ——————————————— B. Ryan, CMA

Note: The medical assistant may sign his or her name in the patient record using only the "CMA" credential if the office has a signature log denoting the entire credential as "CMA(AAMA)."

- The nervous system is complex and works with both conscious and unconscious functions.

  Disorders of the nervous system can be grouped into several types:

  - Infectious
  - Degenerative
  - Convulsive
  - Developmental
  - Traumatic
  - Neoplastic
  - Headache

- Common diagnostic tests include:

  - Radiologic studies (e.g., CT, MRI)
  - EEG

- Physical examination
- Prenatal screening
- Lumbar puncture
- Radiography

- Your responsibilities when working with patients with neurologic disorders may include:

  - Assisting the physician with the neurologic examination
  - Scheduling patients for outpatient procedures
  - Providing emotional support to patients and their families or caregivers

Warm Ups for Critical Thinking

1. Research and prepare a patient education fact sheet about migraine headaches, including the possible triggers, the causes, and the treatments (include abortive headache medications).

2. A 3-year-old girl comes to the office with varicella zoster (chicken pox). She has a fever, and the physician orders acetaminophen. The child's mother asks, "Why can't she have aspirin instead?" How do you respond?

3. Your patient, a 21-year-old man, was in a motor vehicle accident last year, and a spinal cord injury left him paraplegic. Explain how this injury has most likely affected his life, not just physically but emotionally and psychologically. How do you handle any anger or apathy directed at you or the physician?

4. Prepare a presentation for a preschool class on safety, including riding bicycles or riding other toys outside, wearing helmets, and the importance of being in a booster seat while wearing a seatbelt in the car.

5. With cooperation from your instructor, schedule a presentation from a professional at the local health district to discuss communicable diseases such as meningitis and rabies in your community. What questions would you ask about diseases that affect the nervous system?

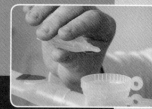

Outline

Common Urinary Disorders
- Renal Failure
- Calculi
- Tumors
- Hydronephrosis
- Urinary System Infections

Common Disorders of the Male Reproductive System
- Benign Prostatic Hyperplasia
- Prostate Cancer

- Testicular Cancer
- Hydrocele
- Cryptorchidism
- Inguinal Hernia
- Infections
- Erectile Dysfunction

Common Diagnostic and Therapeutic Procedures
- Urinalysis
- Blood Tests

- Cystoscopy or Cystourethroscopy
- Intravenous Pyelogram and Retrograde Pyelogram
- Ultrasound
- Rectal and Scrotal Examinations
- Vasectomy

Learning Outcomes

Cognitive Domain

Note: AAMA/CAAHEP 2008 Standards are italicized.

1. Spell and define key terms
2. List and describe the disorders of the urinary system and the male reproductive system
3. Describe and explain the purpose of various diagnostic procedures associated with the urinary system
4. Discuss the role of the medical assistant in diagnosing and treating disorders of the urinary system and the male reproductive system
5. *Identify common pathologies related to each body system*
6. *Describe implications for treatment related to pathology*

Psychomotor Domain

Note: AAMA/CAAHEP 2008 Standards are italicized.

1. Perform a female urinary catheterization (Procedure 19-1)
2. Perform a male urinary catheterization (Procedure 19-2)
3. Instruct a male patient on the testicular self-examination (Procedure 19-3)
4. *Assist physician with patient care*
5. *Prepare a patient for procedures and/or treatments*
6. *Practice standard precautions*
7. *Document patient care*
8. *Document patient education*
9. *Practice within the standard of care for a medical assistant*

Affective Domain

Note: AAMA/CAAHEP 2008 Standards are italicized.

1. *Apply critical thinking skills in performing patient assessment and care*
2. *Use language/verbal skills that enable patients' understanding*
3. *Demonstrate empathy in communicating with patients, family, and staff*
4. *Use appropriate body language and other nonverbal skills in communicating with patients, family, and staff*
5. *Demonstrate awareness of the territorial boundaries of the person with whom you are communicating*

6. Demonstrate sensitivity appropriate to the message being delivered
7. Demonstrate recognition of the patient's level of understanding in communications
8. Recognize and protect personal boundaries in communicating with others
9. Demonstrate respect for individual diversity, incorporating awareness of one's own biases in areas including gender, race, religion, age, and economic status
10. Apply active listening skills
11. Apply local, state, and federal health care legislation and regulation appropriate to the medical assisting practice setting

ABHES Competencies

1. Assist the physician with the regimen of diagnostic and treatment modalities as they relate to each body system
2. Comply with federal, state, and local health laws and regulations
3. Communicate on the recipient's level of comprehension
4. Serve as a liaison between the physician and others
5. Show empathy and impartiality when dealing with patients
6. Document accurately

Key Terms

anuria
blood urea nitrogen (BUN)
catheterization
cryptorchidism
cystoscopy
dialysis
dysuria

enuresis
erectile dysfunction
hematuria
hydrocele
incontinence
intravenous pyelogram (IVP)
lithotripsy

nephrostomy
nocturia
oliguria
prostate-specific antigen (PSA)
proteinuria
psychogenic impotence

pyuria
retrograde pyelogram
specific gravity
ureterostomy
urinalysis
urinary frequency

The process of metabolism creates waste products that must be eliminated from the body. Several body systems contribute to preventing a buildup of the end products of metabolism, including the gastrointestinal system, the respiratory system, and the integumentary system. The urinary system also removes waste from the blood while regulating fluid volume, important electrolytes, blood pressure, and pH (acid-base) balance (Fig. 19-1). Disorders of the filters of the urinary system, the kidneys, are diagnosed through various urine and blood tests and radiographs. Patients with kidney problems are typically referred to a nephrologist, a physician who specializes in the physiology of the kidneys. Patients with disorders of the anatomy, or physical characteristics, of the urinary system are referred to another type of specialist, a urologist. Since the male reproductive system is so inextricably linked to the urinary system, disorders of the male reproductive system are also often referred to the urologist. This chapter does not review the anatomy and physiology of the urinary system but, instead, focuses on common disorders, diagnostic procedures, and treatments associated with the urinary and male reproductive systems.

Common Urinary Disorders

Renal Failure

Renal failure is an acute or chronic disorder of kidney function manifested by the inability of the kidney to excrete wastes, concentrate urine, and aid in homeostatic electrolyte conservation. In acute renal failure, the patient has **oliguria** and a corresponding rise in nitrogen-containing wastes in the blood. The causes of acute renal failure include a serious loss of fluid due to severe burn or hemorrhage, trauma, toxic injury to the kidney, and an obstruction beyond the level of the collecting tubules.

Chronic renal failure is a gradual loss of nephrons with corresponding inability of the kidney to perform its functions. It may result from another disease process,

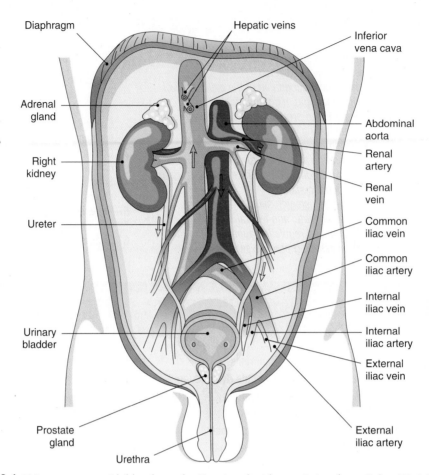

Figure 19-1 Urinary system with blood vessels. (Reprinted with permission from Cohen BJ. Memmler's The Human Body in Health and Disease, 11th ed. Philadelphia: Lippincott Williams & Wilkins, 2009.)

such as systemic lupus erythematosus, diabetic neuropathy, radiation, or renal tuberculosis. The patient has general weakness, edema of the lungs and tissues, and neurologic symptoms such as confusion progressing to seizures and coma as the wastes, or toxins, not filtered by the kidneys build up in the blood.

Treatment for both acute and chronic renal failure may involve renal **dialysis** to remove nitrogenous waste products and excess fluid from the body. Dialysis dependence may be short term in an acute illness or long term in end-stage renal disease. Without functional nephrons, wastes must be filtered through membranes other than those in the renal tissues. Two methods are used: hemodialysis and peritoneal dialysis.

With hemodialysis, toxins are removed from the blood by routing the patient's blood through a dialysis machine containing synthetic filters and a dialysate, a substance used to balance the electrolyte concentration in the blood. The machine can be regulated to remove or retain certain substances as needed for the individual patient. This type of dialysis requires that the patient's circulatory system be accessed as often as three times a week for 3 to 4 hours at a time. Therefore, most patients receive a surgical fistula, or graft, between an artery and

a vein to make entry with a needle during the procedure easier for the patient (Fig. 19-2). The fistula is often placed in one of the arms, and this arm should not be used for taking blood pressures or for blood draws.

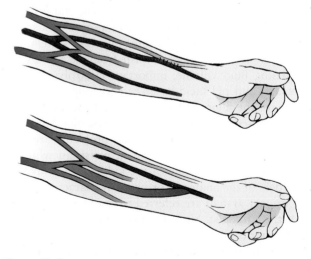

Figure 19-2 Hemodialysis access sites. Arteriovenous fistula (top). Arteriovenous graft (bottom). (Springhouse. Lippincott's Visual Encyclopedia of Clinical Skills. Philadelphia: Wolters Kluwer Health, 2009.)

Patients receiving peritoneal dialysis often perform the procedure at home. An appropriately balanced dialysate is administered through a catheter into the abdominal cavity, allowed to remain in the abdominal cavity for a specified time, and then drained into a collecting bag. As the dialysate flows from the peritoneal cavity, it brings with it filtered wastes and excess fluid removed from the patient's blood through the blood vessels in the abdominal cavity (Fig. 19-3). Patients who have had extensive abdominal surgery with disruption of the peritoneal membranes are not good candidates for this type of dialysis. Peritoneal dialysis allows the patient the freedom to move about and continue a more normal lifestyle at home than with hemodialysis, which requires that the patient go to an outpatient facility several times a week. However, an abdominal catheter may result in an altered body image and psychological depression. The surgical opening on the abdomen can also become infected, leading to peritonitis, a serious infection in the abdominal cavity.

Neither type of dialysis is a cure for the underlying renal dysfunction, but both can prolong life almost indefinitely. Chronic renal failure frequently involves other systems as well as the urinary system and requires treatment for that involvement.

CHECKPOINT QUESTION

1. Which type of dialysis involves the filtering of wastes from the blood directly?

 PATIENT EDUCATION

URINARY TRACT HEALTH

As the medical assistant, you will teach patients about everyday habits related to good general health. Encourage patients with urinary system symptoms to follow these suggestions to avoid urinary tract infections in the future:

For All Patients

- Drink lots of fluids, which help remove waste products from the fluid compartments. We are all generally advised to drink 8 glasses of water a day so that tissues are well hydrated, feces are soft, and infections in the lower urinary system are relatively unlikely.
- Empty your bladder when you feel the need. Urine held beyond comfort causes bladder stress and irritation. Allowing urine to stagnate in the bladder increases the risk of infection.
- Be aware that cranberry juice and vitamin C help acidify the urine and make the urinary system less attractive to bacteria.

Especially for Women

- Avoid using perfumed products in the perineal area. The female urinary meatus is very short and prone to irritation. Urethral infections quickly become bladder infections with irritation.
- Avoid tight-fitting lower garments, especially nylon underwear. Loose-fitting cotton underwear absorbs moisture and allows for airflow, making both bladder and vaginal infections less likely.
- Wipe carefully from front to back after using the toilet. Wash with soap and water, and rinse well if infections are a recurrent problem.
- If you are prone to urinary tract infections, void immediately after sexual intercourse to flush the area of bacteria that might have intruded into the urethra.
- Avoid tub baths, particularly bubble baths; showers are less likely to contribute to infections.

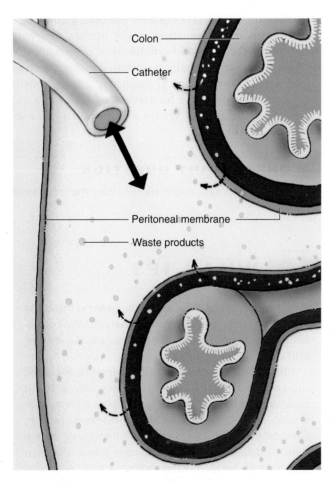

Figure 19-3 Continuous ambulatory peritoneal dialysis. Peritoneal dialysis works through a combination of diffusion and osmosis. (Springhouse. Lippincott's Visual Encyclopedia of Clinical Skills. Philadelphia: Wolters Kluwer Health, 2009.)

Calculi

Calculi are stone formations that may be found anywhere in the urinary system and may range from granular particles to staghorn structures that fill the renal pelvis. Stones seem most likely to form if the urine is alkaline; the symptoms vary with the size and location of the stone. Hematuria may be present if rough edges of calculi abrade the mucous membrane lining the urinary system. The patient has flank pain if a stone lodges in one of the ureters.

Treatment may not be needed if the stones are small enough to be flushed out with increased fluid intake. Large stones may require surgery or **lithotripsy**, a procedure in which ultrasound is used to crush the stones. In either case, the chemical makeup of the stones is evaluated for the forming components, and the patient's diet may be adjusted to prevent recurrence.

Tumors

The urinary system may be a primary or secondary site for tumors. Tumors are more common in the urinary bladder but may also occur in the kidney. Symptoms vary but usually include hematuria and an unexplained abdominal mass. Treatment is based on the extent and type of tumor and may include surgery, chemotherapy, radiation, or a combination.

 CHECKPOINT QUESTION

2. What are calculi, and when are they more likely to form?

Hydronephrosis

Hydronephrosis is distention of the renal pelvis and calyces resulting from an obstruction in the kidney or ureter that causes a backup of urine. The symptoms include flank pain, hematuria, pyuria, fever, and chills. To restore the flow of urine, the stricture must be corrected, if possible, through cystoscopy. If it is not possible to restore the flow of urine to the urinary bladder, it may be necessary to perform a **nephrostomy** (opening the kidney and placement of a catheter in the kidney pelvis) or **ureterostomy** (surgical creation of an opening to the outside of the body from the ureter) (Fig. 19-4).

Urinary System Infections

Glomerulonephritis is inflammation of the glomerulus, or filtering unit, of the kidney. Symptoms range from very mild edema of the extremities, **proteinuria**, **hematuria**, and oliguria to complete renal failure. It is occasionally seen in children 1 to 4 weeks after a streptococcal infection as the large streptococcal antibodies are trapped in the small capillaries of the glomerulus, causing irritation and inflammation. Glomerulonephritis in adults may be chronic, with scarring and hardening of the glomeruli from repeated episodes of acute glomerulonephritis, and may lead to renal failure. Symptoms of the chronic form include proteinuria, casts in the urine (see Chapter 28), and hematuria. Treatment is usually symptomatic, and if an infection is involved, an antibiotic is prescribed.

Pyelonephritis is inflammation of the renal pelvis and the body of the kidney. It usually results from an ascending infection from the ureters and may be acute or chronic. Symptoms include those of any infection, such as chills and fever, nausea, and vomiting, but also include flank pain and **pyuria** (pus in the urine). Medication to acidify the urine and make the system less hospitable to bacteria may be the treatment of choice for pyelonephritis. In addition, an antibiotic may be prescribed.

Cystitis is an inflammation of the urinary bladder. This condition is far more common in women than in men because a woman's urethra is shorter. Symptoms begin with **urinary frequency**, **dysuria**, and urgency and progress to chills, fever, nausea, vomiting, and flank pain. The causative microorganism is identified with a urine culture, and the treatment usually is an antibiotic once the causative microorganism has been identified.

Urethritis is inflammation of the urethra that may occur before the signs and symptoms of cystitis appear, or it may indicate a sexually transmitted disease, such as gonorrhea or nongonococcal urethritis. The treatment for cystitis is also effective for urethritis. Other signs and symptoms of the urinary system and the possible causes are listed in Table 19-1.

 CHECKPOINT QUESTION

3. Why are women more likely than men to have cystitis?

 WHAT IF?

A mother brings her 5-year-old daughter to the office with complaints of burning on urination. What questions do you ask? How do you educate the mother and child?

First, ask if the child urinates when she feels the urge or if she holds her urine. Some young girls are inclined to hold their urine long past the time to void, setting up a perfect situation for bacterial growth. Caution the child to go to the bathroom when the need arises, making sure to use terms she can understand. Next, ask the mother if she uses bubble bath in the child's bath water. Young girls have a very short urethra and are prone to urethritis if they bathe in water with certain types of bubble bath. Finally, explain that the child must learn to wipe from front to back to avoid urinary tract infections.

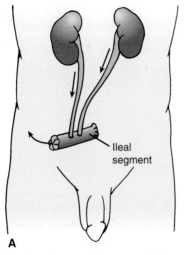

A

Conventional ileal conduit. The surgeon transplants the ureters to an isolated section of the terminal ileum (ileal conduit), bringing one end to the abdominal wall. The ureter may also be transplanted into the transverse sigmoid colon (colon conduit) or proximal jejunum (jejunal conduit).

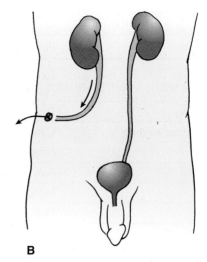

B

Cutaneous ureterostomy. The surgeon brings the detached ureter through the abdominal wall and attaches it to an opening in the skin.

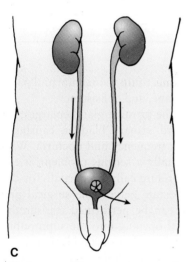

C

Vesicostomy. The surgeon sutures the bladder to the abdominal wall and creates an opening (stoma) through the abdominal and bladder walls for urinary drainage.

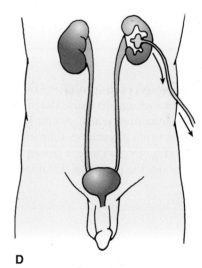

D

Nephrostomy. The surgeon inserts a catheter into the renal pelvis via an incision into the flank or, by percutaneous catheter placement, into the kidney.

Figure 19-4 A ureterostomy. (Reprinted with permission from Smeltzer SC, Bare BG, Hinkle JL, Cheever KH. Brunner & Suddarth's Textbook of Medical-Surgical Nursing. Philadelphia: Lippincott Williams & Wilkins, 2008.)

Common Disorders of the Male Reproductive System

Male patients with disorders of the reproductive system often have signs and symptoms pertaining to the urinary system. If you work in a family practice or internal medicine office, you may care for male patients with reproductive system disorders, or these patients may be referred to urology for specific treatment or surgery. Common disorders are discussed in the following sections.

Benign Prostatic Hyperplasia

As most men reach their middle years, the prostate begins to enlarge, or hypertrophy. Benign prostatic hyperplasia

TABLE 19-1	Symptoms of Urinary Tract Disorders and Possible Causes
Symptoms	Possible Causes
Anuria	Renal failure, acute nephritis, lead or mercury poisoning, complete obstruction of urinary tract
Burning during voiding	Urethritis
Burning during and after voiding	Cystitis
Dysuria	Infection
Enuresis	Normal to age 3 years
Frequency	Infection, diabetes
Hematuria	Diseases of glomeruli, trauma, neoplasm, calculi
Incontinence	Infection, uterine prolapse, nerve damage, neoplasm, senility
Nocturia	Infection, prostatic hypertrophy, abdominal pressure (pregnancy), diabetes
Oliguria	Acute nephritis, dehydration, fever, urinary obstruction, neoplasm
Polyuria	Diabetes mellitus, diabetes insipidus, diuretic use, high fluid intake
Proteinuria	Disease of glomeruli or protein metabolism, infection, nephrotic syndrome
Pyuria	Infection
Renal colic	Calculi
Urgency	Infection, disease of the prostate

is a noncancerous enlargement of the prostate gland that occurs commonly in men over age 40 years. Diagnosis is with a digital rectal examination, which should be performed as part of the routine physical examination in men after age 40 years (Fig. 19-5). Using a gloved hand and water-soluble lubricant, the physician will insert the

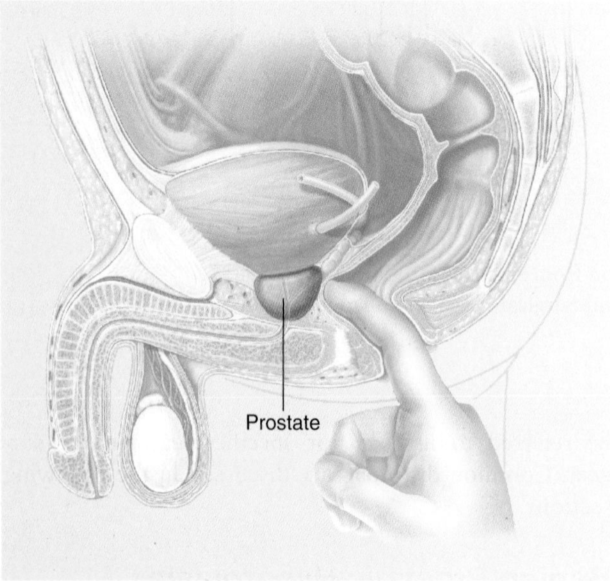

Figure 19-5 Digital rectal exam (DRE).

index finger into the rectum and palpate the prostate for size, shape, and consistency.

As the prostate gland enlarges, it presses on the urethra and urinary bladder, causing urinary symptoms such as frequency and **nocturia**. While this condition is not usually a serious problem, it can be treated medically or surgically by partially or completely removing the prostate gland. The surgical procedure, prostatectomy, can be performed transurethrally or through a surgical opening into the suprapubic area of the lower abdomen. If the prostate is removed transurethrally, the procedure is a transurethral resection of the prostate. Box 19-1 describes the surgical techniques used to treat prostatic hypertrophy in more detail.

Prostate Cancer

Prostate cancer, like most cancers, is best treated when detected early. In the early stages of the disease, many men are asymptomatic. As a result, male patients over age 40 years should be encouraged to have yearly physical examinations that include a digital rectal examination, which often allows the physician to palpate an enlarged gland. If the prostate gland is enlarged, a biopsy of the prostate may be advised to determine the cause of the enlargement.

Another diagnostic test often ordered as part of the routine physical examination is the **prostate-specific**

BOX 19-1

SURGICAL INTERVENTION FOR PROSTATIC HYPERTROPHY

Transurethral Resection of the Prostate
A cystoscope with an electrocautery wire cutting loop, a resectoscope, is inserted through the urethra and rotated through the prostate to remove pieces of the gland. The pieces are washed out with irrigating fluid introduced through the scope. There is no abdominal incision, making this a relatively safe procedure for the high-risk patient. The whole organ is not usually removed for this surgery; therefore, the obstruction frequently returns. This is not a choice for malignancies.

Suprapubic Prostatectomy
Performed through the abdominal wall and bladder, suprapubic prostatectomy allows the surgeon to peel out the whole organ through a wide surgical field and to check the bladder for involvement. This approach is the choice for large prostate glands or for malignancies. As in all surgeries, there are postoperative risks, particularly for the elderly. These include pain, hemorrhage, urinary leakage, and prolonged convalescence.

Perineal Resection
An incision between the scrotum and the anus is a short, direct route to the prostate without interfering with the bladder and is preferred for some large malignancies. It appears to be relatively nontraumatic for the very old or infirm. Surgeons find that the field offers less room to maneuver than with the suprapubic approach. It is not a good choice for young men because erectile dysfunction and urinary and fecal incontinence are frequent postoperative complications. The proximity of the anal area also increases the risk of infection.

Retropubic Resection
A low abdominal incision above the pubis but below the bladder avoids trauma to the bladder and thereby allows a shorter convalescence than with the suprapubic approach. It also provides better removal options than the transurethral approach. It is a good choice if pathology is limited to the prostate, with no bladder involvement.

antigen, or **PSA**, blood test. This antigen is normally found in the blood of all men, but its level increases with any inflammation of the prostate, including cancer. While the cause of prostate cancer is not known, it is most common in men over age 50 years, with 75% of diagnoses in men over age 75 years. Treatment depends on the extent of the malignancy and the patient's age and general health status. Prostate cancer is often treated by a combination of surgery, chemotherapy, and radiation.

 CHECKPOINT QUESTION

4. Does the patient with benign prostatic hyperplasia have an elevated prostate-specific antigen level? Why or why not?

Testicular Cancer

Although testicular cancer accounts for only about 1% of all malignancies, the metastatic and mortality rates are high. This type of cancer is most often seen in men ages 15 to 34 years. The cause of testicular cancer is unknown, but predisposing factors may include cryptorchidism, infection, genetic factors, and endocrine abnormalities. The symptoms are gradual and painless and may initially only involve a vague feeling of scrotal heaviness.

Once a diagnosis of testicular cancer has been made, treatment may be orchiectomy, or surgical removal of the testicle. Chemotherapy and radiation may also be used.

Hydrocele

Hydrocele, a collection of fluid in the scrotum and around the testes, may result from trauma or infection or may simply be due to aging. Diagnosis is based on symptoms and inspection. If the condition is extremely uncomfortable, aspiration of the excessive fluid may be required, and if the condition persists, surgical intervention may be the treatment of choice. In most cases, no treatment is necessary, and the fluid is reabsorbed by the body. Hydrocele is common in male infants but generally subsides without treatment.

Cryptorchidism

Normally, the testes descend from the abdominal cavity into the scrotal sac in the male fetus by the eighth month of gestation. In a small percentage of male infants, one or both of the testes fail to descend by the time of delivery (Fig. 19-6). **Cryptorchidism** refers to either one or both undescended testes. Surgical correction, known as *orchiopexy*, is usually performed before age 4 years, preferably at age 1 or 2 years. If an undescended testis is not surgically corrected, it results in sterility of the undescended organ and may increase the risk of testicular malignancy later in life.

 CHECKPOINT QUESTION

5. What are the causes of hydrocele?

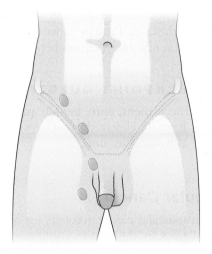

Figure 19-6 Possible locations of undescended testicles.

Inguinal Hernia

After the testes descend in the male fetus and the inguinal canals close, small rings are left open at the anterior base of the abdominal wall as a passage for the spermatic cord. There is no connection between this area and the abdominal contents, but this area remains a possible site for weakness and protrusion of the intestines with age or exertion. The patient with an inguinal hernia is often asymptomatic unless the intestines protrude through the weakened area, which may result in a noticeable bulge and pain. Diagnosis is made in the early stages by having the patient bear down and cough while the physician inserts a finger into a pouch made by the scrotum up into the external and internal inguinal rings. Pressure against the finger indicates weakness of the muscles in this area.

Treatment of an inguinal hernia depends on the patient's physical condition. Surgical correction of a hernia, called a *herniorrhaphy*, repositions the protruding organ and repairs the opening.

Infections

Infections of the male urinary tract are likely to spread to the reproductive system because they share many of the same organs. The most common infections of the male reproductive system are epididymitis, orchitis, and prostatitis. Although not all infections result from a sexually transmitted microorganism, many of the infections of the male reproductive system are caused by sexually transmitted diseases. Refer to Chapter 20 for more information about sexually transmitted diseases that affect both men and women.

Infection in the epididymis usually results from an infected prostate or other inflammation in the urinary tract. Microorganisms that may cause epididymitis include staphylococci, streptococci, *Escherichia coli*, chlamydia, and *Neisseria gonorrhoeae*. Symptoms include a swollen scrotum, pain, tenderness, fever, and malaise. Diagnosis is based on these symptoms and a culture of any drainage from the penis. Treatment includes an antibiotic, bed rest, fluids, and palliative measures for pain.

The microorganisms that cause epididymitis often also cause orchitis, and the treatment is virtually the same. Orchitis may also result in hydrocele, which should be treated if it becomes a severe complication.

Chronic prostatitis is common among the elderly and may be confused with prostatic hypertrophy if repeated infections cause the organs to fibrose. The causative agents are much like those of other infections of the male reproductive system, with the leading cause being *E. coli*. It frequently results from catheterization or cystoscopy. Some pathogens reach the prostate by way of the bloodstream of the lymph system. Signs and symptoms may include inguinal pain, fever, low back and joint pain, burning, dysuria, and urethral discharge. Urine specimens contain blood and pus. Diagnosis is based on signs, symptoms, and urinalysis. Antibiotic treatment is required to treat chronic prostatitis.

 CHECKPOINT QUESTION

6. What are some microorganisms responsible for causing infections in the male reproductive system?

 PATIENT EDUCATION

HIV/AIDS PREVENTION

When providing instructions about AIDS prevention, explain to your patient that it is safest, of course, to abstain from sex. Encourage your patients to have sex only with a partner who is known not to be infected, who has sex with no one but the patient, and who does not use needles or syringes. Also, advise the patient to use a latex condom if it is not known whether the sexual partner is infected. Generally, instruct patients to:

- Avoid contact with another person's blood, body fluids, semen, and vaginal secretions.
- Avoid sharing needles, syringes, and any objects that come into contact with blood or body fluids.
- Avoid using alcohol and drugs. Use of these substances can hinder clear thinking and lead to unwise decision making.

Erectile Dysfunction

Erectile dysfunction, also known as *impotence*, is the inability to achieve or maintain an erection; it may be psychological or organic. **Psychogenic impotence** may be caused by something as simple as exhaustion, anxiety, or depression, and in such cases, it usually disappears with resolution of the underlying cause. Organic erectile dysfunction may result from disease in almost any other body system, including endocrine imbalance, cardiovascular problems, nervous system impairment, or urinary disease. Organic erectile dysfunction may also be caused by injury to the pelvic organs or by medication that impairs any of the systems serving the reproductive system.

Diagnosis is based on a detailed medical and sexual history with an analysis of lifestyle and emotional status. Blood studies and measurements of both penile arterial flow and nerve conduction to this area are usually required. Treatment depends on the cause and may include a vacuum tube system that pulls blood into the penis, creating an erection, or vitamin E injections into the penis. Today, many new drugs, such as sildenafil (Viagra™), stimulate erections in the impotent male. If none of these are effective, a penile implant can be inserted surgically.

Common Diagnostic and Therapeutic Procedures

Urinalysis

The single most important step in diagnosing urinary diseases is the examination of the patient's urine, or **urinalysis.** Tests should always be performed on a fresh specimen and with the first morning specimen when concentrated urine is needed, such as for pregnancy testing. The urinalysis includes a physical and chemical evaluation, **specific gravity**, and a microscopic examination (see Chapter 28). If an infection is suspected, the physician may also order a urine culture.

The patient may produce the urine specimen by performing a clean-catch midstream procedure after receiving instructions from you on the proper procedure for collecting the specimen. In some cases, the physician may order a urine specimen obtained by **catheterization,** which is the introduction of a sterile flexible tube into the urinary bladder (Fig. 19-7). In the medical office, a

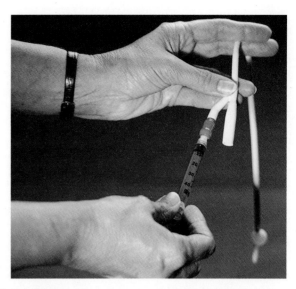

Figure 19-8 Sterile water is inserted into the indicated lumen to inflate the balloon of the indwelling catheter. When the balloon is inflated, the catheter will remain within the bladder.

straight catheter is used for catheterization and removed once the urine specimen is obtained. Some patients have an indwelling catheter inserted at another facility, such as a hospital. Indwelling catheters are similar to straight catheters, but these types are kept in place by a balloon on the end of the catheter inflated after placement in the bladder (Fig. 19-8). Indwelling catheters are not usually inserted in the medical office.

Catheters are sized 8 to 10 fr (French) for children and 14 to 20 fr for adults. (*Note:* French is a unit of measurement to describe the size of the diameter of catheters.) Procedures 19-1 and 19-2 describe the procedure for performing a catheterization in females and males, respectively, in the medical office, and Box 19-2 explains some principles of urinary catheterization.

Blood Tests

Serum levels of uric acid, **blood urea nitrogen (BUN)**, or creatinine may be indicated for diagnosis of some disease processes of the urinary system. It will likely be your responsibility to draw the patient's blood and process it on site or direct it to the proper testing facility (see Chapter 26).

Cystoscopy or Cystourethroscopy

Cystoscopy is direct visualization of the bladder and urethra with a lighted instrument called a *cystoscope* (Fig. 19-9). Cystoscopy allows the physician to diagnose many disorders of the lower urinary tract, such as tumors and inflammation. You may be responsible for providing preoperative instructions to the patient

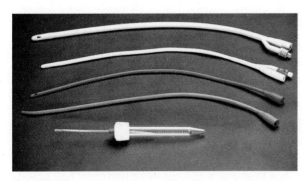

Figure 19-7 Types of catheters. From the top: No. 24 French indwelling catheter; No. 16 French indwelling catheter; No. 16 French straight catheter; Coudé catheter; and self-contained catheterization collection unit.

PRINCIPLES OF CATHETERIZATION

Catheterization is usually a last resort for obtaining a urine specimen. Even under the most aseptic conditions, there is a risk of introducing infection into the urinary system. However, some patients require catheterization when there is no other alternative. For example, catheterization is required in the following circumstances:

- It is impossible to obtain a clean-catch midstream specimen for urinalysis.
- The residual urine, or urine left in the bladder after urination, must be measured.
- Medication must be instilled into the bladder to treat an infection.
- The patient has urinary retention or cannot urinate.

Urinary catheter types and sizes vary. They are made of plastic or rubber. If the patient has prostatic hypertrophy, the physician may order a Coudé catheter (see Fig. 19-7), which is slightly curved and a bit stiffer than the other types so it is easier to advance it beyond the obstructing enlarged prostate gland.

as directed by the physician. This procedure is usually done under local anesthesia and may be performed in the urologist's office, but some physicians prefer to have the patient receive a general anesthetic and outpatient hospitalization.

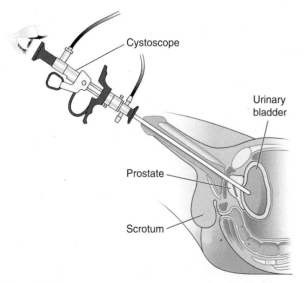

Figure 19-9 The interior of the urinary bladder as seen through a cystoscope. (Modified with permission from Cohen BJ. Medical Terminology: An Illustrated Guide. Philadelphia: Lippincott Williams & Wilkins, 2003.)

 CHECKPOINT QUESTION

7. What is the most common test for disorders of the urinary system performed in the medical office?

Intravenous Pyelogram and Retrograde Pyelogram

An **intravenous pyelogram (IVP)** is radiographic examination of the kidneys and urinary tract using a radiopaque dye injected into the circulatory system. This dye is filtered by the kidneys to serve as a contrast medium and enhance visualization of the renal structures. Although this procedure is not done in the medical office, you will schedule the examination at the appropriate facility and give the patient instructions to be followed before the procedure. Specifically, the patient is required to cleanse the bowels with a laxative the night before the test and to have an enema the morning of the procedure, since feces may prevent adequate visualization of the kidneys. In addition, the patient is asked not to eat or drink anything for at least 8 hours before the dye is injected to increase the blood concentration and visibility of the dye.

You must question the patient carefully about possible iodine allergy, including allergic reactions to seafood, particularly shellfish. Encourage the patient to increase fluid intake after the test to flush out the dye and counteract any dehydration caused by the preliminary cleansing.

A **retrograde pyelogram** is similar to the IVP except that the dye is not injected intravenously but is introduced through a catheter in the ureters through a cystoscope. This test is commonly used when IVP is contraindicated because of poor kidney function. Like IVP, this test is not performed in the medical office, but you may be responsible for making arrangements with the appropriate facility and giving the patient any necessary instructions.

 CHECKPOINT QUESTION

8. How does a retrograde pyelogram differ from an intravenous pyelogram?

 PATIENT EDUCATION

RENAL CALCULI

Clark Watkins, a 45-year-old white man, has severe right flank pain radiating to the suprapubic and inguinal regions of the abdomen. He has a fever of 100.3° F, nausea, and some vomiting. Urinalysis shows gross and microscopic hematuria and calcium crystal casts; it is clear of pyuria and white blood cells. Dr. Brown performs in-office ultrasonography, and the results suggest renal calculi. He orders an IVP, which reveals sand-to-gravel calculi.

Your role is to provide patient education. Demonstrate to Mr. Watkins the procedure for filtering his urine and provide him with the strainer so he can bring in the solid material for analysis. Mr. Watkins's diet will be altered in accordance with the composition of the stones. He may be referred to a dietitian or given a diet list after counseling with Dr. Brown. Encourage Mr. Watkins to increase his fluid intake to flush the stones and to walk frequently to assist peristalsis in the ureters and passing the stones. Urge him to drink fruit juices, especially cranberry juice, in addition to water, and discourage caffeine drinks. He may need an antiemetic if nausea and vomiting interfere with fluid intake. Caution him to watch for signs of infection and obstruction, including cloudy urine, which may contain pus, and fever.

Ultrasound

Ultrasound is noninvasive use of sound waves to show stones and obstructions in the urinary system and tissues. No special preparation is required other than an explanation of the procedure to the patient. If ordered by the physician, you may be responsible for scheduling this procedure with the appropriate facility.

Rectal and Scrotal Examinations

For the male patient seen in the physician's or urologist's office, you will assist with examination of the reproductive organs by instructing the patient to disrobe from the waist down and providing him with appropriate draping. The physician will inspect and palpate the scrotum for lumps and inguinal hernia. Using a gloved hand and water-soluble lubricant, the physician will perform a digital rectal examination, inserting the index finger into the rectum and palpating the prostate for size, shape, and consistency.

At home, male patients should perform the testicular self-examination because this is the best method for early detection of testicular cancer. The American Cancer Society recommends that all men perform this examination frequently, possibly weekly, and you are responsible for teaching the patient about this disease and the self-examination. You should explain that the best time for the self-examination is after a warm shower or bath, when the scrotal sac is relaxed (Procedure 19-3). If lumps or thickened areas are palpated during

the examination, instruct the patient to notify the physician immediately.

 CHECKPOINT QUESTION

9. When is the best time to instruct a patient to perform the testicular self-examination?

Vasectomy

A popular form of reproductive control is the vasectomy, or surgical removal of all or a segment of the vas deferens to prevent the passage of sperm from the testes. This procedure is commonly performed in the medical office, and you will assist by instructing the patient on preoperative orders as indicated by the physician. Some physicians order light preoperative sedation and may require that the patient have nothing by mouth after midnight on the day of the procedure.

On the day of the procedure, you should assist the physician by providing the appropriate surgical tray or instruments and assist the disrobed patient into the lithotomy position with appropriate draping materials to provide privacy. The physician will make two small incisions near the scrotal sac, pull each vas deferens (from the right and left testes) through the incision, clamp each vas deferens proximally and distally, and surgically cut and remove a segment of each. The remaining vas deferens ducts are placed back in the scrotal sac after the clamps are removed, and the site is sutured.

Ejaculation and sexual function are not affected by this procedure. The volume of sperm in the ejaculate is so small that it is not noticeable. The sperm produced by the testes after this procedure are absorbed in the testes. Since sterility may not be immediate, the patient should be advised to use another form of birth control, such as a condom, until sperm counts confirm that the ejaculate is free of sperm. You should advise the patient to return to the office for periodic sperm counts until no sperm are found in the ejaculate.

 AFF TRIAGE

While you are working in a medical office, the following three situations occur:

A. Patient A, a 24-year-old patient, has obtained a urine specimen for a work physical.
B. The physician has asked you to teach patient B, a 30-year-old male, to perform the testicular self-examination before discharging him.

(continued)

C. Patient C is a 67-year-old woman who needs a catheter to relieve bladder distention due to urinary retention.

How do you sort these patients? Who do you see first? Second? Third?

First see patient C, since she has urinary retention and is most likely very uncomfortable. Next, test the urine specimen from patient A. The quality of the urine specimen decreases as the urine specimen sits out, and once it is tested, the results can be given to the physician for diagnosis. Patient B should be addressed last. Patient education should never be rushed, and he should be given an opportunity to ask questions for clarification.

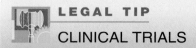

LEGAL TIP
CLINICAL TRIALS

Physicians who participate in clinical trials using new drugs or procedures have an ethical and legal obligation to follow specific guidelines, including:

- Notifying the patient that the drug or procedure is experimental and detailing the risks and benefits of the treatment clearly.
- Obtaining an informed, written consent before beginning the drug or performing the procedure.
- Assuring that the drug or procedure is documented appropriately and reported accurately according to the standards for the research being conducted.
- Providing a high standard of care for all patients regardless of whether or not they are participating in a clinical trial.

Medication Box

Commonly Prescribed Urinary System Medications

Note: The generic name of the drug is listed first and is written in all lowercase letters. Brand names are in parentheses, and the first letter is capitalized.

ciprofloxacin (Cipro)	Oral suspension: 250 mg/mL, 500 mg/mL Tablets: 100 mg, 250 mg, 500 mg, 750 mg	Antibiotic
doxycycline (Oracea)	Capsules: 40 mg	Antibiotic
fesoterodine fumarate (Toviaz)	Tablets: 4 mg, 8 mg	Antimuscarinic
nitrofurantoin (Macrobid, Macrodantin)	Capsules: 25 mg, 50 mg, 100 mg	Antibiotic
oxybutynin chloride (Ditropan)	Syrup: 5 mg/5 mL Tablets: 5 mg Transdermal patch: 36 mg patch, delivers 3.9 mg/day	Antimuscarinic
phenazopyridine hydrochloride (Pyridium)	Tablets: 95 mg, 97.2 mg, 100 mg, 200 mg	Urinary analgesic
sildenafil citrate (Viagra, Revatio)	Tablets: 20 mg, 25 mg, 50 mg, 100 mg	Erectile dysfunction
sulfamethoxazole (Septra)	Tablets: 400 mg, 800 mg	Anti-infective; sulfonamide
tadalafil (Cialis)	Tablets: 2.5 mg, 5 mg, 10 mg, 20 mg	Erectile dysfunction
tamsulosin hydrochloride (Flomax)	Capsules: 0.4 mg	Benign prostatic hyperplasia
testosterone (Depo-Testosterone, Delatestryl)	Injection: 100 mg/mL 200 mg/mL	Androgen hormone
tolterodine tartrate (Detrol, Detrol LA)	Capsules: 2 mg, 4 mg Tablets: 1 mg, 2 mg	Antimuscarinic

español SPANISH TERMINOLOGY

¿Se orina involuntariamente?
  Do you pass water involuntarily?

Necesitamos una muestra de orina.
  Need a urine specimen.

Va a ser un poco incomodo.
  It will be uncomfortable.

¿Tiene dificultades para orinar?
  Do you have burning when urinating?

¿Tiene que levantarse por la noche a orinar?
¿Cuántas veces?
  Do you have to get up to urinate during the night? How many times?

 MEDIA MENU

- **Student Resources on thePoint**
  - **Animation: Renal Function**
  - **Video: Performing a Female Urinary Catheterization (Procedure 19-1)**
  - **CMA/RMA Certification Exam Review**
- **Internet Resources**

  Brady Urological Institute, Johns Hopkins Medical Institutions
  http://urology.jhu.edu

  Urology Channel
  http://www.urologychannel.com

  National Kidney & Urologic Diseases Information Clearinghouse
  http://kidney.niddk.nih.gov

  Prostate Cancer Research Institute
  http://www.prostate-cancer.org/pcricms

  American Cancer Society
  http://www.cancer.org

  National Kidney Foundation
  http://www.kidney.org

PSY **PROCEDURE 19-1:**   **Female Urinary Catheterization**

Purpose: Using sterile aseptic technique, perform a straight catheterization on a female torso model
Equipment: Sterile straight catheterization tray with 14- or 16-French catheter, sterile gloves, antiseptic solution, sterile specimen cup with lid, lubricant, sterile drape, examination light, anatomically correct female torso model

Steps	Reasons
1. Wash your hands.	Handwashing aids infection control.
2. Identify the patient, explain the procedure, and have the patient disrobe completely from the waist down; provide a gown and adequate draping.	Identifying the patient helps prevent errors in treatment. The privacy of the patient should be maintained at all times.
3. Place the patient in the dorsal recumbent or lithotomy position, draping carefully to prevent unnecessary exposure. Carefully open the tray and place it between the patient's legs. Shine the examination light on the perineum.	The dorsal recumbent or lithotomy position allows the best view of the perineum and urinary meatus. Placing the tray between the legs of the patient allows easy access to the catheter and supplies. Adequate lighting is essential.
4. Remove the sterile glove package and put on the sterile gloves without contaminating them.	Contaminating the gloves will contaminate the supplies and may cause the patient to develop a urinary tract infection after the procedure.
5. Carefully remove the sterile drape and place it under the buttocks of the patient without contaminating your gloves.	If the sterile drape is on top of the tray, it may be carefully lifted out of the tray by the edge with clean hands and carefully placed under the buttocks. This drape is a barrier to protect the examination table from spills.
6. Open the antiseptic swabs and place them upright inside the catheter tray. Open the lubricant and squeeze a generous amount onto the tip of the catheter while it lies in the catheter tray.	The antiseptic swabs should be opened before beginning the actual catheterization. Placing the package upright prevents the antiseptic from spilling. Lubricant applied to the catheter allows for easier insertion.
7. Remove the sterile urine specimen cup and lid and place them to the side of the tray without contaminating your gloves.	Urinary catheterization is a sterile procedure.
8. Using your nondominant hand, carefully expose the urinary meatus by spreading the labia. This hand is now contaminated and must not be moved out of position until the catheter is in the bladder.	Moving this hand during the cleaning process will contaminate the area.
9. Cleanse the urinary meatus using the antiseptic swabs by wiping from top to bottom on each side and down the middle of the exposed urinary meatus. Use a separate swab for each side and the middle.	Continue to hold the labia apart with the nondominant hand.

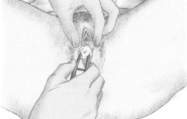

Step 9. Expose the urinary meatus and cleanse from top to bottom.

Steps

Reasons

Steps	Reasons
10. Using your sterile dominant hand, pick up the catheter and carefully insert the lubricated tip into the urinary meatus approximately 3 inches. The other end of the catheter should be left in the tray, which will collect the urine that drains from the bladder.	The adult female urethra is approximately 2 to 3 inches long. Once urine begins flowing into the catheter tray, the catheter is in far enough.

Step 10. Insert the catheter approximately 3 inches with the sterile hand, while continuing to hold the labia apart with the nondominant hand.

Steps	Reasons
11. Once the urine begins to flow into the catheter tray, hold the catheter in position with your nondominant hand by releasing the labia and moving your fingers down onto the catheter. Use your dominant hand to direct the flow of urine into the specimen cup if a specimen is needed.	Once the catheter is inserted into the bladder, the contaminated hand can hold the external part of the catheter in place while the dominant hand can be used to obtain a specimen.
12. When the urine flow has slowed or stopped *or* 1,000 mL has been obtained, carefully remove the catheter by pulling it straight out.	No more than 1,000 mL of urine should be removed from the bladder, since doing so may cause painful spasms of the bladder. Most patients do not have 1,000 mL.
13. Wipe the perineum carefully with the drape that was under the buttocks. Dispose of the urine appropriately and discard the catheter, tray, and supplies in a biohazard container.	Once the catheter is removed, it is not necessary to keep your dominant hand sterile.
14. **AFF** Explain how to respond to a patient who is visually impaired.	Face the patient when speaking to him or her and always let him or her know what you are going to do before touching him or her.
15. If a urine specimen was obtained, properly label the specimen container and complete the laboratory requisition. Process the specimen according to the guidelines of the laboratory.	Specimens obtained to be sent to an outside laboratory should be labeled and accompanied by a completed request form.
16. Remove your gloves and wash your hands.	Standard precautions must be followed throughout the procedure.
17. Instruct the patient to dress and give any follow-up information regarding test results as necessary.	Telling the patient what to do and what to expect will reduce confusion and misunderstanding.
18. Document the procedure in the patient's medical record.	Procedures are considered not to have been done if they are not recorded.

Charting Example:

02/14/2013 9:15 AM Catheterization with a 14-fr straight cath, 300 mL dark amber urine obtained, specimen to Acme lab for C & S —————————————————————————————— S. Strobb, CMA

Note: The medical assistant may sign his or her name in the patient record using only the "CMA" credential if the office has a signature log denoting the entire credential as "CMA(AAMA)."

PSY PROCEDURE 19-2:   Male Urinary Catheterization

Purpose: Using sterile aseptic technique, perform a straight catheterization on a male torso model
Equipment: Sterile straight catheterization tray with 14- or 16-French catheter, sterile gloves, antiseptic solution, sterile specimen cup with lid, lubricant, sterile drape, examination light, anatomically correct male torso model

Steps	Purpose
1. Wash your hands.	Handwashing aids infection control.
2. Identify the patient, explain the procedure, and have the patient disrobe completely from the waist down while providing a gown and adequate draping.	Identifying the patient helps prevent errors in treatment. The privacy of the patient should be maintained at all times.
3. Place the patient supine, draping carefully to prevent unnecessary exposure. Carefully open the tray and place it to the side of the patient on the examination table or on top of the patient's thighs.	The male urinary meatus is on the glans penis. Placing the tray on top of the patient's legs allows easy access to the catheter and supplies.
4. Remove the sterile glove package and put on the sterile gloves without contaminating them.	Contaminating the gloves will contaminate the supplies and may cause the patient to develop a urinary tract infection after the procedure.
5. Carefully remove the sterile drape and place it under the glans penis.	If the sterile drape is the top item in the tray, it may be carefully lifted out of the tray by the edge with clean hands and placed under the penis. This drape is a barrier to protect the examination table and patient from any spills.
6. Open the antiseptic swabs and place them upright inside the catheter tray. Open the lubricant and squeeze a generous amount onto the tip of the catheter as it lies in the bottom of the catheter tray.	The antiseptic swabs should be opened before beginning the catheterization. Placing the package upright helps prevent the antiseptic from spilling. Lubricant on the catheter allows for easier insertion.
7. Remove the sterile urine specimen cup and lid and place them to the side of the tray without contaminating your gloves.	Urinary catheterization is a sterile procedure.
8. Using your nondominant hand, carefully pick up the penis, exposing the urinary meatus. This hand is now contaminated and must not be moved out of position until the catheter is inserted into the urinary bladder.	Moving this hand will contaminate the area.
9. Cleanse the urinary meatus using the antiseptic swabs by wiping from top to bottom on each side and down the middle of the exposed urinary meatus. Use a separate swab for each side and the middle.	Continue to hold the penis with the dominant hand.

Step 9. Expose the urinary meatus and cleanse from top to bottom.

PSY PROCEDURE 19-2:   Male Urinary Catheterization *(continued)*

Steps	Reasons
10. Using your sterile dominant hand, pick up the catheter and carefully insert the lubricated tip into the urinary meatus approximately 4 to 6 inches. The other end of the catheter should be left in the tray, which will collect the urine that drains from the bladder.	The adult male urethra is approximately 4 to 6 inches long. Once urine begins flowing into the catheter tray, the catheter is in far enough.

Step 10. Carefully insert the catheter into the urethra.

Steps	Reasons
11. Once the urine begins to flow, hold the catheter in position with your nondominant hand. Use your dominant hand to direct the flow of urine into the specimen cup if a specimen is needed.	Once the catheter is inserted into the bladder, the contaminated hand can hold the external part of the catheter in place while the dominant hand can be used to obtain a specimen.
12. When the urine flow has slowed or stopped *or* 1,000 mL has been obtained, carefully remove the catheter by pulling it straight out.	No more than 1,000 mL of urine should be removed from the bladder, since doing so may cause painful spasms of the bladder.
13. Wipe the glans penis carefully with the drape and dispose of the urine, catheter, tray, and supplies appropriately in a biohazard container.	Once the urinary catheter has been removed, it is not necessary to keep the dominant hand sterile.
14. AFF Explain how to respond to a patient who has dementia.	Solicit assistance from a caregiver or other staff member to help during the procedure. Give simple directions to the patient about what he or she should do. Speak clearly, not loudly.
15. If a urine specimen was obtained, properly label the container and complete the laboratory requisition. Process the specimen according to the guidelines of the laboratory.	Specimens obtained to be sent to an outside laboratory should be labeled and accompanied by a completed request form.
16. Remove your gloves and wash your hands.	Standard precautions must be followed throughout the procedure.
17. Instruct the patient to dress and give any follow-up information regarding test results as necessary.	Telling the patient what to do and what to expect will reduce confusion and misunderstanding.
18. Document the procedure in the patient's medical record.	Procedures are considered not to have been done if they are not recorded.

Charting Example:

6/17/2013 3:00 PM Catheterization with 14-French straight cath, 600 mL light amber urine obtained, specimen to Acme lab for C & S ———————————————————————————————— J. Jones, CMA

Note: The medical assistant may sign his or her name in the patient record using only the "CMA" credential if the office has a signature log denoting the entire credential as "CMA(AAMA)."

PSY PROCEDURE 19-3: | **Instructing a Male Patient on the Testicular Self-Examination**

Purpose: Teach a male patient to perform the testicular self-examination
Equipment: A patient instruction sheet if available, testicular examination model or pictures

Steps	Purpose
1. Wash your hands.	Handwashing aids infection control.
2. Identify the patient and explain the procedure.	Identifying the patient prevents errors in treatment.
3. Using the testicular model or pictures, explain the procedure, telling the patient to examine each testicle by gently rolling the testicle between the fingers and the thumb with both hands while checking for lumps or thickenings.	Both hands should be used to check each testicle to ensure complete palpation of all areas. Lumps and thickened areas are not normal and should be reported to the physician.

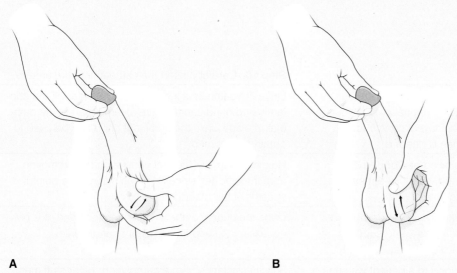

A   B

Step 3. (A) Gently roll the testes in a horizontal plane between the thumb and fingers.
(B) Follow the same procedure and palpate upward along the testis.

4. Explain that the epididymis is a structure on top of each testicle and should be palpated to avoid incorrectly identifying it as an abnormal growth or lump.	If the epididymis is not correctly identified, the patient may palpate it during the examination and erroneously believe it is an abnormal growth.

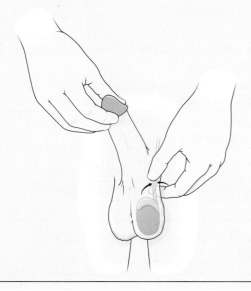

Step 4. Locate the epididymis, a cordlike structure on the top and back of the testicle that stores and transports sperm.

PSY PROCEDURE 19-3:   **Instructing a Male Patient on the Testicular Self-Examination (continued)**

Steps	Purpose
5. Instruct the patient to report any abnormal lumps or thickenings to the physician.	Any abnormalities should be assessed by the physician to determine the cause.
6. Allow the patient to ask questions about the self-examination.	The patient should always be encouraged to ask questions to ensure understanding.
7. **AFF** Explain how to respond to a patient who speaks limited English.	Solicit assistance from anyone who may be with the patient or a staff member who speaks the native language to interpret if available. If no interpreter is available, use hand gestures or pictures to explain the procedure to the patient.
8. Document the procedure in the patient's medical record.	Procedures are considered not to have been done if they are not recorded.

Charting Example:

12/13/2013 10:15 AM Pt. given verbal and written instructions on the testicular self-examination; verbalized
understanding ————————————————————————————— C. Brook, CMA

Note: The medical assistant may sign his or her name in the patient record using only the "CMA" credential if the office has a signature log denoting the entire credential as "CMA(AAMA)."

- The urinary system performs many vital functions to maintain the internal environment of the body. Patients may require an examination of the urinary system for:
  - Signs and symptoms that indicate disorders of the urinary system, especially infection of the urinary bladder and urethra.
  - Evaluation during a complete physical examination even if no symptoms are present.
  - Examination of the male reproductive system, which shares the same organs as the male urinary system, for any disorders of the male reproductive system.

- Your role in working with patients with urologic disorders may include:
  - Assisting the physician as necessary during the physical examination.
  - Preparing the patient for urologic procedures.
  - Performing urologic procedures such as urinary catheterization.
  - Providing patient education as directed by the physician.

Warm Ups for Critical Thinking

1. Differentiate between peritoneal dialysis and hemodialysis. Why are some patients poor candidates for peritoneal dialysis? What can you ask the patient to determine whether or not the peritoneal catheter is functioning or infected?

2. Research the newest pharmacologic agents used to treat erectile dysfunction and explain the method of action, usual dosages, and side effects.

3. A male patient in your office has just been diagnosed with a low sperm count, and the physician has recommended that he switch from briefs to boxer shorts. How do you think this will affect his sperm count, and why?

4. Create a patient education brochure explaining the procedure for performing the testicular self-examination.

5. Identify the resources in your community for patients diagnosed with renal failure.

6. Elderly patients who experience incontinence may be too embarrassed to discuss this condition with anyone. What interpersonal skills can you use to obtain this information from the patient?

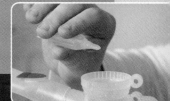

CHAPTER

20 Obstetrics and Gynecology

Learning Outcomes

Cognitive Domain

Note: AAMA/CAAHEP 2008 Standards are italicized.

1. Spell and define key terms
2. List and describe common gynecologic and obstetric disorders
3. Identify your role in the care of gynecologic and obstetric patients
4. Describe the components of prenatal and postpartum patient care
5. Explain the diagnostic and therapeutic procedures associated with the female reproductive system
6. Identify the various methods of contraception
7. Describe menopause
8. *Identify common pathologies related to each body system*

9. *Describe implications for treatment related to pathology*

Psychomotor Domain

Note: AAMA/CAAHEP 2008 Standards are italicized.

1. Instruct the patient on the breast self-examination (Procedure 20-1)
2. Assist with the pelvic examination and Pap smear (Procedure 20-2)
3. Assist with colposcopy and cervical biopsy (Procedure 20-3)
4. *Assist physician with patient care*
5. *Prepare a patient for procedures and/or treatments*
6. *Practice standard precautions*
7. *Document patient care*

8. *Document patient education*
9. *Practice within the standard of care for a medical assistant*

Affective Domain

Note: AAMA/CAAHEP 2008 Standards are italicized.

1. *Apply critical thinking skills in performing patient assessment and care*
2. *Use language/verbal skills that enable patients' understanding*
3. *Demonstrate empathy in communicating with patients, family, and staff*
4. *Use appropriate body language and other nonverbal skills in communicating with patients, family, and staff*
5. *Demonstrate awareness of the territorial boundaries of the person with whom you are communicating*
6. *Demonstrate sensitivity appropriate to the message being delivered*
7. *Demonstrate recognition of the patient's level of understanding in communications*
8. *Recognize and protect personal boundaries in communicating with others*

9. *Demonstrate respect for individual diversity, incorporating awareness of one's own biases in areas including gender, race, religion, age, and economic status*
10. *Apply active listening skills*
11. *Apply local, state, and federal health care legislation and regulation appropriate to the medical assisting practice setting*

ABHES Competencies

1. Assist the physician with the regimen of diagnostic and treatment modalities as they relate to each body system
2. Comply with federal, state, and local health laws and regulations
3. Communicate on the recipient's level of comprehension
4. Serve as a liaison between the physician and others
5. Show empathy and impartiality when dealing with patients
6. Document accurately

Key Terms

abortion	cystocele	hysterosalpingogram	oligomenorrhea
amenorrhea	dysmenorrhea	laparoscopy	parity
amniocentesis	dyspareunia	lightening	pessary
Braxton-Hicks contractions	Goodell sign	lochia	polymenorrhea
Chadwick sign	gravid	menarche	primigravida
colpocleisis	gravida	menorrhagia	primipara
colporrhaphy	gravidity	menses	proteinuria
colposcopy	hirsutism	metrorrhagia	puerperium
culdocentesis	human chorionic	multipara	rectocele
curettage	gonadotropin (HCG)	nulligravida	salpingo-oophorectomy
		nullipara	

The female reproductive system is responsible for the development and maintenance of primary and secondary sexual characteristics and for sexual reproduction. Gynecology and obstetrics are the two medical specialties concerned with female sexual and reproductive functions. Gynecology is a specialty of medicine that deals with development and disorders of the female reproductive system, including the internal and external organs. Obstetrics is the branch of medicine that cares for female patients through pregnancy, childbirth, and the postpartum period. The organs of the female internal reproductive system are shown in Figure 20-1.

Puberty is the onset of production of cyclical hormones that cause secondary sexual characteristics, including

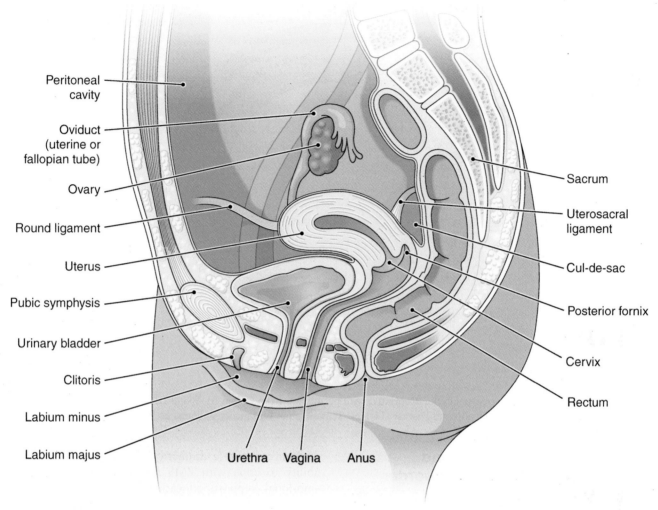

Peritoneal cavity

Oviduct (uterine or fallopian tube)

Ovary

Round ligament

Uterus

Pubic symphysis

Urinary bladder

Clitoris

Labium minus

Labium majus

Sacrum

Uterosacral ligament

Cul-de-sac

Posterior fornix

Cervix

Rectum

Urethra   Vagina   Anus

Figure 20-1 Female reproductive system. (Reprinted with permission from Cohen BJ. Memmler's The Human Body in Health and Disease, 11th ed. Philadelphia: Lippincott Williams & Wilkins, 2009.)

menses, or menstruation. The age at which a girl begins menses is **menarche**. The menstrual cycle, which is about 28 days, comprises a series of complex events in the internal organs controlled by hormones secreted by the anterior pituitary gland and the ovaries (Fig. 20-2). Always remind and encourage patients, especially adolescents, to record and track the menstrual cycle, since the regularity of the cycle is often critical to the physician's assessment of the patient's gynecologic health. In addition, the first day of the last menstrual period (LMP) is necessary for calculating an approximate due date in the pregnant patient. This chapter discusses some of the common disorders of the female reproductive system and caring for the obstetric patient in the medical office before and after delivery.

Gynecologic Disorders

Dysfunctional Uterine Bleeding

Dysfunctional uterine bleeding is abnormal or irregular uterine bleeding, including heavy, irregular, or light bleeding caused by an endocrine imbalance. Abnormal uterine bleeding includes the following:

- Menorrhagia: excessive bleeding during menses
- **Metrorrhagia**: irregular bleeding at times other than menses
- **Polymenorrhea**: abnormally frequent menses
- Postmenopausal bleeding: bleeding after menopause that is not associated with tumor, inflammation, or pregnancy

Diagnosis of dysfunctional uterine bleeding consists of ruling out other causes, such as hormonal imbalance, tumor, or another condition of the endometrial lining of the uterus. Treatment includes hormone therapy and oral contraceptives or curettage (scraping) of the uterine cavity, depending on the cause. Hysterectomy, surgical removal of the uterus, may be the treatment of choice for patients who do not respond to conservative therapy, who are at increased risk for adenocarcinoma, and who do not desire pregnancy.

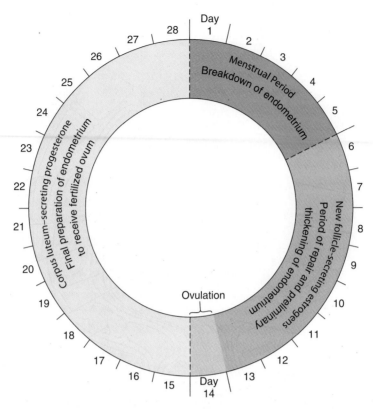

Figure 20-2 The menstrual cycle. (Reprinted with permission from Cohen BJ, Wood DL. Memmler's The Human Body in Health and Disease, 11th ed. Philadelphia: Lippincott Williams & Wilkins, 2009.)

Premenstrual Syndrome and Premenstrual Dysphoric Disorder

Characterized by a wide variety of physical, psychological, and behavioral signs and symptoms, premenstrual syndrome (PMS) and premenstrual dysphoric disorder (PMDD) occur on a regular, cyclic basis. Many women complain of breast tenderness and a tendency to retain fluids 7 to 10 days before the start of the menstrual cycle; however, when symptoms and mood changes affect routine daily activities, the physician may make a diagnosis of PMS (Box 20-1). When symptoms are severe and affect work, social activities, and interpersonal relationships, a diagnosis of PMDD may be made by the physician.

Both PMS and PMDD usually diminish within a few days after the onset of menses, and the cause is idiopathic (unknown). Diagnosis is based on the physician's assessment of the history and physical examination. Patients should chart their symptoms for several months on a calendar that includes the menstrual cycle. The treatment for both include simple lifestyle changes, such as eating healthy foods, getting regular exercise, using birth control medications to stop ovulation, and taking anti-inflammatory medications to help with any physical discomfort. Women who are diagnosed with PMDD may also be prescribed an antidepressant and may be referred to counseling to assist with developing coping strategies.

You can have a dramatic influence on the patient's ability to cope with PMS and PMDD by providing emotional support; educating the patient about the disorders; and encouraging the recommended lifestyle changes, including regular exercise and dietary restrictions, such as eliminating caffeine, salt, and animal fats. Patients also should be encouraged to get adequate rest and avoid unnecessary stress.

PATIENT EDUCATION

PREMENSTRUAL DYSPHORIC DISORDER

Although many women have symptoms of premenstrual syndrome, a few women have a more severe form of PMS known as *premenstrual dysphoric disorder*, or *PMDD*. Diagnosis of PMDD is made when five or more of the following symptoms are present a week before the menstrual cycle begins:

- Feelings of sadness or despair including possible suicidal thoughts
- Feelings of tension or anxiety
- Panic attacks
- Mood swings, crying

- Lasting irritability or anger that affects other people
- Disinterest in daily activities and relationships
- Trouble thinking or focusing
- Tiredness or low energy
- Food cravings or binge eating
- Difficulty sleeping
- Feeling out of control
- Physical symptoms such as bloating, breast tenderness, headaches, and joint or muscle pain

In addition to individual counseling and stress management, the physician may order antidepressants called *serotonin reuptake inhibitors*, which have been shown to help some women.

Source: Office on Women's Health in the Department of Health and Human Services.

 CHECKPOINT QUESTION

1. What is the difference between menorrhagia and metrorrhagia?

Endometriosis

Endometriosis is a condition of unknown cause in which endometrial tissue grows outside the uterine cavity.

Endometrial tissue may be found in the fallopian tubes, the ovaries, the uterosacral ligaments, and in rare cases, in other parts of the abdominal cavity. The patient, who is often of reproductive age, complains of infertility, **dysmenorrhea**, pelvic pain, and **dyspareunia**. The patient's symptoms and physical findings may indicate endometriosis, but the diagnosis and the severity must be confirmed by direct visualization, usually by way of a **laparoscopy** (Fig. 20-3).

Treatment of endometriosis may relieve the pelvic pain, but some treatments reduce fertility. The type of therapy depends on the age of the patient, the severity of the symptoms, and the patient's desire for future pregnancy. Hormone and drug therapy to suppress the growth of the tissue and laparoscopic excision of the tissue using laser or cautery may be used to treat endometriosis. For patients with severe symptoms, the treatment of choice may be a hysterectomy with possible bilateral salpingo-oophorectomy, or surgical removal of the fallopian tubes and ovaries.

Uterine Prolapse and Displacement

Prolapse of the uterus is an abnormal condition in which the uterus droops or protrudes down into the vagina. Often, the condition is accompanied by **cystocele, rectocele**, or both. Cystocele is herniation of the urinary bladder into the vagina, and rectocele is herniation of the rectum into the vagina. The degree of prolapse is usually

---

BOX 20-1

PREMENSTRUAL SYNDROME

The hormonal flux associated with the menstrual cycle may affect body systems other than the reproductive system in some women. The cascade of events results in the following series of symptoms:

- Acne
- Breast swelling and tenderness
- Feeling tired
- Difficulty sleeping
- Upset stomach, bloating, constipation, or diarrhea
- Headache or backache
- Appetite changes or cravings
- Trouble concentrating or remembering
- Tension, irritability, mood swings, or crying spells
- Anxiety or depression

Although no treatment works the same on all women, the following are some common treatments for PMS that the physician may suggest:

- Take a multivitamin every day that includes 400 micrograms of folic acid.
- Include a calcium supplement with vitamin D to keep bones strong.
- Exercise regularly.
- Eat healthy foods, including fruits, vegetables, and whole grains.
- Avoid salt, sugary foods, caffeine, and alcohol.
- Get enough sleep.
- Find healthy ways to cope with stress.
- Don't smoke.

Over-the-counter medications such as ibuprofen, aspirin, or naproxen sodium may be ordered by the physician for the pain associated with PMS. Severe cases may require the physician to prescribe drugs to prevent ovulation such as birth control pills.

From the Office on Women's Health in the Department of Health and Human Services, 2007, http://www.womenshealth.gov.

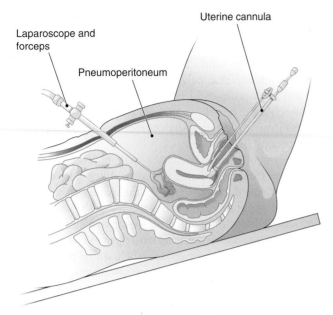

Figure 20-3 Laparoscopy. The laparoscope is inserted through a small incision in the abdomen. A forceps is inserted through the scope to grasp the fallopian tube. To improve the view, a uterine cannula is inserted into the vagina to push the uterus upward. Insufflation of gas creates an air pocket, and the pelvis is raised, which forces the intestines higher into the abdomen. (Reprinted with permission from Cohen BJ. Medical Terminology: An Illustrated Guide. Philadelphia: Lippincott Williams & Wilkins, 2003.)

described as mild, moderate, or severe, or grade I, II, or III. A commonly used method classifies the prolapse in degrees:

- First-degree prolapse occurs when the uterus has descended to the level of the vaginal orifice.
- Second-degree prolapse occurs when the uterine cervix protrudes through the vaginal orifice.

- Third-degree prolapse occurs when the entire cervix and uterus protrude beyond the vaginal orifice.

Diagnosis of uterine prolapse is made during a pelvic examination, at which time the degree of prolapse can be determined. While many women do not have symptoms, others complain of pelvic pressure, dyspareunia, urinary problems, or constipation. Surgical treatment may include vaginal hysterectomy, **colporrhaphy** (suture of the vagina), or **colpocleisis** (surgery to occlude the vagina). Medical management for patients who are elderly or a poor risk for surgery includes hormone therapy to strengthen the muscular floor of the pelvis and the use of a **pessary**. A pessary is a device that is inserted into the vagina and fits around the cervix to support the uterus. You should instruct the patient on the proper procedure for caring for the device by removing it according to the physician's orders and washing it with soap and warm water before reinserting it into the vagina.

The uterus is normally tilted slightly forward over the bladder with the cervix at a right angle to the direction of the vagina. The uterus is movable, and stress on the supporting ligaments occasionally tilts it from its natural position, known as *uterine displacement* (Fig. 20-4). The symptoms of uterine displacement may include pressure in the rectal area or against the bladder that is not usually severe, just troublesome to the patient. Treatment follows the same protocol as required for uterine prolapse. In some instances, the uterus may simply be stitched back into its original position in a hysteropexy.

Leiomyomas

Leiomyomas are benign tumors of the uterus, including fibroid tumors, myomas, and fibromyomas.

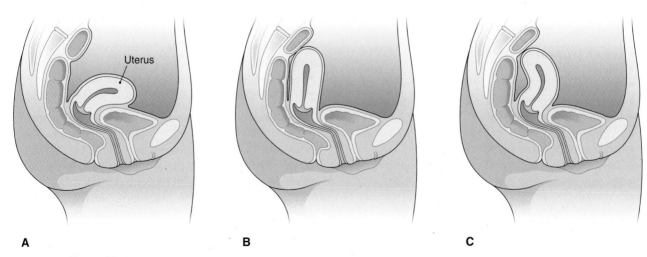

A   **B**   **C**

Figure 20-4 Retrodisplacements of the uterus. (**A**) The normal position of the uterus as detected on palpation. (**B**) In retroversion, the uterus turns posteriorly as a whole. (**C**) In retroflexion, the fundus bends posteriorly above the cervical end.

These tumors may be in any of the uterine tissue layers—endometrium, myometrium, or perimetrium—and they vary greatly in size. Most patients are asymptomatic, but large tumors tend to distort the uterus and are relatively likely to be symptomatic. Symptoms may include abnormal bleeding, pelvic pressure and discomfort, constipation, urinary frequency, and infertility.

A presumptive diagnosis is based on the patient's symptoms and physician's assessment, which initially includes bimanual examination and sounding of the uterus. Sounding of the uterus requires the physician to do a pelvic examination and possibly the insertion of a uterine sound (a long slender instrument; refer to Chapter 6) into the uterine cavity. Obstruction or resistance may be due to the tumor pressing into the uterine cavity. Most physicians request an ultrasound of the uterus to confirm the presence of these tumors.

Treatment of leiomyoma depends on the size of the tumor or tumors. Small asymptomatic tumors are monitored to detect excessive growth. Depending on the patient's age and desire for pregnancy, myomectomy or hysterectomy may be indicated.

 CHECKPOINT QUESTION

2. What are some symptoms of endometriosis?

Ovarian Cysts

Numerous types of ovarian cysts, including functional cysts and polycystic ovaries, are benign. Functional ovarian cysts, which are fairly common, include the follicular cyst. This is a fluid-filled sac that causes few if any problems. The patient is most often asymptomatic unless the cyst is large or ruptures. Functional cysts are usually detected during surgery, and treatment is simply puncture or excision.

In contrast, polycystic ovary syndrome (Stein-Leventhal syndrome) is a more troublesome and complex disorder. It affects both ovaries and is most often found in adolescent girls and young women, who have numerous symptoms of an endocrine imbalance. The signs include anovulation, irregular menses or **amenorrhea** (no menses), and **hirsutism**, an abnormal or excessive growth of hair. Diagnosis is based on pelvic examination, ultrasonography, laparoscopy, or exploratory laparotomy. Treatment is difficult and depends on the signs and symptoms and the patient's desire for future pregnancy. Management of this disorder includes hormone therapy or oral contraceptives.

Gynecologic Cancers

The malignant tumors affecting the female reproductive system and their characteristics, diagnosis, and treatment are outlined in Table 20-1. For patient education, you should know the recommendations regarding the frequency of pelvic and breast examinations and Pap smears. You should obtain current brochures and literature on various types of cancers from either the American Cancer Society or the American College of Obstetrics and Gynecology and have them readily available to patients.

Cervical and breast cancers have an excellent prognosis when detected and treated early, but left untreated or diagnosed in later stages, these cancers are deadly. Instruct and encourage all female patients to perform a breast self-examination every month (Procedure 20-1). Patients should also be encouraged to have a complete physical that includes a breast examination by the physician and a pelvic examination and Papanicolaou (Pap) test, which is a screening test for early detection of cancer of the cervix. The American College of Obstetricians and Gynecologists (ACOG) recommends that the first Pap test and pelvic exam be performed about 3 years after the first sexual intercourse or by age 21 years, whichever comes first, and annually until age 30 years. Women over age 30 years who have had three negative Pap tests can be screened every 2 to 3 years or annually as recommended by the physician.

Initially, the abnormal growth of cancerous cells in the cervix is asymptomatic, which further necessitates early detection during the physical examination and Pap smear. The Pap test is a grading of any abnormal tissue scraped from the cervix using a classification system such as the one described in Table 20-2. Some laboratories use another classification, the Bethesda system, to provide a more descriptive narrative of the abnormal cells. Cervical cells in the Bethesda system are categorized as normal, atypical squamous cells (ASC), squamous intraepithelial lesions (SIL), atypical glandular cells, or cancer. In addition, the squamous intraepithelial lesions may be noted as high grade (HSIL) or low grade (LSIL) (Fig. 20-5). Regardless of the method used by the laboratory to classify the Pap test results, not all abnormal results indicate cancer. However, since this is a deadly disease, it must be ruled out using further diagnostic studies such as **colposcopy**, a magnified examination of the cervical tissue with a special instrument called a *colposcope*. Other reasons for an abnormal Pap result include inflammation of the cervix and some sexually transmitted diseases such as human papilloma virus (HPV) infection.

Infertility

Female infertility is more difficult to diagnose than male infertility. Most testing begins by eliminating the male as the infertile party and then focuses

TABLE 20-1	Cancers of the Female Reproductive System			
Cancer	Warning Signs	Risk Factors	Early Detection	Treatment
Breast	Breast changes: lumps, pain, thickening, swelling, retraction, dimpling	Over age 40, history of breast cancer, early menarche, nulliparity, first birth at late age	Monthly self-examination, mammogram by age 40 and yearly after age 40, yearly clinical breast exam, monthly self-breast exam	Lumpectomy, mastectomy, radiation, chemotherapy
Cervical	Often asymptomatic; irregular bleeding, abnormal vaginal discharge	Intercourse at early age, multiple sex partners, cigarette smoking, history of STDs such as HPV	Annual Pap smear	Cryotherapy; electrocoagulation; surgery, radiation, chemotherapy; new vaccine is available to prevent certain types of HPV that may cause cervical cancer
Endometrial	Irregular bleeding outside menses; unusual vaginal discharge; excessive bleeding during menses; postmenopausal bleeding	Obesity; early menarche; multiple sex partners; late menopause; history of infertility; family history	Endometrial biopsy at menopause for high-risk women	Progesterone therapy; surgery; radiation; chemotherapy
Ovarian	Often asymptomatic; abdominal enlargement; vague digestive disorders, discomfort; gas, distention	Risk increases with age (esp. >60 years), nulliparity, history of breast cancer	Periodic complete pelvic examination	Surgery; radiation; chemotherapy

on the female partner. Testing is usually not started until after 1 year of unprotected intercourse without conception.

The causes of infertility may include uterine or cervical abnormalities, tubal occlusion or scarring, a hormonal imbalance, or psychological factors. Diagnosis requires a complete history and physical examination.

An endometrial biopsy may diagnose anovulation; progesterone blood levels may indicate hormonal deficiencies; or hysterosalpingography may indicate tubal occlusion or uterine abnormalities. Treatment necessitates identifying and correcting the problem. Procedures such as in vitro fertilization may also be recommended, again, depending upon the nature of the problem.

TABLE 20-2	Classification of Papanicolaou Tests
Class	Characteristics
I	Normal test, no atypical cells
II	Atypical cells but no evidence of malignancy
III	Atypical cells possible but not conclusive for malignancy
IV	Cells strongly suggest malignancy
V	Strong evidence of malignancy

 CHECKPOINT QUESTION

3. What two factors greatly affect the prognosis of all cancers?

Sexually Transmitted Diseases

Many of the diseases transmitted through sexual contact have serious consequences and may affect men or women. The most deadly of these is acquired immunodeficiency syndrome (AIDS), although other sexually transmitted diseases (STDs) also continue to be a problem. Since STDs are easily transmitted, all STDs

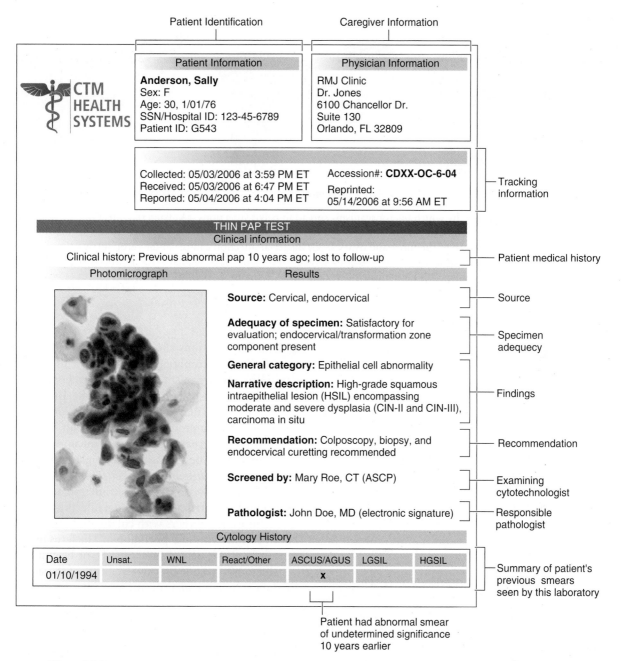

Patient Identification · Caregiver Information

Patient Information
Anderson, Sally Sex: F Age: 30, 1/01/76 SSN/Hospital ID: 123-45-6789 Patient ID: G543

Physician Information
RMJ Clinic Dr. Jones 6100 Chancellor Dr. Suite 130 Orlando, FL 32809

Collected: 05/03/2006 at 3:59 PM ET
Received: 05/03/2006 at 6:47 PM ET
Reported: 05/04/2006 at 4:04 PM ET

Accession#: **CDXX-OC-6-04**
Reprinted:
05/14/2006 at 9:56 AM ET — Tracking information

THIN PAP TEST
Clinical information

Clinical history: Previous abnormal pap 10 years ago; lost to follow-up — Patient medical history

Photomicrograph · Results

Source: Cervical, endocervical — Source

Adequacy of specimen: Satisfactory for evaluation; endocervical/transformation zone component present — Specimen adequecy

General category: Epithelial cell abnormality

Narrative description: High-grade squamous intraepithelial lesion (HSIL) encompassing moderate and severe dysplasia (CIN-II and CIN-III), carcinoma in situ — Findings

Recommendation: Colposcopy, biopsy, and endocervical curetting recommended — Recommendation

Screened by: Mary Roe, CT (ASCP) — Examining cytotechnologist

Pathologist: John Doe, MD (electronic signature) — Responsible pathologist

Cytology History

Date	Unsat.	WNL	React/Other	ASCUS/AGUS	LGSIL	HGSIL
01/10/1994				x		

— Summary of patient's previous smears seen by this laboratory

Patient had abnormal smear of undetermined significance 10 years earlier

Figure 20-5 Typical Pap smear report. (Thomas H. McConnell, The Nature of Disease Pathology for the Health Professions, Philadelphia: Lippincott Williams & Wilkins, 2007.)

must be reported to the local health department by the medical office. This may be your responsibility, or the physician may be required to report the disease according to local policy or the policy of the medical office. In some areas, you may have to file a form or written report; others have a phone reporting system. You need to be familiar with your office policy and procedure manual regarding this requirement and the local laws on reporting. The patient should be encouraged to notify sexual partners so that they may also receive treatment for the appropriate STD. Figure 20-6 outlines the pathway by which microorganisms spread in female pelvic infections regardless of the reason, but especially when sexually transmitted diseases are involved.

AIDS

AIDS is an infectious disease that overwhelms the body's immune system. The pathogen that causes AIDS is the human immunodeficiency virus (HIV), which destroys T-helper cells, lowering the body's ability to fight infection. Transmission of HIV most often occurs through an exchange of blood or body fluids, including a sexual act with an HIV-positive partner. A person who is HIV

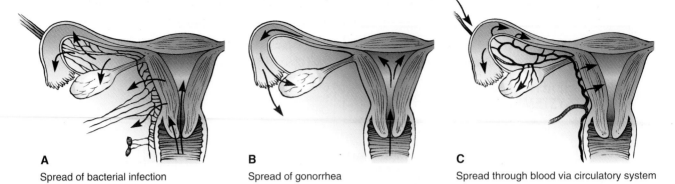

A
Spread of bacterial infection

B
Spread of gonorrhea

C
Spread through blood via circulatory system

Figure 20-6 Pathway by which microorganisms spread in pelvic infections. (**A**) Bacterial infection spreads up the vagina into the uterus and through the lymphatics. (**B**) Gonorrhea spreads up the vagina into the uterus and then to the tubes and ovaries. (**C**) Bacterial infection can reach the reproductive organs through the bloodstream (hematogenous spread). (From Smeltzer SC, Bare BG. Textbook of Medical-Surgical Nursing, 9th Ed. Philadelphia: Lippincott Williams & Wilkins, 2000.)

positive may go through the following stages as the infection progresses to AIDS:

1. Acute infectious state with generally mild flulike symptoms
2. Latent period without symptoms but still infectious
3. Weight loss, lymphadenopathy, fever, diarrhea, anorexia, fatigue, and skin rashes
4. Onset of immunodeficiency disorders, such as Kaposi sarcoma and *Pneumocystis carinii* pneumonia

Although new treatments prolong the HIV-positive individual's life, there currently is no cure; however, research to find more effective treatments and a possible cure is ongoing.

Syphilis

After AIDS, syphilis is the most serious STD. The cause of syphilis is a microorganism known as *Treponema pallidum*, a spirochete. The first sign is a chancre or ulcerated lesion at the primary site of infection on the genitalia. This chancre appears several days to several weeks after infection, heals very quickly, and may not be noticed. Although the chancre heals quickly, the spirochete spreads quickly through the bloodstream and becomes systemic, with far-reaching consequences. The second phase is identified by a rash that may appear anywhere on the body. The patient continues to be infectious at this stage, but treatment with penicillin will stop the progression of the disease to the next, or tertiary, phase. If left untreated, the rash will disappear, and the syphilis may lie dormant for years. At some point, however, the patient will experience cardiovascular damage, central nervous system involvement, and death (Fig. 20-7).

Infants born with syphilis caused by transplacental infection are commonly mentally retarded, deaf, blind, or deformed. Many babies spontaneously abort or are delivered stillborn.

Chlamydia

Chlamydia infections cause urethritis in men, cervicitis in women, and lymphogranuloma venereum in both, all caused by the organism *Chlamydia trachomatis*. Chlamydia is the most common STD in the United States. Female patients may be asymptomatic or may have vague flulike symptoms that are difficult to diagnose without specific reason to suspect infection. In severe cases, there may be extensive lymph gland involvement known as *lymphogranuloma venereum*. Chlamydia is one of the leading causes of pelvic inflammatory disease, causing tubal scarring and eventual infertility in women. Infants born to mothers with chlamydial infections may have conjunctivitis and pneumonia. The fetus may spontaneously abort, deliver prematurely, or be stillborn.

Diagnosis is made by a swab culture of the site sent to the laboratory for identification of the microorganism.

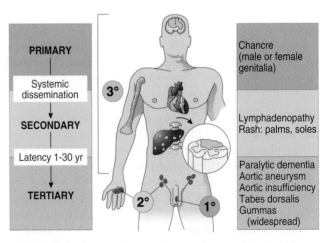

Figure 20-7 Clinical characteristics of the various stages of syphilis. (Image from Rubin E MD and Farber JL MD. Pathology, 3rd Edition. Philadelphia: Lippincott Williams & Wilkins, 1999.)

The disease is treated with an antibiotic such as doxycycline, tetracycline, or sulfamethoxazole until the patient tests negative for the presence of the pathogen.

Condylomata Acuminata

Condylomata acuminata is a viral infection of the genital area causing the growth of soft, papillary warts that appear in a wide variety of places, including the vulva, vagina, cervix, and perineum. The cause is the human papilloma virus, or HPV. The genital warts usually appear about 3 months after exposure. Biopsy of the condyloma is appropriate to rule out the slight possibility of a malignancy. Although HPV is difficult to eradicate, cryotherapy (freezing the involved area) or laser ablation (burning with laser) has moderate success.

HPV has been implicated as a risk for cervical cancer in some women, but currently, there is a vaccine, Gardasil™, to protect against four types of HPV that are responsible for 70% of cervical cancers and 90% of genital warts (Centers for Disease Control and Prevention). The Advisory Committee on Immunization Practices (ACIP) recommends this vaccine for girls over the age of 9; however, there are no current federal laws requiring administration of this vaccine.

 CHECKPOINT QUESTION

4. Which sexually transmitted disease may cause conjunctivitis and pneumonia in newborns born to infected mothers?

Gonorrhea

Gonorrhea is the second most common STD and is caused by a Gram-negative diplococcus, *Neisseria gonorrhoeae*. The symptoms appear in the genitalia 2 to 8 days after exposure. In some female patients, the Bartholin and Skene glands fill with pus, and the infection may spread to the cervix. However, female patients may be asymptomatic and unaware of the disease. The disease may lead to salpingitis with scarring and adhesions or pelvic inflammatory disease. Infants born to mothers infected with gonorrhea may develop purulent conjunctivitis with corneal ulcerations that result in blindness. All infants are now treated prophylactically in the newborn nursery.

Diagnosis is based on the symptoms and through a culture of the drainage if present. Once diagnosed, gonorrhea may be treated with penicillin, although penicillin-resistant strains are now appearing.

Herpes Genitalis

Herpes genitalis is caused by the herpes simplex virus 2 (HSV2) and is characterized by painful vesicular lesions in the vaginal, vulvar, or anorectal area.

This genital infection usually appears within 3 to 7 days after exposure. The infected patient may present with painful vesicles in the genital region that rupture and leave equally painful ulcers that eventually heal in about 10 days. In addition, the patient may have swollen and tender lymph nodes and flulike symptoms. After the lesion heals, the patient may be in remission for years, or the symptoms may recur with each stressful situation. Patients with herpes genitalis should be advised to avoid sexual contact during episodes of vesiculation because the exudate is highly contagious. Although there is no cure, the condition is somewhat controlled with an antiviral agent such as acyclovir.

Infants born vaginally to mothers with active lesions may develop the disease within a few weeks of birth. The virus spreads rapidly to the organs of the infant and up to 90% of infected infants die.

Vulvovaginitis, Salpingitis, and Pelvic Inflammatory Disease

Although vulvovaginitis, salpingitis, and pelvic inflammatory disease can be caused by any type of microorganism, these disorders are commonly caused by sexually transmitted infections (see Fig. 20-6). Vulvovaginitis is an inflammation of the vulva and vagina and is one of the common complaints of female patients. Symptoms often include pruritus, burning of the vulva or the vagina (or both), and increased vaginal discharge. On examination, the vulva and vagina are reddened. The type of discharge often indicates the cause of the disorder, and effective treatment depends on the cause. The causative agent is confirmed by a microscopic examination of a vaginal smear or by culture of the vaginal discharge and may include the following microorganisms:

- *Trichomonas vaginalis*: Known as *trich*, this protozoan causes an STD. The signs are a thin, frothy, greenish or gray vaginal discharge with an odor. Signs and symptoms include dysuria with urinary frequency and intense pruritus. Treatment is oral metronidazole for both partners.
- *Candida albicans*: Also known as *monilia*, this fungus grows best in the presence of glucose. The signs include a thick, curd-like discharge with white patches on the vaginal walls, usually with no odor. Intense itching is usual. The pathogen is found in the intestines and is most likely to affect the patient during the secretory phase of the menstrual cycle. It is very common during pregnancy and in patients receiving antibiotic therapy. Treatment requires nystatin vaginal suppositories, which may be purchased without a prescription.
- *Gardnerella vaginitis*: This Gram-negative bacillus causes a gray discharge with a foul odor. It is treated with metronidazole.

Salpingitis is a bacterial infection of the fallopian tubes that is most often transmitted by sexual intercourse. Young sexually active women, women with multiple sexual partners, and women with intrauterine devices are at increased risk for salpingitis. Numerous microorganisms may cause salpingitis, but the most common microbes include *N. gonorrhoeae*, *C. trachomatis*, genital mycoplasma, and normal flora bacteria. Salpingitis is sometimes called *pelvic inflammatory disease* when the surrounding structures, including the pelvic peritoneum, uterus, ovaries, and surrounding tissues, are inflamed. Signs and symptoms include varying degrees of abdominal pain and tenderness with or without fever and leukocytosis, an abnormal increase in the white blood cell count.

Cultures for gonorrhea and tests for chlamydia are essential for antibiotic therapy. **Culdocentesis** may be necessary to obtain purulent drainage and determine the exact cause of the infection. Laparoscopy may be performed to determine the extent of the infection. Treatment for mild infections includes antibiotic and analgesic therapy, bed rest, and removal of the source of infection. In patients with pyosalpinx (pus in the fallopian tubes), tubal obstruction, abscess, serious inflammation, and edema, treatment may be a hysterectomy with bilateral **salpingectomy-oophorectomy** or an incision and drainage.

 CHECKPOINT QUESTION

5. Which sexually transmitted disease is associated with female reproductive cancer?

Common Diagnostic and Therapeutic Procedures

The Gynecologic Examination

As part of the gynecologic examination, the physician examines the patient's breasts, performs a pelvic examination, and obtains a Pap smear. Because of the risk of contracting infection from body fluids, especially blood, you and the physician must observe standard precautions, wearing protective barriers such as gloves as appropriate during the examination. When scheduling the appointment, instruct the patient not to douche, use vaginal medication, or have sexual intercourse for 24 hours before the examination. If a Pap smear will be performed, the appointment should be scheduled about 1 week after the end of menses. When the patient arrives for the scheduled appointment, spend time with the patient to establish rapport, especially with new patients and patients with special needs, such as the young, elderly, and disabled. A procedure that is rushed or seems hurried to the patient may diminish the professional image of the office and the patient's attitude toward the physician and staff.

The physician usually begins the examination by examining the breast and surrounding tissue, including the axillae and chest tissue up to the clavicle. This tissue is inspected for dimpling or size disparity and palpated for lumps or thickenings. Next, the physician examines the external and internal female genitalia to identify or diagnose any abnormal conditions (Procedure 20-2). Although the dorsal lithotomy position provides the best visibility for the physician, this position may be difficult for elderly or some disabled persons. Elevating the head of the table to 30 degrees may be easier for the patient while allowing the physician to do a thorough examination. The elevation of the table does not seem to have any disadvantages, and often the patient finds this position more comfortable, but consult with the physician if the lithotomy position is not possible. If elevating the head of the examination table is not appropriate, an alternative position, such as the Sims position, may be necessary.

After visually inspecting the external genitalia, the physician examines the internal female structures. To begin, a vaginal speculum is inserted into the vagina. The vaginal speculum may come in a variety of sizes and is made of either stainless steel (Fig. 20-8) or plastic (Fig. 20-9). Selecting an appropriately sized vaginal speculum is important to maintain the patient's comfort and to facilitate the examination. Although the patient's age and size are the primary factors, the largest speculum that is comfortable for the patient provides the best visibility. Two sizes may be set out to give the physician a choice. Vaginal specula come in pediatric, small, medium, and large sizes, and a variety of sizes should be available in each examination room.

In addition to having the correct size vaginal speculum available for the physician, you should make sure

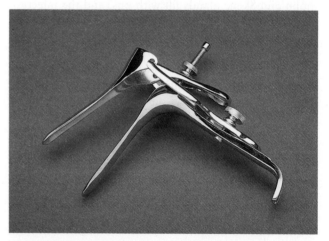

Figure 20-8 A stainless steel vaginal speculum. (LifeART image copyright © 2008 Lippincott Williams & Wilkins. All rights reserved.)

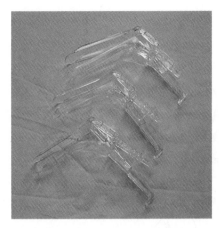

Figure 20-9 A variety of plastic, disposable vaginal specula. (From Weber J, Kelley J. Health Assessment in Nursing. 2nd ed. Philadelphia: Lippincott Williams & Wilkins, 2003.)

the speculum is warmed for patient comfort. Warm the speculum by running it under warm water (Fig. 20-10) or by storing it on an electric heating pad set on a low setting. Some examination tables are equipped with a special warming drawer for the vaginal specula that heats them automatically as long as the examination table is plugged into an electrical outlet. Some physicians prefer that lubricant not be used on the speculum before insertion since it may interfere with obtaining the cells during the Pap smear. The water used to warm the speculum may serve as a lubricant for easier insertion.

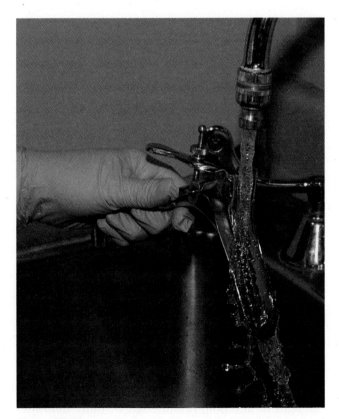

Figure 20-10 Warm the vaginal speculum with warm water.

Always follow the instructions given by your physician to prepare the patient and the equipment and supplies for this examination.

Once the cervical cells are obtained, the physician will remove the vaginal speculum and perform a bimanual examination using gloved hands. During this part of the examination, the physician may want lubricant applied to gloved fingers for easier insertion into the vaginal and rectum. Specifically, the physician will insert fingers into the vagina and the rectum to feel for the position and size of internal organs (Fig. 20-11). Your role during this part of the examination includes assisting the physician as necessary and supporting the patient. When this part of the examination is finished, you should assist the patient to a sitting position, prepare any specimens obtained for transport to the laboratory, and instruct the patient on the procedure for obtaining the results. You should also reinforce any instructions given by the physician before discharging the patient.

 WHAT IF?

The first Pap smear or gynecologic examination for young women may cause great anxiety. What if an 18-year-old woman is to have her first Pap smear today? How should you handle the situation?

Bring the patient into the room and encourage her to talk about her feelings. Do not have her change into an examining gown until she has had an opportunity to speak with the physician or practitioner about the procedure. The physician may require the presence of another health care worker, like the medical assistant, during the examination; however, some physicians feel comfortable performing the examination without assistance. If you remain in the room, you will have an opportunity to provide reassurance and information. Male physicians should have a female health care worker in the room during the examination as a legal precaution.

Colposcopy

Colposcopy is visual examination of the vaginal and cervical surfaces using a stereoscopic microscope called a colposcope. It is often performed to evaluate patients with atypical Pap smear results to locate the origin of abnormal cells; to select areas for cervical, endocervical, or endometrial biopsy; to assess cervical lesions; or for follow-up in patients with a history of cervical dysplasia or cervical cancer.

If a biopsy is to be done, be sure that written consent has been obtained. When possible, label specimen

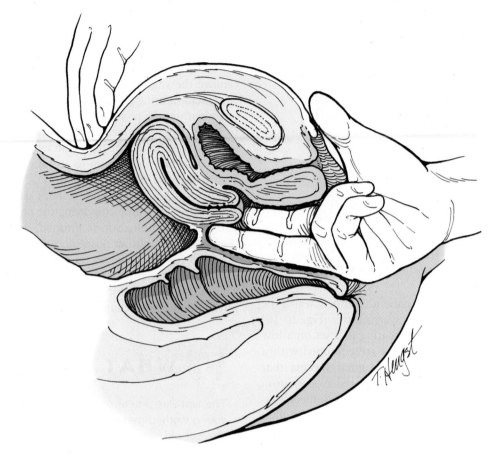

Figure 20-11 The bimanual examination. (LifeART image copyright © 2008 Lippincott Williams & Wilkins. All rights reserved.)

containers and complete laboratory request forms before the procedure. Have the completed forms and labeled containers ready in the examination room for use after the specimen is obtained. Although there is usually very little or no bleeding from the biopsy, chemical cautery using silver nitrate or Monsel solution should be available to control bleeding as necessary. The patient preparation for colposcopy with cervical biopsy is similar to that required for the pelvic examination (Procedure 20-3).

 CHECKPOINT QUESTION

6. What procedures are normally included in the complete gynecologic examination?

Hysterosalpingography

Hysterosalpingography is a diagnostic procedure in which the uterus and uterine tubes are radiographed after injection of a contrast medium. The radiograph is called a **hysterosalpingogram**. This test is often performed to determine the configuration of the uterus and the patency of the fallopian tubes for patients with infertility. Although this test is not usually performed in the physician's office, you may be responsible for scheduling the procedure and explaining to the patient any preparations including where to go and when the procedure will be performed.

Dilation and Curettage

Dilation and **curettage** (D & C) may be performed to remove uterine tissue for diagnostic testing, to remove endometrial tissue, to prevent or treat **menorrhagia**, or to remove retained products of conception after a spontaneous **abortion** or miscarriage. During the procedure, the cervical canal is widened with a uterine sound, and the lining of the uterus is scraped with a curet (see Chapter 6 for a picture of a curet). This procedure usually requires anesthesia and may be performed as an inpatient or outpatient procedure. The patient must sign a preoperative consent form, and you may be asked to give any preoperative instructions as directed by the physician. Preoperative instructions may include advising the patient of the need for a perineal pad, not a tampon, to be worn postoperatively and information regarding the signs of infection, hemorrhage, or other follow-up care according to the specifications of the physician.

CHECKPOINT QUESTION

7. Why would a hysterosalpingography be necessary?

Obstetric Care

Unlike other physicians, obstetricians are frequently called to the hospital to deliver infants during regular office hours. In the absence of the physician, you must use good judgment when pregnant patients come into the office for a scheduled appointment or call with questions and concerns. For instance, you may have to determine whether a situation can wait for the physician's return, whether another physician should be consulted, whether the patient should go to the hospital, or whether, with the physician's permission, you should advise the patient how to manage the problem. Protocols listed in the policy and procedure manual for actions to be taken in specific situations help ensure that, in the physician's absence, safe procedures are followed for your patients and help protect you and your physician from errors in treatment.

 PATIENT EDUCATION

FOLIC ACID BEFORE AND DURING PREGNANCY

Women who are planning to get pregnant and those who are pregnant should take folic acid, a B vitamin to prevent neural tube defects. Although medical experts do not know how folic acid works, it is needed to make healthy new cells, like the ones that make up a baby's brain and spine. Taking folic acid every day, starting before and during pregnancy, can reduce the risk for these serious birth defects by 50% to 70%. Every woman who could possibly get pregnant should take 400 micrograms (400 mcg or 0.4 mg) of folic acid daily in a vitamin or in foods that have been enriched with folic acid. Many foods, including cereals, are enriched with folic acid. Encourage patients to check the label since some cereals provide 100% of the daily amount required.

Diagnosis of Pregnancy

Many patients suspect that they are **gravid**, or pregnant, because they have signs; however, early signs of pregnancy may indicate other disorders and therefore are considered presumptive until a conclusive diagnostic procedure is done. Presumptive signs include amenorrhea, nausea, vomiting, breast enlargement and tenderness, fatigue, and urinary frequency. Probable signs include **human chorionic gonadotropin (HCG)** in the maternal urine or blood, changes in the uterus and cervix, **Braxton-Hicks contractions**, and enlargement of the uterus (Table 20-3). Braxton-Hicks contractions are irregular uterine contractions that occur fairly frequently but do not affect the cervix like the contractions of active labor. These contractions are normal, and although the patient may or may not be aware, the physician can feel the contractions during a bimanual examination or while palpating the abdomen. The diagnosis of pregnancy is confirmed by the physician or the image of a fetus on ultrasonography.

Cervical changes that occur during pregnancy include softening of the cervix, known as **Goodell sign**; increased vascularity of the cervix and vagina causing a bluish-violet color (**Chadwick sign**); and formation of a mucous plug. The mucous plug forms in the cervical os (opening) and protects the developing fetus and the amniotic sac from the external environment. With the onset of labor, the mucous plug is expelled with a small amount of blood and is often referred to as the bloody show.

TABLE **20-3** Signs and Symptoms of Pregnancy		
Presumptive Signs	**Probable Signs**	**Conclusive Signs**
Cessation of menses	HCG in urine, blood	Fetal heart tone
Nausea and vomiting	Braxton-Hicks contrac-	Fetal movement detected by
Breast tenderness	tions	examiner
Breast enlargement	Enlargement of abdomen	Visualization of the fetus
Patient feels quickening or	Uterine changes	
fetal movement	Goodell sign	
Fatigue	Chadwick sign	
Urinary frequency		

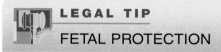

LEGAL TIP

FETAL PROTECTION

Many medications that might be considered beneficial to the pregnant female may be dangerous to the developing fetus. It is important, therefore, for the professional medical assistant to carefully question female patients who might be pregnant or who are known to be pregnant about any medications including drugs purchased over the counter. This information should be passed along to the physician. The U.S. Food and Drug Administration (FDA) has developed a method to classify drugs that are dangerous to the fetus. These categories are listed on package inserts that accompany prescription drugs and in various drug reference books such as the *Physician's Desk Reference*. The categories and a description of dangerous effects on the fetus are listed as follows:

- Category A: Research indicates that there is probably no risk at any point in the pregnancy.
- Category B: Animal research indicates no fetal risk, but human studies are not complete.
- Category C: Research on animals shows this drug to be a danger. Human studies are inconclusive, or no studies are available.
- Category D: There is clear precedence for risk, but the drug may be used if there is no substitution.
- Category X: There is clear evidence of risk, and the drug should not be used by pregnant women.

 CHECKPOINT QUESTION

8. Why are presumptive signs and symptoms of pregnancy not considered to be conclusive?

First Prenatal Visit

A pregnant patient's initial prenatal visit is extensive and critical to the ongoing assessment of the pregnancy. The first examination is done to establish a detailed baseline of the patient's physical condition and includes a confirmation of pregnancy, a complete history and physical, determination of the estimated date of delivery, assessment of gestational age, identification of risk factors, and patient education. To elicit complete and accurate information, the health history interview should be conducted in a private room where there will be no interruptions. This is a complete physical examination with a pelvic examination, screening for *N. gonorrhoeae*, chlamydial

infection, cervical cancer, syphilis, and tuberculosis. The first prenatal visit also includes the following:

- Bloodwork: The Venereal Disease Research Laboratory, rapid plasma reagin, or other test for syphilis; complete blood count with hematocrit, hemoglobin, and white blood cell count with differential; and blood type with Rh factor. Blood for a rubella titer is also collected to determine maternal immunity to German measles, a disease that can result in serious birth defects if contracted during pregnancy.
- Tuberculosis screening: Tine test or purified protein derivative injection.
- Urinalysis: Glucose, albumin, and acetone testing.

The physical and pelvic examination will include laboratory tests such as the Pap smear, urine pregnancy test, clinical pelvimetry, and laboratory blood tests. Also, the estimated date of delivery will be calculated. This is a prediction of the due date, assuming the pregnancy progresses normally (Box 20-2). Normal gestation

BOX 20-2

DETERMINING THE ESTIMATED DATE OF CONFINEMENT OR EXPECTED DATE OF DELIVERY

The Estimated Date of Confinement (EDC) is also called the *expected date of delivery (EDD)*. Because of the negative connotations of the word "*confinement*" and because women are no longer confined during pregnancy or the postpartum period, terminology for the due date is changing to reflect current maternity trends. Many methods are used for determining this projected date. The Nagele rule requires an arithmetic calculation using the following formula:

The first day of the last menstrual period (LMP) − 3 months + 7 days + 1 year

Example: LMP = May 3, 2007

LMP =	5	3	2007
	−3	+7	+1
Due date =	2	10	2008

A simpler method is adding 9 months and 7 days to the first day of the LMP. Try that method with the example.

The third common method is to use a gestational wheel. Using the inner wheel, line up the first day of the LMP on the outer wheel with the appropriate arrow and read around the wheel to the indicated milestones in the pregnancy. Many wheels indicate the date of conception and times recommended for blood work and other testing, and all show the date that delivery is expected.

is 37 to 40 weeks. Infants born before the 37th week are considered to be premature. Those born after the 41st week are postmature.

Patients should be instructed to notify the physician if any of the following occurs:

- Vaginal bleeding or spotting
- Persistent vomiting
- Fever or chills
- Dysuria
- Abdominal or uterine cramping
- Leaking amniotic fluid
- Alteration in fetal movement
- Dizziness or blurred vision
- Other problems

In addition, advise the pregnant patient to avoid taking any medications or drugs, even over-the-counter preparations, without consulting the physician. Many factors, including medications, nicotine, and alcohol can put the developing fetus at risk. Depending on maternal exposure to the substance and the stage of fetal development, development may be so altered as to cause deformities or damage to other internal organs and may threaten the life of the fetus.

Parity Versus Gravidity

You and the physician will obtain a thorough and detailed history of the patient, including information about previous pregnancies to help predict the outcome of this one. The term **parity** refers to the number of live births, and **gravidity** refers to any pregnancy, regardless of its length and outcome. The pregnant, or gravid, woman is a **gravida**, usually with an indicator of the number. A woman who has never been pregnant is a **nulligravida**, while the woman who is pregnant for the first time is a **primigravida**. The number of live births is also given a prefix indicator, such as **nullipara** (has never borne a living child), **primipara** (first living child), and **multipara** (many live births).

These numbers are listed for the physician's review as gr (or simply g), p, pret (preterm or premature), and ab (abortion, spontaneous or induced). For example, a woman who is pregnant for the third time, has lost no pregnancies, and carried her previous pregnancies to term is listed as gr iii, pret 0, ab 0, p ii. (Arabic numbers are also acceptable.) A woman who is pregnant for the fifth time and who has delivered one set of twins and two single infants, has had no premature infants, and has lost one pregnancy spontaneously would be listed as gr v, pret 0, ab i, p iv.

Subsequent Prenatal Visits

If the pregnancy is progressing as expected and without complications (Fig. 20-12), then the patient is scheduled for office visits monthly at 4, 8, 12, 16, 20, 24, and 28 weeks of gestation. The patient is usually seen every 2 weeks during the last 2 months and once a week after the 36th week of gestation. This schedule may be altered according to the patient's condition. Table 20-4 outlines

the specific examination and procedures to be performed during subsequent prenatal visits. The height of the fundus (Fig. 20-13) is also palpated at each visit to assess fetal growth. Typically, the top of the uterus, the fundus, can be palpated at or slightly above the level of the maternal umbilicus when the fetus is at 5 months' gestation. During the third trimester, the abdomen will be palpated to determine fetal presentation and position, which are important details for a normal vaginal delivery.

The fetal heart tones (FHT) will also be recorded at the subsequent prenatal visits. Around the 10th week of gestation, the fetal heart rate can be heard with the aid of a Doppler device (Fig. 20-14), and after the 20th week, a fetoscope can be used. The fetoscope is a special nonelectronic stethoscope (Fig. 20-15). The fetal heart tones should fall within a range of 120 to 160 beats per minute.

CHECKPOINT QUESTION

9. The pregnant patient should be advised to contact the physician when what problems occur?

Onset of Labor

Labor is the physiologic process leading to expelling the fetus from the uterus. About 4 weeks before the onset of labor, **lightening** indicates that the fetus has descended further into the pelvis, and the patient may appear to be carrying the baby lower in the abdomen. The actual onset of labor is characterized by regular uterine contractions that become more intense and more frequent with time. True labor is distinguished from false labor by its effect (dilation and effacement) on the cervix and the increased frequency and intensity of contractions. Another indication of true labor is bloody show, the expulsion of the mucous plug from the cervical os. The patient may call to say her water broke, which indicates rupture of the amniotic sac, another indication of impending labor and delivery.

Whatever signs or symptoms of labor occur, you should know how to advise the patient. The physician makes the decision to send the patient to the hospital, to come to the medical office, or to stay home and wait. You relay the information from the patient to the physician. The office's policy and procedure manual should include specific instructions regarding how the physician wants pregnant patients managed if the physician is not immediately available.

The onset of labor should be discussed with the patient so she knows what to expect and how to manage the situation. Always have the patient's medical record available when talking with the patient or the physician. It is critical to the decision-making process to know the patient's estimated date of delivery and physical

FETAL DEVELOPMENT*

1st Lunar Month (4 weeks)

The embryo is 4 to 5 mm in length.
Trophoblasts embed in decidua.
Chorionic villi form.
Foundations for nervous system,
    genitourinary system, skin,
    bones, and lungs are formed.
Buds of arms and legs begin to form.
Rudiments of eyes, ears, and nose appear.

2nd Lunar Month (8 weeks)

The fetus is 27 to 31 mm in length
    and weighs 2 to 4 g
Fetus is markedly bent.
Head is disproportionately large as
    a result of brain development.
Sex differentation begins.
Centers of bone begin to ossify.

3rd Lunar Month (3 months)

The fetus' average length is 6 to 9
    cm, and weight is 45 g.
Fingers and toes are distinct.
Placenta is complete.
Fetal circulation is complete.

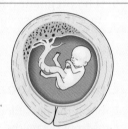

4th Lunar Month (4 months)

The fetus is 12 cm in length and
    weighs 110 g.
Sex is differentiated.
Rudimentary kidneys secrete urine.
Heartbeat is present.
Nasal septum and palate close.

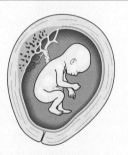

5th Lunar Month (5 months)

The fetus is 19 cm in length and
    weighs approximately 300 g.
Lanugo covers entire body.
Fetal movements are felt by mother.
Heart sounds are perceptible by
    auscultation.

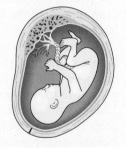

6th Lunar Month (6 months)

The fetus is about 23 cm in length
    and weighs 630 g.
Skin appears wrinkled.
Vernix caseosa appears.
Eyebrows and fingernails develop.

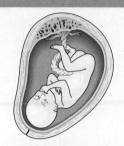

7th Lunar Month (7 months)

The fetus is about 27 cm in length
    and weighs about 1100 g.
Skin is red.
Pupillary membrane disappears
    from eyes.
The fetus has an excellent chance
    of survival.

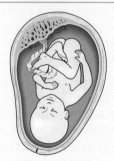

8th Lunar Month (8 months)

The fetus is 28 to 30 cm in length
    and weighs 1.8 kg.
Fetus is viable.
Eyelids open.
Fingerprints are set.
Vigorous fetal movement occurs.

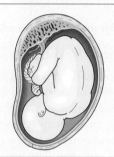

9th Lunar Month (9 months)

The fetus' average length is 32 cm;
    weight is about 2500 g.
Face and body have a loose
    wrinkled appearance because
    of subcutaneous fat deposit.
Lanugo disappears.
Amniotic fluid decreases.

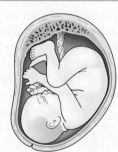
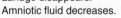

10th Lunar Month

The average fetus is 36 cm in length
    and weighs 3000 to 3600 g.
Skin is smooth.
Eyes are uniformly slate colored.
Bones of skull are ossified and
    nearly together at sutures.

* All lengths given are crown to rump.

Figure 20-12 Fetal development.

TABLE 20-4	Schedule of Prenatal Visits
Month	**Frequency**
1–6	Monthly
7–8	Every 2 weeks
9	Weekly
Included in Visit:	**When Done:**
Weight	Each visit
Blood pressure	Each visit
Fundal height	Each visit
Fetal heart rate	Each visit
Check of edema	Each visit
Pelvic examination	First visit, middle of ninth month, weekly as indicated
Inquiry about symptoms, signs, problems	Each visit
Prenatal education	Each visit
Nutrition and appetite	Each visit
Urinalysis for glucose, albumin	Each visit
Hematocrit, hemoglobin	First visit, at 32–34 weeks (more often for anemia)
Urine culture	Per signs, symptoms
Rh titer	First visit
AFP	15–20 weeks
Blood glucose	First visit, 24–28 weeks
Ultrasonography	For fetal age, best 8–16 weeks

From Reeder SJ, Martin LL, Koniak D. Maternity Nursing. 17th ed. Philadelphia: Lippincott Williams & Wilkins, 1992:403.

condition. Many patients today are choosing options for delivery other than a standard hospital delivery with the physician present. Options include midwife assistance, a birthing center, water birth, and home delivery. The patient must be informed about the advantages and risks of all of these and, together with the physician, make a decision that takes into account the well-being of the mother and the newborn.

Cesarean Section

Sometimes a normal vaginal delivery is not possible or advisable, such as in the following situations:

- Cephalopelvic disproportion: the baby's head is too large for the birth canal
- Placenta previa

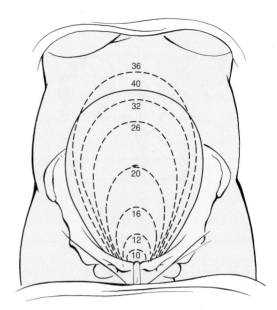

Figure 20-13 Height of the fundus at corresponding gestational dates varies greatly from patient to patient. Those shown are most common. A convenient rule of thumb is that at 5 months of gestation, the fundus is usually at or slightly above the umbilicus. (Reprinted with permission from Weber J. Health Assessment in Nursing. Philadelphia: Lippincott Williams & Wilkins, 2003.)

- Poor presentation other than an occipital presentation, such as transverse (the baby lying across the cervix) or breech (a buttocks first presentation)
- Failure to progress: inefficient labor or the cervix will not dilate
- Infant or maternal distress

In these situations, the infant is delivered by cesarean section. An incision is made through the abdominal wall into the uterus, and the infant is removed. It was once believed that women who had delivered by cesarean section should not be allowed to deliver vaginally because it was feared that the uterine scar might rupture. Current surgical techniques have lessened that fear, and many women now deliver vaginally after a cesarean delivery.

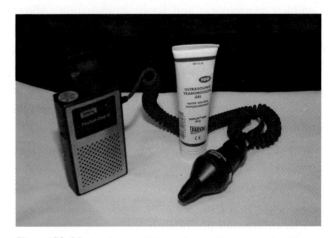

Figure 20-14 An electronic Doppler used to assess fetal heart tones before the 20th gestational week.

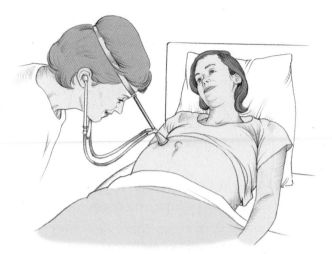

Figure 20-15 A fetoscope. (From Nursing Procedures. 4th ed. Ambler, PA: Lippincott Williams & Wilkins, 2004.)

Postpartum Care

The postpartum period, the **puerperium**, runs from childbirth until involution, when the reproductive structures return to normal. It may take as long as 6 weeks. Once the patient is discharged from the hospital, her care will be managed at the medical office. Hospital reports received in the medical office for the patient's record usually contain certain acronyms and abbreviations related to labor and delivery and the postpartum period. Box 20-3 explains these special terms.

The time for the first postpartum visit depends on the type of delivery and the patient's condition when discharged from the hospital. The needs of postpartum patients today may be greater than in the past because the length of stay in the hospital is typically shorter, with some patients discharged within 24 hours after delivery. Usually the patient is scheduled for the postnatal visit within 4 to 6 weeks of delivery if there were no complications.

At the postpartum visit, the physician performs a complete gynecologic and breast examination. Allow plenty of time for counseling the patient regarding her new role as a parent. Many patients have questions and concerns regarding breastfeeding, birth control, menstruation, and parenting. Before the examination, obtain the patient's weight and vital signs and samples for urinalysis and possibly hematocrit and hemoglobin. During the examination, the physician assesses any uterine discharge. **Lochia**, a discharge from the uterus after delivery, progresses through the following stages:

- *Lochia rubra*: Blood-tinged discharge within 6 days of delivery
- *Lochia serosa*: Thin, brownish discharge lasting about 3 to 4 days after the lochia rubra
- *Lochia alba*: White postpartum discharge that has no evidence of blood and may last up to week 6

BOX 20-3

ACRONYMS AND ABBREVIATIONS USED IN LABOR AND DELIVERY AND THE POSTPARTUM PERIOD

Following is a brief list of terms frequently used in the medical record.

AROM	Artificial rupture of membranes
AVD	Assisted vaginal delivery
CPD	Cephalopelvic disproportion
L & D	Labor and delivery
NSVD	Normal spontaneous vaginal delivery
PROM	Premature rupture of membranes
SROM	Spontaneous rupture of membranes
VBAC	Vaginal birth after cesarean

Terms for presentations

LOA	Left occiput anterior
LOP	Left occiput posterior
ROA	Right occiput anterior
ROP	Right occiput posterior

Fetal descriptors

AGA	Appropriate for gestational age
LBW	Low birth weight
LGA	Large for gestational age
SGA	Small for gestational age

The amount of lochia should diminish considerably during the puerperium. The patient should be instructed to notify the physician if there is any abnormality of the lochial progression.

 PATIENT EDUCATION

KEGEL EXERCISES

The patient's age, gravidity, and past childbearing take their toll on the muscles of the perineum. Kegel exercises can increase the tone of this area. Stronger perineal support helps eliminate stress incontinence and supports the vaginal walls to avoid uterine prolapse.

These exercises should be performed three times every day for 5 minutes each time. In addition, the exercises should be done in three positions: lying down, sitting, and standing. Explain to the patient that she can do Kegel exercises at any time, such as when standing in the grocery line, waiting at a stop light, or sitting in class. Essentially, the exercises involve tightening the pelvic muscles as if stopping the flow of urine. Advise the patient not to tighten the stomach, legs, or other muscles. Also, most patients do not feel bladder control results for 3 to 6 weeks.

CHECKPOINT QUESTION

10. What is lochia? Name and describe the three types.

Obstetric Disorders

Ectopic Pregnancy

Gestation in which a fertilized ovum implants somewhere other than in the uterine cavity is an ectopic pregnancy. Usually an ectopic pregnancy occurs in the fallopian tube, and when it does, it may be called a tubal pregnancy. Other sites of implantation include the abdomen, the ovaries, and the cervical os. The patient may have signs of early pregnancy, including breast enlargement or tenderness, nausea, and absent or delayed menses. Pelvic pain, syncope, abdominal symptoms, painful sexual intercourse, and irregular menstrual bleeding begin fairly early in the pregnancy. If an ectopic pregnancy is not diagnosed early, there is the potential for rupture of the fallopian tube, which causes hemorrhage into the abdominal cavity and the possibility of shock and death. Diagnostic procedures include urine or serum human chorionic gonadotropin pregnancy test, ultrasound to determine the location of the pregnancy, laparoscopy to visualize the enlarged tube, and perhaps culdocentesis to confirm abdominal bleeding. Treatment is surgical excision of the ectopic pregnancy through either a laparoscopy or laparotomy.

Hyperemesis Gravidarum

Nausea and vomiting, commonly called morning sickness, are expected during early pregnancy and usually can be treated with small frequent meals, adequate hydration, and reassurance. However, if the vomiting becomes unrelenting and leads to dehydration, electrolyte imbalance, and weight loss, the diagnosis is hyperemesis gravidarum. Occasionally the patient must be hospitalized. At early prenatal visits, you may have to discern between morning sickness and the more serious hyperemesis gravidarum by obtaining a complete description of the nausea and vomiting. Of course, the physician makes the diagnosis and orders appropriate treatment, including antiemetics or intravenous fluids if necessary.

Abortion

One of the common disorders of pregnancy is first-trimester spontaneous abortion, also called an early pregnancy loss or miscarriage. With early diagnosis of pregnancy, it is now known whether the spontaneous abortion occurs more often than previously thought. An induced abortion is intentional, whereas a spontaneous abortion occurs because of fetal or maternal conditions without any outside interference in the pregnancy.

A spontaneous abortion is defined as the loss of pregnancy before the fetus is viable. You need to be familiar with the early signs and symptoms of an impending spontaneous abortion to advise a patient who calls until the physician can be contacted. The first symptom is usually vaginal bleeding, followed by uterine cramps and low back pain. Without telling the patient that she may be in danger of spontaneously aborting her pregnancy (this is diagnosing), you may instruct the patient to come to the medical office, go to the emergency room, or remain at home on bed rest until the physician returns the call, depending on the office policy and procedure.

CHECKPOINT QUESTION

11. Where is the most common site of implantation for an ectopic pregnancy?

Preeclampsia and Eclampsia

Hypertension that is directly related to the pregnancy is termed pregnancy-induced hypertension (PIH). The two types of PIH are preeclampsia and eclampsia. Preeclampsia is characterized by **proteinuria**, edema of the lower extremities, and hypertension after the 20th week of gestation. As the condition progresses, the patient may complain of blurred vision, headaches, edema, and vomiting. Medical management includes restricted activities, increased bed rest, sexual abstinence, antihypertensive therapy, and well-balanced meals with an increase in protein and a decrease in sodium. Close monitoring of the patient is important, and it requires scheduling the patient for more frequent office visits. The risk of developing eclampsia increases as the pregnancy advances.

Eclampsia is almost always preceded by preeclampsia but has a sudden onset. In eclampsia, the clinical signs of preeclampsia are still present but become more extreme. Eclampsia is always characterized by seizures that may be followed by coma, hypertensive crisis, and shock. The progression of preeclampsia to eclampsia constitutes a medical emergency. Management of eclampsia includes stabilizing the patient and may require induced delivery of the baby, regardless of gestational age.

Placenta Previa and Abruptio Placentae

Placenta previa is a condition in which the placenta is implanted either partially or completely over the internal cervical os, making delivery of the fetus before the placenta difficult. During the second or third trimester of pregnancy, the patient may have painless vaginal bleeding, which may be minimal, such as spotting, or profuse. Placenta previa is easily diagnosed by prenatal ultrasound. Medical management includes bed rest and drug therapy if the patient is preterm. If the patient is near term and if the bleeding is severe and poses a danger to the mother or fetus, then delivery of the baby is essential, usually by cesarean.

The premature separation or detachment of the placenta from the uterus is abruptio placentae. Depending on the severity of the separation, symptoms include pain, uterine tenderness, bleeding, signs of impending shock, and fetal distress or death. If abruptio placentae is confirmed, the baby is usually delivered by cesarean section.

 CHECKPOINT QUESTION

12. What is placenta previa, and how is it managed in a preterm patient?

Common Obstetric Tests and Procedures

Pregnancy Tests

Many over-the-counter pregnancy tests check for HCG in the urine. Chapter 29 has more information about urine pregnancy tests.

Alpha-Fetoprotein

Blood levels of alpha-fetoprotein (AFP) are obtained from maternal serum to screen the fetus for defects in the neural tube, a part of the fetus that develops into the brain and spinal cord. The test is performed at 16 to 18 weeks of gestation and is used for screening purposes. Elevated AFP levels may indicate nervous system deformities, including spina bifida, but falsely elevated tests can be caused by more than one fetus or incorrect gestational dates. AFP results that are below the normal range may indicate Down syndrome in the developing fetus. Abnormal results indicate the need for further studies, including **amniocentesis** and fetal ultrasound.

Amniocentesis is insertion of a needle through the abdomen and into the gravid uterus to remove fluid from the amniotic sac. This fluid is analyzed for a variety of nervous system disorders. It can also be used to diagnose genetic problems, estimate gestational age, or assess lung maturity of the fetus. It may be performed in the office, and if so, you are responsible for preparing the patient, assisting the physician, preparing the specimen for transportation to the laboratory, and giving the patient any postprocedural instructions from the physician.

Fetal Ultrasonography

An ultrasound of the fetus is performed using high-frequency sound waves to create an image of internal structures. Fetal ultrasound is performed to assess the size, gestational age, position, and number of fetuses as well as fetal structures and development (Fig. 20-16). Some abnormal maternal and fetal conditions, such as ectopic pregnancy, placenta previa, neural tube defects, and cardiac defects may be diagnosed by ultrasound. The gender of the fetus may also be determined, although this is not typically a justification

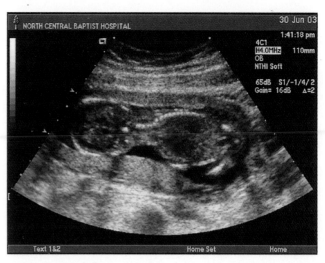

Figure 20-16 Fetus viewed via ultrasound. The outline of the fetal head and trunk can be clearly seen in the transverse position.

for performing an ultrasound. Although some obstetric offices have a sonographer on staff, fetal ultrasounds may have to be scheduled in an outpatient facility.

Contraction Stress Test and Nonstress Test

A contraction stress test (CST) is performed in the third trimester to determine how the fetus will tolerate uterine contractions. Uterine contractions may be induced by the woman stimulating her nipples, known as the nipple-stimulating CST, or the contractions can be induced by the administration of oxytocin, called an oxytocin-stimulated CST. In both tests, the fetal heart tones and movement are monitored in relation to the uterine contractions. Although the contractions are meant to be temporary, the CST is usually performed in the hospital in case continued contractions and delivery occur.

The nonstress test (NST) is a noninvasive obstetric procedure used to evaluate the fetal heart tones and movement in relation to spontaneous uterine contractions. The NST may be safely performed in the medical office, whereas the CST is usually performed in the hospital setting.

 CHECKPOINT QUESTION

13. In what instances might a fetal ultrasonography be ordered by the physician?

Contraception

Numerous methods of contraception (birth control) are available (Table 20-5). The decision to practice contraception and the selection of an appropriate method involves many factors, including the patient's religious, cultural, and personal beliefs. In addition, the health history, financial situation, and motivation of the patient

TABLE 20-5	Main Methods of Contraception		
Method	**Description**	**Advantages**	**Disadvantages**
Surgical Vasectomy, Tubal	Tubes carrying gametes cut	Nearly 100% effective; no chemical or mechanical devices	Not easily reversible; rare surgical complications
Hormonal Pill	Oral estrogen or progesterone to prevent ovulation	Highly effective; requires no last-minute preparation	Alters physiology; serious side effects possible
Injection	Inject synthetic progesterone every 3 months to prevent ovulation	Highly effective; lasts 3–4 months	Alters physiology; possible side effects are menstrual irregularity and amenorrhea; expensive
Patch	Patch with progesterone, estrogen worn on skin 3 out of 4 weeks to prevent ovulation	Use is simple; does not require pill or injection	Should be replaced same day of week; pregnancy can occur if patch off for more than 24 hours or left on more than 1 week
Ring	Small, flexible ring in vagina releases synthetic progesterone, estrogen to prevent pregnancy for 1 month	Does not require pill or injection; does not interfere with sexual intercourse	Side effects may include bleeding between periods, breast tenderness, other symptoms associated with hormone therapy
IUD	T-shaped plastic device with copper or progesterone	Spontaneous sexual intercourse	Heavy or long menstrual periods; cramping during and after insertion; periodic check for placement by feeling for string
Barrier Male condom	Sheath fits over erect penis, contains ejaculate	Easily available; does not affect physiology; protects from STDs	Must be applied before intercourse; may slip or tear
Female condom	Sheath that fits into vagina, held in place with rings	Easily available; protects from STDs	More expensive than male condom; must be inserted before intercourse
Diaphragm	Rubber cap fits over cervix; prevents entrance of sperm	Does not affect physiology; some protection from STDs	Must be inserted before intercourse; requires fitting by physician
Other Spermicide	Chemical to kill sperm; best used with a barrier method	Easily available; does not affect physiology; some protection from STDs	Local irritation; must be used just before intercourse
Fertility awareness	Abstinence while fertile per menstrual history, basal temperature, quality of cervical mucus	Does not affect physiology; accepted by certain religions	High failure rate; requires careful record keeping
Emergency contraception	Morning-after pill reduces risk of pregnancy up to 120 hours after unprotected sexual intercourse	May prevent pregnancy after unprotected sexual intercourse	Nausea, vomiting; no protection from STDs; may not prevent ectopic pregnancy; the closer to ovulation, the greater the chance of pregnancy

Adapted from Cohen BJ. Memmler's The Human Body in Health and Disease. 11th ed. Baltimore: Lippincott Williams & Wilkins, 2009.

may be important considerations for the patient, the spouse or partner, and the physician. To reinforce the physician's advice and instructions, you should understand the various methods, including the indications, risk factors, cost, and effectiveness. Both you and the physician should be prepared to educate and advise the patient regarding the choice of contraception.

Menopause

Menopause, also called the climacteric period, is the stage of life during which ovulation ceases because of decreasing ovarian function. This period, characterized by the cessation of the menstrual cycle, usually occurs around 45 to 50 years of age. Changes in the menstrual cycle in early menopause include **oligomenorrhea**, amenorrhea, dysfunctional uterine bleeding, and hot flashes, flushing, or perspiration.

The use of supplemental estrogen, or hormonal replacement therapy (HRT), was prescribed a few years ago to relieve menopausal symptoms such as hot flashes and depression and was believed to also protect against cardiovascular and skeletal disorders. However, in 2002, a research study was published that revealed elevated health risks for women who took hormone replacement therapy. As a result, fewer women today are taking HRT, and most physicians only recommend these medications for women with severe symptoms of menopause. For women with only minor menopausal symptoms, weight-bearing exercises, a healthy diet, and vitamin and mineral supplements have eased the transition through the menopausal stage without the use of hormone replacement medications. In either case, women in this stage of life should continue to have regular pelvic examinations, Pap smears, breast examinations, and mammograms and should speak with the physician about any questions or concerns.

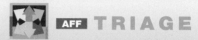 **TRIAGE**

While you are working in a gynecology medical office, the following three situations arise:

A. Patient A calls wanting information about the vaginal ring contraception.

B. Patient B is pregnant, and this is the first prenatal visit.

C. Patient C has been seen by the physician and needs to have a hysterosalpingography scheduled at the outpatient ambulatory center.

How do you sort these situations? What do you do first? Second? Third?

First, have the receptionist take a message from patient A and call her back later. This is clearly not an emergency, and you can call her back at a more convenient time. Next you should discharge patient C, letting her know that you will schedule the outpatient procedure later today and call her with the details tomorrow. Finally, call patient B to the examination room and take a thorough medical history and vital signs. Since patient B is new, she may require additional time and reassurance. She may also have questions and concerns about her pregnancy, and you do not want to be rushed during the patient education part of this initial visit.

Medication Box

Commonly Prescribed Female Reproductive System Medications

Note: The generic name of the drug is listed first and is written in all lowercase letters. Brand names are in parentheses, and the first letter is capitalized.

acyclovir (Zovirax)	Capsules: 200 mg Suspension: 200 mg/5 mL Tablets: 400 mg, 800 mg	Antiviral
citalopram hydrobromide (Celexa)	Tablets: 10 mg, 20 mg, 40 mg	Antidepressant
clomiphene citrate (Clomid; Milophene)	Tablets: 50 mg	Fertility
clindamycin phosphate (Cleocin; Clindesse)	Vaginal cream: 2% Vaginal suppositories: 100 mg	Antibiotic
doxycycline hyclate (Atridox; Doryx; Vibramycin)	Capsules: 50 mg, 100 mg Tablets: 20 mg, 100 mg	Antibiotic
drospirenone and ethinyl estradiol (Yasmin; YAZ)	Tablets (Yasmin): 3 mg drospirenone and 0.03 mg ethinyl estradiol as 21 yellow tablets and 7 white (inert)	Contraception

Commonly Prescribed Female Reproductive System Medications *(continued)*		
	Tablets (YAZ): 3 mg drospirenone and 0.02 mg ethinyl estradiol as 24 light pink tablets and 4 white (inert)	
escitalopram oxalate (Lexapro)	Tablets: 5 mg, 10 mg, 20 mg	Antidepressant
estradiol (Estrace: tablets) (Climara: patches)	Tablets: 0.5 mg, 1 mg, 1.5 mg, 2 mg Transdermal: 0.014 mg/24 hours to 0.075 mg/24 hours	Hormone replacement
estrogen, conjugated (Premarin)	Injection: 25 mg/5 mL Tablets: 0.3 mg, 0.45 mg, 0.625 mg	Hormone
etonogestrel and ethinyl estradiol (NuvaRing)	Vaginal ring: delivers 0.12 mg etonogestrel and 0.015 mg ethinyl estradiol daily	Contraception
fluoxetine hydrochloride (Prozac; Sarafem)	Capsules: 90 mg (delayed release) Capsules: 10 mg, 20 mg, 40 mg Tablets: 10 mg, 15 mg, 20 mg	Antidepressant
human papillomavirus recombinant vaccine (Gardasil)	Injection: 0.5 mL single-dose vial	Vaccine
imiquimod (Aldara)	Cream: 5% single-use packets, containing 12.5 mg	Immune response modifier
medroxyprogesterone acetate (Depo-Provera)	Injection: 104 mg/0.65 mL; 150 mg/mL; 400 mg/mL	Contraceptive
paroxetine hydrochloride (Paxil)	Tablets: 10 mg, 20 mg, 30 mg, 40 mg	Antidepressant
valacyclovir hydrochloride (Valtrex)	Tablets: 500 mg, 1,000 mg	Antiviral

español SPANISH TERMINOLOGY

¿Cuál fue el primer día de su último periodo menstrual?
  When was the first day of your last menstrual period?

¿Usa algun método anticonceptivo?
  Do you use a contraceptive device?

¿Cuándo fue su ultima mamografía?
  When was your last mammogram?

¿Ha alcanzado la menopausia?
  Have you gone through menopause?

MEDIA MENU

- **Student Resources on thePoint**
  - **CMA/RMA Certification Exam Review**
- **Internet Resources**

  American College of Obstetricians and Gynecologists
  http://www.acog.org

  Center for Disease Control and Prevention, STDs
  http://www.cdc.gov/std/general

  American Social Health Association
  http://www.ashastd.org/sitemap.cfm

  American Fertility Association
  http://www.theafa.org

  American Cancer Society
  http://www.cancer.org

  National Women's Health Information Center
  http://www.womenshealth.gov

PSY **PROCEDURE 20-1:** **Instructing the Patient on the Breast Self-Examination**

Purpose: Properly instruct the female patient on the procedure for performing a breast self-examination
Equipment: Patient education instruction sheet if available; breast examination model if available

Steps	Purpose
1. Wash your hands.	Handwashing aids infection control.
2. Explain the purpose and frequency of examining the breasts.	The purpose is to check for lumps, dimples, and thickened areas that can indicate malignancy and allow for early diagnosis and treatment. The patient should be encouraged to examine her breasts at the same time each month, about a week after the menstrual cycle.
3. Describe the three positions necessary for the patient to examine the breasts: in front of a mirror, in the shower, and lying down.	Inspecting and palpating the breasts in a variety of positions allows for a thorough examination of all breast tissue.
4. Explain that she should disrobe and inspect the breasts in front of a mirror with her hands on her hips and with her arms raised above her head. Advise the patient to look for any changes in contour, swelling, dimpling of the skin, or changes in the nipple.	Regular inspection shows what is normal and gives the patient confidence for the examination.

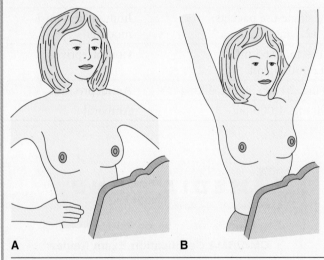

A   B

Step 4 **(A)** Inspect both breasts in front of a mirror with the hands on the hips.
(B) Inspect both breasts with the arms raised over the head. (Reprinted with permission from Pillitteri A. Maternal and Child Health Nursing. Philadelphia: Lippincott Williams & Wilkins, 2007.)

5. In the shower, the patient should feel each breast with her hands over wet skin, using the flat part of the first three fingers. Instruct her to use her right hand to lightly press over all areas of her left breast and her left hand to examine her right breast, checking for any lumps, hard knots, or thickenings.	Palpating the breasts in the shower allows the hands to glide more easily over wet skin.

PSY PROCEDURE 20-1: | **Instructing the Patient on the Breast Self-Examination** *(continued)*

Steps	Purpose

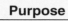

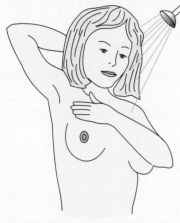

Step 5. Examine the breasts in the shower. (Reprinted with permission from Pillitteri A. Maternal and Child Health Nursing. Philadelphia: Lippincott Williams & Wilkins, 2007.)

6. After showering, the patient should lie down and examine her right breast after placing a pillow or folded towel under her right shoulder and placing her right hand behind her head. With her left hand, she should use the flat part of the fingers to palpate the breast tissue, using small circular motions beginning at the outermost top of her right breast and working clockwise around the breast.

Placing a pillow or folded towel under the right shoulder distributes the breast tissue more evenly on the chest.

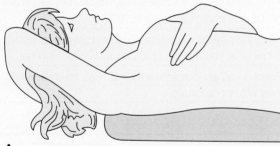

A

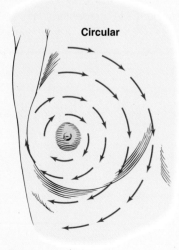

Circular

B

Step 6. (A) While lying down, palpate each breast carefully. (Reprinted with permission from Pillitteri A. Maternal and Child Health Nursing. Philadelphia: Lippincott Williams & Wilkins, 2007.) **(B)** Palpate the breast using the flat part of the fingers in a circular motion. (Reprinted with permission from Weber J, Kelley J. Health Assessment in Nursing. Philadelphia: Lippincott Williams & Wilkins, 2003.)

(continued)

PSY PROCEDURE 20-1:   Instructing the Patient on the Breast Self-Examination (continued)

Steps	Purpose
7. Encourage the patient to palpate the breast carefully by moving her fingers in toward the nipple, while palpating every part of the breast, including the nipple.	Breast tissue extends from the clavicle to the end of the rib cage and from the sternum to underneath the axilla.
8. Repeat the procedure for the left breast, placing a pillow or folded towel under the left shoulder and the left hand behind the head.	Both breasts should be examined at the same time.
9. Gently squeeze each nipple between the thumb and index finger. Report any discharge to the physician.	Unless the patient is lactating, discharge from the nipple is not normal.

Step 9. Squeeze each nipple gently. (Reprinted with permission from Pillitteri A. Maternal and Child Health Nursing. Philadelphia: Lippincott Williams & Wilkins, 2007.)

Steps	Purpose
10. Explain to the patient that she should promptly report any abnormalities to the physician.	Early detection of problems may mean early treatment of disease and, possibly, a cure.
11. **AFF** Explain how to respond to a patient who is visually impaired.	Face the patient when speaking and always let her know what you are going to do before touching her.
12. Document the patient education.	Procedures are considered not to have been done if they are not recorded.

Charting Example:

4/12/2014 2:15 PM Pt. given written and verbal instructions on performing the monthly breast self-examination.
She verbalized understanding. Advised to contact the office for any problems or abnormalities——————E. Smith, CMA

Note: The medical assistant may sign his or her name in the patient record using only the "CMA" credential if the office has a signature log denoting the entire credential as "CMA(AAMA)."

PSY PROCEDURE 20-2: Assisting with the Pelvic Examination and Pap Smear

Purpose: Prepare the examination room and the female patient for a pelvic examination and Pap smear and assist the physician as needed

Equipment: Gown and drape; appropriate size vaginal speculum; cotton-tipped applicators; water-soluble lubricant; examination gloves; examination light; tissues; materials for Pap smear: cervical spatula and/ or brush, glass slides and fixative solution *or* container with liquid medium to preserve the cells, laboratory request form, identification labels, and other materials that may be required by laboratory; biohazard container

Steps	Purpose
1. Wash your hands.	Handwashing aids infection control.
2. Assemble the equipment and supplies.	The vaginal speculum can be warmed under warm running water (see Fig. 20-10), on a heating pad set on warm, or in a warming drawer found on some examination tables. Lubricant must not be used on the vaginal speculum before insertion because this will cause inaccurate Pap smear results.
3. If slides are used, label each slide with the date and type of specimen on the frosted end with a pencil. For liquid medium, label the outside of the container.	Each slide should be labeled C for cervical, V for vaginal, or E for endocervical, depending on where the physician obtains the cells for examination. This is not necessary when liquid medium is used.
4. Greet and identify the patient. Explain the procedure.	Identifying the patient prevents errors. Explaining the procedure may reduce anxiety.
5. Ask the patient to empty her bladder and, if necessary, collect a urine specimen.	An empty bladder will make the examination more comfortable.
6. Provide the patient with a gown and drape and ask her to disrobe from the waist down.	If the patient is also having a breast examination, she should be instructed to disrobe completely and put the gown on with the opening in the front. This allows easier access for the breast examination. Allow the patient privacy for changing into the examination gown.

Step 6. Give the patient a gown and drape while explaining what to remove and how to put the gown on.

Steps	Purpose
7. Position the patient in the dorsal lithotomy position with her buttocks at the bottom edge of the table.	Because this position is embarrassing and may stress the legs and back, assist the patient into this position only when the physician is ready to do the examination.
8. Adjust the drape to cover the patient's abdomen and knees, exposing the genitalia, and adjust the light over the genitalia for maximum visibility.	Good visibility is essential for a thorough examination.
9. Assist the physician with the examination by handing instruments and supplies as needed.	Anticipating the physician's needs during the procedure promotes a more thorough and efficient examination

(continued)

PSY PROCEDURE 20-2: **Assisting with the Pelvic Examination and Pap Smear** *(continued)*

Steps	Purpose
10. After applying examination gloves, hold the microscope slides or container of liquid medium while the physician obtains the specimen. 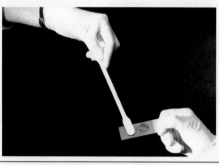 **Step 10.** Hold the slide by the frosted end to receive the smears if glass slides are used.	The physician may want you to assist once the specimen is obtained.
11. If glass slides are used, spray or cover each slide with fixative solution by holding the slide 4 to 6 inches from the can and spraying lightly once across the slide or dropping the fixative onto the slide.	Spraying the fixative solution too close to the slide will distort the cells or blow them off the slide. The fixative is necessary to preserve the cervical scrapings for cytology analysis. If a liquid medium is used, no fixative is necessary.
12. When the physician removes the vaginal speculum, have a basin or other container ready to receive it. 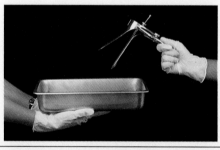 **Step 12.** Receive the used instruments in a basin or other container to transfer to the soaking solution for sanitizing.	Disposable specula may be put into a biohazard trash container. Nondisposable specula need to be sanitized and sterilized between patients.
13. Apply lubricant across the physician's two manual fingers without touching the end of the lubricant container to the physician's gloves. 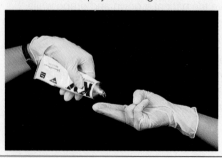 **Step 13.** Apply about 1 to 2 inches of water-soluble lubricant to the physician's gloved fingers.	Water-soluble lubricant helps make the examination more comfortable.

PSY PROCEDURE 20-2: **Assisting with the Pelvic Examination and Pap Smear (continued)**

Steps	Purpose
14. Encourage the patient to relax during the bimanual examination as needed.	The patient may be more relaxed during the examination if you are supportive.

Step 14. Technique for bimanual examination of the pelvic organs in women. (Reprinted with permission from Smeltzer SC, Bare BG. Textbook of Medical-Surgical Nursing. Philadelphia: Lippincott Williams & Wilkins, 2008.)

Steps	Purpose
15. After the examination, help the patient slide up to the top of the examination table and remove both feet at the same time from the stirrups.	Injury can be prevented if the patient moves up the table before removing feet from the stirrups. Removing both feet at the same time puts less strain on the patient.
16. Offer the patient tissues to remove excess lubricant, and help her sit if necessary, watching for signs of vertigo.	Excess lubricant can be uncomfortable. Some patients, especially older adults, may be dizzy on sitting up.
17. Ask the patient to get dressed and assist as needed. Provide for privacy as the patient dresses.	Telling the patient what to do will reduce confusion and misunderstanding.
18. Reinforce any physician instructions regarding follow-up appointments and advise the patient on the procedure for obtaining the laboratory findings from the Pap smear.	For quality management, let the patient know when to schedule follow-up appointments and when and how laboratory findings will be obtained.
19. **AFF** Explain how to respond to a patient who has dementia.	Solicit assistance from the caregiver or other staff member to help during the procedure. Give simple directions to the patient about what she should do. Speak clearly, not loudly.
20. Properly care for or dispose of equipment and clean the examination room. Wash your hands.	Follow standard precautions when handling contaminated supplies and equipment.
21. Document your responsibilities during the procedure, such as routing the specimen and patient education.	Procedures are considered not to have been done if they are not recorded.

Charting Example:

2/27/2014 3:00 PM Pap and pelvic today per Dr. Todd. Thin Prep sent to Acme lab for cytology. Pt. given written and oral instructions on obtaining results ———————————————————— B. Lewis, CMA

Note: The medical assistant may sign his or her name in the patient record using only the "CMA" credential if the office has a signature log denoting the entire credential as "CMA(AAMA)."

PSY PROCEDURE 20-3:   **Assisting with the Colposcopy and Cervical Biopsy**

Purpose: Prepare the examination room and the female patient for a colposcopy with cervical biopsy
Equipment: Gown and drape, vaginal speculum, colposcope, specimen container with preservative (10% formalin), sterile gloves in appropriate size, sterile cotton-tipped applicators, sterile normal saline solution, sterile 3% acetic acid, sterile povidone-iodine (Betadine), silver nitrate sticks or ferric subsulfate (Monsel solution), sterile biopsy forceps or punch biopsy instrument, sterile uterine curet, sterile uterine dressing forceps, sterile 4 × 4 gauze, sterile towel, sterile endocervical curet, sterile uterine tenaculum, sanitary napkin, examination gloves, examination light, tissues, biohazard container

Steps	Purpose
1. Wash your hands.	Handwashing aids infection control.
2. Verify that the patient has signed the consent form.	Colposcopy with biopsy is an invasive procedure that requires written consent.
3. Assemble the equipment and supplies.	Anticipate and plan for necessary equipment and supplies before the procedure starts to avoid having delays during the procedure.
4. Check the light on the colposcope.	Properly functioning equipment is crucial to the quality of the examination.
5. Set up the sterile field without contaminating it.	A biopsy is an invasive procedure requiring surgical asepsis.
6. Pour sterile normal saline and acetic acid into their sterile containers. Cover the field with a sterile drape.	Items that can be placed on the sterile field include the sterile cotton-tipped applicators and sterile containers for the solutions. Covering the sterile field maintains sterility as you prepare the patient.
7. Greet and identify the patient. Explain the procedure.	Identifying the patient prevents errors. Explaining the procedure may ease anxiety.
8. When the physician is ready to proceed, assist the patient into the dorsal lithotomy position. If you are to assist the physician from the sterile field, put on sterile gloves after positioning the patient.	Correct positioning is essential for a clear view of the cervix.
9. Hand the physician the applicator immersed in normal saline, followed by the applicator immersed in acetic acid.	Acetic acid swabbed on the area improves visualization and aids in identifying suspicious tissue.

Step 9. Hand the physician an applicator that has been immersed in normal saline.

Steps	Purpose
10. Hand the physician the applicator with the antiseptic solution.	The area to be sampled for biopsy must be swabbed with an antiseptic solution to reduce microorganisms and pathogens in the area.

PSY PROCEDURE 20-3: **Assisting with the Colposcopy and Cervical Biopsy** *(continued)*

Steps	Purpose
11. If you did not apply sterile gloves to assist the physician, apply clean examination gloves and receive the biopsy specimen into the container of 10% formalin preservative.	Because the specimen may be hazardous, standard precautions must be observed. The specimen container with preservative may be obtained from the laboratory.
12. Provide the physician with Monsel solution or silver nitrate sticks to stop any bleeding.	If bleeding occurs, a coagulant, such as Monsel solution or silver nitrate, may have to be applied if necessary.
13. When the physician is finished with the procedure, appropriately assist the patient from the stirrups and to a sitting position. Explain to the patient that a small amount of bleeding may occur. Have a sanitary napkin available.	Bleeding with a cervical biopsy is usually minimal, and a small sanitary pad should be sufficient.
14. Label the specimen container with the patient's name and date and prepare the laboratory request.	The specimen must be properly identified, and the laboratory request must be complete or the specimen may not be processed at the lab.

Step 14. Always label the specimen container before sending it to the lab.

Steps	Purpose
15. Ask the patient to get dressed and assist as needed. Provide for privacy as the patient dresses.	Telling the patient what to do will reduce confusion and misunderstanding.
16. Reinforce any physician instructions regarding follow-up appointments and how to obtain the biopsy findings.	For quality management, let the patient know when to schedule follow-up appointments, and tell the patient when and how laboratory findings will be provided.
17. **AFF** Explain how to respond to a patient who does not speak English or is ESL.	Solicit assistance from anyone who may be with the patient or a staff member who speaks her native language to interpret if available. If no interpreter is available, use hand gestures or pictures to explain procedure to the patient.
18. Properly care for or dispose of equipment and clean the examination room. Wash your hands.	Standard precautions should be followed during and after this procedure.
19. Document your responsibilities during the procedure, such as routing the specimen and patient education.	Procedures are considered not to have been done if they are not recorded.

Charting Example:

10/15/2014 10:45 AM Colposcopy performed per Dr. Lyttle; cervical biopsy obtained and sent to Acme lab for cytology. Minimal bleeding post procedure; pt. given sanitary pad, oral and written instructions on postprocedure care. Verbalized understanding ——————————————————— J. Pratt, CMA

Note: The medical assistant may sign his or her name in the patient record using only the "CMA" credential if the office has a signature log denoting the entire credential as "CMA(AAMA)."

- Assisting in obstetrics and gynecology is a challenging and fascinating area of medicine. This chapter:
  - Describes the examination of the female reproductive system
  - Explains your role in assisting the patient and the physician in the examination of the female reproductive system
  - Describes a variety of disorders related to the female reproductive system
  - Discusses normal physiologic functions such as menarche and menopause
  - Addresses the care of the pregnant patient including disorders or conditions sometimes seen in pregnancy

- As a professional medical assistant, you will be responsible for:
  - Providing reassurance and emotional support to the gynecologic patient
  - Assisting the physician during the gynecologic exam if needed
  - Processing any specimens for the laboratory using standard precautions
  - Maintaining the examination room, equipment, and supplies

Warm Ups for Critical Thinking

1. A multiparous patient who is married and has a history of cigarette smoking desires a highly effective method of contraception. What are her best choices for contraception? Explain which choice is best and why.
2. Your patient has both genital herpes and condylomata acuminata. She wants to know whether these disorders are contagious and how they can be cured. How do you respond to these questions?
3. Research the effects of maternal exposure to alcohol, tobacco, and nicotine and prepare a poster describing your findings that could be used to educate pregnant women and those considering pregnancy.
4. In addition to the contraceptives listed in this chapter, list the contraceptives available today, including the advantages and risks associated with each.
5. Using a drug reference book, research some of the newer drugs on the market to treat and/or prevent osteoporosis that may occur after menopause. What are the side effects of these medications?
6. Prepare a patient education poster for your medical office about breast cancer awareness.

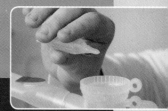

CHAPTER 21

Endocrinology

Learning Outcomes

Cognitive Domain

Note: AAMA/CAAHEP 2008 Standards are italicized.

1. Spell and define key terms
2. Identify abnormal conditions of the thyroid, pancreas, adrenal, and pituitary glands
3. Describe the tests commonly used to diagnose disorders of these endocrine system glands
4. Explain your role in working with patients with endocrine system disorders
5. *Identify common pathologies related to each body system*
6. *Describe implications for treatment related to pathology*

Psychomotor Domain

Note: AAMA/CAAHEP 2008 Standards are italicized.

1. Manage a patient with a diabetic emergency (Procedure 21-1)
2. *Assist physician with patient care*
3. *Prepare a patient for procedures and/or treatments*
4. *Practice standard precautions*
5. *Document patient care*
6. *Document patient education*
7. *Practice within the standard of care for a medical assistant*

Affective Domain

Note: AAMA/CAAHEP 2008 Standards are italicized.

1. *Apply critical thinking skills in performing patient assessment and care*
2. *Use language/verbal skills that enable patients' understanding*
3. *Demonstrate empathy in communicating with patients, family, and staff*
4. *Use appropriate body language and other nonverbal skills in communicating with patients, family, and staff*
5. *Demonstrate awareness of the territorial boundaries of the person with whom you are communicating*
6. *Demonstrate sensitivity appropriate to the message being delivered*
7. *Demonstrate recognition of the patient's level of understanding in communications*
8. *Recognize and protect personal boundaries in communicating with others*
9. *Demonstrate respect for individual diversity, incorporating awareness of one's own biases in areas including gender, race, religion, age, and economic status*
10. *Apply active listening skills*

11. *Apply local, state, and federal health care legislation and regulation appropriate to the medical assisting practice setting*

ABHES Competencies

1. Assist the physician with the regimen of diagnostic and treatment modalities as they relate to each body system
2. Comply with federal, state, and local health laws and regulations

3. Communicate on the recipient's level of comprehension
4. Serve as a liaison between the physician and others
5. Show empathy and impartiality when dealing with patients
6. Document accurately

Key Terms

acromegaly	glycosuria	insulin-dependent diabetes mellitus	polyuria
Addison disease	goiter		pruritus
Cushing syndrome	Graves disease	ketoacidosis	radioimmunoassay (RAI)
diabetes insipidus	Hashimoto thyroiditis	ketones	
dwarfism	hormones	non-insulin-dependent diabetes mellitus	thyrotoxicosis
endocrinologist	hyperglycemia		
exophthalmia	hyperplasia	polydipsia	
gigantism	hypoglycemia	polyphagia	

Together with the nervous system, the endocrine system regulates most body functions. Although the control exerted by the nervous system is immediate and usually elicits a short-term response, the endocrine system regulates chemical metabolism for a longer acting, more widespread response. **Hormones** are the chemical regulators, or messengers, of the endocrine glands. Some hormones stimulate system-wide metabolic processes, whereas others target specific tissues or organs (Table 21-1).

The endocrine glands differ from the body's other glands, such as sweat glands, because they are ductless (Fig. 21-1). Endocrine glands secrete hormones directly into the bloodstream for transmission rather than having direct access to target tissues. The body regulates the release of hormones through negative feedback, which "tells" the appropriate gland how much hormone to release based on the need for increased or decreased secretion. Some endocrine glands release hormones to maintain a specific range in the blood (thyroid hormones), whereas others have cyclic or rhythmic fluctuations (estrogen or progesterone).

Although you may see patients with endocrine system disorders in any medical practice specialty, physicians who specialize in the treatment of these disorders specifically are known as **endocrinologists**. Many disorders of the endocrine system result from an oversecretion or undersecretion of hormones. This chapter will focus on some common disorders of the endocrine system and the role of the medical assistant in caring for these patients in the medical office.

COG Common Disorders of the Endocrine System

Disorders of the Thyroid

Hyperthyroidism

The most common form of hyperthyroidism, **Graves disease**, results from the hypersecretion of thyroid hormones. This condition, also known as **thyrotoxicosis** (Box 21-1), causes an increase in metabolism. In addition to elevated blood levels of thyroid hormones (thyroxine [T_4] and triiodothyronine [T_3]), the patient may have an enlarged thyroid gland known as a **goiter** (Fig. 21-2) and unusual protrusion of the eyeballs known as **exophthalmia** (Fig. 21-3). Additional signs and symptoms of Graves disease include:

- Increased heart rate
- Increased body temperature

TABLE **21-1**	The Major Endocrine Glands and Their Hormones	
Gland	Hormone	Principal Functions
Anterior pituitary	HGH (human growth hormone)	Promotes growth of all body tissues
	TSH (thyroid-stimulating hormone)	Stimulates the thyroid gland to produce thyroid hormones
	ACTH (adrenocorticotropic hormone)	Stimulates adrenal cortex to produce cortical hormones
	FSH (follicle-stimulating hormone)	Stimulates growth and hormone activity of ovarian follicles; stimulates growth of testes
	LH (luteinizing hormone)	Causes development of corpus luteum in ruptured ovarian follicle in females; stimulates secretion of testosterone in males
Posterior pituitary kidney	ADH (antidiuretic hormone; vasopressin)	Promotes reabsorption of water in tubules
	Oxytocin	Causes contraction of uterus; causes ejection of milk from mammary glands.
Thyroid	Thyroid hormone (thyroxine [T_4] and triiodothyronine [T_3])	Increase metabolic rate; required for normal growth
	Calcitonin	Decreases calcium level in blood
Adrenal medulla	Epinephrine and norepinephrine	Increase blood pressure and heart rate
Adrenal cortex	Cortisol (95% of glucocorticoids)	Aids in metabolism of carbohydrates, proteins, fats; active during stress
	Aldosterone (95% of mineralocorticoids)	Aids in regulating electrolytes and water balance
Pancreatic islets	Insulin	Aids transport of glucose into cells; required for cellular metabolism of foods, especially glucose; decreases blood glucose levels
	Glucagon	Stimulates liver to release glucose, increasing blood glucose levels
Testes	Testosterone	Stimulates growth and development of male sexual organs
Ovaries	Estrogen	Stimulates growth of primary female sexual organs and development of secondary sexual characteristics

- Excessive sweating
- Inability to sleep
- Increased appetite
- Weight loss
- Excitability and nervousness

The treatment for hyperthyroidism includes destruction of part or all of the thyroid gland through the use of radioactive iodine or surgery. When seen in the medical office, these patients require frequent blood tests to check the thyroid hormone levels as ordered by the physician.

Hypothyroidism

Hypothyroidism results from an undersecretion of thyroid hormones, which may be congenital or acquired. Infants with congenital hypothyroidism are usually diagnosed at birth and treated with appropriate thyroid hormones. However, if a diagnosis is not made in the infant, irreversible mental retardation will occur. In adults, hypothyroidism may occur because of surgical removal of thyroid tissue, radioactive destruction of the gland, the use of antithyroid medications, or a deficiency of iodine in the diet. One form of hypothyroidism,

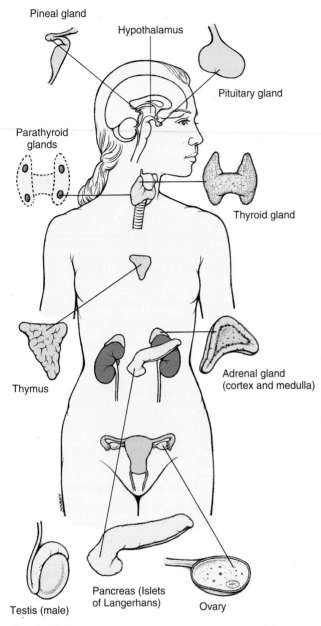

Figure 21-1 The main hormone-secreting glands of the endocrine system.

CHECKPOINT QUESTION

1. Why does the patient with hyperthyroidism have an increased appetite with weight loss?

Disorders of the Pancreas

Diabetes Mellitus

Dysfunction of the islets of Langerhans cells within the pancreas results in diabetes mellitus, a disorder affecting

Hashimoto thyroiditis, is actually a disease of the immune system in which the tissue of the thyroid gland is replaced with fibrous tissue. Regardless of the cause, treatment of hypothyroidism is replacement of thyroid hormones, which must be taken by the patient for the remainder of his or her life.

Your role in the medical office includes assisting the physician with any tests or procedures to diagnose and treat thyroid disorders. These tasks may include performing venipuncture for blood specimens and sending these to the lab for testing, obtaining referrals as needed, and scheduling patients for thyroid surgery with a head or neck surgeon, educating patients about their disease, and encouraging compliance with any medications ordered by the physician.

Toxic goiter (Graves disease)

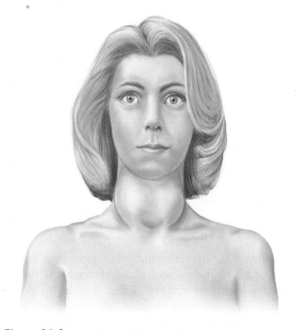

Figure 21-2 An enlarged thyroid gland or goiter. (Asset provided by Anatomical Chart Co.)

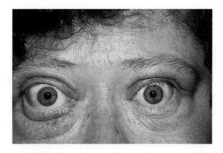

Figure 21-3 Exophthalmia. (From Goodheart HP. Goodheart's Photoguide of Common Skin Disorders. 2nd ed. Philadelphia: Lippincott Williams & Wilkins, 2003.)

carbohydrate metabolism. Although the exact cause of diabetes mellitus is not known, the result is a decrease in the production and secretion of insulin from the pancreas. Because insulin is necessary to carry glucose into the cells of the body, a decrease in insulin results in **hyperglycemia** (an elevated blood glucose), which ultimately results in **glycosuria** (glucose in the urine).

Type 1 Diabetes Mellitus

Type 1 diabetes mellitus is sometimes referred to as **insulin-dependent diabetes mellitus** and occurs most often in children and young adults. The signs and symptoms of hyperglycemia include the following:

- **Polydipsia** (increased thirst)
- **Polyuria** (excessive urination)
- **Polyphagia** (abnormal hunger)
- Weight loss

Usually, the young patient with type 1 diabetes develops symptoms abruptly without warning and may require hospitalization with intravenous insulin and frequent monitoring of blood glucose. Once diagnosed, these patients will require daily insulin and blood glucose monitoring for the remainder of their lives. Because these patients are often young, active, and still growing physically, managing blood glucose and diet may be challenging for both the patient and their caregivers. These patients should be encouraged to understand and manage their disease as independently as possible (Fig. 21-4).

Type 2 Diabetes Mellitus

Type 2 diabetes mellitus may be referred to as **non–insulin-dependent diabetes mellitus**; however, many patients with this condition do require insulin to control elevated blood glucose levels. This type of diabetes mellitus occurs most often in adults over the age of 40 years and has a gradual onset. Although insulin is produced by the pancreas, it cannot exert its effect on cells because of a deficiency of insulin receptors on cell membranes. Risk factors for developing type 2 diabetes are obesity and a family history of diabetes mellitus.

The patient with type 2 diabetes will have symptoms of hyperglycemia similar to patients with type 1

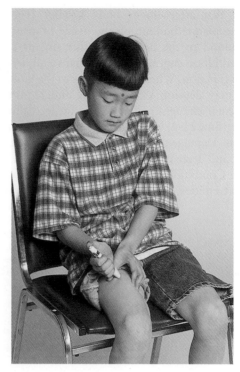

Figure 21-4 A young child with diabetes mellitus.

diabetes including polydipsia and polyuria. However, patients with type 2 diabetes mellitus will also have **pruritus** (severe itching) and neuropathy (disorders of the nervous system). Usually, the physician will recommend that the patient lose weight and eat a well-balanced diet, which may help to control the elevated blood glucose levels and reduce the need for parenteral insulin. Oral medications that enable insulin to react with the remaining cell membrane receptors are used as necessary; however, elevated blood glucose that does not respond to diet control and oral medications must be treated with insulin, which is injected subcutaneously.

Gestational Diabetes Mellitus

Another type of diabetes mellitus occurs only during pregnancy and is known as *gestational diabetes mellitus*. Although the pregnant patient may have all the signs and symptoms of type 1 or 2 diabetes mellitus, this condition disappears after the patient delivers the baby. It is important that the patient's urine be checked at every medical office visit for the presence of glucose; a blood specimen for glucose should be taken between 24 and 28 weeks of gestation. Early diagnosis of this condition is important to reduce complications, such as fetal abnormalities and death.

Managing Diabetes Mellitus

Long-term complications from uncontrolled hyperglycemia include damage to the heart, kidneys, and eyes, usually resulting from vascular system (blood vessel) changes that affect many body systems (Fig. 21-5). Increased plaque buildup on the inside of arteries supplying blood to the heart and other organs causes a decreased blood supply to those organs and, over time, a loss of function. When this happens to the kidneys, the patient may develop kidney failure and require dialysis. Vascular changes to the eyes result in diabetic retinopathy (Box 21-2) with a decrease in visual acuity and blindness. Damage to the nervous system results in neuropathy and decreased sensation, particularly in the legs and feet. Combined with the decreased blood flow to the lower extremities, this neuropathy could result in ulcers on the feet and legs that do not heal, become infected, and require eventual limb amputation (Fig. 21-6). These complications are not only debilitating, but they can also be life threatening.

In addition to the dietary restrictions including carbohydrate intake, insulin injections are necessary for patients with type 1 diabetes and may be necessary for patients with type 2 diabetes. Insulin is measured in units and administered subcutaneously (refer to Chapter 9). An insulin syringe is identified by the calibration in units, not milliliters (mL), and the orange cap. When administering insulin, use only an insulin syringe

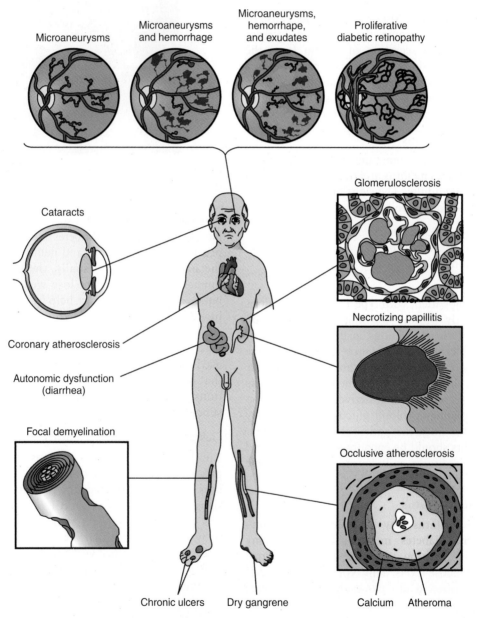

Figure 21-5 Secondary complications of diabetes. The effects of diabetes on a number of vital organs result in complications that may be incapacitating (cerebral and peripheral vascular disease), painful (neuropathy), or life threatening (coronary artery disease, pyelonephritis with necrotizing papillitis). (Raphael Rubin, David S. Strayer, Rubin's Pathology: Clinicopathologic Foundations of Medicine, Fifth Edition. Philadelphia: Lippincott Williams & Wilkins, 2008.)

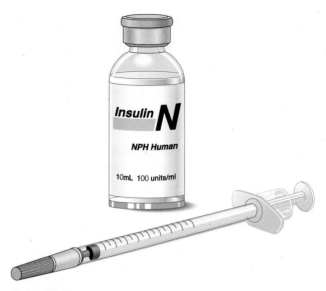

Figure 21-7 Only use an insulin syringe and needle to administer insulin. (LifeART image copyright © 2011. Lippincott Williams & Wilkins. All rights reserved.)

BOX 21-2

DIABETIC RETINOPATHY

Diabetic retinopathy is seen in patients with a history of diabetes mellitus and is caused by small hemorrhages from the capillaries supplying blood to the eye. After the capillaries rupture, scarring occurs that decreases the amount of oxygen to the eye. Over time, this scarring and decrease in oxygen results in permanent damage, causing a decrease in vision and eventual blindness. Controlling blood glucose levels can help control this devastating disease, which is currently the leading cause of blindness in the United States.

and needle that are calibrated to the concentration of insulin ordered by the physician. Do not use an insulin syringe and needle for anything other than insulin (Fig. 21-7). Depending on the needs of the patient, the action of insulin may vary from rapid acting (onset 5 to 15 minutes), short-acting (onset 30 minutes), intermediate acting (onset 2 hours), and long acting (onset 2 hours). Some diabetic patients may require more than one type of insulin to manage their blood glucose. Insulin can also be administered subcutaneously via an insulin pump (Fig. 21-8).

The role of the medical assistant includes working with the physician to diagnose and treat patients with diabetes mellitus while providing support and education to the patient and family members about this disease (Fig. 21-9). The lifestyle changes (e.g., dietary restrictions, weight management, exercise, frequent blood

monitoring) that are necessary to control blood glucose levels are often new to the patient and difficult to manage alone. Once diagnosed, the medical record must clearly identify the diagnosed patient's diabetes because many other health care problems and treatments may exacerbate this disease. You should also be alert for patients who may be having a diabetic emergency and react according to physician orders and office policy and procedure with regards to these situations.

You may be asked by the physician to obtain frequent blood specimens, schedule patients to speak with a dietician as necessary, and educate patients about their oral hypoglycemic medications or insulin. Because of the decreased sensation and possibility of painless sores or ulcers on the feet that can lead to infection and amputation, it is important that diabetic patients remove

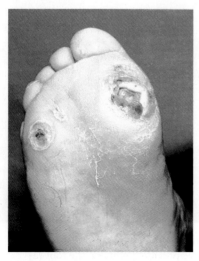

Figure 21-6 Neuropathic ulcers occur on pressure points in areas with diminished sensation in diabetic polyneuropathy. Because pain is absent the ulcer may go unnoticed. (Bates B.B. A guide to physical examination and history taking. 6th ed. 1995. Philadelphia: J.B. Lippincott.)

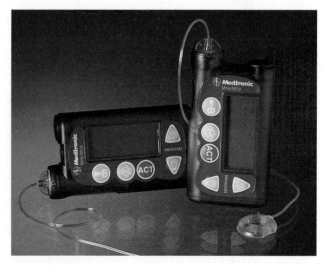

Figure 21-8 Medtronic (Northridge, CA) insulin pump system.

Foot Care Tips

1.	Check your bare feet every day. Look for cuts, sores, bumps, red spots. Use a mirror or ask a family member for help if you have trouble seeing the bottoms of you feet.
2.	Wash your feet in warm - not hot - water every day. Use a mild soap. Do not soak your feet. Dry your feet with a soft towel. Dry between your toes.
3.	Cover your feet with a lotion or petroleum jelly after washing them, before putting on your shoes and socks. Do not put the lotion or jelly between your toes.
4.	Cut your toenails straight across. Do not leave sharp edges that could cut the next toe.
5.	Use a dry towel to rub away dead skin.
6.	Do not try to cut calluses or corns yourself with a razor blade or knife. Do not use wart removers on your feet. If you have warts or painful corns or calluses, see a doctor who treats foot problems. This kind of doctor is called a podiatrist.
7.	Wear thick, soft socks. Do not wear mended socks or stockings with holes or seams that might rub into your feet.
8.	Check your shoes before you put them on to be sure they have no sharp edges or objects in them.
9.	Wear shoes that fit well and let your toes move. Break in new shoes slowly. Do not wear flip-flops, shoes with pointed toes or plastic shoes. Never go barefoot.
10.	Wear socks if your feet are cold at night. Do not use heating pads or hot water bottles on your feet.
11.	Have your doctor check your bare feet at least every visit. Take off your shoes and socks when you go in the exam room. This will remind the doctor to check your feet.
12.	See a podiatrist for help if you can't take care of your feet yourself.

Figure 21-9 Foot care tips for people with diabetes.

their shoes and socks at each office visit so that a visual inspection may be made of the feet and lower legs. In some offices, the medical assistant may be asked to assist with evaluating sensation in the feet (Fig. 21-10A–C).

WHAT IF?

What if your older adult patient is having difficulty seeing the numbers on the insulin syringe?

Although many elderly patients have visual difficulties that occur naturally with age, the patient with diabetes may have increased visual difficulties from the vascular changes in the eyes that result from the disease. Although you should always discuss these problems with the physician before advising the patient, there are visual aids that the patient can get from the pharmacist that fit onto the side of the syringe and magnify the image, making the numbers for "units of insulin" larger in appearance and easier to see. Perhaps a friend, neighbor, or other family member can assist the patient with filling the syringes. In some cases, the physician may want a visiting nurse to come to the patient's house during the week to prefill the syringes for the patient. Whatever the solution, always ask older adult patients about their medications and any difficulties they may be having with administering those medications, and work with the physician to come up with the best plan for the patient.

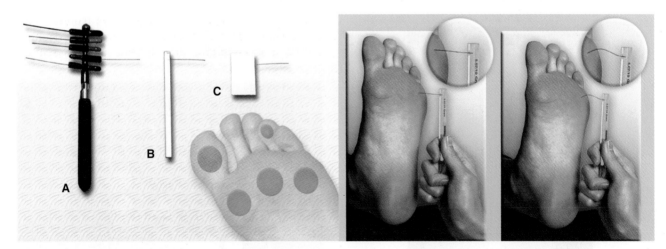

Figure 21-10 The monofilament test is used to assess the sensory threshold in patients with diabetes. The test instrument—a monofilament—is gently applied to about five pressure points on the foot (as shown in image on *left*). (**A**) Example of a monofilament used for advanced quantitative assessment. (**B**) Semmes-Weinstein monofilament used by clinicians. (**C**) Disposable monofilament used by patients. The examiner applies the monofilament to the test area to determine whether the patient feels the device. (Adapted with permission from Cameron B. L. 2002. Making diabetes management routine. American Journal of Nursing *102*(2) 26–32.)

Diabetic Emergencies

When glucose cannot be used for energy by the cells, the body turns to fats and proteins, which are converted to **ketones** by the liver. These ketones accumulate in the blood because the cells cannot use them rapidly. As these acids build up, they lower the pH of the blood, a condition known as **ketoacidosis**. Left untreated, ketoacidosis and hyperglycemia will progress to diabetic coma and death. The treatment is immediate intervention with parenterally administered fast-acting insulin. Symptoms of ketoacidosis and impending diabetic coma include:

- Flushed, dry skin
- A fruity (acetone) smell on the breath
- Thirst
- Deep respirations
- Rapid, weak pulse
- Abdominal pain
- Elevated blood glucose

Occasionally, a patient with diabetes mellitus has too much insulin in the blood, resulting in **hypoglycemia**, or a decreased blood glucose level. This can result when the patient skips a meal or increases physical activity without making adjustments in insulin. The result can produce a condition known as *insulin shock* and includes the following symptoms:

- Pale, moist skin
- Shallow respirations
- Rapid, bounding pulse
- Subnormal blood glucose levels

Procedure 21-1 describes the management of a patient having a diabetic emergency, such as hyperglycemia and ketoacidosis or insulin shock.

 CHECKPOINT QUESTION

2. What is the difference between type 1 and type 2 diabetes mellitus?

 PATIENT EDUCATION

CONTROLLING DIABETES MELLITUS

Use every opportunity to educate patients with diabetes about the importance of regulating blood glucose and eating sensibly. Also explain that, although these measures can control diabetes, the long-term effects of hyperglycemia can result in vascular changes that may cause blindness and kidney damage. Specifically, instruct patients how to:

- Maintain good personal hygiene to reduce secondary infections

- Manage their dietary intake of calories and carbohydrates
- Care for their feet properly because peripheral circulation may be poor
- Check blood glucose levels frequently and keep a log of the results
- Dispose of insulin syringes correctly
- Be aware of the signs and symptoms of diabetic ketoacidosis and insulin shock

Disorders of the Adrenal Glands

Addison disease

Hypoadrenocorticalism, or **Addison disease**, results from a deficiency of hormone secretion (mineralocorticoids and glucocorticoids) from the adrenal cortex. A decrease in these hormones causes an imbalance of electrolytes, specifically a loss of sodium and an increase in potassium. Other symptoms include weakness, lethargy, weight loss, hypotension, anemia, and a poor tolerance to stress.

The adrenal insufficiency of this disease results in an increase in the release of adrenocorticotropic hormone (ACTH) from the anterior pituitary gland. As this hormone becomes elevated in the blood, the patient will have hyperpigmentation of the skin (Fig. 21-11). Treatment includes oral replacement of the deficient mineralocorticoid and glucocorticoid hormones.

Cushing Syndrome

Hyperadrenocorticalism, also known as **Cushing syndrome**, may be caused by **hyperplasia** of the adrenal cortex or a tumor, resulting in an increased production of ACTH from the pituitary. Excessive cortisol promotes

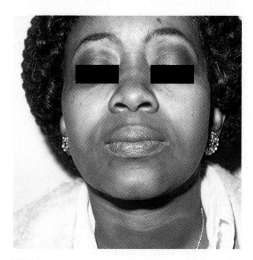

Figure 21-11 Hyperpigmentation seen in Addison disease. (From Goodheart HP. Goodheart's Photoguide of Common Skin Disorders. 2nd ed. Philadelphia: Lippincott Williams & Wilkins, 2003.)

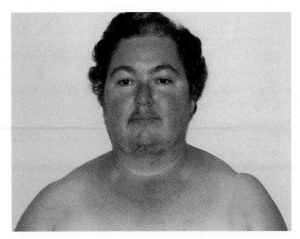

Figure 21-12 The round face of Cushing syndrome. (From Weber J, Kelley J. Health Assessment in Nursing. 2nd ed. Philadelphia: Lippincott Williams & Wilkins, 2003.)

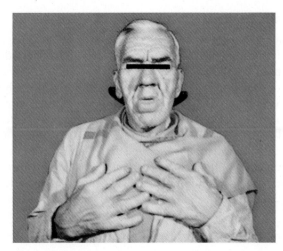

Figure 21-13 Acromegaly. (From Willis MC. Medical Terminology: A Programmed Learning Approach to the Language of Health Care. Baltimore: Lippincott Williams & Wilkins, 2002.)

fat deposits in the trunk of the body, with the extremities remaining thin. Osteoporosis is accelerated, whereas the skin is fragile and heals slowly after injuries. The face is characteristically round (Fig. 21-12).

Cushing syndrome may also be present in patients who are taking corticosteroids for medical reasons. Patients who may be prescribed corticosteroids include transplantation recipients and those with severe asthma or rheumatoid arthritis. Treatment for hyperadrenocorticalism requires removal of the cause of the hypersecretion, which could be either a pituitary or an adrenal tumor.

The role of the medical assistant in assisting with the diagnosis and treatment of disorders of the adrenal glands includes performing venipuncture for blood levels of the hormones secreted by the adrendal glands and supporting glands such as the pituitary. Diagnostic imaging tests may also be ordered by the physician and require you to obtain any preauthorizations or referrals if necessary and schedule the appropriate tests. Although the physician is responsible for advising patients on their diagnosis and treatment for adrenal gland disorders, your responsibilities may include supporting them through education and exhibiting a caring attitude to ensure compliance with any treatment prescribed by the physician.

 CHECKPOINT QUESTION

3. Which disorder of the adrenal gland results in elevated cortisol levels?

Disorders of the Pituitary Gland

Gigantism and Acromegaly

The pituitary gland, also known as the *hypophysis*, is the master gland responsible for controlling many aspects of the endocrine system. Hyperpituitarism is marked by an excess production of human growth hormone (HGH) secreted from the anterior lobe of the pituitary gland. Normally, HGH is secreted only up to the time of maturity when the epiphyseal lines on the long bones seal; however, hyperpituitarism during childhood or adolescence will result in an increase in bone length and a final height of 7 or 8 feet. This condition is called **gigantism** and is noted by excessive size and stature.

If hyperfunction of the anterior pituitary occurs near the end of puberty or during adulthood after epiphyseal closure, bone length does not change, but bone width increases, resulting in a condition known as **acromegaly** (Fig. 21-13). The patient with this disorder will have physical features such as a prominent jaw, an enlarged nose, and unusual thickening of the hands, feet, and skin. Unusual hyperactivity of the pituitary gland is associated with a tumor of the gland. Treatment of acromegaly requires surgical removal of the tumor or its destruction by radiation.

Dwarfism

Hypopituitarism is a deficiency of the anterior pituitary hormones, which may be caused by injury, atrophy of the gland, or certain types of tumors. If this condition occurs early in life, growth will be retarded, and **dwarfism** will result. A person with dwarfism is extremely short but has normal body proportions. Children who are diagnosed with this disorder can be given HGH to stimulate growth.

Adult hypopituitarism may be classified according to whether the various anterior pituitary hormones are selectively or completely deficient. If all the hormones are deficient, the condition is called *panhypopituitarism*, and if only certain hormones are deficient, the condition is named for the specific deficiency.

CHECKPOINT QUESTION

4. How are hypopituitarism and hyperpituitarism different?

Diabetes Insipidus

Diabetes insipidus results from a deficiency of antidiuretic hormone (ADH) secreted by the posterior pituitary gland. A deficiency in this hormone causes the renal tubules in the kidneys to reabsorb water and salts, resulting in polyuria with an increased urine output between 5 to 10 liters a day. Other clinical symptoms include polydipsia as the body tries to compensate for the dehydration caused by the increased urine production. Although the cause may be unknown, damage to the posterior pituitary gland from trauma or a pituitary tumor may result in this condition. Treatment involves correction of the causative factor if known and the administration of synthetic ADH by tablets, injection, or nasal spray.

As with other glandular disorders, your role in the medical office will be supportive, obtaining a thorough and complete history from the patient and performing any procedures or tests ordered by the physician to help with making an accurate diagnosis. Patients diagnosed with disorders of the pituitary gland will require patient education and emotional support to encourage compliance with any treatment prescribed by the physician.

WHAT IF?

What if your patient asks you if he or she should purchase and wear a medic alert bracelet?

Many of the diseases of the endocrine system are chronic and require monitoring and appropriate administration of hormones for the remainder of the patient's life. Unfortunately, if these patients become unresponsive or unable to verbalize their condition in an emergency, the appropriate treatment may be overlooked and have serious consequences for the patient. Always encourage any patient with a chronic disease to wear a medic alert necklace or bracelet to avoid a delay in treatment should an emergency arise.

COG Common Diagnostic and Therapeutic Procedures

A variety of laboratory tests and diagnostic procedures may be ordered by the physician to assist in the correct identification of endocrine disorders. Your assistance with performing or scheduling these laboratory or other

diagnostic procedures is important so that treatment may be initiated as quickly as possible. In most cases, testing of blood and urine can be used to measure the various hormone levels. Although the procedures for collecting these specimens are discussed in the clinical laboratory section of this text, you should be familiar with the procedures for collecting the specimen in addition to the procedure for processing the specimen appropriately. In some situations, you may have to schedule the patient for specimen collection at an outside laboratory facility.

Some examples of commonly performed tests for diabetes mellitus include the fasting glucose test and the glucose tolerance test (GTT), both using blood samples to check the levels of glucose. Although the urine glucose test is not used to diagnose or monitor diabetes mellitus, it is commonly part of the reagent strips used to check a variety of substances in the urine when performing a urinalysis (see Chapter 28). The glycohemoglobin, or hemoglobin A1C, blood test may be ordered by the physician to determine how well the blood glucose has been controlled in a patient with type 1 or type 2 diabetes mellitus during the previous 2 to 3 months. Ideally, a hemoglobin A1C level of 7% or lower is generally a good sign that the average blood glucose levels have been 170 mg/dL or less over the past 6 to 12 weeks. Table 21-2 describes the hemoglobin A1C levels and the corresponding mean glucose levels, and Table 21-3 describes other blood tests used to diagnose disorders of the endocrine system.

Thyroid functions tests measure the levels of T_4, T_3, and thyroid-stimulating hormone in the blood. In addition, the physician may order diagnostic imaging procedures to diagnose abnormalities with the thyroid gland. Specifically, a thyroid scan and the radioactive iodine uptake are ordered to diagnose thyroid disorders. During a thyroid scan, a radioactive compound is administered and localizes in the thyroid gland. The gland is then visualized with a scanner device to detect tumors or

TABLE **21-2**	Correlation of Hemoglobin A1C Values and Mean Blood Glucose Levels
Hemoglobin A1C (%)	**Mean Blood Glucose Levels (mg/dL)**
6	135
7	170
8	205
9	240
10	275
11	310
12	345

TABLE 21-3	Laboratory Tests for Endocrine System Disorders	
Endocrine Gland	**Blood Test**
Thyroid	Thyroxine (T4) Triiodothyronine (T3)
Anterior pituitary	TSH (thyroid-stimulating hormone) GH (growth hormone) FSH (follicle-stimulating hormone) LH (luteinizing hormone)
Pancreas	Glucose Hemoglobin A1C
Adrenal cortex	Corticoids

nodules. The radioactive iodine uptake procedure determines the amount of thyroid function by having the patient take an oral dose of radioactive iodine and measuring the absorption of this iodine in the thyroid gland.

Another test for endocrine disorders is the **radioimmunoassay (RAI)**, which measures hormone levels in blood by introducing radioactive substances into the body. The test is based on the ability of antibodies to bind specifically to radioactively labeled hormone molecules and to nonradioactive molecules. Computed tomography (CT) scans, magnetic resonance imaging (MRI), and ultrasonography are also used in the diagnosis of pathologic conditions of the endocrine system. Although you will not be performing the imaging procedures used in diagnosing endocrine system disorders, your role will include scheduling the patient for these procedures as ordered by the physician.

 CHECKPOINT QUESTION

5. What is the purpose of the hemoglobin A1C blood test?

 AFF TRIAGE

While you are working in a medical office, the following three situations occur at the same time:

A. Patient A is a 62-year-old man who is waiting for you to obtain a blood specimen that the physician has ordered for T_3 and T_4.

B. Patient B is a new patient who has just been taken back to an examination room and needs to have vital signs taken.

C. Someone from the laboratory is on the phone with the results for a diabetic patient who had a hemoglobin A1C drawn yesterday.

How do you sort these patients? What do you do first? Second? Third?

First, have someone take the message from the laboratory personnel. Anyone from the clinical staff can take these results. Patient B should have his vital signs taken and recorded. After checking for completion of the necessary new patient paperwork, you should notify the physician that he is ready to be seen. While the physician is examining patient B, you should perform a venipuncture on patient A. Unless the physician has indicated a need to speak with patient A, he can be discharged after the blood specimen is taken.

Medication Box		
Commonly Prescribed Endocrine System Medications		
Note: The generic name of the drug is listed first and is written in all lowercase letters. Brand names are in parentheses, and the first letter is capitalized.		
desmopressin acetate (DDAVP; Minirin)	Nasal solution: 0.1 mg/mL, 1.5 mg/mL Tablets: 0.1 mg, 0.2 mg	Posterior pituitary hormone
glyburide (DiaBeta)	Tablets: 1.25 mg, 2.5 mg, 5 mg	Oral hypoglycemic
glimepiride (Amaryl)	Tablets: 1 mg, 2 mg, 4 mg	Oral hypoglycemic
glucagon (Glucagen)	Powder for injection: 1 mg vial (mix with 1 mL of diluent)	Antihypoglycemic
hydrocortisone (Cortef)	Tablets: 5 mg, 10 mg, 20 mg	Glucocorticoid
insulin (Humulin R)	Injection: 100 units/mL	Antidiabetic/pancreatic hormone
insulin (Lispro; Humalog)	Injection: 100 units/mL	Antidiabetic/pancreatic hormone

Commonly Prescribed Endocrine System Medications *(continued)*		
insulin glargine (Lantus)	Injection: 100 units/mL	Antidiabetic/pancreatic hormone
levothyroxine sodium (Synthroid; Levoxyl)	Tablets: 25 mcg to 300 mcg	Thyroid hormone
metformin hydrochloride (Glucophage; Fortamet)	Tablets: 500 mg, 850 mg, 1,000 mg	Oral hypoglycemic
methylprednisolone (Medrol; Medrol Dosepak)	Tablets: 2 mg to 32 mg	Glucocorticoid
methylprednisolone acetate (Depo-Medrol)	Injection: 20 mg/mL; 40 mg/mL; 80 mg/mL	Glucocorticoid
somatropin (Accretropin; Genotropin; Humatrope)	Injection: 5 mg/mL (Accretropin) Injection: 1.5 mg to 13.8 mg/vial Injection: 5 mg to 24 mg/vial	Anterior pituitary hormone
triamcinolone acetonide (Kenalog-10; Kenalog-40)	Injection: 10 mg/mL, 40 mg/mL	Glucocorticoid

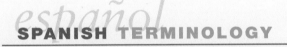

SPANISH TERMINOLOGY

¿Padece de sed excesiva?
   Do you have excessive thirst?

Necesitouna muestra de orina.
   I need a urine specimen.

¿Cómo está su apetito?
   How is your appetite?

Necesito tomarle una muestra de sangre.
   I need to take a blood sample.

MEDIA MENU

- **Student Resources on thePoint**
  - **Animation: Diabetes**
  - **CMA/RMA Certification Exam Review**
- **Internet Resources**

  The Hormone Foundation
  http://www.hormone.org

  National Graves Disease Foundation
  http://www.ngdf.org

  American Diabetes Association
  http://www.diabetes.org

  American Dietetic Association
  http://www.eatright.org

  The Thyroid Foundation of America
  http://www.allthyroid.org

PSY PROCEDURE 21-1:   **Manage a Patient with a Diabetic Emergency**

Purpose: Respond to a patient who comes into the office with signs and symptoms consistent with a diabetic emergency, either hyperglycemia or hypoglycemia
Equipment: Gloves, blood glucose monitor and strips, fruit juice or oral glucose tablets

Steps	Reasons
1. Wash your hands.	Handwashing aids infection control.
2. Recognize the signs and symptoms of hyperglycemia and hypoglycemia. *Hyperglycemia:* • Flushed, dry skin • A sweet, fruity smell on the breath • Thirst • Deep respirations • Rapid, weak pulse • Abdominal pain *Hypoglycemia:* • Pale, moist skin • Shallow, fast respirations • Rapid, bounding pulse • Weakness • Shakiness	
3. Identify the patient and escort him or her into the examination room. 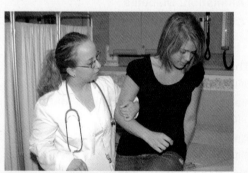 **Step 3.** Assist the patient to the examination room.	This prevents error in treatment, helps gain the patient's compliance, and eases anxiety.
4. Determine whether the patient has been previously diagnosed with diabetes mellitus. 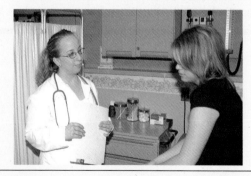 **Step 4.** Determine if the patient is known to have diabetes.	You may ask a patient if he or she is diabetic. However, if patients are confused, they may say "no" when they are, in fact, diabetic. You may also check the medical record or look for a medic alert bracelet or necklace, but the absence of a medic alert tag is not evidence that the patient is not diabetic.

PSY PROCEDURE 21-1:   Manage a Patient with a Diabetic Emergency (continued)

Steps	Reasons
5. Ask the patient if he or she has eaten today and taken any medication.	The signs and symptoms of hyperglycemia or hypoglycemia may be difficult to distinguish. A patient who has eaten but has not taken insulin may be hyperglycemic. A patient who has not eaten but has taken insulin may be hypoglycemic.
6. Notify the physician about the patient and perform a stick for a blood glucose and measure as directed. **Step 6.** Perform a finger stick as directed by the physician or office policy and procedure.	A patient experiencing hyperglycemia will have a capillary blood glucose between 250 and 800 mg/dL. A patient experiencing hypoglycemia will have a blood glucose of less than 70 mg/dL.
7. Notify the physician of blood glucose results and treat the patient as ordered by the physician. A. Administer insulin subcutaneously to a patient with hyperglycemia. B. Administer a quick-acting sugar, such as an oral glucose tablet or fruit juice, for a patient with hypoglycemia.	It is important to act quickly while remaining calm when treating a patient having a diabetic emergency.
8. **AFF** Explain how to respond to a patient who is developmentally challenged.	Solicit information from anyone who may have accompanied the patient to the office. To avoid injury, assess for safety before completing a procedure when there is the possibility that the patient may not cooperate.
9. Be prepared to notify emergency medical services as directed by the physician if the symptoms do not improve or worsen.	In some situations, the patient requires insulin to be administered intravenously.
10. Document any observations and treatments given.	Procedures are considered not to have been done if they are not recorded.

Charting Example:

10/14/2014 11:00 AM Pt. presented to office with complaint of weakness since last evening that has gotten worse this morning. Awake and answers questions appropriately, but seems lethargic. BP 110/62 (R) sitting, pulse 122. Skin pale, skin cool, moist. Denies being diabetic, but wearing a medic alert bracelet indicating that she is diabetic. Dr. Smith notified ———————————————————————————————— J. Jones, CMA

10/14/2014 11:05 AM Blood glucose 65 mg/dL. Pt. given 8 oz. orange juice orally and a glucose tablet as ordered ———————————————————————————————— J. Jones, CMA

10/14/2014 11:10 AM Pt. states he "feels better" but continues to look pale, pulse 110, BP 120/72. Given another 8 oz. orange juice as ordered ———————————————————————————————— J. Jones, CMA

Note: The medical assistant may sign his or her name in the patient record using only the "CMA" credential if the office has a signature log denoting the entire credential as "CMA(AAMA)."

- The endocrine system controls many bodily processes indirectly through chemical messengers called *hormones*.
- Hormones are secreted directly into the blood stream.
- Disorders of the endocrine system include alterations in hormone secretion, and either too much hormone is secreted (hypersecretion or excess) or not enough hormone is secreted (hyposecretion or deficiency).
- Disorders of the thyroid gland include Graves disease and Hashimoto thyroiditis.

- Diabetes mellitus is a disorder of the pancreas involving the production of insulin and its ability to take glucose into the cells of the body.
- Depending on when the anterior pituitary gland secretes too much growth hormone, the patient may have gigantism or acromegaly.
- Your role in working with patients with endocrine system disorders includes emotional support to ensure compliance with treatments that are often required for the life of the patient.

Warm Ups for Critical Thinking

1. A 40-year-old female patient is seen in the office with a complaint of weight gain and hair loss. After the physical examination, she asks you why the physician felt the front of her neck. How would you respond? What gland is located there?

2. Your 56-year-old patient with diabetes cannot understand why his blood glucose levels are above 200 mg/dL, and he tells you that he "does not eat candy or sweets." Upon furthering questioning, you find out his diet consists of pasta and diet soda. What education does this patient need, if any? Create a brochure that would help this patient understand diabetes mellitus using language a patient would understand.

3. Research the transphenoidal hypophysectomy surgical procedure used to remove pituitary gland tumors. How is this procedure performed? What hormone replacement medications will the patient have to take postoperatively?

4. Your patient is concerned about the thyroid function tests that the physician has ordered and asks you to explain what these tests involve. What could you say to this patient? Would you tell the patient that this test would determine the presence of a thyroid tumor? Why or why not?

5. Create a brochure for the newly diagnosed diabetic patient explaining the hemoglobin A1C test.

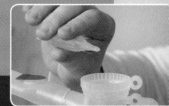

22 Pediatrics

Outline

The Pediatric Practice
Safety
Types of Pediatric Office Visits
Child Development
Psychological Aspects of Care
Physiologic Aspects of Care
Role of the Parent
The Pediatric Physical Examination
The Pediatric History
Obtaining and Recording Measurements and Vital Signs

Administering Medications
Oral Medications
Injections
Collecting a Urine Specimen
Understanding Child Abuse
Pediatric Illnesses and Disorders
Impetigo
Meningitis
Encephalitis
Tetanus
Cerebral Palsy

Croup
Epiglottitis
Cystic Fibrosis
Asthma
Otitis Media
Tonsillitis
Obesity
Attention Deficit Hyperactivity Disorder

Learning Outcomes

Cognitive Domain

Note: AAMA/CAAHEP 2008 Standards are italicized.

1. Spell and define key terms
2. List safety precautions for the pediatric office
3. Explain the difference between a well-child and a sick-child visit
4. List types and schedule of immunizations
5. Describe the types of feelings a child might have during an office visit
6. List and explain how to record the anthropometric measurements obtained in a pediatric visit
7. Identify two injection sites to use on an infant and two used on a child
8. Describe the role of the parent during the office visit
9. List the names, symptoms, and treatments for common pediatric illnesses
10. *Identify common pathologies related to each body system*

11. *Describe implications for treatment related to pathology*

Psychomotor Domain

Note: AAMA/CAAHEP 2008 Standards are italicized.

1. Obtain an infant's length and weight (Procedure 22-1)
2. Obtain the head and chest circumference (Procedure 22-2)
3. Apply a urinary collection device (Procedure 22-3)
4. *Assist physician with patient care*
5. *Prepare a patient for procedures and/or treatments*
6. *Practice standard precautions*
7. *Document patient care*
8. *Document patient education*
9. *Practice within the standard of care for a medical assistant*

Affective Domain

Note: AAMA/CAAHEP 2008 Standards are italicized.

1. *Apply critical thinking skills in performing patient assessment and care*
2. *Use language/verbal skills that enable patients' understanding*
3. *Demonstrate empathy in communicating with patients, family, and staff*
4. *Use appropriate body language and other nonverbal skills in communicating with patients, family, and staff*
5. *Demonstrate awareness of the territorial boundaries of the person with whom you are communicating*
6. *Demonstrate sensitivity appropriate to the message being delivered*
7. *Demonstrate recognition of the patient's level of understanding in communications*
8. *Recognize and protect personal boundaries in communicating with others*
9. *Demonstrate respect for individual diversity, incorporating awareness of one's own biases in areas including gender, race, religion, age, and economic status*
10. *Apply active listening skills*
11. *Apply local, state, and federal health care legislation and regulation appropriate to the medical assisting practice setting*

ABHES Competencies

1. Assist the physician with the regimen of diagnostic and treatment modalities as they relate to each body system
2. Comply with federal, state, and local health laws and regulations
3. Communicate on the recipient's level of comprehension
4. Serve as a liaison between the physician and others
5. Show empathy and impartiality when dealing with patients
6. Document accurately

Key Terms

aspiration	immunization	pediatrics	sick-child visit
autonomous	neonatologist	psychosocial	well-child visit
congenital anomaly	pediatrician	restrain	

Medical assistants who work in an office where infants and children are seen must understand that the needs of children and adolescents are often different from those of adult patients. **Pediatrics** is the medical specialty devoted to the care of infants, children, and adolescents. This care includes diagnosis and treatment of childhood diseases, prevention of accidents and trauma, and monitoring the physical and **psychosocial**, or mental and emotional, development of the child. These patients are not simply small adults; however, they may contract some of the illnesses that are seen in adult patients. Pediatric patients are also susceptible to a unique array of illnesses and problems not present in adults. Some young patients have **congenital anomalies** that are life threatening or debilitating. Because children have immature nervous systems, faster metabolism, and accelerated growth patterns, they are subject to complications that may not occur in adult patients.

A **pediatrician** is a physician who is specially trained to care for both the well child and diseases of infants, children, and adolescents. While most traditional pediatricians treat all children up through the teen years, pediatric specialists include **neonatologists**, physicians who treat only newborns, and physicians who specialize in the treatment of adolescents. In addition, the medical assistant working in the family practice office will see patients of all ages, including children.

COG The Pediatric Practice

Safety

A pediatric office decorated and furnished in a manner appropriate to the physical and psychosocial needs of children creates an unthreatening and possibly even inviting environment. Child-size furniture helps these patients feel comfortable and welcome. Popular toys evoke happy associations. Safe toys allow for hands-on activity while the child is waiting to see the physician. Popular storybooks and magazines give parents an opportunity to read quietly to a child who may not feel well enough to play. Some offices provide waiting rooms that are designed to separate sick and well children to prevent the transmission of communicable diseases between patients.

Safety should be a prime concern for choosing toys and equipment for a pediatric office. Waiting room toys should be examined frequently and replaced when damaged or soiled. All toys should be washable and should be cleaned according to office policy to reduce the risk of disease transmission. Try to see the office from a child's viewpoint. If necessary, get down to a child's level to discover dangers, such as sharp table corners and exposed electrical outlets, that an adult standing to observe and evaluate the environment might overlook.

The examination room should also be designed for children's safety. Keep all medical equipment out of a child's reach, and never leave a young child alone in the examining room. Follow these tips to ensure your patient's safety:

- Place infant scales on a sturdy table, and never leave an infant alone on a scale.
- Store any disinfectants away from patient care areas.
- Store and dispose of all sharps in proper containers.
- Practice stringent handwashing and standard precautions with every patient. Many childhood diseases are highly contagious and can be transmitted by poor medical asepsis.

 CHECKPOINT QUESTION

1. What are three safety precautions that should be used in a pediatric office?

 WHAT IF?

What if you have an uncooperative infant or child?

During the examination and certain procedures, you may need to help restrain the child. Restraining is sometimes necessary to protect the child from injury and to help the physician complete the examination in a timely manner. Many children understandably resist the examination or procedure because they are frightened and do not want to be touched. Calm and gentle restraint is in the best interest of everyone involved.

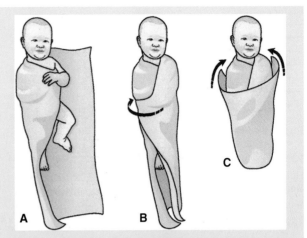

Mummy restraint. Place the child diagonally on a small receiving blanket. **(A)** Wrap the right corner across the torso, covering the right arm and shoulder. Pull it snugly under the child's left arm and tuck it under the child's body. **(B)** Pull the left corner across the child's left arm and shoulder and tuck it snugly under the torso at the back so that the child's weight secures the end. **(C)** Wrap the end of the blanket up around the child.

Types of Pediatric Office Visits

The Well-Child Office Visit

Well-child visits are regularly scheduled office visits whose goal is to maintain the child's optimum health. Although these visits are typically scheduled to correspond with immunizations, the first newborn visit is often required within 1 week after birth. At this visit, you may be required to obtain a blood specimen from the newborn patient to check for the absence of the enzyme phenylalanine hydroxylase, also known as a *PKU test*. This test must be performed between 1 and 7 days after birth because an absence of this enzyme may result in mental retardation if not treated by 3 to 4 weeks of age. Treatment of the newborn with this deficiency includes a diet low in phenylalanine.

In addition to including a complete examination and an evaluation of the child's neurologic and psychosocial development, any other concerns on the part of the caregiver are also addressed at these visits (Fig. 22-1). The neurologic examination consists of the physician checking for the presence or absence of various reflexes. Table 22-1 describes various infant reflexes and the normal responses typically assessed at the well-child infant visit. In addition to the reflexes, the physician observes for development appropriate for the age of the infant or child. The child is observed or the caregiver is questioned about areas such as social development, fine motor development, gross motor development, language, and nutrition using a guide such as the Denver II Developmental Screening Test (DDST).

The well-child visit also provides an opportunity to administer **immunizations** to protect children from

History

→ Demographic data
→ Chief concern
→ History of chief concern
→ Health and family profile
→ Past health history
→ Family health history
→ Review of systems

Physical examination

→ General appearance
→ Vital signs

Height

Head
Head circumference

Ears and hearing

Nose

Neck

Lungs

Breasts

Mental status

Neurologic function

Intelligence

Temperament

Eyes and vision

Mouth and speech

Heart

Chest
Chest circumference

Abdomen
Abdominal circumference

Back

Genitorectal area

Extremities

Skin

Developmental appraisal
Stage of development

Weight

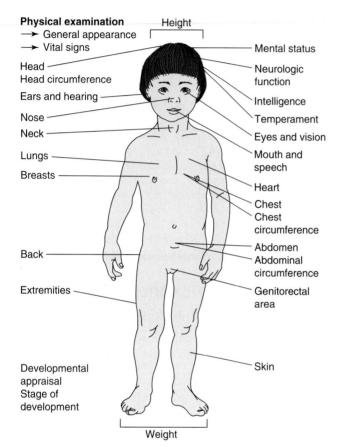

Figure 22-1 Assessing the Child Overview: History and Examination. (From Pillitteri, A. 2003, Maternal and Child Nursing, 4th Ed., Philadelphia: Lippincott, Williams & Wilkins.)

diseases that in the past caused early death or long-term health problems. Immunizations produce immunity by slowly introducing an altered form of the disease-producing bacteria or virus into the body, which stimulates the body to produce antibodies to protect against the specific disease. Immunization schedules are developed by the American Academy of Pediatrics (AAP) and the Centers for Disease Control and Prevention, and they change periodically as new vaccines become available (Figs. 22-2 and 22-3). These schedules include one for children ages 0 to 6 years and another for children ages 7 to 18 years. You should post these schedules prominently in the office and replace as necessary with the latest information. All children must be current with their immunizations before they are permitted to attend public school.

Vaccine manufacturers have established protocols that must be followed to ensure full immunity to the specific diseases. If you are responsible for administering

vaccines, you must read all package inserts and become familiar with the correct administration and possible adverse effects before administering the medication. In addition, you must give the parent or caregiver of the child the written vaccine information statement (VIS) about each vaccine you are administering (Fig. 22-4) detailing the benefits and risks that may be associated with each vaccine. In some cases, it may be necessary to obtain written consent before administering the vaccine. The VIS for individual vaccines describes the disease and provides information specific to the immunization, such as recommended ages and adverse reactions (Fig. 22-5). The most current vaccine schedules and information sheets for all vaccines can be found on the Centers for Disease Control and Prevention website.

The Sick-Child Office Visit

A **sick-child visit** occurs whenever an infant or child requires medical treatment for signs or symptoms of illness or injury. The goal of these visits is diagnosis and treatment of the child's immediate illness or injury. After examining the child, the physician may pursue diagnostic tests and treatments including radiography, laboratory tests, medication, or simply the reassurance that the illness will run a predictable and manageable course. Table 22-2 lists three common childhood illnesses and their causes, signs and symptoms, and treatments.

CHECKPOINT QUESTION

2. What is the difference between well-child and sick-child visits?

WHAT IF?

What if a child's mother complains that her baby vomits everything he eats?

If the vomiting is projectile, the child may have pyloric stenosis, a disorder usually seen in infants several days to several months old. Diagnosis is usually made by parental history, physical examination, and radiography. The physician often can palpate an olive-shaped lump in the right upper quadrant of the abdomen while the child is supine. Surgery (pyloroplasty) is the treatment. Although pyloric stenosis is not an emergency, surgery is usually scheduled promptly to prevent dehydration. Inform the parents about the disorder and reassure them as needed.

Vomiting may also be caused by gastroenteritis, or an infection of the stomach and intestines caused by a bacterium or virus. These infants may also have diarrhea. Regardless of the cause, infants may dehydrate very quickly and should be seen by the physician without delay.

TABLE 22-1	Infant Reflexes and Responses
Reflex	**Response**
Sucking or rooting	Stroking the cheek causes the infant to turn toward the stroke with its mouth open to suck. This reflex subsides by 3–6 months.
Moro or startle	A loud noise or sudden change in position causes the infant to look startled; the back arches, the arms and legs fly out and then quickly come back close to the body, and the infant cries. The Moro reflex results in the thumbs and forefingers forming a C while the other fingers spread open (in the startle reflex, the fingers remain clenched). Both reflexes disappear by 6 months.
Grasp	Stroking the infant's palm causes the fingers to grasp; stroking the plantar surface causes the toes to flex to grasp. The palmar grasp disappears by 3 months. The plantar grasp disappears by 9–12 months.
Tonic neck or fencing	With the infant supine, the physician turns the head to either side. The arm and leg on the side the infant is facing will flex, and the limbs on the opposite side will extend. This reflex disappears by 3–4 months.
Placing or stepping	The physician holds the infant upright at the edge of the examining table with the heel just below the edge. When the tops of the feet touch the table edge, the infant will place each foot up on the table and make walking movements. This reflex disappears by 6 weeks.
Babinski	When the plantar surface of the foot is stroked, the toes flare outward. This reflex disappears by 12 months.

COG Child Development

Psychological Aspects of Care

Understanding a child's psychological needs and development helps you provide safe and effective care. During an office visit, the patient may have the same feelings as adults: fear and powerlessness. However, depending on the child's age and ability to understand, the behaviors associated with these feelings are different from those of the adult patient. Specifically, children may have these feelings:

• Fear that something painful and frightening will be done
• Anxiety about repetition of a previous bad experience
• Guilt and feelings of being punished for being bad or misbehaving
• Powerlessness and loss of physical autonomy
• Curiosity about new surroundings and experiences

Some children verbalize these feelings, whereas others can express them only by crying and resisting the approach of the medical staff. As a professional medical assistant, you can reassure patients and family members by demonstrating your understanding of the child's feelings and displaying a kind and gentle manner. Include the child in the explanation of procedures on an age-appropriate level. Children who are encouraged to "help" during the examination or procedure (such as holding the adhesive bandage before receiving an injection) may also feel part of the examination and may be more cooperative.

Physiologic Aspects of Care

To anticipate age-appropriate behavior and to provide proper psychological support and physical care, you must have a broad knowledge of child growth and development patterns. Never expect a child to react or respond beyond his or her developmental age. For example, a 2-year-old child is naturally reluctant to be examined and may resist your advances. Many 4- or 5-year-old children are curious and willing to cooperate if you turn the examination into a game. Children older than 4 years should understand the need to comply, but this age group may still have to be restrained during some procedures, such as injections. A normal child's growth and development of mind, body, and personality follow an orderly progression. Table 22-3 describes the stages of growth and development and lists special considerations for the medical assistant.

At birth, the nervous system is complete but immature. During regular visits to the pediatrician, the infant is tested for infantile automatisms—reflexes found in the newborn that disappear later in childhood (Fig. 22-6). Examples include the stepping reflex, the Moro (or startle) reflex, and the rooting reflex. The absence of infantile automatisms after birth or the continuation of these reflexes beyond infancy suggests central nervous system dysfunction and requires further testing. A popular tool for evaluating specific gross and fine motor coordination in infants and children up to 6 years of age is the DDST II. This tool assists with evaluating children from the most basic reflexes to complex interpersonal reactions. If you perform the assessment, you should be trained in proper testing to evoke the most diagnostic response. Children should register within the normal range for their age. The DDST II does not measure intelligence levels.

Recommended Immunization Schedule for Persons Aged 0 Through 6 Years—United States • 2011
For those who fall behind or start late, see the catch-up schedule

Vaccine ▼ Age ►	Birth	1 month	2 months	4 months	6 months	12 months	15 months	18 months	19–23 months	2–3 years	4–6 years	
Hepatitis B[1]	HepB	HepB				HepB						
Rotavirus[2]			RV	RV	RV[2]							
Diphtheria, Tetanus, Pertussis[3]			DTaP	DTaP	DTaP	see footnote[3]	DTaP				DTaP	
Haemophilus influenzae type b[4]			Hib	Hib	Hib[4]	Hib						
Pneumococcal[5]			PCV	PCV	PCV	PCV				PPSV		
Inactivated Poliovirus[6]			IPV	IPV		IPV					IPV	
Influenza[7]						Influenza (Yearly)						
Measles, Mumps, Rubella[8]						MMR		see footnote[8]			MMR	
Varicella[9]						Varicella		see footnote[9]			Varicella	
Hepatitis A[10]						HepA (2 doses)				HepA Series		
Meningococcal[11]										MCV4		

Range of recommended ages for all children

Range of recommended ages for certain high-risk groups

This schedule includes recommendations in effect as of December 21, 2010. Any dose not administered at the recommended age should be administered at a subsequent visit, when indicated and feasible. The use of a combination vaccine generally is preferred over separate injections of its equivalent component vaccines. Considerations should include provider assessment, patient preference, and the potential for adverse events. Providers should consult the relevant Advisory Committee on Immunization Practices statement for detailed recommendations: **http://www.cdc.gov/vaccines/pubs/acip-list.htm**. Clinically significant adverse events that follow immunization should be reported to the Vaccine Adverse Event Reporting System (VAERS) at **http://www.vaers.hhs.gov** or by telephone, **800-822-7967**. Use of trade names and commercial sources is for identification only and does not imply endorsement by the U.S. Department of Health and Human Services.

1. **Hepatitis B vaccine (HepB).** (Minimum age: birth)
   At birth:
   • Administer monovalent HepB to all newborns before hospital discharge.
   • If mother is hepatitis B surface antigen (HBsAg)-positive, administer HepB and 0.5 mL of hepatitis B immune globulin (HBIG) within 12 hours of birth.
   • If mother's HBsAg status is unknown, administer HepB within 12 hours of birth. Determine mother's HBsAg status as soon as possible and, if HBsAg-positive, administer HBIG (no later than age 1 week).
   Doses following the birth dose:
   • The second dose should be administered at age 1 or 2 months. Monovalent HepB should be used for doses administered before age 6 weeks.
   • Infants born to HBsAg-positive mothers should be tested for HBsAg and antibody to HBsAg 1 to 2 months after completion of at least 3 doses of the HepB series, at age 9 through 18 months (generally at the next well-child visit).
   • Administration of 4 doses of HepB to infants is permissible when a combination vaccine containing HepB is administered after the birth dose.
   • Infants who did not receive a birth dose should receive 3 doses of HepB on a schedule of 0, 1, and 6 months.
   • The final (3rd or 4th) dose in the HepB series should be administered no earlier than age 24 weeks.
2. **Rotavirus vaccine (RV).** (Minimum age: 6 weeks)
   • Administer the first dose at age 6 through 14 weeks (maximum age: 14 weeks 6 days). Vaccination should not be initiated for infants aged 15 weeks 0 days or older.
   • The maximum age for the final dose in the series is 8 months 0 days
   • If Rotarix is administered at ages 2 and 4 months, a dose at 6 months is not indicated.
3. **Diphtheria and tetanus toxoids and acellular pertussis vaccine (DTaP).** (Minimum age: 6 weeks)
   • The fourth dose may be administered as early as age 12 months, provided at least 6 months have elapsed since the third dose.
4. **Haemophilus influenzae type b conjugate vaccine (Hib).** (Minimum age: 6 weeks)
   • If PRP-OMP (PedvaxHIB or Comvax [HepB-Hib]) is administered at ages 2 and 4 months, a dose at age 6 months is not indicated.
   • Hiberix should not be used for doses at ages 2, 4, or 6 months for the primary series but can be used as the final dose in children aged 12 months through 4 years.
5. **Pneumococcal vaccine.** (Minimum age: 6 weeks for pneumococcal conjugate vaccine [PCV]; 2 years for pneumococcal polysaccharide vaccine [PPSV])
   • PCV is recommended for all children aged younger than 5 years. Administer 1 dose of PCV to all healthy children aged 24 through 59 months who are not completely vaccinated for their age.
   • A PCV series begun with 7-valent PCV (PCV7) should be completed with 13-valent PCV (PCV13).
   • A single supplemental dose of PCV13 is recommended for all children aged 14 through 59 months who have received an age-appropriate series of PCV7.
   • A single supplemental dose of PCV13 is recommended for all children aged 60 through 71 months with underlying medical conditions who have received an age-appropriate series of PCV7.

   • The supplemental dose of PCV13 should be administered at least 8 weeks after the previous dose of PCV7. See MMWR 2010:59(No. RR-11).
   • Administer PPSV at least 8 weeks after last dose of PCV to children aged 2 years or older with certain underlying medical conditions, including a cochlear implant.
6. **Inactivated poliovirus vaccine (IPV).** (Minimum age: 6 weeks)
   • If 4 or more doses are administered prior to age 4 years an additional dose should be administered at age 4 through 6 years.
   • The final dose in the series should be administered on or after the fourth birthday and at least 6 months following the previous dose.
7. **Influenza vaccine (seasonal).** (Minimum age: 6 months for trivalent inactivated influenza vaccine [TIV]; 2 years for live, attenuated influenza vaccine [LAIV])
   • For healthy children aged 2 years and older (i.e., those who do not have underlying medical conditions that predispose them to influenza complications), either LAIV or TIV may be used, except LAIV should not be given to children aged 2 through 4 years who have had wheezing in the past 12 months.
   • Administer 2 doses (separated by at least 4 weeks) to children aged 6 months through 8 years who are receiving seasonal influenza vaccine for the first time or who were vaccinated for the first time during the previous influenza season but only received 1 dose.
   • Children aged 6 months through 8 years who received no doses of monovalent 2009 H1N1 vaccine should receive 2 doses of 2010–2011 seasonal influenza vaccine. See MMWR 2010;59(No. RR-8):33–34.
8. **Measles, mumps, and rubella vaccine (MMR).** (Minimum age: 12 months)
   • The second dose may be administered before age 4 years, provided at least 4 weeks have elapsed since the first dose.
9. **Varicella vaccine.** (Minimum age: 12 months)
   • The second dose may be administered before age 4 years, provided at least 3 months have elapsed since the first dose.
   • For children aged 12 months through 12 years the recommended minimum interval between doses is 3 months. However, if the second dose was administered at least 4 weeks after the first dose, it can be accepted as valid.
10. **Hepatitis A vaccine (HepA).** (Minimum age: 12 months)
    • Administer 2 doses at least 6 months apart.
    • HepA is recommended for children aged older than 23 months who live in areas where vaccination programs target older children, who are at increased risk for infection, or for whom immunity against hepatitis A is desired.
11. **Meningococcal conjugate vaccine, quadrivalent (MCV4).** (Minimum age: 2 years)
    • Administer 2 doses of MCV4 at least 8 weeks apart to children aged 2 through 10 years with persistent complement component deficiency and anatomic or functional asplenia, and 1 dose every 5 years thereafter.
    • Persons with human immunodeficiency virus (HIV) infection who are vaccinated with MCV4 should receive 2 doses at least 8 weeks apart.
    • Administer 1 dose of MCV4 to children aged 2 through 10 years who travel to countries with highly endemic or epidemic disease and during outbreaks caused by a vaccine serogroup.
    • Administer MCV4 to children at continued risk for meningococcal disease who were previously vaccinated with MCV4 or meningococcal polysaccharide vaccine after 3 years if the first dose was administered at age 2 through 6 years.

The Recommended Immunization Schedules for Persons Aged 0 Through 18 Years are approved by the Advisory Committee on Immunization Practices (**http://www.cdc.gov/vaccines/recs/acip**), the American Academy of Pediatrics (**http://www.aap.org**), and the American Academy of Family Physicians (**http://www.aafp.org**).
Department of Health and Human Services • Centers for Disease Control and Prevention

Figure 22-2 A 2011 immunization schedule, ages birth to 6 years.

Recommended Immunization Schedule for Persons Aged 7 Through 18 Years—United States • 2011

For those who fall behind or start late, see the schedule below and the catch-up schedule

Vaccine ▼ Age ▶	7–10 years	11–12 years	13–18 years	
Tetanus, Diphtheria, Pertussis[1]		Tdap	Tdap	Range of recommended ages for all children
Human Papillomavirus[2]	see footnote [2]	HPV (3 doses)(females)	HPV Series	
Meningococcal[3]	MCV4	MCV4	MCV4	
Influenza[4]	Influenza (Yearly)			
Pneumococcal[5]	Pneumococcal			Range of recommended ages for catch-up immunization
Hepatitis A[6]	HepA Series			
Hepatitis B[7]	Hep B Series			
Inactivated Poliovirus[8]	IPV Series			
Measles, Mumps, Rubella[9]	MMR Series			Range of recommended ages for certain high-risk groups
Varicella[10]	Varicella Series			

This schedule includes recommendations in effect as of December 21, 2010. Any dose not administered at the recommended age should be administered at a subsequent visit, when indicated and feasible. The use of a combination vaccine generally is preferred over separate injections of its equivalent component vaccines. Considerations should include provider assessment, patient preference, and the potential for adverse events. Providers should consult the relevant Advisory Committee on Immunization Practices statement for detailed recommendations: **http://www.cdc.gov/vaccines/pubs/acip-list.htm**. Clinically significant adverse events that follow immunization should be reported to the Vaccine Adverse Event Reporting System (VAERS) at **http://www.vaers.hhs.gov** or by telephone, **800-822-7967.**

1. **Tetanus and diphtheria toxoids and acellular pertussis vaccine (Tdap).**
   (Minimum age: 10 years for Boostrix and 11 years for Adacel)
   - Persons aged 11 through 18 years who have not received Tdap should receive a dose followed by Td booster doses every 10 years thereafter.
   - Persons aged 7 through 10 years who are not fully immunized against pertussis (including those never vaccinated or with unknown pertussis vaccination status) should receive a single dose of Tdap. Refer to the catch-up schedule if additional doses of tetanus and diphtheria toxoid–containing vaccine are needed.
   - Tdap can be administered regardless of the interval since the last tetanus and diphtheria toxoid–containing vaccine.

2. **Human papillomavirus vaccine (HPV).** (Minimum age: 9 years)
   - Quadrivalent HPV vaccine (HPV4) or bivalent HPV vaccine (HPV2) is recommended for the prevention of cervical precancers and cancers in females.
   - HPV4 is recommended for prevention of cervical precancers, cancers, and genital warts in females.
   - HPV4 may be administered in a 3-dose series to males aged 9 through 18 years to reduce their likelihood of genital warts.
   - Administer the second dose 1 to 2 months after the first dose and the third dose 6 months after the first dose (at least 24 weeks after the first dose).

3. **Meningococcal conjugate vaccine, quadrivalent (MCV4).** (Minimum age: 2 years)
   - Administer MCV4 at age 11 through 12 years with a booster dose at age 16 years.
   - Administer 1 dose at age 13 through 18 years if not previously vaccinated.
   - Persons who received their first dose at age 13 through 15 years should receive a booster dose at age 16 through 18 years.
   - Administer 1 dose to previously unvaccinated college freshmen living in a dormitory.
   - Administer 2 doses at least 8 weeks apart to children aged 2 through 10 years with persistent complement component deficiency and anatomic or functional asplenia, and 1 dose every 5 years thereafter.
   - Persons with HIV infection who are vaccinated with MCV4 should receive 2 doses at least 8 weeks apart.
   - Administer 1 dose of MCV4 to children aged 2 through 10 years who travel to countries with highly endemic or epidemic disease and during outbreaks caused by a vaccine serogroup.
   - Administer MCV4 to children at continued risk for meningococcal disease who were previously vaccinated with MCV4 or meningococcal polysaccharide vaccine after 3 years (if first dose administered at age 2 through 6 years) or after 5 years (if first dose administered at age 7 years or older).

4. **Influenza vaccine (seasonal).**
   - For healthy nonpregnant persons aged 7 through 18 years (i.e., those who do not have underlying medical conditions that predispose them to influenza complications), either LAIV or TIV may be used.
   - Administer 2 doses (separated by at least 4 weeks) to children aged 6 months through 8 years who are receiving seasonal influenza vaccine for the first time or who were vaccinated for the first time during the previous influenza season but only received 1 dose.
   - Children 6 months through 8 years of age who received no doses of monovalent 2009 H1N1 vaccine should receive 2 doses of 2010-2011 seasonal influenza vaccine. See *MMWR* 2010;59(No. RR-8):33–34.

5. **Pneumococcal vaccines.**
   - A single dose of 13-valent pneumococcal conjugate vaccine (PCV13) may be administered to children aged 6 through 18 years who have functional or anatomic asplenia, HIV infection or other immunocompromising condition, cochlear implant or CSF leak. See *MMWR* 2010;59(No. RR-11).
   - The dose of PCV13 should be administered at least 8 weeks after the previous dose of PCV7.
   - Administer pneumococcal polysaccharide vaccine at least 8 weeks after the last dose of PCV to children aged 2 years or older with certain underlying medical conditions, including a cochlear implant. A single revaccination should be administered after 5 years to children with functional or anatomic asplenia or an immunocompromising condition.

6. **Hepatitis A vaccine (HepA).**
   - Administer 2 doses at least 6 months apart.
   - HepA is recommended for children aged older than 23 months who live in areas where vaccination programs target older children, or who are at increased risk for infection, or for whom immunity against hepatitis A is desired.

7. **Hepatitis B vaccine (HepB).**
   - Administer the 3-dose series to those not previously vaccinated. For those with incomplete vaccination, follow the catch-up schedule.
   - A 2-dose series (separated by at least 4 months) of adult formulation Recombivax HB is licensed for children aged 11 through 15 years.

8. **Inactivated poliovirus vaccine (IPV).**
   - The final dose in the series should be administered on or after the fourth birthday and at least 6 months following the previous dose.
   - If both OPV and IPV were administered as part of a series, a total of 4 doses should be administered, regardless of the child's current age.

9. **Measles, mumps, and rubella vaccine (MMR).**
   - The minimum interval between the 2 doses of MMR is 4 weeks.

10. **Varicella vaccine.**
    - For persons aged 7 through 18 years without evidence of immunity (see *MMWR* 2007;56[No. RR-4]), administer 2 doses if not previously vaccinated or the second dose if only 1 dose has been administered.
    - For persons aged 7 through 12 years, the recommended minimum interval between doses is 3 months. However, if the second dose was administered at least 4 weeks after the first dose, it can be accepted as valid.
    - For persons aged 13 years and older, the minimum interval between doses is 4 weeks.

The Recommended Immunization Schedules for Persons Aged 0 Through 18 Years are approved by the Advisory Committee on Immunization Practices (**http://www.cdc.gov/vaccines/recs/acip**), the American Academy of Pediatrics (**http://www.aap.org**), and the American Academy of Family Physicians (**http://www.aafp.org**).
Department of Health and Human Services • Centers for Disease Control and Prevention

Figure 22-3 A 2011 immunization schedule, ages 7 to 18 years. (Accessed at http://www.cdc.gov/vaccines/recs/schedules/downloads/child/7-18yrs-schedule-pr.pdf.)

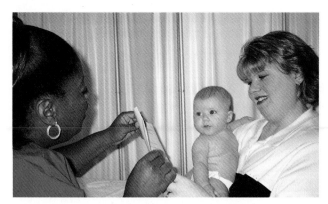

Figure 22-4 Provide VIS to the caregiver before administering any vaccines.

Role of the Parent

Parents are a source of support and comfort to a child. Their presence minimizes stress in unfamiliar surroundings. Encourage parents to remain with young children and to assist in care when appropriate. For instance, ask the parent to stand beside the child as you weigh him or her. Many children are more compliant if much of the preliminary workup is performed while the parent **restrains,** or holds, the child (Fig. 22-7).

As a child develops and becomes more **autonomous,** or independent, a parent's immediate presence may be less meaningful as long as the child knows that the parent is close by. Many adolescent patients prefer to be alone with the physician to demonstrate their independence and to discuss matters that they may not be comfortable talking about with the parent present. Depending on the maturity of the adolescent, ask the patient, not the parent, if the parent should be present during the examination.

 CHECKPOINT QUESTION

3. What kinds of feelings might a pediatric patient experience during an office visit?

 LEGAL TIP

MAKE SURE YOUR INTERVIEW QUESTIONS ARE APPROPRIATE

Some states require obtaining parental permission before treating a minor patient. The exceptions to this rule may include:

- Pregnancy or prenatal care
- Sexually transmitted disease
- Rape
- Life-threatening injury

Emancipated minors (children under age 18 years who support themselves financially), minors enlisted in the armed services, and married minors may obtain treatment without parental consent. You are responsible for knowing your state's laws regarding the treatment of minors.

COG The Pediatric Physical Examination

Typically, you prepare the pediatric patient for examination, and you may also assist with the examination by restraining the child. Often, you are responsible for documenting much of the history and the chief complaint and for collecting specimens for diagnostic testing. When approaching the patient, you should have a calm and cheerful manner and use a firm, but gentle, touch to increase the patient's feeling of security. Involve the parents as much as possible during the examination and keep them in the infant or child's view to reduce anxiety for both the patient and the parent.

During the examination, the physician will systematically review the body systems of the patient. The general appearance of the infant or child is assessed; the heart and lungs are auscultated; the eyes, ears, nose, and throat are inspected; and developmental issues appropriate for the age of the child are discussed with the parent or caregiver. The child who is preschool age or older will have vision and hearing tested. Your role includes obtaining relevant data from the parent, obtaining anthropometric measurements, and performing hearing and vision screening tests as appropriate. Of course, you will be responsible for recording this information in the patient's medical record.

The Pediatric History

A child's medical history differs greatly from an adult patient's history. During the early years, it is important to know the prenatal history, including details of the mother's pregnancy, labor, and delivery. The length of the pregnancy, any maternal illnesses or complications, neonatal complications, and risk factors must be recorded as predictors of the infant's health and development. Most newborn charts contain a copy of the delivery record or birth summary outlining the delivery with the Apgar score and progress notes from the newborn nursery (Box 22-1). As the child grows, the history expands to include childhood illnesses, developmental milestones, immunizations, and nutritional status.

MEASLES, MUMPS & RUBELLA (MMR) VACCINES

WHAT YOU NEED TO KNOW

Many Vaccine Information Statements are available in Spanish and other languages. See www.immunize.org/vis.

1 | Why get vaccinated?

Measles, mumps, and rubella are serious diseases.

Measles
- Measles virus causes rash, cough, runny nose, eye irritation, and fever.
- It can lead to ear infection, pneumonia, seizures (jerking and staring), brain damage, and death.

Mumps
- Mumps virus causes fever, headache, and swollen glands.
- It can lead to deafness, meningitis (infection of the brain and spinal cord covering), painful swelling of the testicles or ovaries, and, rarely, death.

Rubella (German Measles)
- Rubella virus causes rash, mild fever, and arthritis (mostly in women).
- If a woman gets rubella while she is pregnant, she could have a miscarriage or her baby could be born with serious birth defects.

You or your child could catch these diseases by being around someone who has them. They spread from person to person through the air.

Measles, mumps, and rubella (MMR) vaccine can prevent these diseases.

Most children who get their MMR shots will not get these diseases. Many more children would get them if we stopped vaccinating.

2 | Who should get MMR vaccine and when?

Children should get 2 doses of MMR vaccine:

– The first at **12-15 months of age**
– and the second at **4-6 years of age**.

These are the recommended ages. But children can get the second dose at any age, as long as it is at least 28 days after the first dose.

Some **adults** should also get MMR vaccine:

Generally, anyone 18 years of age or older who was born after 1956 should get at least one dose of MMR vaccine, unless they can show that they have had either the vaccines or the diseases.

Ask your provider for more information.

MMR vaccine may be given at the same time as other vaccines.

> Note: A "combination" vaccine called **MMRV**, which contains both MMR and varicella (chickenpox) vaccines, may be given instead of the two individual vaccines to people 12 years of age and younger.

3 | Some people should not get MMR vaccine or should wait

- People should not get MMR vaccine who have ever had a life-threatening allergic reaction to gelatin, the antibiotic neomycin, or to a previous dose of MMR vaccine.

- People who are moderately or severely ill at the time the shot is scheduled should usually wait until they recover before getting MMR vaccine.

- Pregnant women should wait to get MMR vaccine until after they have given birth. Women should avoid getting pregnant for 4 weeks after getting MMR vaccine.

- Some people should check with their doctor about whether they should get MMR vaccine, including anyone who:
  - Has HIV/AIDS, or another disease that affects the immune system
  - Is being treated with drugs that affect the immune system, such as steroids, for 2 weeks or longer.
  - Has any kind of cancer
  - Is taking cancer treatment with x-rays or drugs
  - Has ever had a low platelet count (a blood disorder)

- People who recently had a transfusion or were given other blood products should ask their doctor when they may get MMR vaccine

Ask your provider for more information.

Figure 22-5 2011 Measles, Mumps, & Rubella (MMR) Vaccine Information Statement. (Accessed at http://www.cdc.gov/vaccines/pubs/vis/downloads/vis-mmr.pdf.)

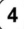
4 | What are the risks from MMR vaccine?

A vaccine, like any medicine, is capable of causing serious problems, such as severe allergic reactions. The risk of MMR vaccine causing serious harm, or death, is extremely small.

Getting MMR vaccine is much safer than getting any of these three diseases.

Most people who get MMR vaccine do not have any problems with it.

Mild Problems

- Fever (up to 1 person out of 6)
- Mild rash (about 1 person out of 20)
- Swelling of glands in the cheeks or neck (rare)

If these problems occur, it is usually within 7-12 days after the shot. They occur less often after the second dose.

Moderate Problems

- Seizure (jerking or staring) caused by fever (about 1 out of 3,000 doses)
- Temporary pain and stiffness in the joints, mostly in teenage or adult women (up to 1 out of 4)
- Temporary low platelet count, which can cause a bleeding disorder (about 1 out of 30,000 doses)

Severe Problems (Very Rare)

- Serious allergic reaction (less than 1 out of a million doses)
- Several other severe problems have been known to occur after a child gets MMR vaccine. But this happens so rarely, experts cannot be sure whether they are caused by the vaccine or not. These include:
  - Deafness
  - Long-term seizures, coma, or lowered consciousness
  - Permanent brain damage

> Note: The first dose of **MMRV** vaccine has been associated with rash and higher rates of fever than MMR and varicella vaccines given separately. Rash has been reported in about 1 person in 20 and fever in about 1 person in 5.
> Seizures caused by a fever are also reported more often after MMRV. These usually occur 5-12 days after the first dose.

5 | What if there is a moderate or severe reaction?

What should I look for?

- Any unusual condition, such as a high fever, weakness, or behavior changes. Signs of a serious

allergic reaction can include difficulty breathing, hoarseness or wheezing, hives, paleness, weakness, a fast heart beat or dizziness.

What should I do?

- **Call** a doctor, or get the person to a doctor right away.
- **Tell** your doctor what happened, the date and time it happened, and when the vaccination was given.
- **Ask** your provider to report the reaction by filing a Vaccine Adverse Event Reporting System (VAERS) form.
  Or you can file this report through the VAERS website at **www.vaers.hhs.gov**, or by calling **1-800-822-7967**.

VAERS does not provide medical advice.

6 | The National Vaccine Injury Compensation Program

A federal program has been created to help people who may have been harmed by a vaccine.

For details about the National Vaccine Injury Compensation Program, call **1-800-338-2382** or visit their website at **www.hrsa.gov/vaccinecompensation**.

7 | How can I learn more?

- Ask your provider. They can give you the vaccine package insert or suggest other sources of information.
- Call your local or state health department.
- Contact the Centers for Disease Control and Prevention (CDC):
  - Call **1-800-232-4636 (1-800-CDC-INFO)**
  - Visit CDC website at: **www.cdc.gov/vaccines**

DEPARTMENT OF HEALTH AND HUMAN SERVICES
CENTERS FOR DISEASE CONTROL AND PREVENTION

Vaccine Information Statement (Interim)
MMR Vaccine (3/13/08) 42 U.S.C. §300aa-26

Figure 22-5 *(continued)*

TABLE 22-2	Common Childhood Illnesses		
Illness	**Signs and Symptoms**	**Cause**	**Treatment**
Common cold	Congestion, cough, malaise, sore throat, fever	Virus	Increase oral fluids, rest, mist humidifier, cold medications if ordered by the physician
Gastroenteritis	Vomiting, diarrhea, fever	Virus *or* bacteria	Increase oral fluids, medications if ordered by the physician
Otitis media	Earache (may accompany or follow a cold), reduced the hearing, fever, tugging at the affected ear in infants	Virus *or* bacteria	Increased oral fluids, medications if ordered by physician

TABLE 22-3	Pediatric Growth and Developmental Stages			
Age	**Growth**	**Stage**	**Development**	**Medical Assistant Considerations**
Infancy (0–1 yr)	Triples birth weight; increases physical control of body; may walk by first birthday	Trust	Newborn can see, hear, smell, feel pain, and communicate. Protective mechanisms include blink reflex, pulling in for warmth, and pulling away from pain or restraint. Development cephalic to caudal: head control; then full-body control (e.g., rolling over, crawling, walking); then motor (e.g., picking up small objects). Fastest period of growth and development, from total dependence to walking and talking.	Involve parent; keep parent in child's view; approach child slowly; use soft, soothing voice; speak reassuringly. Advise parents to call for fever over 100.5°F, diarrhea, vomiting, failure to nurse or take a bottle. Encourage appropriate use of car seat as required by law in most states.
Toddler (1–3 yr)	Growth rate slows; body proportions change; language skills begin	Autonomy	Growth levels off but exploration and social development continue. Negativism precedes autonomy. The child will begin to seek relationships and is acutely aware of strangers.	Use all skills above; explain procedures so child can understand; expect resistance; use firm, direct approach; ignore negative behavior; restrain to maintain child's safety; allow child to hold security object. Warn parents of increased potential for accidents. Continue to encourage use of car seat and proper restraint in motor vehicle.

(continued)

TABLE **22-3**			**Pediatric Growth and Developmental Stages** *(continued)*	
Age	**Growth**	**Stage**	**Development**	**Medical Assistant Considerations**
Preschool (3–6 yr)	Language and self-control develop; motor skills increase	Initiative	Socialization continues, with fairly clear-marked stages of social development in next 10 years. Many early-stage problems resolve. Except for usual communicable diseases, generally a time of good health. Diseases such as leukemia, Hodgkin disease, and various sarcomata may present, but these are usually years spent establishing relationships with peers, exercising autonomy, and completing growth process.	Use all skills above. Encourage child to speak about feelings; explain why procedure is being done; have child help as much as possible (e.g., hold equipment). Advise parents to be alert for risks of accidents and trauma with riding toys such as tricycles and bicycles. Encourage the use of helmets. *Children over 40 pounds or 4 years can use booster seat until 8 years or 4 ft. 9 in. tall. Check your state laws.*
School age (6–12 yr)	Social skills develop; peer group becomes important; self-concept develops	Industry		Involve child in decision making; involve child in care (e.g., collecting specimens, choosing which procedure is done first; encourage and support questions). Children may indicate what hurts and how they feel, so include child when asking questions. *Encourage use of booster seat to age 8 years and seatbelt thereafter, according to state law.*
Adolescent (12–18 yr)	Emotional changes; identity, place in world being defined	Identity		Discuss procedures so adolescent can understand; adolescents may resist authority figures; be sure patient education includes smoking, alcohol, and perhaps birth control and sexually transmitted diseases. At physician's discretion, this information may be discussed without parent. As children in this age group begin to drive, encourage use of seatbelts for self and passengers.

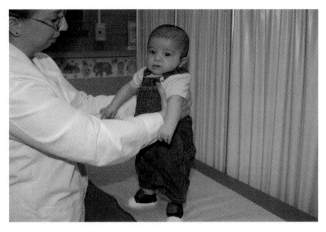

Figure 22-6 The presence or absence of reflexes is determined during the pediatric examination.

Obtaining and Recording Measurements and Vital Signs

Before the physical examination is conducted, you should obtain some or all of the following measurements: height or length, head and chest circumference, weight, temperature, and the pulse and respiratory rate. The blood pressure may or may not be required, depending on the child's age and the preference of the examiner. The measurements and schedule for obtaining them should be detailed in the office policy and procedure manual.

For a well-child visit, you typically measure the child's height or length, head and chest circumference, and weight. These measurements show the child's growth and development patterns and are good indicators of health status. Weight is the most frequently obtained

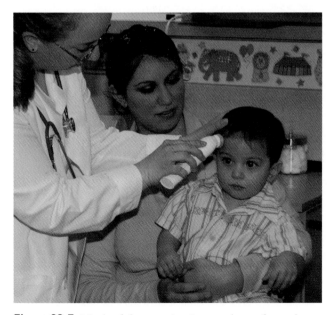

Figure 22-7 Much of the examination can be performed while the caregiver holds the baby.

BOX 22-1

THE APGAR SCORE

Named for pediatrician Virginia Apgar, the Apgar score is a method for describing the general health of newborns at 1 minute and 5 minutes after delivery. Signs assessed include:

- Heart rate
- Respiratory effort
- Muscle tone
- Response to a suction catheter in the nostril
- Color

A perfect score for each sign is 2; a total absence of any sign is 0. A perfect score of 10 indicates the following:

- Heart rate is greater than 100 beats per minute.
- Respirations are eupneic, or the baby is crying.
- Muscle tone is good, and the baby is active.
- Baby coughs or sneezes in response to suction catheter.
- Skin is completely pink, with no acrocyanosis.

Most babies have 1-minute scores of 7 to 9 because many have a bit of acrocyanosis until respiration is fully established. Babies with 1-minute scores below 4 usually require medical assistance, particularly respiratory intervention with oxygen.

The Apgar score is not considered an indicator of future intelligence or health problems. Rather, it is used by the obstetrician, pediatrician, and delivery room personnel to assess newborns who may require closer observation or intervention.

---

measurement in pediatrics; it is often needed by the physician to assess nutritional status and determine medication dosages. Head and chest measurements may alert the physician to cardiac or intracranial abnormalities. Procedures 22-1 and 22-2 describe the steps for obtaining the weight, length, and head and chest circumference.

After obtaining these measurements, you may be required to graph the weight, height or length, and head circumference on a separate growth chart that is placed into the patient's medical record (Fig. 22-8A,B). These charts are designed to show the child's growth patterns using data obtained at each well-child visit. Once the measurements are plotted, the child's percentile can be determined. The percentile is used to compare the patient's growth with those of children of the same age. The head circumference is not included on growth charts for children older than 36 months, and chest circumference is usually not graphed.

Birth to 36 months: Girls
Head circumference-for-age and
Weight-for-length percentiles

NAME _____

RECORD # _____

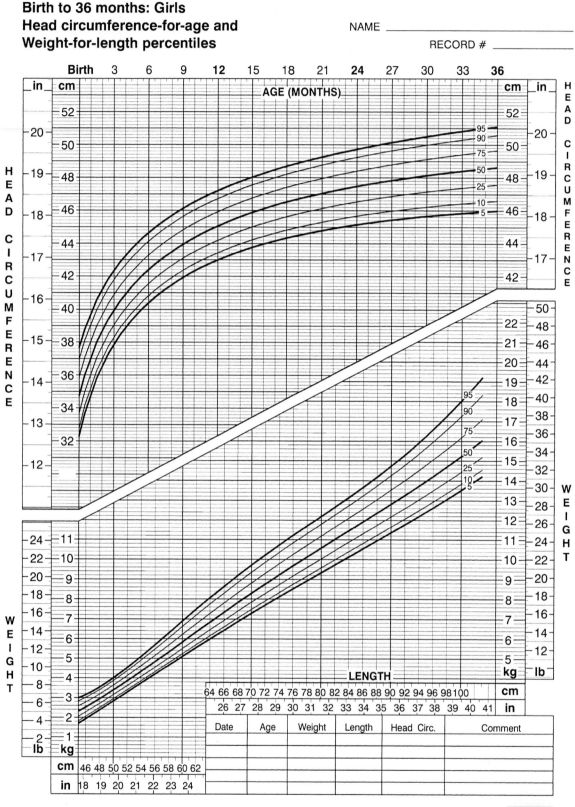

Published May 30, 2000 (modified 10/16/00).
SOURCE: Developed by the National Center for Health Statistics in collaboration with
the National Center for Chronic Disease Prevention and Health Promotion (2000).
http://www.cdc.gov/growthcharts

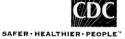

SAFER · HEALTHIER · PEOPLE™

A

Figure 22-8 Growth charts. (**A**) Birth to 36 months, girls.

2 to 20 years: Boys
Stature-for-age and Weight-for-age percentiles

NAME _____

RECORD # _____

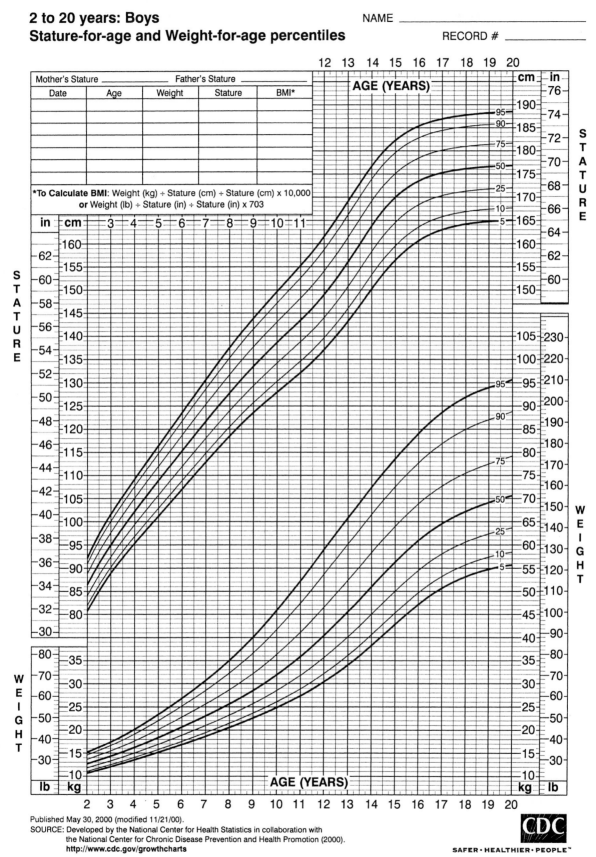

Published May 30, 2000 (modified 11/21/00).

SOURCE: Developed by the National Center for Health Statistics in collaboration with
the National Center for Chronic Disease Prevention and Health Promotion (2000).
http://www.cdc.gov/growthcharts

CDC
SAFER · HEALTHIER · PEOPLE™

B

Figure 22-8 *(continued)* Growth charts. (**B**) Age 2 to 20 years, boys.

CHECKPOINT QUESTION

4. Why is it important to track a child's anthropometric measurements?

Pediatric Vital Signs

Temperature

A child's temperature may be measured by the axillary, oral, rectal, tympanic, or temporal artery method. If the child is compliant, the axillary route is satisfactory, but the tympanic and temporal artery methods have gained popularity because they are rapid, reliable, and most readily accepted at all ages (see Fig. 22-7). Oral measurement may be used with an older child but should not be used if the child is congested, coughing, vomiting, or uncooperative. The rectal route should not be used for newborns and small infants or if the child has diarrhea.

Pulse and Respirations

The pulse rate reflects the heart rate and usually is easily measured. Pulse rate can be affected by activity, body temperature, emotion, and illness. The pulse of children under 2 years of age should be assessed apically. To do this, place the stethoscope on the chest between the sternum and left nipple. Count the rate for 1 full minute. For children older than 2 years, take the radial pulse. Expect the child's heart rate to be considerably higher than an adult's rate. A newborn may have a pulse rate of 100 to 180 beats per minute, and with fever, a rate of 200 beats per minute or more is not unusual. As the child matures, the rate will slow. By age 2, a child's rate may range from 70 to 100 beats per minute. By puberty, the rate is comparable to that of an adult. Table 22-4 details normal pulse rates for children.

Measure respiratory rate by observing the rise and fall of the child's chest. It is not necessary to disguise the fact that you are counting respirations as with adults. Because infants breathe using the abdominal muscles more than the chest, observe abdominal movements and count for 1 full minute. For children over age 2 years, use the same method as adults: count the respiratory rate for 30 seconds and multiply by two. Expect a newborn's respiratory rate to be as high as 35 per minute (Table 22-5). Like the pulse rate, the respiratory rate

TABLE 22-4	Normal Pulse Rates for Children
Age	**Rate/Minute**
Newborn	100–180
3 mo–2 yr	80–150
2–10 yr	65–130
10 yr and older	60–100

TABLE 22-5	Normal Respiratory Rates for Children
Age	**Rate/Minute**
Newborn	30–35
1–2 yr	25–30
4–6 yr	23–25
8 yr and older	16–20

will slow as the child matures. At age 2 years, it will be about 25, and by puberty, it will be comparable to an adult's rate.

Blood Pressure

Blood pressure measurements are not required for most pediatric patients but may be appropriate at times. Blood pressure is the most difficult measurement to obtain in an infant or child because it is so difficult to prevent movement. Infants and children have smaller extremities than adults and require a smaller cuff. Because of their soft, nonresistant vessels and smaller bodies, children have lower blood pressure than adults. You may have problems determining the diastolic pressure in some children using a standard sphygmomanometer. In children less than 1 year of age, expect a blood pressure of about 90/50. The blood pressure will gradually rise as the child matures. By age 10, a child's blood pressure will be in the low normal range of 110/60 (Table 22-6). Blood pressure checks become routine when children are about school age.

CHECKPOINT QUESTION

5. How does a child's pulse and respiratory rate differ from an adult's?

COG Administering Medications

Administering medications to children challenges you and the parents who are responsible for home administration. Medication dosages for children are calculated

TABLE 22-6	Normal Blood Pressure for Children	
Age	**Systolic**	**Diastolic**
Newborn	<90	<70
1–5 yr	<110	<70
10 yr and older	<120	<84

Blood pressure measured in millimeters of mercury.

by weight or by body surface area. However, because children vary in weight, age, and fat-to-muscle ratio, they metabolize and absorb medication at varying rates. As a result, the physician prescribes medication according to how much the child weighs, and you must give only the amount prescribed. To prevent errors, always check drug dosage calculations for an infant or child with another staff member. The formulas for calculating pediatric dosages are described in Chapter 9. Before administering any medication, you should know the safe amount, correct administration procedure, intended actions, and side effects. In most pediatric practices, the physician uses only 50 or so medications that are suitable for children, making it relatively easy for you to learn all that is necessary about each medication. As for any medication, the seven "rights" of drug administration remain the same: the *right patient*, *right drug*, *right dose*, *right route*, *right time*, *right method*, and *right documentation*.

Oral Medications

Use caution when administering oral medications to a child to prevent **aspiration**. Hold infants in a semi-reclining position, not lying down. Place the medication in the mouth beside the tongue. Depending on the child's age, use a medication spoon, syringe, dropper, or medicine cup. Many children will suck medication from a syringe easily and safely. Administer small amounts of medication, allowing the child time to swallow. Always explain to children who are old enough to understand why medications are important, and then proceed in a swift and safe manner to give the medication.

Injections

Medications are given to infants and children by injection when there is no choice. Children commonly fear injections more than any other medical procedure. You should approach the child in a calm and firm manner, but never lie to the child or say that the injection will not hurt. Although it is important for the child to know that an injection is about to be given, you can prevent some anxiety by not letting the child see the syringe. Offer the child an age-appropriate explanation, and then quickly give the medication. After administering any medication, praise and comfort the child.

Most children's injections are given in the vastus lateralis, at least until age 2 years (Fig. 22-9). The dorsogluteal site is not used for children under age 2 years because the muscles have not developed well. Chapter 9 lists the steps in administering an intramuscular injection.

 CHECKPOINT QUESTION

6. How is medication dosage calculated for children?

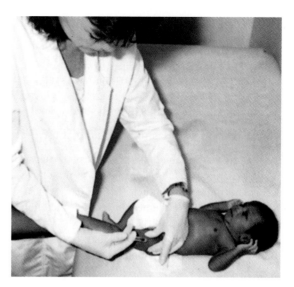

Figure 22-9 The vastus lateralis is the site of choice for infant injections.

COG **Collecting a Urine Specimen**

Because infants and small children cannot void into a specimen container on command, you must use a collection device if a urine specimen is needed. Procedure 22-3 describes the procedure for applying a urinary collection device. Once applied, the device should be left in place until the infant urinates. The infant may wear a diaper over the collection device until the specimen is obtained.

COG **Understanding Child Abuse**

A child's social and physical well-being may be compromised by physical or emotional abuse or neglect or by sexual abuse. Abuse is thought to be the second most common cause of death in children under age 5 years. Although many children are permanently disabled or seriously injured as a result of physical abuse, many more carry emotional scars that will never heal. Medical assistants should be aware of the signs of abuse—either obvious indications or subtle warnings—that must be pursued for the child's safety.

These are the *obvious* indications of child abuse:

- Reports of physical or sexual abuse by the child
- Previous reports of abuse in the family with current indicators
- Conflicting stories about the "accident" or injury from the parents and the child
- Injuries inconsistent with the history
- Injuries blamed on siblings or someone other than the parent
- Repeated emergency room visits for injuries
- Fractures, burns, or skeletal injuries of a suspicious nature

These indications of child abuse are *hidden* or not apparent:

- Dislocations
- Nervous system trauma, particularly shaken baby syndrome
- Internal injuries, particularly to the abdominal area

These are *behavioral* indications of child abuse:

- Too-willing compliance, overeagerness to please
- Passive avoidance, such as refusing to make eye contact, shrinking from contact
- Extremely aggressive, demanding, rage-filled behavior
- Role reversal, parenting the parent
- Developmental delay (the child may be using energy needed for maturation to defend against abuse)

These are the *warning signs* of child abuse:

- Malnutrition
- Poor growth pattern
- Poor hygiene
- Gross dental disorders
- Unattended medical needs

If you suspect a child is being abused, approach the child and the parent in a calm and supportive manner. Discuss any suspicions about the cause of a child's injuries privately with the physician right away. State laws vary regarding the procedure for reporting abuse; local regulations should be outlined in the policies and procedures manual. As a medical assistant, you have an ethical and moral responsibility to report suspected cases of abuse or neglect.

LEGAL TIP

REPORTING SUSPECTED CHILD ABUSE

The Federal Child Abuse Prevention and Treatment Act mandates that threats to a child's physical and mental welfare be reported by anyone having contact with children in a professional or employment setting (e.g., teachers, physicians, nurses, medical assistants, daycare workers). Health care workers, teachers, social workers, and others who work with children are protected against liability if they report their suspicions in good faith.

COG Pediatric Illnesses and Disorders

Because children do not have a well-developed immune system, they are particularly susceptible to viral and bacterial infections. As a result, sick-child visits occur frequently during early childhood. Some infants and small children have febrile seizures during illness because of the child's immature nervous system. This does not mean that the child will be prone to seizures as he or she matures. Parents should be instructed how to obtain a child's temperature and be encouraged to call the office for any evidence of a fever. All parents should be advised never to give aspirin to young children with viral fever, since aspirin has been associated with Reye syndrome. This syndrome causes encephalopathy and fatty infiltration of the internal organs and may cause either mental retardation or death. Check with the physician about the type of medication to use before suggesting any medication or antipyretic, including over-the-counter medications.

Impetigo

A common skin disorder in children is impetigo, a contagious bacterial infection that may be caused by either the *Staphylococcus* or *Streptococcus* bacteria. The lesions commonly occur on the face, neck, and other exposed areas of the body (Fig. 22-10). Patches of exudative vesicles produce honey-colored crusts. These vesicles leave red areas when the crusts are removed.

The treatment for impetigo is washing the area two to three times a day and applying a topical antibiotic. An oral antibiotic may be prescribed for severe cases. Discourage scratching and advise parents to keep separate and wash frequently any towels, washcloths, and bed linens to prevent the spread of the disease.

Meningitis

Inflammation of the meninges covering the spinal cord and the brain, termed meningitis, can result from either a bacterial or a viral infection. Viral meningitis is usually not life threatening and is short lived, but bacterial meningitis is often severe and may be fatal. The infectious process is usually precipitated by an upper respiratory, sinus, or ear infection, and since these infections commonly occur in children under age 5 years, they are the most likely age group to develop this disease.

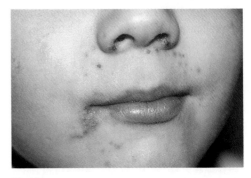

Figure 22-10 Impetigo lesions are commonly found on the face and neck.

Meningitis can also result from head trauma in which an open area allows the microorganisms to enter the nervous system. Older adolescents living in college dormitories or residence halls are also at high risk for meningitis and should be immunized before leaving for college.

The signs and symptoms of meningitis include nausea, vomiting, fever, headaches, and a stiff neck. A rash with small, reddish-purple dots may appear on the body. As the patient becomes sicker, he or she may become comatose and develop seizures. To diagnose suspected meningitis, the patient is often sent to the emergency room where the physician orders a complete blood count. If the white blood cell count is elevated, a lumbar puncture is performed to withdraw cerebrospinal fluid for analysis. The treatment of meningitis is based on the microorganism. Bacterial and viral meningitis are treated with oral fluids and bed rest, and antibiotics are prescribed if the causative micoorganism is bacterial. Although hospitalization is always required for bacterial meningitis, children with viral meningitis may also be admitted to the hospital for supportive care.

CHECKPOINT QUESTION

7. How does treatment of viral meningitis differ from that of bacterial meningitis?

Encephalitis

Encephalitis is inflammation of the brain that frequently results from a viral infection following chickenpox, measles, or mumps. A strain of the virus is transmitted by mosquitoes. This type is primarily seen on the East and Gulf coasts. Symptoms of all forms include drowsiness, headache, and fever in the early stages; however, seizures and coma may occur in the later stages. As with meningitis, patients suspected of having encephalitis are usually sent to the hospital emergency room for evaluation, including a lumbar puncture and analysis of the cerebrospinal fluid. A diagnosis of encephalitis requires hospitalization for intravenous therapy and supportive care, but the prognosis is usually good if the diagnosis is made early and treatment begins quickly.

Tetanus

Tetanus, commonly called *lockjaw*, is an infection of nervous tissue caused by the tetanus bacillus, *Clostridium tetani*, which lives in the intestinal tract of animals and is excreted in their feces. The organisms are found in almost all soil. The bacilli enter the body through a puncture wound or open area in the skin. Wounds caused by farm equipment in which manure is present

are especially susceptible to tetanus. All deep, dirty wounds should be treated as high risk for tetanus. You should make it a habit to always ask about previous tetanus immunization in patients with any type of accidental laceration or puncture wounds. The vaccine for tetanus is included in the schedule of pediatric immunizations as the diphtheria and tetanus toxoids and acellular pertussis vaccine (DTaP).

CHECKPOINT QUESTION

8. What is the best way to prevent tetanus?

Cerebral Palsy

Cerebral palsy is a term for a group of neuromuscular disorders that result from central nervous system damage sustained during the prenatal, neonatal, or postnatal period of development. Although cerebral palsy is not progressive, the damage may become more obvious as developmental delays are discovered. Impairment may range from slight motor dysfunction to catastrophic physical and mental disabilities. Prognosis varies with the site of the damage and its severity, and, unfortunately, there is no cure. Treatment for patients with cerebral palsy is supportive and rehabilitative. Although the physical impairments may be obvious, you must determine the developmental level of each child individually and interact with the child accordingly. In addition, the physical challenges exhibited by the child with cerebral palsy may not reflect the cognitive abilities. These children may acquire the same pediatric illness and diseases of any child and require immunizations and follow-up expected for any patient. You may also be involved in obtaining preauthorizations and referrals for rehabilitative and supportive care as ordered by the physician.

Croup

Laryngotracheobronchitis, also known as *croup*, is a disease primarily seen in children 3 months to 3 years of age. This disease is caused by a viral infection of the larynx resulting in swelling and narrowing of the airway, which results in dyspnea (difficulty breathing). A child exhibiting signs of possible croup will often have stridor (high-pitched crowing wheeze) on inspiration and a sharp, barking cough. Although children diagnosed with croup may be seen in the office, some children may require hospitalization as determined by the physician. Whether treated at home or in the hospital, antibiotics are usually not ordered unless a secondary bacterial infection is suspected. A cool mist vaporizer and medication to decrease the swelling are often prescribed by the physician.

Epiglottitis

Swelling of the epiglottis may resemble croup, but it is usually more serious and may be life threatening if it progresses to complete obstruction of the airway. It occurs most frequently in children aged 2 to 6 years, although it can be seen in all age groups. It is caused by a bacterial infection, usually *Haemophilus influenzae*. A child diagnosed with epiglottitis in the medical office must be transported immediately to the hospital, since the first priority is maintaining and possibly establishing an airway. As with any medical emergency in the office, you must be prepared to assist the physician as needed while contacting the emergency medical services for transport. In addition, the parents of the sick child will need support and guidance during this emotional time.

Cystic Fibrosis

Cystic fibrosis is an inherited disease that affects the exocrine glands of the body, changing their secretions and making the mucus extremely thick and sticky. Although the disease affects several areas of the body, the most serious complications of cystic fibrosis are usually respiratory. Children with cystic fibrosis are prone to repeated respiratory infections because of the difficulty in clearing the mucus from their airways. Treatment of cystic fibrosis includes medication to reduce the thickness of secretions and frequent breathing treatments to maintain open airways. Many new treatments are being developed, and much exciting research into prevention and cure is underway.

 CHECKPOINT QUESTION

9. Why is epiglottitis considered a medical emergency?

Asthma

As discussed in Chapter 15, asthma is a reversible inflammatory process of the bronchi and bronchioles. When a patient with asthma has dyspnea, it is due to bronchospasm and constriction of the smooth muscle lining the airways. Patients have an increase in mucus production with a productive cough. It becomes difficult for the patient to move air into and out of the lungs. In children, asthma attacks may be triggered by exposure to an allergen in the environment such as mold or dust, an inhaled irritant such as cigarette smoke, or upper respiratory infection. Many children who develop asthma outgrow it by adulthood.

The treatment for asthma includes the administration of bronchodilators through an inhaler, which may not be appropriate for a small child or infant, or through a nebulizer machine (see Chapter 15 for more information about nebulized breathing treatments). An infant

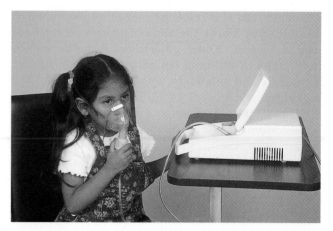

Figure 22-11 Breathing treatments may be administered through a mask.

or small child will not be able to hold the mouthpiece tightly between the lips during the treatment; however, masks are available (Fig. 22-11). As with adult patients taking bronchodilators, the pulse rate should be monitored before, during, and after the treatment.

Otitis Media

Otitis media, an inflammation or infection of the middle ear, is frequently caused by an upper respiratory infection (URI) in infants and children (Fig. 22-12). This disorder is particularly common in infants and children because of the relatively horizontal position of the eustachian tube between the nasopharynx and middle ear (see Chapter 14). Symptoms include severe pain, fever of varying degrees, and mild to moderate hearing loss. Infants may be fussy and tug at their ears. Any elevation in a child's temperature should be a warning to check for otitis media.

Diagnosis is usually made by inspecting the tympanic membrane with an otoscope, which reveals a reddened,

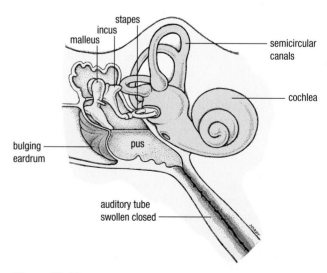

Figure 22-12 Internal structures of the ear with otitis media.

bulging tympanic membrane. If the suspected pathogen is bacterial, an antibiotic may be prescribed. With the exception of aspirin, analgesics are often recommended for the relief of the pain. If nasal congestion is present, a decongestant may reduce some of the swelling. In severe chronic cases, surgery may be performed to relieve pressure, and tubes may be inserted through the tympanic membrane to equalize the pressure.

PATIENT EDUCATION

MIDDLE EAR INFECTIONS

Explain to the child's parents that children have short, straight eustachian tubes. Upper respiratory infections, particularly with coughing, may force microorganisms into the middle ear spaces. As the infection grows, the eustachian tubes swell and eventually close. Exudate from the mucous membrane continues to be produced, causing fluid to build with resulting pressure and pain.

Although the infecting microorganism can be bacterial or viral, bacterial otitis media may be caused by putting the child to bed with a bottle of milk, juice, or formula. The drink and bacteria from the mouth set up a medium for growth within the eustachian tube. Provide patient education to caregivers whenever possible.

Tonsillitis

Pharyngitis, or a sore throat, may be caused by inflammation of the tissues of the throat and/or the tonsils (see Chapter 14). Inspection of the throat may reveal the tissue to be red and swollen, possibly with pustules on the tonsils or in the throat. When a diagnosis of tonsillitis is made, you may be asked to take a sample for a throat culture to rule out *Streptococcus* bacteria as the causative pathogen. (Chapter 29 describes the steps for obtaining a throat culture.) If the throat culture is positive for *Streptococcus*, an antibiotic will be ordered. If the throat culture is negative but the infection appears bacterial, an antibiotic may still be prescribed. Chronic tonsillitis may be treated by surgical removal of the tonsils—a tonsillectomy—by a surgeon who specializes in disorders of the ears, nose, and throat. The medical assistant will often be responsible for obtaining a preauthorization and referral if needed and scheduling the consultation appointment with the referring ear, nose, and throat surgeon.

CHECKPOINT QUESTION

10. Why is otitis media more common in children than adults?

Obesity

According to the American Academy of Pediatrics (AAP), obesity in children has become an epidemic. The importance of assessing the weight and length of infants and children and plotting this information on the appropriate growth chart is essential in assisting the physician in early recognition; however, prevention of obesity is even more important in preventing long-term complications, such as heart disease and diabetes. You must ask parents or caregivers during each visit to the office about the eating patterns, nutrition status, and activity levels of the child and offer education and support when necessary or as indicated by the physician. Since children develop eating habits early in life and take these habits into adulthood, you should teach parents about eating in moderation and increasing physical activity as a means to reduce the weight of an overweight child or prevent abnormal gains in weight. If the physician prescribes a specific diet or reduces caloric intake, you should offer support and guidance to the caregiver as needed.

Attention Deficit Hyperactivity Disorder

Attention deficit hyperactivity disorder (ADHD) is a condition of the brain affecting boys more frequently than girls and causing difficulty in controlling behavior. The problematic behavior in children with ADHD includes the following *signs of inattention* in the school-age child:

- Daydreaming or difficulty paying attention
- Easy distraction
- Inability to complete tasks
- Forgetfulness
- Reluctance to perform tasks that require mental effort
- Low grades in school

The *signs of hyperactivity* are often seen in the following behaviors:

- Excessive talking
- Inability to sit quietly for any length of time
- Breaking rules regarding running or jumping

In addition to inattention and hyperactivity, children with ADHD are often impulsive and behave irrationally to others, even after being repeatedly warned about a specific behavior, dangerous or not. These children have difficulty taking turns and may be disruptive, shouting out answers before being called on in the classroom.

The diagnosis for a child with ADHD is often based on a thorough history of the child's behaviors, including reports from teachers or other professionals who work with the child. The AAP publishes guidelines for diagnosing ADHD in children ages 6 to 12 years. There is no one test for diagnosing this disorder; instead, the diagnosis is based on certain behaviors in several settings (i.e., school and home). Once the physician has made the diagnosis, an individual treatment plan is devised; it may include behavior therapy, psychological counseling for the child and the family, education about ADHD, coordination of the treatment plan with the family and involved teachers, and medications.

AFF TRIAGE

While working in a family practice office, you have to complete the following three tasks:

A. Patient A is a 2-month-old child who has just been placed in examination room 1. You are to take the vital signs and measurements, including length, weight, and head circumference.
B. Patient B is a 14-month-old child who was seen today and diagnosed with otitis media. The physician has asked you to give the parent a prescription for an antibiotic and schedule a referral with an ear, nose, and throat physician for possible myringectomy and tubes.
C. A mother is on the phone and is concerned because patient C, her newborn, is vomiting.

How do you sort these tasks? What do you do first? Second? Third?

First, speak to the mother of patient C. This infant will dehydrate very quickly, and the situation must be assessed promptly and efficiently. Give advice about increasing fluids or giving pediatric electrolyte solutions *only* after assessing the situation, consulting with the physician, and receiving instructions from the physician to pass along to the mother. Next, deal with patient B by giving the parent the prescription and clarifying any other orders from the physician. The information regarding the referral can be given to the parent to make the arrangements, or you may make the appointment later in the day, when time permits. Of course, the required paperwork for the referral must be faxed to the referral physician, and this may be delegated to an administrative assistant according to the office policy and procedure manual.

See patient A after patient B is discharged. When obtaining a history for a well-child checkup, you want to give the parent your undivided attention and take extra time to establish rapport with the parent and the infant.

Medication Box

Commonly Prescribed Pediatric Medications

Note: The generic name of the drug is listed first and is written in all lowercase letters. Brand names are in parentheses, and the first letter is capitalized.

acetaminophen (Tylenol)	Oral syrup: 16 mg/mL Oral solution: 48 mg/mL Oral suspension: 80 mg/0.8 mL Suppositories: 80 mg, 120 mg, 125 mg, 300 mg	Antipyretic, Analgesic
acetylsalicylic acid (ASA, aspirin) (Bayer, St. Joseph's)	Tablets (chewable): 325 mg Suppositories: 120 mg, 200 mg	Antipyretic, Analgesic (*do not give* to children with viral illness)
amoxicillin trihydrate (Amoxil)	Oral suspension: 50 mg/mL, 125 mg/5 mL, 200 mg/5 mL Tablets (chewable): 125 mg, 200 mg, 250 mg, 400 mg	Antibiotic
atomoxetine (Strattera)	Capsules: 10 mg, 18 mg, 25 mg, 40 mg, 60 mg, 80 mg, 100 mg	Attention deficit hyperactivity disorder
ceftriaxone sodium (Rocephin)	Injection: 250 mg, 500 mg, 1 g, 2 g	Antibiotic
diphtheria and tetanus toxoids and acellular pertussis vaccine (DTaP) (Daptacel; Infanrix)	Injection: 0.5 mL	Vaccine (intramuscular [IM])
Haemophilus b conjugate vaccine, meningococcal protein conjugate (PedvaxHIB)	Injection: 0.5 mL	Vaccine (IM)

Commonly Prescribed Pediatric Medications *(continued)*		
Haemophilus b conjugate vaccine, meningococcal protein conjugate (PedvaxHIB)	Injection: 0.5 mL	Vaccine (IM)
Hepatitis B vaccine recombinant (Engerix-B; Recombivax HB)	Injection: 0.5 mL	Vaccine (IM)
ibuprofen (Children's Motrin; Children's Advil; PediaCare Fever)	Oral drops: 40 mg/mL Oral suspension: 100 mg/5 mL Tablets (chewable): 50 mg, 100 mg	Antipyretic; analgesic
measles, mumps, and rubella virus, live (M-M-R II)	Injection: 0.5 mL	Vaccine (subcutaneous)
methylphenidate (Concerta; Ritalin)	Tablets: 5 mg, 10 mg, 20 mg Tablets: 18 mg, 27 mg, 36 mg, 54 mg	Attention deficit hyperactivity disorder
pancreatin (Kutrase)	Capsules: 2,400 units lipase, 30,000 units protease, 30,000 units amylase	Pancreatic enzyme
poliovirus vaccine, inactivated (IPV) rotavirus, live (Rotarix, Rota Teq)	Injection: 0.5 mL Oral suspension: (Rotarix) 1 mL at age 6 weeks, 1 mL after 4 weeks (2 doses) Oral suspension: (Rota Teq) 2 mL at at age 6 weeks, 2 mL after 4 weeks, and 2 mL at 10 weeks (3 doses)	Vaccine (IM) Vaccine
simethicone (Mylicon)	Drops: 40 mg/0.6 mL	Antiflatulent

español SPANISH TERMINOLOGY

¿ El niño/la niña ha estado enfermo o se ha hecho algun daño?
Has the child had any illnesses or injuries?

Necesitamos una muestra de orina.
We need a urine specimen.

¿Qué vacunas ha recibido el nino/la nina?
Which immunizations has the child received?

¿Tose el niño por la noche?
Does the child cough at night?

¿Con qué frecuencia evacua el niño/la niña?
How often does the child have a bowel movement?

MEDIA MENU

- **Student Resources on thePoint**
  - **CMA/RMA Certification Exam Review**
- **Internet Resources**

  American Academy of Pediatrics
  http://www.aap.org

  About Pediatrics
  http://pediatrics.about.com

  Centers for Disease Control and Prevention, Vaccines and Immunizations
  http://www.cdc.gov/vaccines

  Denver Developmental Materials
  http://denverii.com/home.html

  United Cerebral Palsy
  http://www.ucp.org

  U.S. Department of Health and Human Services
  http://www.childwelfare.gov/can

  Mayo Clinic: Childhood Obesity
  http://www.mayoclinic.com/health/childhood-obesity/DS00698

PSY PROCEDURE 22-1:   **Obtaining an Infant's Length and Weight**

Purpose: Accurately determine the length and weight of an infant
Equipment: Examination table with clean paper, tape measure, infant scale, protective paper for the scale, appropriate growth chart

Steps	Reasons
1. Wash your hands.	Handwashing aids infection control.
2. Explain the procedure to the parent and ask him or her to remove the infant's clothing except for the diaper.	Explaining procedures encourages compliance. The diaper should be left on infants who involuntarily urinate.
3. Place the child on a firm examination table covered with clean table paper. If using a measuring board, cover the board with clean paper.	Measurements may not be correct if the surface is not firm. Clean paper prevents cross infection.
4. Fully extend the child's body by holding the head in the midline. Grasp the knees and press flat onto the table gently but firmly. Make a mark on the table paper with your pen at the top of the head and at the heel of the feet.	Most infants assume a flexed position, requiring you to extend the legs for accurate measurement. If you need assistance, ask the parent or a coworker to hold the child in position. A foot board against the soles will give the most accurate measurement.

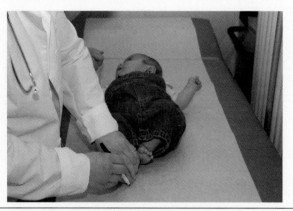

Step 4. Straighten the infant's leg.

5. Pick up the infant and give him or her to the caregiver, or ask the caregiver to pick the baby up.	Measurements cannot be taken with the baby lying on the paper. If a measuring board is used, it may not be necessary to move the baby.
6. Measure between the marks in either inches or centimeters, according to the preference of the physician.	The length measured between the marks made at the infant's head and feet will determine the length.
7. Record the child's length on the growth chart and in the patient's chart.	Procedures are considered not to have been done if they are not recorded. To plot the measurement on the growth chart, find the child's measurement in inches or centimeters and move in that line across to the age column. Make a mark where the two values intersect.

PSY PROCEDURE 22-1: **Obtaining an Infant's Length and Weight (continued)**

Steps	Purpose
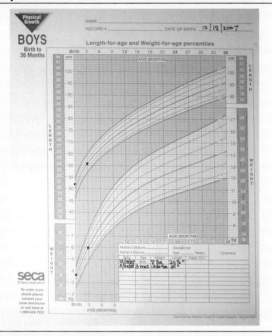	**Step 7.** Make a mark where the child's length and age intersect.
8. Either carry the infant or have the parent carry the infant to the scales.	The medical office may have only one infant scale located in a common area.
9. Place protective paper on the scale and microbalance the scale.	Protective paper prevents transmission of organisms. The balance beam must be centered before each use.
10. Remove the diaper just before laying the infant on the scale.	For the most accurate weight, infants should be weighed without any clothing. However, cool air against the infant's skin may cause the infant to void. Some offices permit the infant to be weighed in the diaper as long as it is dry and clean.
11. Place the child gently on the scale. Keep one of your hands over or near the child on the scale at all times.	Anticipate infant movement and prevent the infant from flipping off of the scale by having your hand ready to stop him or her. Avoid actually touching the infant as this will cause an inaccurate weight.

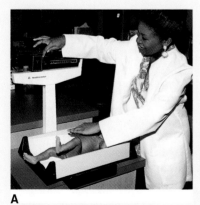
A

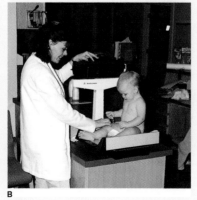
B

Step 11. (A) Infants are weighed lying down. **(B)** Infants who can sit may be weighed while sitting if this is less frightening for them.

(continued)

PSY PROCEDURE 22-1: **Obtaining an Infant's Length and Weight** *(continued)*

Steps	Purpose
12. Quickly but carefully move the counterweights to balance the apparatus exactly.	This will ensure accurate measurement.
13. Pick up the infant and give to parent or have the parent pick up the child. Instruct the parent to replace the diaper if removed for the weight.	Parents should be encouraged to participate in the procedure whenever possible.
14. Record the weight on the growth chart and in the patient's chart.	Procedures are considered not to have been done if they are not recorded. To plot the measurement on the growth chart, find the child's measurement in pounds or kilograms, and then move in that line across to the age column. Make a mark where the two values intersect.

Charting Example:

02/08/2013 10:00 AM 12-month-old, length 30 inches, wt. 22 lb. 6 oz. ——————————— J. DeBard, CMA

Note: The medical assistant may sign his or her name in the patient record using only the "CMA" credential if the office has a signature log denoting the entire credential as "CMA(AAMA)."

PSY PROCEDURE 22-2: **Obtaining the Head and Chest Circumference**

Purpose: Accurately determine the head and chest circumference of an infant
Equipment: Paper or cloth measuring tape, growth chart

Steps	Reasons
1. Wash your hands.	Handwashing aids infection control.
2. Place the infant supine on the examination table or ask the parent to hold the child.	This measurement does not require the infant to lie flat.
3. Measure around the head above the eyebrow and posteriorly at the largest part of the occiput. For an accurate reading, measure the largest circumference.	Placing the tape measure low on the skull will result in an inaccurate head circumference.

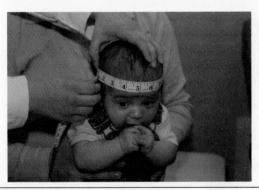

Step 3. Measure around the head above the eyebrow and posteriorly at the largest part of the occiput.

Steps	Reasons
4. Record the child's head circumference on the growth chart and in the patient's chart.	Procedures are considered not to have been done if they are not recorded. To plot the measurement on the growth chart, find the child's measurement in inches or centimeters, and then move in that line across to the age column. Make a mark where the two values intersect.

PSY PROCEDURE 22-2: | **Obtaining the Head and Chest Circumference (continued)**

Steps	Reasons
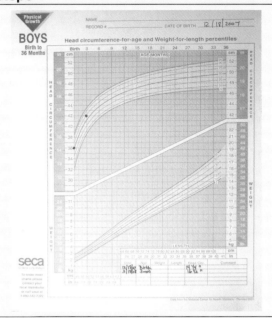	**Step 4.** Make a mark where the child's head circumference in inches or centimeters and age intersect.
5. With the clothing removed from the chest, measure around the chest at the nipple line, keeping the measuring tape at the same level anteriorly and posteriorly.	The tape should be at the same level to ensure the most accurate reading.
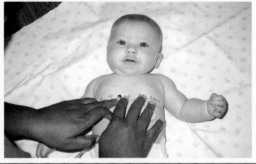	**Step 5.** Measure around the chest at the nipple line, keeping the measuring tape at the same level anteriorly and posteriorly.
6. Record the child's chest circumference on the growth chart and in the patient chart.	Procedures are considered not to have been done if they are not recorded. To plot the measurement on the growth chart, find the child's measurement in inches or centimeters, and then move in that line across to the age column. Make a mark where the two values intersect.

Note: If the head and chest growth are within normal limits, this measurement is not usually required after 12 months.

Charting Example:

10/15/2013 9:45 AM Wt. 14 lb. Length 24 in., Head 15 in., Chest 17 in. ———————— B. Brady, CMA

Note: The medical assistant may sign his or her name in the patient record using only the "CMA" credential if the office has a signature log denoting the entire credential as "CMA(AAMA)."

PSY PROCEDURE 22-3: Applying a Urinary Collection Device

Purpose: Correctly apply a urinary collection device to a child
Equipment: Gloves, personal antiseptic wipes, pediatric urine collection bag, completed laboratory request slip, biohazard transport container

Steps	Reasons
1. Wash your hands.	Handwashing aids infection control.
2. Explain the procedure to the caregivers.	Informing caregivers of procedures aids in compliance and cooperation.
3. Place the child supine. Ask for help from the parents as needed.	The child may be more cooperative if a parent helps.
4. After putting on gloves, clean the genitalia with the antiseptic wipes: A. For girls: Cleanse front to back with separate wipes for each downward stroke on the outer labia. The last clean wipe should be used between the inner labia. B. For boys: Retract the foreskin if the baby has not been circumcised. Cleanse the meatus in an ever-widening circle. Discard the wipe and repeat the procedure. Return the foreskin to its proper position.	For girls, cleansing front to back will remove debris from the area and avoid introducing bacteria into the urethra. For boys, cleansing outward will avoid introducing bacteria into the urethra. Returning the foreskin to the correct position will prevent constriction of the penis.
5. Holding the collection device, remove the upper portion of the paper backing and press it around the mons pubis. Remove the second section and press it against the perineum. Loosely attach the diaper.	The collection device must be securely attached to ensure collection of the next voiding. Reattaching the diaper will avoid soiling if the child has a stool.

Step 5. The collection device fits over the genitalia.

Steps	Reasons
6. Give the baby fluids unless contraindicated, and check the diaper frequently.	Giving the child fluids may stimulate voiding.
7. When the child has voided, remove the device, clean the skin of residual adhesive, and diaper.	Adhesive left on the skin may be irritating.
8. Prepare the specimen for transport to the laboratory or process it according to the office policy and procedure manual.	The specimen cannot be analyzed at the laboratory without proper processing.

PSY PROCEDURE 22-3: **Applying a Urinary Collection Device** *(continued)*

Steps	Reasons
9. Remove your gloves and wash your hands.	Standard precautions must be followed when handling body fluids.
10. Record the procedure.	Procedures are considered not to have been done if they are not recorded.

Charting Example:

08/16/2013 11:45 AM Urine collection device applied; approximately 50 mL clear amber urine obtained after
20 minutes. Specimen sent to Acme Laboratory for urinalysis ——————————————— S. Schein, CMA

Note: The medical assistant may sign his or her name in the patient record using only the "CMA" credential if the office has a signature log denoting the entire credential as "CMA(AAMA)."

Working with children offers many rewards; however, the special developmental needs and unique physiology of children make these patients challenging and must always be taken into consideration. This chapter focuses on:

- The skills necessary to assist with a well-child visit including obtaining and recording normal growth information. It is important to record this information carefully to assist the physician in detecting problems as early as possible.
- Caring for the child who comes to the office for a sick-child visit. This includes maintaining the reception area by separating sick and well children if possible and disinfecting any toys to avoid cross-contamination in other children.
- Common diseases that may be seen in childhood including ear infections, upper respiratory infections, and gastrointestinal problems. Although these diseases are common, they are not pleasant for the child

or the caregiver. You will have a role in reassuring anxious parents while caring for their sick children competently and professionally.

- Education of the pediatric patient caregiver including vaccine information. Parents should always be encouraged to ask questions and should expect to get honest and clear answers.
- Legal and ethical issues related to immunizations, child abuse, and neglect. You must always be alert for signs of neglect and/or abuse and be ready to report your suspicions to the physician.
- Your role in preventing disease in the pediatric patient and assisting with pediatric procedures. In addition to caring for children, you must also provide patient education to caregivers and older children to prevent the spread of disease. Also, your expertise in working with pediatric patients will be appreciated by the physician and the other staff who may find it necessary to have you assist with a variety of pediatric procedures.

Warm Ups for Critical Thinking

1. During years of practice, Dr. Hernandez has found that many new parents are unfamiliar with basic child care needs. He decides to publish a short booklet for his new parents describing various aspects of child care. The booklet should be informative and professional and show genuine concern for children. Using your creativity and your knowledge of child care, develop a sample booklet for Dr. Hernandez's patients after choosing two of the following topics:
   - General safety tips
   - Types of office visits
   - Immunizations (what they are, why they are important, at what ages they are given, side effects and adverse effects)
   - What a parent can expect during an office visit
   - Brief explanation of child development
   - Tips for administering oral medications to children
2. You obtained the weight on Lillian Parks, a 7-month-old girl. She weighs 16½ pounds according

to your balanced pediatric scales. What percentile is this patient according to the growth chart? How would you explain a percentile to the mother of the infant?

3. The father of a toddler is insistent that you give the child an immunization in the arm rather than the thigh. How would you handle this situation?
4. Research one of the following conditions that may be found in pediatric patients and prepare a poster detailing the causes, signs and symptoms, and treatment. Include information for the caregivers or school personnel who may have questions about these conditions:
   - Strep throat
   - Pediculosis
   - Conjunctivitis
5. Compare the developmental skills of a 3-year-old and 5-year-old child. What are the similarities? What are the differences?

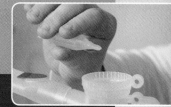

23 Geriatrics

Learning Outcomes

Cognitive Domain

Note: AAMA/CAAHEP 2008 Standards are italicized.

1. Spell and define key terms
2. Explain how aging affects thought processes
3. Describe methods to increase compliance with health maintenance programs among older adults
4. Discuss communication problems that may occur with the older adult and list steps to maintain open communication
5. Recognize and describe the coping mechanisms used by the older adult to deal with multiple losses
6. Name the risk factors and signs of elder abuse
7. Explain the types of long-term care facilities available
8. Describe the effects of aging on the way the body processes medication
9. Discuss the responsibility of medical assistants with regard to teaching older adult patients
10. List and describe physical changes and diseases common to the aging process
11. *Identify common pathologies related to each body system*

12. *Describe implications for treatment related to pathology*

Psychomotor Domain

Note: AAMA/CAAHEP 2008 Standards are italicized.

1. *Assist physician with patient care*
2. *Prepare a patient for procedures and/or treatments*
3. *Practice standard precautions*
4. *Document patient care*
5. *Document patient education*
6. *Practice within the standard of care for a medical assistant*

Affective Domain

Note: AAMA/CAAHEP 2008 Standards are italicized.

1. *Apply critical thinking skills in performing patient assessment and care*
2. *Use language/verbal skills that enable patients' understanding*
3. *Demonstrate empathy in communicating with patients, family, and staff*
4. *Use appropriate body language and other nonverbal skills in communicating with patients, family, and staff*

5. *Demonstrate awareness of the territorial boundaries of the person with whom you are communicating*
6. *Demonstrate sensitivity appropriate to the message being delivered*
7. *Demonstrate recognition of the patient's level of understanding in communications*
8. *Recognize and protect personal boundaries in communicating with others*
9. *Demonstrate respect for individual diversity, incorporating awareness of one's own biases in areas including gender, race, religion, age, and economic status*
10. *Apply active listening skills*
11. *Apply local, state, and federal health care legislation and regulation appropriate to the medical assisting practice setting*

ABHES Competencies

1. Assist the physician with the regimen of diagnostic and treatment modalities as they relate to each body system
2. Comply with federal, state, and local health laws and regulations
3. Communicate on the recipient's level of comprehension
4. Serve as a liaison between the physician and others
5. Show empathy and impartiality when dealing with patients
6. Document accurately

Key Terms

activities of daily living (ADL)	compliance	Kegel exercises	presbycusis
biotransform	degenerative joint disease (DJD)	keratosis (senile)	presbyopia
bradykinesia	dementia	kyphosis (dowager's hump)	senility
cataracts	dysphagia	lentigines	syncope
cerebrovascular accident (CVA)	gerontologists	osteoporosis	transient ischemic attack (TIA)
	glaucoma	potentiation	vertigo

As the older adult population has increased, established concepts about aging have also changed. The greeting card image of a cozy, gray-haired grandmother in her rocking chair is being replaced by a trim, active woman rushing out the door with a briefcase or tennis racket under her arm. **Gerontologists**, specialists in aging, describe many older adults today as healthy enough to maintain homes well into their 80s and 90s. The branch of medicine that deals with the older adult population is geriatrics, and while some physicians today are treating only geriatric patients, a family practice or internal medicine physician also treats older adult patients. Other specialties, such as ophthalmology, also see many geriatric patients daily. Box 23-1 outlines some myths and stereotypes about the older adult. How many are far from typical of this age group today?

Stereotyping the older adult is a subtle and usually unconscious way to disassociate ourselves from the prospect of growing old. Although other cultures respect their older adults for their wealth of wisdom and experience, the American media perpetuate myths and stereotypical reactions by implying that graying hair and wrinkles in the skin are repulsive and should be avoided at all costs. Those costs include billions of dollars spent on delaying the physical signs of aging. Consider how the following situations take on new meaning when applied to different age groups.

- You are running late again. Dashing out of the door, you remember that you left the keys to the car on the kitchen table—again.
- You stride purposefully from the bedroom into the kitchen with a specific goal in mind, only to reach the kitchen without any idea why you were in such a hurry to get there.

We have all done these things and will no doubt do them again. However, if these things are done by an older adult

MYTHS AND STEREOTYPES ABOUT THE OLDER ADULT

Myths
- Old people are weak and sick.
- Old people can no longer learn.
- Old people have no more contributions to make.
- Old people are boring.
- Old people are a drag on the economy.
- Old people are always lonely.
- Old people cannot live alone.
- Old people cannot be trusted to make rational decisions.
- Old people have lost all interest in life.

Stereotypes
- Old people have sensory losses.
- Old people have erratic sleep patterns and nap a lot.
- Old people do everything slower.
- Old people have lost stature and slump a lot.
- Old people cannot remember what happened this morning but can recall everything that happened 40 years ago.

person, they are considered to be a sign of approaching **senility** or **dementia**. While some memory loss and difficulty with thought processes are inevitable as a result of aging, memory loss in the older adult is often the result of various disease processes and medications. The next section describes some techniques that you can use to enhance **compliance** with patients who have difficulty with thought processes, whether the cause is natural aging or a specific disease or medication regimen. You have a responsibility as a professional medical assistant to ensure that your interactions with older adults demonstrate dignity and respect, keeping in mind their individual abilities and uniqueness.

COG Reinforcing Medical Compliance in the Older Adult

Working with older adult patients who may have problems with memory loss or thought processes is extremely important to ensure that they take their medications as prescribed and follow the physician's instructions precisely. A patient who has good rapport with the office staff is likely to be truthful about the need for memory aids, and compliance may be increased. A patient who has difficulties with memory may benefit from the following approaches:

- Write out instructions in easy-to-understand terms.
- Use large print.

- Have the patient repeat instructions to you for reinforcement.
- Ask the patient to show you how he or she will perform a procedure before leaving the office.
- Give the patient a copy of a large appointment calendar and list the times and days for treatments and medications, which should be crossed off as completed.

Many chronic illnesses that affect the older adult require medication or treatment for the remainder of the patient's life. In these situations, the patient may not notice much improvement, making compliance over a long period problematic. You should reinforce the fact that, although the patient may not return to his or her former health status, the prescribed treatment will maintain health at a manageable level. A patient's diabetes or heart disease will not be cured, but treatment will help the patient maintain a reasonable standard of health and independence.

It is important that, each time a patient visits the medical office, you ask for a complete account of all medications being taken, including prescribed and over-the-counter (OTC) medications, herbal supplements, and vitamins. To maintain a complete and accurate list of these medications, you may have patients bring all medications to the office at each visit and ask the patient to state how often each is taken (Fig. 23-1). If you ask, "Mrs. Jones, are you still taking your heart medicine?" she may answer yes whether or not she is actually taking the medication as prescribed. In addition to difficulty with thought processes and occasional forgetfulness, some patients simply grow tired of the constraints that illness and medications impose on their lives, and some must make the financial choice between medication and food on the table. Assisting the patient to find ways to fit health requirements into a fairly normal lifestyle or coordinating with community resources to relieve financial constraints will help to ensure that treatment plans are followed and that the patient achieves the best level of health possible.

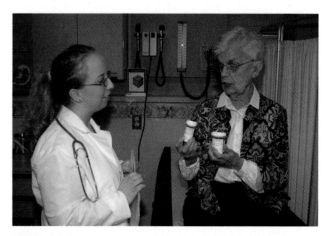

Figure 23-1 Ask patients about medications at every visit.

CHECKPOINT QUESTION

1. What are some reasons a patient may not comply with a prescribed treatment plan?

PATIENT EDUCATION

TIPS FOR IMPROVING MEMORY IN THE OLDER ADULT

Many research studies have been done regarding improving the forgetfulness that sometimes results from aging and that is not associated with an organic brain disorder such as Alzheimer disease or cerebrovascular disease. The factors that seem to play an important role in maintaining and improving memory include many of the same factors necessary for general good health:

- Regular physical exercise
- Maintaining a healthy body weight
- Eating a healthy diet that includes a variety of foods (grains, fruits, vegetables, etc.) and is low in fats

In addition, eating breakfast and regularly exercising the brain with puzzles, word searches, and other activities that require thinking skills may also affect cognitive function.

COG Reinforcing Mental Health in the Older Adult

With the recognized correlation between physical and mental health, we must be acutely aware of the patient's mental status in patients who have acute or chronic physical problems. Some older adult patients are adapting to new roles of dependency after a lifetime of social interaction, career objectives, and family development. Some have been relieved of social responsibility whether they welcome it or not, and if they are ill, they must take on a dependent role. Adjusting to pain or disability is often easier than adjusting to loss of social interaction or dependency.

Paradoxically, if you open yourself to patients, including older adults, and you are accessible and caring, you are likely to be the object of anger simply because you are seen as a safe outlet for venting frustrations. A suffering patient is less likely to release pent-up anger at someone who may respond with hostility or corresponding anger; consequently, the patient may hold these feelings in, and the problem is compounded. Making yourself available to field these emotions can be as therapeutic as any treatment administered to this patient. To do this effectively:

1. Maintain open communication, freely discussing hopes and fears realistically, listening attentively, and offering advice without diagnosing or offering false hope.

2. By listening and being supportive to the patient and family members, help the patient to cope with and express feelings of guilt for being ill, anger at self and others nearby, and the loss of health and independence.

3. Work toward maintaining the patient's positive self-image by reinforcing the positive qualities of the patient's physical health or personal situation as appropriate.

4. Assist family members to maintain a positive support system by listening to concerns and possibly serving as a liaison for outside social services or resources if available.

5. Without being discouraging or offering false hope, prepare the patient for the possibility that a return to the previous state of health may not be feasible.

6. Direct the patient and family to specific support groups, such as the American Heart Association, the American Cancer Society, or another group specific to the patient's problem, to assist them with acquiring information about the patient's condition.

 CHECKPOINT QUESTION

2. How can you help promote good mental health in your older adult patients?

COG Coping with Aging

Although many older adult people are generally healthy and satisfied with their lives, those who live in long-term care facilities or whose health and economic situation are unstable have every right to feel overwhelming stress and grief. Stress will compromise the immune system, raise the blood pressure and blood sugar level, and strain the heart and lungs—all at a time when the patient needs all available resources to fight a debilitating disease process. You can help patients to cope with stress by listening to their fears and concerns, respecting their right to have these feelings, and helping them to reduce the stressors in their lives. Keep in mind that the coping mechanisms (e.g., denial, projection, repression) used to protect ourselves from stress may become more pronounced with age.

The ability of patients to cope with their losses is in direct relation to the importance of the losses and their own personal habits for coping with loss in the past. Be aware of a patient's loss of specific senses, abilities, or important things in life, such as sight, hearing, movement, perception, health, employment, home, and spouse. Also, be alert to the loss of nonspecific things, such as life purpose, goals, a sense of achievement, self-worth, recognition, and security. Some older adult patients react to these losses by disengaging emotionally and relinquishing all decision making to family members. This may compound their grieving and lead to a sense of hopelessness and resignation. To prevent this reaction, involve older adult patients, like all patients, as much as possible by allowing them to have a voice in decisions that will affect their care. The older adults who are encouraged to make decisions and take responsibility for themselves are happier, more sociable, and live longer than those who are not part of the decision-making process in issues that affect their lives.

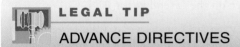

LEGAL TIP
ADVANCE DIRECTIVES

An advance directive is a legal document outlining the wishes of an adult should he/she become mentally incompetent or otherwise unable to communicate decisions about end-of-life care. Although physicians as medical professionals are dedicated to sustaining life, a patient's autonomy must be respected at all times, including decisions to avoid or terminate life-sustaining procedures or equipment. As unpleasant as the prospect of death may be, documenting and communicating the wishes of the patient to the physician will assist with avoiding any confusion about the wishes of the patient should a life-threatening situation arise. Also, if the patient has an advanced directive on file somewhere other than the medical office, this should be noted in the patient's medical record.

Alcoholism

Some older adults, like individuals at any age, cope with loss and life changes by turning to alcohol. Because alcohol slows brain activity and impairs mental processes, coordination, and judgment, a patient who comes to the office under the influence of alcohol may be mistaken for having dementia (mental deterioration), a **transient ischemic attack (TIA)**, or central nervous system impairment. Also, many medications taken by the older adult affect the central nervous system and react badly with alcohol, compounding the problem. For example, alcohol increases the effect of opioids, barbiturates, and depressants of all types, and caretakers may not recognize this reason for the **potentiation.**

Identifying an older adult patient who is using or abusing alcohol may require the entire office to work as a team with the patient's family or caregiver to seek causes of various symptoms, such as impaired judgment or coordination. As often as necessary, you should reinforce with older adult patients and their caregivers the effects of alcohol on mental processes and undesirable interactions with medications. In addition, the patient and

responsible caregivers may require a referral to a mental health professional or other community resource to deal effectively with alcohol abuse. You may be required to make this referral as ordered by the physician.

Suicide

When ill health, multiple losses, and deep depression become too much for the patient to bear, suicide may seem preferable to life. Unlike suicide among younger people, suicide among the older adult is likely to be well planned and successful. Most older adult suicides are white men over age 65, especially those who have recently lost a spouse to death or divorce. These suicides are not usually a cry for help but a genuine effort to end life. Watch for these signs of intent:

- Deepening confusion and scattered attention
- Increasing anger, hostility, or isolation
- Increase in alcoholism or requests for opioids or sedatives
- Marked loss of interest in matters of health
- Secretive behavior
- Sharp mood swings from deep depression to euphoria
- Giving away favored objects

Always take seriously a patient who expresses an intent to commit suicide, and communicate this to the physician. You should work with the health care team to restore mental health as aggressively as to restore physical health.

 CHECKPOINT QUESTION

3. What are some signs of suicidal intent?

COG Long-Term Care

Although many older adults are able to live in their own homes, some enter long-term care facilities if they cannot return to health and independence or are simply tired of the tasks required to maintain a house. There are three main types of long-term care:

- *Group homes* or *assisted living facilities* are for the older adults who are able to tend to their own **activities of daily living (ADL)** (e.g., bathing, dressing, eating) but who may need companionship and light supervision for safety. Often, these facilities allow independent adults access to activities such as golf, swimming, and trips for those who are ready to enjoy life in the later years.
- *Long-term care facilities* are for those who need help with most areas of personal care and moderate medical supervision. Many of these patients are ambulatory but have a chronic disease that makes living at home difficult or impossible.

• *Skilled nursing facilities* are for those who are ill and need constant supervision or rehabilitation before returning home. If the illness is acute and short term, the patient may return to an intermediate stage of care after recovery and possibly to full independence. However, these facilities also provide support and resources to patients who may need end-of-life care.

Although fully independent adults moving to an assisted living facility may be relieved to leave behind the pressures of life and excited to remain active with fewer responsibilities, expect some older adult patients to react to a move to long-term care with sorrow and a deep sense of loss. The patient may show the signs and symptoms of grief: poor appetite, headaches, insomnia, deep depression, and vague aches and pains. Report all signs and symptoms to the physician. Many physicians continue to care for patients residing in long-term care facilities. You may be responsible for blocking time in the daily schedule for the physician to visit these patients, and you may receive phone calls at the medical office from facilities regarding changes in patient's care and physical condition.

 CHECKPOINT QUESTION

4. How are long-term facilities and skilled nursing facilities different?

 WHAT IF?

What if a patient's relative asks you about options for home care for an older adult parent?

Explain that many options allow patients to remain in their home. One option is the use of home health aides. Some insurance plans pay for this service. Home health aides do light housecleaning and cooking and promote patient safety. A second option is a community resource center. Some communities have senior citizen programs that provide transportation for shopping, doctor appointments, and entertainment. These programs get the older patient out of the house, preventing boredom and enhancing self-esteem. A third option is daycare for the older adult. These programs keep the patient safe, entertained, and cared for during the day. The advantages of day care are that it relieves the caregiver of the need to place a parent in a long-term care facility, keeps the patient safe during the day, and allows the relative the freedom to continue employment or attend to personal needs. Community programs for senior citizens are good sources of information for caregivers or for relatives searching for respite or permanent care.

COG Older Adult Abuse

Although older adult abuse is not as widely publicized as child abuse, it is thought to be almost as prevalent. The following are common risk factors for older adult abuse:

• Multiple chronic illnesses that stress the family's physical, emotional, and financial resources
• Senile dementia that precludes reasoning or interaction
• Bladder or bowel incontinence
• Age-related sleep disturbances that interfere with the caretaker's rest
• Dependence on the caretaker for ADL

Older adult abuse and neglect may take several forms, but family members (adult children and spouses) are the typical perpetrators.

• Passive neglect may result from the caretaker's ignorance regarding the patient's physiologic and psychological needs.
• Active neglect may take many forms, including over-medicating to render the patient passive and easier to care for or depriving the victim of adequate nutrition to decrease physical resources.
• Psychological abuse may include threatening imprisonment in the home, perhaps locking in a room, or physical abuse, withholding food or medication, or physical isolation.
• Financial abuse may involve only small amounts of money or entire substantial estates. The patient's financial resources may be embezzled, squandered, or frankly stolen, leaving the victim destitute.
• Physical abuse may be as simple as pinches and slaps or may be life threatening, sexual, or so well concealed that even perceptive health care providers do not suspect it (Fig. 23-2).

Some older adult patients fear reprisal or abandonment by their caregivers, just as children do, and are reluctant to complain of any improprieties. Separate the caregiver from the patient for the examination if possible, and treat the patient with the utmost compassion and care. Document all findings with full descriptions. It may be necessary to photograph the suspected injuries

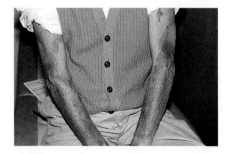

Figure 23-2 You should always be alert to signs of older adult abuse. (From Weber J, Kelley J. Health Assessment in Nursing. 2nd ed. Philadelphia: Lippincott Williams & Wilkins, 2003.)

and report any suspicions to the local adult protective services. Always communicate your concerns with the physician, and, together, make decisions regarding how to proceed with any suspected abuse.

 CHECKPOINT QUESTION

5. What are the types of older adult abuse?

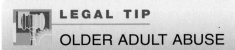

LEGAL TIP

OLDER ADULT ABUSE

If you suspect abuse or neglect, you are responsible ethically and legally for bringing it to the attention of the physician, who should assess the situation and, if it is confirmed, notify the proper authorities. Most states require that health care professionals report all suspected cases of older adult abuse to the department of social services, just as is required for suspected child abuse. The entire medical staff may be held responsible if the abuse is not reported immediately. The following signs may indicate older adult abuse:

- Wound of suspicious origin in various stages of healing
- Signs of restraints having been used, such as wrist or ankle abrasions or bruising
- Neglected large, deep pressure ulcers
- Poor hygiene or poor nutrition with little or no effort at correction
- Dehydration not caused by a disease process
- Untreated injury or medical condition
- Excessive and unwarranted agitation or apathetic resignation

COG Medications and the Older Adult

The need to teach some older adult patients about self-medication is a challenge that will become increasingly common as the general population ages. At the same time that older adult patients need more medications for various disorders, the body is coping with the stress of illness, disease, or injury along with slowing of many bodily functions. The gastrointestinal system is no longer moving medications along as efficiently because peristalsis has slowed. The circulatory system is not absorbing the dissolved medication from the intestines or the injection site and delivering it to the target tissue as quickly. The liver does not **biotransform** (convert) the medication as quickly, so that it remains in the body longer than might be desirable and possibly adds to cumulative effect. Finally, the kidneys are receiving less blood,

so that less medication is filtered and removed from the body. All of these decreases in body systems can result in possible toxic effects of medications in the older adult.

Your responsibility is to elicit information from the patient about all medications they are taking, including prescribed and OTC medications and herbal or vitamin supplements. Follow these guidelines to help ensure that your older adult patient adheres to the prescribed medication regimen:

1. Explain all side effects, precautions, interactions, and expected actions in a manner the patient can understand.
2. Explain the proper dosage and how to measure it. For patients with failing eyesight, mark plastic measuring cups with indelible ink at the correct level so they can easily see it.
3. Write out a schedule and suggest methods to help the patient remember. Suggestions may include a daily dose pack available at pharmacies, an egg carton with hours for taking the medications marked on the cups, and a calendar marked with the medications and hours, to be checked off after taking the medication.
4. Tell the patient to take the most important medication first and space out the other medications according to the physician's order. Medications that are ordered to be taken once a day may not have to be taken in the morning.
5. Encourage the patient not to rush when taking medications. The patient should be sitting or standing, not reclining. One pill should be taken at a time with lots of water. If the medication is difficult to swallow, have the patient try putting the pill on the back of the tongue and drinking water with a straw.
6. A patient who has difficulty reading or has failing eyesight can ask the pharmacist for large print on the label (Fig. 23-3). This makes medication errors less likely. Childproof containers are not necessary if there are no children in the home, and the patient may find them difficult to open.

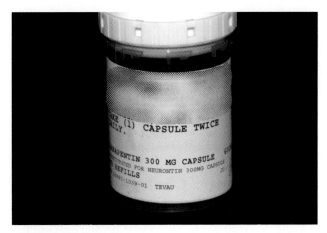

Figure 23-3 Large print on a medication label.

7. Explain that the medication must be taken until it is gone (if this is the case). No medication should be taken by other family members or saved for another illness.

8. Encourage patients to take an active role in therapy. Teach them to apply ointments or transdermal patches or to give themselves injections. A patient who feels in charge is more likely to complete a course of medication or to remain on the medication for the long term than one who feels passive.

 CHECKPOINT QUESTION

6. How can you help your older adult patients follow the medication regimen prescribed by the physician?

 PATIENT EDUCATION

HERBAL SUPPLEMENTS

The herb ginkgo, also known as *ginkgo biloba*, *maidenhair tree*, *kew tree*, *fossil tree*, *ginkyo*, and *yinhsing*, is advertised in the United States as a natural way to improve memory and concentration. It is for this reason that older adults have been targeted for the purchase of this product. After all, it can be purchased over the counter at many pharmacies and health food stores, and so many patients do not consider it a medication. However, it is extremely important that you obtain a thorough history from your patients each time they visit the office and specifically ask about any OTC medications, including herbs and vitamin supplements. This drug may improve memory in some patients, but it causes an increase in clotting time in anyone who takes it and should not be used by patients with bleeding or clotting disorders. Any patient being scheduled for a surgical procedure must also be asked about the use of herbs. Patients who are taking the following medications should avoid taking ginkgo:

- Warfarin (Coumadin)
- Aspirin
- Nonsteroidal anti-inflammatory drugs, such as ibuprofen, naproxen, and indomethacin

The physician should be informed of any patient taking this herbal supplement because reactions with other medications in addition to those listed could have serious consequences.

COG ## Systemic Changes in the Older Adult

Although longevity is considered largely hereditary, environmental factors play a significant part in how long and how well we will live. An obese, physically inactive smoker is much less likely to be in good health than a nonsmoker whose diet is well balanced and who exercises. In addition, certain occupational hazards, such as black lung disease from coal mining, may shorten a life that should have lasted for decades longer.

The aging changes are thought to be programmed into our cells along with our genetic material. Some experts suggest that when cells reach a specific reproduction level, they either do not replace themselves or replicate more slowly or ineffectively. These changes manifest themselves at varying rates for all persons but follow a recognized order as outlined in Table 23-1.

Some older adult patients develop disorders involving communication (Fig. 23-4); however, diseases affecting sight and hearing are common and may interfere with ADL for aging adults. Visually, conditions such as **presbyopia, cataracts,** and, possibly, **glaucoma** become evident with aging (refer to Chapter 14). All of these can affect sight, ranging from a decrease in visual acuity (presbyopia) to blindness if left untreated (cataracts and glaucoma). Having print materials available in large print, obtaining preauthorizations and referrals to an ophthalmologist as ordered by the physician, and being alert for safety issues when assisting older adult patients is your responsibility in the medical office.

Generalizing that all older adults cannot hear is not appropriate; however, as people age, conditions such as ceruminosis and prebycusis (see Chapter 14) are more common and cause hearing loss. Irrigating the ear and instilling otic solution to soften cerumin may be ordered by the physician to treat ceruminosis. Prebycusis is treated with a referral to an audiologist for evaluation and hearing aids (Fig. 23-5).

 WHAT IF?

You are organizing your charts at the beginning of the day and you notice that one of your patients, an 88-year-old man, has HOH (hard of hearing) stamped inside his chart. How can you best communicate with him?

When speaking to an older adult patient who is hearing impaired, it is important not to shout. Instead, get closer to the patient, face the patient directly, and speak slowly and distinctly. Try to give written instructions whenever possible, and encourage the patient to ask questions for clarification. Avoid speaking to the hard-of-hearing patient with your back to the light, since this may cast shadows and prevent the patient from being able to lip read.

TABLE **23-1**	Effects of Aging on Body Systems		
System	**Physiologic Effects**	**Signs and Symptoms**	**Suggestions**
Integumentary	Loss of subcutaneous fat Loss of pigment Loss of elasticity Receding capillaries Slower reproduction of hair, skin cells Diminished oil, sweat production Erratic pigment, cell production	Wrinkling, sagging, decreased ability to maintain hydration, reduced protection against temperature change Less protection against sun damage, paler skin, graying hair Increased skin dryness, risk of trauma Sallow skin, thickened nails Balding; thin, fine hair; slower healing Dry, fragile skin; intolerance to heat Senile lentigines, keratoses	Encourage drinking plenty of fluids, dressing appropriately for weather. Encourage use of sunscreen with appropriate UV protection. Suggest good lubricating lotion and bathing less often; caution to guard against injuries. Suggest ways to avoid overheating. Teach patient to conduct skin checks and to notify the physician of concerns.
Musculoskeletal	Loss of muscle strength, size Loss of bone density, loss of height with osteoporosis Degenerative joint cartilage	Loss of strength, flexibility, endurance Vertebral compression with diminished height, kyphosis, osteoporosis with frequent fractures Less clear margins with spurs of bone that restrict movement, degenerative joint disease (DJD), arthritis	Suggest frequent exercise appropriate to age and ability. Explain weight-bearing exercises. Encourage home safety check to avoid falls. Physician may recommend calcium supplement, dietary consultation, estrogen replacement. Physician may limit phosphorus intake.

A 10 years postmenopause **B** 15 years postmenopause Height loss 1.5" **C** 25 years postmenopause Height loss 3.5"

Typical loss of height associated with osteoporosis and aging.

(continued)

TABLE **23-1**	Effects of Aging on Body Systems *(continued)*		
System	**Physiologic Effects**	**Signs and Symptoms**	**Suggestions**
Nervous	Slow nerve conduction Reduced cerebral reaction times Referred circulatory problems	Slow reaction time, slow learning, slow perception of pain with resulting increase in injuries Loss of balance, vertigo, frequent falls Increase in cardiovascular diseases (atherosclerosis, arteriosclerosis) reflected as cerebrovascular accident (CVA), cerebral hypoxia, TIA	Allow extra time as needed and teach about hazards of delayed circulation. Aim at teaching to comprehension level. Encourage home safety checks. Have patient install bath rails, remove throw rugs. Encourage use of walking aid. Teach patient and family about danger signs for CVA, TIA.
Cardiovascular	Atherosclerosis, arteriosclerosis, narrowing of blood vessels Slow response to demands for increased output Diminished function	Loss of peripheral circulation, fatty plaques with risk of MI, CVA, cold extremities, slow healing time, hypertension Complaints of fatigue on exertion Pulmonary involvement with edema, dyspnea	Encourage exercise; balanced low-fat, low-salt diet; dressing appropriately for weather; home safety check. Help patient pace exercise and exertion. Explain about low-salt diets and orthopneic positions. Explain about smoking hazards, emphysema. Encourage moderate exercise.
Respiratory	Stiffening costal cartilage Decreased gas exchange General loss of muscle mass	Decreased expansion, contraction; barrel chest; decreased lung capacity Fatigue, breathlessness on exertion; impaired healing due to insufficient oxygen, syncope Difficulty coughing deeply, may lead to pneumonia	Encourage exercise as appropriate and use of walking aid. Caution about upper respiratory infection; encourage home safety check. Encourage drinking adequate fluids to liquify respiratory secretions.
Gastrointestinal (GI)	Drying of secretions, including saliva Decreased enzyme activity Slower peristalsis Loss of teeth	Dry mouth, dysphagia Incomplete digestion, poor conversion of nutrients with malnourishment Constipation, flatulence, indigestion Poor chewing, choking on large pieces, loss of appetite, poor nutrition	Teach oral hygiene, adequate fluid intake. Encourage small, frequent well-balanced meals. Refer to a dentist. Suggest dietary counseling.
Urinary	Decreased bladder capacity Decreased bladder muscle tone Fewer functioning nephrons	Urinary frequency Urinary retention with urinary tract infection or incontinence Less blood flowing through kidneys to be cleaned of wastes, creating possibly lethal levels of medications or normal body wastes	Encourage patient to respond to initial urge to void. Suggest exercises for strengthening pelvic floor. Urge patient to empty bladder completely when voiding. Suggest increase in fluid intake to maintain hydration.

TABLE 23-1	Effects of Aging on Body Systems (continued)		
System	**Physiologic Effects**	**Signs and Symptoms**	**Suggestions**
Endocrine	Decreased enzyme activity	Menopause, glucose intolerance with non-insulin-dependent diabetes mellitus, slower metabolism Loss of resistance to illness	Physician will supplement as needed. Encourage compliance with any prescribed medications.
Immune	Diminished production of T cells, B cells Diminished ability of body to distinguish self from foreign substances Diminished other defenses (e.g., GI enzymes)	Increase in autoimmune illnesses Overload on compromised immune system	Encourage age-appropriate immunizations, guarding against communicable diseases. Explain symptoms of autoimmunity.
Eyes	Less time spent in deep sleep Diminished lens accommodation Lens cloud Loss of ciliary function	Less restful sleep, more frequent naps Presbyopia Cataracts (lens opacity) that dim vision as less light reaches the retina Glaucoma (increased intraocular pressure), intolerance to light or glare, poor night vision	Encourage rest periods as needed. Obtain referral to ophthalmologist. Recommend adequate lighting, large-print books, brochures, pamphlets. Avoid night driving.
Ears	Loss of auditory hair cells (organ of Corti) Ossicle becomes fixed	Hearing loss in upper frequencies, problems distinguishing sounds Presbycusis	Obtain referral to otologist, audiologist. Speak clearly, facing patient, in area with few distractions.
Other senses	Diminished sense of smell Diminished sense of taste	Loss of appetite, poor nutrition Increased use of salt, other seasonings	Suggest dietary consultation. Encourage use of seasonings other than salt.
Reproductive (Female)	Decreased egg production system Decreased estrogen production Poor perineal muscle tone Rectocele, cystocele, stress incontinence	Menopause Hot flashes; thinner, drier vaginal walls with itching Painful intercourse; osteoporosis	Physician may prescribe supplemental estrogen. Suggest **Kegel exercises** to strengthen pelvic floor.
Reproductive (Male)	Smaller penis, testicles Atherosclerosis, arteriosclerosis Benign prostatic hypertrophy (BPH)	Loss of libido Erectile dysfunction Urgency, frequency, nocturia, retention	Physician may refer patient for counseling. Explain good nutrition to avoid atherosclerosis. Encourage patient to have yearly checks for BPH.

COG Diseases of the Older Adult

The degenerative conditions noted in Table 23-1 are typically part of the aging process. Many of these changes cause problems that must be managed by the health care team; others are mere inconveniences for the patient. Diseases related to aging are described in the preceding chapters on specialties and the disorders described previously also apply to older adults. However, there are some disorders that affect older

SPEECH, LANGUAGE, AND HEARING DISORDERS

APHASIA:
Aphasia is a complex problem which may result, in varying degrees, in a reduced ability to understand what others are saying, to express oneself, or to be understood. Some individuals with this disorder may have no speech, while others may have only mild difficulties recalling names or words. Others may have problems putting words in their proper order in a sentence. The ability to understand oral directions, to read, to write, and to deal with numbers may also be disturbed. Strokes are the major cause of aphasia in the older population. It has been estimated that there are over one million adults with aphasia in the United States today. Many can be helped to communicate more effectively.

DYSARTHRIA:
Dysarthria interferes with normal control of the speech mechanism. Speech may be slurred or otherwise difficult to understand due to lack of ability to produce speech sounds correctly, maintain good breath control, and coordinate the movements of the lips, tongue, palate, and larynx. Diseases such as parkinsonism, multiple sclerosis, and bulbar palsy, as well as strokes and accidents, can cause dysarthria. Many individuals with dysarthria are over 65. Their communication skills often may be improved by appropriate treatment.

HEARING PROBLEMS: It is estimated that of the approximately 27 million Americans over the age of 65, as many as 50 percent may be affected by hearing impairment. The hearing loss observed as a part of the aging process is called "presbycusis." Many of those with presbycusis describe the problem as being able to "hear" what others are saying, but being unable to understand what is being said. This condition can lead to withdrawal from personal interactions of all types. Family or friends may confuse the disorder with "forgetfulness" or "senility." A hearing aid can often improve communication for older people with hearing loss.

VOICE PROBLEMS: Laryngectomy, the surgical removal of the larynx (voice box) due to cancer, affects approximately 9,000 individuals each year, most of whom are older. They can usually learn to speak again by learning esophageal speech, by using an electronic device or by surgical implant of voice prosthesis. Other forms of disease may result in complete or partial loss of the voice. Most of these problems can be treated.

OTHER COMMUNICATION PROBLEMS: Brain diseases that result in progressive loss of mental faculties may affect memory, orientation to time, place and people, and organization of thought processes, all of which may result in reduced ability to communicate.

Figure 23-4 Focus on the older adult. What are the disorders of communication that most frequently affect older people? (From Communication Disorders and Aging. American Speech-Language-Hearing Association, Rockville, MD. Reprinted with permission.)

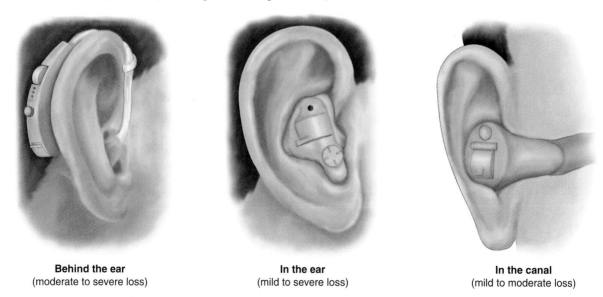

Behind the ear
(moderate to severe loss)

In the ear
(mild to severe loss)

In the canal
(mild to moderate loss)

Figure 23-5 Several types of hearing aids. (From Carol R. Taylor, Carol Lillis, RN, et al. Fundamentals of Nursing: The Art And Science of Nursing Care, Sixth Edition. Philadelphia: Lippincott Williams & Wilkins, 2008.)

patients more often than adults at younger ages. The following sections describe two conditions commonly associated with aging that may appear in the middle years as well.

Parkinson Disease

Parkinson disease is a slow, progressive neurologic disorder affecting specific cells of the brain that produce the neurotransmitter dopamine. The initial symptoms frequently include muscle rigidity, involuntary tremors, and difficulty walking. Parkinson disease affects men more than women and is estimated to affect in some form approximately 1 in 100 persons over age 60 years. This disease may progress for 10 years or more before resulting in complete debilitation or death.

Normally, dopamine and acetylcholine, another neurotransmitter, are in balance and produce smooth, controlled muscle movement. With lower levels of dopamine, acetylcholine is not counterbalanced. This leads to involuntary movements of muscles and inability to control these movements. While the causes of Parkinson disease are unknown, researchers are working to determine whether there is a genetic component. Some evidence suggests that certain toxins may cause the disease. These toxins may be environmental or related to certain medications. The following are the signs and symptoms of Parkinson disease:

• Muscle rigidity
• **Bradykinesia** (abnormally slow voluntary movements)
• Difficulty walking, with a shuffling, mincing gait
• Forward-bending posture with no normal arm swing

• Laryngeal rigidity with a monotone voice
• Pharyngeal rigidity with dysphagia and drooling
• Facial muscle rigidity with a masklike, expressionless face and infrequent blinking reflex, causing frequent eye infections
• Small tremors in the fingers in a characteristic pill-rolling action. These start unilaterally and stop with purposeful action in the affected hand. Tremors are greatest during times of stress and anxiety and are diminished at sleep or rest. Muscles resist passive stretching and become rigid with passive manipulation (Fig. 23-6).

The diagnosis of Parkinson disease is usually made by excluding other causes; however, testing may show decreased levels of dopamine in the urine. A symptomatic history is the primary method of diagnosing after all other possibilities have been ruled out. Parkinson's disease has no cure. Treatment is symptomatic, supportive, and palliative. Medications include the following:

• Levodopa (L-dopa). Dopamine replacement crosses the blood–brain barrier to restore balance with acetylcholine. Individualized doses are gradually increased as symptoms progress. Levodopa is fairly effective for a time but gradually loses its effectiveness. Unfortunately, levodopa has serious side effects, including nausea, vomiting, tachycardia, and arrhythmias. It has severe adverse reactions with alcohol.
• Anticholinergics. These drugs decrease the levels of acetylcholine so that depleted levels of dopamine are not so out of balance. This method works best in mild, early stages.

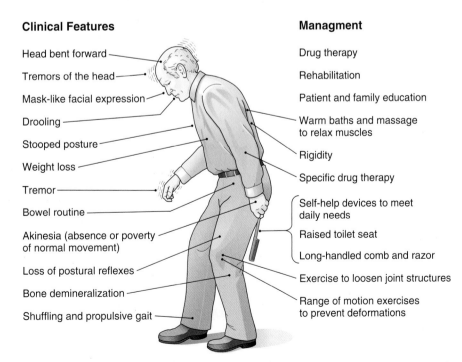

Clinical Features

Head bent forward
Tremors of the head
Mask-like facial expression
Drooling
Stooped posture
Weight loss
Tremor
Bowel routine
Akinesia (absence or poverty of normal movement)
Loss of postural reflexes
Bone demineralization
Shuffling and propulsive gait

Managment

Drug therapy
Rehabilitation
Patient and family education
Warm baths and massage to relax muscles
Rigidity
Specific drug therapy
Self-help devices to meet daily needs
Raised toilet seat
Long-handled comb and razor
Exercise to loosen joint structures
Range of motion exercises to prevent deformations

Figure 23-6 The Parkinson disease patient.

- Antihistamines with anticholinergic action. In the early, mild stages, this method of lowering acetylcholine levels to balance with low levels of dopamine alleviates symptoms.

A procedure known as *deep-brain stimulation* is used to treat tremor and rigidity. In this procedure, electrodes are surgically placed in certain areas of the brain and are connected by wires to an impulse generator that is implanted under the skin of the chest. This transmitter sends electrical impulses to the electrodes in the brain, blocking the impulses that cause the tremors. Although this procedure is effective for controlling involuntary movements and tremors, it is generally not used if medication can control the patient's symptoms. Like all other methods, this treatment is palliative and not curative.

Parkinson patients retain their mental and cognitive functions unless an organic brain disturbance is also present. They are aware of the outward signs of the disease and may be embarrassed and emotionally depressed. They require great psychological support from the medical staff, family, and support groups. You can help in the following ways:

- Encourage the patient to participate in all ADL.
- Promote independence.
- Be aware that, because rigidity extends to the gastrointestinal tract, the patient may have dysphagia and constipation. Suggest that the patient increase fluid intake, eat a balanced diet, and increase fiber intake.
- Tell the patient that a decreased cough reflex can lead to choking. Suggest that the patient take small bites and chew each mouthful of food carefully before attempting to swallow.
- Encourage the patient to use eating aids such as a no-spill cup, plate with high sides, and special utensils. High toilet seats and handrails in the bath also help increase the patient's independence and safety.
- Listen to the patient. Intelligence is still intact and needs to be stimulated.
- Educate the patient about safety factors. The forward-bending posture and altered gait frequently lead to falls. Encourage these patients to hold on to handrails and pick up feet carefully to avoid falling. Also, the home should be free from rugs and loose cords that may cause accidental tripping.
- Enlist the help of support groups. Include the caregiver and urge respite care when exhaustion and stress become overwhelming.

 CHECKPOINT QUESTION

7. How can you assist a patient with Parkinson disease?

Alzheimer Disease

Roughly half of the cases of dementia in the older adult are due to Alzheimer disease. The symptoms of Alzheimer disease may be similar to those caused by TIA, cerebral tumor, and dementia other than Alzheimer disease. Unfortunately, the cause of Alzheimer disease is not known.

The symptoms of Alzheimer disease may begin as early as age 40 years, with a gradual loss of memory and slight personality changes. The changes may occur over as long as 15 years and are frequently so gradual that diagnosis is difficult and may be made only by ruling out all other possibilities. Autopsy reveals organic brain changes, including a loss of neurons and neurotransmitters. Plaques or deposits may be present as a residue of the neural cell deterioration.

Alzheimer disease has seven recognized stages. The progression from one stage to the next may be gradual. Some stages may last for years, but a patient may pass through other stages so quickly that the progression goes unnoticed. Expect varying levels of response from patients in these different levels (Table 23-2). When caring for Alzheimer disease patients, you must remember that anger and hostility are often symptoms of the disease and should not to be taken personally. Be sure to do the following:

- Respond with the utmost patience and compassion.
- Speak calmly and without condescension.
- Never argue with the patient, even if the patient blames you unfairly for something the patient forgot.
- Do not expect the patient to remember you from previous visits. Reintroduce yourself.
- Explain even common procedures as if the patient has never had them explained.
- Approach the patient quietly and professionally in an unthreatening manner, and remind the patient who you are and what you must do.
- Speak in short, simple, direct sentences, and explain only one action at a time.
- Keep a list of support contacts for family members to call.

Home care agencies usually offer respite care, which can be vitally important for caregivers, who need to maintain their own mental and physical health. An exhausted, distraught family member may not be thinking clearly. The most therapeutic action may be for you to assist the family with proper contacts to help make caring for a family member with this devastating disease less traumatic.

Maintaining Optimum Health

No one realistically expects to have the same strength and agility at age 70 years as at age 20 years. With attention to exercise and good nutrition, however, it is

TABLE **23-2**	Levels of Alzheimer Disease
Level	**Description**
I, II	Presenile dementia may end here, with no further progression. Brain changes insignificant; only remarkable symptom may be forgetfulness. ADL done with reasonable ease.
III	Patient losing ability to remember facts, faces, and names but still aware enough to recognize problem and becomes increasingly frustrated and angry. Most ADL still performed reasonably well.
IV	Late confusional or mild Alzheimer disease. Patient beginning to misplace things, has increasing difficulty remembering, and neglects ADL. Most patients aware of a problem but deny any concern.
V	Early dementia or moderate Alzheimer disease. Patient must have custodial care, has severe memory lapses, disorientation, anger, and great frustration.
VI	Middle dementia or moderately severe Alzheimer disease with severe memory loss, no self-care at any level, disoriented most of the time with immense anger, hostility, and combativeness. Fear of water.
VII	Late dementia. Patient requires full-time care and is rarely seen in the office. Unless home care is an option, physician will probably visit long-term care facility. Patient rarely speaks, almost never intelligibly; incontinent; may require tube feeding.

possible to maintain a good level of fitness that adds to quality of life.

Exercise

Exercise plays a vital role in maintaining overall physical and mental health (Table 23-3). Older patients should begin an exercise program only after a thorough physical examination and should follow the physician's recommendation. Provide the following guidelines for older adult patients who are starting an exercise program with the physician's approval:

TABLE **23-3**	Benefits of Exercise
System	**Benefits**
Cardiovascular	Increases endurance Lowers cholesterol to avoid atherosclerosis Maintains vascular elasticity to delay arteriosclerosis
Musculoskeletal	Increases bone mass to reduce osteoporosis Decreases fat–muscle ratio and increases metabolism Retains strength and flexibility to ensure mobility, improve posture
Nervous	Improves mental health by reducing stress, fatigue, tension, boredom Maintains or restores balance to reduce risk of falls
Endocrine	May decrease need for insulin or oral hypoglycemic medication in diabetes

1. Before exercise, always warm up cold muscles for at least 10 minutes. Slow and rhythmic movements, such as walking, raise the heart rate and increase metabolism. Then do slow, easy stretching to lengthen sluggish muscles.
2. Begin by exercising for brief periods. Exercise only 5 to 10 minutes a day the first week, then progress to 10 to 15 minutes a day the next week. Gradually work up to about 30 to 45 minutes of a pleasantly challenging strength and cardiovascular endurance activity after about a month. This routine reduces the chance of injury and is likely to be an attainable goal.
3. Stop if you feel pain, shortness of breath, or dizziness. Never try to work through pain.
4. Breathe deeply and evenly. If you cannot carry on a conversation, slow down. Never hold your breath while you exercise.
5. Rest when you get tired. Do not try to exercise to the point of exhaustion.
6. Keep a record of your progress. It is motivational to watch your performance improve.
7. Exercise with a friend, with a group, or to music that you enjoy (Fig. 23-7).
8. Make exercise a part of your daily routine, but do not make it a chore. Do something vigorous every day and take pride in it.

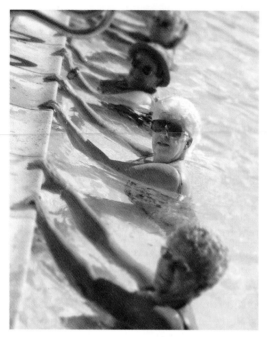

Figure 23-7 Participating in group exercise helps to maintain overall physical and mental health.

 CHECKPOINT QUESTION

8. What are the physical signs that indicate a patient should stop exercising?

Diet

Many older adult patients have difficulty maintaining good nutrition. Reduced activity means a corresponding decrease in hunger. Decaying teeth or poorly fitting dentures cause pain, making it hard to chew. Saliva production decreases, making it harder to swallow. The senses of smell and taste diminish, interfering with the cephalic phase of digestion. Many older adult patients eat alone or are not able to enjoy the socializing that adds immeasurably to the pleasure of eating.

A balanced diet is vital to good health at any age. Although activity levels, and hence calorie requirements, are lower among older adults, vitamin and mineral requirements do not decrease with age. Efforts must be made to increase the nutritional level of older adults. Smaller, more frequent meals may be easier to digest than infrequent large meals. Water should be encouraged to maintain hydration and to aid digestion and elimination.

Talk to patients or their families about valuable social services that may deliver nutritious meals to the home daily or 5 days a week. These programs may ensure that at least one well-balanced meal a day is available. Most services prepare meals to meet special dietary needs, such as low sodium or low fat. The program volunteer is alert to the needs of the patient and will report to a

coordinator if the patient does not answer the door or seems ill or confused. These resources will help to reassure the family that the patient's nutritional and social needs are being met.

 PATIENT EDUCATION

LIQUID DIETARY SUPPLEMENTS

There are many liquid dietary supplements available on the market today, and some are specifically marketed for the older adult. When interviewing the older adult, always assess their nutritional status by asking about the frequency of meals and types of food eaten and obtaining a weight at each visit. Let the physician know if you notice a trend in weight loss or other signs of poor nutrition. With permission of the physician, encourage your patient with nutritional problems to get a liquid supplement in his or her favorite flavor; most come in vanilla, chocolate, and strawberry. Advise your patient that these supplements should not replace a meal, but rather provide extra nutrition between meals.

Safety

Alert the patient and caregivers to hazards in the home of an older adult patient and offer the following suggestions:

- Remove any scatter rugs, especially on highly polished floors.
- Never allow electrical cords to cross passageways.
- Remove or reduce clutter as much as possible.
- Strengthen handrails on stairs and install them in tubs and near the commode.
- Install a telephone by the bedside and near a favorite chair.
- Install and carefully maintain smoke alarms and carbon monoxide detectors throughout the house.
- Establish a system in which someone calls and checks on the patient every day.

Many communities have programs in which volunteers call the sick or older adult daily to check on their needs and offer a few minutes of conversation. If the patient fails to answer, someone goes to the home to check on the patient. This service ensures that the patient is never without contact for long. Lifeline, an emergency service, is another option that increases the feeling of safety for patients who live alone.

 CHECKPOINT QUESTION

9. What are some reasons an older adult patient may have poor nutritional status?

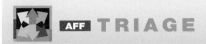 **AFF** TRIAGE

While you are working in a medical office, the following three patients are waiting to be seen:

A. Patient A is a 76-year-old woman who is active but underweight, with a history of osteoporosis. She is here for a physical examination, and the doctor has just instructed you to obtain some blood work for laboratory analysis.

B. Patient B is an 87-year-old man brought in by his daughter, who takes care of him in her home since his stroke 3 years ago. His wife is deceased, and his daughter is concerned because his memory seems to be failing him.

C. Patient C is a 90-year-old man residing in an assisted-living facility with his wife, who is 88. They were brought to the office today because the husband is due for a blood pressure check and possible medication adjustment. They are alert and sharp mentally, although both move more slowly than usual and the wife requires a walker.

How would you sort these patients? Who do you see first? Second? Third?

When working with older adult patients, it is important to remember not to rush them or appear inattentive. Since patient B is having new symptoms and may require a longer time with the physician, you should check him in first and get vital signs and any appropriate medical information from both the patient and his daughter. The husband and wife should be seen next, since all that is required is a brief chief complaint and obtaining vital signs. When both the husband and wife are comfortable and safely seated, you may leave them alone until the doctor is available to see them. Patient A should be seen last because obtaining blood from the older adult requires special attention to detail and patience. Once the blood sample is obtained, patient A may be discharged after checking the medical record to assure that no physician orders have been missed.

Medication Box

Commonly Prescribed Geriatric Medications

Note: The generic name of the drug is listed first and is written in all lowercase letters. Brand names are in parentheses, and the first letter is capitalized.

adalimumab (Humira)	Injection: 40 mg/0.8 mL (subcutaneous [SC])	Antirheumatic
alendronate sodium (Fosamax)	Tablets: 5 mg, 10 mg, 35 mg, 40 mg, 70 mg Oral solution: 70 mg/75 mL	Antiresorptive
allopurinol (Zyloprim)	Tablets: 100 mg, 300 mg	Antigout
alprazolam (Xanax)	Tablets: 0.25 mg, 0.5 mg, 1 mg, 2 mg Oral solution: 1 mg/mL	Antianxiety
benztropine mesylate (Cogentin)	Tablets: 0.5 mg, 1 mg, 2 mg Injection: 1 mg/mL (intramuscular [IM])	Anti-parkinsonian
celecoxib (Celebrex)	Capsules: 50 mg, 100 mg, 200 mg, 400 mg	Nonsteroidal anti-inflammatory
diazepam (Valium)	Tablets: 2 mg, 5 mg, 10 mg Oral solution: 5 mg/5mL	Antianxiety
donepezil hydrochloride (Aricept)	Tablets: 5 mg, 10 mg	Alzheimer disease
enoxaparin (Lovenox)	Prefilled syringe: 60 mg/0.6 mL, (SC) Injection: 80 mg/0.8 mL, 100 mg/mL, Injection: 120 mg/0.8 mL, 150 mg/mL Vial: 300 mg/3 mL	Anticoagulant

(continued)

Medication Box *(continued)*

Commonly Prescribed Geriatric Medications

estrogen (Premarin, Cenestin)	Tablets: 0.3 mg, 0.45 mg, 0.625 mg Vaginal cream: 0.625 mg/g	Hormone
galantamine hydrobromide (Razadyne)	Capsules: 8 mg, 16 mg, 24 mg Tablets: 4 mg, 8 mg, 12 mg Oral solution: 4 mg/mL	Alzheimer disease
gold sodium thiomalate (Aurolate; Myochrysine)	Injection: 50 mg/mL (IM)	Antirheumatic
ibandronate sodium (Boniva)	Tablets: 2.5 mg, 150 mg Injection: 3 mg/3 mL (intravenous)	Antiresorptive
lorazepam (Ativan)	Tablets: 0.5 mg, 1 mg, 2 mg Oral solution: 2 mg/mL	Antianxiety
naproxen (Naprosyn)	Tablets: 200 mg, 250 mg, 375 mg, 500 mg Oral suspension: 125 mg/5 mL	Nonsteroidal anti-inflammatory
raloxifene hydrochloride (Evista)	Tablets: 60 mg	Antiresorptive
sildenafil citrate (Viagra)	Tablets: 20 mg, 25 mg, 50 mg, 100 mg	Erectile dysfunction
tadalafil (Cialis)	Tablets: 2.5 mg, 5 mg, 10 mg, 10 mg, 20 mg	Erectile dysfunction
warfarin sodium (Coumadin)	Tablets: 1 mg, 2 mg, 2.5 mg, 3 mg, 4 mg, 5 mg, 6 mg, 7.5 mg, 10 mg	Anticoagulant
zoster vaccine, live (Zostavax)	Injection: one vial (SC)	Vaccine

español SPANISH TERMINOLOGY

Este medicamento se toma de esta manera.
  This is how you take this medication.

¿Tiene dolor además de la rigidez?
  Do you have pain with the stiffness?

La/el asistente médico/medica domiciliaria le ayudara con su cuidado personal.
  The home health aide will help with your personal care.

¿Ha notado algún cambio en su habilidad para recordar las cosas?
  Have you noticed a change in your memory?

MEDIA MENU

- **Student Resources on thePoint**
  - **CMA/RMA Certification Exam Review**
- **Internet Resources**

  The Center for Social Gerontology
  http://www.tcsg.org
  American Association of Retired Persons
  http://www.aarp.org
  National Center on Elder Abuse
  http://www.ncea.aoa.gov/NCEAroot/Main_Site/Index.aspx
  National Institute on Aging
  http://www.nia.nih.gov
  Centers for Medicare and Medicaid Services
  http://www.cms.hhs.gov

Regardless of the type of specialty you work in, you will encounter the older adult patient. Some important things to remember about the older adult include:

- Avoid stereotyping the older adult into passive, dependent roles.
- Be alert to the normal physiologic changes of aging and adjust your communication techniques accordingly.

- Not all older adult patients are affected by diseases such as dementia, Alzheimer disease, or Parkinson disease.
- Having patients who are diagnosed with Parkinson or Alzheimer disease will require you to understand the disease process and develop excellent interpersonal skills.
- Use patient education opportunities to discuss issues of safety whenever possible.

Warm Ups for Critical Thinking

1. Mrs. Moss, age 78 years, lives with her son and daughter-in-law and their two school-age children. She has dysphagia and a poor appetite. Identify ways in which Mrs. Moss can improve or maintain her nutritional status while participating in the family meals.

2. Mr. Brown is 90 years old, and his wife is 86 years old. They live alone, and Mrs. Brown is the primary caregiver. During the physical examination, Mr. Brown is found to have several large decubital ulcers. Summarize the various types of elder abuse or neglect. What is likely the problem in this case? Explain how you would handle this situation.

3. The pharmacist calls you at the office and says he has an older adult patient waiting to have a prescription for a high blood pressure medication filled. This prescription was filled just 2 weeks ago, but the patient says he is "all out of my medicine." What do you advise the pharmacist to do?

4. Your 68-year-old male patient tells you that he is thinking about joining the senior citizens exercise group at the local community college. He appears to be healthy and is not currently on any medications. How would you respond?

5. The daughter of an older adult woman comes to the office with her 76-year-old mother who lives alone. Would it be permissible to have the daughter present during the interview and physical exam? What about confidentiality?

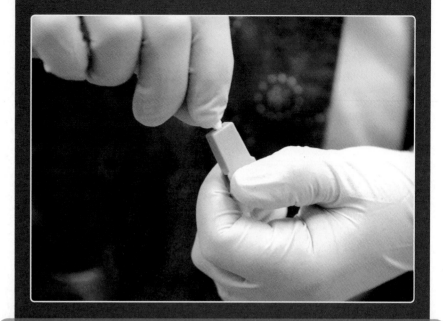

The Clinical Laboratory

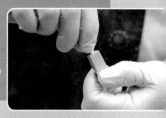

UNIT THREE
Fundamentals of Laboratory Procedures

CHAPTER 24
Introduction to the Clinical Laboratory

Outline

Types of Laboratories
- Referral Laboratory
- Hospital Laboratory
- Physician Office Laboratory

Laboratory Departments
- Hematology
- Coagulation
- Clinical Chemistry
- Toxicology
- Urinalysis
- Immunohematology
- Immunology

Microbiology
Anatomic and Surgical Pathology

Laboratory Personnel
- The Medical Assistant's Responsibility in the Clinical Laboratory
- Scope of Practice for the Medical Assistant in the Clinical Laboratory

Body Systems and Laboratory Testing
- Laboratory Test Panels

Ordering Laboratory Tests
- Laboratory Request Forms
- Laboratory Test Panels

Physician Office Laboratory Testing

Point-of-Care Testing

Laboratory Equipment
- Cell Counter
- Microscope
- Chemistry Analyzer
- Centrifuge
- Incubator
- Refrigerators and Freezers

Learning Outcomes

Cognitive Domain

Note: AAMA/CAAHEP 2008 Standards are italicized.

1. Spell and define key terms
2. Identify the kinds of laboratories where medical assistants work and the functions of each
3. Identify the types of departments found in most large laboratories and give their purposes
4. Identify the types of personnel in laboratories and describe their jobs
5. Describe the medical assistant's responsibility in the clinical laboratory
6. Define scope of practice for the medical assistant and comprehend the conditions

for practice within the state that the medical assistant is employed
7. Identify body systems
8. Describe the panels defined by the American Medical Association for national standardization of nomenclature and testing and list the test results provided in each panel
9. Identify the equipment found in most small laboratories and give the purpose of each
10. Describe the parts of a microscope

Psychomotor Domain

Note: AAMA/CAAHEP 2008 Standards are italicized.

1. Care for the microscope (Procedure 24-1)

571

aliquots	cytogenetics	oncology	reference intervals
analytes	cytology	panels	referral laboratory
autoimmunity	hematology	pathogen	serum
biohazard	histology	physician office	specimens
centrifugation	hypersensitivities	laboratory (POL)	surgical pathology
clinical chemistry	immunodeficiency	procedure manual	toxicology
Centers for Medicare	immunohematology	product insert	unitized test device
and Medicaid	immunology	quality assurance	urinalysis
Services (CMS)	kit	(QA)	whole blood
coagulopathies	microbiology	quality control (QC)	

The medical laboratory staff analyze blood, urine, and other body samples to measure **analytes** (the substances a laboratory tests) that contribute to the diagnosis and treatment of disease. Results of laboratory testing are compared with normal or **reference intervals** (acceptable ranges for a healthy population) to determine the health of body systems or organs. Blood levels of medications are measured to adjust dosages. Bacteria, viruses, parasites, and other microorganisms are identified to begin the treatment process. (See Appendix I for a list of commonly performed laboratory tests and their reference intervals.)

CHECKPOINT QUESTION

1. What are reference intervals? How are they significant to patient care?

Laboratory testing is most commonly used for the following:

- Diagnosing disease
- Monitoring a patient's medication and treatment
- Identifying the cause of an infection
- Preventing disease

COG Types of Laboratories

Laboratory testing is performed in three different kinds of laboratories:

- referral laboratories
- hospital laboratories
- **physician office laboratories (POLs)**

Referral Laboratory

A reference or **referral laboratory** is a large facility in which thousands of tests of various types are performed each day. Referral laboratories employ scientists and technicians who are approved to perform testing. Referral laboratories perform tests that may be too expensive for other labs to offer. Because the referral lab performs such high volumes of each test, it can cost less to perform them at that site.

Referral labs have their own blood drawing stations. They also receive specimens from smaller laboratories and clinics. Some specimens are delivered by courier or the mail. Specimens sent to referral laboratories must be packaged to withstand rough handling, pressure changes, and temperature extremes during shipment. Packaging includes placement in a special leak-proof secondary transport container (Fig. 24-1) approved for biohazardous specimens.

Employees of referral laboratories have specific job descriptions. Specimen processors receive the specimens, and log patient data and specimen information into the laboratory information system. Processors also centrifuge, separate, and prepare **aliquots** (portions of specimens used for testing) if indicated and send them to the correct departments for analysis. Medical assistants may work as specimen processors.

Testing personnel are responsible for **quality control (QC)** procedures, the procedures used to detect and correct errors that occur. There are several different errors that can cause QC to fail. Acceptable quality control results must be achieved before laboratory tests can be reported.

Hospital Laboratory

The medical assistant may also be involved in sending specimens to a hospital laboratory rather than a referral laboratory.

Even in large hospitals, the laboratory performs only the most commonly requested tests and those requiring immediate results. Less commonly ordered tests are sent often performed with unitized devices. The **unitized test device** is used to add a specimen and allow all steps of the testing process to occur in that container. A unitized device is used for a single test and must be discarded after testing.

In the POL, medical assistants perform laboratory duties, such as collecting samples, performing tests, managing QC, maintaining instruments, keeping accurate records, and reporting results.

 CHECKPOINT QUESTION

3. What POL laboratory duties are performed by the medical assistant in addition to testing patient specimens?

COG **Laboratory Departments**

Larger laboratory facilities, such as referral or hospital laboratories, include various departments that require special equipment. Following is a list of common laboratory specialties and the kinds of testing performed in each.

Hematology

Hematology is the study of blood and blood-forming tissues. The laboratory work that goes into the study of blood is performed by a medical laboratory scientist. Hematology can sometimes include the specialty of **oncology**, the medical treatment of cancer. Hematology tests are performed to evaluate blood diseases. Testing in the hematology laboratory includes evaluating blood smears and bone marrow slides under the microscope. Bone marrow is a blood-forming tissue.

Disease processes managed primarily with hematology testing are:

- bleeding disorders, such as hemophilia and platelet disorders
- malignancies, such as lymphoma and leukemia
- bone marrow transplants

Hematologists perform most of their tests on whole blood specimens. The various types of cells in the blood are counted using automated cell counters. Common tests include the white blood cell (WBC) count, red blood cell (RBC) count, platelet count, hemoglobin and hematocrit.

Coagulation

Coagulation testing includes evaluating how well the body's blood clotting process is performing. Coagulation studies include the measurement of prothrombin

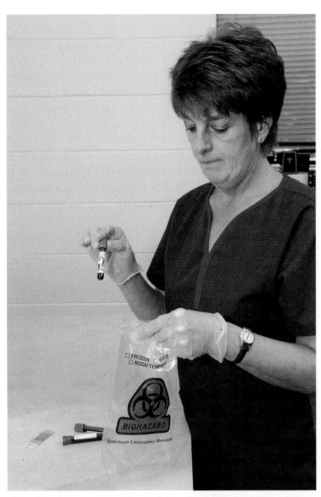

Figure 24-1 Transport containers are constructed to maintain the integrity of the specimen and to protect those who are responsible for the care and handling of possibly hazardous bodily fluids and substances.

to referral laboratories. Whether the test is performed onsite or sent to a referral laboratory, results generally are available within 24 to 48 hours.

 CHECKPOINT QUESTION

2. List duties in a referral or hospital laboratory that can be performed by a medical assistant.

Physician Office Laboratory

The most common type of laboratory is the POL. Samples for less common tests may be obtained, but are sent to hospital or referral laboratories for testing. The most common tests performed at a POL are urinalysis, blood cell counts, hemoglobin and hematocrit, and blood glucose levels. In POLs, pregnancy tests and quick screening tests for diseases such as mononucleosis and strep throat are also available. These screening tests are time (PT) and activated partial thromboplastin time (APTT). Both tests are used to monitor levels of **anticoagulant** drugs, such as heparin and Coumadin, during medication therapy. An anticoagulant is anything that prevents or delays blood clotting.

Hemophilia is a familial disorder of blood clotting. Coagulation specialty labs exist in medical university centers to further investigate the causes and treatments for **coagulopathies**, the diseases associated with abnormal blood-clotting functions. Plasma specimens are used for testing the coagulation process in the laboratory.

 CHECKPOINT QUESTION

4. What are the two most common tests performed in the coagulation laboratory?

Clinical Chemistry

Clinical chemistry (also known as *chemical pathology*) is the area of the laboratory that analyzes body fluids. Most chemistry laboratories are automated and use test methods that are closely monitored and quality controlled. The tests are performed on any kind of body fluid but mostly on serum or plasma. Serum is the yellow liquid part of blood that is left after blood has been allowed to clot, and all blood cells have been removed. Separation of the serum from the cells is most easily done by **centrifugation**. Centrifuging packs the blood cells and platelets to the bottom of the centrifuge tube and leaves the serum sitting on top of packed cells. Plasma is like serum, but the blood does not clot first.

Chemistry tests can be further subcategorized into subspecialities of:

- General or routine chemistry
- Endocrinology—the study of hormones
- **Immunology**—the study of the immune system and antibodies
- Pharmacology—the study of drugs
- **Toxicology**—the study of drugs and poisons

Toxicology

Toxicology is often a separate department in the chemistry laboratory. Toxicology is a branch of chemistry that studies the effects of chemicals. In addition to detecting drugs of abuse, it is also used to detect poisoning.

Drugs of abuse testing performed in the toxicology laboratory may be for either medical purposes or "for cause" scenarios. For cause scenarios include testing required by an employer. For cause specimens and forensic specimens require a legal chain of custody. For this reason, toxicology laboratories testing these specimens are secured with limited access.

Urinalysis

The **urinalysis** department may stand alone or be a part of one of the other laboratory sections. A routine urinalysis usually includes the following tests: color, transparency, specific gravity, pH, protein, glucose, ketones, blood, bilirubin, nitrite, urobilinogen, and leukocyte esterase. Some laboratories include a microscopic examination of urinary sediment with all routine urinalysis tests. If not, the microscopic examination is performed if the specimen's transparency, glucose, protein, blood, nitrite, or leukocyte esterase is abnormal. Urine pregnancy tests also may be performed in this department.

Routine urine testing is performed for several reasons:

- to detect renal and metabolic diseases
- to diagnose diseases of the kidneys or urinary tract
- to monitor patients with diabetes

 CHECKPOINT QUESTION

5. What testing limitations are required for medical assistants in urinalysis?

Immunology

Clinical immunology is the study of diseases caused by disorders of the immune system. Testing in the immunology department is based on the reactions of antibodies, proteins formed in the body in response to foreign substances, such as bacteria or viruses. The foreign substances are proteins called *antigens*. Increased need for testing to evaluate the body's cellular immune response has resulted from treating autoimmune diseases and AIDS.

The diseases caused by disorders of the immune system fall into two categories: **immunodeficiency** and **autoimmunity**. In immunodeficiency, parts of the immune system fail to respond as they should. In autoimmunity, the immune system attacks the patient's own body. Examples of autoimmunity are systemic lupus erythematosus and rheumatoid arthritis. Other immune system disorders include different **hypersensitivities**. In hypersensitivity, the immune system responds too much to harmless compounds. An example of hypersensitivity is asthma.

Immunohematology

Commonly called the *blood bank*, this department is found only in hospitals and blood donor centers. The **immunohematology** department involves a wide variety of procedures used in donor selection and techniques used to detect **antigen** or **antibody** reactions that can harm a patient receiving a transfusion. Blood products that are prepared, stored, and dispensed from the blood bank include whole blood, packed red cells, platelets, fresh-frozen plasma, and Rh immune globulin, such as RhoGAM. Other services may include autologous donation (donation of blood by prospective patients for their own use). The autologous service is not available in all blood banks.

The most common testing taking place in an immunohematology laboratory is crossmatching for compatibility of blood for transfusion in patients and for detection and identification of antibodies.

Immunohematology can also provide testing to detect hemolytic disease of the newborn.

 CHECKPOINT QUESTIONS

6. What is another name for the immunohematology laboratory?
7. Testing in the immunology laboratory is based on what two types of proteins?

Microbiology

The **microbiology** department identifies the microorganisms that cause disease. Sensitivity tests the antibiotics that will successfully treat **pathogens** grown from patients' specimens. A bacterial species that causes a disease is a pathogen. Microbiology may include one or more of the following:

- Bacteriology—the study of bacteria
- Virology—the study of viruses
- Mycology—the study of fungi and yeasts
- Parasitology—the study of parasites

 CHECKPOINT QUESTION

8. Define the term *pathogen*.

Anatomic and Surgical Pathology

Anatomic and surgical pathology are involved in the diagnosis of disease using the gross inspection and microscopic examination of tissues removed from the body during surgery. In **surgical pathology**, the pathologist gives a diagnosis of the presence or absence of disease in tissue that is surgically removed from a patient.

Histology

Histology is the study of the microscopic structure of tissue. Histotechnologists prepare and stain samples of tissue for the pathologist to review under a microscope to determine whether disease is present.

Types of histology specimens include tissue obtained through biopsy and surgical frozen sections that must be evaluated immediately to determine whether further surgery is needed.

Cytology and Cytogenetics

Cytology is the study of the microscopic structure of cells. In cytology, the individual cells in body fluids and other specimens are evaluated microscopically for the presence of disease such as cancer. The most common cytology test is the Papanicolaou (Pap) test, in which vaginal cells scraped from the cervix are evaluated. **Cytogenetics** is a type of cytology used to test the genetic structure of the cells obtained from fluids such as amniotic fluid. These cells are examined for chromosome deficiencies related to genetic disease. Cytotechnologists prepare the specimens for review, and screen the slides for the test results. Pathologists review a percentage of patient slides reviewed by the cytotechnologist to confirm accuracy of the cytologists' reports.

COG Laboratory Personnel

Each professional position in a laboratory requires a particular level of education and training and has specific responsibilities (Box 24-1). The medical assistant may have an important role in laboratories other than the medical office. In general, medical assistants may be responsible for the following:

- Informing patients of the proper procedure or preparation for obtaining laboratory **specimens** (which are samples, such as blood or urine, used to evaluate a patient's condition)
- Obtaining a quality specimen
- Arranging for appropriate specimen transport
- Performing common laboratory tests using standards to ensure the accuracy, reliability, and timeliness of patient test results
- Documenting and maintaining a **quality assurance (QA)** program that ensures thorough patient care
- Maintaining laboratory instruments and equipment to manufacturers' standards

 CHECKPOINT QUESTION

9. What standards must be maintained when performing laboratory testing?

Medical assistants may control purchase of laboratory supplies and selection of reagents. Reagents are the substances used to test a patient specimen to measure an analyte. As the medical assistant, you may be in charge of **biohazard** safety and waste disposal for the workplace. Biohazards are biological agents that have the

BOX 24-1

LABORATORY PERSONNEL

- Pathologist. A physician who studies disease processes. Commonly, a pathologist oversees the technical aspects of a laboratory.
- Chief technologist or laboratory manager. A supervisor who manages the day-to-day operations of a laboratory, including staffing, test menu and pricing, purchasing, and QC.
- Medical technologist or clinical laboratory scientist. A graduate of a bachelor's (4-year) degree program (or equivalent) in medical laboratory science, who has been certified by the American Society of Clinical Pathology. Laboratory technologists perform all levels of testing and supervise laboratory departments.
- Medical laboratory technician or clinical laboratory technician. A graduate of an associate (2-year) degree program (or equivalent) in medical laboratory science who is nationally certified.
- Laboratory assistant. A person with a high school diploma or equivalent who is a graduate of a vocational or on-the-job laboratory assistant training program. Laboratory assistants collect and process specimens and can perform some designated testing.
- Phlebotomist. A professional trained to draw blood and to process blood and other samples. A phlebotomist may be a laboratory assistant, medical assistant, or person trained specifically in phlebotomy. A nationally certified phlebotomist has a high school diploma or equivalent and either is a graduate of an approved training program or has a minimum of 1 year of full-time work in phlebotomy.
- Histologist. A technician trained to process and evaluate tissue samples, such as biopsy or surgical samples.
- Cytologist. A professional trained to examine cells under the microscope and to look for abnormal changes; Pap smears are generally examined by cytologists.
- Specimen processor or accessioner. A professional trained to accept shipments of specimens and to centrifuge, separate, or otherwise process the samples to prepare them for testing. In addition, this position usually includes numbering and labeling the specimens and entering specimen information into a computer.

capacity to harm humans. Medical assistants may work in specimen processing. You must be aware of boundaries in your scope of practice in medical laboratory technology.

WHAT IF?

What if the patient asks you why his physician is ordering a specific laboratory test?

It is beyond any health care professional's scope of practice to answer a clinical question for a physician. The only exception is when the physician instructs the professional with a response for that particular patient. Some credible responses that can be shared with the patient include:

- "Your physician has ordered these tests to find out what is causing your symptoms."
- "These are the tests physicians order when you have a physical to be certain you are healthy."
- "This test is important to watch when you are taking this medication."

COG Body Systems and Laboratory Testing

Laboratory tests exist to help identify the cause of a person's illness. Sometimes a test reveals the specific cause. Sometimes a test will only suggest the possibility of a specific cause. A laboratory test also can eliminate a suspected cause. Understanding the significance of a laboratory result as it relates to a disease or body system is the key to ordering the test(s) most significant for the patient's symptoms. Appendix J lists highlights of the body systems, associated diseases, and laboratory tests used in diagnosis. Use the information in Appendix J to answer the following Checkpoint Questions.

CHECKPOINT QUESTION

10. What laboratory tests are performed when a diagnosis of acute appendicitis is being considered?

COG Ordering Laboratory Tests

Laboratory Request Forms

Laboratories provide and utilize request forms appropriate to their individual operations (Fig. 24-2). All forms should be convenient to use, with clear instructions for complete patient and physician identification. Most request forms cover a variety of tests, so that a single form can be used for tests in hematology, chemistry, immunology, and so on. Some forms serve as both a request and report form, listing expected values by test (Fig. 24-3). Many requisitions now contain bar codes

THIRD SHEET PHYSICIANS OFFICE   ☐ A   ☐ B   ☐ C   ☐ D

VISIT NUMBER						DATE OF SERVICE					
MRN #								DR. NAME				
CPI #								DR #				
PATIENT NAME				US PROVIDER NAME	
DATE OF BIRTH						SUB PROVIDER NO.		BILLING AREA

DATE OF INJURY | | | | | | LOCATION | | | | SPECIAL FSC | | |

INJURY TYPE: ☐ ACCIDENTAL   ☐ CAR   ☐ WORKER'S COMP

EMPLOYER'S NAME & ADDRESS

PRE-AUTH. #/CAROLINA ACCESS #

R E F   P H Y S

UPIN #   DOCTORS NAME

ADDRESS

CITY   STATE

TELEPHONE NO.
(   )

ONSET DATE | | | |

I authorize any holder of medical or other information about me to release to my healthcare provider, third party processor, the Health Care Financing Administration or its intermediaries or carriers any information needed for this health care encounter or a related claim. I permit a copy of this authorization to be used in place of the original, and request payment of authorized insurance benefits be made on my behalf to the WFU Physicians. I understand I am responsible for payment of these charges. I am also responsible for payment if my insurance carrier decides this is a non-covered service or requires prior authorization which I did not obtain.

X _____

SIGNATURE   DATE

IF ACCIDENTAL, *
DATE OF ONSET

OTHER DIAGNOSIS

789.00	Abdominal Plan	700	Corns and Calluses	684	Impetigo	601.01	Prostatitis, Chronic
706.1	Acne	733.6	Costochrondritis	487.1	Influenza	569.3	Rectal Bleeding
314.00	ADD - w/o hyperactivity	595.0	Cystitis, Acute	780.52	Insomnia	714.0	Rheumatoid Arthritis
314.01	ADD - w/hyperactivity	331.0	Dementia, NOS	564.1	Irritable Bowel	477.9	Rhinitis, Allergic
309.0	Adjust React. Breif Depression	311	Depressive Disorder	702.0	Keratosis, Actinic	472.0	Rhinitis - Chronic
995.2	Adverse Drug Reaction	691.8	Dermatitis, Atopic	702.19	Keratosis, Seborrheic	460	Rhinitis - Purulent
331.0	Alzheimer's Disease	691.0	Dermatitis, diaper	386.35	Labyrinthitis	133.0	Scabies
626.0	Ameorrhea	692.6	Dermatitis, Poison Ivy*		Laceration, Uncomp. (Specify Site)*	706.2	Sebaceous Cyst.
280.0	Anemia, Fe defic., Blood loss	692.9	Dermatitis & Eczema			345.10	Seizure Gen. Convul. Epileptic
280.1	Anemia, Fe defic., Dietary Def.	250.01	Diabetes Mellitus, Insulin dep.	464.0	Laryngitis, Acute	461. __	Sinusitis, Acute (Specify sinus)
281.0	Anemia, pernicious	250.00	Diab. Mellitus, Non-insulin dep.	132. __	Lice (Specify Site)		
300.02	Anxiety Disorder, Generalized	780.4	Dizziness/Vertigo, Light-headedness			473. __	Sinusitis, Chronic (Specify sinus)
308.0	Anxiety Reaction to Stress		Drug Dependence (Specify Drug)	214.1	Lipoma, skin		
414.00	A.S.H.D.			785.6	Lymph Nodes, Enlargement	701. __	Skin Tags (Specify Sites)
493.00	Asthma, childhood	995.2	Drug Reaction, Adverse	627.2	Menopausal Symptoms		
493.00	Asthma, extrinsic	625.3	Dysmenorrhea	626.1	Menstruation, Infrequent	845.00	Sprain, Ankle*
493.10	Asthma, intrinsic	536.8	Dyspepsia	626.2	Menstrucation, Excess or Freq.	847.2	Sprain, Lumbar*
427.31	Atrial Fibrillation	788.1	Dysuria	424.0	Mitral Valve Prolapse		Sprain/Strain (Specify Site, Lig.)*
724.2	Back Pain, Low	692.9	Eczema and Dermatitis	075	Mononucleosis		
596.0	Bladder Neck Obstruction	345.10	Epilepsy, General Convulsive		Nevus/Mole (Specify Site)	034.0	Strep Throat
	Boil & Carbuncle (Specify Site)	784.7	Epistaxis			438. __	Stroke, s/p, specific
		381.81	Eustachian Tube Dysfunction	278.00	Obesity, NOS		
610.0	Breast, fibrocycstic	780.7	Fatigue	715. __	Osteoarthritis (Specify Site)		Tendonitis (Specify Site)
611.72	Breast, Mass	610.1	Fibrocystic Breast Disease				
466.0	Bronchitis, Acute	729.1	Fibromyalgia	380.22	Otitis Externa, Acute	110.5	Tinea Corporis
491.20	Bronchitis, Chronic	729.0	Fibrositis	382.00	O.M., Acute Suppurative	V15.82	Tobacco Use
727.3	Bursitis	535.00	Gastritis, Acute Non-alcoholic	381.10	O.M., Chronic Serous	703.0	Toenail, Ingrown
3544.0	Carpal Tunnel Syndrome	008.8	Gastroenteritis, Viral	719.	Pain In Joint (Specify Joint)	463	Tonsillitis, Acute
	Cellulitis (Specify Site)	530.81	GERD			465.9	Upper Respiratory Infection
		274.0	Gout, arthropathy	729.5	Pain in Limb	099.40	Urethritis, non-GC
380.4	Cerumen in Ear	309.0	Grief Reaction	723.1	Pain, Neck	788.41	Urinary Frequency
616.0	Cervicitis	346.00	Headache, Migraine, Classical	785.1	Palpitations	599.0	UTI, Site Not Specified
786.51	Chest Pain	346.10	Headache, Migraine Common	300.01	Panic Attack	623.8	Vaginal Bleeding
052.9	Chicken Pox, no complications	784.0	Headache, Muscle Tension	795.0	Pap Smear, Abnormal	627.3	Vaginitis, Post Menopausal Atrophic
078.11	Condyloma Acumination	599.7	Hematuria	533.30	Peptic Ulcer, acute, no compl.	112.1	Vulvo Vaginitis, Monilial
428.0	Congestive Heart Failure	455.44	Hemorrhoids, Ext. Thrombosed	533.70	Peptic Ulcer, chronic, no compl.	131.01	Vulvo Vaginitis, Trichomonal
372.03	Conjunctivitis	455.5	Hemorrhoids, Ext. c-Comp.	462	Pharyngitis	616.10	Vulvo Vaginitis, Other
564.0	Constipation	455.2	Hermorrhoids, Int. c-Complication	614.0	PID, Acute	078.19	Warts, Plantar
V25.01	Contraception, Birth Control Pills	054.10	Herpes, Genital	614.1	PID, Chronic	078.10	Warts, Viral
V25.02	Contraception, Other	553.3	Hiatal Hernia	486	Pneumonia	783.1	Weight Gain, Abnormal
	Contusion (Specify Site)*	272.0	Hypercholesterolemia	V22.0	pregnancy, Normal, G1	783.2	Weight Loss, Abnormal
		272.2	Hyperlipidemia	V22.1	Pregnancy, Normal, not G1	V70.0	Well Adult Physical
491.20	C.O.P.D. w/o Acute Exacerbation	401.1	Hypertensionn, Benign Essential	625.4	Premenstrual Tension Syn.	V72.3	Well Woman Gyne.
491.21	C.O.P.D. w/Acute Exacerbation	402.10	Hypertensive H.D. w/o CHF	600	Prostate, Hyperpl.		
918.1	Corneal Abrasion*	244.9	Hypothyrodism, Acquired	601.0	Prostatitis, Acute		

Figure 24-2 Laboratory requisition. (Courtesy of Quest Diagnostics, 2007.)

Time Order Received:	**Third Street**	Doctor:
Time Collected:	**PHYSICIAN'S OFFICE, INC.**	
Time Reported:	123 Main Street Baltimore, MD 21201	Date:

LABORATORY

| Patient Name | Chart No. |

URINALYSIS

PHYSICAL

Color _____

Clarity_____

CHEMICAL

Leuk. Esterase _____

Nitrite _____

Urobilinogen _____

Protein _____

pH _____

Specific Gravity _____

Blood _____

Bilirubin _____

Ketones _____

Glucose _____

PREGNANCY

Urine HCG _____

Serum HCG _____

PROTHROMBIN TIME

Seconds _____

INR _____

SEDIMENTATION RATE

_____ Males 0-10

_____ Females 0-20

GLUCOSE

_____ 80-110 mg/dl

MONO

_____ NEG

STREP SCREEN

_____ NEG

PROVIDER PERFORMED MICROSCOPY

URINE MICROSCOPIC

Epis _____

WBCs_____

RBCs _____

Bacteria _____

Mucus _____

Amorphous _____

Other _____

KOH

_____

_____

WET PREP

_____

_____

_____

_____

Performed by: _____

Figure 24-3 Laboratory result form. Reference values are provided for the various tests.

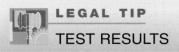

LEGAL TIP
TEST RESULTS

While working in a laboratory, you will have access to the results of many confidential blood tests, such as tests for HIV, drugs, pregnancy, and sexually transmitted diseases. You have an ethical responsibility not to communicate any results to unauthorized persons. Only patients and their physicians are entitled to the results. The only exception is the provision in state laws requiring the reporting of certain test results for public safety. Confidentiality is a HIPAA requirement in addition to an ethical responsibility.

that allow fast, accurate processing and reduce specimen identification errors. Most hospitals use computer-generated forms that also contain specimen labels. Box 24-2 lists the information required on all laboratory request forms.

PATIENT EDUCATION
SPECIMEN COLLECTION

Before collecting a specimen, instruct the patient on the proper preparation for testing. For instance, does the test require that the patient fast or follow a specific dietary regimen? Does the test require stopping any medications or modifying dose patterns? Is the timing of collection imperative, or will a random sample be sufficient? Failure to inform the patient properly before testing may result in erroneous (invalid) test results, which can cause a delay in treatment or incorrect diagnosis.

At the time of specimen collection, tell the patient:

- the name of the test (e.g., blood cell count), and
- the type of specimen required (e.g., blood, stool, urine).

Be sure to tell the patient approximately how long it will take for the results to be available and how and by whom the patient will be contacted regarding the results.

Patient education requirements for drawing an HIV test vary from state to state, although most require pretest and posttest counseling. Most states do not allow HIV test results to be given over the telephone.

Laboratory Test Panels

Common laboratory tests are organized into standard groups or **panels**. The **Centers for Medicare and Medicaid Services (CMS)** require the use of panels defined by the American Medical Association (AMA). The tests included in the comprehensive metabolic, basic metabolic, electrolyte, hepatic function, and lipid panels are defined in Table 24-1.

BOX 24-2

LABORATORY REQUEST FORMS: COMMONLY REQUIRED INFORMATION

- Patient's database. This includes name, address, and the medical office identification number to avoid errors with identical names. Other identifying information may be included.
- Patient's birth date and gender. Many test results vary with age and sex.
- Date and time of collection. Often test results are affected by the passage of time or the time of day the specimen was collected.
- Physician's name and address or identification number. Results may have to be reported immediately; this information also avoids errors in reporting.
- Checklist of the test or tests to be performed. These may be grouped under one heading as a panel, such as a renal panel or liver panel, which includes more than one test to determine the state of health of one organ, or a general health profile such as a complete blood count.
- Other required information may include the source of the specimen, such as culture swabs for microbiology tests; medications the patient is taking that may alter certain test results (e.g., anticoagulants affecting prothrombin time); directions for reporting (e.g., an immediate need should be marked "STAT"); and total volume of a 24-hour urine specimen.

TABLE 24-1 Test Panels Defined by the AMA and Mandated by CMS				
Comprehensive Metabolic	**Basic Metabolic**	**Electrolyte**	**Hepatic Function**	**Lipid**
Glucose	Glucose	Sodium	Albumin	Cholesterol
Calcium	Calcium	Potassium	Total protein	Triglycerides
Sodium	Sodium	Chloride	ALP	HDL
Potassium	Potassium	CO_2	ALT	LDL
Chloride	Chloride		AST	
CO_2	CO_2		Total bilirubin	
BUN	BUN		Direct bilirubin	
Creatinine	Creatinine			
Albumin				
Total protein				
ALP				
ALT				
AST				
Total bilirubin				

CO_2, carbon dioxide; BUN, blood urea nitrogen; ALP, alkaline phosphatase; ALT, alanine aminotransferase; AST, aspartate aminotransferase; HDL, high-density lipoprotein; LDL, low-density lipoprotein.

COG Physician Office Laboratory Testing

Most tests performed in the POL fall into one of two general categories: tests performed on a semiautomated machine and tests conducted with a self-contained kit. Tests in these categories vary among manufacturers.

The best source of information for safe and accurate testing is the **product insert**. In a product insert, the manufacturer provides the instructions and details for performing that test. It is shipped inside the test kit or the instrument reagents. Box 24-3 outlines the type of information contained in test product inserts. A test **kit** is a packaged set of supplies needed to perform a test. The package insert information should be used to write a procedure. The procedure will go in the **procedure manual** of all the tests performed at that medical office. Having a manual like this is suggested by the United States Department of Health and Human Services (HHS) and the Centers for Disease Control and Prevention (CDC). The CDC provides step-by-step instructions for writing a clinical procedure.

LEGAL TIP

ORDERS FOR LABORATORY TESTS

- A written request authorized by a practitioner licensed to order laboratory tests is required before a medical assistant can proceed with collection of a specimen for any laboratory procedure.
- In the communication of a laboratory order, the licensed provider (not a delegated representative) must obtain the patient's informed consent to undergo the procedure prior to referring the patient to the laboratory for testing.
- A licensed provider must be one of three people: the physician, the physician's assistant, or the nurse practitioner (not an RN, BSN, or MSN).
- This ordering process is both an ethical and a legal requirement in all 50 states.
- Depending on institutional policy, phoned orders from the licensed provider may be accepted only if their authenticity is later documented in the patient's record by the practitioner responsible for the verbal order.
- A licensed provider may write one single order for laboratory testing to be repeated at the ordered time interval lasting up to 6 months. This is called a *Standing Order* and must be renewed by the licensed provider every 6 months.

BOX 24-3

UNDERSTANDING KIT PACKAGE INSERTS

Test package inserts provide the following basic pieces of information:

- Procedure. Explains the test method in numbered steps, usually with illustrations.
- Test principles. Outlines the test.
- Specimen required. Tells whether the test is done on blood, urine, or other body fluids and what collection method is acceptable. Indicates if the specimen may be stored for later testing and, if so, under what conditions.
- Reagents needed (or included). Lists the reagents in the kit and any other reagents or materials necessary to perform the test.
- Quality control. States recommendations for testing procedures to ensure that test results are accurate.
- Expected values. Lists normal values for comparison to results obtained.
- Interferences. Explains any factors that may alter test results or compromise test accuracy.

 CHECKPOINT QUESTION

11. Who is authorized to order a laboratory test on a patient?

COG Point-of-Care Testing

Point-of-care tests (POC tests, or POCT) have become available because computer chip technology allows small, handheld devices to be carried to the patient's bedside, the pharmacy, the physician's office, the patient's home, and to other nonlaboratory sites. POC testing is defined as testing at the point where patient care is given.

Some people may think that because using a POC instrument is so easy, all that is needed is to turn the instrument on and start doing tests on patient specimens. However, good laboratory practice is defined by the HHS and the CDC.

Good laboratory practices for POLs performing POCT direct the POL to define:

- the people responsible for method selection and development, training, QC, etc.
- the procedure for staff training
- the procedure for reporting of results
- QA monitoring, including QC procedures

COG Laboratory Equipment

Laboratory equipment and supplies for performing physician office tests come in a variety of types and sizes. It is not necessary to become familiar with every possible type of laboratory equipment. However, a few basic pieces are common to most small laboratories. These include the following:

- Automated cell counter
- Microscope
- Chemistry analyzer
- Centrifuge
- Incubator
- Refrigerator or freezer

Cell Counter

A cell counter is an automated analyzer used to count and size blood cells. The simplest cell counter counts only RBCs and WBCs and performs hemoglobin and hematocrit testing. Specimens are inserted individually, and results may be printed or read from a screen (see Chapter 27). Cell counters also include more complex analyzers that accept hundreds of specimens and perform 12 to 15 tests, calculations, and cell differentials on each specimen.

Microscope

The microscope is used to identify and count cells and microorganisms in blood and other body specimens. Learning how to use a microscope properly requires time and repeated practice. The compound microscope is the type most commonly used in the medical office. The compound microscope is a two-lens system in which ocular and objective lenses together provide the total magnification. A light source illuminates the objects as they are magnified. Figure 24-4 shows a microscope and its various parts.

The *frame*, which consists of the arm and base, is the basic structural component of the microscope. The oculars at the top of the instrument are for the user's eyes. Each is marked with its magnification, usually ×10. Binocular microscopes (two eyepieces) minimize eyestrain and have adjustments to allow for variations in spacing between the user's eyes.

To bring the object to be viewed into focus, the *coarse adjustment knob* is used with the lower-powered objective to focus on the object; the *fine adjustment knob* is used with the higher-powered objective or the oil immersion lens for the greatest definition. Always focus in two steps. First look at the slide and objective from the side (not through the ocular or oculars), bringing the slide very close to the lens. Then look through the ocular or oculars while moving the slide farther from the lens to bring it into focus. This procedure will prevent damage to the lens from contact with the slide.

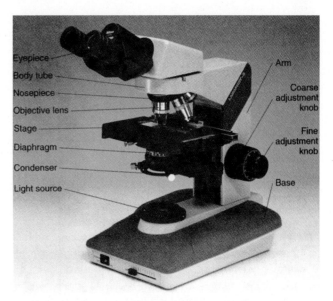

Figure 24-4 Basic components of the standard light microscope. (Courtesy of Nikon, Melville, NY.)

The *nosepiece* houses three or four objective lenses and rotates to bring the objective into working position. Pressure to the objectives should never be used to rotate lenses. Only the grip should be used to make this adjustment. The magnification power is marked on each objective. The shorter, or low-power, objective magnifies ×10. The higher power magnifies ×40 for closer observation. With the use of oil, the third objective, called the *oil immersion lens*, magnifies ×100. Some microscopes have a fourth objective with a ×4 lens to scan larger specimens. To determine the total magnification of a specimen, multiply the magnification of the working objective by the magnification of the ocular lens (×10):

- Low power: $10 \times 10 = 100$
- High power: $40 \times 10 = 400$
- Oil immersion: $100 \times 10 = 1,000$

The *stage* is the flat surface that holds the slide for viewing. An opening in the solid surface allows illumination of the slide from below. Many stages have clips to hold the slide in place and to allow manual movement of the slide as needed. Some stages mechanically adjust the position vertically or horizontally by moving adjustment knobs, also called *X-* and *Y-axis knobs*.

The *condenser* concentrates the light rays to focus on the slide. The condenser is adjustable. In the lower position, the light focus is reduced; in the higher position, it is increased.

The *diaphragm*, in the condenser, consists of interlocking plates that adjust into a variable-sized opening, or iris, to regulate the amount of light from the source in conjunction with the condenser. The more highly magnified the slide must be, the greater the need for light.

The *light source* is housed in the base.

PROPER HANDLING OF A MICROSCOPE

- Always lift your microscope with one hand holding the "arm" and the other hand under the base; avoid bumping or jarring the scope. This delicate instrument can easily go out of alignment if it is handled roughly. You will only be able to carry one microscope or lamp at a time if you are to avoid the possibility of damage.
- Use your microscope on a sturdy, solid surface and away from the edge. Vibrations can also cause the microscope to go out of alignment.
- Never touch the lenses of the eyepieces and objectives with your finger. Keep all glass and optical lenses clean. Use lens paper dipped in a lens cleaning solution to gently wipe dust and oils off the eyepieces, objectives, condenser, and illumination glass. (Never use a paper towel or tissue to wipe a lens—the fibers in them will scratch the lenses.)
- Keep the stage and the other metal parts free of excess oil. An alcohol wipe is best but is not recommended for use on the lenses.
- To keep your microscope in top condition for years, have the microscope professionally serviced once a year.
- When you are finished using your microscope, rotate the nosepiece so that it is on the low-power objective, roll the nosepiece so that it is all the way down to the stage, and then replace the dust cover.
- Always keep the dust cover on your scope when it is not in use.

Microscopes are delicate, expensive instruments. To ensure that the microscope used in the clinical laboratory is kept in good working order, it must be handled properly (Box 24-4) and maintained according to the manufacturer's standards (Procedure 24-1). Be sure to place it in a low-traffic area and away from any source of vibration such as a centrifuge. It should always be covered when not in use. Check out the skills video included in this textbook to see the process of maintaining a microscope.

Chemistry Analyzer

Chemistry analyzers vary from simple instruments that perform from a single to a few tests and require manual operation to complex analyzers that perform 30 or more tests per sample and are operated by computer.

A number of bench-top chemistry analyzers are suitable for POL testing. Several use dry reagent technology, in which all reagents are impregnated into a special strip or card. The strip or card is inserted into the analyzer, and a drop of whole blood or serum is applied to the strip with an automated pipette. Other analyzers use wet reagent systems with special reagent packs required for each type of test. Whatever the analyzer, the operator must follow the specific manufacturer's instructions for proper care and use.

Centrifuge

A centrifuge swings its contents in a circle to separate liquids into their component parts. Centrifugation is the process of separating blood or other body fluid cells from liquid components using a centrifuge. A specimen of **whole blood** (blood containing all its cellular components), when centrifuged, is separated into a bottom layer of heavy RBCs, a thin middle layer of platelets and WBCs called the *buffy coat* (Fig. 24-5), and a top liquid layer that is the lightest of the components. The top layer is **serum,** if the specimen was allowed to clot before centrifuging, or **plasma** if the specimen was anticoagulated and not allowed to clot.

Tubes must always be balanced in the centrifuge (Box 24-5). If an uneven number of tubes is to be spun, a tube with water must balance the odd tube. Try to place tubes with approximately the same level of liquid in opposing spaces. All tubes must be securely capped. Never start centrifugation until the lid is locked. Never open the centrifuge until all motion has stopped, and

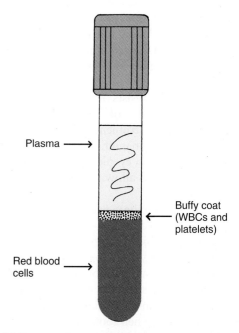

Plasma →

Buffy coat → (WBCs and platelets)

Red blood → cells

Figure 24-5 Centrifuged blood specimen. (Reprinted with permission from McCall R. Phlebotomy Essentials. Baltimore: Lippincott Williams & Wilkins, 2003.)

BOX 24-5

QUICK TIPS FOR SAFE CENTRIFUGE OPERATION

1. Wear appropriate PPE.
2. Use the centrifuge on a solid, level work surface.
3. Avoid unbalanced loads; immediately stop the centrifuge if it is vibrating more than normal.
4. Always keep the lid closed while the rotor is spinning, and do not disturb the centrifuge while it is operating.
5. Properly dispose of any broken or damaged centrifuge tubes.

(Source: 6 Safety Tips for Operating a Centrifuge, www. labmanager.com/stips.asp?ID=105 Posted: 2/24/2010.)

never stop the spin by hand. Follow the manufacturer's recommendations for cleaning, oiling, and maintaining the centrifuge. As with all equipment, read the instructions before operation.

A special type of centrifuge called a *microhematocrit centrifuge* is used to perform hematocrit testing, further discussed in Chapter 27.

CHECKPOINT QUESTION

12. How does the centrifuge work, and what is its purpose?

Incubator

Microbiology specimens require a suitable environment to thrive and reproduce. Culture media inoculated with specimens are stored in an incubator for approximately 24 hours to allow microbes to reproduce to a large enough quantity to be identified. The incubator is set at about body temperature (99°F or 37°C), and a daily log is maintained to record the incubator temperature.

Refrigerators and Freezers

Laboratory refrigerators and freezers are similar to those used in the home, but their uses are very different. They store reagents, kits, and specimens. The temperature is critical and must be measured and recorded daily. The refrigerator should be able to maintain a constant temperature of 4°C to 8°C to remain in service. Food should never be stored in these refrigerators because of the possibility of biohazard contamination.

WHAT IF?

What if a specimen tube breaks in the centrifuge?

- If a specimen tube breaks in a centrifuge, do not open the lid. Avoid disturbing the centrifuge for 30 minutes so any aerosols can settle.
- Put on personal protective equipment (PPE), including face shield, impervious gown, and gloves.
- Remove rotors and buckets, seal in a plastic bag, and move aside to perform the cleaning procedure described below.
- Dispose of any sharp debris in a sharps container.
- Clean the inside of the centrifuge with paper towels and chemical disinfectant. (*Note:* Avoid bleach solution, which may be corrosive.)
- Soak removable parts in disinfectant for 30 minutes, rinse, dry and replace them in the centrifuge.
- Discard liquid and other wastes using proper procedures.
- Clean the face shield and gown per lab protocol, and dispose of gloves appropriately.

MEDIA MENU

- **Student Resources on thePoint**
  - **Video: Caring for a Microscope (Procedure 24-1)**
  - **CMA/RMA Certification Exam Review**
- **Internet Resources**

  Commission on Office Laboratory Accreditation
  http://www.cola.org

  Centers for Medicare and Medicaid Services
  http://www.cms.hhs.gov

  Center for Disease Control and Prevention
  http://www.cdc.gov

  United States Department of Health and Human Services
  http://www.hhs.gov

PSY PROCEDURE 24-1:   **Caring for a Microscope**

Purpose: To protect the integrity and function of the microscope
Equipment: Lens paper, lens cleaner, gauze, mild soap solution, microscope, hand disinfectant, surface disinfectant

Steps	Reasons
1. Wash your hands.	Handwashing aids infection control.
2. Assemble the equipment.	Equipment must be readily accessible in order for the procedure to be done.
3. If you need to move the microscope, carry it in both hands, one holding the base and the other holding the arm. (See Box 24-4.)	Jarring or dropping the microscope will damage the optics.
4. Clean the optical areas following these steps: A. Place a drop or two of lens cleaner on a piece of lens paper. B. Wipe each eyepiece thoroughly with lens paper and lens cleaner. Do not touch the optical areas with your fingers.	Do not use tissue or gauze because either may scratch the lenses. Direct contact will transfer oils from your skin to the optical surfaces.

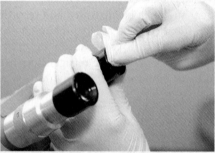

Step 4B. Wipe each eyepiece with lens paper and lens cleaner.

C. Wipe each objective lens starting with the lowest power and continuing to the highest power (usually an oil immersion lens). If the lens paper appears to have dirt or oil on it, use a clean section of the lens paper or a new piece of lens paper with cleaner.

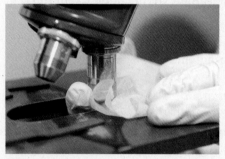

Step 4C. Wipe each objective lens with lens paper and lens cleaner. Clean the oil objective last so you won't carry its oil to the other objective lenses.

D. Using a new piece of dry lens paper, wipe eyepiece and the objective lens so that no cleaner remains.

Removing the cleaner completely prevents distortion by residue.

E. With a new piece of lens paper moistened with lens cleaner, clean the condenser and illuminator optics.

PSY PROCEDURE 24-1: **Caring for a Microscope (continued)**

Steps	Reasons

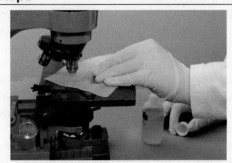

Step 4E. Clean and dry the condenser and illuminator optics.

5. Clean areas other than the optics:
  A. Moisten gauze with mild soap solution or use an alcohol wipe and wipe all areas other than the optics including the stage, base, and adjustment knobs.
  B. Moisten another gauze with water and rinse the washed areas.

This removes oil and dirt from mechanical and structural surfaces.

6. To store the cleaned microscope, ensure that the light source is turned off. Rotate the nosepiece so that the low-power objective is pointed down toward the stage. Cover the microscope with the plastic dust cover that came with it or a small trash bag.

This protects the mechanism and surfaces between uses.

7. Document microscope cleaning on the microscope maintenance log sheet.

Documentation of instrument service history is required for all laboratory equipment.

NAME OF LABORATORY:		INSTRUMENT NAME AND ID:		
Date of Maintenance	Action Performed	Comments	OK to Use?	Initials

Step 7. Sample instrument log sheet.

Note: To maintain precision focusing, the microscope should be used in a low-traffic area and away from any source of vibration such as a centrifuge.
Note: Follow the manufacturer's recommendations for changing the light bulb and servicing the microscope.

Charting Example:

8/26/2012 11:30 AM Microscope cleaned according to manufacturer's recommendations —————— D. Howell, CMA

- Laboratory analysis of blood, urine, and other body samples provides the physician with powerful diagnostic tools to identify diseases and disorders.
- Hospital and referral laboratories are divided into departments named for the specialty testing done in that department. Knowledge of each of the specialty categories makes it easier to understand the nature of the tests and the diagnostic information they provide. Specialty categories include: hematology, coagulation, clinical chemistry, toxicology, urinalysis, immunohematology, immunology, microbiology, and anatomic and surgical pathology.
- Just like the specific academic and clinical experience required to be eligible for the CMA exam, there are specific academic and clinical experiences required for the various types of laboratory professionals to be eligible for their certification exams.
- The product insert is the key tool for accurate testing and QC instructions. To obtain an accurate result from a test kit or reagent, the instructions in the product insert must be strictly followed.
- Laboratory test panels defined by the AMA and mandated by CMS provide national standardization of nomenclature and testing to evaluate disease processes and organ systems.
- Instead of testing in a central laboratory, POCT is performed, usually with a handheld instrument, wherever the patient is receiving care. Use of POCT equipment appears very simple, but errors with POCT have the same serious outcomes as errors that occur in general laboratory testing. Adhering to good laboratory practice standards will reduce the risk of erroneous patient test results.
- There are a few basic pieces of laboratory equipment that are standard from laboratory to laboratory. Each laboratory may have some or all of this equipment. There are a variety of companies that manufacturer instruments in each category described.
- The medical assistant has the responsibility to maintain a safe work environment. Following manufacturers' instructions for operating their instruments is a required safety precaution. Pay special attention to the safety guidelines for operating a centrifuge.

Warm Ups for Critical Thinking

1. Review Box 24-2 on understanding package inserts. Ask your instructor for a copy of a package insert from a test kit you will be using in class. Locate each bulleted item listed in the box and find the corresponding information on your sample package insert.
2. Review the section of this chapter describing referral laboratories. The physician requests a laboratory test that is unfamiliar to you. You do not find the test listed in the referral laboratory's test catalogue. How would you get the appropriate patient preparation and specimen collection, processing, and transport instructions for the requested test?

CLIA Compliance and Laboratory Safety

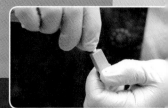

Clinical Laboratory Improvement Amendments

Laws Governing the Clinical Laboratory

Laboratory Quality Assessment

Laboratory Safety

Occupational Safety and Health Administration

Adherence of Health Care Personnel to Recommended Guidelines

Hand Hygiene

Personal Protective Equipment for Health Care Personnel

Safe Work Practices to Prevent Exposure to Bloodborne Pathogens

Biohazard Waste Disposal

General Safety Guidelines

Incident Reports

Cognitive Domain

Note: AAMA/CAAHEP 2008 Standards are italicized.

1. Spell and define the key terms
2. Explain the significance of the CLIA and describe how to maintain compliance in the physician office laboratory
3. Discuss the practices physician office laboratories must define to assure good performance of waived testing
4. Using CLIA guidelines, identify laboratory tests that are and are not within the scope of practice for a medical assistant
5. *Identify disease processes that are indications for CLIA-waived tests*
6. Identify the consequences of practicing outside CLIA guidelines
7. *Identify the role of the Centers for Disease Control (CDC) regulations in health care settings*
8. Define critical values and document the proper notification to the health care professional
9. Identify results that require follow-up and document action in chart
10. Identify how to handle all test results whether inside or outside the reference interval and document on a flow sheet
11. Identify and use quality control methods

12. Define proficiency testing and describe why CLIA requires it to maintain laboratory quality
13. Identify the source of instrument maintenance and calibration instructions
14. *Analyze charts, graphs, and/or tables in the interpretation of health care results*
15. Define OSHA and state its purpose
16. *Discuss the application of standard precautions with regard to: a) all body fluids, secretions, and excretions; b) blood; c) non-intact skin; and d) mucous membranes*
17. *Identify safety techniques that can be used to prevent accidents and maintain a safe work environment*
18. List the types and uses of personal protective equipment
19. *Identify safety signs, symbols, and labels*
20. Describe the reasons to file an incident report
21. Describe the Needlestick Safety and Prevention Act and list its requirements

Psychomotor Domain

Note: AAMA/CAAHEP 2008 Standards are italicized.

1. *Practice standard precautions*
2. *Participate in training on standard precautions*

3. *Comply with safety signs, symbols, and labels*
4. *Evaluate the work environment to identify safe versus unsafe working conditions*
5. Screen and follow up test results and document laboratory results appropriately (Procedure 25-1)
6. Use methods of quality control (Procedure 25-2)
7. *Document accurately in the patient record*
8. Perform routine maintenance of clinical equipment (Procedure 25-3)
9. *Perform patient screening using established protocols*
10. *Assist physician with patient care*

2. Document accurately
3. Understand the various medical terminology for each specialty
4. Comply with federal, state, and local health laws and regulations
5. Apply principles of aseptic techniques and infection control
6. Screen and follow up patient test results
7. Use standard precautions
8. Advise patients of office policies and procedures
9. Practice quality control
10. Dispose of biohazardous materials

ABHES Competencies

1. Define scope of practice for the medical assistant, and comprehend the conditions for practice within CLIA regulations

Key Terms

aerosol	confirmatory test	material safety data sheet (MSDS)	shifts
calibration	control	nonwaived testing	specificity
bloodborne pathogens	critical values	personal protective equipment (PPE)	standard precautions
chemical hygiene plan (CHP)	Department of Health and Human Services (HHS)	proficiency testing	transmission-based precautions
CLIA certification	direct microscopic examination	provider-performed microscopy (PPM, or PPMP)	therapeutic range
Clinical and Laboratory Standards Institute (CLSI)	external control	qualitative test	trends
Commission on Office Laboratory Accreditation (COLA)	Food and Drug Administration (FDA)	quantitative test reconstitution	universal precautions
	internal control	sensitivity	

COG Clinical Laboratory Improvement Amendments

"CLIA" stands for the **Clinical Laboratory Improvement Amendments Act of 1988**. CLIA is a federal regulatory program that sets standards for the quality of laboratory testing. Every facility that performs laboratory procedures on human specimens, even just a single test per year, requires appropriate certification under the CLIA program.

Even if a laboratory does tests at no cost, it must have a CLIA certificate to meet federal requirements. To help POLS with CLIA compliance, the **Commission on Office Laboratory Accreditation (COLA)** was established. COLA is one of the organizations CLIA approves to do laboratory inspections. COLA works to support the health care industry by providing knowledge and resources for maintaining quality laboratory operations.

Laws Governing the Clinical Laboratory

The goals of CLIA are to standardize laboratory testing and enforce quality protocols anywhere tests are performed on patients. The Centers for Medicare and

Medicaid Services (CMS) regulate all laboratory testing performed on humans through CLIA.

There may be state regulations for laboratory testing. When state requirements are stricter than federal requirements, the state requirements must be followed.

 CHECKPOINT QUESTION

1. What is the purpose of CLIA?

Levels of Testing

CLIA regulations established three levels of testing based on the complexity of the test. These levels include waived tests, moderate-complexity tests, and high-complexity tests. Laboratory personnel are required to have specific education or training in order to perform certain tests.

The levels of testing are monitored for compliance by agencies of the federal government.

Waived Tests

Waived tests are simple, one-step tests. However, performing them incorrectly can cause errors and endanger patient health. Consequently, the government requires a Certificate of Waiver (CW) to perform waived tests.

Oversight of waived testing and Certificates of Waiver are controlled by the **Department of Health and Human Services (HHS)**. HHS is the U.S. government's agency for protecting the health of all Americans and providing essential human services. The **Centers for Disease Control and Prevention (CDC)** is the U.S. federal agency under HHS that works to protect public health and safety. CDC sets standards for good laboratory practices. CDC's job is to focus national attention on:

- disease prevention
- environmental health
- occupational safety and health
- prevention and education activities to improve the health of the people of the United States

Waived testing includes many tests simple enough for the patient to perform at home (e.g., dipstick urinalysis and glucose monitoring). Even with the waiver, the physician office laboratory (POL) must still follow all manufacturers' recommendations for each piece of equipment or product used for testing. Medical assistants may perform waived tests.

The following are a few of the tests listed in the waived category:

- Urine dipstick or reagent tablets
- Fecal occult blood packets
- Urine pregnancy testing kits using color comparison charts
- Centrifuged microhematocrits
- Point-of-care blood glucose determination testing

Disease processes that are indications for CLIA-waived tests are described in Table 25-1.

TABLE 25-1 Disease Processes That Indicate CLIA-Waived Tests	
Waived Test	**Some Related Disease Processes**
Urine dipstick or reagent tablets	Hematuria; metabolic disorders; kidney disorders; multiple myeloma; inflammation; diabetes mellitus; liver disease; urinary tract infection; hepatitis; hemolytic anemia
Fecal occult blood packets	Colon cancer
Urine pregnancy testing kits using color comparison charts	Pregnancy
Nonautomated erythrocyte sedimentation rate tests	Inflammation
Nonautomated copper sulfate testing for hemoglobin	Anemia; polycythemia; dehydration
Centrifuged microhematocrits	Anemia; polycythemia; dehydration
Low-complexity blood glucose determination testing	Hyperglycemia; hypoglycemia; diabetes; pre-diabetes
Hemoglobin by single analyte instruments with self-contained reagent and specimen interaction and direct measurement and readout	Anemia; polycythemia; dehydration
CLIA-waived strep test kits	Group A streptococcal infection
CLIA-waived mono test kits	Infectious mononucleosis
CLIA-waived influenza test kits	Influenza A or B

CHECKPOINT QUESTIONS

2. Can a medical assistant perform waived testing on a POL patient?
3. Identify disease processes that are indications for urine dipstick testing.

Other tests, including those for rapid strep, have waived methodologies available, but the **Food and Drug Administration (FDA)** has not provided waived status for every lab test. The FDA is an agency of the HSS. The FDA is responsible for protecting and promoting public health through the regulations and supervision of laboratory and blood transfusions products. The most up-to-date listing of available waived tests can be found on the Center for Medicare and Medicaid (CMS) Web site. The CMS is an agency within HHS. It is responsible for administering the Medicare and Medicaid programs. CMS is important in this discussion because for the POL to receive Medicare and Medicaid funds, it must be compliant with CLIA.

Box 25-1 lists criteria to help understand waived testing.

CHECKPOINT QUESTION

4. Give the full name and responsibility or purpose for the HHS, CDC, CMS, and FDA.

BOX 25-1

DETERMINE IF YOUR TESTING SITE PERFORMS WAIVED LABORATORY TESTING

The complexity of laboratory testing can be overwhelming. The information provided here is designed to help you understand waived testing and good laboratory practices that will help ensure accurate patient test results.

If your laboratory draws patient specimens but does not perform any testing on site and refers them to another laboratory for testing, you do not need to determine whether the testing is classified as waived or nonwaived. Compliance with testing requirements is the responsibility of the testing laboratory. However, good laboratory practices should be followed to ensure that the patient has been properly prepared for testing and that the correct specimen(s) are obtained. Specimen storage and transportation to the testing site are very important to assure that the specimen is acceptable for testing when it reaches the testing site so that the test results are reliable.

Who decides if I am doing waived testing?

The oversight of laboratory testing is CLIA. These regulations require that all laboratories that examine materials derived from the human body for diagnosis, prevention, or treatment purposes, regardless of location or size, be certified by the HHS.

The CMS administers the CLIA laboratory certification program for HHS in conjunction with the CDC and the FDA.

What are waived tests?

Waived tests are determined by FDA to be so simple that there is little risk of error. Even though waived tests are described as simple to perform, erroneous results are possible and can produce untoward patient outcomes if acted upon.

What tests are considered waived?

Tests and methods that are waived are listed on the Web site: http://www.cms.hhs.gov/CLIA/downloads/CR5600.waivedtble.pdf.

What are the requirements for laboratories that perform waived testing?

According to the CLIA law, laboratories that perform waived testing must meet the following requirements:

• Enroll in the CLIA program
• Pay applicable certificate fees biennially
• Follow manufacturers' test instructions

What do I need to do if I perform PPMP in my laboratory?

Laboratories that perform PPMP testing must follow the following requirements under CLIA:

• Enroll in the CLIA program
• Pay applicable certificate fees biennially
• Meet certain quality and administrative requirements

Will laboratories that only perform waived testing be inspected by CMS?

CMS makes onsite visits to approximately 2% of CW laboratories. The visits are educational and focused on information gathering. CMS has indicated that it is important that every CW site receive education about good laboratory practices and how to understand and follow manufacturer's instructions.

ETHICAL TIP

Common Issues of Laboratory Noncompliance with CLIA Standards

Efforts to reduce medical errors, improve health care quality, and increase patient safety have been gaining national attention. As a part of the POL survey by a CMS surveyor, the CMS surveyor provides observations of noncompliance in the CW POL and to CMS. It is the ethical responsibility of anyone performing laboratory tests to be informed of what testing he or she is allowed to perform and the performance requirements of each laboratory test.

The most common issues of noncompliance include:

- Performing nonwaived testing without using CLIA-required quality measures
- Performing nonwaived tests without proper credentials
- Not meeting CLIA requirements for personnel, quality control (QC), proficiency testing, or instrument maintenance; not having adequate records
- Not having the most recent instructions for the waived-test systems in use
- Not routinely checking the product insert for changes
- Not using correct terminology when reporting results
- Using expired reagents or control materials
- Not storing products as described in the product insert
- Not following up with **confirmatory tests** as specified in the test instructions (*Note:* A confirmatory test is an additional, more specific test performed to rule out or confirm a preliminary test result to provide a final result.)
- Not performing function checks or **calibration** checks to ensure the test system's operation (*Note:* Calibration is a method provided by the manufacturer to standardize a test or laboratory instrument.)

Moderate-Complexity Tests

Most of the testing performed in large laboratories is considered moderate complexity. Moderate-complexity testing has one or more of these characteristics:

- It uses complex manual methodologies or instrumentation.
- It is suitable for use only by highly trained scientists inside the clinical laboratory.
- It requires detailed quality assurance (QA) and QC procedures.

Moderate-complexity testing laboratories are subject to unannounced inspections from either CMS or CMS-approved agencies. The following are some moderate-complexity tests that may be performed in POLs with moderate-complexity certification and medical laboratory scientists qualified to perform the tests:

- Urine and throat cultures
- Automated testing for cholesterol, high-density lipoproteins, and triglycerides
- Gram staining
- Microscopic urinalysis
- Automated hematology procedures
- Manual white blood cell count differentials
- Automated coagulation procedures
- Automated chemistry procedures
- Automated urinalyses

One category of testing is called **provider-performed microscopy** (**PPM or PPMP**). PPM is **direct microscopic examination**, the direct examination of a patient specimen using a microscope. PPM is a type of **nonwaived testing**. Nonwaived tests are tests at a level of complexity that does not meet the CLIA criteria for waiver. PPM testing is outside of the scope of practice for medical assistants. In any laboratory from POL to large referral laboratories, PPM can be performed only by a physician, dentist, nurse midwife, nurse practitioner, or physician assistant under the direct supervision of a physician. Any qualified person may perform PPM in the clinical laboratory where the microscope is housed. PPM tests include:

- All direct wet-mount preparations
- All potassium hydroxide preparations
- Pinworm examinations
- Urine sediment examinations

High-Complexity Tests

High-complexity tests, which are rarely performed in medical offices, include:

- Advanced cell studies (cytogenetics)
- Cytology (e.g., Pap tests)
- Histopathology
- Manual cell counts

If the level of testing is in question, it must be considered high complexity. CMS publishes a list of all tests in all complexity categories. States may establish stricter rules than those set by the governing body, but they may not adopt less strict rules.

 CHECKPOINT QUESTION

5. List the three levels of laboratory testing defined by CLIA. Which level of testing is approved for performance by medical assistants?

CLIA Certification

Medical assistants who are asked to prepare a medical office to perform laboratory testing will first need to apply for **CLIA certification**. CLIA certification is required by any group that performs even one test, including a waived test.

The CLIA application collects information about a laboratory's operation, which is necessary to determine the type of certificate to be issued and the fees to be assessed. The application for a CLIA CW may be accessed at https://www.cms.gov/cmsforms/downloads/cms116.pdf. Information to be submitted with the application includes:

• Verification of state licensure, as applicable
• Documentation of qualifications: education (copy of diploma, transcript from accredited institution, continuing medical education units)
• Credentials
• Laboratory experience

There are penalties for a laboratory that does not comply with CLIA regulations.

CHECKPOINT QUESTION

6. How does the POL find the forms to apply for a CLIA CW?

Laboratory Quality Assessment

CLIA requires a QA plan. This is a plan for ensuring the quality of all areas of the laboratory's technical and support functions. QA should monitor the following laboratory functions:

• Patient preparation
• Specimen collection, processing, preservation, and transportation
• Test analysis, reporting and interpretation

The laboratory must have a written QA policy that is communicated to all of the laboratory staff. The purpose of the QA policy is to prevent problems before they occur. When there is an error or problem, corrective action must begin and be documented. When the lab is inspected, the inspector will expect to see a well-written QA policy.

As a part of the QA plan, the laboratory must have a training and continuing education plan for the laboratory personnel. There must be evaluations to ensure that workers are competent. The qualifications and responsibilities of all laboratory workers are specified by CLIA.

Personnel Training

Although a medical assistant receives training in laboratory procedures in the classroom and school laboratory, the exact tests performed in a POL are taught as a part of orientation to the POL.

CHECKPOINT QUESTION

7. Why does a POL need a QA plan? What should be included in the plan?

Competency Assessment

Competency assessment is the evaluation of a person's ability to perform a test and to use a testing device. Periodic evaluation of competency is a CLIA requirement. The evaluation must focus on education and promoting good testing practices.

Proficiency testing provides evaluation of the laboratory. Proficiency testing programs provide unknown samples to test as if they were patient specimens. The POL sends the results to the proficiency testing service, and the results are graded on how close they are to the target values. The testing agency grades the laboratory's results and reports them both to the laboratory and to CMS. Laboratory inspectors require proficiency testing results for review during the inspection.

Patient Test Management

The laboratory must have a policy to keep specimens properly treated and identified. The policy must provide for the results to be accurately reported. Policy and procedure manuals will instruct the medical assistant in the laboratory to correctly:

• prepare the patient,
• handle the specimen,
• perform the test, and
• know what to do if the test results are questionable.

The procedure manual should give the instructions on performing a laboratory test from beginning to end.

CLIA Standards for Laboratory Procedure Manuals

The laboratory procedure manual is the primary reference in operating the POL. CLIA regulations require each laboratory to have a procedure for every test in the laboratory. Procedures must follow the manufacturer's testing instructions. The instructions are in the product insert.

Procedures require reagents and controls. A **control** is a device or solution used to monitor the test to correct test results. A reagent is a substance that produces a reaction with a patient specimen so the analyte can be detected or measured. Requirements for using the controls are listed in the product insert.

Product inserts contain most of the needed information (Table 25-2) to write a procedure. The POL must add the instructions to make the test results available within that office. A procedure manual can also include examples of forms used.

TABLE **25-2**	**Components of a Manufacturer's Product Insert**
Component	**Information provided**
Intended use	Describes the test purpose, the substance being detected or measured, testing methodology, appropriate specimen, and the FDA-cleared conditions for use. It may address if the test is to be used for diagnosis or screening.
Summary	Explains what the test detects and a short history of the methodology, including the disease process or health condition being detected or monitored.
Test principle	States the methodology of the test. Details the technical aspects of the test. Explains how the components of the test system interact with the patient's specimen to detect or measure a specific substance.
Precautions	Alerts the user of practices or conditions that might affect the test and warns of potential hazards. Might address conditions for specimen acceptability.
Storage/stability	Specifies conditions for storing reagents and test systems to protect their stability. It includes recommended temperature ranges and any physical requirements (e.g., protection from light or humidity.) Also addresses the stability of reagents and test systems when opened or after reconstitution. Describes indicators of reagent deterioration.
Reagents and materials supplied	Lists the reagents and materials provided in the test system kit, and the concentration and major ingredients used to make the reagents.
Materials required but not provided	Lists materials needed to perform the test, but not provided in the test system kit.
Specimen collection and preparation	Details the procedures for specimen collection, handling, storage, and stability, including (as needed) the directions for performing a fingerstick, appropriate anticoagulant or swab type, and directions for specimen preparation. Might address conditions for specimen acceptability.
Test procedure	Provides step-by-step instructions for performing the test, often with pictures or graphs. Includes critical information (e.g., the order of reagent addition, timing of test steps, mixing and temperature requirements, and reading of the test results).
Interpretation of results	Describes how to read and interpret the test results, often including visual aids. Alerts the user when results are invalid and gives instructions on what to do when the results cannot be interpreted. Might include precautions against reporting results unless supplementary and/or confirmatory testing is performed.
Quality control	Explains what parts of the test system are monitored by QC procedures and provides instructions on how to perform QC. Includes recommendations on how frequently QC should be performed, acceptable QC results, and what to do when QC values are not acceptable. Might include information about external QC, and, if applicable, internal QC.
Limitations	Describes conditions that might influence the test results or for which the test is not designed. Limitations should include: • Possible interferences from medical conditions, drugs, or other substances. • Warning that the test is not approved with alternate specimen types or in alternate populations (e.g., pediatric). • Indications of the need for additional testing that might be more specific or more sensitive. **Specificity** is the ability of a test to detect a particular substance or constituent without interference or false reactions by other substances. **Sensitivity** is the lowest concentration of an analyte that can reliable be detected or measured by a test system. • Warning that the test does not differentiate between infection and the carrier state. • Statement that the test result should be considered in the context of clinical signs and symptoms, patient history, and other test results.

(continued)

TABLE 25-2	Components of a Manufacturer's Product Insert *(continued)*
Component	**Information provided**
Expected values	Describes the test result the user should expect. Explains how results might vary. Might contain study results conducted to derive the information.
Performance characteristics	Details the results of studies conducted to evaluate test performance. Included are data used to determine accuracy, precision, sensitivity, specificity, and reproducibility of the test and results of studies of the impact of interfering substances.

Department of Health and Human Services and Centers for Disease Control Prevention. Morbidity and Mortality Weekly Report. November 11, 2005.

Some suggestions for developing a procedure manual are listed in Box 25-2.

CHECKPOINT QUESTION

8. What does a laboratory procedure manual contain, and why is it necessary?

BOX 25-2

SUGGESTED SHORTCUTS FOR DEVELOPING A LABORATORY PROCEDURE MANUAL

- Use test package inserts and operator's manuals as the primary reference.
- Use a template with a standard format so all procedures contain the essential elements.
- Keep a computer file and a hard copy of your manual.
- Use a binder with tabs and sheet protectors so that it is easy to update the manual as changes occur.
- You may use package inserts in your manual if you supplement them with instructions for reporting patient results, protocols for reporting panic values, actions if the test becomes inoperable, and criteria and procedures for referring the specimens to another laboratory including specimen submission and handling. When using package inserts, the physician laboratory director must review and approve any modifications in the procedure.
- Describe actions to take when the test does not perform as expected.
- Integrate control procedures with the steps for performing patient testing to assure control testing is performed.
- Include established reference intervals and critical values for the test.
- Describe how to record and report results and how to handle critical values.

Screen and Follow-Up Test Results

The medical assistant's responsibilities do not stop with being familiar with the laboratory tests performed in the POL. Test results must be screened for needed follow-up actions. The follow-up actions on any report must be documented on the report. The step-by-step instructions for this process are described in Procedure 25-1.

Screening a test result includes checking how it compares to the reference interval. The reference interval for the test or tests included in the report will be listed on the report form. They are the test results usually seen in a healthy population. The best place to find the reference interval for a test is the manufacturer's package insert for the test being reported. When screening a laboratory report, start by noting test results that fall outside the listed normal values.

Critical values are also known as *alert values* or *critical limits*. Critical values are considered to be life-threatening test results. See Table 25-3 for results considered to be critical values in some offices. The medical assistant must notify the physician of critical results measured in the POL or reported back from the referral laboratory. Documentation of the notification of critical test results is essential. Each medical office should establish a list of critical values agreed upon by the physician(s) in that office. A protocol for alerting the physician and documenting this communication is needed.

For reviewing the test results, the medical assistant must have instructions on office policy for the types of test results that require follow up and the process for the follow up. A policy for result reviews will ensure that the physician is alerted to all the conditions that require action or intervention.

CHECKPOINT QUESTION

9. What are the two essential steps in following up on a critical value?

Each state has laws for reporting communicable diseases. The Department of Public Health for each state requires medical assistants to notify them of the occurrence of

TABLE 25-3	Example Critical Values for Some Common Laboratory Tests	
Analyte	**Critical Values**	
(Lab Test)	**Low**	**High**
Serum glucose	40 or 45 mg/dL	>500 mg/dL
Serum sodium	<120 mEq/L	>160 mEq/L
Serum potassium	<2.5 mEq/L	>6.0 mEq/L
Serum calcium (total)	<7.0 mg/dL	>13.0 mg/dL
White blood cell count	$<2 \times 10^{-9}$/L	$>50 \times 10^{-9}$/L
Platelet count	$<20 \times 10^{-9}$/L	$>1{,}000 \times 10^{-9}$/L
Prothrombin time	Not applicable	International normalized ratio (INR) >5
Partial thromboplastin time	Not applicable	>100 seconds

a reportable disease. The local health department can provide a list of all conditions that should be reported in a particular city or county. Some conditions must be reported within 24 hours of suspected or confirmed diagnosis by the most rapid method available, and others can be reported within 3 days of suspected or confirmed diagnosis. Notification must be thoroughly documented.

Using Flow Sheets to Improve Patient Care

A flow sheet is a form used to collect important data regarding a patient's condition. It is a type of documentation and is identified in the CLIA regulations. Patients' results not recorded elsewhere in the chart may be documented here. The flow sheet stays in the patient's chart and serves as a record of whether care expectations have been met. This documentation is a method of CLIA compliance. Each time the patient makes an office visit, the doctor will look at the flow sheet and address the patient's condition on the flow sheet. When a new test is performed, the medical assistant adds the newest results to the flow sheet. This allows the patient's progress to be monitored at a glance, as in Figure 25-1.

An example of a test often monitored by a flow sheet is the prothrombin time tested in hematology. Test results are monitored on a patient on anticoagulant therapy. The flow sheet monitors the patient's levels to maintain a certain **therapeutic range**. The therapeutic range is the test result range the physician wants for the patient. Using a flow sheet to record the result at each testing allows monitoring the stability of the result within the therapeutic range. Medication can be adjusted to an appropriate dose.

Quality Control

QC testing is designed to detect problems that can happen because of:

- operator error,
- reagent or test kit deterioration,
- instrument malfunction, and
- improper environmental conditions.

The POL must have written policies and procedures for monitoring the accuracy, precision, and quality of each test in place. If a test has good precision, the medical assistant will get similar results if asked to repeat the test. If similar results are not obtained, the method is not in control and results cannot be reported. The medical assistant must investigate the problem with the test. Finding and resolving problems is called *troubleshooting*. When the problem is corrected, the patient specimen and controls can be tested again.

There are two typical types of controls in waived testing. One is called an **internal control**. The internal control is built into the testing device. It verifies that the device is in good working order. The internal control must measure acceptable results to get accurate test results on a patient specimen. The internal control results must be recorded each time they are measured.

An internal control does not prove that the results will be accurate when the specimen is added, whereas the **external control** acts just like a patient specimen. The external control monitors the test from applying the specimen to result interpretation. External controls are usually liquids similar to patient specimens. Documenting external control results is also a requirement.

✓ CHECKPOINT QUESTION

10. Why would a physician want a medical assistant to record a patient's test results on a flow sheet?

✓ CHECKPOINT QUESTION

11. Explain the differences between internal and external controls. Why do you have to test both?

ANTICOAGULATION FLOWSHEET

Patient's name: _____   Date of Birth: ___/___/_____

Target International Normalized Ratio (INR):   ☐ 2.0-3.0   ☐ 2.5-3.5   ☐ Other: _____

Date	Current Dose	INR	Complications	New Dose	Next INR	Initials

Figure 25-1 Anticoagulant flow sheet.

The product insert or instrument manual describes the minimum requirement for control testing. The frequency for testing them cannot be less than what is specified by the manufacturer. At the very least, test external controls with each new shipment of reagents or kits, with each new lot number, and with each new operator.

Companies that make the controls make the specimens that test like human specimens. These control samples come with known reference ranges. Documenting and monitoring control testing results provides an indication that the test was properly performed by the medical assistant. QC results that read within the known reference ranges indicate that the test system (reagents, instruments, or any components) and the medical assistant performed as expected. CLIA requires that a record be kept of each control sample result. The control log must show the:

- date and time of the test;
- results expected;
- results obtained;
- action taken for correction, if any; and
- initials of the person performing the test.

Documentation must be consistent, and the records must be retained for at least 2 years.

Records of control results should be reviewed monthly to detect shift and trend changes in performance over time. The **Clinical and Laboratory Standards Institute (CLSI)** establishes rules to ensure the safety, standards, and integrity of all testing performed on human specimens. Figure 25-2 is an example of a form containing information recommended by CLSI on which control sample testing can be recorded. If the controls do not test as expected, then patient testing should not be performed or reported until the problem is identified and corrected.

The product insert will provide information for troubleshooting. Start by checking the reagents and controls for expiration dates, accurate **reconstitution**, and expiration dates once reconstituted. Not all controls and test reagents come in liquid form. Those that do not must be reconstituted. Reconstitution is adding water to bring a material back to its liquid state. The water added must be measured precisely when added. Next check to see that the testing instrument is clean and functioning properly.

If all of this has been done, reconstitute or open a new control sample or reagent and begin the process again. Use manufacturer contact information to get technical assistance. If there is a delay in correcting the problems, specimens for this test can be sent to a referral laboratory for timely results.

Qualitative and Quantitative Quality Control

Some laboratory tests are **qualitative tests**. A qualitative test has positive or negative results. Other laboratory tests are **quantitative tests**. The results of quantitative tests are measured and reported in a numeric value.

The tool for manually recording quantitative quality control is the Levey-Jennings QC Chart (Fig. 25-3). Using the chart builds a picture of how the test is performing over time. Monitoring the charts for **shifts** and **trends** will warn that a test may not be performing correctly. A test is exhibiting a shift when QC results make an obvious change in results. A test is exhibiting a trend when results increase or decrease over time. See examples of shifts and trends

| | | | QUALITATIVE QC LOG SHEET FOR _____ | | | | | |
| | | | RECORD LOT NUMBER IF DIFFERENT FROM LAST LOT NUMBER. | | | | | |
TEST DATE	KIT LOT	POSITIVE CONTROL LOT #	NEGATIVE CONTROL LOT #	POSITIVE CONTROL RESULT	NEGATIVE CONTROL RESULT	OK TO USE?	IF NO, CORRECTIVE ACTION	INITIALS

Figure 25-2 QC log sheet.

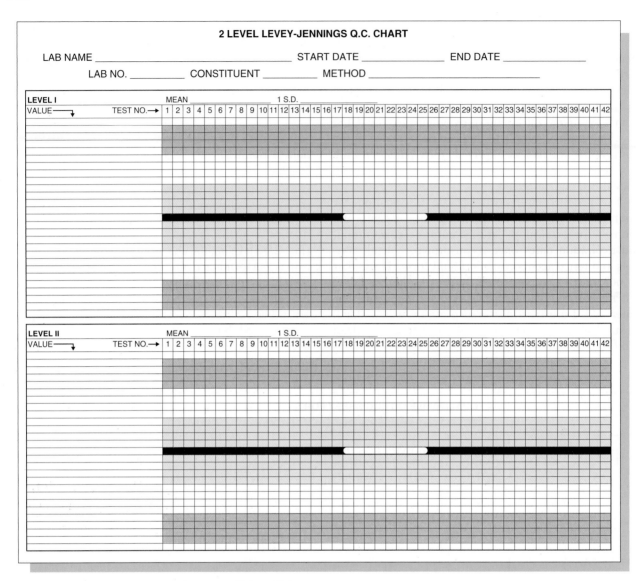

Figure 25-3 Levey-Jennings Chart.

in Figure 25-4 Being alert for shifts or trends will allow you to investigate a potential reagent problem and prevent having controls fail, causing repeat testing and delayed reporting of patient results. Procedure 25-2 describes how to perform quality control monitoring using a QC chart.

 CHECKPOINT QUESTION

12. How does the medical assistant determine when to run controls on a test?

Reagent Management

Reagents are chemicals used to perform a test. When the reagent reacts with the patient's specimen, it provides a test result. All reagents have a manufacturer's lot number and expiration date. These must be recorded on the QC log sheet when quality control is tested. The date the package is opened and the initials of the person who opened the package should be documented on the outside of each package.

CLIA requires each laboratory to test new reagents (or kit lots) for acceptability before using them to perform patients' tests. The new reagent must be tested against the reagent in use to ensure that the results of both are comparable to each other. Documentation of this verification process is required. Measuring the external controls is used to test this acceptability.

Some test kits contain several reagents. The reagents in a test kit have to be used with the kit they came in. They cannot be mixed with reagents from other kits. An example of this is fecal blood testing. It is unacceptable to use fecal occult blood test cards from one kit lot and developer reagent from a different kit lot together for patient testing.

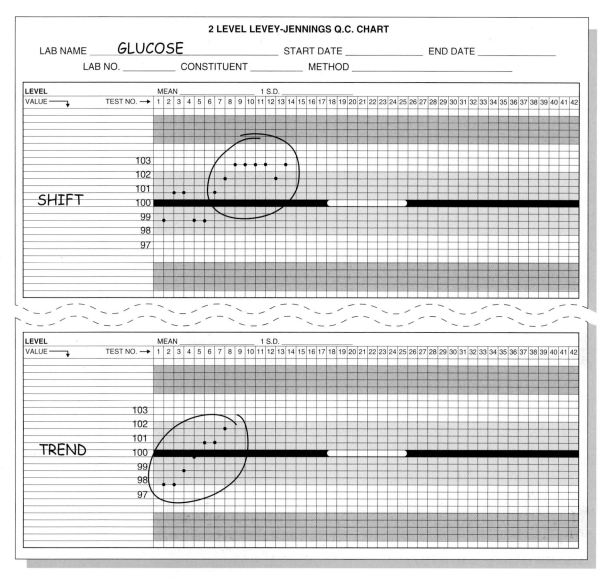

Figure 25-4 QC charts representing a shift and a trend.

 CHECKPOINT QUESTION

13. What action does the medical assistant take when controls are not acceptable?

Instrument Calibration and Maintenance

Laboratory instruments come with maintenance schedules and methods for evaluating performance provided by the manufacturer. Maintenance of equipment and supplies must be documented in the QC logbook. Any troubleshooting must be documented.

If the QC results are not within their printed ranges, the instrument's calibration (standardization) should be checked by the manufacturer's instructions. After that, the patient and QC specimens must be retested. If the calibration is correct and the new QC results are within the printed range, the patient's results are correct and may be reported.

Documentation must show the troubleshooting done and by whom.

Procedure 25-3 describes the steps for performing routine maintenance of clinical equipment.

 CHECKPOINT QUESTION

14. What is the source of instrument maintenance and calibration instructions?

ETHICAL TIP

Laboratory Code of Ethics

I. Duty to the Patient

Laboratory professionals are accountable for the quality of the laboratory services they provide. This includes maintaining individual competence in judgment and performance and striving to

(continued)

safeguard the patient from incompetent or illegal practice by others.

Laboratory professionals exercise sound judgment in establishing, performing, and evaluating laboratory testing.

Laboratory professionals maintain confidentiality of patient information and test results. They safeguard the dignity and privacy of patients and provide accurate information to other health care professionals about the patient services they have provided.

II. Duty to Colleagues and the Profession

Laboratory professionals strive to maintain a reputation of honesty, integrity, and reliability.

Laboratory professionals actively strive to establish cooperative and respectful working relationships with other health care professionals with the primary objective of ensuring a high standard of care for the patients they serve.

III. Duty to Society

Laboratory professionals have the responsibility to contribute to the general well-being of the community.

Laboratory professionals comply with laws and regulations pertaining to the practice of laboratory medicine and seek with conscience to change those that do not meet high standards of care and practice.

Source: The American Society for Clinical Laboratory Science: http://www.utmem.edu/ascls/Region3/Ethics.Html.

COG **Laboratory Safety**

All medical assistants want to avoid exposure to health and safety risks. Injuries affect morale and threaten the emotional and physical health of the injured person. Safe laboratory practice boils down to four skills:

* common sense
* safety-focused attitude
* good personal behavior
* good housekeeping

Learning about safety requirements prepares the medical assistant to use these four skills.

Occupational Safety and Health Administration

The **Occupational Safety and Health Administration** (**OSHA**) is a federal agency in the U.S. Department of Labor that monitors and protects the health and safety of workers (see Chapter 2). Two OSHA standards of particular importance to medical laboratories are the Occupational Exposure to Bloodborne Pathogens Standard

and the Hazardous Communication (HazCom) Standard, or the "right to know law."

Prevention of disease transmission in a medical facility is often called *infection control* or *biohazard risk management*. The OSHA Bloodborne Pathogens Standard requires all medical employers to provide training for their employees in techniques that will protect them from occupational exposure to infectious agents, including bloodborne pathogens.

In addition, OSHA standards require that all workers who are at risk for exposure to potentially hazardous material wear **personal protective equipment (PPE)** supplied by the employer.

Workers who are sensitive to allergens, such as latex, must be supplied with latex-free equipment. Box 25-3 provides a review of the symptoms of latex allergies and evaluation criteria to determine their level of severity.

BOX 25-3

THREE MAJOR TYPES OF LATEX REACTIONS

1. *Irritant dermatitis*—skin irritation that is not an allergic response. Some causes include inadequate drying after handwashing, aggressive scrubbing technique or detergents, abrasive effect of glove powder, climatic irritation (cold climates can cause dry, chapped skin, and hot weather can cause excessive sweating), and emotional stress. Irritant hand dermatitis can cause breaks in the skin, which can allow easier entry of the sensitizing latex protein or glove chemicals, and, in turn, lead to latex allergy.

2. *Delayed cutaneous hypersensitivity (type IV allergy)*—contact (hand) dermatitis that is generally due to the chemicals used in latex glove production. It is mediated via T cells. The skin reaction is seen 6–48 hours after contact. The reaction is local and limited to the skin that has contacted the glove. Those with type IV allergy are at increased risk of developing type I allergy. One route of sensitization is that latex proteins more easily enter the body if the skin barrier is broken.

3. *Immediate reaction (type I allergy)*—systemic allergic reactions caused by circulating IgE antibodies to the proteins in natural latex. Symptoms include hives; rhinitis; conjunctivitis; asthma due to bronchoconstriction; and, in severe cases, anaphylaxis and hypotension. Symptoms occur within about 30 minutes of exposure to latex. Several routes of exposure that can lead to type I sensitivity are cutaneous, mucosal, parenteral, and aerosol (from inhaling latex glove powder).

A medical assistant performing phlebotomy or assisting with collection of most samples is safe with glove protection. Situations that may result in splashes, splatters, or spreading of an **aerosol** (particles suspended in gas or air), however, require full coverage, including a face shield and footwear.

OSHA requires employers to provide free immunization against hepatitis B virus. Medical assistants carry the risk of exposure to bloodborne pathogens. Exposure can occur if the skin is pierced or if any body fluid splashes into the eyes, nose, mouth, other opening, or abrasion.

Another component of the Bloodborne Pathogen Standard is that all equipment and working surfaces be cleaned and decontaminated with disinfectant after contact with blood or other potentially infectious materials. OSHA requires use of a hypochlorite solution (diluted 1:10 with water). Hypochlorite is bleach.

The OSHA HazCom Standard requires hazardous chemicals be labeled. A warning, such as "danger," "flammable," precautions to avoid exposure, and first-aid measures for exposure (Figure 25-5) are requirements of the manufacturer. In addition, manufacturers must supply a **material safety data sheet** (**MSDS**) for their products. MSDS provide the manufacturer's instructions for storage, handling, and disposal of the chemical. They describe the risks associated with the product and indicate steps necessary to prevent exposure. These sheets should be maintained in a binder near the site of use and should be reviewed routinely by all office staff (Box 25-4).

An up-to-date volume of MSDS for all chemicals used in the laboratory is part of the facility's chemical hygiene plan. The plan should also include chemical safety requirements specific to that medical office.

 CHECKPOINT QUESTION

15. What are the major pieces of information provided on a material safety data sheet?

OSHA requires that a **Chemical Hygiene Plan** (**CHP**) be available to employees exposed to chemical hazards. A Chemical Hygiene Plan is a part of the HazCom standard and must address the following concerns:

1. Procedures to be used when working with hazardous chemicals
2. Control measures to reduce exposure to hazardous chemicals
3. Measures to check that protective equipment is functioning properly
4. The employee information and training program

You must always be safety conscious when using laboratory equipment. All specimens studied in the laboratory should be considered hazardous and must be treated as such. A medical assistant who is aware of the types of hazards in the clinical laboratory is likely to work safely and avoid injury.

 CHECKPOINT QUESTION

16. Define OSHA and describe its purpose.

Adherence of Health Care Personnel to Recommended Guidelines

Adherence to recommended infection control practices decreases transmission of infectious agents in health care settings. The medical assistant should easily recognize the safety symbol for a biohazard. In health care facilities, education and training on standard and transmission-based precautions are typically provided at the time of orientation. Training should be repeated to maintain competency. (Standard precautions and transmission-based precautions are discussed in more detail below.)

Hand Hygiene

It is well known that washing hands is important for reducing transmission of infectious agents in medical offices and is a basic element of **standard precautions**. Handwashing with soap and water and using alcohol-based products are both effective. Standard precautions are used in medical offices to reduce the risk for transmission of pathogens.

Universal precautions has been expanded to include feces, nasal secretions, saliva, sputum, sweat, tears, urine, and vomitus, even when no blood is evident. Universal precautions are used to control infection. In using universal precautions, human blood and most body fluids are handled as if they are infectious for HIV, hepatitis B virus (HBV), hepatitis C virus (HCV), and other **bloodborne pathogens**. HBV and HCV are considered bloodborne pathogens because when they are present in human blood they cause disease. **Human immunodeficiency virus** (**HIV**) is a bloodborne pathogen that causes acquired immunodeficiency syndrome (AIDS). With AIDS, the patient's immune system fails, allowing opportunistic infections.

The type and length of fingernails can reduce the benefits of washing hands. Artificial nails provide a place for pathogens to live and grow. Artificial nails do this more than natural nails. CDC recommends that medical assistants not wear artificial fingernails and extenders because they are associated with infections. Medical offices may prohibit medical assistants from wearing artificial nails or extenders.

Personal Protective Equipment for Health Care Personnel

PPE refers to a variety of barriers used alone or in combination to protect medical assistants from contact with

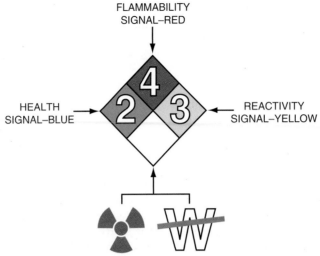

Figure 25-5 Hazardous material rating system. (Reprinted with permission from McCall R. Phlebotomy Essentials. Baltimore: Lippincott Williams & Wilkins, 2007.)

Identification of Health Hazard Color Code: **BLUE**		Identification of Flammability Color Code: **RED**		Identification of Reactivity (Stability) Color Code: **YELLOW**	
	Type of possible injury		Susceptibility of materials to burning		Susceptibility to release of energy
SIGNAL		SIGNAL		SIGNAL	
4	Materials that on very short exposure could cause death or major residual injury even though prompt medical treatment was given.	4	Materials that will rapidly or completely vaporize at atmospheric pressure and normal ambient temperature, or that are readily dispersed in air and that will burn readily.	4	Materials that in themselves are readily capable of detonation or of explosive decomposition or reaction at normal temperatures and pressures.
3	Materials that on short exposure could cause serious temporary or residual injury even though prompt medical treatment was given.	3	Liquids and solids that can be ignited under almost all ambient temperature conditions.	3	Materials that in themselves are capable of detonation or explosive reaction but require a strong initiating source or that must be heated under confinement before initiation or that react explosively with water.
2	Materials that on intense or continued exposure could cause temporary incapacitation or possible residual injury unless prompt medical treatment is given.	2	Materials that must be moderately heated or exposed to relatively high ambient temperatures before ignition can occur.	2	Materials that in themselves are normally unstable and readily undergo violent chemical change but do not detonate. Also materials that may react violently with water or that may form potentially explosive mixtures with water.
1	Materials that on exposure would cause irritation but only minor residual injury even if no treatment is given.	1	Materials that must be preheated before ignition can occur.	1	Materials that in themselves are normally stable, but that can become unstable at elevated temperatures and pressures or that may react with water with some release of energy, but not violently.
0	Materials that on exposure under fire conditions would offer no hazard beyond that of ordinary combustible material.	0	Materials that will not burn.	0	Materials that in themselves are normally stable, even under fire exposure conditions, and that are not reactive with water.

infectious agents. Medical assistants use different types of PPE based on the type of patient interaction and likely kinds of transmission.

The employer measures how much occupational exposure exists and provides training to recognize tasks and activities that may result in exposure to infectious materials. Training must include an explanation of the use and limitations of PPE.

Gloves

Gloves are used to prevent contamination of your hands when they may be in direct contact with potentially

BOX 25-4

MATERIAL SAFETY DATA SHEET

An MSDS is required for each of the hazardous materials at a particular site. In the laboratory, these can include disinfectants, cleaning compounds, laboratory chemicals, and some office supplies (e.g., toners, printing compounds). All of these must be labeled as hazardous, with the contents listed on the label. Protocols for each hazardous agent used on site must be listed on the MSDS with the following information:

- *Product name and identification.* Include all names (trade and generic) by which it may be known.
- *Hazardous components.* List all hazardous components if the agent contains more than one.
- *Health hazard data.* Note the risks to those using the agent.
- *Fire and explosive data.* If this is a volatile agent, note what precautions are necessary to prevent an accident.
- *Spill and disposal procedures.* Note how to handle spills and disposal to avoid danger.
- *Recommendations for PPE.* Note whether gloves, gown, face shield, or other equipment should be worn during use of this agent.
- *Handling, storage, and transportation precautions.* List any special precautions that must be observed.

infectious material, may have direct contact with patients who are infected with pathogens transmitted by the contact route, or are handling or touching visibly or potentially contaminated patient care equipment and surfaces.

The FDA approves gloves used for health care purposes. Gloves vary a lot. Vinyl gloves fail more than latex or nitrile gloves. Either latex or nitrile gloves are better than vinyl because they provide manual dexterity and hold up longer for procedures that involve more than brief patient contact.

Discarding gloves between patients prevents transmission of infectious material. Gloves cannot be washed and reused. Glove reuse has been associated with transmission of infections. When gloves are worn with other PPE, they are put on last. Gloves that are removed properly will prevent hand contamination. Washing hands following glove removal further ensures that the hands will not carry infectious material. Infectious material can penetrate through tears and can contaminate hands during glove removal.

Lab Coats

The employer is required to provide lab coats to medical assistants when it is going to be used as PPE.

The practice of medical assistants washing their own lab coats at home is not allowed by OSHA.

If you want to wear a personal lab coat, then an additional employer-handled lab coat would be required when anticipating the possibility of exposure.

 CHECKPOINT QUESTION

17. Why does policy require the health care worker to wash his or her hands after removing gloves?

Face Protection

Masks

Masks are used for three primary purposes in medical offices:

1. To protect medical assistants from contact with infectious material (standard precautions and droplet precautions)
2. To protect patients from exposure to infectious agents carried in a medical assistant's mouth or nose.
3. Placed on coughing patients to limit the spread of infectious respiratory secretions from the patient to others

Masks may be used in combination with goggles to protect the mouth, nose, and eyes.

Goggles and Face Shields

A medical assistant may use a face shield instead of a mask and goggles, for more complete face protection. Goggles protect the eyes but do not provide splash or spray protection to other parts of the face. Wearing eye protection and face shields when blood or body fluid exposures may occur is required by the OSHA Bloodborne Pathogens Standard. Personal eyeglasses and contact lenses are not considered adequate protection.

Respirators

Medical assistants exposed to patients with tuberculosis are recommended by CDC to use respirators. They are recommended for other diseases, such as smallpox, that could be transmitted through the airborne route. When the understanding of inhalation transmission of other diseases is better, the use of PPE can be more precise.

 CHECKPOINT QUESTION

18. List the types and uses of PPE.

Safe Work Practices to Prevent Exposure to Bloodborne Pathogens

Prevention of Needlesticks and Other Sharps-Related Injuries

Medical assistants may be injured by sticks from needles and other sharps that can transmit HBV, HCV, and

HIV. The OSHA Bloodborne Pathogen Standard states that having sharps disposal containers, self-sheathing needles, and needleless systems helps prevent dangerous needlesticks (Fig. 25-6).

The Needlestick Safety and Prevention Act became a law because sharps injuries are a serious problem. The act requires medical offices to keep an injury log to record the details of sharps injuries. You must

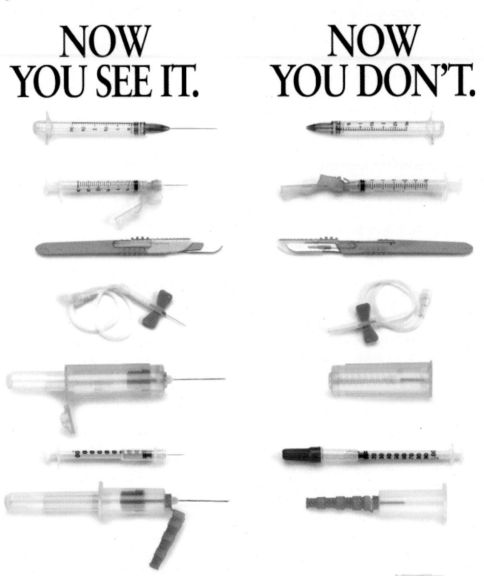

NOW YOU SEE IT. NOW YOU DON'T.

PROTECT YOURSELF AND OTHERS— USE SHARPS WITH SAFETY FEATURES

BE PREPARED. Anticipate injury risks and prepare the patient and work area with prevention in mind. Use a sharps device with safety features whenever it is available.

BE AWARE. Learn how to use the safety features on sharps devices.

DISPOSE WITH CARE. Engage safety features immediately after use and dispose in sharps safety containers.

  sharps

Support for printing this poster came from an unrestricted educational grant provided by Safety Institute, Premier, Inc. DISCLAIMER: Mention or depiction of any company or product does not constitute endorsement by CDC.

Figure 25-6 CDC sharps safety.

be trained to use the safety devices provided by the employer.

WHAT IF?

What if you stick yourself with a contaminated needle?

- Cleanse the wound thoroughly with soap and water or substance for tissue cleaning.
- Report the incident to the practice manager or appropriate person for documentation.
- Complete the required institutional incident report form.
- Ask the practice manager any questions about follow up on the patient source of contamination.

It is also recommended that you:

- Seek care from the nearest emergency room or health care facility.
- Have blood drawn as soon as possible for HBsAg, antibody to hepatitis B surface antigen (anti-HBs), hepatitis C antibody, and anti-HIV.

If health care providers at the facility have questions about appropriate care, they can call the national HIV Post-Exposure Prophylaxis Hotline for Clinicians at 1-888-HIV-4911, which is open 24 hours a day.

Prevention of Mucous Membrane Contact

Exposure of mucous membranes of the eyes, nose, and mouth to blood and body fluids can transmit infectious material to medical assistants. Preventing these exposures is part of standard precautions. Safe work practices, including PPE, are used for protection from contact with infectious material. These practices include keeping hands from touching the mouth, nose, eyes, or face and positioning patients to direct sprays and splatter away from the face of the medical assistant. Adjusting the PPE while working with the patient will cause face or mucous membrane contamination.

Precautions to Prevent Transmission of Infectious Agents

Two types of precautions are used to prevent exposure to infectious material: standard precautions and transmission-based precautions. *Standard precautions* apply to all patients in medical offices. **Transmission-based precautions** are for patients who come to the office infected with pathogens. There are transmission-based precautions for different categories of diseases. Because the exact disease may not be known when the patient comes to the medical office, the type of transmission-based precaution most closely related to the clinical symptoms and potential pathogen is used.

WHAT IF?

What if your laboratory is not in compliance with OSHA's safety regulations?

In such a situation, your health and that of your colleagues is in jeopardy. OSHA developed the guidelines to protect you from serious injury or death. OSHA can impose significant fines for noncompliance. Continued noncompliance may result in loss of the laboratory's license. In some situations, the physician may not be allowed to file for Medicare compensation. Other situations may incur large fines. To bring the laboratory back into compliance, any citations must be addressed and corrected. OSHA inspectors will revisit the site and reconsider licensure.

Standard Precautions

Over the years, the CDC published documents suggesting methods for protection from infectious diseases in the laboratory. As more was learned about disease transmission, the CDC recommended that blood and body fluid precautions be used for all patients. This expanded coverage is called *universal precautions*. Universal precautions require that the blood and body fluids of all patients be treated as infectious. This includes blood and body fluids taken as specimens to the laboratory. Universal precautions do not eliminate the need for transmission-based precautions.

Standard precautions assume that all blood, body fluids, secretions, excretions (except sweat), nonintact skin, and mucous membranes may contain transmissible infectious agents. Therefore, when handling these specimens in the laboratory, standard precautions are critical to employee safety and laboratory compliance with federal regulations. These precautions include:

- Handwashing
- Using PPE
- Using safe needle practices

New Element of Standard Precautions: Respiratory Hygiene/Cough Etiquette

Transmission of SARS (severe acute respiratory syndrome) brought about the need for infection control measures in a medical office. Respiratory hygiene/cough etiquette has been added to standard precautions. Any person with signs of illness including cough and congestion is being reminded to use cough etiquette while in the medical office.

Elements include:

1. Posted signs (Fig. 25-7)
2. Covering the mouth/nose with a tissue when coughing and prompt disposal of used tissues

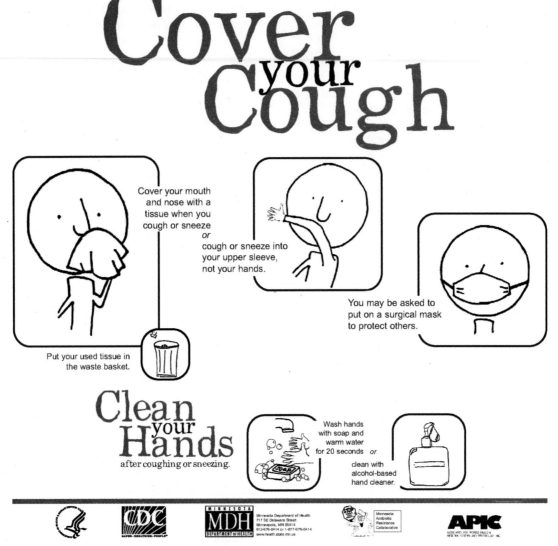

Figure 25-7 CDC cough etiquette.

3. Using surgical masks on the coughing person
4. Washing hands after contact with respiratory secretions
5. Separation, ideally greater than 3 feet, of persons with respiratory infections in waiting areas

Transmission-Based Precautions

There are three categories of transmission-based precautions

- Contact precautions
- Droplet precautions
- Airborne precautions

For some diseases that have multiple routes of transmission, more than one transmission-based precautions category may be used. They are all used in addition to standard precautions.

Contact Precautions

Contact precautions are used to prevent transmission of diseases spread by direct or indirect contact with the patient or the patient's environment. Medical assistants wear a gown and gloves for all interactions that may involve contact with the patient or potentially contaminated areas in the patient's environment.

Droplet Precautions

Droplet precautions are used to prevent transmission of diseases spread through close respiratory or mucous membrane contact with respiratory secretions. Medical assistants wear a mask for close contact with infectious patients.

Airborne Precautions

Airborne precautions prevent transmission of infectious agents that remain infectious over long distances in the air. Medical assistants caring for patients on airborne precautions wear a mask or respirator. In medical offices, the patient must be masked and placed in a private room with the door closed.

Transmission-Based Precautions prior to Laboratory Confirmation

Use of transmission-based precautions at the time a patient arrives at a medical office for care reduces transmission. The precautions remain in place until specimen culture results are available.

Discontinuation of Transmission-Based Precautions

Transmission-based precautions remain in place as long as the patient is infectious. For some diseases, state laws dictate the duration of precautions. In immunocompromised patients, the virus can be contagious for weeks or months. Contact and/or droplet precautions should continue for this time.

Biohazard Waste Disposal

Biohazardous waste, also called *infectious waste* or *biomedical waste*, is any waste containing infectious materials such as blood. The POL must comply with state and OSHA regulations for its disposal. Most medical offices use medical waste disposal companies who provide complete custody documentation, essential for regulatory compliance.

General Safety Guidelines

The following guidelines are some important safety factors required in all laboratories. Follow them carefully to protect yourself, your coworkers, and your patients.

1. Never eat, drink, or smoke in the laboratory area.
2. Never touch your face, mouth, or eyes with your gloves or with items such as a pen or pencil used in the laboratory.
3. Do not apply makeup or lipstick or insert contact lenses in the laboratory.
4. Wear gloves and appropriate protective barriers whenever contact with blood, body fluids, secretions, excretions, broken skin, or mucous membranes is possible. If a splatter, splash, spill, or exposure to aerosols is possible, wear appropriate PPE.
5. Label all specimen containers with biohazard labels.
6. Store all chemicals according to the manufacturer's recommendations. Discard any container with an illegible label. Never store chemicals in unlabeled containers.
7. Wash hands frequently for infection control. Always wash hands before and after gloving and before leaving the work site.

8. Clean reusable glassware with recommended disinfectant or soap and dry thoroughly before reuse. Wear gloves to prevent cuts.
9. Avoid inhaling the fumes of any chemicals found in the laboratory or wearing contact lenses when working with these types of chemicals.
10. Know the location and operation of all safety equipment such as fire extinguishers.
11. Use safe practices when operating laboratory equipment. Read the manuals and know how to operate the equipment. Avoid contact with damaged electrical equipment.
12. Disinfect all laboratory surfaces after use and at the end of the day with a 10% bleach solution or appropriate disinfectant. Never allow clutter to accumulate.
13. Dispose of needles and broken glass in sharps containers. Use biohazard containers for any other contaminated articles.
14. Use mechanical pipetters, but never the mouth, to apply suction to a pipette (Fig. 25-8).
15. Use the proper procedure for removing chemical or biological spills. If the spill is biological:
    - Put on gloves and other PPE as indicated by the size of the spill.
    - Cover the area with absorbent material, such as paper towels, to soak up the spill; discard in a biohazard container.
    - Flood the area with disinfecting solution, such as a 10% bleach solution, and allow it to sit for 10 to 15 minutes.
    - If a spill contains broken glass, use a mechanical means of picking up the glass. Do not use your hands.
    - Wipe up the solution with disposable material.

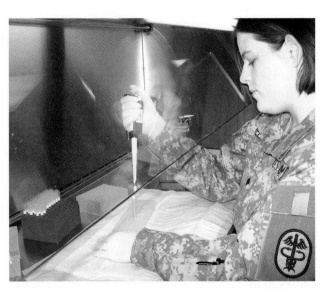

Figure 25-8 Use mechanical pipetters, but never the mouth, to apply suction to a pipette. (Image courtesy U.S. Army.)

- Dispose of all waste in a biohazard container.
- With gloves on, remove eyewear and discard or disinfect per office policy. Remove remaining PPE and place in a biohazard container or the biohazard laundry bag (for reusable linen).
- Remove and dispose of gloves. Wash your hands.

16. Avoid spills:
    - Pour carefully (palm the label).
    - Pour at eye level if possible or practical; never pour close to the face.
    - Tightly cap all containers immediately after use.

17. Use a splatter guard or splash shield whenever there is any risk of splatter or exposure to aerosols. Spills, splatters, and exposure to aerosols commonly occur in the following circumstances:
    - Taking the stopper off of a blood collection tube
    - Transferring blood from a collection syringe to a specimen receptacle
    - Conducting centrifugation
    - Preparing a smear
    - Flaming the inoculation loop

18. When removing a stopper, hold the opening away, use gauze around the cap, and twist gently. Avoid glove contact with the specimen.

19. Immediately report to your supervisor any work-related injury or biohazard exposure.

20. Follow all guidelines for standard precautions and the requirements of the various types of transmission-based precautions.

21. When opening a tube or container, hold the mouth away from you to avoid aerosols, splashes, and spills.

 CHECKPOINT QUESTION

19. How would you clean up a biological spill?

Incident Reports

An incident report is indicated if a patient, employee, or visitor is injured, if an employee is stuck with a contaminated needle, in case of medication error, or if blood is drawn from the wrong patient. The incident report should be completed by the medical assistant involved or closest to the patient or visitor involved in the incident. In addition to the signature of the person completing the form, a supervisor or doctor should review and sign the form in accordance with the office incident report policy.

 CHECKPOINT QUESTION

20. Describe the reasons to file an incident report.

SPANISH TERMINOLOGY

Buenos días. Le habla _____ de la oficina del doctor/ de la doctora _____.
> Hello. This is ___*name*___ from doctor ___*name*___'s office.

¿Necesito hablar con _____?
> May I speak with _____*name*_____?

_____, el doctor/la doctora _____ me pidió que lo/la llamara con las resultados de su prueba.
> ___*name*___, Dr. ___*name*___ asked me to call you about your test results.

Su _____ fue demasiado alto (o bajo).
> Your ___*test name*___ was too high (or too low).

El médico quiere que usted siga estas instrucciones.
> The doctor wants you to follow these instructions.

Tiene que llamar a la oficina mañana para sacar una cita para la próxima semana.
> You need to call the office tomorrow to schedule a follow-up appointment next week.

¿Entiende usted lo que le pido que haga?
> Do you understand what I am asking you to do?

MEDIA MENU

- **Student Resources on thePoint**
  - **Video: Perform Routine Maintenance of Laboratory Equipment (Glucose Meter Example) (Procedure 25-3)**
  - **CMA/RMA Certification Exam Review**
- **Internet Resources**

  Commission on Office Laboratory Accreditation
  http://www.cola.org

  Centers for Medicare and Medicaid Services
  http://www.cms.hhs.gov

  Clinical and Laboratory Standards Institute
  http://www.clsi.org

  Occupational Safety and Health Administration
  http://www.osha.gov
  http://www.gpoaccess.gov/fr/index.html

  CLIA Web site to access certificate application
  http://www.cms.hhs.gov/cmsforms/downloads/cms116.pdf

PSY PROCEDURE 25-1: Screen and Follow Up Laboratory Test Results and Document Appropriately

Purpose: To alert physician to a patient's critical lab results as soon as possible and document appropriately
Equipment: Patient laboratory results, critical values list for office, patient's chart, telephone (as needed)

Steps	Reasons
1. Review laboratory reports received from reference laboratory.	Laboratory reports may contain results that require immediate intervention for patient safety.
2. Note which reports may be placed directly on the patient's chart for the physician's routine review and which require immediate notification due to critical results.	Critical results must be reported to the physician in a timely manner so that action can be taken to modify the patient's condition.
3. Notify the physician of the result. Take any immediate instructions from the physician. The physician will want to contact the patient for immediate action.	Lab results requiring immediate follow-up should be reported to the physician by the most direct method.
4. Follow instructions and document notification and follow-up.	Relaying instructions to the patient is the first priority. Documenting physician notification and, if directed, patient notification verifies that the process was completed.
5. Chart remaining reports appropriately.	All laboratory results should be routed according to laboratory policy for timely follow up with the patient.

Charting Example:

02/12/2012 10:00 AM Critical level glucose of 597 mg/dL reported to Dr. Peters. Dr. will follow up with patient. ———
——— M. Miller, CMA

Note: The medical assistant may sign his or her name in the patient record using only the "CMA" credential if the office has a signature log denoting the entire credential as "CMA(AAMA)."

PSY PROCEDURE 25-2: Quality Control Monitoring Using a QC Chart

Purpose: To determine the acceptability of quality control results in compliance with CLIA standards
Equipment: Instrument test results and quality control charts

Steps	Reasons
1. Assemble the charts and data.	
2. On the QC chart (see Fig. 25-3), plot the control.	Levey-Jennings charts list the acceptable control results obtained for the test run. Results and their evaluation provide an ongoing report of test performance.
3. Evaluate chart for acceptability of results.	For waived testing, CLIA requires that quality control procedures be performed in compliance with the manufacturer's instructions.
4. If results are within accepted limits, report patient test results.	
5. If results are not within accepted limits, do not report patient results. Troubleshoot the test. Repeat testing on the patient and control specimens.	If control results are not acceptable, the patient results are not valid.
6. If results are within accepted limits, report patient results. Document corrective action and acceptable control results.	For waived testing, CLIA requires that quality control procedures be performed in compliance with the manufacturer's instructions.
7. If control results are not within accepted limits, notify the physician of the test malfunction.	Provide the physician information to be aware of the delay in testing.
8. Arrange to have the patient specimen referred for testing or store the specimen appropriately until repairs can be made.	The specimen may deteriorate if left at room temperature for too long.
9. Troubleshoot within manufacturer's guidelines for operator troubleshooting. Document this in the maintenance log. If this is not successful, arrange for repairs on the instrument. Document any manufacturer-supplied repairs in the maintenance log.	CLIA requires that all maintenance on an instrument be documented in the maintenance log.
10. Keep physician informed of testing status.	The physician needs to know the status of test availability.
11. Before returning the instrument to service, validate calibration and quality control. Document appropriately.	For waived testing, CLIA requires that quality control procedures be performed in compliance with the manufacturer's instructions.

Charting Example:

02/12/2012 10:00 AM QC results plotted and within acceptable limits ————————CDH, CMA

Note: The medical assistant may sign his or her name in the patient record using only the "CMA" credential if the office has a signature log denoting the entire credential as "CMA(AAMA)."

PSY PROCEDURE 25-3:

Perform Routine Maintenance of Laboratory Equipment (Glucose Meter Example)

Purpose: To meet CLIA standards for quality performance by maintaining clinical equipment according to manufacturer's instructions

Equipment: Laboratory instrument to be maintained, instrument manual from manufacturer, instrument maintenance log, maintenance supplies as indicated in the instrument manual, PPE, hand sanitizer, surface sanitizer, contaminated waste container

Steps	Reasons
1. Wash your hands. Put on gloves.	The meter is used for patient testing. In maintaining it, you will be exposed to remaining specimen residue.
2. Read or review the maintenance section of the instrument manual.	CLIA requires that maintenance be performed according to manufacturer recommendations.
3. Follow the manufacturer's step-by-step instructions for maintaining the instrument.	Following the manufacturer's instructions ensures optimum instrument performance.
4. Turn on the instrument and ensure that it is calibrated.	Calibration of the instrument is essential for accurate test results.
5. Perform the test on the quality control material. Record results. Determine whether QC is within control limits. If yes, proceed with patient testing. If no, take corrective action and recheck controls. Document corrective action. Proceed with patient testing when acceptable QC results are obtained.	For waived testing, CLIA requires that quality control procedures be performed in compliance with the manufacturer's instructions.
6. Document maintenance procedures performed in instrument maintenance log.	Maintenance is not considered performed unless procedures are documented.
7. Properly care for or dispose of equipment and supplies.	Proper disposal is protection from potential exposure to pathogens.
8. Clean the work area. Remove personal protective equipment and wash your hands.	Attention to infection control is important when working with the parts of an instrument that analyze patient specimens.

Charting Example:

02/12/2012 10:00 AM Routine maintenance performed on glucose meter per manufacturer's instructions. Meter was then calibrated and quality control material was tested with acceptable results————————— DHW, CMA

Note: The medical assistant may sign his or her name in the patient record using only the "CMA" credential if the office has a signature log denoting the entire credential as "CMA(AAMA)."

- The goals of CLIA are standardization of laboratory testing and enforcement of quality protocols.
- Only CLIA-waived tests are within the scope of practice for a medical assistant. A comprehensive list of waived tests is available at http://www.cms.gov.
- Urgent clinician notification of critical results is a responsibility of the laboratory. Documentation of the proper notification of such test results to the health care professional responsible for the patient is essential.
- QC testing is designed to detect problems that might arise because of operator error, reagent or test kit deterioration, instrument malfunction, or improper environmental conditions. A comprehensive quality control program monitors each phase of the laboratory process.
- OSHA monitors and protects the health and safety of workers. OSHA standards are federal regulations that protect workers by eliminating or minimizing chemical, physical, and biological hazards and preventing accidents.
- Standard precautions are based on the principle that all blood, body fluids, secretions, excretions (except sweat), nonintact skin, and mucous membranes may contain transmissible infectious agents. Standard precautions include a group of infection prevention practices that apply to all patients.
- The Needlestick Safety and Prevention Act was signed into law because occupational exposure to blood-borne pathogens from accidental sharps injuries in health care is a serious problem.
- An incident report is indicated if a patient, employee, or visitor is injured, if an employee is stuck with a contaminated needle, in case of medication error, or if blood is drawn from the wrong patient.

Warm Ups | for Critical Thinking

1. List all items that must be documented in the laboratory. Design a form to meet these requirements. Who should complete the form? Where should it be kept? Explain your responses.
2. Working with another student, develop a plan of action to use in case your controls do not come into range and how to go about correcting a problem.
3. Review the laboratory safety rules and create a poster summarizing these rules for display in the classroom.
4. Obtain a unitized test device for a test you will perform in your laboratory training. Demonstrate the internal control and the external control. Describe the purpose of each and why it is necessary to have both.

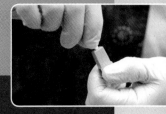

Outline

Learning Outcomes

Cognitive Domain

Note: AAMA/CAAHEP 2008 Standards are italicized.

1. Spell and define the key terms
2. Describe the proper patient identification procedures
3. Identify equipment and supplies used to obtain a routine venous specimen and a routine capillary skin puncture
4. Describe proper use of specimen collection equipment
5. List the major anticoagulants, their color codes, and the suggested order in which they are filled from a venipuncture

6. Describe the location and selection of the blood collection sites for capillaries and veins
7. Describe specimen labeling and requisition completion
8. Differentiate between the feel of a vein, tendon, and artery
9. Describe the steps in preparation of the puncture site for venipuncture and skin puncture
10. Describe care for a puncture site after blood has been drawn
11. Describe safety and infection control procedures

12. Describe quality assessment issues in specimen collection procedures
13. List six areas to be avoided when performing venipuncture and the reasons for the restrictions
14. Summarize the problems that may be encountered in accessing a vein, including the procedure to follow when a specimen is not obtained
15. List several effects of exercise, posture, and tourniquet application upon laboratory values

Psychomotor Domain

Note: AAMA/CAAHEP 2008 Standards are italicized.

1. *Demonstrate proper use of sharps disposal containers*
2. *Practice standard precautions*
3. *Participate in training on standard precautions*
4. *Perform handwashing*
5. Obtain a blood specimen by evacuated tube or winged infusion set (Procedure 26-1)
6. Obtain a blood specimen by capillary puncture (Procedure 26-2)
7. *Use medical terminology, pronouncing medical terms correctly, to communicate information*
8. *Prepare a patient for procedures and/or treatments*
9. *Document patient care*
10. *Respond to issues of confidentiality*
11. *Perform within scope of practice*
12. *Perform patient screening using using established protocols*

Affective Domain

Note: AAMA/CAAHEP 2008 Standards are italicized.

1. *Display sensitivity to patient rights and feelings in collecting specimens*
2. *Explain the rationale for performance of a procedure to the patient*
3. *Show awareness of patients' concerns regarding their perceptions related to the procedure being performed*

4. *Demonstrate sensitivity to patients' rights*
5. *Apply critical thinking skills in performing patient assessment and care*
6. *Use language/verbal skills that enable patients' understanding*
7. *Demonstrate respect for diversity in approaching patients and families*
8. *Demonstrate empathy in communicating with patients, family, and staff*
9. *Apply active listening skills*
10. *Demonstrate awareness of the territorial boundaries of the person with whom you are communicating*
11. *Demonstrate sensitivity appropriate to the message being delivered*
12. *Demonstrate recognition of the patient's level of understanding in communications*
13. *Demonstrate respect for individual diversity, incorporating awareness of one's own biases in areas including gender, race, religion, age, and economic status*

ABHES Competencies

1. Define and use entire basic structure of medical words and be able to accurately identify in the correct context, i.e. root, prefix, suffix, combinations, spelling, and definitions
2. Build and dissect medical terms from roots/ suffixes to understand the word element combinations that create medical terminology
3. Document accurately
4. Comply with federal, state, and local health laws and regulations
5. Identify and respond appropriately when working/caring for patients with special needs
6. Maintain inventory equipment and supplies
7. Communicate on the recipient's level of comprehension
8. Use pertinent medical terminology
9. Recognize and respond to verbal and nonverbal communication
10. Use standard precautions
11. Dispose of biohazardous materials
12. Collect, label, and process specimens
13. Perform venipuncture
14. Perform capillary puncture

Key Terms

anchor	barrier precautions	butterfly	edematous
antecubital space	bevel	cultured	evacuated tube
anticoagulant	blood cultures	distal	fasting
antiseptic	breathing the syringe	diurnal rhythms	flanges

gauge	hemolysis	order of draw	sharps container
gauze sponges	luer adapter	palpate	syringe
gel separator	lumen	peak level	taut
hemachromatosis	lymphedema	polycythemia vera	therapeutic phlebotomy
hematocrit	multisample needle	probing	thrombosed
hematoma	needle disposal unit	prophylaxis	trough level
hemoconcentration	NPO	requisition	

This chapter describes blood collection equipment and procedures for safe venipuncture and skin puncture. Although collection of arterial specimens is another type of specimen collection, it is limited to the evaluation of respiratory function and not performed by medical assistants.

Blood is a biohazardous material. It should be handled with standard precautions and appropriate **barrier precautions**. Barrier precautions are physical products, equipment, or methods used specifically for the purpose of protecting the patient and the medical assistant from exposure to potentially infectious material.

Medical assistants are exposed to pathogens like HIV, hepatitis B, and hepatitis C from needlestick injuries. A medical assistant's risk of disease may be reduced by the use of **prophylaxis** (protective treatment for the prevention of disease once exposure has occurred). Know the instructions for immediate action from the Centers for Disease Control and Prevention (CDC) in case of a needlestick injury (Box 26-1).

Obtaining blood specimens requires knowledge, skill, practice, and empathy for patients. A comfortable routine that complies with office policy is established by each phlebotomist. The quality of a laboratory test result is only as good as the quality of the specimen collected for testing. The quality of the specimen starts with the phlebotomist's attention to several factors:

- Patient identification
- Verifying patient compliance with preparation requirements
- Checking the test requisition form for requested tests, patient information, and any special requirements and verifying appropriate action
- Timing of collections
- Selecting a suitable site for the venipuncture
- Preparing the equipment, the patient, and the puncture site
- Collecting the sample in the appropriate container
- Recognizing complications from the phlebotomy
- Assessing the need for sample recollection and/or rejection

- Labeling the collection tubes at the drawing area
- Provision of any special handling techniques

COG Blood Drawing Station

A blood drawing station is equipped for performing phlebotomy procedures (Fig. 26-1). The station should be out of the regular office traffic pattern for safety. The station should include a table close at hand for supplies and a chair or bed for the patient. The table should be at a convenient height for working and have enough space to hold all of the phlebotomy supplies. Phlebotomy chairs should be comfortable and have adjustable armrests to allow proper positioning of either arm. A safety device locks the armrest in place in front of the patient to prevent falling from the chair if fainting occurs. A bed

---

BOX 26-1

IMMEDIATE ACTION AFTER NEEDLESTICK INJURY

If you are exposed to the blood or other body fluid of a patient by needlestick or other means during the course of your work, immediately follow these steps:

- Wash needlesticks and cuts with soap and water.
- Flush splashes to the nose, mouth, or skin with water.
- Irrigate eyes with clean water, saline, or sterile irrigant.
- Report the incident to your supervisor.
- Initiate written documentation of the incident as directed by facility procedure.
- Immediately seek medical treatment.

Source: Courtesy of the Centers for Disease Control and Prevention.

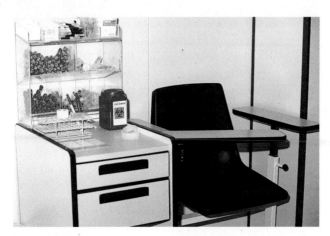

Figure 26-1 A well-stocked blood drawing station.

or reclining chair should be available for patients with a history of fainting and to perform heelsticks or other procedures on infants and small children.

COG Requisition

The **requisition** is an order form for laboratory tests. A requisition form must accompany each sample submitted to the laboratory. For a patient having the specimen collection in the laboratory, there must be a requisition for the tests the physician is requesting. The required data for the requisition form are:

- Patient's first and last names
- Patient's identification (ID) number
- Patient's date of birth
- Requesting physician's name
- Sources of specimen—when requesting microbiology, cytology, fluid analysis, or other testing where analysis and reporting is body site specific
- Date and time of collection
- Initials of the phlebotomist/collector

COG Labeling the Sample

The properly labeled sample is essential so that the results of the test match the patient. The key elements on the label are

- Patient's first and last names
- Patient's ID number
- Date, time, and initials of the phlebotomist on the label of each tube

Note: All patient information *must* match the same on the requisition form.

Automated systems may include labels with bar codes.

COG Equipment

The following equipment is needed for routine venipuncture.

Evacuated Collection Tubes

The **evacuated tube** system consists of a tube holder (adapter) (Fig. 26-2), a **multisample needle** specifically for use with the evacuated tube, and the evacuated tube. This is a closed system allowing the patient's blood to flow from the vein through the needle and into the collection tube without exposure to the air. This allows collecting multiple tubes with a one venipuncture. Evacuated tubes are designed to fill with a predetermined volume of blood because of the vacuum inside the tube. The vacuum is premeasured by the manufacturer to draw the precise amount of blood into the tube. The tube fills until the vacuum is exhausted. A tube that has lost all or part of its vacuum will not fill completely, if at all. *Troubleshooting tip:* If, while drawing a patient blood specimen, the tube should not fill, try another evacuated tube before withdrawing from the vein.

The rubber stoppers sealing the tubes are color coded according to the additive in the tube. These tubes are made of glass or plastic and range in size from 2 to 15 mL. Tube size is selected according to the patient's age, amount of blood needed, and the size and condition of the patient's vein. The tubes are sterile to prevent contamination of the specimen and the patient. Blood should *never* be poured from one tube to another because the tubes can have different additives or coatings.

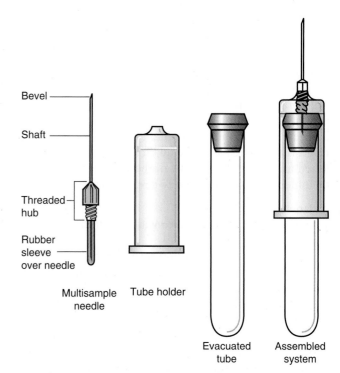

Figure 26-2 Traditional components of the evacuated tube system. (Reprinted with permission from McCall R. Phlebotomy Essentials. Baltimore: Lippincott Williams & Wilkins, 2007.)

CHECKPOINT QUESTION

1. How does the evacuated tube fill with the correct measurement of blood?

Tube Additives

Different laboratory tests require different types of blood specimens. For tests requiring serum samples, the blood is drawn into a tube that allows clotting. The clotting process takes 30 to 60 minutes at 22°C to 25°C. The specimen should be allowed to complete the clotting process prior to being centrifuged for separation of the serum from the clot; this is required to attain the optimum specimen. Other tests require whole blood or plasma, and these samples are drawn into a tube that contains an **anticoagulant** additive because it prevents clotting. An additive is any substance that is placed in a tube. Additives have specific functions. The following is a list of the most common additives and their functions:

- Anticoagulants prevent the blood from clotting.
- Clot activators speed up coagulation.
- **Gel separators** form a barrier between the cells and the serum or plasma portion after the specimen has been centrifuged. This protects the serum from interaction with the red blood cells (RBCs) that would alter test results.

The evacuated tube system uses color-coded stoppers to identify the additive contained in each type of tube (Table 26-1). It is necessary to use the correct anticoagulant because improper anticoagulant use can alter test results. It is also necessary to fill the tube until the vacuum is exhausted. Underfilled tubes will alter patient test results due to overdilution of the specimen by the tube additive.

WHAT IF?

What if, while drawing a blood specimen, the blood flow stops before collection of the required tubes is complete?

While drawing a blood specimen, the blood flow may stop leaving a partially filled tube. The following steps may restart the blood flow. They should be gently tried before discontinuing the collection and resticking the patient. Try each step, allowing a few seconds in between for the blood flow to respond. There should be no excessive or aggressive jabbing of the patient.

- Gently nudge the needle forward.
- Slightly pull the needle backward.
- Very slightly rotate the needle in the vein.
- Remove the vacuum tube and replace it with another tube.

If these attempts do not restart the blood flow, terminate the stick and follow-up with postcare of the phlebotomy site. Another attempt should be made to complete the collection. Look for a site on the opposite arm. Do not tie the tourniquet around the same arm the second time. Perform the phlebotomy and complete the specimen collection.

Should the second attempt fail, *do not pour the specimen form tube to tube*. There is a reason why—it will critically ruin all test results.

Should a choice to pour off the specimen go unnoticed, there are several negative outcomes for the patient:

- If the tube collected contained no anticoagulant, the blood had begun to clot. What is poured off will be falsely diluted. The results of tests performed on that specimen will be abnormally low. The results of the tests performed on the original tube will be falsely elevated.
- If the tube collected contained no anticoagulant, again, the blood had begun to clot. Platelets are removed from the liquid part of the blood to make the clot. If the specimen is poured from a partially clotted tube into a lavender-top tube, it will be used to count blood cells. All of the cell counts will be abnormally low because some of the cells in the specimen have been tied up in the clot forming in the red-top tube. The platelet count will be critically low.
- The light-blue-top tube is used to test for blood clotting factors. If the specimen just described is poured into a light-blue-top tube, the tests for clotting factors will be falsely abnormal because some of the clotting factors were left behind in the original tube with the forming clot.
- If the partially filled tube collected did contain an anticoagulant, the blood has been chemically altered. The poured-off blood will probably not clot and will require that the patient have another unnecesary stick. If the blood should clot and testing proceeds, the anticoagulant chemicals in the blood will ruin any chemistry tests that were ordered.

The patient is at risk from any testing performed on specimens poured off from the original tube.

CHECKPOINT QUESTION

2. Describe four errors that can occur when part of a whole blood specimen is poured from one collection tube into another collection tube.

TABLE 26-1 **Evacuated Tube System: Color Coding**

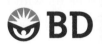

BD Helping all people live healthy lives

BD Vacutainer® Order of Draw for Multiple Tube Collections

Designed for Your Safety

Reflects change in CLSI recommended Order of Draw (H3-A5, Vol 23, No 32, 8.10.2)

Closure Color	Collection Tube	Mix by Inverting
BD Vacutainer® Blood Collection Tubes *(glass or plastic)*		
	• Blood Cultures - SPS	8 to 10 times
	• Citrate Tube*	3 to 4 times
or	• BD Vacutainer® SST™ Gel Separator Tube	5 times
	• Serum Tube *(glass or plastic)*	5 times (plastic) none (glass)
	• BD Vacutainer® Rapid Serum Tube (RST)	5 to 6 times
or	• BD Vacutainer® PST™ Gel Separator Tube With Heparin	8 to 10 times
	• Heparin Tube	8 to 10 times
or	• EDTA Tube	8 to 10 times
	• BD Vacutainer® PPT™ Separator Tube K₂EDTA with Gel	8 to 10 times
	• Fluoride (glucose) Tube	8 to 10 times

* When using a winged blood collection set for venipuncture and a coagulation (citrate) tube is the first specimen tube to be drawn, a discard tube should be drawn first. The discard tube must be used to fill the blood collection set tubing's "dead space" with blood but the discard tube does not need to be completely filled. This important step will ensure proper blood-to-additive ratio. The discard tube should be a nonadditive or coagulation tube.

Note: Always follow your facility's protocol for order of draw

Handle all biologic samples and blood collection "sharps" (lancets, needles, luer adapters and blood collection sets) according to the policies and procedures of your facility. Obtain appropriate medical attention in the event of any exposure to biologic samples (for example, through a puncture injury) since they may transmit viral hepatitis, HIV (AIDS), or other infectious diseases. Utilize any built-in used needle protector if the blood collection device provides one. BD does not recommend reshielding used needles, but the policies and procedures of your facility may differ and must always be followed. Discard any blood collection "sharps" in biohazard containers approved for their disposal.

= 1 inversion

BD Technical Services
1.800.631.0174
BD Customer Service
1.888.237.2762
www.bd.com/vacutainer

1 Becton Drive
Franklin Lakes, NJ 07417
www.bd.com/vacutainer

BD, BD Logo and all other trademarks are property of Becton, Dickinson and Company. © 2010 BD
Franklin Lakes, NJ, 07417   1/10   VS5729-6

Courtesy and © Becton, Dickinson and Company.

Order of Draw

There are several concerns for the medical assistant collecting blood specimens:

- Microbial contamination of specimens that are required to be sterile
- Cross contamination between the various anticoagulant additives to the tubes
- Tissue thromboplastin

Specimens drawn to culture the blood for pathogens (**blood cultures**) require additional skin preparation with iodine solution. This extra preparation is required to sterilize the site of the venipuncture. Bacteria are present on all skin. These bacteria can contaminate blood drawn for culture. If the physician has requested blood-culture testing, the skin must be prepared, and the specimen for blood-culture testing must be drawn first. Blood cultures are not a routine request in most medical offices.

The chemicals added to blood tubes to preserve the blood for various types of testing have a possibility of carryover from one tube to the next. This possibility is low, but must be considered because of the serious errors it can cause in test results.

The third concern in phlebotomy is tissue fluid. Tissue fluid contains *tissue thromboplastin*. Tissue thromboplastin is present in tissue fluid so that if the skin is punctured or cut, it can start the clotting process to stop blood loss. This is a positive protection mechanism for the body. It can also cause a lot of problems when a specimen is being drawn for coagulation testing.

Coagulation testing is performed to determine if the patient's blood contains adequate factors to clot in a normal length of time. It is also performed to identify causes of abnormally long clotting times. If a specimen is contaminated with tissue thromboplastin, the blood in the tube will be activated to clot. None of the clotting factors in the specimen are going to measure the true coagulation factors in the body. The times will all be shorter, so a patient with an abnormally long coagulation time could appear normal. For this reason, a small amount of blood must be drawn in a red-top tube to remove tissue thromboplastin prior to collecting blood into the light-blue-top coagulation tube. Probing with the needle releases additional amounts of tissue thromboplastin.

A specific **order of draw** of the tubes avoids these concerns. The Clinical and Laboratory Standards Institute (CLSI) is an organization of representatives from the health care community, industry, and government who develop voluntary guidelines and standards for the laboratory. CLSI recommends one order of draw for both collection of evacuated tubes and filling evacuated tubes from a syringe. Recommended protocols from various manufacturers and the CLSI, as well as policies of individual laboratories, may slightly differ. The protocol for the facility should be the order used.

Note: Tubes must be thoroughly mixed. Erroneous test results may be obtained when the blood is not thoroughly mixed with the additive. Refer back to Table 26-1 for the most recent CLSI-designated order of draw and suggested inversions required to thoroughly mix each tube. Table 26-2 lists the rationale for the standard order of draw.

If a mistake is made in the order of draw, record the actual order of draw on the request form or in the computer so that it is visible in the laboratory testing area. Findings are reviewed for evidence of contamination before they are reported. If interference is suspected, the laboratory can suggest recollection of the specimen to validate the original test results.

CHECKPOINT QUESTION

3. What is the proper order of draw when using the evacuated tube system? Why is this important?

Needles

Multisample needles with safety features are shown in Figure 26-3. Figure 26-4 is a traditional needle and tube holder. A safety needle–retracting device in the needle holder allows the safety to be provided as part of the needle holder rather than as a part of the needle (Fig. 26-5A). The Needlestick Safety and Prevention Act requires needles to have safety features to minimize accidental needlesticks. Users can select products that both meet requirements and provide ease of use. Figure 26-5B pictures various sharps devices prior to use and with the safety mechanism in place.

Sterile, disposable, single-use-only needles are used for venipuncture. They are silicon coated, so they penetrate the skin smoothly. The end of the needle that pierces the vein is cut on a slant or **bevel**. The bevel allows the needle to penetrate the vein easily and prevents coring (removal of a portion of skin or vein). The long, cylindrical portion of the needle is called the *shaft*, and the end that connects to the blood-drawing apparatus is called the *hub*.

The **gauge** of a needle indicates the size of the **lumen** (opening) of the needle. The larger the gauge number is, the smaller the diameter of the needle (i.e., 20 gauge is larger than 25 gauge). Selection of the gauge is based on the size and condition of the patient's vein. A 21- or 22-gauge needle is used for most routine blood collection. Never use a needle smaller than 23 gauge to collect blood, because the lumen is too small and will rupture RBCs, causing hemolysis of the specimen.

With beveled points on both ends, multisample needles are threaded in the middle to screw into the needle holder. One end of the needle is longer and is exposed for piercing the patient's skin and entering the vein.

TABLE 26-2 CLSI Order of Draw and Rationale for Collection Order

Order of Draw	Tube Stopper Color	Rationale for Collection Order
Blood cultures (sterile collections)	Yellow, culture bottles (sterile media containers [SPS])	Minimizes chance of microbial contamination.
Plain (nonadditive) tubes	Red	Prevents contamination by additives in other tubes. Must be drawn prior to a light-blue top as a "throw away tube" if not ordered.
Coagulation tubes	Light blue	Second or third position in order of draw; prevents tissue thromboplastin contamination. Must be the first additive tube in the order because all other additive tubes affect coagulation tests.
Serum separator gel tubes	Red and gray rubber; gold plastic	Prevents contamination by additives in other tubes. Comes after specimens drawn for coagulation tests because it contains silica particles to activate clotting in the tube. Carryover of the silica particles into the coagulation specimen would activate clotting and affect coagulation tests. Carryover of silica into subsequent tubes can override the anticoagulant in them.
Plasma tubes and plasma separator gel tubes	Green and light-green top	Contains heparin, which affects coagulation tests and interferes in collection of serum specimens. Causes the least interference in tests other than coagulation tests.
Ethylenediaminetetraacetic acid tubes	Lavender; white	EDTA tubes have more carryover (EDTA) problems than any other additive. Elevates sodium and potassium levels. Chelates and decreases calcium and iron levels. Elevates prothrombin time and partial thromboplastin time results.
Oxalate/fluoride tubes	Gray	Sodium fluoride and potassium oxalate elevate sodium and potassium levels, respectively. Comes after hematology tubes because oxalate damages cell membranes and causes abnormal red blood cell morphology.

The shorter end penetrates the rubber stopper of the collection tube and, with its retractable rubber sleeve, prevents leakage of blood during tube changes. The sleeve is pushed back when it goes into the stopper, allowing blood to flow into the tube, and re-covers the end of the needle when the tube is removed.

CHECKPOINT QUESTION

4. Why is a 23-gauge needle too small to draw a blood specimen for laboratory testing?

Winged Infusion Set (Butterfly)

To attach the winged infusion set (Fig. 26-6), thread or attach the end of the set to the tube holder. Use the smallest evacuated collection tube available. This puts less pressure on small, fragile veins.

A drawback in using the winged infusion system is that the bevel cut may be more blunt than the multisample needle, resulting in more painful punctures. Because the needle part of the system is much shorter than the multisample needle, it cannot reach deep veins.

Studies have shown that winged sets cause more needlesticks to phlebotomists. After withdrawing the needle from the patient, it tends to hang loose on the end of the tubing. Phlebotomists should use extra caution and activate the safety device as quickly as possible.

Due to their limitations, winged sets should be used only for small, fragile veins in pediatrics and geriatrics. A winged infusion set is also known as a **butterfly**. Figure 26-7A–D demonstrates the procedure for using the butterfly in a hand vein.

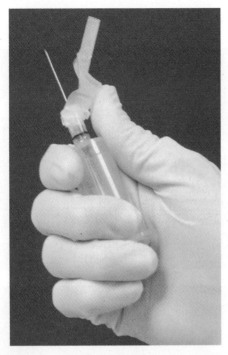

Figure 26-3 BD Eclipse multisample safety needle attached to traditional tube holder. (Courtesy of Becton-Dickinson, Franklin Lakes, NJ.)

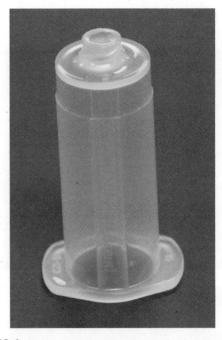

Figure 26-4 Traditional needle and tube holder. (Reprinted with permission from McCall R. Phlebotomy Essentials. Baltimore: Lippincott Williams & Wilkins, 2003.)

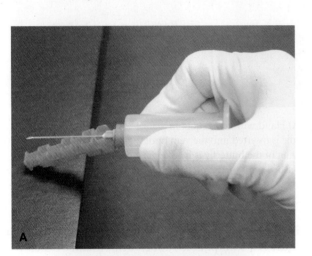

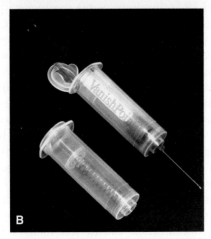

Figure 26-5 Safety tube holder. (**A**) Venipuncture Needle-Pro with needle-sheathing device. (**B**) Vanish point tube syringe with needle-retracting device. (Retractable Technologies, Little Elm, TX.)

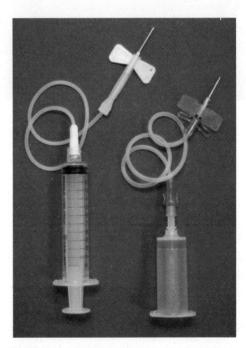

Figure 26-6 Winged infusion sets. *Left:* Attached to a syringe. *Right:* Attached to evacuated tube holder by means of a Luer adapter. (Reprinted with permission from McCall R. Phlebotomy Essentials. Baltimore: Lippincott Williams & Wilkins, 2003.)

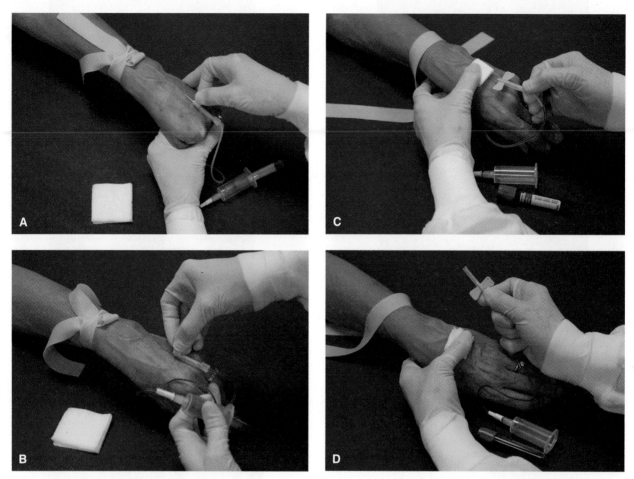

Figure 26-7 Procedure for using butterfly in a hand vein. (**A**) Hand with tourniquet in place reveals prominent vein. (**B**) With the skin pulled taut over the knuckles, the needle is inserted into the vein until there is a flash of blood in the tubing. (**C**) Using the nondominant hand, a wing of the butterfly is held against the patient's hand to steady the needle while the blood collecting tube is pushed onto the blood collecting needle. (**D**) Once the proper tubes have been drawn, gauze is placed over the vein, and the needle is removed. (Reprinted with permission from McCall R. Phlebotomy Essentials. Baltimore: Lippincott Williams & Wilkins, 2003.)

 CHECKPOINT QUESTION

5. Why might the butterfly result in a more painful stick for the patient?

Holder/Adapter

The holder is sometimes called a **luer adapter.** The open end of the holder accepts the blood collection tube. There are **flanges** (extensions) on the sides of the rim of the holder to aid in tube placement and removal. Holder safety features may include a shield that covers the needle or a device that retracts the needle into the holder after it is withdrawn from the vein.

Tourniquet

The tourniquet constricts the flow of venous blood in the arm and makes the veins more prominent so that they are easier to find and penetrate with a needle. The tourniquet is a soft, pliable rubber strip, usually 1 inch wide and 15 to 18 inches long. Some tourniquets are made of latex. Rubber or other nonlatex tourniquets must be used for patients with latex allergies. The tourniquet, tied correctly, can easily be released with one hand, does not cut into the patient's arm, and is inexpensive enough that a new tourniquet can be used for each patient. The maximum time limit for leaving the tourniquet in place is 2 minutes. More time can cause **hemoconcentration** (decrease of the fluid content of blood) and **hemolysis** (rupturing of RBCs, causing release of intracellular contents into the plasma). Hemoconcentration and hemolysis cause errors in test results. If the tourniquet is released before completing of the venipuncture procedure, reapplication should be delayed for at least 2 minutes.

Hemoconcentration causes too many cells to be present for the amount of serum or plasma. This false elevation results in inaccurate laboratory measurement of iron, calcium, and some enzymes.

To avoid hemoconcentration, the phlebotomist should:

1. Ensure that the tourniquet is not on too tight or left on too long.
2. Instruct the patient to avoid pumping his or her hand and to just make a fist.
3. Avoid probing with the needle ("fishing" for a vein).
4. Avoid sclerosed or occluded veins.

 CHECKPOINT QUESTION

6. If the tourniquet is left on the arm too long, what is the effect on the test results?

By taking similar precautions, the phlebotomist will also avoid hemolysis. Hemolysis contamination is not always visible. Alterations of patient test results occur long before hemolysis reaches the level of a visible color change of plasma or serum from slightly yellow to pink or red. When cells are hemolyzed, they are not recognized as RBCs by hematology cell counters, resulting in falsely decreased results in cell counts and hemoglobin determinations. When the RBCs rupture, all of their intracellular contents are released into the serum or plasma. Fluid inside the cell contains components different from regular plasma.

An example is the electrolyte, potassium. The fluid inside the cell has much more potassium than the plasma. Even hemolysis that cannot be seen can cause significant increases in the patient's potassium level. The phlebotomist can avoid hemolysis by using a needle with a large enough diameter to not cause rupture of RBCs as they pass through the needle into the collection tube.

Reusable tourniquets have been found to be contaminated with blood and bacterial pathogens. Bacterial pathogens have been **cultured** (grown in the laboratory) from sampling blood stains on used tourniquets. These comprise methicillin-resistant *Staphylococcus aureus*, *Escherichia coli*, *Pseudomonas aeruginosa*, and other bacterial antigen contaminants. Because it is impossible to disinfect tourniquets, disposable tourniquets are useful in minimizing patient and health care worker infections.

 CHECKPOINT QUESTION

7. Can hemolysis and its effects be present in a specimen that does not appear hemolyzed?

Alcohol Wipes

Antiseptics inhibit the growth of bacteria. They are used to clean the skin before venipuncture. The most commonly used antiseptic for routine blood collection is 70% isopropyl alcohol. Alternatives are required when collecting blood specimens for tests that may be inaccurate if contaminated with alcohol. These tests are identified in the medical office specimen collection procedure or manual. Iodine wipes or swabs are used if a blood culture is to be drawn.

Gauze Sponges

Gauze sponges are gauze pads that come in multiple sizes depending upon their use in various clinical areas. Cotton or rayon balls may be used but are not recommended because of their tendency to stick to the site and cause bleeding when removed.

Bandages

An adhesive bandage (e.g., Band-Aid™) is used to cover the site once the bleeding has stopped. Patients may be allergic to the adhesive or latex in the bandage. If a patient is allergic, use paper, cloth, or knitted tape over a folded gauze square. Do not use a bandage on infants under age 2 years because of the danger of aspiration and suffocation. Latex-free bandages are available.

Needle Disposal Unit

A **needle disposal unit** may also be called a **sharps container**. Even with safety features, immediately dispose of used needles, lancets, and other sharp objects in the puncture-resistant, leak-proof, disposable sharps container. These containers are marked as *biohazard* and are red or bright orange for easy identification. Needles should never be cut, bent, or broken before disposal.

Gloves

A new pair of gloves must be used for each patient. Nonsterile, disposable latex, nitrile, vinyl, or polyethylene gloves are acceptable.

Standard precautions require handwashing after glove removal. Good glove fit enhances safe manipulation. Gloves that are dusted with powder can be a source of contamination for some tests, especially those collected by capillary puncture. Gloves are not required to be sterile.

Some users have allergic responses to glove powder. Powder in latex gloves puts latex particles in the air, posing danger to those with latex allergy. Gloves are available powder free and/or latex free. The best practice for the medical assistant is to ask the patient whether he or she has a latex allergy before starting the phlebotomy procedure. The phlebotomist can avoid gloves, tourniquets, and bandages containing latex before exposing the patient.

CHECKPOINT QUESTION

8. What phlebotomy equipment might cause allergic reactions from the patient?

Syringe System

As discussed previously, evacuated tubes remove the blood from the vein because they contain a vacuum. A **syringe** is helpful with fragile veins because the vacuum can be applied slowly and gently, rather than all at once as with vacuum tubes. Syringes are made of disposable plastic and vary in volume from 1 to 50 mL. Choose the smallest syringe volume that will accommodate the total amount of blood necessary for the tests the physician has requested.

The plunger of the syringe often sticks and is hard to pull. A technique called "**breathing the syringe**" makes the plunger easier to move. To do this, pull back the plunger to about halfway up the barrel, and then push it back. This makes the plunger move more smoothly and reduces the tendency to jerk when it is first pulled after insertion into the vein. The vacuum created by pulling on the plunger while a needle is in a patient's vein fills the syringe with blood. Pulling the plunger slowly and resting between pulls allows the vein time to refill with blood.

Using a syringe for blood collection requires transfer of blood to a collection tube. Various brands of devices ensure safety during the transfer of blood from a syringe into an evacuated tube. When performing this transfer, force on the syringe plunger is not required because the vacuum in the tube will draw the specimen from the syringe. Blood specimens collected by syringe must be transferred to evacuated tubes following proper order of draw.

CHECKPOINT QUESTIONS

9. What is the benefit of using a new tourniquet for each patient?
10. What is the benefit of using a syringe to collect a blood specimen from a delicate vein?

COG Patient Relations and Identification

The phlebotomist's role requires a professional, courteous, and understanding manner in all contacts with the patient. The medical assistant should greet the patient, identify himself or herself, and indicate the procedure that will take place. Effective communication—both verbal and nonverbal—is essential.

Ask the patient for a full name and verify it with the test requisition. Using the requisition for reference, ask a patient to provide additional information such as birthdate.

If possible, speak with the patient during the process. The patient who is at ease will be less focused on the procedure. You should always thank the patient and excuse yourself courteously when finished.

Remember to respect the rights of the patient as addressed in the Patient Bill of Rights. The Patient Bill of Rights was created to try to reach the following three major goals:

1. To help patients feel more confident about their care—that their needs are cared about, that there is a way they can report their problems, and that they need to work on taking care of their health.
2. To emphasize the relationship between patients and their health care providers.
3. To emphasize the patients' need to take responsibility for their part of making the health care system work for them.

WHAT IF?

What if your patient feels faint while you are drawing blood?

1. Remove the tourniquet and withdraw the needle as quickly as possible.
2. Talk to the patient to divert attention from the procedure and to help keep him or her alert.
3. Have the patient lower his or her head and breathe deeply while you physically support him or her to prevent injury in case of collapse.
4. Loosen a tight collar or tie if possible.
5. Apply a cold compress or washcloth to the forehead and back of the patient's neck.
6. Call for the physician if the patient does not respond.

Modified with permission from McCall R. Phlebotomy Essentials. Baltimore: Lippincott Williams & Wilkins, 2003.

COG Venipuncture Site Selection

The procedure should start with washing hands and putting on gloves. Equipment and supplies should be assembled near the phlebotomy chair. Many patients know from experience where it is easiest to find an accessible vein. Using the patient's experience and your own knowledge and skill, help to choose the best site. Talk quietly with the patient and progress through the procedure with confidence.

The forearm veins in the **antecubital space** (the inside of the elbow) are commonly used for venipuncture. The three main veins in this area are the cephalic, median cubital, and basilic (Fig. 26-8A,B). Hand veins are also acceptable

Right arm in anatomic position

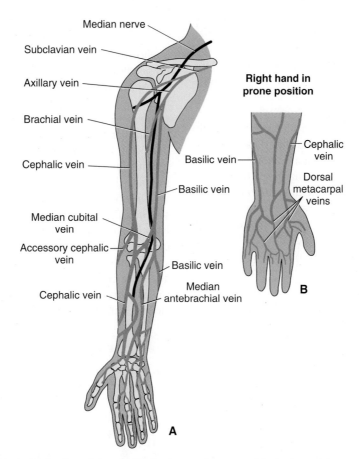

Figure 26-8 (**A**) Principal veins of the arm, including major antecubital veins subject to venipuncture. (**B**) Forearm, wrist, and hand veins subject to venipuncture. (Reprinted with permission from McCall R. Phlebotomy Essentials. Baltimore: Lippincott Williams & Wilkins, 2003.)

if a forearm vein cannot be found. Foot veins are a last resort because they are more likely to have complications.

Following are certain areas to be avoided when choosing a site.

- Burns or scars should be avoided.
- Areas with a hematoma or bruising should also be avoided. If another site is not available, collect the specimen **distal** (away from the origin) to the hematoma.
- **Thrombosed** veins feel like rope or cord and roll easily.
- **Edematous** tissue contains tissue fluid accumulation that alters test results.
- Intravenous (IV) therapy/blood transfusions contain fluid that may dilute the specimen, so collect from the opposite arm if possible.
- The upper extremity on the side of a previous mastectomy may result in test results affected by **lymphedema** (lymphatic obstruction).

Although some veins are visible, the best choice for venipuncture is found by touch. Use the tip of the index finger to **palpate** veins to determine their suitability. Palpating helps locate veins and determine their size,

depth, and direction. Do not slap the arm when trying to locate a vein because this can cause bruising in addition to altering test results from the specimen. Trace the path of veins with the index finger. Arteries pulsate, are most elastic, and have a thick wall. Thrombosed veins lack resilience, feel cordlike, and roll easily. If no suitable antecubital vein can be found, repeat the procedure to this point on the other arm.

If veins are not found, force blood into the vein by massaging the arm from wrist to elbow; tap the site with the index and second fingers; apply a warm, damp washcloth to the site for 5 minutes; or lower the arm to allow the veins to fill.

☑ CHECKPOINT QUESTIONS

11. What areas are to be avoided when selecting the venipuncture site. Why?
12. Why should the practice of slapping the patient's arm to make a vein more palpable be avoided?

COG Performance of the Venipuncture

The medical assistant needs to be thoroughly familiar with each step of the venipuncture procedure. To maintain the patient's confidence, the phlebotomist must be confident and accurate with each step of the procedure. Procedure 26-1 is Obtaining a Blood Specimen by Evacuated Tube or Winged Infusion Set. Those who have witnessed or actually experienced a venipuncture personally may have seen these steps performed differently than in the procedure. Each step does have a reason, and more explanation may help in understanding the differences.

If the patient indicates that fasting instructions or dietary restrictions were not followed, notify the physician for a decision whether or not to proceed with the venipuncture. If the physician cannot be reached, or you are instructed to proceed in obtaining the specimen, "nonfasting" should be written on both the test requisition and the specimen label.

The patient may become defensive on being questioned about compliance with preparations prior to collecting the specimen. If the patient has not complied with pretesting requirements, the medical assistant may be questioned and challenged that the requirements are too strict or not necessary. The patient may also say that he or she has not been questioned like this before. The patient's frustration may increase on learning that he or she will have to reschedule the procedure and not complete it on the current visit. You should educate the patient while answering the patient's questions, explaining the reasons for the requirements. Some patients can be consoled by learning the negative effects to test results that come from not following pretesting requirements.

Verify that the necessary collection tubes are available at hand and be prepared for special sample handling (i.e., protect from light, place immediately on ice, etc.). Always have extra supplies at hand as well since equipment can fail. If you are alone with the patient in the phlebotomy area, the only recourse to equipment problems may be to discontinue the phlebotomy, correct the situation, and stick the patient again for the specimen. Resticking the patient should be avoided.

Cleansing the site selected for the blood draw should be in a circular direction, beginning at the site and working outward. Working outward from the center drags contaminants away from the puncture site. Some phlebotomists use the gauze to wipe over the site a few times. This wipes contaminants directly onto the puncture site.

Allow the cleansed site to air dry. Do not blow on the site or wave the air with the hand above the site. This directs bacteria back to the area that was just cleaned. Blowing on the site may be a natural instinct or a gesture to the patient that the medical assistant is not wasting his or her time. Instructing the patient through the procedure will give the patient understanding of the steps and the medical assistant's concern for his or her care.

A venipuncture site should not be palpated again after cleansing. This reintroduces bacteria to the clean site. For personal protection, the medical assistant must not use the forefinger above the selected phlebotomy site to anchor the vein. This increases risk of a possible accidental needlestick.

Apply adequate pressure to the site to avoid the formation of a hematoma. Rushing to complete the steps of the venipuncture can lead to a hematoma due to inadequate pressure at the site. Asking the patient may be useful, but does not limit the medical assistant's responsibility for monitoring pressure on the site. The medical assistant must monitor that the patient is applying adequate pressure.

Do not apply a bandage to the patient's arm until the site has completely stopped bleeding. The patient may have bleeding abnormalities or anticoagulant therapy that cause prolonged bleeding at the puncture site. The bandage should only be applied after the site has been monitored for adequate clotting. Pressure will increase on the site when the patient stands and puts his or hands down. Inadequate clotting can allow the site to start bleeding again.

 CHECKPOINT QUESTION

13. How do the patient instructions for fasting differ from having nothing by mouth?

PATIENT EDUCATION

INSTRUCTING PATIENTS ON DIETARY RESTRICTIONS

Fasting and NPO are two common dietary restrictions. Because most patients will not understand the differences between these requirements, the medical assistant must provide clear explanations.

Fasting

Fasting, the most common dietary restriction, requires the patient to not eat for a certain period, usually from midnight until specimen collection the following morning. Fasting allows the patient to drink water; in fact, adequate hydration is necessary to ensure that veins are palpable and accessible for venipuncture. Dehydration by abstaining from all fluids can falsely elevate some test results, making them appear abnormal when they really are not.

NPO

NPO orders require that the patient have absolutely nothing by mouth for a certain period. This type of order is usually used if the patient is scheduled for surgery or for some radiology procedures. The purpose of an NPO order is to minimize secretions by reducing the body's fluid level.

COG Troubleshooting Guidelines

Probing is *not* the way to troubleshoot blood drawing problems.

If an Incomplete Collection or No Blood Is Obtained

- Change the position of the needle. Move it forward (it may not be in the lumen). Or, move it backward (it may have penetrated too far). Figure 26-9A–G shows proper and improper needle positions.
- Adjust the angle (the bevel may be against the vein wall).
- Loosen the tourniquet; it may be obstructing blood flow.
- Try another tube. There may be no vacuum in the one being used.
- Re-anchor the vein. Veins sometimes roll away from the point of the needle and puncture site.

If Blood Stops Flowing into the Tube

If blood stops flowing into the tube, the vein may have collapsed. The medical assistant should resecure the tourniquet to increase venous filling. This will require assistance. If resecuring the tourniquet is not successful, the medical assistant should remove the needle, take care of the puncture site, and draw the specimen from another site. Another cause of this problem may be the needle pulling out of the vein when switching tubes. Holding the equipment firmly and placing fingers against patient's arm, will provide leverage when using the flanges when withdrawing and inserting tubes.

Problems Other Than an Incomplete Collection

- The most common complication of venipuncture is **hematoma** formation, caused by blood leaking into the tissues during or after venipuncture. Hematomas are

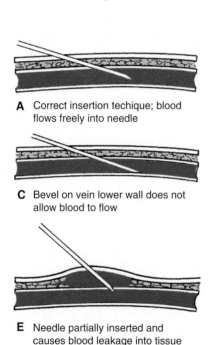

A Correct insertion techique; blood flows freely into needle

C Bevel on vein lower wall does not allow blood to flow

E Needle partially inserted and causes blood leakage into tissue

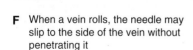

F When a vein rolls, the needle may slip to the side of the vein without penetrating it

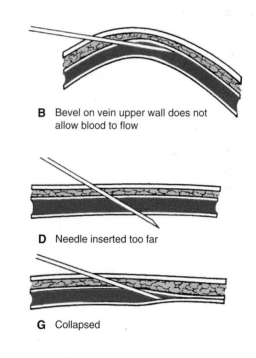

B Bevel on vein upper wall does not allow blood to flow

D Needle inserted too far

G Collapsed

Figure 26-9 Proper and improper needle positioning. (**A**) Needle correctly positioned in a vein; blood flows freely into the needle. (**B**) Bevel on the upper wall of the vein prevents blood flow. (**C**) Bevel on the lower wall of the vein prevents blood flow. (**D**) Needle inserted too deep runs through the vein. (**E**) Partially inserted needle causes blood to leak into tissue. (**F**) Needle slipped beside the vein, not into it; this occurs when a vein rolls to the side. (**G**) Collapsed vein prevents blood flow. (Reprinted with permission from McCall R. Phlebotomy Essentials. Baltimore: Lippincott Williams & Wilkins, 2007.)

painful, cause bruising, and can cause injuries to nerves. Box 26-2 describes situations that may trigger hematoma formation. If a hematoma begins to form during the venipuncture, release the tourniquet immediately, withdraw the needle, and hold pressure on the site for at least 2 minutes. Cold compresses reduce pain and swelling. Hematoma formation is especially a problem in older patients.

- Accidental puncture of an artery is recognized by the blood's bright red color and the pulsing of the specimen into the tube. In this case, it is important to hold pressure over the site for a full 5 minutes after the needle is removed.

Permanent nerve damage may result from poor site selection, patient movement during needle insertion, inserting the needle too deeply or quickly, or excessive blind probing.

COG Additional Considerations

To Prevent Hematoma

- Puncture only the uppermost wall of the vein.
- Remove the tourniquet before removing the needle.
- Use the major superficial veins.
- Make sure the needle fully penetrates the uppermost wall of the vein. (Partial penetration may allow blood to leak into the soft tissue surrounding the vein by way of the needle bevel.)
- Apply pressure to the venipuncture site.

To Prevent Hemolysis

Note: Hemolysis can interfere with many tests.
- Gently mix tubes with anticoagulant additives.
- Avoid drawing blood from a hematoma.
- If using a needle and syringe, avoid drawing the syringe plunger back too forcefully, and avoid frothing the sample.

- Make sure the venipuncture site is dry.
- The venipuncture is not traumatic.

Causes of Hemoconcentration

Hemoconcentration can be caused by prolonged tourniquet application; massaging, squeezing, or probing a site; and/or sclerosed or occluded veins.

Prolonged Tourniquet Application

The primary effect of prolonged tourniquet application is hemoconcentration of the specimen. Significant increases can be found in total protein, aspartate aminotransferase (AST), total lipids, cholesterol, and iron from prolonged tourniquet application. It also affects **hematocrit** (packed cell volume).

 LEGAL TIP

ASSESS THE RISK OF PHLEBOTOMY LIABILITY

To reduce a laboratory's exposure to phlebotomy liability, address the following issues in your policy manual, your new employee training program, and in your employee competency assessments.

- Put the proper information on every tube of blood, including the time and date of collection and the phlebotomist's initials.
- Note that phlebotomy textbooks set a range between 15° and 30° for the angle of needle insertion.
- Require adherence to facility protocol regardless of an employee's experience.
- Perform regular competency evaluations on all phlebotomy staff members.
- In vein selection, the vein of choice is the medial vein, which typically lies in a depression in the center of the antecubital area. It is the vein of choice because it is usually larger, more stationary, closer to the surface of the skin, and more isolated from other underlying structures than the other veins.
- The error considered most critical for a medical office is misidentifying a patient. Avoiding this risk requires strict adherence to the facility's patient identification policy.

Patient Preparation Factors

- *Therapeutic drug monitoring*: Drugs have different patterns of administration, body distribution, metabolism, and elimination that affect their concentration as measured in the blood.

Many drugs will have **peak** (the highest serum level of drug in a patient based on a dosing schedule) and **trough** (the lowest levels drawn immediately before a dose) levels. Check for timing instructions for drawing the appropriate specimens.

- *Effects of exercise*: Muscular activity has effects. The creatine kinase (CK), AST, lactate dehydrogenase (LDH), and platelet count may increase.
- *Stress*: Stress may cause elevation in white blood cells (WBCs). Anxiety that results in hyperventilation may cause acid–base imbalances.
- *Diurnal rhythms*: **Diurnal rhythms** are fluctuations during the day. Serum iron levels tend to drop during the day. Check the timing of these variations for the desired collection point.
- *Posture*: Postural changes (supine to sitting, etc.) are known to vary the laboratory results of some analytes. The difference in these lab values have been attributed to shifts in body fluids. Fluids tend to stay in the bloodstream when the patient is recumbent or supine. This tends to dilute the blood. There is a shift of fluids to the interstitial spaces upon standing or ambulation. The lab tests that are the most affected by this phenomenon are enzymes, albumin, triglycerides, cholesterol, calcium, and iron.

Box 26-3 lists some common errors in venipuncture to guard against.

 CHECKPOINT QUESTION

14. Why should the forefinger not be used above the selected phlebotomy site to anchor the vein?

COG **Capillary Puncture (Microcollection) Equipment**

Capillary puncture or skin puncture requires penetration of the capillary bed in the dermis of the skin with a puncture device. The small specimen volumes required by point-of-care (POC) instruments allow more laboratory tests to be collected by skin puncture. The equipment used to collect the specimen depends on the patient's age and condition and on the test being performed.

Puncture Devices

A sterile disposable puncture device is used to pierce the skin to obtain drops of blood for testing. These devices are designed to control depth of puncture and have a spring-loaded point or blade to reduce accidental sharps injuries. Manufacturers offer puncture devices in a range of lengths and depths to facilitate varying puncture situations and sample requirements. Figure 26-10A–C shows several types of puncture devices used for microcollection.

Microhematocrit Tubes

Microhematocrit tubes are narrow glass or plastic disposable capillary tubes used for hematocrit determinations. They fill by capillary action and hold 50 to 75 μL of blood. Capillary action is a scientific principal that explains how the blood can flow upward. Microhematocrit tubes for sampling specimens directly from a lavender-top tube are plain; those used for collecting hematocrit specimens directly from a capillary puncture

---

BOX 26-3

SOURCES OF ERROR IN VENIPUNCTURE

Errors in Venipuncture Preparation
- Improper patient identification
- Failure to check patient adherence to dietary restrictions
- Failure to calm patient prior to blood collection
- Use of improper equipment and supplies
- Inappropriate method of blood collection
- Failure to dry the site completely after cleansing with alcohol

Errors in Venipuncture Procedure
- Inserting needle bevel side down
- Use of needle that is too small, causing hemolysis of specimen
- Venipuncture in an unacceptable area
- Prolonged tourniquet application
- Wrong order of tube draw

- Failure to immediately mix blood collected in additive-containing tubes
- Pulling back on syringe plunger too forcefully
- Failure to release tourniquet prior to needle withdrawal

Errors After Venipuncture Completion
- Failure to apply pressure immediately to venipuncture site
- Vigorous shaking of anticoagulated blood specimens
- Forcing blood through a syringe needle into tube
- Mislabeling of tubes
- Failure to label appropriate specimens with infectious disease precaution
- Failure to put date, time, and initials on requisition
- Slow transport of specimens to laboratory

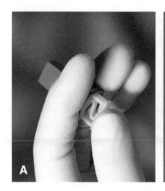
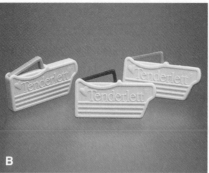
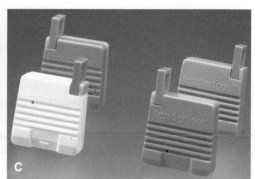

Figure 26-10 Several types of finger and heel puncture lancets. (**A**) Vacutainer Genie lancets. (Courtesy of Becton-Dickinson, Franklin Lakes, NJ.) (**B**) Tenderlett toddler, junior, and adult lancet devices. (Courtesy of ITC, Edison, NJ.) (**C**) Tenderfoot toddler, newborn, preemie, and micropreemie heel incision devices. (Courtesy of ITC, Edison, NJ.)

are coated with heparin. Plain tubes have a blue band on one end of the capillary tube, and ammonium tubes have a red band. A plastic or clay sealant is used to close one end of the tube (Fig. 26-11).

Microcollection Containers

Microcontainers are small plastic tubes with color-coded stoppers that indicate the additive. The color coding is the same as that for the tubes used in venipuncture, but the microcontainer contains no vacuum to remove the blood from the patient. Samples for light-sensitive analytes, such as bilirubin, are collected in amber-colored plastic tubes that protect the blood from light exposure. Microcontainers are filled by blood droplets from a capillary puncture.

Filter Paper Test Requisitions

Microcollection may also be accomplished using filter paper attached to a test requisition. Filter paper is a special paper product made to be thick and absorbent. It is used to collect blood specimens to test newborns for genetic defects, such as hypothyroidism and phenylketonuria. The filter paper is printed with circles that must be filled with blood. Figure 26-12A,B shows an example of how the requisition and attached filter paper could look. The lateral surface of the newborn's heel

is punctured, and the blood droplet is absorbed into individual circles on a filter paper card. A large drop of blood must be applied from one side of the paper, and the blood must soak through to the other side. The specimen should air-dry in a horizontal position and not be stacked with other collection requisitions.

Warming Devices

For heelsticks, warmers increase blood flow before the skin is punctured. Heel-warming devices (Fig. 26-13) provide a temperature not exceeding 42°C. Alternatively, a diaper or towel may be wet with warm tap water and used to wrap the hand or foot before skin puncture. Do not use water that is hot enough to burn the patient.

COG Performing a Capillary Puncture

Adult skin punctures are performed when no veins are accessible, to save veins for procedures such as chemotherapy, and for POC testing. Technology now allows some tests to be performed on very small blood samples. However, some results are more accurate on venipuncture specimens than on capillary specimens. Tests that cannot be performed on skin puncture specimens include erythrocyte sedimentation rate methods, coagulation studies on plasma, cultures, and tests that require large blood volumes.

The skin puncture is the preferred method to obtain blood from infants and children. Venipuncture on infants and children can damage veins and surrounding tissues.

Selection of the Capillary Puncture Site

The location of the puncture must be carefully considered in addition to the patient's age, accessibility of

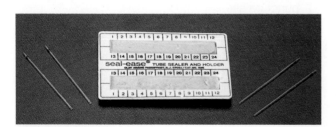

Figure 26-11 Microcollection tubes and clay sealant.

A

1

Newborn Screening - Initial Specimen Form

SUBMITTER CODE

Prior Transfusion may invalidate results

Not Used For Repeat Testing

SPECIMEN NOT SATISFACTORY Code

*** LAB USE ONLY ***

NMS LAB ID NUMBER

DATE AND TIME STAMP

HOSPITAL OR LAB SUBMITTING SPECIMEN

SUBMITTER'S NAME

SUBMITTER'S ADDRESS

CITY STATE ZIP CODE

PHONE

DOCTOR

PCP NAME

PHONE

CONTACT NAME #

MEDICAL STATUS

TRANSFUSED DATE

PREMATURE SICK / I.C.U.

TYPE OF FEEDING

BREAST PROTEIN IV

FORMULA NONPROTEIN

1 2 2 3 6 7 5

NEWBORN INFORMATION

LAST NAME

FIRST NAME

BIRTH

Month # Day Year HOUR Military Time

DATE DRAWN

Month # Day Year HOUR Military Time

MOTHER

MAIDEN NAME

FIRST NAME

MOM'S DATE OF BIRTH Month # Day Year

ADDRESS AGE

CITY STATE ZIP CODE

PHONE

MEDICAL RECORD NUMBER

OTHER

ETHNICITY

HISPANIC

NON-HISPANIC

RACE

ASIAN / PACIFIC ISLANDER

BLACK WHITE

NATIVE AMERICAN OTHER

SEX

MALE

FEMALE

TWINS/MULTIPLE ABC

ABNORMAL RESULTS

BIRTHWEIGHT

GRAMS * ONLY *

STATE OF NEW MEXICO

Scientific Laboratory Division

700 Camino de Salud NE / P.O. Box 4700

Albuquerque, NM 87196-4700

Phone (505) 841-2581

Expires: 02/04 SLD 601 2/01

L-8967302

RESULTS WILL NOT BE ISSUED IF THE REQUESTED INFORMATION IS NOT COMPLETED

B

2

Newborn Screening - Second Specimen Form

SUBMITTER CODE

Prior Transfusion may invalidate results

May Be Used For Repeat Testing

SPECIMEN NOT SATISFACTORY Code

*** LAB USE ONLY ***

NMS LAB ID NUMBER

DATE AND TIME STAMP

HOSPITAL OR LAB SUBMITTING SPECIMEN

SUBMITTER'S NAME

SUBMITTER'S ADDRESS

CITY STATE ZIP CODE

PHONE

DOCTOR

PCP NAME

PHONE

CONTACT NAME #

MEDICAL STATUS

TRANSFUSED DATE

PREMATURE SICK / I.C.U.

TYPE OF FEEDING

BREAST PROTEIN IV

FORMULA NONPROTEIN

1 2 2 3 6 7 6

NEWBORN INFORMATION

LAST NAME

FIRST NAME

BIRTH

Month # Day Year HOUR Military Time

DATE DRAWN

Month # Day Year HOUR Military Time

MOTHER

MAIDEN NAME

FIRST NAME

MOM'S DATE OF BIRTH Month # Day Year

ADDRESS AGE

CITY STATE ZIP CODE

PHONE

MEDICAL RECORD NUMBER

OTHER

ETHNICITY

HISPANIC

NON-HISPANIC

RACE

ASIAN / PACIFIC ISLANDER

BLACK WHITE

NATIVE AMERICAN OTHER

SEX

MALE

FEMALE

TWINS/MULTIPLE ABC

ABNORMAL RESULTS

BIRTHWEIGHT

GRAMS * ONLY *

STATE OF NEW MEXICO

Scientific Laboratory Division

700 Camino de Salud NE / P.O. Box 4700

Albuquerque, NM 87196-4700

Phone (505) 841-2581

Expires: 02/04 SLD 601 2/01

L-8967302

RESULTS WILL NOT BE ISSUED IF THE REQUESTED INFORMATION IS NOT COMPLETED

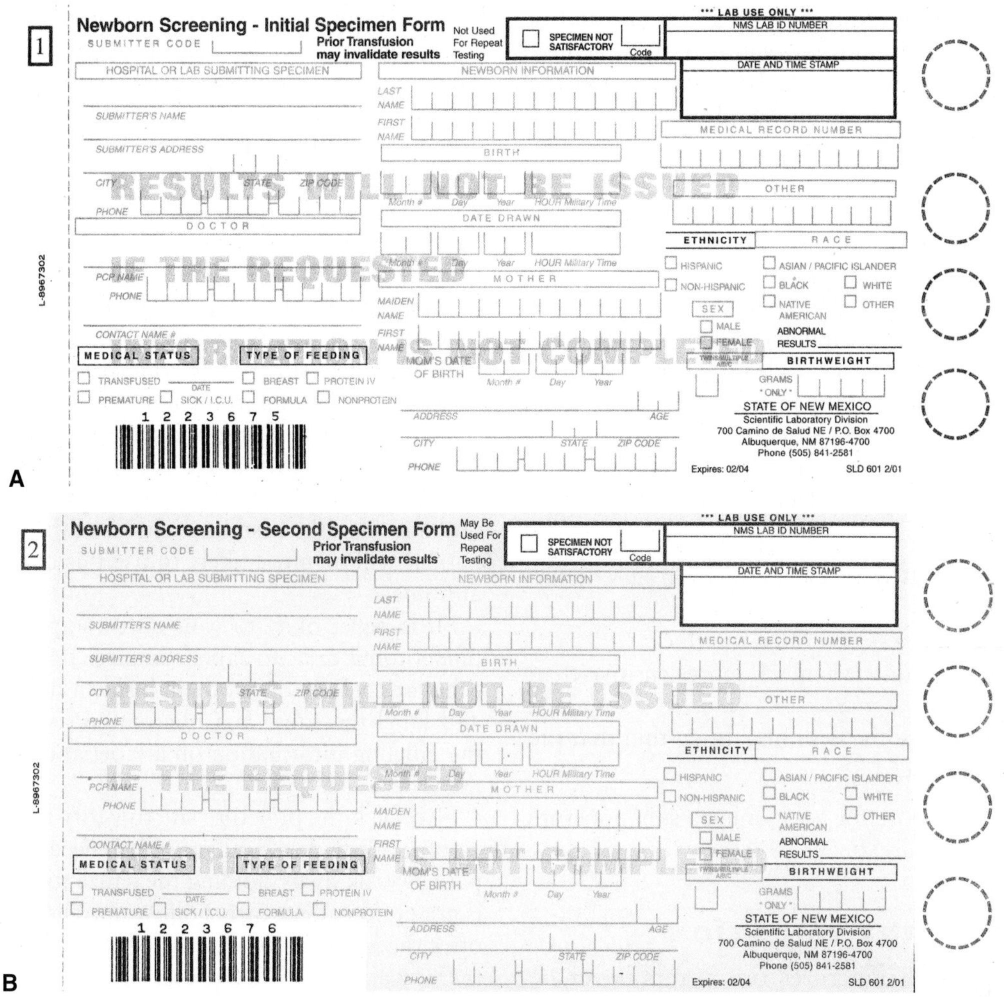

Figure 26-12 Newborn screening specimen forms. (**A**) Initial specimen form. (**B**) Second specimen form. (Courtesy of Daniel Gray, State of New Mexico Scientific Laboratory, Albuquerque, NM.)

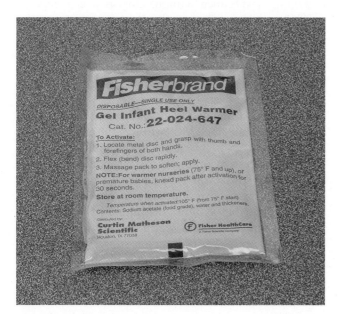

Figure 26-13 Infant heel warmer. (Reprinted with permission from McCall R. Phlebotomy Essentials. Baltimore: Lippincott Williams & Wilkins, 2007.)

acceptable sites, and the tests ordered. Skin puncture in adults and older children most often involves one of the fingers. Recommended sites are the fleshy pad of the third or fourth finger of the patient's nondominant hand only. For finger puncture sites, it is best to have the hand below the heart. Do not use the tip of the finger or the center of the finger. Avoid the side of the finger where there is less soft tissue, where vessels and nerves are located, and where the bone is closer to the surface. If the patient has cold hands, warm them by holding them under warm running water or by vigorously rubbing them.

Prepare the skin as for a venipuncture. When the puncture and collection are complete, place a clean gauze sponge on the puncture site and hold it in place until the bleeding has stopped. Dispose of contaminated material appropriately and completely wash your hands.

For infant heel punctures in children under age 1 year, the CLSI (described earlier in this chapter) set the standard of a maximum of 2 mm for heel punctures to avoid hitting bone. Because the thickness of the tissue on the side of an infant's heel can be as little as 2.0 mm and as little as 1.0 mm at the positive curvature of the heel, heel punctures on infants must never be performed on the back of the heel. If performed on the side of the heel, they must be no deeper than 2.0 mm. Prewarming the infant's heel (42°C for 3–5 minutes) increases the flow of blood for collection of heel punctures. Monitor the warming temperature to avoid burns to infants' thin skin.

Hold the baby's foot firmly to avoid sudden movement while performing the heel puncture. Follow standards for obtaining a capillary specimen. When finished, elevate the heel, place a clean gauze sponge on the puncture site, and hold it in place until the bleeding has stopped. Dispose of contaminated material appropriately and complete hand hygiene.

Specific sites not recommended for capillary puncture are:

- Bruised, infected, swollen, or traumatized sites on fingers or heels
- Thumb, because the skin is often too thick
- Second finger, because it is much more sensitive than other fingers
- Fifth finger, because the flesh may be so thin that the bone could be pierced

The complete procedure for performing a skin puncture is outlined in Procedure 26-2.

 CHECKPOINT QUESTION

15. Why must heel punctures on infants never be performed on the back of the heel?

Performance of a Capillary Puncture

The introductory steps on the capillary collection process are the same as those for the venipuncture. As in the venipuncture procedure, the medical assistant needs to be thoroughly familiar with each step of the procedure. To maintain the patient's confidence, the phlebotomist must be confident and accurate with each step of the procedure.

Procedure 26-2 is Obtaining a Blood Specimen by Capillary Puncture. Those who have witnessed or actually experienced a capillary puncture personally may have seen these steps performed differently than in the procedure. Each step does have a reason, and more explanation may help in understanding the differences.

Cleansing the site selected for the blood draw should be in a circular direction, beginning at the site and working outward. Allow the cleansed to site to air dry. Do not blow on the site or wave the air with the hand above the site. This directs bacteria back to the area that was just cleaned.

Placement of the puncture on the finger is considerate to the patient's comfort on leaving the medical office. The puncture should be made perpendicular to the ridges of the finger print so that the drop of blood does not run down the ridges. Making the puncture perpendicular to the ridges of the finger print also prevents the pain of using that finger for touch. Making the puncture horizontal with the ridges of the finger print causes using that finger to feel like it just had a paper cut.

Wipe away the first drop of blood, which tends to contain excess tissue fluid. Explaining this to the patient reduces surprise on seeing the first drop of blood "wasted." It is important not to skip this step due to rushing or from feeling pressure from the patient. It is helpful to teach the patient the step of wiping away the first drop of blood. If the patient understands that contamination in the first drop can harm the test results, the patient will be more likely to use this correct technique at home.

It is never okay to wait until the patient leaves the phlebotomy area to label samples. If microhematocrit tubes are collected, put them inside a plain red-top tube and label the tube. If a microtainer is collected, write the labeling information on a label and wrap it around the tube.

Recheck the puncture site to verify that bleeding has stopped. Provide a bandage only if necessary. Letting the patient walk away holding the gauze to his or her finger is not good patient care. Follow up. The patient may not offer the information that he or she is on anticoagulant therapy and may bleed excessively.

Complications of Capillary Puncture

Obtaining a specimen without clots is a challenge in capillary puncture. The capillary puncture activates the body's clotting system to stop the bleeding as soon as the skin is punctured. If an anticoagulated specimen is required, it should be drawn first to get an adequate volume before the blood begins to clot. Any other additive specimens are collected next, and clotted specimens are collected last. If the blood has begun to produce microscopic clots while filling the last tube, this is not a problem because clotting is required in this tube.

Avoid excessive squeezing of the fingertip or heel because the RBCs will rupture and contaminate the specimen. If excessive squeezing is required because of inadequate blood flow, discontinue the puncture. Choose another site and warm the site prior to the puncture. Box 26-4 lists common sources of errors in microcollection that should be avoided.

 CHECKPOINT QUESTION

16. Why must anticoagulated specimens be drawn first when performing a capillary puncture?

> **BOX 26-4**
>
> ## SOURCES OF ERROR IN SKIN PUNCTURE
>
> - Misidentification of patient
> - Puncturing wrong area of infant heel
> - Puncturing bone in infant heel
> - Puncturing fingers of infants
> - Puncturing wrong area of adult finger
> - Contaminating specimen with alcohol or Betadine™
> - Failure to discard first blood drop
> - Excessive massaging of puncture site
> - Collecting air bubbles in pH or blood gas specimen
> - Hemolyzing specimen
> - Failure to seal specimens adequately
> - Failure to chill specimens requiring refrigeration
> - Erroneous specimen labeling
> - Failure to document skin puncture collection on the requisition or in the computer
> - Failure to warm site
> - Delaying specimen transport
> - Bruising site as a result of excessive squeezing

COG Phlebotomy Quality Control

Many factors must be addressed to ensure specimen quality. Phlebotomy errors may cause serious harm to patients. Quality control consists of methods practiced in every capillary puncture or venipuncture to optimize the quality of each specimen. The list includes:

- Patient identification
- Patient preparation
- Communicating with the patient
- Diet
- Medications
- Specimen collection
- Selection of the venipuncture or capillary puncture site
- Type of collection and amount of specimen to be collected
- Need for special timing for collection
- Types and amounts of preservatives and anticoagulants
- Patient posture
- Duration of tourniquet use
- Actual time of specimen collection
- Choosing the correct equipment
- Order of draw
- Need for special handling between time of collection and time received by the laboratory (e.g., refrigeration, protection from light)
- Specimen labeling
- Specimen processing and storage
- Time

- Temperature
- Needed clinical data when indicated

Quality control begins with a thorough specimen collection manual that specifies the instructions for collecting every type of specimen. The phlebotomist must meet the written standards at all times. The supervisor observes phlebotomists at work to verify compliance with facility protocol. In the absence of a phlebotomy supervisor, coworkers can observe each other to validate compliance.

 CHECKPOINT QUESTION

17. What is included in phlebotomy quality control?

COG Safety and Infection Control

Protect Yourself

- Practice standard precautions
- Dispose of needles immediately upon removal from the patient's vein. Do not bend, break, recap, or resheath needles to avoid accidental needlestick or splashing contents.
- Clean up any blood spills with a disinfectant such as freshly made 10% bleach (sodium hypochlorite) solution. All surfaces should be cleaned daily with freshly made 10% bleach solution.
- If stuck with a contaminated needle:
  1. Remove gloves and dispose of them properly.
  2. Allow site to bleed for several minutes.
  3. Wash the area well with soap and water.
  4. Record the patient's name and ID number.
  5. Follow the institution's guidelines regarding documentation (incident report), treatment, and follow-up.

Protect the Patient

- Place blood collection equipment away from patients.
- Practice hygiene for the patient's protection. When wearing gloves, change them between each patient and wash your hands frequently. Always wear a clean lab coat.

 CHECKPOINT QUESTION

18. What steps should be taken if stuck with a contaminated needle?

Spill Kit Supplies and Instructions

The supplies available in a biohazard spill kit should include but are not limited to the following:

- A copy of the biohazardous spill cleanup instructions
- Nitrile disposable gloves

- Lab coat
- Absorbent material, such as absorbent paper towels or granular absorbent material
- All-purpose disinfectant such as normal household bleach (diluted 1:10)
- Bucket for diluting disinfectant
- Dustpan and broom
- Sharps disposal container
- Biohazard waste bags

When cleaning blood spills, wear disposable gloves of sufficient sturdiness so they will not tear while cleaning. If the gloves develop holes, tears, or splits, remove them, wash your hands immediately, and put on fresh gloves. Disposable gloves must never be washed or reused.

Spills of blood and blood-contaminated fluids should be properly cleaned using sodium hypochlorite (household bleach) diluted 1:10 with water. Steps for cleaning a biological spill are outlined in Chapter 25.

COG **Therapeutic Phlebotomy**

Phlebotomy may be a treatment for a disease. Used this way, it is called a **therapeutic phlebotomy**. It is used to treat **polycythemia vera**. Polycythemia vera causes the patient's RBC count to be too high. A disease with too much iron in the RBCs is called **hemachromatosis**. This disease may also be treated with a therapeutic phlebotomy.

MEDIA MENU

- **Student Resources on thePoint**
  - **Animation: Intramuscular Injection**
  - **Animation: Intravenous Injection**
  - **Video: Obtaining a Blood Specimen by Evacuated Tube or Winged Infusion Set (Procedure 26-1)**
  - **Video: Obtaining a Blood Specimen by Capillary Puncture (Procedure 26-2)**
  - **CMA/RMA Certification Exam Review**
- **Internet Resources**

  The University of Utah Eccles Health Sciences Library
  http://library.med.utah.edu/WebPath/TUTORIAL/PHLEB/PHLEB.html
  Phlebotomy Pages
  http://www.phlebotomypages.com
  Austin Community College—Phlebotomy Quizzes
  http://www2.austin.cc.tx.us/kotrla/phlebquiz.htm
  Centers for Disease Control and Prevention—Phlebotomy Information
  http://www.cdc.gov/ncbddd/hemochromatosis/training/pdf/phlebotomy_info.pdf

español SPANISH TERMINOLOGY

Le voy a tomar una muestra de sangre de su brazo.
I will be drawing blood from your arm.

¿Cuándo fue la última vez que se comió o tomó algo?
When did you last eat or drink anything?

Gracias
Thank you

Le voy a pinchar el dedo.
I will be sticking your finger.

PSY PROCEDURE 26-1:

Obtaining a Blood Specimen by Evacuated Tube or Winged Infusion Set

Purpose: To obtain blood for diagnostic purposes and/or monitoring of prescribed treatment
Equipment: Multisample needle and adaptor or winged infusion set, evacuated tubes, tourniquet, sterile gauze pads, bandages, sharps container, 70% alcohol pad, permanent marker or pen, appropriate PPE (e.g., gloves, impervious gown, face shield)

Steps	Reasons
1. Check the requisition slip to determine the tests ordered and specimen requirements.	This ensures proper specimen collection.
2. Wash your hands.	Handwashing aids infection control.
3. Assemble the equipment. Check the expiration date on the tubes. Discard expired supplies.	Assembling the equipment ensures that everything you need is available.
4. **AFF** Greet and identify the patient. Explain the procedure. Ask for and answer any questions.	Identifying the patient maintains sample integrity. Explaining the procedure helps ease anxiety and ensure compliance.
5. **AFF** If your patient is visually impaired, you will take extra steps such as touching the patient at the point you intend to perform the venipuncture and reaffirm that the patient understands that you will be obtaining a blood specimen at that point. Reassure the patient with more detailed verbal explanations of each step you take because he or she cannot see you performing the step. Tell the patient when you put on your gloves and when you are getting your supplies together. Help the patient by explaining the next step before you do it.	A visually impaired patient cannot see actions taken to prepare for a phebotomy. Talking through each step builds the patient's confidence level by keeping him or her informed of what you are doing and why.
6. If a fasting specimen is required, ask the patient for the last time he or she ate or drank anything.	For fasting specimens, the patient should not have eaten or drunk anything other than water within at least the last 8 hours.
7. Put on nonsterile latex or vinyl gloves. Use other personal protective equipment as defined by facility policy.	Standard precautions protect the phlebotomist and the patient.
8. *For evacuated tube collection*: Break the seal of the needle cover and thread the sleeved needle into the adaptor, using the needle cover as a wrench. *For winged infusion set collection*: Extend the tubing. Thread the sleeved needle into the adaptor. *For both methods*: Tap the tubes that contain additives to ensure that the additive is dislodged from the stopper and wall of the tube. Insert the tube into the adaptor until the needle slightly enters the stopper. Do not push the top of the tube stopper beyond the indentation mark. If the tube retracts slightly, leave it in the retracted position.	This ensures proper needle placement and tube positioning and prevents loss of vacuum in the evacuated tubes.
9. Instruct the patient to sit with a well-supported arm.	Veins in the antecubital fossa are most easily located when the arm is straight.

(continued)

PSY PROCEDURE 26-1: **Obtaining a Blood Specimen by Evacuated Tube or Winged Infusion Set** *(continued)*

Steps	Reasons
10. Apply the tourniquet around the patient's arm 3–4 inches above the elbow.	The tourniquet makes the veins more prominent.

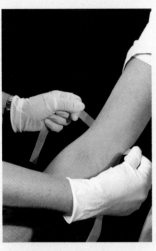

A. Apply the tourniquet snugly, but not too tightly.

Step 10. Apply the tourniquet 3–4 inches above the elbow.

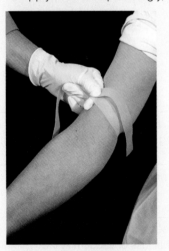

B. Secure the tourniquet by using the half-bow knot.

Step 10A. Apply the tourniquet snuggly, but not tightly.

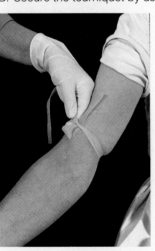

Step 10B. Secure the tourniquet by using a half-bow knot.

PSY PROCEDURE 26-1: | **Obtaining a Blood Specimen by Evacuated Tube or Winged Infusion Set (continued)**

Steps	Reasons
C. Make sure the tails of the tourniquet extend upward to avoid contaminating the puncture site. 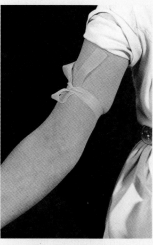	
D. Ask the patient to make a fist and hold it but not to pump the fist.	**Step 10C.** The tourniquet should extend upward. Making a fist raises the vessels out of the underlying tissues and muscles.
11. Select a vein by palpating. Use your gloved index finger to trace the path of the vein and judge its depth. 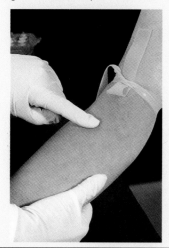	The index finger is the most sensitive for palpating. **Step 11.** Trace the path of the vein.
12. Release the tourniquet after palpating the vein if it has been left on for more than 1 minute. Have the patient release the fist.	The tourniquet should not be left on for more than 1 minute at a time during the procedure.
13. Cleanse the venipuncture site with an alcohol pad, starting in the center of the puncture site working outward in a circular motion. Allow the site to dry, or dry the site with sterile gauze. Do not touch the area after cleansing.	The circular motion helps avoid recontamination of the area. Puncturing a wet area stings and can and cause hemolysis of the sample.

(continued)

Obtaining a Blood Specimen by Evacuated Tube or Winged Infusion Set *(continued)*

Steps	Reasons
14. If blood being drawn for culture will be used in diagnosing a septic condition, make sure the specimen is sterile. To do this, apply alcohol to the area for 2 full minutes. Then apply a 2% iodine solution in ever-widening circles. Never move the wipes back over areas that have been cleaned; use a new wipe for each sweep across the area.	Ensuring sterility of the specimen will add in accurate identification of the pathogen, if present.
15. Reapply the tourniquet if it was removed after palpation. Ask the patient to make a fist.	Tourniquet time greater than 1 minute may alter test results.
16. Remove the needle cover. Hold the needle assembly in your dominant hand, with your thumb on top of the adaptor and your fingers under it. Grasp the patient's arm with the other hand, using your thumb to draw the skin taut over the site. This anchors the vein about 1–2 inches below the puncture site and helps keep it in place during needle insertion.	Anchoring the vein allows easier needle penetration and less pain.
17. With the bevel up, line up the needle with the vein approximately one quarter to half an inch below the site where the vein is to be entered. At a 15° to 30° angle, rapidly and smoothly insert the needle through the skin. Use a lesser angle for winged infusion set collections. Place two fingers on the flanges of the adapter, and with the thumb, push the tube onto the needle inside the adapter. Allow the tube to fill to capacity. Release the tourniquet and allow the patient to release the fist. When blood flow ceases, remove the tube from the adapter by gripping the tube with your nondominant hand and place your thumb against the flange during removal. Twist and gently pull out the tube. Steady the needle in the vein. Avoid pulling up or pressing down on the needle while it is in the vein. Insert any other necessary tubes into adapter and allow each to fill to capacity.	The sharpest point of the needle is inserted first. Proper tube filling ensures correct ratio of blood to additive. Removal of the tourniquet releases pressure on the vein and helps prevent blood from seeping into adjacent tissues and causing a hematoma.

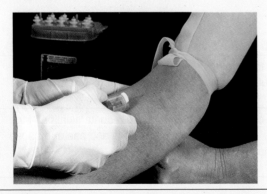

Step 17. Insert the needle at a 15°–30° angle.

| 18. With the tourniquet released, remove the tube from the adapter before removing the needle from the arm. | Removing the last tube from the adapter before removing the needle from the vein prevents excess blood from dripping from the tip of the needle onto the patient. |

PSY PROCEDURE 26-1: **Obtaining a Blood Specimen by Evacuated Tube or Winged Infusion Set (continued)**

Steps	Reasons
19. Place a sterile gauze pad over the puncture site. Do not apply any pressure to the site until the needle is completely removed. 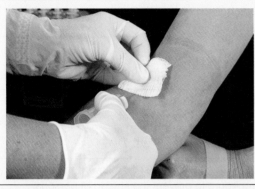 **Step 19.** Place a guaze pad over site.	Applying pressure before completely removing the needle will cause pain to the patient and most likely cause a hematoma.
20. After the needle is removed, immediately activate the safety device and apply pressure, or have the patient apply direct pressure for 3–5 minutes. Do not bend the arm at the elbow. 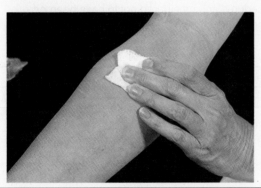 **Step 20.** Apply pressure for 3–5 minutes.	Pressure decreases the amount of blood escaping at the time of needle withdrawal. Bending the arm increases the chance of blood seeping into subcutaneous tissues. Unfolding the bent arm disturbs the clot forming at the puncture site and causes bleeding.
21. Activate needle safety device. Discard the used needle in a sharps container. 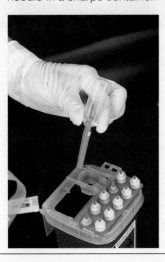 **Step 21.** Properly dispose of sharps.	

(continued)

PSY PROCEDURE 26-1: **Obtaining a Blood Specimen by Evacuated Tube or Winged Infusion Set (continued)**

Steps	Reasons
22. If the vacuum tubes contain an anticoagulant, they must be mixed immediately by gently inverting the tube 8–10 times. Do not shake the tube.	Mixing anticoagulated tubes prevents clotting of blood.
23. Label the tubes with patient information as defined in facility protocol.	Proper labeling of blood specimens maintains accurate sample identification.
24. Check the puncture site for bleeding. Apply a dressing, a clean 2 × 2 gauze pad folded in quarters, and hold in place using an adhesive bandage or 3-inch strip of tape.	
25. **AFF** Thank the patient. Instruct the patient to leave the bandage in place for at least 15 minutes, not to carry a heavy object (such as a purse) or lift heavy objects with that arm for 1 hour.	Courtesy helps the patient have a positive attitude about the procedure and the physician's office.
26. Properly care for or dispose of all equipment and supplies. Clean the work area. Remove protective equipment and wash your hands.	Standard precautions must be followed throughout the procedure to prevent the spread of personal microorganisms.
27. Test, transfer, or store the blood specimen according to the medical office policy.	
28. Record the procedure.	Procedures are considered not to have been performed if they are not recorded.

Charting Example:

05/31/2012 10:00 AM OP venipuncture for platelet count, dx code ###.## per Dr. Jacobs

——— *J. DeBard, CMA*

Note: The medical assistant may sign his or her name in the patient record using only the "CMA" credential if the office has a signature log denoting the entire credential as "CMA(AAMA)."

 PSY PROCEDURE 26-2: **Obtaining a Blood Specimen by Capillary Puncture**

Purpose: To obtain blood for diagnostic purposes and/or monitoring of prescribed treatment
Equipment: Skin puncture device, 70% alcohol pads, 2 × 2 gauze pads, microcollection tubes or containers, heel-warming device if needed, small bandages, pen or permanent marker, and PPE (e.g., gloves, impervious gown, face shield)

Steps	Reasons
1. Check the requisition slip to determine the tests ordered and specimen requirements.	This ensures proper specimen collection.
2. Wash your hands.	Handwashing aids infection control.
3. Assemble the equipment.	Having the equipment ready will speed collection Identifying the patient maintains sample integrity.
4. **AFF** Greet and identify the patient. Explain the procedure. Ask for and answer any questions.	Explaining the procedure helps ease anxiety and ensure compliance.

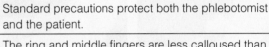

PSY PROCEDURE 26-2: **Obtaining a Blood Specimen by Capillary Puncture** *(continued)*

Steps	Reasons
5. **AFF** Many of your patients for capillary puncture will be infants and small children. Some children respond well to distractions. Most children become more upset the longer you drag out the procedure. Speak softly and move gently and with confidence. This will calm the child and the parent(s). If the parent appears upset, suggest that the parent let another medical assistant hold the child while the blood is collected.	The medical assistant will be more focused on positioning the child and maintaining that position than will an upset parent.
6. Put on gloves.	Standard precautions protect both the phlebotomist and the patient.
7. Select the puncture site (the lateral portion of the tip of the middle or ring finger of the nondominant hand or lateral curved surface of the heel of an infant). The puncture should be made in the fleshy central portion of the second or third finger, slightly to the side of center and perpendicular to the grooves of the fingerprint.	The ring and middle fingers are less calloused than the forefinger. The lateral part of the tip is the least sensitive part of the finger. A puncture made across the fingerprints will produce a large, round drop of blood. In an infant skin puncture, the area and the depth designated reduces the risk of puncturing the bone.

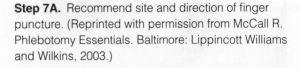

Step 7A. Recommend site and direction of finger puncture. (Reprinted with permission from McCall R. Phlebotomy Essentials. Baltimore: Lippincott Williams and Wilkins, 2003.)

Perform heel puncture only on the plantar surface of the heel, medial to an imaginary line extending from the middle of the great toe to the heel and lateral to an imaginary line drawn from between the fourth and fifth toes to the heel. Use the appropriate puncture device for the site selected.

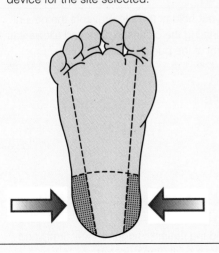

Step 7B. Acceptable areas for heel punctures on newborns. (Reprinted with permission from McCall R. Phlebotomy Essentials. Baltimore: Lippincott Williams and Wilkins, 2003.)

(continued)

Steps	Reasons
8. Make sure the site chosen is warm and not cyanotic or edematous. Gently massage the finger from the base to the tip, or massage the infant's heel.	Massaging the area increases the blood flow. Good circulation at the chosen site yields a better blood sample for analysis.
9. Grasp the finger firmly between your nondominant index finger and thumb, or grasp the infant's heel firmly with your index finger wrapped around the foot and your thumb wrapped around the ankle.	The area must be dry to eliminate alcohol residue, which can cause the patient discomfort and interfere with test results.

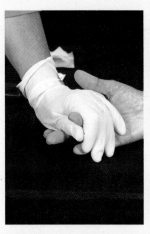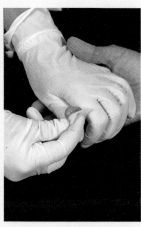

Cleanse the selected area with 70% isopropyl alcohol and allow to air dry.

Step 9A. Grasp the finger firmly.

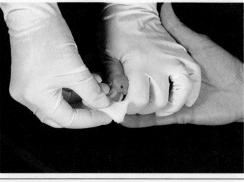

Step 9B. Cleanse the site with alcohol and allow to air dry.

10. Hold the patient's finger or heel firmly and make a swift, firm puncture. Perform the puncture perpendicular to the whorls of the fingerprint or footprint. Dispose of the used puncture device in a sharps container.	Maintaining your hold at the site prevents the patient from contaminating the cleansed area and allows you to have control of the puncture site.

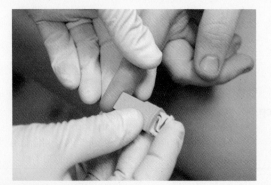

Step 10. Hold the patient's finger or heel firmly and make a swift, firm puncture.

PSY PROCEDURE 26-2: **Obtaining a Blood Specimen by Capillary Puncture (continued)**

Steps	Reasons
11. Obtain the first drop of blood and wipe it away with dry gauze. Apply pressure toward the site but do not milk the site.	The first discarded drop may be contaminated with tissue fluid or alcohol residue. Milking the site will dilute the specimen with tissue fluid.

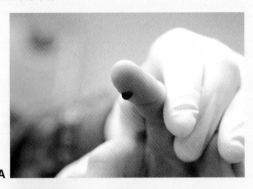

A

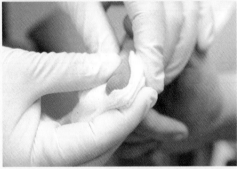

B

Step 11A. Obtain the first drop of blood.
Step 11B. Wipe it away.

Steps	Reasons
12. Collect the specimen in the chosen container or on a slide. Touch only the tip of the collection device to the drop of blood. Blood flow is encouraged if the puncture site is held downward and gentle pressure is applied near the site. Cap microcollection tubes with the caps provided and mix the additives by gently tilting or inverting the tubes 8–10 times.	Scraping the collection device on the skin activates platelets and may cause hemolysis. Mixing the specimens prevents clotting. Touching the tube to the site may cause contamination.
13. When collection is complete, apply clean gauze to the site with pressure. Hold pressure or have the patient hold pressure until bleeding stops. Label the containers with the proper information. Do not apply a dressing to a skin puncture of an infant under age 2 years. Never release a patient until the bleeding has stopped.	Proper labeling of blood specimens maintains accurate sample identification. Younger children may develop a skin irritation from the adhesive bandage. Also, a young child may put the bandage in his or her mouth and choke.

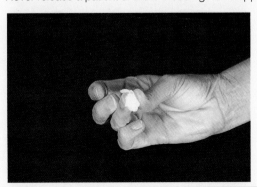

Step 13. Apply pressure with clean gauze.

(continued)

PSY **PROCEDURE 26-2:** **Obtaining a Blood Specimen by Capillary Puncture** *(continued)*

Steps	Reasons
14. Thank the patient. Instruct the patient to leave the bandage in place for at least 15 minutes.	Courtesy helps the patient have a positive attitude about the procedure and the physician's office.
15. Properly care for or dispose of equipment and supplies. Clean the work area. Remove gloves and wash your hands.	Standard precautions protect the phlebotomist and the patient.
16. Test, transfer, or store the specimen according to the medical office policy.	Specimens require immediate attention.
17. Record the procedure.	Procedures are considered not to have been done if they are not recorded.

Note: Several precautions should be observed to produce the most accurate specimen. The greatest concern with microcollection specimens is hemolysis, the rupture of erythrocytes with the release of hemoglobin. Do not squeeze or milk the heel or finger to increase blood flow. Never scrape the microcollection device on the skin. Allow the container to touch only the drop of blood. Also, be careful to avoid additional sources of errors, which are listed in Box 26-4.

Charting Example:

07/12/2012 9:00 AM OP fingerstick for prothrombin time dx ###.## per Dr. Robins
——*S. Smith, CMA*

Note: The medical assistant may sign his or her name in the patient record using only the "CMA" credential if the office has a signature log denoting the entire credential as "CMA(AAMA)."

- The properly labeled sample is essential to the results of the test matching the patient. The key elements in labeling are the patient's first and last names, the patient's ID number, the date and time of the collection, and the phlebotomist's initials.
- The forearm veins in the antecubital space (the inside of the elbow) are commonly used for venipuncture. The three main veins in this area are the cephalic, median cubital, and basilic. Certain areas are to be avoided when choosing a site including burns or scars, areas with a hematoma or bruising, thrombosed veins, edematous tissue, and the upper extremity on the side of a previous mastectomy.
- Skin puncture in adults and older children most often involves one of the fingers. Recommended sites are the fleshy pad of the third or fourth finger of the patient's nondominant hand only. Do not use the tip or the center of the finger. For infant heel punctures in children under age 1 year, the maximum of 2 mm for heel punctures is necessary to avoid hitting bone.
- Contraindications for using a specific site for capillary puncture are bruised, infected, swollen, or traumatized sites on fingers or heels; the thumb, because the skin is often too thick; the second finger, because it is much more sensitive than other fingers; and the fifth finger, because the flesh may be so thin that the bone could be pierced.
- Because the first step in quality of any laboratory test result is in the procurement of the specimen, quality assurance is critical in specimen collection procedures.
- The maximum time limit for leaving the tourniquet in place is 2 minutes.
- Maintain a professional attitude and be sympathetic to the fears and anxieties of the patient in all areas of patient care. For many patients, venipuncture is particularly frightening. Demonstrate compassion and understanding to allay their fears.

Warm Ups for Critical Thinking

1. What effects do hemoconcentration and hemolysis of the specimen have in test results?
2. Your patient complains of serious pain when you insert the needle into the vein. Explain the steps to improve the patient's comfort.
3. How can you help ease patient anxiety about venipuncture? List the steps to take.
4. Your patient asks you how long you have been drawing blood and whether you are "good"? How do you respond? Justify your response.
5. Describe the steps you would take if you started a venipuncture and got no specimen in the tube.

Explain how each step could result in a successful blood collection.

6. Your patient has come from the doctor with an order for you to draw and refer a specimen for HIV testing. The patient knows the doctor has specifically ordered a test for HIV. The patient wants to discuss with you all the questions she has about HIV testing. You are in a room with other medical assistants. What do you say to your patient?
7. Serious risk is created when specimens are poured from one collection tube to another. Describe these risks and how they are created.

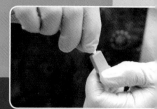

27 Hematology

What is Blood?

Plasma

Formation and Pathophysiology of Blood Cells

Erythrocytes and Their Functions

Types of Leukocytes and Their Functions

Platelets and Their Functions

Hematologic Testing

Complete Blood Count

Erythrocyte Sedimentation Rate

Hemostasis, Thrombosis, Coagulation, and Fibrinolysis

Coagulation (Hemostasis) Tests

Point-of-Care Hematology Testing

The Medical Assistant's Responsibilities in the Hematology Laboratory

Cognitive Domain

Note: AAMA/CAAHEP 2008 Standards are italicized.

1. Spell and define the key terms
2. List the parameters measured in the complete blood count and their normal ranges
3. State the conditions associated with selected abnormal complete blood count findings
4. Explain the functions of the three types of blood cells
5. Describe the purpose of testing for the erythrocyte sedimentation rate
6. List the leukocytes seen normally in the blood and their functions
7. *Analyze charts, graphs, and/or tables in the interpretation of health care results*
8. *Distinguish between normal and abnormal test results*
9. Explain the hemostatic mechanism of the body
10. List and describe the tests that measure the body's ability to form a fibrin clot
11. Explain how to determine the prothrombin time and partial thromboplastin time

Psychomotor Domain

Note: AAMA/CAAHEP 2008 Standards are italicized.

1. Make a peripheral blood smear (Procedure 27-1)
2. Stain a peripheral blood smear (Procedure 27-2)
3. Perform a hemoglobin determination (Procedure 27-3)
4. Perform a microhematocrit determination (Procedure 27-4)
5. Determine a Westergren erythrocyte sedimentation rate (Procedure 27-5)
6. Obtain information on proper collection methods for hematology testing
7. *Practice standard precautions*
8. *Use medical terminology, pronouncing medical terms correctly, to communicate information*
9. *Instruct patients according to their needs to promote disease prevention*
10. *Prepare a patient for procedures and/or treatments*
11. *Document patient care*
12. *Respond to issues of confidentiality*

13. *Perform within scope of practice*
14. *Practice within the standard of care for a medical assistant*
15. *Document accurately in the patient record*
16. *Perform quality control measures*
17. Perform hematology testing
18. *Screen test results*

Affective Domain

Note: AAMA/CAAHEP 2008 Standards are italicized.

1. *Display sensitivity to patient rights and feelings in collecting specimens*
2. *Explain the rationale for performance of a procedure to the patient*
3. *Show awareness of patients' concerns regarding their preceptions related to the procedure being performed*

ABHES Competencies

1. Apply principles of aseptic techniques and infection control
2. Collect, label, and process specimens
3. Perform selected CLIA-waived tests that assist with diagnosis and treatment
4. Dispose of biohazardous materials
5. Use standard precautions
6. Perform hematology testing
7. Document accurately
8. Practice quality control
9. Adhere to OSHA compliance rules and regulations

Key Terms

adhesion
band
basophils
coagulation
complete blood count (CBC)
eosinophils

erythrocytes
erythrocyte indices
erythrocyte sedimentation rate (ESR)
erythropoietin
folate
hematocrit

hemoglobin
leukocytes
lymphocytes
monocytes
morphology
neutrophils
plasma

platelets
point-of-care testing (POC or POCT)
sickle cell anemia
thrombocytes
thrombosis
WBC differential

There are three primary functions of the hematology laboratory. Hematology analyzes the blood cells. Anemias, leukemias, and infections are detected and managed in hematology. Hematology includes the study of **hemostasis**. Hemostasis is the patient's blood making clots.

COG What is Blood?

Bone marrow is the site of blood cell production. Until age 3 years, bones are filled with active marrow. Active marrow makes the blood cells. After age 3 years, inactive marrow begins to take over. At about age 22 years, active marrow is mainly present in the sternum and ends of the femur and humerus. These are the sites used for sampling bone marrow.

Hemopoiesis is red blood cell (RBC) production. In the bone marrow cells mature into different types for different needs in the body. (Fig. 27-1). Hemopoiesis requires hormones and nutrients such as iron. When cells are mature, they move from the bone marrow into the bloodstream.

Blood comprises three types of cells: **erythrocytes** (RBCs), **leukocytes** (white blood cells [WBCs]), and **thrombocytes** (platelets) (Fig. 27-2A–H). Most cells are erythrocytes; exposure to oxygen makes the blood red. WBCs are infection-fighting cells, and platelets are tiny pieces of cell that make clots.

 CHECKPOINT QUESTION

1. Where does hemopoiesis take place?

COG Plasma

Plasma is the yellowish, liquid part of blood. Spinning a tube of fresh, anticoagulated blood in a centrifuge separates the plasma from the blood cells. The plasma is poured off for some types of tests.

Plasma contains substances, including:

- Glucose
- Vitamins

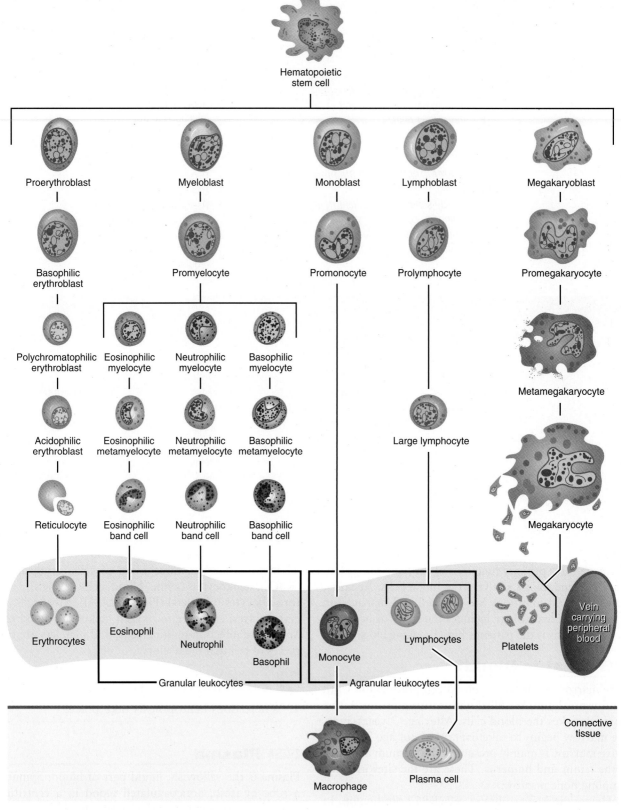

Figure 27-1 Maturation of blood cell lines. (From Eroschenko V. diFiore's Atlas of Histology, With Functional Correlations. 12th ed. Baltimore: Lippincott Williams & Wilkins, 2012.)

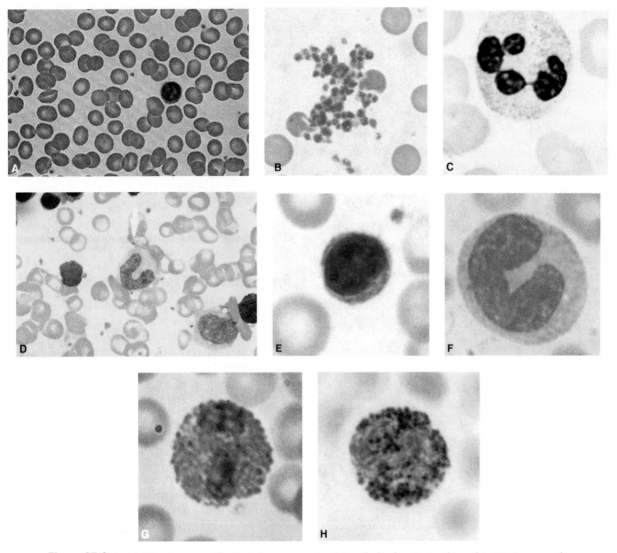

Figure 27-2 (**A**) A blood smear. (**B**) RBCs (large, round cells) and platelets (stained purple). (**C**) Segmented neutrophil. (**D**) Neutrophil band. (**E**) Lymphocyte. (**F**) Monocyte. (**G**) Eosinophil. (**H**) Basophil.

- Hormones
- Antibodies
- Urea (waste)
- Phospholipids
- Fats

COG Formation and Pathophysiology of Blood Cells

Erythrocytes and Their Functions

RBCs carry oxygen and carbon dioxide. The **hemoglobin** in the RBCs actually carries the gases. The RBCs release carbon dioxide and pick up oxygen.

When the blood filters through the kidneys, the kidneys detect how much oxygen is present. The kidneys send a hormone called **erythropoietin** to the bone marrow. When the erythropoietin reaches the bone marrow, it stimulates the bone marrow to produce more RBCs to carry more oxygen. When the kidneys detect more oxygen, they stop making erythropoietin.

There has to be enough Vitamin B_{12} and folate in the body for the RBCs to be healthy. An RBC is a red disk that curves inward on both sides. It can squeeze through tiny capillaries.

PATIENT EDUCATION

IRON DEFICIENCY ANEMIA

Patients who have iron deficiency anemia must eat a special diet.

They should eat foods high in iron, such as liver, oysters, kidney beans, lean meats, turnips, egg yolks, whole-wheat bread, carrots, raisins, and dark greens. A vitamin supplement with iron can be added to the diet. Patients should be warned that iron supplements can cause constipation and dark stools.

Types of Leukocytes and Their Functions

Leukocytes defend against bacteria and viruses. There are five major types of WBCs:

- Basophils
- Eosinophils
- Lymphocytes (T cells and B cells)
- Monocytes
- Neutrophils

Basophils

On a stained blood smear, **basophils** have round, purple-black granules in their cytoplasm. Basophils release histamine when there is an immune response. Histamine makes them part of inflammatory reactions, such as asthma and allergies.

Eosinophils

On a stained blood smear **eosinophils** have red granules. Eosinophils are active in allergies and parasite infestations.

 CHECKPOINT QUESTION

2. Elevated eosinophils and basophils are both seen with what condition?

Lymphocytes

Lymphocytes recognize cells foreign to the body. They make antibodies to destroy the foreign cells. The antibodies coat the cells. The antibodies may cause the foreign cells to destroy the pathogen or to destroy the cells by puncturing holes in their membranes. Increased lymphocyte counts usually signal a viral infection such as infectious mononucleosis.

Monocytes

Monocytes also recognize foreign cells. Monocytes are part of the body's immune response. They engulf the foreign cell and kill the antigens.

Neutrophils

Neutrophils also fight foreign cells by engulfing them. Digestive enzymes in the cells kill the foreign material and the neutrophil itself at the same time.

A **band** is a young neutrophil. When the bands are increased, they usually indicate an acute infection that needs immediate treatment.

 CHECKPOINT QUESTION

3. What is the function of neutrophils?

PATIENT EDUCATION

DIETARY FOLATE

The blood must contain enough folate to produce healthy RBCs. When there is not enough folate present, anemia develops. Folate in the blood comes from a person's diet. Some foods with folate are:

- Leafy green vegetables
- Citrus fruits and juices
- Dried beans and peas

Folate may also be taken as a dietary supplement.

Platelets and Their Functions

The body uses **platelets** to form clots and control bleeding. When there is an internal or external injury, platelets stick together on the injured vessel to stop the bleeding. They do this by forming a plug. The bleeding is usually from many small capillaries. There is more bleeding when there are fewer platelets.

COG Hematologic Testing

Common hematology tests include **complete blood count (CBC), erythrocyte sedimentation rate (ESR, or** *sed rate*), and coagulation tests. Clinical Laboratory Improvement Amendment (CLIA) regulations limit the types of hematology testing medical assistants can perform. The list of hematology tests medical assistants can perform, updated regularly by the Centers for Medicare and Medicaid Services (CMS), includes the following:

- ESR (not automated)
- Hematocrit (all spun microhematocrit procedures)
- Hemoglobin (selected methods)
- Prothrombin time (selected methods)

Complete Blood Count

More than just for hematology, the CBC is the most frequently ordered test in the entire laboratory. (Box 27-1). It consists of a number of parameters, including the following:

- WBC count and differential
- RBC count
- Hemoglobin
- Hematocrit
- Mean cell volume (MCV)
- Mean corpuscular hemoglobin (MCH)
- Mean corpuscular hemoglobin concentration (MCHC)
- Platelet count

AUTOMATED BLOOD CELL COUNTERS

A number of biotechnology companies have instruments that can count and size blood cells. Although each has its own specific method, the main operating principles are similar.

A portion of whole blood (anticoagulated with EDTA) is taken in and diluted. These dilutions are moved into counting chambers, where they are drawn through tiny holes (apertures). As the cells pass through the holes, an electrical current, a light beam, or a laser beam is interrupted. The instrument registers the interruption as a cell. It can tell the size of the cell by the length of time the beam is interrupted or the amount of light scatter.

These instruments have become so sophisticated that a WBC differential now can be reported accurately. Hemoglobin is also measured, along with other parameters, such as mean corpuscular hemoglobin, adding to the diagnostic value of the complete blood count.

White Blood Cell Count and Differential

WBCs defend the body from bacteria and viruses. The normal range for a WBC count is 4,300 to 10,800/mm³. A patient's WBC count can be determined by use of an automated cell counter. Most common automated cell counters are not CLIA waived and not in the scope of practice for the medical assistant.

Patients with low WBC counts may be susceptible to infections.

To view WBCs, a drop of blood is smeared on a glass slide and then stained so that they can be seen with a microscope (Procedures 27-1 and 27-2). From the smear, the types of WBCs are counted and reported by type. This count is known as the **WBC differential**. WBC differentials are not CLIA waived.

The WBC types and their approximate percentage of the WBC count include the following:

- Neutrophils (see Fig. 27-2, C and D) = 59%
- Lymphocytes (see Fig. 27-2E) = 34%
- Monocytes (see Fig. 27-2F) = 4%
- Eosinophils (see Fig. 27-2G) = 2%
- Basophils (see Fig. 27-2H) = 1%

CHECKPOINT QUESTION

4. How are the types of WBCs counted and reported?

Red Blood Cell Count

RBCs are counted by hematology cell counter instruments. Anemia can be caused by a low RBC count (as in iron deficiency) (Fig. 27-3) or blood loss. The normal range of RBCs for men is 4.6 to 6.2 million/mm³; for women, it is 4.2 to 5.4 million/mm³.

When the WBC differential is counted on the blood smear, RBC **morphology** or appearance is evaluated and reported. This report contains comments on the variation classifications that appear due to the disease conditions:

- Variations in size
- Variations in shape
- Alterations in color
- Alterations in how the RBCs are spread out on the blood smear

Table 27-1 describes some common erythrocyte abnormalities and their associated conditions.

Hemoglobin

Hemoglobin contains four chains called *globins*. Defects in the globin chains cause abnormal hemoglobins. **Sickle cell anemia** is caused by a defective globin chain. Iron is found in the globin and gives RBCs their red color. The normal range for hemoglobin is 13 to 18 g/dL (or g/100 mL) in men and 12 to 16 g/dL in women. Measuring the hemoglobin is used to diagnose anemia (Procedure 27-3). There are also point-of-care (POC) methods approved for use by medical assistants. An example is the HemoCue System Hemoglobin Plasma/Low Hemoglobin Analyzer.

Hematocrit

The **hematocrit** is the percentage of RBCs in whole blood. Microhematocrit tubes are collected and spun in a special microcentrifuge to separate the cells from the

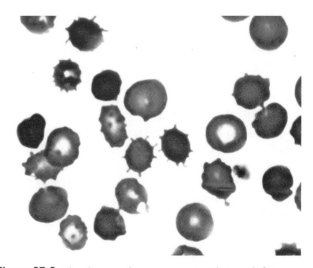

Figure 27-3 Blood smear from a patient with iron deficiency anemia showing RBCs that are hypochromic and microcytic. (From Rubin R, Strayer D. Rubin's Pathology. 4th ed. Baltimore: Lippincott Williams & Wilkins, 2005.)

TABLE **27-1** Erythrocyte Abnormalities	
Abnormality	**Associated Conditions**
Hypochromia—diminished hemoglobin in RBCs; appear paler with more area of central pallor	Anemias (especially iron deficiency), thalassemia, hemolytic anemia
Hyperchromia—increased hemoglobin in RBCs; appear to have less or no area of central pallor (condition in which nearly all the RBCs are spherocytes)	Megaloblastic anemia (characterized by large, dysfunctional RBCs), hereditary spherocytosis
Polychromasia—some RBCs have a blue color	Hemolysis, acute blood loss
Microcytosis—RBCs are smaller than usual	Iron deficiency anemia, thalassemia
Macrocytosis—RBCs are larger than normal	Vitamin B_{12} and folate deficiencies, megaloblastic anemias
Elliptocytes/ovalocytes—RBCs are distinctly oval in shape	Hereditary elliptocytosis, iron deficiency anemia, myelofibrosis (disorder in which bone marrow tissue develops in abnormal sites), sickle cell anemia (hereditary anemia characterized by the presence of sickle-shaped RBCs)
Target cells—RBCs resemble a target with light and dark rings	Liver impairment, anemias (especially thalassemia), hemoglobin C disease (genetic blood disorder)
Schistocytes—RBCs are fragmented	Hemolysis, burns, intravascular coagulation (clot formation within the vessels)
Spherocytes—RBCs show no area of central pallor	Hereditary spherocytosis, hemolytic anemias, burns
Burr cells—RBCs have small, regular spicules (sharp points)	Artifact as blood dries, hyperosmolarity (a condition of increased numbers of dissolved substances in the plasma)

plasma. After the tubes are spun, they are measured to determine the percentage of RBCs present.

The purpose of measuring the hematocrit is also to detect types of anemia. The normal range is 45% to 52% in men and 37% to 48% in women (Procedure 27-4).

 CHECKPOINT QUESTION

5. A patient has a hematocrit of 20%. What does this percentage signify?

Erythrocyte Indices

Erythrocyte indices, MCV, MCH, and MCHC are calculations. The hematology cell counter measures the size of the RBCs and how much hemoglobin they hold. The calculations help diagnose and treat anemias. There are different types of anemia, and knowing the type is required to plan a treatment. The MCV, MCH, and MCHC help identify the actual type of anemia.

Mean Cell Volume

The MCV is the average size of the RBCs in categories:

• Normal-size cells are called *normocytic*.
• Smaller-size cells are called *microcytic*.
• Larger-size cells are called *macrocytic*.

The MCV can indicate anemias caused by nutritional deficiencies. The normal range for MCV is 80 to 95 fL.

Microcytosis (MCV below 80 fL) indicates iron deficiency.

Macrocytosis (MCV above 95 fL) indicates deficiency of vitamin B_{12} and folate.

Mean Cell Hemoglobin and Mean Cell Hemoglobin Concentration

RBCs with inadequate amounts of hemoglobin are termed hypochromic. The MCH calculation measures the amount of hemoglobin in a single RBC. The normal range for MCH is 27 to 31 picograms.

The MCHC is the average amount of hemoglobin per RBC. The normal range for MCHC is 32 to 36 g/dL. MCHC is decreased in the same conditions as the MCV.

Decreased MCHC values, termed **hypochromia**, may be due to:

• Iron deficiency anemia
• Thalassemia
• Blood loss
• Vitamin B_6 deficiency

There are disorders in which the MCV and the MCHC differ: in an anemia called *pernicious anemia*, the MCV is high, but the MCHC is normal.

CHECKPOINT QUESTION

6. When reviewing a patient's test results, you see that the patient's RBCs are noted to be very small. What is a possible diagnosis for this condition?

A patient's anemic condition may be investigated for its cause and for potential treatment. A test used in this investigation is ferritin. Ferritin stores iron in the body. If the body is deficient in iron, an iron supplement may be ordered as a treatment for the anemia. Measurements of the iron, total iron binding capacity (TIBC), and % Saturation are also useful in this investigation. The TIBC reveals how much iron the body could hold if the patient consumed enough iron in diet and/or supplements. If the TIBC is low, the body could hold more iron if more was ingested. The TIBC can be normal, but the patient can still be anemic if the patient does not have enough iron to bind. The % Saturation result tells how much iron is bound in the body. This also reveals how much is not bound that could be corrected with increased iron intake. These tests are performed to identify iron-deficiency anemia from the other types of anemia.

See Box 27-2 for an Introduction to Laboratory Case Studies.

WHAT IF?

What if a patient asks you about the criteria for donating blood?

The American Red Cross bases criteria for donating blood on recommendations from government agencies and the Centers for Disease Control and Prevention (CDC) and findings of research projects. In addition, each state has its own laws regulating blood donors. Generally, blood donors must meet the following criteria:

- Age 16 years or older (donors who are age 16 years require a parent's permission; donors who are age 65 years or older require a physician's consent)
- Weight of 110 lbs or more
- Hemoglobin at least 12.5 g/dL (women) or 13.5 g/dL (men)
- Pulse of 50 to 110 beats per minute
- Blood pressure lower than 180/100

The donor also must provide a brief history. The entire procedure lasts approximately 1 hour; the actual blood donation time is about 10 minutes. Blood can be donated every 56 days. Only 1 unit (pint) will be taken at a time. All blood will be tested by the American Red Cross for HIV, hepatitis, and syphilis.

Platelet Count

The normal range for platelets is 200,000 to 400,000/mm³. Low platelet counts are associated with increased bleeding. The bleeding is usually from many small capillaries.

Table 27-2 illustrates how CBC results would appear on a laboratory report. The normal values are required to be listed for each result on the report.

CHECKPOINT QUESTION

7. Using Table 27-2, list the abnormal results. What is a common diagnosis for this combination of abnormal values?

TABLE 27-2 Patient CBC Report		
Analyte	**Patient Result**	**Normal Range**
White blood cells	9,200 μ/L	4,300–10,800 μ/L
Red blood cells	3.9 million/μL ↓	men: 4.6–6.2 million/μL women: 4.2–5.4 million/μL
Hemoglobin	10.2 g/dL ↓	men: 13–18 g/dL women: 12–16 g/dL
Hematocrit	35% ↓	men: 45%–52% women: 37%–48%
Mean cell volume	74 μL/red cell ↓	80–95 μL/red cell
Mean cell hemoglobin	23 pg/red cell ↓	27–31 pg/red cell
Mean cell hemoglobin concentration	27 g/dL ↓	32–36 g/dL
Platelets	279,000/μL	200,000–400,000/μL

INTRODUCTION TO LABORATORY CASE STUDIES

Case studies allow comparison of patient symptoms, laboratory results, and diagnoses. Laboratory case studies begin with data collection. RIs (normal or expected ranges) listed in the case are found in tables in this chapter and in the textbook appendices. In the medical office, reference intervals will be listed in the laboratory procedure manual as well.

Patient history:
70-year-old female.

Symptoms of dyspnea on exertion, easy fatigability, and lassitude for past 2 to 3 months.

Denied hemoptysis or gastrointestinal or vaginal bleeding. Claimed diet was good, but appetite varied.

Physical exam:
Other than pallor, no significant physical findings were noted. Occult blood was negative.

Laboratory Results:
CBC (with microscopic
differential):   *RBC morphology:*
WBC 5.9 × 10⁹/L   2+ hypochromasia
HGB 5.9 g/dL   3+ microcytosis
HCT 20.9 %   2+ anisocytosis
MCV 56.2 fL   2+ elliptocytes and
                                        target cells
MCH 15.9 pg   occ teardrops and
                                        fragments
MCHC 28.3 g/dL
RDW 20.2
Platelets 383 × 10⁹/L

White Blood Cell Differential
Neutrophils   82%
Lymphocytes   13%
Monocytes   1%
Eosinophils   4%
Basophils   0%

PLT morphology: Within normal limits
Look for relationships in symptoms, laboratory values, and potential patient diagnoses.
Use this patient evaluation for the case study investigation in Warm Ups for Critical Thinking #6.

end of the hour, the distance the RBCs have fallen is measured. The method used in POLs to measure ESR is called the *Westergren method.* Other methods have a much higher risk of exposure to blood. The Westergren method has a closed system that reduces the medical assistant's exposure to the patient's blood. Procedure 27-5 and Figure 27-4 outline the steps for the Westergren method.

Always verify the following conditions to ensure accurate ESR results:

- Test should be started within 2 hours of specimen collection.
- Test should be conducted at room temperature.
- The blood column must contain no bubbles.
- The tube must remain completely vertical during testing.
- The sedimentation rack must be placed on a counter with no vibrations. (Do not place near a centrifuge.)
- The sedimentation rack must be away from all drafts and direct sunlight.
- Test results should be read at exactly 60 minutes.

The normal range for men is 0 to 10 mm/hr, and for women, it is 0 to 20 mm/hr. ESR values do not diagnose a specific disease. They measure how much inflammation is present in the body. The more rapidly the RBCs fall in the tube, the more inflammation is present. An example of a disease monitored by the ESR is fibromyalgia.

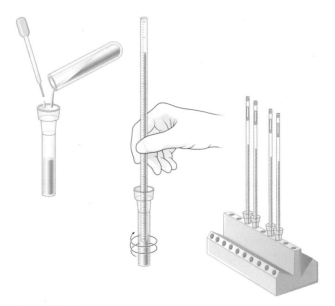

Figure 27-4 Westergren Dispette System for ESR determination. *Left:* EDTA-anticoagulated whole blood is poured into a vial containing 3.8% sodium citrate. *Center:* Dispette is placed in vial using a twisting motion until blood reaches bottom of safety autozeroing plug. *Right:* Vial and Dispette are placed upright in a special rack for 60 minutes before reading the ESR. (Courtesy of Ulster Scientific, Highland, NY.)

Erythrocyte Sedimentation Rate

The ESR measures how quickly RBCs settle out in a tube. The blood is placed in a specially made tube and allowed to settle undisturbed for 1 hour. At the

COG Hemostasis, Thrombosis, Coagulation, and Fibrinolysis

Coagulation tests measure the ability of blood to clot. Coagulation proteins are activated in the body from an internal or external cut or tear. The proteins initiate the formation of the clot. As the clot gets bigger, it forms a plug that stops bleeding.

The steps in coagulation are:

1. *Vasoconstriction.* The vein constricts to reduce blood loss.
2. *Platelet plug formation.* The platelets stick to each other and the wound to form a plug.
3. *Fibrin clot formation.* The coagulation factors make the plug stable. (The two most common tests for testing clotting are prothrombin time and partial thromboplastin time.)
4. *Clot lysis and vascular repair.* The clot must lyse or it will cause other problems. The clot dissolving is called lysis. While the clot dissolves, the blood vessel heals.

Platelets sticking together over the injury is **adhesion.** While the platelets are sticking together, a substance in the blood called *fibrinogen* helps strengthen the plug. Platelets begin to stick together about 20 seconds after the injury.

Thrombosis is blood clotting inside a vessel. When the thrombosis blocks the vessel, it stops the blood flow. There are two types of thromboses:

- *Venous thrombosis* is a blood clot that develops in a vein.
- *Arterial thrombosis* is a blood clot that develops in an artery.

When the thrombosis is in an artery to the heart, the result is a heart attack. When the thrombosis is an artery of the brain, the result is a stroke. If a thrombosis comes loose from one site and moves from the bloodstream to another part of the body, it is called an *embolism.*

Coagulation (Hemostasis) Tests

The two most common laboratory coagulation tests are the prothrombin time (PT) and the partial thromboplastin time (PTT). There are waived testing analyzers for measuring the PT as seen in Figures 27-5 and 27-6.

Prothrombin Time

The patient's PT is measured by adding two reagents to the patient's specimen. If the substances were inside the body, they would start a clot. Adding the substances to the blood and measuring the clotting time gives a PT result. The normal range is 12 to 15 seconds, but each laboratory establishes its own range. This is the test used to monitor a patient taking Coumadin™.

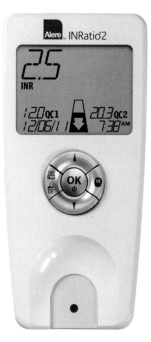

Figure 27-5 INRatio2 Monitor. The INRatio2 monitor for PT/INR testing from HemoSense. INRatio2 provides PT and INR results in less than 1 minute using one drop of blood from a fingerstick. (Courtesy of Alere Inc., Waltham, MA.)

The PT is reported along with an international normalized ratio (INR). The INR is a standardized result. The INR is a calculation from the patient's PT result and a reference standard. The INR is reported because it is similar from lab to lab. PT results can very a lot from lab to lab. The INR will be comparable in any lab the patient might choose.

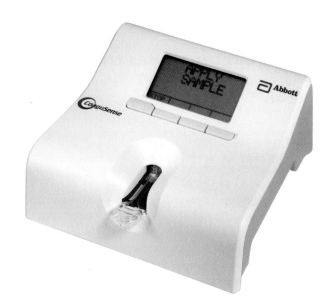

Figure 27-6 Abbott CoaguSense PT/INR Monitoring System. CoaguSense provides PT and INR by directly detecting clot formation. (Courtesy of Abbott Point of Care.)

Several POC instruments allow medical assistants to determine PT and INR in the office.

CHECKPOINT QUESTION

8. Why is the INR a better result than the PT?

Partial Thromboplastin Time

The PTT test is similar to a PT test. The same reagents are added to the patient's specimen. This time, however, they are added in a different sequence with an incubation period in between. The clotting time is then determined. The normal range is 32 to 51 seconds, but each laboratory establishes its own range, so there may be a slight variation. The PTT test identifies different factor deficiencies than the PT test. A hemophilia patient will have a long PTT time because of its missing coagulation factor.

CHECKPOINT QUESTION

9. What are the two most common tests used to determine how well a fibrin clot will form?

Coagulation Factor Levels

The body uses several coagulation factors to successfully clot blood. When a patient has a bleeding problem, the coagulation factors can be measured to identify if one of them is low. In some cases, the coagulation factor can be added to the patient's blood to restore normal clotting. Periodic replacements may be required to maintain the normal level. Coagulation factors are usually measured after a patient has an abnormal PT or PTT result.

CHECKPOINT QUESTION

10. Why measure a patient's coagulation factor levels?

WHAT IF?

Your patient is taking Coumadin and does not return for scheduled prothrombin tests. What should you do?

Let the physician know. Document all phone conversations with the patient, including the date, time, and message. Also document the patient's responses. The patient should be informed of the dangers of taking too much or too little Coumadin. The dangers are bleeding from an overdose or clotting with an underdose. Help the patient understand that without having his blood checked, the overdosing or underdosing can happen. Make sure the patient understands the purpose of the medication and why blood tests are so important.

COG Point-of-Care Hematology Testing

Point-of-care testing is performed near the patient instead of going to a laboratory. POC tests may include waived and moderately complex tests. To perform within the scope of practice, the medical assistant should verify that the test being performed is waived. POC tests are included on the laboratory's CLIA certificate and must be performed within CLIA guidelines. A current listing of all of the POC waived testing methods and analyzers approved by CLIA may be found at this Web site: http://www.cms.gov/CLIA/downloads/waivetbl.pdf.

This Web site is updated several times each year.

CHECKPOINT QUESTION

11. Are all POCT waived tests?

COG The Medical Assistant's Responsibilities in the Hematology Laboratory

Standard precautions are required in hematology as well as all other areas of the medical practice. There are no pretesting requirements for basic hematology procedures. Drawing blood specimens with too small a needle will hemolyze specimens, destroying the blood cells. The resulting cell counts will be inaccurate and may result in inappropriate treatment for the patient based on those results. Professionalism in the hematology laboratory includes the correct use of medical terminology. Refer to tests by their appropriate names. Pronounce those names correctly. Not only does this portray professionalism, it also is reassuring to the patient to hear you use medical terminology accurately. In all patient concerns, you are responsible for patient confidentiality.

You will note that some procedures in this chapter specify that CLIA does not qualify medical assistants to perform them. This limits those procedures from the medical assistant's scope of practice. Medical assistants may perform hematology procedures approved for their scope of practice once they are trained and documented to be proficient.

Individual testing procedures will identify the quality control measures that must be documented prior to reporting a patient result. Until these results are acceptable and documented, the test result is not approved for reporting. The test result(s) should be screened quickly for reporting status. Any values within the critical ranges posted within that practice should be reported immediately as instructed in the office policy for critical test results.

 CHECKPOINT QUESTION

12. What is the best reference for determining if a laboratory assay is within the medical assistant's scope of practice?

 MEDIA MENU

- **Student Resources on thePoint**
  - **Animation: Hemostasis**
  - **Video: Performing a Microhematocrit Determination (Procedure 27-4)**
  - **CMA/RMA Certification Exam Review**
- **Internet Resources**
  American Society of Hematology
  http://www.hematology.org

  Lab Tests Online
  http://www.labtestsonline.org/understanding/analytes/esr/test.html

  The Medical Biochemistry Page
  http://web.indstate.edu/thcme/mwking/blood-coagulation.htmltop

  University of Minnesota Hematography
  http://www1.umn.edu/hema

PSY PROCEDURE 27-1:   Making a Peripheral Blood Smear

Purpose: To prepare a blood sample for microscopic examination
Equipment: Clean glass slides with frosted ends, pencil, well-mixed whole blood specimen, transfer pipette, hand disinfectant, surface disinfectant, gloves, biohazard container

Steps	Purpose
1. Wash your hands.	Handwashing aids infection control.
2. Assemble the equipment.	Equipment must be readily accessible for the procedure to be done.
3. **AFF** Greet and identify the patient. Explain the procedure. Ask for and answer any questions.	
4. Put on gloves.	PPE prevents exposure to biohazards.
5. Obtain an ethylenediaminetetraacetic acid ([EDTA] lavender-top tube) blood specimen from the patient, following the steps for venipuncture described in Chapter 26.	The EDTA tube is the anticoagulated blood tube used for hematology testing.
6. Place a drop of blood 1 cm from the frosted end of the slide.	Doing so leaves adequate room to spread the specimen.

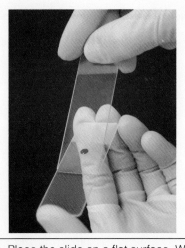

Step 6. Drop of blood on slide with spreader placed in front. (Reprinted with permission from McCall R. Phlebotomy Essentials. Baltimore: Lippincott Williams & Wilkins, 2003.)

7. Place the slide on a flat surface. With the thumb and forefinger of the dominant hand, hold the film second (spreader) slide against the surface of the first at a 30° angle. Draw the spreader slide back against the drop of blood until contact is established. (*Note:* The angle of the spreader slide may have to be greater than 30° for large or thin drops of blood and less than 30° for small or thick drops.) Allow the blood to spread under the edge, and then push the spreader slide at a moderate speed toward the other end of the slide, keeping contact between the two slides at all times.	A flat surface allows for smooth movements. A 30° angle allows the blood to be spread thinly for viewing.

PSY PROCEDURE 27-1: **Making a Peripheral Blood Smear (continued)**

Steps	Purpose
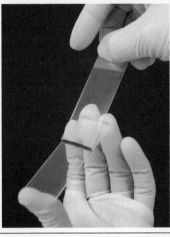	**Step 7.** Spreader slide with drop of blood spreading to its edges. (Reprinted with permission from McCall R. Phlebotomy Essentials. Baltimore: Lippincott Williams & Wilkins, 2003.)
8. Label the slide on the frosted area.	The slide must be labeled with the patient's name or identification number; the frosted end will retain the markings.
9. Allow the slide to air-dry.	Heating will distort cells.
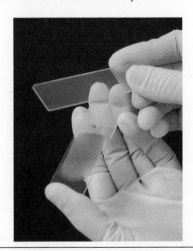	**Step 9.** A properly prepared smear will yield a slide that is easy to read. (Reprinted with permission from McCall R. Phlebotomy Essentials. Baltimore: Lippincott Williams & Wilkins, 2003.)
10. Properly care for or dispose of equipment and supplies. Clean the work area. Remove gloves and wash your hands.	Too much blood will make the smear too thick to identify the cells.

Note: Too much blood will make the smear invalid.

PSY PROCEDURE 27-2: Staining a Peripheral Blood Smear

Purpose: To aid in identifying the types of blood cells in a patient sample for diagnosis and treatment of infectious processes and blood dyscrasias

Equipment: Staining rack, Wright stain materials, prepared slide, tweezers, hand disinfectant, surface disinfectant, gloves, impervious gown and face shield

Steps	Purpose
1. Wash your hands.	Handwashing aids infection control.
2. Assemble the equipment.	Equipment must be readily accessible for the procedure to be done.
3. Put on gloves, impervious gown, and face shield.	PPE prevents exposure to biohazards.
4. Obtain a recently made dried blood smear. Verify that the slide is labeled with identification of the appropriate patient.	A smear that is more than 2 hours old may have deteriorated.
5. Place the slide on a stain rack blood side up. Place staining solution(s) onto slide according manufacturer's instructions. 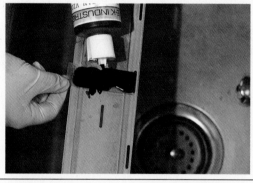	This provides a stable surface for staining. Wright stain contains alcohol to fix blood to the to slide and to stain the cells according to their characteristics. **Step 5.** Place slide on stain rack and apply stain onto slide.
6. Holding the slide with tweezers, gently rinse slide with water. Wipe off the back of the slide with gauze. Stand the slide upright and allow it to dry. 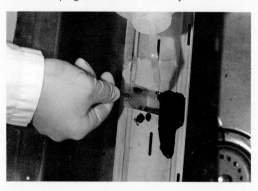	This rinses and removes the excess stain for the viewing under a microscope. **Step 6.** Rinse slide, and then wipe the unstained side with gauze.
7. Properly care for or dispose of equipment and supplies. Clean the work area. Remove gloves, gown, and face shield and wash your hands.	Maintaining a clean work space limits exposure to biohazards.

Note: Some manufacturers provide a simple one-step method that consists of dipping the smear in a staining solution and then rinsing. Directions provided by the manufacturer vary with the specific test.

PSY PROCEDURE 27-3:   Performing a Hemoglobin Determination

Purpose: To determine the oxygen-carrying capacity of the blood in a patient sample for diagnosis and treatment of anemia

Equipment: Hemoglobinometer, applicator sticks, whole blood, hand disinfectant, surface disinfectant, gloves, biohazard container

Steps	Purpose
1. Wash your hands.	Handwashing aids infection control.
2. Assemble the necessary equipment.	Equipment must be readily accessible for the procedure to be done.
3. Put on gloves.	PPE prevents exposure to biohazards.
4. Obtain a blood specimen from the patient by capillary puncture following the procedures in Chapter 26. An EDTA (lavender-top tube) blood specimen from the patient is also acceptable.	EDTA is the anticoagulant required for hematology testing.
5. Place well-mixed whole blood into the hemoglobinometer chamber as described by the manufacturer.	This prepares the sample for the hemoglobin determination.
6. Slide the chamber into the hemoglobinometer.	The chamber must be in the receiving slot for the reading.
7. Record the hemoglobin level from the digital readout.	Doing so provides a record of testing and results.
8. Clean the work area with surface disinfectant. Dispose of equipment and supplies appropriately. Remove gloves and wash your hands.	Maintaining a clean work space limits exposure to biohazards.

Note: This procedure may vary with the instrument. Some manufacturers offer a digital readout that is less subjective and is therefore considered more accurate and easier to use.

Charting Example:

12/02/2012 10:30 AM Cap puncture L ring finger. Hgb 9.5. Dx code ###.## per Dr. Royal. Dr. Royal notified of results

———————————————————————————————————— R. Smith, CMA

Note: The medical assistant may sign his or her name in the patient record using only the "CMA" credential if the office has a signature log denoting the entire credential as "CMA(AAMA)."

PSY **PROCEDURE 27-4:** **Performing a Microhematocrit Determination**

Purpose: To determine the quantity of erythrocytes in a centrifuged blood specimen for diagnosis and treatment of anemia

Equipment: Microcollection tubes, sealing clay, microhematocrit centrifuge, microhematocrit reading device, hand disinfectant, surface disinfectant, gloves, biohazard container, sharps container

Steps	Purpose
1. Wash your hands.	Handwashing aids infection control.
2. Assemble the equipment.	Equipment must be readily accessible for the procedure to be done.
3. Put on gloves.	PPE prevents exposure to biohazards.
4. Draw blood into the capillary tube by one of these methods: A. Directly from a capillary puncture (see Chapter 26) in which the tip of the capillary tube is touched to the blood at the wound and allowed to fill to three quarters or the indicated mark. B. From a well-mixed EDTA tube of whole blood; again, the tip is touched to the blood and allowed to fill three quarters of the tube.	Whole blood from a capillary puncture has not clotted and is acceptable. If blood from a tube is not well mixed, the reading is likely to be inaccurate.
5. Place the forefinger over the top of the tube, wipe excess blood off the sides, and push the bottom into the sealing clay.	Holding the finger over the tip stops blood from dripping out the bottom. The clay seals one end of the tube to contain it during centrifugation.
6. Draw a second specimen in the same manner.	A second tube is necessary for duplicate testing as a quality control measure.
7. Place the tubes, clay-sealed end out, in the radial grooves of the microhematocrit centrifuge opposite each other. Put the lid on the grooved area and tighten by turning the knob clockwise. Close the centrifuge lid. Spin for 5 minutes or as directed by the centrifuge manufacturer.	Specimens should always be placed opposite each other to balance the centrifuge. Read the manufacturer's directions for the specific centrifuge used in your facility; a 5-minute spin is normal.
8. Remove the tubes from the centrifuge and read the results; instructions are printed on the device. Results should be within 5% of each other. Take the average and report as a percentage.	Results with greater than 5% variation have been found to offer unreliable results.

Step 8. Read results from the centrifuge reading device.

PSY PROCEDURE 27-4: **Performing a Microhematocrit Determination (continued)**

Steps	Purpose
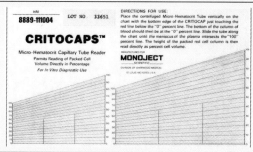	
Step 8. Hematocrit reader.	
9. Dispose of the microhematocrit tubes in a biohazard container. Properly care for or dispose of other equipment and supplies. Clean the work area. Remove gloves and wash your hands.	Maintaining a clean work space limits exposure to biohazards.

Note: Some microhematocrit centrifuges have the scale printed in the machine at the radial grooves.

Charting Example:

> *03/28/2012 4:20 PM Capillary puncture, left ring finger. Hct: 42%. Dx code XXX.XX per Dr. Erikson.*
>
> *Dr. notified of results ——————————————————————————— M. Mays, CMA*

Note: The medical assistant may sign his or her name in the patient record using only the "CMA" credential if the office has a signature log denoting the entire credential as "CMA(AAMA)."

PSY PROCEDURE 27-5: **Westergren Erythrocyte Sedimentation Rate**

Purpose: To determine the rate at which erythrocytes separate from plasma and settle in a tube for diagnosis of nonspecific inflammatory processes

Equipment: Hand disinfectant, gloves, EDTA blood sample less than 2 hours old, ESR kit, sedimentation rack, pipette, timer, surface disinfectant, biohazard disposal container, sharps container, impervious gown, face shield

Steps	Purpose
1. Wash your hands.	Handwashing aids infection control.
2. Assemble the necessary equipment.	Equipment must be readily accessible for the procedure to be done.
3. Put on gloves, impervious gown, and face shield.	PPE prevents exposure to biohazards.
4. Verify that the patient information on the specimen tube is that of the appropriate patient. Gently mix the EDTA lavender-stoppered anticoagulation tube for 2 minutes.	The blood must not be allowed to clot; it must be drawn into an anticoagulation tube.
5. Using a vial from the ESR kit and a pipette, fill vial to the indicated mark. Replace stopper and invert vial several times to mix (see Fig. 27-5).	Mixing the tube allows the specimen to thoroughly combine with the diluents in the vial.

(continued)

PSY PROCEDURE 27-5: **Westergren Erythrocyte Sedimentation Rate** *(continued)*

Steps	Purpose
6. Using an ESR calibrated pipette from the kit, insert the pipette through the tube's stopper with a twist and push down slowly but firmly until the pipette meets the bottom of the vial (see Fig. 27-5). The pipette will autozero with the excess flowing into the holding area. If the blood column does not reach the autozero point, discard used materials and start again at Step 4.	Presence of the full calibrated volume is necessary for an accurate test result. Bubbles and incorrect filling will alter the test results.
7. Place the tube in a holder that will keep the tube vertical (see Fig. 27-5).	Any deviation from being absolutely vertical will produce inaccurate test results.
8. Wait exactly 1 hour; use a timer for accuracy. Keep the tube straight upright and undisturbed during the hour.	
9. Record the level of the top of the RBCs after 1 hour. Normal results for men are 0–10 mL/hr; for women, normal results are 0–20 mL/hr.	Never use a shorter time and multiply the reading; less time will give inaccurate results.
10. Properly care for or dispose of equipment and supplies. Clean the work area. Remove gloves, gown, and face shield. Wash your hands.	Maintaining a clean work space limits exposure to biohazards.

Charting Example:

02/21/2012 12:30 PM ESR performed Dx code XXX.XX per Dr. North's order. Westergren ESR test results 12 mL/hr.

Dr. North notified ——————————————————————————————— J. Howell, RMA

- There are three types of blood cells:
  - RBCs transport gases (mainly oxygen and carbon dioxide) between the lungs and the tissues.
  - WBCs (leukocytes) provide the main line of defense against foreign invaders such as bacteria and viruses.
  - Platelets are critical elements of clot formation.
- Elevations in ESR values are not specific for any disorder but indicate inflammation.
- Basophils release histamine when the immune response is triggered. They contribute to inflammatory reactions and are often associated with asthma and allergies.
- Eosinophils are active at the end of allergic responses and with parasite elimination.
- Lymphocytes recognize that a particular cell or particle is foreign to the body andmake antibodies specific to its destruction.

- Monocytes engulf foreign material. As crucial elements of immune responses, monocytes capture, process, and nonspecifically kill antigens.
- Neutrophils defend against foreign invaders by engulfing them. Their numbers increase in patients with bacterial infections as the bone marrow releases them to fight the bacteria.
- A test result is abnormal if it is not within the reference interval listed on the laboratory report.
- Coagulation factors are produced by the liver and circulate in the blood (plasma) until the hemostasis begins.
- The PT is the primary monitor of Coumadin anticoagulant therapy.
- PTT may be prolonged in certain factor deficiencies, especially those that cause hemophilia. Heparin (anticoagulant) therapy also prolongs the PTT. Thus, it is used to monitor dosages.

Warm Ups for Critical Thinking

1. A patient was taking a medication that caused him to become neutropenic. To what might he be susceptible?
2. A patient lives at a very high elevation, where there is less oxygen than at sea level. Would you expect her hemoglobin to be greater than, less than, or the same as if she lived at sea level?
3. On microscopic review, a patient's RBCs are described as macrocytic. What impact would that characteristic have on the patient's MCV?
4. A patient with rheumatoid arthritis has an ESR of 77 mm/hr when she has her blood tested at the doctor's office; 2 weeks later, she returns, and now the rate is 31 mm/hr. With her condition in mind, would you expect that she is improving or not?
5. A patient has a platelet count of 75,000/mm^3. How would that impact the patient's coagulation studies?
6. Using the patient information in the Box 27-2, use these steps to complete the exercise as a case study.

To begin your evaluation:
*** *Research* the definitions of the morphology terms
Because of the initial test results, these tests were performed:

Iron studies:

serum ferritin <10 ng/mL	(12–86)
serum iron 24 µg/dL	(RI, 65–175)
TIBC 729 µg/dL	(RI, 250–410)
Saturation 3%	(RI, 20–55)

A. Define the symptoms in the patient history and physical exam.
B. Use those definitions to develop areas of concern.
C. Why did the physician order a CBC with differential?
D. What are the RIs for the tests included in the CBC?
E. Define the terms used to describe the red cell morphology.
F. What are the possible causes of this morphology?
G. Why did the doctor choose the follow-up tests listed?
H. Predict the diagnosis for the patient.
Let's take this to the next step:
- The history and exam lead to exploring a cause that would be the same for fatigue and for pallor. What causes can you list?
- Looking at the causes you listed, which ones would be evaluated using a CBC count?
- Which tests on the CBC count are abnormal? Are they elevated or decreased? Do these results eliminate any causes you listed?
- The patient's WBCs appear normal, so they are not involved in this disease process.
- After defining the terms used to describe the RBCs in the RBC morphology, the cells are determined to have very abnormal shapes with very little hemoglobin.
- Have you narrowed your list to iron deficiency anemia?
- For more information from this case study, evaluate the follow-up tests ordered by the physician. Do the results confirm the diagnosis of iron deficiency anemia?

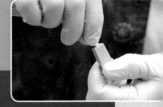

CHAPTER
28

Urinalysis

Learning Outcomes

Cognitive Domain

Note: AAMA/CAAHEP 2008 Standards are italicized.

1. Spell and define the key terms
2. Describe the methods of urine collection
3. List and explain the physical and chemical properties of urine
4. List confirmatory tests available and describe their use
5. List and describe the components that can be found in urine sediment and describe their relationships to chemical findings
6. *Analyze charts, graphs, and/or tables in the interpretation of health care results*
7. *Identify disease processes that are indications for CLIA-waived testing*

Psychomotor Domain

Note: AAMA/CAAHEP 2008 Standards are italicized.

1. Explain to a patient how and/or assist a patient to obtain a clean-catch midstream urine specimen (Procedure 28-1)
2. Explain the method of obtaining a 24-hour urine collection (Procedure 28-2)
3. Determine color and clarity of urine (Procedure 28-3)
4. Accurately interpret chemical reagent strip reactions (Procedure 28-4)
5. Prepare urine sediment for microscopic examination (Procedure 28-5)
6. *Practice standard precautions*
7. *Perform handwashing*

8. *Use medical terminology, pronouncing medical terms correctly, to communicate information*
9. *Instruct patients according to their needs to promote health maintenance and disease prevention*
10. *Prepare a patient for procedures and/or treatments*
11. *Document patient care*
12. *Respond to issues of confidentiality*
13. *Perform within scope of practice*
14. *Practice within the standard of care for a medical assistant*
15. *Document accurately in the patient record*
16. *Perform quality control measures*
17. Perform urinalysis
18. *Screen test results*
19. *Perform patient screening using established protocols*
20. *Report relevant information to others succinctly and accurately*

Affective Domain

Note: AAMA/CAAHEP 2008 Standards are italicized.
1. *Distinguish between normal and abnormal test results*
2. *Display sensitivity to patient rights and feelings in collecting specimens*
3. *Explain the rationale for performance of a procedure to the patient*
4. *Show awareness of patients' concerns regarding their perceptions related to the procedure being performed*

5. *Demonstrate empathy in communicating with patients, family, and staff*
6. *Apply active listening skills*
7. *Use appropriate body language and other nonverbal skills in communicating with patients, family, and staff*
8. *Demonstrate awareness of the territorial boundaries of the person with whom you are communicating*
9. *Demonstrate sensitivity appropriate to the message being delivered*
10. *Demonstrate recognition of the patient's level of understanding in communications*
11. *Recognize and protect personal boundaries in communicating with others*
12. *Demonstrate respect for individual diversity, incorporating awareness of one's own biases in areas including gender, race, religion, age, and economic status*
13. *Demonstrate awareness of the consequences of not working within the legal scope of practice*

ABHES Competencies

1. Use standard precautions
2. Screen and follow up patient test results
3. Perform selected CLIA-waived urinalysis testing that assist with diagnosis and treatment
4. Instruct patients in the collection of a clean-catch, midstream urine specimen

Key Terms

acidic pH	diurnal variation	microalbumin	specific gravity
acidosis	glucose oxidase	microhematuria	sulfosalicylic acid (SSA)
albumin	glycosuria	myoglobin	supernatant
bacteriuria	gross hematuria	neutral pH	Tamm-Horsfall mucoprotein
basic pH	hematuria	nitrite	threshold
Benedict reaction	hyperglycemia	nitroprusside	turbidity
bilirubin	Ictotest	phagocytic	urethral meatus
bilirubinuria	ketoacidosis	proteinuria	urine dipstick
chain-of-custody procedure	ketones	pyuria	urobilinogen
Clinitest	leukocyte esterase	reducing sugars	
conjugated bilirubin	lyse	sediment	

A urinalysis is a physical and chemical examination of urine to assess renal function and other possible problems. Because so many urinalyses are done in the office laboratory, proficiency in this skill is essential for the medical assistant. As indicated by clinical symptoms or physical and chemical findings in the urine, a microscopic examination may be added. The medical assistant may prepare urine sediment for microscopic examination (see Procedure 28-5). The microscopic examination may be performed by the physician under the Clinical Laboratory Improvement Amendments (CLIA) category physician-performed microscopy.

The physician may order a urinalysis for several reasons:

- To assess overall health
- To diagnose a medical condition
- To monitor a medical condition

The urinalysis to assess overall health is usually a screen for disorders such as diabetes, kidney disease, or liver disease. The urinalysis to diagnose a medical condition may be ordered if the patient has symptoms such as abdominal pain, back pain, frequent or painful urination, or blood in the urine. The urinalysis can also be used to monitor the patient's condition and treatment.

As with all body fluids, urine must be handled using Occupational Safety and Health Administration–mandated personal protective equipment (PPE) and safety guidelines.

 CHECKPOINT QUESTION

1. For what reasons might the physician order a urinalysis?

COG Specimen Collection Methods

Urine specimens are tested for a variety of analytes. How the specimen is collected depends on the test that has been requested. Most often a random urine is collected for urine specimens. A *random urine* is voided into a clean, dry container. To diagnose a urinary tract infection (UTI), the specimen is collected either as a clean-catch midstream or by catheter and submitted to the laboratory in a sterile container with a lid (Fig. 28-1). These methods are used to be sure any bacteria identified came from the urinary tract and not specimen contamination. If the physician needs to know the microorganism causing disease, a culture must be performed. A culture is a laboratory test in which microorganisms are grown in a nutrient medium to be identified and tested for antibiotic susceptibility. All cultures require the specimen not be contaminated during the preliminary testing process. Proper patient instruction in the clean-catch procedure avoids contamination, which would produce misleading results in urine culture or microscopic analysis.

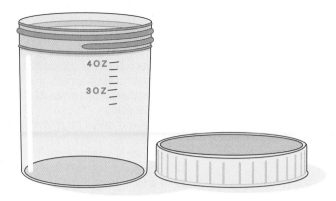

Figure 28-1 Sterile specimen cup with lid.

Once the urine is collected, many of its elements deteriorate within 1 hour. If testing cannot be performed within this time, the specimen is refrigerated at 4° to 8°C for up to 4 hours. Multiplication of microorganisms in an unrefrigerated specimen changes the pH from acidic to alkaline. Glucose in the urine may be used as a nutrient by the microorganisms, resulting in a false-negative or lowered glucose result.

The timing of collection can be an important consideration. First morning urine specimens are the most concentrated and are useful for many tests that are more easily determined with concentrated components (e.g., pregnancy testing); 2-hour postprandial (after a meal) specimens are used for glucose testing.

Random Specimen

When a random specimen is indicated, the patient voids the urine into a clean, dry container. No precautions are taken for any kind of contamination. The sample may contain white blood cells (WBCs), bacteria, and squamous epithelium cells as contaminants. Label all specimens directly on the container and not on the lid, because the lid may become separated from the specimen. Check the office policy manual for minimum label requirements. In female patients, the specimen may contain vaginal contaminants, such as trichomonads and yeast. Always check with female patients and note on the test requisition if the patient is menstruating because the specimen may be contaminated with blood.

First Morning Void

It is easiest to identify urine abnormalities in a more concentrated urine specimen. A first morning void reflects the ability of the kidney to concentrate urine during dehydration, which occurs overnight. Urine formed over a 6- to 8-hour period provides the preferred concentration. This is called a *first morning specimen* or an *early morning void*. It may be necessary to clarify this term for the patient with alternative sleep patterns.

Postprandial Specimen

A postprandial urine specimen is one that is collected exactly 2 hours after the patient eats a meal. The patient should be instructed to empty the bladder prior to eating the meal. This will ensure that the collected urine is entirely postprandial.

Clean-Catch Midstream Urine Specimen

A clean-catch midstream urine is useful when the physician suspects an infection. This specimen can be used for a culture if nothing has been allowed to contaminate the urine, such as a pipette or reagent strip. Collection is done after the urinary meatus and surrounding skin have been cleansed. The urine is voided into a sterile container. See Figure 28-2.

 Clean-Catch

A clean-catch specimen is necessary to confirm the presence or absence of infecting organisms in the urine. The specimen must be free of any contaminating matter that might be present on the genital organs. Most patients are not familiar with aseptic technique. Procedure 28-1 outlines the specific patient education instructions for both male and female patients. The container must not touch the genital area. Disabled or elderly patients may require assistance with the procedure. The specimen must be labeled as established by office procedures and refrigerated immediately.

Instructions for the Female Patient:
• The patient should begin by washing her hands.
• If menstruating, insert a fresh tampon (or use cotton to stop the flow).
• Separate the skin folds around the urinary opening.
• Wash the urinary opening and its surroundings from front to back with a sterile antiseptic pad.
• Keep the skin folds apart with the fingers of one hand.

Instructions for the Male Patient:
• The patient should begin by washing his hands.
• Wash the end of the penis with an antiseptic wipe.
• Allow it to dry.

Midstream

Collection begins after cleansing the external **urethral meatus** (the external opening of the urethra). Midstream specimen collection avoids contaminants from the urethra or the urinary meatus and ensures that the specimen represents bladder contents. Instruct the patient to begin the void directly into the toilet. The patient stops the flow and voids the middle third of the urine stream into the collection container. Once the patient has collected about 25 mL of urine, the bladder may be emptied into the toilet.

24-Hour Collection

Because some substances, such as proteins, are excreted with **diurnal variation** (variation during a 24-hour period), a 24-hour collection is a better indicator of values than a random specimen. To obtain this kind of specimen, the

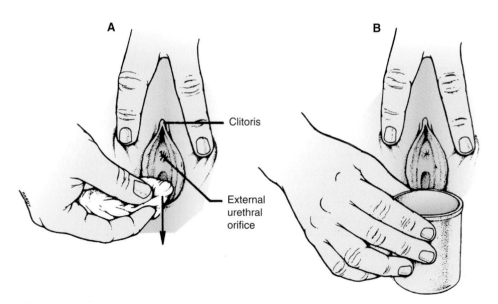

Figure 28-2 Obtaining a clean-catch midstream urine specimen in the female patient. Obtaining a clean-midstream urine specimen in the female patient. (**A**) Instruct the patient to hold the labia apart and wash from high up front toward the back with gauze soaked in soap. (**B**) The collection cup is held so that it does not touch the body, and the sample is obtained only while the patient is voiding with the labia held apart.

patient collects all voided urine within a 24-hour period (Procedure 28-2). Providing an information sheet with written instructions for collecting a 24-hour urine specimen helps ensure the patient's compliance.

PATIENT EDUCATION

INSTRUCTIONS FOR 24-HOUR URINE COLLECTION

The following instructions can be given to patients to ensure proper collection:

Instructions to Patients

- Instructions must be followed exactly. Your test results are based on the total amount of urine excreted by your body over a 24-hour period. Not following instructions will result in inaccurate results reported to your physician.
- The medical assistant will instruct you if the test has drug or diet requirement.
- The medical assistant will give you a container to collect the urine. A preservative may be in the container. Do not throw away the preservative. Preservatives may be toxic. Do not void directly into the container. Be very careful not to spill the preservative. Refrigerate the container during collection.

Day 1

- Empty your bladder into the toilet. Record the specific date and time on your 24-hour urine container.
- Collect all specimens during the day, evening, and night for the entire 24-hour period. Add all of the specimens to the container. Gently shake the container after each urine specimen is added. Keep the urine container refrigerated during the collection period and until you take it to the physician or laboratory for testing.

Day 2

- Exactly 24 hours later, completely empty your bladder and add this specimen to the container. This last specimen completes your 24-hour collection. Record the ending date and time on the container. Replace the cap and tighten firmly. Refrigerate the specimen until you can take it to the physician or laboratory.
- If you were on a special diet for this test, you may resume your normal diet after the specimen is collected.

If you do spill the preservative, immediately wash with large amounts of water. You will have to get a new container from your physician or laboratory to collect the specimen.

Other Specified Number of Hours

There may be circumstances that prompt the physician to order a specimen over a timeframe that is less than 24 hours. Such collections may be requested as 2-hour, 6-hour, or 12-hour specimens. The basic protocol described in Procedure 28-2 applies with modifications made in timing.

1. Void into the toilet and note this time and date as the beginning.
2. After the first voiding, collect each void, and add it to the urine container for the number of hours indicated by the physician.
3. At precisely the number of hours indicated by the physician after beginning the collection, empty the bladder even if there is no urge to void, and add this final volume of urine to the container.
4. Note on the label the ending time and date.

Bladder Catheterization

Another method for aseptic urine collection is catheterization. The catheter is inserted into the bladder through the urethra. Some medical assistants may be trained to perform catheterizations. Bladder catheterization is recommended when the patient cannot give a urine specimen in a sterile manner using the clean-catch method. The specimen must not be collected from a drainage bag.

Suprapubic Aspiration

Suprapubic aspiration is the least common method of urine collection. A needle is inserted into the bladder through the skin of the abdominal wall above the symphysis pubis, and urine is withdrawn (aspirated) as shown in Figure 28-3. This method is not common and is performed by a physician. You may be asked to assist with the procedure.

CHECKPOINT QUESTION

2. What is the time frame for testing urine that is not refrigerated? Why is this important?

WHAT IF?

A patient asks you what drugs can be detected in the urine. What do you say?

Many employers are requiring routine urine drug testing for their employees. Urine tests are preferred to blood tests because they are less expensive and are noninvasive. The following drugs can be detected in the urine: amphetamines, barbiturates, benzodiazepines, cocaine, marijuana, opioids, phencyclidine (also known as *PCP*), and methadone. You may tell or show the patient a list of these tests. If you must obtain urine specimens for drug testing, it is essential that you ensure security of the urine and confidentiality of the results.

COG Drug Testing

Each urine specimen submitted for drug testing must be analyzed using an initial test approved for commercial use by the U.S. Food and Drug Administration. Several techniques are available to screen for the five drug classes. Two tests are required to prove a positive drug result. The initial test eliminates negative urine specimens from further testing. A negative specimen either contains no drug or has a concentration less than a specified cutoff level. If the result of the first specimen is positive, gas chromatography/mass spectrometry (GC/MS) technology is used for confirmation testing.

Chain of Custody

The **chain-of-custody** process is used to document that the sample has been in possession of, or secured by, a responsible person at all times. See Box 28-1. Performed correctly, it eliminates doubt about sample identification or that the sample has been tampered with. The chain-of

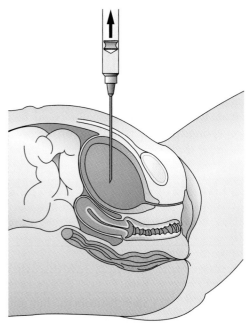

Figure 28-3 Suprapubic aspiration of urine. The full bladder is easily accessible by an abdominal puncture.

BOX 28-1

WHEN IS SOMETHING IN YOUR CUSTODY?

Samples are considered to be in your custody when:

1. They are in your physical possession.
2. They are in your view, after being in your physical possession.
3. They are in your physical possession and then sealed so that tampering is visibly evident.
4. They are kept in a secure area, with access restricted to authorized personnel only.

---

custody document should include the name or initials of the individual collecting the specimen, each person who subsequently had custody of it, and the date the specimen was received at the testing facility. General guidelines of chain-of-custody procedures are listed in Box 28-2.

Patient Processing and Specimen Collection

To perform a chain-of-custody specimen collection, the collector must first escort the subject from the waiting area to the collection area. The collector should be aware of body language and potential efforts to conceal a device to deliver clean urine. The collector and the subject must be the only people present in the collection area during the collection process.

The collector should obtain the necessary supplies: chain-of-custody form, specimen identification labels, tamper seals, and specimen bottle from a secured area or kit in view of the subject. The collector fills out the top portion of the Chain-of-Custody for Drug Analysis form. The subject is required to produce a form of photo identification (ID) issued by the subject's employer or the federal, state, or local government (e.g., a driver's license).

BOX 28-2

CHAIN-OF-CUSTODY GUIDELINES

1. Keep the number of people involved in collecting and handling samples to a minimum.
2. Always document the transfer of samples on a chain-of-custody form.
3. Always keep the chain-of-custody form together with the sample.
4. Identify samples legibly and written in permanent ink.

Faxes or photocopies of ID are not acceptable. Positive ID by an employer representative (not a coworker or another employee being tested) is also acceptable. If the subject cannot produce positive ID, the specimen collection procedure cannot be continued.

The medical assistant instructs the subject to remove outer clothing. Outer garments can conceal substances that could be used to tamper with a specimen. All personal belongings must remain with the medical assistant. The subject must show the medical assistant everything in his or her pockets to identify anything that could be used to contaminate the specimen. The subject may return the items to his or her pockets once they are examined and approved by the medical assistant.

1. The subject selects an individually wrapped or sealed collection container. The subject must witness the container being unwrapped and seal broken. The subject signs a specimen ID label, places it on the specimen container, and places the matching ID label on the chain-of-custody form.
2. No water can be available to the subject in the restroom. Blue dye is added to the toilet bowl turning toilet water blue to discourage specimen tampering. The subject is required to rinse and dry hands in front of the collector prior to specimen collection.
3. The patient can take nothing but the collection container into the room used for urination. The collector escorts the subject into the restroom. If the subject is wearing long sleeves, the collector instructs him or her to roll up the sleeves. The collector directs the subject to provide a specimen of at least 45 mL, to not flush the toilet, and to return to the medical assistant with the specimen as soon as he or she has completed the void. The subject snaps the cap tightly on the specimen to prevent leakage. The collector should never accept an uncapped specimen container from the subject.
4. If the subject cannot provide a sample, all forms and containers must be destroyed. New supplies will be used if the subject returns to perform the collection again.
5. The subject places the tamper seal over the top of the specimen container. One end of the seal must attach to the ID label. The medical assistant instructs the subject to write his or her initials on the seal after it is attached. The subject reads, signs, and dates the custody form. After the subject completes his or her part, the medical assistant records the specimen temperature, reviews the form for completeness, and signs and dates the form as the collector.
6. The subject must place the specimen into the specimen bag. The medical assistant refrigerates the specimen. Depending on office policy, the bagged specimen may be boxed and shipped to the testing laboratory or transported via courier. If a courier picks up

the specimen, the courier signs the chain-of-custody form to document taking possession of the specimen. The form is placed in the bag with the specimen prior to leaving the laboratory.

This chain-of-custody procedure is used in the following situations:

- Post-accident testing: testing of an employee who is involved in an on-the-job accident.
- Pre-employment testing: testing a candidate for employment.
- Random testing: testing of employees chosen for immediate testing randomly.
- Reasonable suspicion/cause testing: testing an employee if there is objective, factual, or individualized basis for testing.
- Return-to-duty/follow-up testing: testing of employees who failed a previous drug test before allowing them to return to the job.

COG Physical Properties of Urine

The physical properties of the urine specimen include the urine's color, appearance (such as clarity or **turbidity**), specific gravity, and odor. The first part of a urinalysis is direct visual observation. Color and clarity are assessed visually and are subjective, which means the individual performing the testing will determine whether these properties can be considered within the normal range (Table 28-1).

Color

Urine color can be affected by many things including diet, drugs, diseases, and the concentration of the urine. Normal, fresh urine is pale to dark yellow or amber in color. The yellow color is due to the pigment urochrome. Pale urine is typically very dilute and is seen after high fluid intake. Dark yellow color can signify highly concentrated urine such as when the patient is dehydrated. Red or red-brown color could be from a food dye, eating fresh beets, a drug, or the presence of

TABLE 28-1	Expected Ranges for Urine Physical Properties
Property	**Expected Range**
Color	Pale yellow to amber
Clarity	Clear
Odor	Slightly aromatic but not fruity, no ammonia
Specific gravity	1.001–1.035

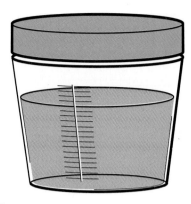

Figure 28-4 Hematuria in a urine specimen.

either hemoglobin or **myoglobin** (a protein in heart and skeletal muscle) (Fig. 28-4).

 Clarity

Normal, freshly voided urine is usually clear. Haziness or turbidity (cloudiness) may be caused by cellular material or protein in the urine. It may also develop from precipitation of salts while standing. Red blood cells, WBCs, bacteria, or mucus can also cause turbidity. These are not considered normal.

Laboratories vary in terminology used to express clarity or turbidity of urine. Common terminology dictates that when a small amount of turbidity is present so that black lines on white paper can be seen through the specimen, it is hazy. As turbidity increases and these black lines can no longer be seen, it is called *cloudy* (Procedure 28-3). The three terms most commonly used to describe clarity are *clear, hazy,* and *cloudy.*

Table 28-2 summarizes the common causes of variations in the color and clarity of urine.

Specific Gravity

The **specific gravity** reflects the ability of the kidney to concentrate or dilute the urine. Specific gravity is the weight of the urine compared to the weight of water. Urine, which contains cells and elements such as sodium, potassium, and chloride, is heavier than water. Specific gravity for a normal urine specimen is 1.001 to 1.035.

Urine with low specific gravity is dilute, probably as the result of high fluid intake. Abnormal conditions that produce dilute urine are diabetes insipidus and kidney infection or inflammation. In end-stage renal disease, the kidney cannot concentrate urine above a specific gravity of 1.007–1.010.

Urine with high specific gravity is concentrated. A patient with a high specific gravity is dehydrated. Sweating, vomiting, or diarrhea may produce a concentrated specimen because the body is trying to conserve water. High specific gravity can occur in diabetes mellitus. A urine specimen with a specific gravity of over 1.035 is either contaminated, contains very high levels of glucose, or contains contrast media from radiographic studies.

Specific gravity can be determined by a variety of methods. The specific gravity pad on the reagent strip takes a drop of urine, and the color change is compared to a chart to determine the value. This allows specific gravity to be determined in combination with the other chemical assays on the reagent strip and is the most common and efficient method of measurement. An older tool for measuring specific gravity is the refractometer or total solids meter, which requires a drop of urine and is read using a scale that measures the amount of light

TABLE 28-2	Common Causes of Variations in the Color and Clarity of Urine
Color and Clarity	**Possible Causes**
Yellow-brown or green-brown	Bile in urine (as in jaundice)
Dark yellow or orange	Concentrated urine, low fluid intake, dehydration, inability of kidney to dilute urine, fluorescein (intravenous dye), multivitamins, excessive carotene
Bright orange-red	Pyridium (urinary tract analgesic)
Red or reddish brown	Hemoglobin pigments, pyrvinium pamoate (Povan™) for intestinal worms, sulfonamides (sulfa-based antibiotics)
Green or blue	Artificial color in food or drugs
Blackish, grayish, smoky	Hemoglobin or remnants of old RBCs (indicating bleeding in upper urinary tract), chyle, prostatic fluid, yeasts
Cloudy	Phosphate precipitation (normal after sitting for a long time), urates (compound of uric acid), leukocytes, pus, blood, epithelial cells, fat droplets, strict vegetarian diet

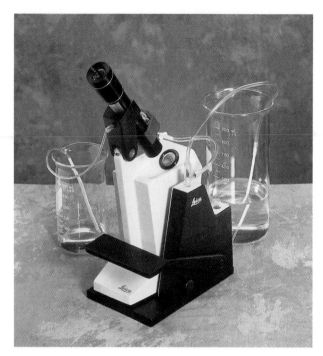

Figure 28-5 Determining specific gravity of urine using a refractometer. The advantage of this is that only one drop of urine is required.

bent by the particles in the urine (Fig. 28-5). With the refractometer, the urine that contains more particles, bends more light. That raises the specific gravity value registered by the refractometer.

 CHECKPOINT QUESTION

3. What are the three physical properties of urine, and which two are assessed visually?

COG Chemical Properties of Urine

Urine contains chemicals produced in the body and ingested from the environment. The reagent strip performs 10 chemical measurements. Table 28-3 gives the expected value for each chemical property. Detecting and measuring chemical properties allows urine testing to be used in diagnosis.

Reagent strips that can be dipped into urine have chemicals embedded in pads. The chemicals in the pads react with the chemicals in the urine. A reagent pad will change color as the chemical reaction takes place. All reagent pad colors are compared with a color chart to interpret the reactions at the specific time indicated for each reaction (Procedure 28-4). This color measurement may be performed visually or with a semi-automated strip-reading instrument (Fig. 28-6).

TABLE 28-3	Expected Ranges of Chemical Properties
Property	**Expected Range**
Glucose	Negative
Bilirubin	Negative
Ketones	Negative
Blood	Negative
pH	5.0–8.0
Protein	Negative to trace
Urobilinogen	0.1–1.0 mg/dL
Nitrite	Negative
Leukocyte esterase	Negative

Precautions for Using Reagent Strips

1. Reagent strips should be tested with positive and negative controls on each day of use. Each reagent pad on the strip must give a positive or negative test result as appropriate.
2. Failure to observe color changes at the appropriate time intervals may cause inaccurate results.
3. Reagents and reagent strips must be stored properly to retain reactivity.
4. Observe color changes and color charts under good lighting.

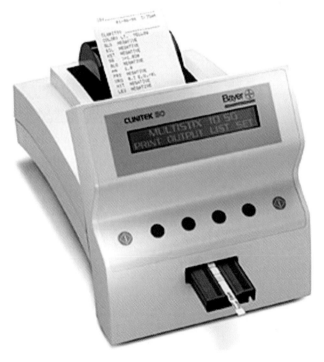

Figure 28-6 Bayer Clinitek Dipstick Reader.

5. Proper collection and storage of urine is necessary to ensure preservation of components, such as bilirubin and ketones.
6. Do not allow the reagent pads of the strip to touch the fingers or other surfaces.

pH

The kidney helps maintain the acid–base balance of the body. To keep a stable pH, the kidney must control the change of pH of the urine to balance the pH that results from diet and metabolism. If there is too much acid in the body (**acidosis**), then the kidney will excrete the acid. When the body does not contain enough acid, the kidney does not excrete much acid.

The more acid there is present in a specimen, the lower the pH will be. **Acidic pH** is from 1–6. The less acid there is present in a specimen, the higher the pH will be. Nonacidic pH (**basic pH**) is 8–12. That leaves 7 in the middle. 7 is **neutral pH**, neither an acid or a base.

Expected patient values for urine pH can range from 5.0 to 8.0. The typical pH value for freshly voided urine is 6.0. Blood moving through the kidneys is usually acidified by renal tubules and collecting ducts. Slightly acidic urine is normal. It also occurs with a high-protein diet and uncontrolled diabetes. A pH above 7.0 can occur after meals and with a vegetarian diet, certain renal diseases, and UTI.

Glucose

Glucose is filtered and reabsorbed in the kidneys. The renal **threshold** level for glucose is 180 g/dL. When the blood glucose goes over the threshold, the kidneys will not reabsorb all of it. The glucose that the kidney does not reabsorb into the blood is released into the urine. This causes a positive result for the presence of glucose in the urine, or **glycosuria**. The threshold can vary and requires measuring the actual blood level in addition to the urine level for a diagnostic assessment. Normal urine does not contain glucose. When the glucose measured on the dipstick indicates that no glucose is present, the patient's blood level of glucose will be less than 180 mg/dL. A blood glucose level of 180 mg/dL is still an abnormally high level (**hyperglycemia**). Glycosuria can occur if blood levels are greater than 180 mg/dL (Box 28-3). An example of hyperglycemia is diabetes mellitus.

The reagent test strip (**urine dipstick**) uses a reaction called **glucose oxidase** to detect glucose in urine. It measures only glucose. Glucose is not the only kind of sugar present in urine. Most laboratories test newborn and infant urines for the sugars other than glucose. These are called **reducing sugars**. Examples of reducing sugars are galactose and fructose. The most common test for reducing sugars is called the **Clinitest**™ method. The presence of these other reducing sugars in the urine may indicate

---

RENAL THRESHOLD AND GLYCOSURIA

Glucose is resorbed in the proximal convoluted tubule. When blood glucose levels exceed 180 mg/dL, depending on the individual, not all of the glucose can be reabsorbed into the bloodstream. Rarely does a healthy person's blood glucose level exceed this threshold value. Diabetic patients, however, may pass some glucose in their urine because of the high level in their blood. A frequently used term, "spilling sugar," means that not all of the sugar is reabsorbed and some is excreted in the urine.

metabolism abnormalities in the infants. These abnormalities must be identified early for the infant to thrive.

CHECKPOINT QUESTION

4. In what disease process would monitoring glycosuria be useful?

Ketones

Ketones are chemicals produced during fat metabolism. Energy is derived from carbohydrate metabolism. Without enough carbohydrates, as in starvation, low-carbohydrate diet, and inadequately managed diabetes, fats are used by the body for energy. Using up the body's fat results in the body using protein for energy, thus producing ketones.

In normal urine, ketones are typically too low to be measurable. A positive ketone test indicates that the body is burning more fat than normal. One disorder resulting in **ketoacidosis** (too much ketone in the blood and urine) is diabetes mellitus. If ketosis occurs in a diabetic patient, it is a serious sign that the disease is out of control. Quick response of the physician to alter the patient's medication is required to avoid diabetic coma.

CHECKPOINT QUESTION

5. Why would a person on a low-carbohydrate weight loss plan want to monitor the ketones in his or her urine?

Proteins

It is not abnormal to have a small amount of protein in one's urine. The medical assistant would report this amount as "trace." Proteinuria is an increased amount of protein present in urine. Proteinuria is diagnostic of kidney disease. Strenous exercise can cause a temporary increase in urine protein. Proteinuria is present in pregnancy, infection, **hematuria** (blood in urine), **pyuria** (WBCs in urine), and multiple myeloma. The presence of vaginal discharge, semen, heavy mucus, pus, and blood in the urine can cause a false-positive urine protein result. This cause of false-positive results can be avoided by teaching the patient the proper method for collecting a clean-catch specimen.

 CHECKPOINT QUESTION

6. What factors may cause a false positive urine protein test result?

Blood

There are two ways that blood appears in the urine. Small numbers of RBCs are occasionally observed in urine. Hematuria not due to contamination from menstrual flow indicates bleeding in the urinary tract that may result from renal disorders, certain neoplasms, UTI, or trauma to the urinary tract. See Figure 28-4 for an example of the appearance of hematuria in a urine specimen.

The second way blood appears in urine is as the contents of the RBCs rupture or **lyse**. The reagent strip reacts to hemoglobin, which is the primary constituent of RBCs. Hemoglobinuria may occur with transfusion reactions, chemical toxicity, or burns. The strip also reacts to myoglobin, a protein found in muscles. Myoglobin may be released into the bloodstream from a crushing injury or other trauma and may then be excreted in the urine.

In **microhematuria**, the amount of blood in the urine is so small that the color of the specimen is not affected. Microhematuria can only be detected with the reagent strip. A large amount of urine is the blood is known as **gross hematuria**. Gross hematuria alters the color of the urine to a red or brownish red color. The presence of RBCs in the urine can result from multiple variations of kidney disorders, kidney stones, kidney trauma, and bleeding disorders.

 CHECKPOINT QUESTION

7. A patient arrives in the physicians' office doubled over in pain. The physician orders a STAT urinalysis. The patient submits a specimen that is brownish red in color. The patient has a history of kidney stones. What is the likely result for the reagent dipstick test for blood?

Bilirubin

Bilirubin is formed during breakdown of hemoglobin. It is processed in the liver before being excreted into the intestines. Most bilirubin cannot dissolve, so urine contains very low levels of bilirubin. A normal reagent strip test result for bilirubin is negative. **Bilirubinuria** (bilirubin in the urine) can occur with hepatitis, biliary tract obstruction, and hemolytic states such as transfusion reactions. One type of bilirubin does dissolve into the bloodstream. This bilirubin is called **conjugated bilirubin**. It is easily fitered by the kidneys but is only high enough to detect in the urine if the bilirubin in the blood is elevated.

The reagent strip is designed to react to bilirubin; however, dark yellow urine can make it difficult to read the reaction because bilirubin is a yellow pigment.

Note: Bilirubin is a highly unstable substance and will break down with exposure to light. Specimens must be shielded from light and processed as soon as possible to avoid deterioration of the specimen.

 CHECKPOINT QUESTION

8. A patient is in the office for a repeat visit. She was just diagnosed with hepatitis B. What reagent strip test would be positive strictly because of liver disease?

Urobilinogen

The bilirubin that goes to the intestines mixes with bacteria already in the intestinal tract. The enzymes in the bacteria break bilirubin into parts. One of the parts is called **urobilinogen**. Most urobilinogen is eliminated in the feces. About 15% of it is reabsorbed into the blood, goes back to the liver, and is re-excreted into the intestines. A small amount is excreted by the kidneys. The diagram in Figure 28-7 shows the normal pathway of bilirubin and urobilinogen.

Small amounts of urobilinogen are normally found in urine, usually 0.1 to 1.0 mg/dL. As with bilirubin, increased levels of urobilinogen can be found with conditions that have a high rate of RBC destruction. Bowel obstructions cause the feces to remain in the intestines for longer periods. While it remains, it reabsorbs urobilinogen. Urobilinogen levels rise both in urine and in serum when this occurs. Liver impairment can also lead to increased levels of urobilinogen because some of the urobilinogen that is reabsorbed from the intestinal tract is processed by the liver and excreted in the feces.

Nitrite

Some types of bacteria that infect the urinary tract have an enzyme that can reduce nitrate to **nitrite**.

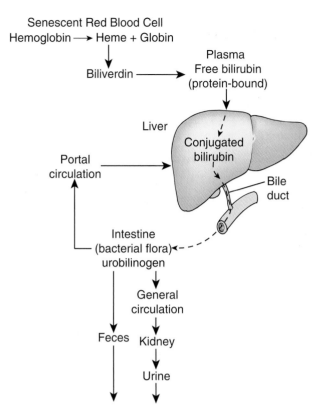

Figure 28-7 Process of bilirubin formation.

9. A patient has a negative result on the nitrite reaction on the urine dipstick. Could the patient still possibly have a positive leukocyte esterase result on that specimen?

Microalbumin

Some urine reagent test strips contain a reagent pad for measuring microalbumin.

One of the proteins measured in the protein reagent pad is **albumin**. When the kidneys are healthy, almost no proteins pass out of the kidneys and into the urine. However, if a person's kidneys become diseased or damaged some proteins begin to filter through and appear in the urine. In the very early stages of kidney disease, tiny bits of albumin, **microalbumin**, begin to appear in the urine. Once the microalbumin goes above 150 mg, the patient has reached early glomerular damage.

Normal random urine protein results equal 0 to 20 mg/dL. Normal random urine albumin results equal 0 to 23 mg/dL. Kidney function is normal within these ranges. Higher values on protein and albumin indicate kidney disease.

COG Confirmatory Testing

Reasons for Performing Confirmatory or Secondary Macroscopic Urine Tests

Individual medical offices have policies to confirm certain dipstick test results. Office choices are not always the same. Part of training in a new laboratory is learning which dipstick test results are confirmed in that office. See Box 28-4 for a list of confirmatory tests that may be used in any laboratory.

Common bacteria that can cause UTIs are *Escherichia coli, Enterobacter, Klebsiella,* and *Proteus* species. These bacteria contain enzymes that convert the nitrate in them to nitrite. This factor is used to assess the presence of bacteria in urine. If these types of bacteria are present, nitrates will be converted to nitrites, and the resulting pink color development can be observed on the reagent pad. A positive nitrite test result indicates **bacteriuria**, which occurs with UTIs. Bacteriuria is the presence of bacteria in urine. A negative nitrite test result does not indicate the absence of bacteriuria because not all types of bacteria reduce nitrate to nitrite.

Leukocyte Esterase

Leukocytes in the urine indicate a UTI. A positive leukocyte esterase test indicates that WBCs are present in the specimen. **Phagocytic** WBCs, such as neutrophils, are called to the kidney to fight the infection. Phagocytic cells can engulf bacteria, dead cells, or harmful foreign particles. These leukocytes contain an enzyme called *esterase*. This enzyme is detected with the **leukocyte esterase** reaction on the reagent strip. Normal urine may contain a few WBCs but not in sufficient numbers to produce a positive leukocyte esterase test. A negative leukocyte esterase test means that an infection is not likely.

BOX 28-4

URINE CONFIRMATORY TESTING

Reagent strip tests are screening tests. Confirmation with a more sensitive and/or specific method may be requested to follow up some positive results. Your laboratory will have a specific procedure outlining the performance of confirmation tests.

Analyte	Common Confirmatory Test
Protein	SSA test
Ketones	Acetest™
Bilirubin	Ictotest™
Glucose	Clinitest™

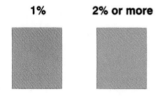

5-Drop Method Standard Procedure

DIRECTIONS FOR TESTING:

1. Collect urine in clean container. With dropper in upright position, place **5 drops** of urine in test tube. Rinse dropper with water and add 10 drops of water to test tube.

2. Drop one tablet into test tube. Watch while complete boiling reaction takes place. Do not shake test tube during boiling, or for the following 15 seconds after boiling has stopped.

3. At the end of this 15-second waiting period, shake test tube gently to mix contents. Compare

color of liquid to Color Chart below. Ignore sediment that may form in the bottom of the test tube. Ignore changes after the 15-second waiting period.

4. Write down the percent (%) result which appears on the color block that most closely matches the color of the liquid.

NEGATIVE	1/4%	1/2%	3/4%	1%	2% or more

Figure 28-8 Clinitest™ for reducing sugars.

Confirmatory procedures are usually performed for one or more of these reasons:

- to validate a dipstick test result,
- to do a test that cannot be done with a dipstick because of the specimen's intense color, or
- to do a more specific test than the method on the dipstick.

Box 28-4 lists several types of confirmation tests. Check the laboratory procedure manual for the confirmation testing used in the laboratory.

Copper Reduction Test

The copper reduction method, or Clinitest™ (Fig. 28-8), discussed earlier, is used as a confirmatory test for glucose measured on the urine dipstick. *Note:* the reaction produces heat, so always use a glass tube.

Another name for the copper reduction test is the **Benedict reaction.** Any reducing substances in the urine react with the copper sulfate in the reagent. This results in a color change that goes from blue through green to orange. The change is proportional to the amount of reducing substance in the urine sample. The color change must be watched throughout the entire reaction. If the amount of reducing substances is really high, the color change moves quickly through orange and back to blue again. If the entire reaction is not observed, the return to the blue color could be interpreted as a negative result.

Nitroprusside Test

A **nitroprusside** reaction is used to detect ketone. (Nitroprusside is a compound that reacts with ketones to produce a purple reaction.) This is the method used on both reagent strips and tablet tests. Many laboratories choose to confirm results with the nitroprusside tablet

(Acetest™). The lactose present in the tablet method serves to enhance the color reaction with that method.

Precipitation Test

Turbidity or precipitation tests confirm a positive protein result on the reagent test strip. The most common confirmation test is observing the amount of cloudiness when equal amounts of urine and **sulfosalicylic acid** (**SSA**) are mixed. The urine used must be centrifuged to remove all particulate matter before adding the acid.

If the amount of protein is negligible and produces a negative reagent strip reaction, there should be no cloudiness when the SSA is added to the urine. When the concentration of urine protein reaches approximately 20 mg/dL, turbidity will result because SSA combines with the protein in the urine. As protein levels increase, so will the degree of turbidity during the reaction with the acid. A protein dipstick result that is greater than a trace may be an indication of proteinuria.

Diazo Test

Many laboratories confirm a positive bilirubin result on the urine test strip result using a diazo tablet method, called the **Ictotest™** (Fig. 28-9). The diazo tablet

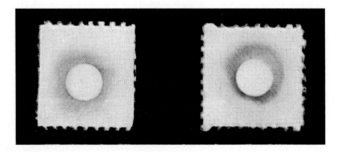

Figure 28-9 Diazo tablet test for bilirubin.

procedure is good for confirmation because it is more sensitive than the strip procedure. The tablet method can detect as little as 0.05 to 0.1 mg/dL of bilirubin in a urine sample. The Ictotest™ is a specific test for bilirubin and is four times as sensitive as the reagent strip pad. This color change is much easier to detect than the one on the reagent test strip.

▶ COG Urine Sediment

The microscopic examination of urine can corroborate the findings of the urinalysis and may produce additional data with diagnostic value. Cells and other structures are noted and counted during a microscopic examination. Microscopic examination of urine is not a CLIA-waived procedure, so examining and reporting results of the microscopic examination of urine is outside the scope of practice for a medical assistant. Urine **sediment** is prepared by centrifuging urine and saving the button of cells and other particulate matter that collects in the bottom of the tube. This button is resuspended in the residual **supernatant** (urine above the sediment when the tube of urine is centrifuged), and a drop of this suspension is placed on a slide and viewed with a microscope. Making a sediment button concentrates all of the structures in the urine so that it is unlikely that any components will be missed (Procedure 28-5).

A slide system used in conjunction with a unique centrifuge tube is available to examine sediments. This provides some standardization of the procedure so that the numbers in the findings have meaning with regard to abnormal results. Glass slides, with or without coverslips, may still be used by some laboratories.

Structures Found in Urine Sediment

The following structures may appear in the urine: RBCs, WBCs, bacteria, epithelial cells, crystals, casts, and others, as shown in Figure 28-10. Correlations with chemical properties of the urine are described as appropriate.

Red Blood Cells

Hematuria is the presence of RBCs in urine. This may indicate glomerular damage, tumors of the urinary tract, kidney trauma, urinary stones, renal infarcts, acute tubular necrosis, upper and lower UTIs, nephrotoxins, and physical distress. RBCs may also appear as a contaminant in urine from the vagina in menstruating women or from trauma from a bladder catheterization. When the urine sediment contains RBCs, the reagent strip should be positive for blood. Protein may also be positive if hemolysis is occurring because hemoglobin is a protein. A positive reagent strip test for blood with no RBCs seen microscopically may occur with various kinds of hemolysis. In hemolysis, the RBCs have ruptured and spilled their contents into the urine. The hemoglobin that remains turns the test blood positive.

White Blood Cells

Leukocytes in urine sediment indicate a UTI. The leukocyte esterase test on the reagent strip will be positive when WBCs are present. The protein test may be

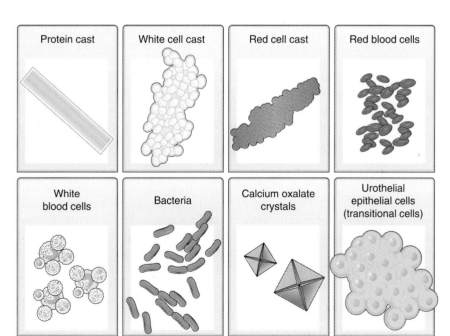

| Protein cast | White cell cast | Red cell cast | Red blood cells |
| White blood cells | Bacteria | Calcium oxalate crystals | Urothelial epithelial cells (transitional cells) |

Figure 28-10 Microscopic examination of urinary sediment. Some of the more common formed elements found in urine are shown here.

positive if some of the WBCs lyse, or if the infection is damaging the renal tubules, as in glomerulonephritis.

Bacteria

Bacteria are always present on the skin but not usually in the bladder. Urine normally does not contain bacteria if a clean-catch specimen is collected properly. The presence of significant amounts (more than a trace) of bacteria in a urine specimen is considered an indication of a UTI. A positive nitrite result may be obtained when bacteria are seen.

Bacteria are common if the clean-catch procedure is inadequate. There is abundant normal microbial flora of the vagina or external urethral meatus. Any trace bacteria present rapidly multiply in urine left standing at room temperature. Microbial organisms should be considered in relationship to the patient's clinical symptoms. The diagnosis of UTI requires a culture.

Epithelial Cells

Epithelial cells cover the skin and organs and line the urinary tract. Their shapes vary according to their location of origin. Epithelial cells are normally found in urine, but increased amounts can indicate an irritation such as inflammation somewhere in the urinary system. The three types of epithelial cells in the urine are squamous, transitional, and renal. *Squamous epithelial cells* cover external skin surfaces and are considered a normal finding in urine, because urine comes in contact with skin during urination. *Transitional epithelial cells* line the bladder and are seen with infections of the lower urinary tract such as cystitis. *Renal epithelial cells* line the nephrons and are seen with infections and inflammations of the upper urinary tract. The presence of renal epithelial cells can elevate the protein in the urine.

 CHECKPOINT QUESTION

10. A urinalysis report notes that renal epithelial cells were present when the specimen was examined microscopically. What reagent strip test may be positive?

Crystals

Crystals are made up of a chemical substance in the urine in sufficient quantities to form a solid three-dimensional structure that can be seen microscopically. The three most common crystals found in urine sediment—calcium oxalate, uric acid, and triple phosphate are not independently pathologic. However, uric acid crystals can be seen with fever, leukemia, or gout. Crystals can contribute to the formation of stones in the urinary tract.

 PATIENT EDUCATION

WHAT CAN I DO TO AVOID A KIDNEY STONE?

Kidney stone prevention is primarily a function of diet.

- *Drink more fluid.* Unless instructed by a physician, drink enough fluid to make your urine clear or pale yellow. In concentrated urine, crystals are more likely. Crytals continue to grow and form a stone.
- *Eat less protein.* Americans eat much more protein than the body needs. The extra protein that the body does not need turns to fat. Fat makes kidney stones more likely.
- *Cut the salt.* The average American consumes about twice the recommended amount of salt and five times more than the body needs. Sodium causes urine calcium levels to increase, making it more likely to have a kidney stone.
- *Take in more citrate.* Citrate is a chemical that inhibits the production of kidney stones. The more you have in your urine, the less likely the formation of a stone. Citrate is in lemons, oranges, and grapefruit.

Casts

Cast formation occurs in the distal convoluted tubule of the nephron or the collecting duct (Fig. 28-11). When protein is present in sufficient quantities, it will cement together whatever solutes or cells are in the tubule as well; this is called a *cast*. See the diagram of various casts (Fig. 28-12). The mucoprotein that cements urinary casts together is called **Tamm-Horsfall mucoprotein**. Most casts eventually break free and flow into the urine. The type of cast can indicate certain pathologies. For instance, in pyelonephritis, WBCs that are present to combat the infection become trapped in the protein network and form WBC casts (Fig. 28-13).

Other Structures

Other structures can be found in urine sediment. Yeast in the urine can result from vaginal contamination of the specimen or may be the causative agent of a UTI, especially in a diabetic patient. The parasite *Trichomonas vaginalis* is a contaminant from the genital tract of an infected person. See yeast and *T. vaginalis* in Figure 28-14. Mucus may be present if there is an inflammation in the urinary tract. Mucus threads are usually reported in quantities such as few, moderate, or many. Spermatozoa may be found when there has been a recent emission (Fig. 28-15).

KIDNEY CORTEX

Figure 28-11 here shows labels: Dilute interstitial fluid, Glomerular capsule, Proximal convoluted tubule, Distal convoluted tubule, Collecting duct, Descending limb, Loop of Henle, Ascending limb, Concentrated interstitial fluid.

KIDNEY MEDULLA

⟹ Sodium (Na$^+$)   ⟶ Water (H$_2$O)

Figure 28-11 Distal convoluted tubule and collecting duct of the kidney. The distal convoluted tubule (DCT) (3) includes the macula densa and juxtaglomerular (JG) apparatus. The collecting duct (4) consists of the cortical collecting duct (CCD), outer medullary collecting duct (OMCD), and inner medullary collecting duct (IMCD). (From Cohen BJ, Taylor JJ. Memmler's The Human Body in Health and Disease, 10th edition. Baltimore: Lippincott Williams & Wilkins, 2005.)

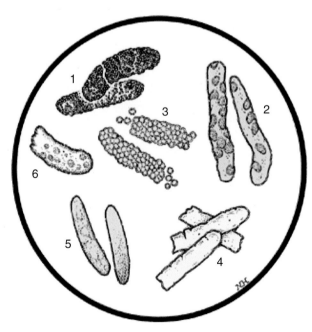

Figure 28-12 Urinary casts. (1) Coarse granular casts. (2) Epithelial casts. (3) RBC casts. (4) Waxy casts. (5) Hyaline casts. (6) Casts with pyocytes (pus corpuscles). (Neil O. Hardy. Wesport, CT. From Stedman's Medical Dictionary, 27th Edition. Baltimore: Lippincott Williams & Wilkins, 2000.)

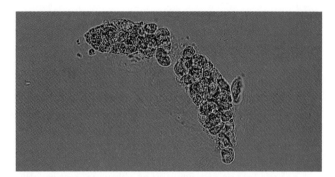

Figure 28-13 WBC cast. The cast depicted in the photomicrograph is a hyaline cast to which polymorphonuclear neutrophils have adhered. The leukocytes on the cast surface show a granular cytoplasm and multilobed nuclei (bright-field microscopy).

COG **Reviewing Patient Results**

From evaluation of the patient urinalysis results in Figure 28-16, what can be said about this patient? All of the results in this report are within normal or expected ranges. These results do not indicate specific disease, and they do not indicate the lack of disease.

COG **The Medical Assistant's Responsibilities in the Urinalysis Laboratory**

As in all areas of the physician office laboratory or any laboratory, practice standard precautions as discussed in earlier chapters.

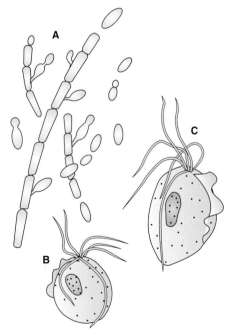

Figure 28-14 Organisms that cause vaginal infections. (**A**) *Candida albicans* (blastospores and pseudohyphae). (**B,C**) *T. vaginalis*.

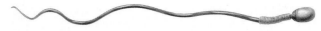

Figure 28-15 Spermatozoan.

In the collection of specimens for urinalysis, display sensitivity to patient rights and feelings in collecting specimens. There are no pretesting requirements for basic urine testing. Be professional in responding to the patient's questions about the reason his or her doctor ordered the test or the meaning of abnormal test results. These are questions to be answered by the patient's physician. You may understand the basic uses of the test but not know how or why the physician plans to use this test in diagnosing the patient. Refer to the physician to instruct the patient according to his or her needs to promote disease prevention.

Another requirement for professionalism in the urinalysis laboratory is the correct use of medical terminology. Refer to tests by their appropriate names. Pronounce those names correctly. Not only does this portray professionalism, it also is reassuring to the patient to hear accurate use of medical terminology.

Procurement of a patient specimen must be documented in the patient's chart. Follow the laboratory's policies on the documentation of test results.

CENTRAL MEDICAL CENTER

211 Medical Center Drive • Central City, US 90000-1234 • PHONE: (012) 125-6784 • FAX: (012) 125-9999

11//02/20xx
13:49

NAME : TEST, PATIENT	LOC: TEST	DOB: 2/2/XX	AGE: 38Y
MR# : TEST-221			SEX: M
ACCT # : H111111111			

M63560 COLL: 11/2/20xx 13:24   REC: 11/2/20xx 13:25

URINE BASIC

Color	STRAW		
Appearance	CLEAR		
Specific Gravity	1.010	[1.003 - 1.035]	
pH	5.5	[5.0 - 9.0]	
Protein	NEG	[0 - 10]	MG/DL
Glucose	NEG	[NEG]	
Ketones	NEG	[NEG]	
Bilirubin	NEG	[NEG]	
Urine Occult Blood	NEG	[NEG]	
Nitrites	NEG		

URINE MICROSCOPIC

Epithelial Cells	3 to 4	/HPF
WBCs	0 to 1	/HPF
RBCs	0	/HPF
Bacteria	0	
Mucous Threads	0	

TEST, PATIENT   TEST-221   END OF REPORT   PAGE 1
11/02/20xx   13:49   INTERIM REPORT
INTERIM REPORT COMPLETED

Figure 28-16 Sample urinalysis report.

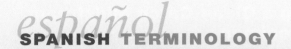

SPANISH TERMINOLOGY

Necesitamos que nos dé una prueba de orina.
> You will collect a urine specimen.

Orine en el inhodoro por algunos segundos.
> Urinate in the toilet a few seconds.

Pare, y orine en el envase para la muestra.
> Stop and urinate in the specimen cup.

Necesita tomar una muestra de todo el orín que haga por 24 horas.
> You are going to save all of your urine for 24 hours.

Devuelva la muestra de orina a la oficina tan pronto sea posible, luego de que haya terminado de tomar las muestras.
> Return the specimen to the office as soon as possible after collection is complete.

MEDIA MENU

- **Student Resources on thePoint**
  - **Video: Obtaining a Clean-Catch Midstream Urine Specimen (Procedure 28-1)**
  - **Video: Determining Color and Clarity of Urine (Procedure 28-3)**
  - **Video: Chemical Reagent Strip Analysis (Procedure 28-4)**
  - **Video: Preparing Urine Sediment (Procedure 28-5)**
  - **CMA/RMA Certification Exam Review**
- **Internet Resources**
  - **National Institutes of Health—Urinalysis**
    http://www.nlm.nih.gov/medlineplus/ency/article/003579.htm
  - **Lab Tests Online**
    http://www.labtestsonline.org/understanding/analytes/urinalysis/test.html
  - **Medical Technology**
    http://www.irvingcrowley.com/cls/urin.htm

PSY **PROCEDURE 28-1:** **Obtaining a Clean-Catch Midstream Urine Specimen**

Purpose: To minimize contamination of a voided urine specimen
Equipment: Sterile urine container labeled with patient's name, cleansing towelettes (two for male patients, three for female patients), gloves if you are to assist patient, hand sanitizer

Steps	Reasons
1. Wash your hands. If you are to assist the patient, put on gloves.	Handwashing aids infection control.
2. Assemble the equipment.	Equipment must be readily accessible to perform the procedure.
3. **AFF** Identify the patient and explain the procedure. Display sensitivity to patient rights and feelings in collecting specimens. Explain the rationale for performance of a procedure to the patient.	Show awareness of patients' concerns regarding their perceptions related to the procedure being performed. Ask for and answer any questions.
4. **AFF** If the patient is hearing impaired, you may need to face the person and speak clearly, not loudly. You should have an easy-to-read instruction guide for the patient to follow and point out where there are questions. If the patient can sign and you cannot, have someone proficient in sign language assist you in instructing the patient.	Understanding the instructions is critical to obtaining a quality specimen.
5. If the patient is to perform the procedure, provide the necessary supplies.	The patient will need the appropriate materials in order to do the collection properly.

6. Have the patient perform the procedure.
A. Instruct the male patient:
   i. If uncircumcised, expose the glans penis by retracting the foreskin, then clean the meatus with an antiseptic wipe. The glans should be cleaned in a circular motion away from the meatus. A new wipe should be used for each cleaning sweep.
   ii. Keeping the foreskin retracted, initially void a few seconds into the toilet or urinal.
   iii. Bring the sterile container into the urine stream and collect a sufficient amount (about 30–60 mL). Instruct the patient to avoid touching the inside of the container with the penis.
   iv. Finish voiding into the toilet or urinal.
 	
B. Instruct the female patient:
   i. Kneel or squat over a bedpan or toilet bowl. Spread the labia minora widely to expose the meatus. Using an antiseptic wipe, cleanse on either side of the meatus, and then cleanse the meatus itself. Use a wipe only once in a sweep from the anterior to the posterior surfaces, and then discard it.
   ii. Keeping the labia separated, initially void a few seconds into the toilet.
   iii. Bring the sterile container into the urine stream and collect a sufficient amount (about 30–60 mL).
   iv. Finish voiding into the toilet or bedpan.
	The antiseptic solution removes bacteria from the urinary meatus and the surrounding skin. Wiping away from the meatus with an antiseptic wipe will remove bacteria from the area; wiping toward the meatus or returning to the area with a used wipe will reintroduce bacteria to the site. Organisms in the lower urethra and at the meatus will be washed away.
	Collecting the middle of the stream ensures the least contamination with skin bacteria. Touching the inside with the penis may contaminate the specimen.
	Prostatic fluid may be expressed at the end of the stream and may contaminate the specimen.
	
	The antiseptic solution removes bacteria from the urinary meatus. Bringing a wipe back to the surface already cleaned will recontaminate the area. The antiseptic solution is washed away before the specimen is collected at midstream.
	
	Organisms remaining in the meatus will be washed away.

PSY PROCEDURE 28-1: **Obtaining a Clean-Catch Midstream Urine Specimen (continued)**

Steps	Reasons
7. Cap the filled container and place it in a designated area.	Cap the container to protect the specimen from contamination and to protect the handler from exposure.
8. **AFF** Demonstrate recognition of the patient's level of understanding in communications. Apply active listening skills.	As this topic and the explanation are uncomfortable to most people, you must be sensitive to the patient's feelings. The instructions should be given in a professional manner. At the same time, you must apply active listening skills to recognize the patient's level of understanding.
9. Transport the specimen in a biohazard container for testing.	Transporting in a biohazard container will protect those who handle it in transit.
10. Properly care for or dispose of equipment and supplies. Clean the work area. Remove gloves and wash your hands.	Caring for supplies and the work area provide a safe environment and a clean environment for future testing. Washing hands is the key step of standard precautions.

Charting Example:

05/31/2012 1:30 PM Pt instructed in midstream collection of urine with antiseptic wipe. U/A: Color, straw; clarity, clear; specific gravity, 1.020; dipstick negative; pH 7.0. ——————————————————— S. Miller, CMA

Note: The medical assistant may sign his or her name in the patient record using only the "CMA" credential if the office has a signature log denoting the entire credential as "CMA(AAMA)."

PSY PROCEDURE 28-2: **Obtaining a 24-Hour Urine Specimen**

Purpose: To determine the quantity and proportion of substances in a 24-hour urine sample
Equipment: Patient's labeled 24-hour urine container (some patients require more than one container), preservatives required for the specific test, chemical hazard labels, graduated cylinder that holds at least 1 L, serologic or volumetric pipettes, clean random urine container, fresh 10% bleach solution, gloves, impervious gown, face shield, hand disinfectant, surface disinfectant

Steps	Reasons
1. Wash your hands.	Handwashing aids infection control.
2. Assemble the equipment.	Equipment must be readily accessible to perform the procedure.
3. **AFF** Identify the patient and explain the procedure. Display sensitivity to patient rights and feelings in collecting specimens. Explain the rationale for performance of the procedure to the patient. Show awareness of patients' concerns regarding their perceptions related to the procedure being performed. Ask for and answer any questions.	Explaining the procedure in an atmosphere of reassurance allows the patient to ask questions. Answering patient questions improves the probability of a quality specimen collection.
4. **AFF** If your patient is developmentally challenged, check with the individual who transported the patient to the office. Identify if this person is the caregiver or how to contact the caregiver to provide the instructions for collection.	Providing the caregiver with accurate, detailed instructions will improve the quality of the specimen.

(continued)

PSY PROCEDURE 28-2: **Obtaining a 24-Hour Urine Specimen** *(continued)*

Steps	Reasons
5. Identify the type of 24-hour urine collection requested and check for any special requirements, such as any acid or preservative that should be added. Label the container appropriately. 	Proper identification avoids errors. Special additives protect the integrity of the specimen. **Step 5.** 24–hour urine containers containing hazardous chemicals should be labeled appropriately.
6. Put on gloves, impervious gown, and face shield.	PPE protects you from exposure to biohazards.
7. Add to the 24-hour urine container the correct amount of acid or preservative using a serologic or volumetric pipette. Some reference laboratories provide these specimen containers to clients with the preservative already added.	This prevents altered findings due to incorrect preparation.
8. Use the provided label or make a label with spaces for the patient's name, beginning time and date, and ending time and date so that the patient can fill in the appropriate information.	This ensures that the patient documents the testing times.
9. Instruct the patient to collect a 24-hour urine sample as an follows: A. Void into the toilet, and note this time and date as the beginning. B. After the first voiding, collect each void and add it to the urine container for the next 24 hours. C. Precisely 24 hours after beginning collection, empty the bladder even if there is no urge to void and add this final volume of urine to the container. D. Note on the label the ending time and date.	Instructing the patient is required for accurate specimen collection.
10. **AFF** Explain to the patient that, depending on the test requested, the 24-hour urine may have to be refrigerated the entire time. Instruct the patient to return the specimen to you as soon as possible after collection is complete.	Proper care of the specimen prevents degradation of the urine components, which may alter findings.
11. **AFF** Demonstrate recognition of the patient's level of understanding in communications. Apply active listening skills.	As this topic and the explanation are uncomfortable to most people, you must be sensitive to the patient's feelings. The instructions should be given in a professional manner. At the same time, the medical assistant must apply active listening skills to recognize the patient's level of understanding.
12. Record in the patient's chart that supplies and instructions were given to collect a 24-hour urine specimen and the test that was requested.	This documents patient education and instructions.

PSY PROCEDURE 28-2: **Obtaining a 24-Hour Urine Specimen (continued)**

Steps	Reasons
13. When you receive the specimen, verify beginning and ending times and dates before the patient leaves. Check for any acids or preservatives to be added before the specimen goes to the testing laboratory.	This protects the integrity of the specimen.
14. Wearing gloves, impervious gown, and face shield, pour the urine into a cylinder to record the volume. Pour an aliquot of the urine into a clean container to be sent to the laboratory. (Label the specimen with the patient's ID.) Record the volume of the urine collection and the amount of any acid or preservative added on the sample container and on the laboratory requisition. If permitted, you may dispose of the remainder of the urine. Note that some reference labs will accept the entire 24-hour specimen and make this measurement at the laboratory.	PPE is required for protection from biohazards.
15. Record the volume on the patient's test requisition and chart.	Specimen volume is required in test calculations for providing test results.
16. Clean the cylinder with fresh 10% bleach solution and then rinse with water. Let it air dry. If you are using a disposable container, be sure to dispose of it in the proper biohazard container.	Adequate cleaning and disposal of contaminated equipment and supplies maintains a clean, safe environment.
17. Clean the work area and dispose of waste properly. Remove PPE and wash your hands.	Adequate cleaning of the work area is required to minimize exposure to biohazards and contamination. Washing hands is the key factor of standard precautions.

Note: Some containers come with the preservative already added. In either case, be sure the patient is instructed not to discard preservative and not to allow it to be handled. Instruct the patient not to void directly into the container.
Warning! Use caution when handling acids and other hazardous materials. Be familiar with the material safety data sheets for each chemical in your site.
Note: Depending on the type of office and laboratory, you may not need the aliquot.

Charting Example:

3/8/2012 9:30 am Pt instructed to collect urine for 24 hours and verbalized understanding. Pt was given container and written instructions to begin collecting at 8:00 am on 3/9 and to end on 3/10 at 8:00 am. Will bring specimen in on 3/10. ———————————————————————————————— *M. Smith, CMA*

3/10/2012 10:10 am Pt returned with 24-hour specimen collection. Total volume is 1850 mL. Labeled 50-mL aliquot to reference laboratory. ———————————————————————————————— *M. Smith, CMA*

Note: The medical assistant may sign his or her name in the patient record using only the "CMA" credential if the office has a signature log denoting the entire credential as "CMA(AAMA)."

PSY PROCEDURE 28-3: **Determining Color and Clarity of Urine**

Purpose: To determine the visible characteristics of a urine specimen
Equipment: Gloves, impervious gown, 10% bleach solution, patient's labeled urine specimen, clear tube, white paper scored with black lines, hand disinfectant, surface disinfectant, and usually a centrifuge.

Steps	Reasons
1. Wash your hands.	Handwashing aids infection control.
2. Assemble the equipment.	Equipment must be readily accessible to perform the procedure.
3. Put on PPE.	PPE is required for protection from biohazards.
4. Verify that the name on the specimen container and the name on the report form are the same.	This prevents reporting errors.
5. Pour about 10 mL of urine into the tube. If the specimen is less that 10 mL, note this on the test result form.	This provides an adequate quantity for testing and allows for visual assessment of the urine.
6. In bright light against a white background, examine the color. The most common colors are straw (very pale yellow), yellow, dark yellow, and amber (brown–yellow).	The intensity of the yellow color, which is due to urochrome, depends on urine concentration. (Table 28-2 has information about other urine colors).
7. Determine clarity. Hold the tube in front of the white paper scored with black lines. If you see the lines clearly (not obscured), record as clear. If you see the lines but they are not well delineated, record as hazy. If you cannot see the lines at all, record as cloudy.	The lines help discern clarity by providing contrast.
8. Properly care for or dispose of equipment and used supplies. Clean the work area using disinfectant. Remove PPE. Wash your hands.	Adequate cleaning of the work area is required to minimize exposure to biohazards and contamination. Washing hands is the key factor of standard precautions.
9. Report relevant information to others succinctly and accurately.	Reporting testing information clearly and accurately is required for records.

Note: Rapid determination of color and clarity is necessary because some urine turns cloudy if left standing. Bilirubin, which may be found in urine in certain conditions, breaks down when exposed to light. Protect the specimen from light if urinalysis is ordered but testing is delayed. If further testing is to be done but is delayed for more than an hour, refrigerate the specimen to avoid alteration of chemistry.

Charting Example:

05/31/2012 2:45 pm Random urine collected. Yellow/clear ———————————————— H. Henderson, CMA

Note: The medical assistant may sign his or her name in the patient record using only the "CMA" credential if the office has a signature log denoting the entire credential as "CMA(AAMA)."

PSY **PROCEDURE 28-4:** **Chemical Reagent Strip Analysis**

Purpose: To determine the level of constituents in a patient's urine to aid in the diagnosis of urinary or metabolic disorders

Equipment: Patient's labeled urine specimen, chemical strip (such as Multistix™ or Chemstrip™), manufacturer's color comparison chart, stopwatch or timer, PPE, hand disinfectant, surface disinfectant

Steps	Reasons
1. Wash your hands.	Handwashing aids infection control.
2. Assemble the equipment.	Equipment must be readily accessible to perform the procedure.
3. Put on PPE.	PPE is required for protection from biohazards.
4. Verify that the name on the specimen container and the name on the report form are the same.	This prevents reporting errors.
5. Mix the patient's urine by gently swirling the covered container.	Mixing the specimen is required to get a representation sample of the entire collection.
6. Remove the reagent strip from its container and replace the lid to prevent deterioration of the strips by humidity.	Urine dipsticks are extremely sensitive to moisture. They will not provide accurate test results without protection from the moisture in the environment.
7. Immerse the reagent strip in the urine completely, immediately remove it, sliding the edge of the strip along the lip of the container to remove excess urine. Pooling of excess urine on the dipstick causes cross-contamination among the reactions, possibly obscuring accurate color detection.	Immediate removal of the strip prevents colors from leaching during prolonged exposure to urine.
8. Start your stopwatch or timer immediately.	Reactions must be read at specific intervals as directed on the package insert and on the color comparison chart.
9. Compare the reagent pads to the color chart, determining results at the intervals stated by the manufacturer. Example: Glucose is read at 30 seconds. To determine results, examine that pad 30 seconds after dipping and compare with color chart for glucose.	This adheres to strict time-sensitive protocol.

(continued)

PSY PROCEDURE 28-4: Chemical Reagent Strip Analysis *(continued)*

Steps	Reasons

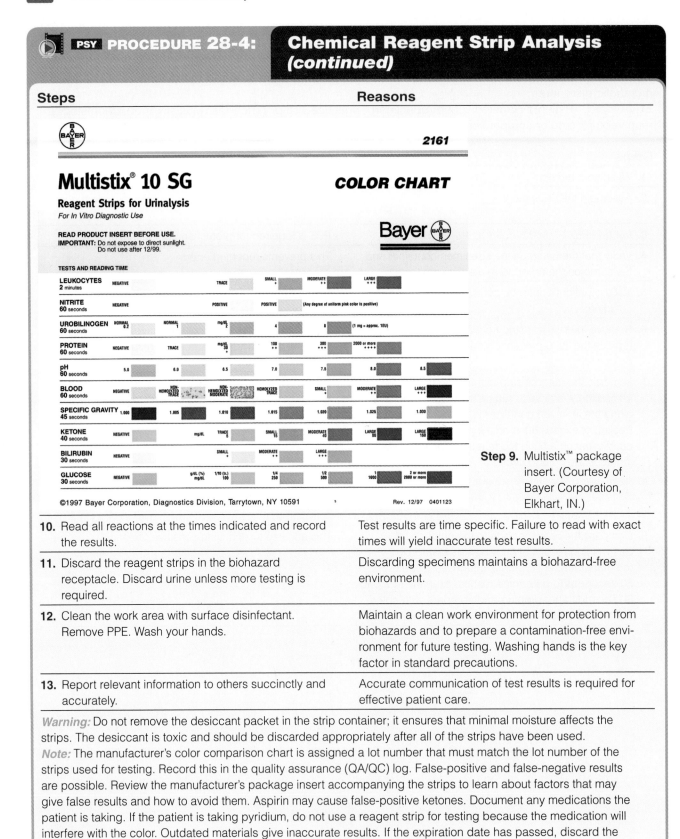

Step 9. Multistix™ package insert. (Courtesy of Bayer Corporation, Elkhart, IN.)

Steps	Reasons
10. Read all reactions at the times indicated and record the results.	Test results are time specific. Failure to read with exact times will yield inaccurate test results.
11. Discard the reagent strips in the biohazard receptacle. Discard urine unless more testing is required.	Discarding specimens maintains a biohazard-free environment.
12. Clean the work area with surface disinfectant. Remove PPE. Wash your hands.	Maintain a clean work environment for protection from biohazards and to prepare a contamination-free environment for future testing. Washing hands is the key factor in standard precautions.
13. Report relevant information to others succinctly and accurately.	Accurate communication of test results is required for effective patient care.

Warning: Do not remove the desiccant packet in the strip container; it ensures that minimal moisture affects the strips. The desiccant is toxic and should be discarded appropriately after all of the strips have been used.

Note: The manufacturer's color comparison chart is assigned a lot number that must match the lot number of the strips used for testing. Record this in the quality assurance (QA/QC) log. False-positive and false-negative results are possible. Review the manufacturer's package insert accompanying the strips to learn about factors that may give false results and how to avoid them. Aspirin may cause false-positive ketones. Document any medications the patient is taking. If the patient is taking pyridium, do not use a reagent strip for testing because the medication will interfere with the color. Outdated materials give inaccurate results. If the expiration date has passed, discard the materials.

PSY PROCEDURE 28-5: **Preparing Urine Sediment**

Purpose: To aid in the determination and identification of formed elements and solid particles in a urine specimen

Equipment: Patient's labeled urine specimen, urine centrifuge tubes, transfer pipette, centrifuge (1,500–2,000 rpm), gloves, impervious gown, face shield, hand disinfectant, surface disinfectant

Steps	Reasons
1. Wash your hands.	Handwashing aids infection control.
2. Assemble the equipment.	Equipment must be readily accessible to perform the procedure.
3. Put on PPE.	PPE is required for protection from biohazards.
4. Verify that the name on the specimen container and the name on the report form are the same.	This prevents reporting errors.
5. Swirl specimen to mix. Pour 10 mL of well-mixed urine into a labeled centrifuge tube or standard system tube. Cap the tube with a plastic cap or parafilm.	Capping the tube prevents a biohazardous aerosol when the centrifuge is running.
6. Centrifuge the sample at 1,500 rpm for 5 minutes.	Centrifugation ensures that cellular and particulate matter is pulled to the bottom of the tube.
7. When the centrifuge has stopped, remove the tubes. Make sure no tests are to be performed first on the supernatant. Remove the caps and pour off the supernatant, leaving 0.5–1.0 mL of it. Suspend the sediment again by aspirating up and down with a transfer pipette, or follow the manufacturer's directions for a standardized system.	The concentrated urine is now prepared for microscopic examination.
8. Properly care for and dispose of equipment and supplies. Clean the work area with surface disinfectant. Remove PPE. Wash your hands.	A clean environment is required for removal of biohazards. Washing hands is the key factor of standard precautions.

Note: If the urine is to be tested by chemical reagent strip, perform the dip test before spinning the urine. Preparing a urine specimen of less than 3 mL for sediment is not recommended because that is not enough urine to create a true sediment. However, some patients cannot provide a large amount of urine. In such cases, document the volume on the chart to ensure proper interpretation of results. Centrifuge maintenance requires periodic checks to ensure that the speed and timing are correct. Document this information on the maintenance log.

- Proper collection of a urine specimen varies with the test to be performed. Unless otherwise specified by the physician, a freshly voided specimen is all that is necessary. This is called a *random urine*. To diagnose a UTI, the specimen is collected either as a clean-catch midstream or by catheter and submitted to the laboratory in a sterile container with a lid. Detecting the microorganism causing the disease may require that a culture be performed. All cultures require that the specimen not be contaminated during the preliminary testing process.

- Once the urine is collected, many of its elements deteriorate within 1 hour. If testing cannot be performed within this time, the specimen is refrigerated at 4° to 8°C for up to 4 hours.

- The physical properties of urine include color, appearance (such as clarity or turbidity), specific gravity, and odor.

- The specific gravity reflects the ability of the kidney to concentrate or dilute the urine. Specific gravity for a normal urine specimen is 1.001 to 1.035.

- Urine contains chemicals produced in the body and ingested from the environment. The reagent strip produces 10 chemical measurements. Detecting and measuring chemical properties can facilitate the diagnosis of many conditions.

- The kidney helps maintain the acid–base balance of the body. To maintain a constant pH, the kidney must control the change of pH of the urine to balance the pH that results from diet and metabolism.

- Ketones are a group of chemicals produced during fat metabolism. In normal circumstances, energy is derived primarily from carbohydrate metabolism. In conditions of insufficient carbohydrates, as in starvation, low-carbohydrate diet, and inadequately managed diabetes, fats are used by the body for energy, and ketones are produced.

- Small quantities of proteins are found in normal urine. Proteinuria is an important indicator of renal disease.

- Bilirubin is formed during breakdown of hemoglobin. It is processed in the liver before being excreted into the intestines. A normal reagent strip test result for bilirubin is negative. Bilirubinuria can occur with certain liver diseases (e.g., hepatitis), biliary tract obstruction, and hemolytic states such as transfusion reactions.

- The bilirubin that goes to the intestines mixes with the enzymes from bacteria already in the intestinal tract. The enzymes break bilirubin into parts. One of the parts is called *urobilinogen*. Most urobilinogen is eliminated in the feces. A small amount is excreted by the kidneys. Small amounts of urobilinogen are normally found in urine, usually 0.1 to 1.0 mg/dL.

- A positive nitrite test result indicates bacteriuria, which occurs with UTIs. A negative nitrite test result does not indicate the absence of bacteriuria since all types of bacteria do not reduce nitrate to nitrite.

- Leukocytes in the urine indicate a UTI. A positive leukocyte esterase test indicates that WBCs are present in the specimen. Normal urine may contain a few WBCs but not in sufficient numbers to produce a positive leukocyte esterase test.

- Turbidity or precipitation tests confirm a positive protein result on the reagent test strip. The most common confirmation test is observing the amount of cloudiness when equal amounts of urine and SSA are mixed.

- Many laboratories confirm a positive bilirubin result on the urine test strip result using a diazo tablet method (Ictotest™). The diazo tablet procedure is good for confirmation because it is more sensitive than the strip procedure.

- The following structures may appear in the urine: RBCs, WBCs, bacteria, epithelial cells, crystals, casts, and others.

- Hematuria is the presence of RBCs in urine. This may indicate glomerular damage, tumors of the urinary tract, kidney trauma, urinary stones, renal infarcts, acute tubular necrosis, upper and lower UTIs, nephrotoxins, and physical distress.

- Bacteria are always present on the skin but not usually in the bladder. The presence of significant amounts (more than a trace) of bacteria in a urine specimen is considered an indication of a UTI.

- A urinalysis is a physical and chemical examination of urine to assess renal function and other possible problems. Because so many urinalyses are done in the office laboratory, proficiency in this skill is essential for the medical assistant.

1. A patient was taking a medication that changed the color of his urine. How did this impact urine testing? What action should the medical assistant take?

2. What effects on test results are caused by leaving the urine specimen at room temperature for an extended length of time? How does this impact the usefulness of the test results?

3. Physicians frequently send orders back to the laboratory to have a culture and sensitivity done on a urine specimen that was collected earlier for urinalysis. What actions are necessary for the urine to still be acceptable for additional testing?

4. Create a patient education brochure for collecting a clean catch, midstream urine specimen. Remember that all patients may not understand clinical terms for laboratory specimens.

5. A urine specimen is left in the light for an extended period of time. What chemistry may be affected by this? Why?

6. A patient with kidney disease has a urinalysis. Which dipstick chemistry test will be elevated for this reason?

Microbiology and Immunology

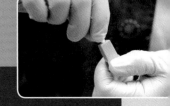

Outline

**Standard Precautions and
Safety in the Microbiology
Laboratory**
Biohazards
Chemical Hazards
Equipment
**Microbiology Specimen
Collection and Handling
Techniques**
Quality Control in Handling
Microbiological
Specimens
Demonstrate Effective
Communication Skills
during Patient Education
Transporting the Specimens
Culture Techniques
Types of Specimens
Culture Media
Physical States of Media

Functional Types of Media
Caring for the Media
Incubation
**Slide Preparation and
Staining**
Identification by Staining
Bacterial Morphology
Susceptibility Testing
Microbiology Test Reports
Rickettsia and Chlamydia
Mycoplasma
Viruses
Eukaryotic Microorganisms
Fungi
Protozoa and Helminths
Nematodes and Arthropods
Infections of Body Systems
Integumentary
Respiratory

Gastrointestinal
Nervous
Genitourinary
Reproductive
Host Defense Mechanisms
**Physical and Chemical
Methods of Control**
Fecal Blood Testing
The Immune System
Diseases Caused by the
Immune System
Immunological Testing
Principles
Waived Tests Based on
Immunological Testing
Principles
**The Medical Assistant's
Responsibilities in
the Microbiology and
Immunology Laboratories**

Learning Outcomes

Cognitive Domain

*Note: AAMA/CAAHEP 2008 Standards are
italicized.*
1. Spell and define the key terms
2. *List major types of infectious agents*
3. *Compare different methods of controlling
   the growth of microorganisms*
4. *Discuss quality control issues related to
   handling microbiological specimens*
5. Describe the medical assistant's
   responsibilities in microbiological testing
6. *Analyze charts, graphs, and/or tables in the
   interpretation of health care results*

Psychomotor Domain

*Note: AAMA/CAAHEP 2008 Standards are
italicized.*
1. Collect throat specimens (Procedure 29-1)
2. Collect nasopharyngeal specimens
   (Procedure 29-2)
3. Collect wound specimens (Procedure 29-3)
4. Collect sputum specimens (Procedure 29-4)
5. Collect stool specimens (Procedure 29-5)
6. Collect blood specimens for culture
   (Procedure 29-6)
7. Collect genital specimens (Procedure 29-7)

8. Test stool specimens for occult blood (Procedure 29-8)
9. Prepare a smear for microscopic evaluation (Procedure 29-9)
10. Perform a Gram stain (Procedure 29-10)
11. Inoculate a culture (Procedure 29-11)
12. Perform mononucleosis testing (Procedure 29-12)
13. Perform human chorionic gonadotropin pregnancy testing (Procedure 29-13)
14. Perform rapid group A strep testing (Procedure 29-14)
15. *Prepare patient for procedures and/or treatments*
16. *Document patient care*
17. *Respond to issues of confidentiality*
18. *Perform within scope of practice*
19. *Perform quality control measures*
20. *Screen test results*
21. *Practice standard precautions*
22. *Perform handwashing*
23. *Perform CLIA-waived microbiology testing*
24. *Practice within the standard of care for a medical assistant*

Affective Domain

Note: AAMA/CAAHEP 2008 Standards are italicized.

1. *Distinguish between normal and abnormal test results*
2. *Display sensitivity to patient rights and feelings in collecting specimens*
3. *Explain the rationale for performance of a procedure to the patient*
4. *Show awareness of patient's concerns regarding their perceptions related to the procedure being performed*

5. *Demonstrate empathy in communicating with patients, family, and staff*
6. *Apply active listening skills*
7. *Use appropriate body language and other nonverbal skills in communicating with patients, family, and staff*
8. *Demonstrate awareness of territorial boundaries of the person with whom you are communicating*
9. *Demonstrate sensitivity appropriate to the message being delivered*
10. *Demonstrate recognition of the patient's level of understanding in communications*
11. *Recognize and protect personal boundaries in communicating with others*
12. *Demonstrate respect for individual diversity, incorporating awareness of one's own biases in areas including gender, race, religion, age, and economic status*

ABHES Competencies

1. Document patient care
2. Perform quality control measures
3. Screen test results
4. Perform immunology testing
5. Practice standard precautions
6. Perform handwashing
7. Obtain specimens for microbiology testing
8. Perform CLIA-waived microbiology testing
9. Perform pregnancy test
10. Perform Strep A test
11. Instruct patients in the collection of fecal specimens

Key Terms

aerobes	differential stain	immunity	opportunistic
agar	diplococci	inoculum	pilosebaceous unit
anaerobes	endometrium	isolate	resistant
bacilli (singular, bacillus)	erector pili muscle	Kirby-Bauer method	sensitive
biological agent	erythrasma	media	sensitivity testing
biohazard symbol	eyewashes	mordant	smears
broth	folliculitis	mycology	specificity
carbuncle	furuncle	mycoses	spirochetes
cervix	Gram negative	normal flora	subcutaneous
cocci	Gram positive	nosocomial infection	superficial
cultures	Gram stain	ophthalmia neonatorum	systemic
	impetigo		

Microbiology is the study of small life. The "micro" part of the name specifies that the part of life in this study is microscopic. In microbiology, the goal is to identify pathogens in the specimens submitted to the department. **Normal flora** are bacteria that normally live on the body and do not cause disease. In microbiology, the specimens that are submitted contain the pathogen (if one is present) along with the normal flora growing at the site that was cultured. Microbiology's job is to separate the pathogen and identify it from the midst of all the bacteria growing on the culture. The use of standard precautions in microbiology is to protect the medical assistant, the physician, patients, and all coworkers from **nosocomial infections**. Nosocomial infections are infections acquired in a medical setting.

Bacteria require the following five elements for survival: nutrients, warmth, moisture, darkness, and oxygen (**aerobes**) or lack of oxygen (**anaerobes**). The microbiology laboratory uses culture media, incubators, and techniques to control the specimen's exposure to oxygen to provide these conditions.

Specimens submitted to the microbiology laboratory are collected from wounds, the throat, vagina, urethra, or skin, using a swab. Specimens may be collected during surgery and also by venipuncture. Sputum, stool, or urine are other possible specimens. In all instances, aseptic technique must be practiced to ensure the integrity of the specimen (see Chapter 2).

COG **Standard Precautions and Safety in the Microbiology Laboratory**

Biohazards

As in all other laboratories, standard precautions are the primary source of safety against biological agents. **Biological agents** are the bacteria, viruses, fungi that are submitted to microbiology as specimens. The **biohazard symbol** (Fig. 29-1) is a universal warning of the presence of biological agents. The biological agents can cause rashes, illness, and even death. Always be reminded that the most effective standard precaution is handwashing (Fig. 29-2).

 CHECKPOINT QUESTION

1. What are the possible adverse effects from exposure to some biological agents?

Chemical Hazards

The Occupational Safety and Health Administration (OSHA) safety standards for the use of chemicals is important for safety in microbiology, too. The same chemical hygiene plan that includes material safety

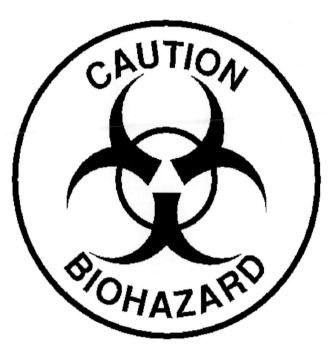

Figure 29-1 Biohazard symbol.

data sheets for each chemical are required for microbiology also.

 CHECKPOINT QUESTION

2. What is the document the physicians' office prepares to outline its plan for chemical safety?

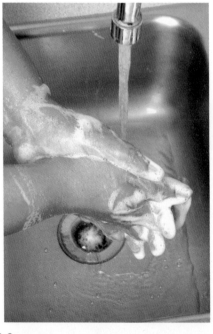

Figure 29-2 Good handwashing skills are essential to prevent disease transmission. (From Molle EA, Durham LS, West-Stack C. LWW's Textbook for Administrative Medical Assisting. Baltimore: Lippincott Williams & Wilkins, 2004.)

Equipment

Safety equipment in microbiology is the same safety equipment used throughout the laboratory.

Eyewashes are used to irrigate and flush the eyes following a hazardous exposure. They are a safety tool available in some laboratories. If eyewashes are present, employees must be trained in their proper use, and, as with the fire extinguishers, training must be documented and the records retained in the safety manual. Eyewashes should be clearly marked so that they may be accessed within the first seconds after the exposure. If an MSDS indicates that first aid response to an exposure requires flushing for 15 or more minutes, then an eyewash station or safety shower is required. Requirements less than 15 minutes require no special equipment. This applies to all sections of the laboratory.

 CHECKPOINT QUESTION

3. How is the need for an eyewash station in a physicians' office laboratory determined?

Personal protective equipment (PPE) is used in the microbiology laboratory to protect from biohazardous and chemical exposures as it is throughout the clinical areas. Shoes worn in the laboratory should not be sandals or any type of open-toed shoe to avoid exposure to spills.

COG Microbiology Specimen Collection and Handling Techniques

Microbiology reports give the physician a snapshot of the condition of the site used to obtain the specimen. For instance, a throat culture will identify pathogens present in the throat. For meaningful results, the specimen must be collected from the appropriate site using the proper method. The specimen must also be handled so that test results will be accurate (Box 29-1).

Most microbiology specimens for culture in a physicians' office laboratory are referred to a reference laboratory. To identify the correct method for collecting and transporting these specimens, refer to the laboratory's specimen manual. Table 29-1 is an example of an excerpt from a specimen manual. The medical assistant must follow the guidelines listed in the charts to identify the correct methods for the specific specimen being referred.

 CHECKPOINT QUESTION

4. What is the appropriate transport media for dialysis fluid? Use Table 29-1 to determine your answer.

BOX 29-1

GUIDELINES FOR SPECIMEN COLLECTION AND HANDLING

- Follow standard precautions for specimen collection as outlined by the Centers for Disease Control and Prevention.
- Review the requirements for collecting and handling the specimen, including the equipment, the type of specimen to be collected (e.g., exudate, blood, mucus), the amount required for laboratory analysis, and the procedure to be followed for handling and storage.
- Assemble the equipment and supplies. Use only the appropriate specimen container as specified by the medical office or laboratory.
- Ensure that the specimen container is sterile to prevent contamination of the specimen by organisms not present at the collection site.
- Examine each container before use to make sure that it is not damaged, the medium is intact and moist, and it is well within the expiration date.
- Label each tube or specimen container with the patient's name and/or identification number, the date, the name or initials of the person collecting the specimen, the source or site of the specimen, and any other information required by the laboratory. Use an indelible pen or permanent marker. Make sure you print legibly, document accurately, and include all pertinent information.

Quality Control in Handling Microbiological Specimens

The result of a laboratory test is only as good as the specimen.

- Specimen collection
  1. Positively identify the patient before collecting a specimen.
  2. Label the specimen according to laboratory procedure. All information described previously must be included. If the specimen is not fully and correctly labeled, the laboratory may be required to dispose of the specimen and cancel the request. This is critical for specimens that cannot be resampled such as a surgical specimen.
  3. Prepare the patient for the collection procedure. This may include instructing the patient of the preparation procedure before the day of the collection.
  4. Verify use of correct collection container, required volume of specimen, and appropriate timing of specimen collection.

TABLE **29-1**	Specimen Collection Guidelines by Specimen Type or Site	
A list of common specimens with the recommended method of collection and transport.		
Specimen Type or Site	**Volume or Method of Collection**	**Container or Transport**
Abscess		
Bacteria, fungal	1–5 ml aspirate swab	Sterile no-additive tube, culturette, or transport medium
Acid-fast bacillus (AFB) (tuberculosis)	1–5 ml aspirate	Sterile no-additive tube
Blood		
Bacteria (1 culture = 1 set)	10 ml	Aerobe (silver-top bottle)
Adult	10 ml	Anaerobe (purple-top bottle)
Peds/short draw	1–3 ml	Aerobe (blue-top bottle)
Fungal	10 ml, adult	Isolator tube
	1.5 ml, infant	
AFB	10 ml	Isolator tube; can combine with fungal request
Body fluids (sterile)		
Joint, pericardial, peritoneal, pleural, vitreous, etc. Bacteria, fungal, AFB	5 ml, optimal 1 ml, minimum	Sterile no-additive tube
Bronchial washing		
Bacteria, fungal, AFB	1–5 ml	Sterile container
Cervix		
Bacteria, fungal, AFB	Swab	Transport medium
Cerebrospinal fluid		
Bacteria	0.5 ml minimum	Sterile no-additive tube
Fungal (includes Cryptococcal Antigen)	2 ml minimum	Sterile no-additive tube
AFB	1 ml minimum	Sterile no-additive tube
Cyst fluid		
Bacteria, fungal, AFB	1–5 ml aspirate optimal, swab	Sterile tube; transport medium
Dialysis fluid		
Bacteria	1 ml minimum for Gram stain 10 ml per blood culture bottle	Sterile no-additive tube One aerobic (silver top) tube and one anaerobic (purple top) tube
Ear		
Bacteria, fungal, AFB	Swab	Transport medium
Exudate (pus)		
Bacteria, fungal, AFB Fungal, AFB	Aspirate optimal, swab Aspirate, tissue, bone, pus, aspirated fluid	Sterile no-additive transport medium
Eye		
Bacteria, fungal, AFB	Swab, ocular specimen	Transport medium
Hair	Hair shaft and base	Dry, sterile container
Nail	Nail shavings and debris	Dry, sterile container
Skin scrapings	Edge of lesion	Dry, sterile container

Specimen Type or Site	Volume or Method of Collection	Container or Transport
<u>Skin scrapings</u>	Edge of lesion	Dry, sterile container
<u>Sinus</u>		
Bacteria, fungal, AFB Fungal, AFB	Aspirate optimal, swab Aspirate, tissue, pus, bone	Sterile tube; transport medium
<u>Sputum:</u> Three to five specimens, *collected on separate days*, will be accepted for culture (preferably first morning sputum). Additional specimens submitted after bronchoscopy or after therapy is initiated will be accepted Bacteria, fungal AFB	5 ml 5 ml, minimum	Sterile screw-capped Sterile screw-capped
<u>Stool</u> Bacteria (intestinal tract culture [ITC])	10-gm minimum if delivery will be delayed	Container with sterile, leak-proof lid; deliver to lab within 1 hour via Cary Blair Transport (not suitable if looking for yeast)
Ova and parasite	10-gm minimum if delivery will be delayed	Container with sterile, leak-proof lid. Deliver to lab within 1 hour Formalin/polyvinyl alcohol (PVA) vials
C. difficile toxin	10 gm, minimum	Container with sterile, leak-proof lid; deliver to lab within 1 hour
Fecal specimens for WBCs, occult, fecal fat	10 gm, minimum	Container with sterile, leak-proof lid; deliver to lab within 1 hour
<u>Throat</u> Bacteria, fungal	Swab	Transport medium
<u>Tracheal aspirate</u> Bacteria, fungal, AFB	5 ml, minimum	Sterile screw-capped container
<u>Transtracheal</u>	As much as possible	Sterile tube or container; deliver to lab immediately
<u>Ulcer</u> Bacteria, fungal, AFB Fungal, AFB	Aspirate optimal, swab Aspirate, pus, tissue	Sterile tube; transport medium
<u>Urethral cultures</u> Bacteria, fungal, AFB	Exudate or drainage, swab	Sterile tube; transport medium
<u>Urine</u> Bacteria, fungal	10 ml, minimum	Urine-specific Vacutainer Tube or a sterile screw-capped container
<u>Uterine cultures</u> Bacteria, fungal	Exudate or drainage, swab	BD vacutainer urine C&S Preservative Plus plastic tube
<u>Vaginal</u> Bacteria Fungal	Swab Tissue, pus, aspirate	Transport medium
<u>Wound</u> Bacteria Fungal, AFB	Aspirate optimal, swab Aspirated fluid, pus, tissue, bone, ocular specimens	Sterile tube; transport medium

BOX 29-2

SPECIAL STOOL SPECIMENS

Follow these tips when collecting stool specimens to test for pinworms or parasites or to obtain a swab for culture. Remember to follow standard precautions.

- *Pinworms:* Schedule the appointment early in the morning, preferably before a bowel movement or bath. Pinworms tend to leave the rectum and lay eggs around the anus during the night. Press clear adhesive tape against the anal area. Remove it quickly and place it sticky side down on a glass slide for the physician to inspect.
- *Parasites:* Caution the patient not to use a laxative or enema before the test to avoid destroying the evidence of parasites. If the stool contains blood or mucus, include as much as possible in the specimen container because these substances are most likely to contain the suspected organism.
- *Stool culture:* A sterile cotton-tipped swab is passed into the rectal canal beyond the sphincter and rotated carefully. Place it in the appropriate culture container or process as directed for smear preparation.

5. See Box 29-2 for tips when collecting stool specimens to test for pinworms or parasites or to obtain a swab for culture. Remember to follow standard precautions.
6. Check the laboratory procedure manual for requirements for preserving the specimen. Use the appropriate transport media, if indicated (Fig. 29-3).
7. Collect the required specimen for each test ordered.

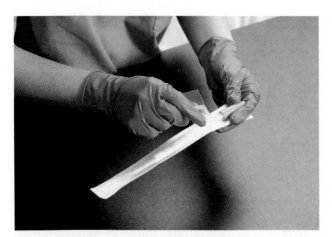

Figure 29-3 Preparing transport media for use.

8. Follow any special handling requirement. Among other instructions, these may include refrigeration, freezing, and/or protection from light.
- Specimen transport
  1. Train transporting personnel in appropriate safety and packaging procedures.
  2. Package and preserve specimens appropriately and securely for travel.
  3. Transport specimens at the appropriate temperature.
  4. Determine acceptable transport time.
  5. Determine mode of transport.

These steps are important for keeping the pathogen alive until it reaches the laboratory.

- Specimen handling
  The steps for handling a specimen for testing in microbiology are detailed and specific. It is detrimental to the patient if a specimen is mishandled or lost. Most specimens for culture cannot be simply recollected. Each step in the process is to keep the pathogen alive and the patient source correctly identified throughout the handling, transporting, testing, and reporting process.

  1. Handle all specimens as if infectious. Follow standard precautions.
  2. Track all specimens. The laboratory needs to be aware of any delays in transportation.
     Follow with ID and a sample number.
     Confirm specimen receipt within the medical office.
     Confirm date and time of specimen receipt.
- Specimen referral
  1. Document the time lapse before referral. Record:
     Tests/specimens referred
     Date of referral
     Name of person referring test
  2. Monitor/track and record:
     Turnaround time
     Results delivery
     Problems with referral
- Specimen storage
  1. Follow laboratory procedures for:
     Storage requirements
     Specimen retention time
     Storage location
- Specimen disposal for any specimen remnants remaining at the collection site
  1. Follow laboratory disinfection and disposal policies
  2. Comply with local regulations
  3. Review all stored specimens per the laboratory schedule for timely disposal

See Box 29-3 for the responsibilities of the medical assistant receiving the specimen at the reference laboratory.

RESPONSIBILITIES OF THE MEDICAL ASSISTANT RECEIVING THE SPECIMEN AT THE REFERRAL LABORATORY

- Verify completeness of the test requisition.
- Verify the integrity of the specimen:
  1. Determine adequate amount and condition of specimen.
  2. Determine that specimen is legibly and appropriately labeled.
  3. Determine if appropriate specimen was submitted for the requested test.
  4. Determine notation of collector identification.
  5. Enforce procedures for rejecting specimens.

CHECKPOINT QUESTION

5. Why are there so many steps for handling a specimen for culture?

Demonstrate Effective Patient Communication Skills during Patient Education

Demonstrate effective communication skills during patient education. In order for you to obtain a good specimen, the patient needs to understand the collection instructions and why they are important to him or her. Display sensitivity to patient rights and feelings in collecting specimens. Patients may be sensitive to the sites and collection methods for some specimens. Be aware that patients may have concerns about what they think having a test means. The medical assistant must use active listening skills to recognize when a patient does not understand the instructions and may be intimidated to say so. Demonstrate empathy in clarifying instructions to avoid embarrassing the patient. Smile and use a relaxed body posture to set a relaxed atmosphere. Respect the patient's need for personal space when discussing intimate body parts.

Keep in mind that communication techniques may need to be adjusted out of respect for individual diversity, gender, race, religion, age, and economic status.

CHECKPOINT QUESTION

6. Why is accurate communication necessary in instructing patients on specimen collection?

Transporting the Specimens

Care must be taken to transport or process the specimen as soon as possible so the organisms do not die. The sooner the specimen is processed, the sooner the pathogen can be identified and treatment can begin. Some microorganisms, such as *Neisseria gonorrhoeae*, are very fragile and must be cultured under controlled conditions as quickly as possible.

Specimens to be processed in outside or regional laboratories must be placed in transport medium such as Culturette (Marion Scientific) (Fig. 29-4) or Precision Culture CATS (Precision Dynamics). All directions appropriate for the specimen are stated on the package. Most transport systems are designed to be self-contained and include a plastic tube with a sterile swab and transport medium appropriate for the type of specimen. Most are stored at room temperature.

Special care must be taken in filling out all identification slips and information.

Properly prepared transport media may be mailed or routed by a courier. The reference laboratory may provide a mailing or shipping container, either cardboard or plastic foam, to protect the specimen during transport. A label indicating the presence of a biohazardous biological specimen is attached to the outside of the container. In many instances, specimens are collected and transported on days that ensure their arrival during the business week to avoid having them remain in transit until the start of a new week. Delays in testing may cause some of the microorganisms to die or to overproliferate, possibly compromising the results of the test. Communication with the testing laboratory is necessary to accomplish this coordination.

For the most reliable results, laboratory tests should be performed on fresh specimens within 1 hour after collection. When this is not possible, the specimen must be stored properly to preserve the physical and chemical properties necessary for accurate diagnosis. Specimens should never be subjected to extreme temperature changes. Table 29-2 lists general guidelines for handling and storing specimens commonly collected in the medical office.

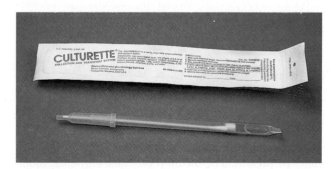

Figure 29-4 Transport media.

TABLE 29-2	Handling and Storing Commonly Collected Specimens	
	Handling	**Storage**
Urine	Clean-catch midstream with care to avoid contaminating the inside of the container; must not stand more than 1 hour after collection.	Refrigerate if cannot be tested within 1 hour; add preservative at direction of laboratory; preservatives not usually used for urine culture.
Blood	Handle carefully, as hemolysis may destroy microorganisms; collect in anticoagulant tube at room temperature; specimen must remain free of contaminants; see laboratory manual for proper anticoagulant.	For most specimens, refrigerate at 4°C (39°F) to slow changes in physical and chemical composition.
Stool	Collect in clean container. To test for ova and parasites, keep warm.	Deliver to laboratory immediately. If delayed, mix with preservative provided or recommended by laboratory, or use transport medium.
Microbiology specimens	Do not contaminate swab or inside of specimen container by touching either to surface other than site of collection. Protect anaerobic specimens from exposure to air.	Transport specimen as soon as possible. If delayed, refrigerate at 4°C (39°F) to maintain integrity.

Observe standard precautions while handling any of these specimens.

 CHECKPOINT QUESTION

7. List three reasons that culture specimens must be handled as soon as possible after collection.

COG **Culture Techniques**

To identify a microorganism, the first requirement is to put it in a place it can grow. That supportive environment is created in bacterial **cultures**. To culture a specimen, a small sample, the **inoculum**, is placed into or onto the culture medium using a wire probe. The organisms will replicate under controlled conditions. After incubation, the colonies of the pathogen can be separated from normal flora and removed from the agar for identification. Procedure 29-11 describes the steps for culture inoculation.

Types of Specimens

Procedures for patient instruction, collection, and assisting physician collection of specimens for microbiology testing are outlined in Procedures 29-1 through 29-7.

Culture Media

Media support the growth of microorganisms for identification. Various types of **media** are prepared with a mixture of substances that nourish pathogens. All of the suspected microorganism's requirements for growth must be present. The medium provides nutrients, moisture, and the proper pH.

Physical States of Media

Liquid media are solutions that do not solidify at temperatures above freezing. The liquid media is most often poured into glass tubes or bottles and refered to as **broth**. A commonly used liquid media is nutrient broth, which contains beef extract and other nutrients.

Semisolid media have more agar or gelatin than the liquid media. Semisolid media provide information about the bacteria by observing its motility and growth pattern.

Solid media are most often poured into Petri dishes. When they gel, they offer a flat surface for growing bacteria or fungi. The plate's lid maintains the integrity of the specimen. Petri plates are clear and allow visual examination of a culture as it grows. **Agar** is the most widely used solid media. The basic component of agar comes from red algae. Various nutrients are added to agar to support growth of different organisms. These agars are named in relation to their nutrients, for example, *nutrient agar* and *blood agar*. Observing the response of the organism to various agars offers information helpful in determining the organism's identity.

Functional Types of Media

General purpose media are used to support the growth of a wide variety of bacteria that do not have special growth requirements. The special media are enriched, selective, and differential media.

- *Enriched media* contain added nutrients such as blood, serum, hemoglobin, or specific growth factors. Chocolate agar has heat-treated blood added. It turns a brown, chocolate color giving it that name.

• *Selective media* allow some organisms to grow by limiting the growth of other organisms. This is helpful in separating the pathogen from the normal flora. An example is mannitol salt agar. The salt additive inhibits most human pathogens other than *Staphylococcus*. So, if bacterial colonies grow on a mannitol salt agar plate when it is cultured from a specimen with mixed bacteria, those colonies are most likely one of the *Staphylococcus* species.

• *Differential media* grow several different organisms allowing them to show visible differences. Some of the differences make identification easier. Colonies of different bacteria grow a different color, different bacteria cause the agar to change color, some bacteria form gas bubbles in the agar. An example is MacConkey agar. This agar contains neutral red, a dye that is yellow at a neutral pH and pink or red at an acidic pH. *Escherichia coli*, usually found in the intestinal tract, becomes acidic growing on this agar, so it appears pink or red. *Salmonella* remains a neutral pH growing on this agar, so it appears a natural off-white color.

Caring for the Media

Culture media in disposable plastic petri dishes can be purchased from medical supply companies. The plates are supplied in a plastic sleeve and must be stored in the refrigerator with the side containing the medium on top (Fig. 29-5). The plates should be stored in the plastic wrapper to keep the medium moist. Petri plates stored with the medium down may form condensation on the lids that will drip onto the surface, making it too moist for an accurate culture. Check the expiration date and the condition of the medium surface before using the plates. Discard any plates that are past the expiration date or any medium that has dried or cracked. When the shipment arrives, date each sleeve.

When a new shipment of media is received, move the oldest media to the front so it is used first. Media come with an expiration date just as other laboratory reagents do. Use the oldest first, based on the date it expires, not the date it was received. Note that the temperature of the refrigerator should be checked and recorded daily. Be sure not to overfill the refrigerator or allow media to be placed against the back wall or sides. This will raise the temperature.

Agar must be refrigerated until needed and then warmed to room temperature before use. A cold plate or tube will kill many microorganisms. A warmer temperature for growth is provided by an incubator set at about 99°F (37°C), or just about body temperature. Check and record the incubator temperature daily.

Incubation

The inoculated media are incubated in an incubator with the temperature set between 20° and 40° C. The temperature and darkness are maintained by an incubator (Fig. 29-6). The incubator maintains optimal temperature; humidity; and other conditions, such as the carbon dioxide and oxygen content of the atmosphere inside.

Incubation containers designed for anaerobic bacteria (bacteria that live without oxygen) may contain a tablet that generates carbon dioxide and eliminates oxygen in the closed environment of the medium container. Figure 29-7 displays one type of anaerobic culture setup.

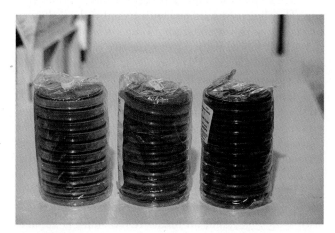

Figure 29-5 Solid media are supplied on Petri plates wrapped in a plastic sleeve. Petri plates are always stored medium side up.

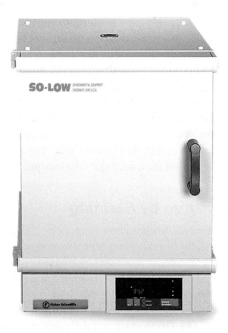

Figure 29-6 Standard laboratory incubator. (Courtesy of So-Low Environmental Equipment, Cincinnati, OH.)

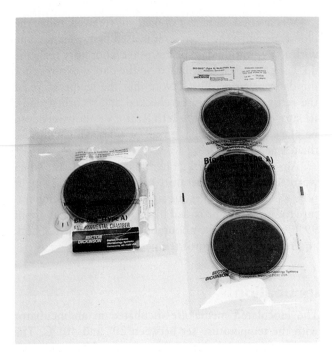

Figure 29-7 The Bio-Bag anaerobic culture set. It includes a plate of CDC-anaerobic blood agar in an oxygen-impermeable bag. The system contains its own gas-generating kit and cold catalyst. (Courtesy of Becton Dickinson, Franklin Lakes, NJ.)

COG Slide Preparation and Staining

To observe microorganisms with a microscope, the specimen requires preparation on a slide and staining as described in Procedure 29-9. Some pathogens are more easily identified if they are allowed to move freely in a wet mount. For more information about wet mounts, see Box 29-4. These are best viewed immediately, but at the latest, they should be viewed within 30 minutes of collection. To preserve the specimen for longer-term evaluation, the technique described in Procedure 29-9 should be used. Materials that have been dried on glass slides are called **smears**. The specimen is fixed to the slide by a short exposure to heat. Once fixed to the slide, the smear must be stained to be visible under the microscope.

Identification by Staining

Staining the microorganisms may help the physician narrow the field of possible pathogens and initiate treatment before a culture has been incubated. Most bacteria are hard to see or identify without special treatment such as staining.

The primary stain used in the microbiology lab is the **Gram stain**. The Gram stain is a **differential stain**. In the Gram stain process four-steps prepare the slide in a process that differentiates bacteria into **Gram-negative** and

---

BOX 29-4

PREPARING A WET MOUNT SLIDE

To prepare a wet mount, follow these steps:

1. Place a drop of the specimen on a glass slide with sterile saline or 10% potassium hydroxide (KOH).
2. Place a coverslip over the specimen to reduce evaporation.
3. To decrease evaporation, coat the rim of the coverslip with petrolatum.
4. Inspect the slide by microscope using the high-power objective lens with diminished light.

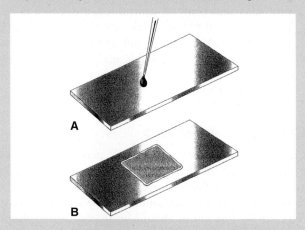

Wet mount slide preparation. **(A)** A drop of fluid containing the organism is placed on a glass slide. **(B)** The specimen is covered with a coverslip ringed with petroleum jelly.

Gram-positive groups. The procedure for Gram staining is detailed in Procedure 29-10.

Each step of the staining procedure has a specific reason. The slide is first stained with crystal violet, followed by rinsing with water. Gram's iodine is applied. Gram's iodine is a **mordant** used to fix the dye on the smear to make is more intense. The iodine is removed from the slide with a water rinse. If viewed under the microscope at this point, the bacteria would appear purple. Next, 95% ethyl alcohol is applied to the slide to remove the color. Gram-positive bacteria will keep the purple color even when exposed to the ethyl alcohol. Gram-negative bacteria will lose the purple color when exposed to the ethyl alcohol. If viewed under the microscope now, the Gram-negative bacteria would be difficult to detect because they will be almost colorless. The slide is again rinsed with water. Safranin, an intensely red stain, is applied. The slide is rinsed one last time with water to remove the excess safranin. Bacteria that retain the primary purple color of the crystal violet stain are called *Gram-positive*

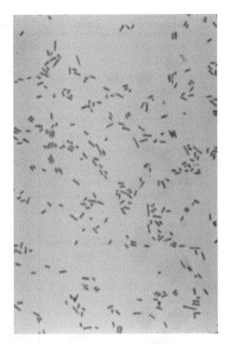

Figure 29-8 Gram-negative bacteria. (From Sweet RL, Gibbs RS. Atlas of Infectious Diseases of the Female Genital Tract. Philadelphia: Lippincott Williams & Wilkins, 2005.)

TABLE 29-3	Categorizing Bacteria
Morphology	**Types**
Round (spherical)	Cocci
Grapelike clusters	Staphylococci
Chain formations	Streptococci
Paired	Diplococci
Rod shaped	Bacilli
Somewhat oval	Coccobacilli
End-to-end chains	Streptobacilli
Spiral	Spirochetes
Flexible (usually with flagella, whip-like extremities that aid movement)	Spiralla
Rigid, curved rods (comma-shaped)	Vibrios

bacteria. The remaining bacteria appear red or pink due to the safranin stain. These are said to be *Gram negative* (Fig. 29-8). They are red because the crystal violet was lost. The mordant did not hold the purple color onto the smear when the ethyl alcohol was applied. Procedure 29-10 details the steps for Gram staining a smear.

Clinical Laboratory Improvement Amendments (CLIA) regulations allow the medical assistant to prepare the Gram stain to be read and reported by the physician. It is beyond the scope of practice for a medical assistant to perform the microscopic evaluation of the stained smear.

Bacterial Morphology

The size, shape, and arrangement of bacteria, and other microbes, is a defining characteristic called **morphology**. Bacteria come in a variety of sizes and shapes. The most common bacterial shapes are rod, spherical, and spiral. Within each of these groups are hundreds of variants. Bacteria may exist as single cells or with other groupings such as chains, uneven clusters, pairs, tetrads, etc. Table 29-3 lists categories of bacteria by morphology. Figure 29-9 is a diagram of **cocci** in these groupings. The fact that bacteria have different shapes provides a factor to use in identification. Figure 29-10 shows diagrams of bacterial morphology.

Organisms have both a genus and species name. The genus is always spelled with a capital letter, and the species begins with a lowercase letter (e.g., *Staphylococcus aureus*). In print, the name is in italics or underlined.

Cocci are spherical in shape. One species of cocci, the *Staphylococci*, are found on all surfaces of the skin and many mucous membranes. They are generally not pathogenic unless they reach an area that is usually sterile, where they may cause some form of infection. Species of *Streptococci* may cause sore throat, scarlet fever, rheumatic fever, many pneumonias, and various skin infections. **Diplococci**, spherical cocci in pairs, cause bacterial meningitis, gonorrhea, and some of the pneumonias (Fig. 29-11).

Bacilli are a rod shape and are usually aerobic (requiring oxygen to live). Most bacteria are bacilli and often found in soil. Diseases caused by bacilli include tetanus, botulism, gas gangrene, tuberculosis, pertussis, salmonellosis, certain pneumonias, and otitis media.

Spirochetes are long, spiral, flexible organisms. Spirochetes are responsible for syphilis and Lyme disease. *Vibrio* is a very motile comma-shaped bacteria. These bacteria cause cholera.

COG Sensitivity Testing

When microorganisms are unable to grow in the presence of one or more antimicrobial drugs, they are said to be *susceptible* to that drug. **Sensitivity testing** determines if an antibiotic will be effective in stopping growth of an organism. It also identifies antibiotics that will *not* stop the growth of an organism. Organisms that are inhibited by an antimicrobial agent are called **sensitive**. Organisms that grow even in the presence of an antimicrobial agent are said to be **resistant** to that antimicrobial agent. The results of this test can be used to predict the potential effect in the patient.

Bacteria can become resistant to an antibiotic at any time. When bacteria become resistant to the antibiotic

Figure 29-9 Morphologic arrangements of cocci. (From Engelkirk P. Burton's *Microbiology for the Health Professions.* 8th ed. Baltimore: Lippincott Williams & Wilkins, 2007.)

Arrangement	Description	Appearance	Example	Disease
Diplococci	Cocci in pairs	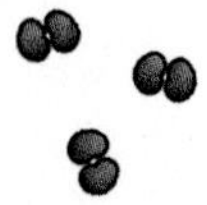	*Neisseria gonorrhoeae*	Gonorrhea
Streptococci	Cocci in chains	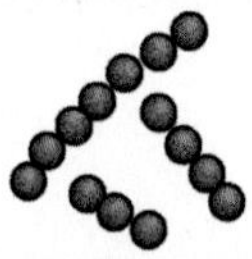	*Streptococcus pyogenes*	Strep throat
Staphylococci	Cocci in clusters	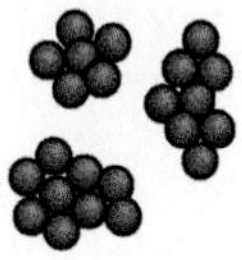	*Staphylococcus aureus*	Boils
Tetrad	A packet of 4 cocci	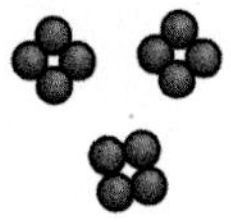	*Micrococcus luteus*	Rarely pathogenic
Octad	A packet of 8 cocci	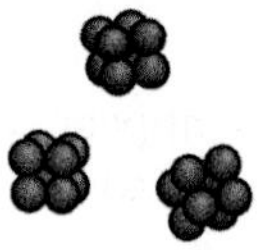	*Sarcina ventriculi*	Rarely pathogenic

once used to kill it, that antibiotic may no longer be effective. Testing a pathogen begins with identifying the pathogen causing the infection.

In microbiology, the first step in testing for antibiotic sensitivity is to **isolate** (separate from any other microorganisms present) the pathogen and identify it. Once it has been identified, a decision can be made on whether sensitivity testing is required. The pathogen identified may respond to treatments that have already been established. If this is not case, once that pathogen has been indentified, the physician will order the antibiotic that is effective.

To perform the sensitivity testing, the isolated pathogen is inoculated to a large agar plate. Paper disks impregnated with antibiotics are applied to the culture plate containing the organism, and the prepared plate is incubated for 24 hours. When the plate is observed for growth, the antibiotic disks that exhibit a margin with no bacterial growth indicate that the pathogen is sensitive or susceptible to this medication. If there is no zone around the disk, the organism is said to be *resistant* to that antibiotic. If there is a small zone, it may be reported as *intermediate*. The antibiotic of choice will be the one with the largest zone

of inhibition (no growth). Multiple antibiotics can be tested on one plate. This is the manual technique for sensitivity testing. The name of the technique is the **Kirby-Bauer method**. Figure 29-12 diagrams the steps used to perform the manual disc antibiotic sensitivity test. Automated instruments perform this testing in large laboratories.

COG Microbiology Test Reports

The presence of pathogenic bacteria is considered a positive culture.

A culture that is reported as "no growth in 24 hours" will be incubated another 24 hours to confirm there is no growth. Some pathogens require more than 24 hours to demonstrate growth on the culture medium.

A culture that is reported as "no growth in 24 or 48 hours" usually indicates that there is no infection. If the symptoms persist, however, a culture may be repeated if specimen resampling is possible.

If a culture is positive, susceptibility testing may be performed to guide antimicrobial treatment.

Box 29-5 describes the responsibilities of the medical assistant when reviewing patients' laboratory results.

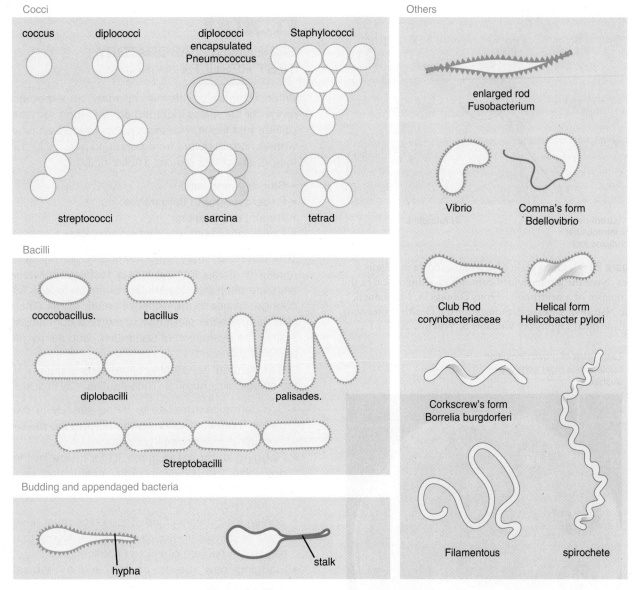

Figure 29-10 Bacterial morphology diagram.

CHECKPOINT QUESTIONS

8. Why can a microbiology test result not be ordered STAT?

9. What test result is indicated if the culture report reads: "no growth in 24 to 48 hours"?

⊙ Rickettsias and Chlamydias

Specialized forms of bacteria that fit in a category of their own are the rickettsias and chlamydiae. They are smaller than bacteria but larger than viruses. Both stain negatively with the Gram stain. They cause disease in both animals and humans. Because they require a living host for replication and survival, they are referred to as **obligate intracellular parasites**. Due to this, neither will grow on laboratory culture media.

Organisms of the genus *Rickettsia* are carried on arthropods. Arthropods include lice, fleas, and ticks. Diseases caused by *Rickettsia* species include Rocky Mountain spotted fever. These organisms transfer by inhalation or direct contact. *Chlamydia* species may cause blindness, pneumonia, and lymphogranuloma venereum, a prevalent sexually transmitted disease.

CHECKPOINT QUESTION

10. What organism causes Rocky Mountain spotted fever?

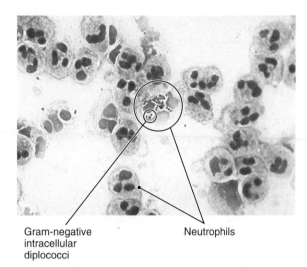

Gram-negative intracellular diplococci

Neutrophils

Figure 29-11 Gram stain of urethral exudate in gonorrhea. Note the intracellular Gram-negative diplococci in the cytoplasm of a neutrophil. (From Thomas H. McConnell, The Nature of Disease Pathology for the Health Professions, Philadelphia: Lippincott Williams & Wilkins, 2007.)

Large area of growth inhibition – bacterium is <u>most sensitive</u> to antibiotic C

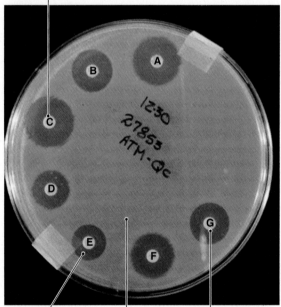

Small area of growth inhibition – bacterium is <u>least sensitive</u> to antibiotic E

Pure growth of bacteria from a single colony

Antibiotic disc – each disc contains a different antibiotic

Figure 29-12 Antibiotic sensitivity testing. The surface of the culture plate is overgrown by bacteria that were collected from a single colony and evenly spread across the surface. White paper discs soaked with different antibiotics are placed on the plate, and the plate is incubated 24 hours. Clear areas around discs are where bacterial growth has been inhibited. Bacterial sensitivity to a particular antibiotic is related to the size of the zone of inhibited: a large zone suggests the antibiotic may be effective in treating the patient's infection. (From Thomas H. McConnell, The Nature Of Disease Pathology for the Health Professions, Philadelphia: Lippincott Williams & Wilkins, 2007.)

BOX 29-5

SCREENING LABORATORY TEST RESULTS

When a laboratory test is reported, an expected range for the test is included on the report with the patient test result. The tests use a range because what is normal differs from person to person. Many factors affect test results. These include:

- Sex, age and race
- Recent food and fluid intake
- Recent medications
- Compliance with any pretest instructions

The physician may also compare current test results to those from previous tests. Laboratory tests are often part of a routine checkup to look for changes in health the patient's health status. They also help with the diagnosis of medical conditions, plan or the evaluation of treatments, and the monitoring of diseases.

The medical assistant will screen test results per the office policy manual. These duties may include:

- Comparing test results to those already in the patient's medical record and notifying the physician per his or her instructions.
- Flagging abnormal tests results for review by the physician. The physician may designated how abnormal the results must be to indict the need for follow-up.
- Screen for critical values. Each office must have a list of physician-approved critical levels that require immediate physician notification.
- Flagging new results posted in the medical record notifying the physician of the need to review and document.
- Documentation of these functions must be noted on the report or in the medical record.
- Documentation must included the screener's initials and date.

 PATIENT EDUCATION

LYME DISEASE

The deer tick is an arthropod capable of transmitting *Borrelia burgdorferi*, the spirochete responsible for Lyme disease (Fig. 29-13). When the infected deer tick (Fig. 29-14) bites a human, the organism enters the body and can produce mild to severe symptoms, including a rash, joint aches, fever, general body aches, and alterations in neurologic and cardiac function.

Lyme disease can be prevented. Instruct patients to avoid tick habitats, to apply insect repellent, and to wear shoes and light-colored clothing when working outside in wooded areas. Clothing should be checked for ticks and washed in hot water with strong soap. Stress the importance of looking for ticks and removing them properly when they are found.

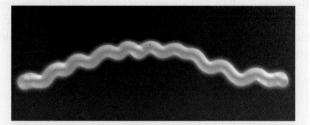

Figure 29-13 Lyme disease organism, the *B. burgdorferi* spirochete. (Asset provided by Anatomical Chart Co.)

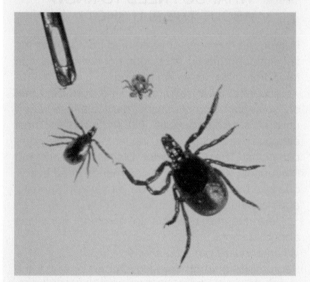

Figure 29-14 Deer ticks at the larval, nymphal, and adult stages. A sewing needle in the upper-left corner of the picture provides scale. (Photo provided by the American Lyme Disease Foundation.)

COG Mycoplasma

Mycoplasma are Gram negative, and the ones that are pathogenic to humans cause atypical pneumonia and genitourinary (GU) infections. Figure 29-15 is a picture of colony of *Mycoplasma pneumoniae*. Figure 29-16 is an electron micrograph of *M. pneumoniae*. Figure 29-17 is the picture of a patient with a *Mycoplasma* infection.

Viruses

Virology is the study of viruses, the smallest microorganisms. Viruses cause influenza, infectious hepatitis, rabies, polio, and AIDS. They are so small that they

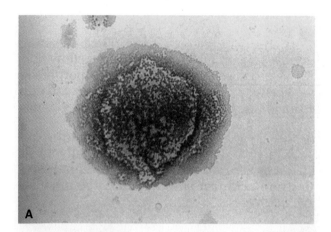

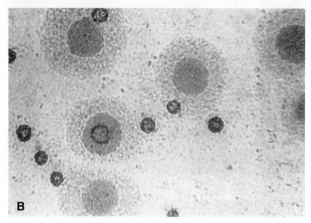

Figure 29-15 Colonies of *M. pneumoniae*. (From Koneman EW et al. Diagnostic Microbiology, 5th Ed. Baltimore: Lippincott Williams & Wilkins, 1997.)

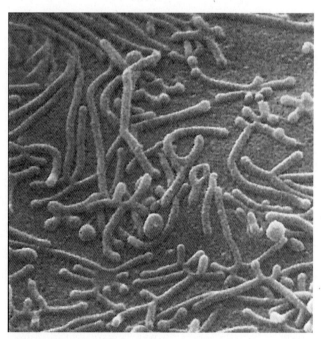

Figure 29-16 Scanning electron micrograph of *M. pneumoniae*. (Strohl WA, et al. Lippincott's Illustrated Reviews: Microbiology. Philadelphia: Lippincott Williams & Wilkins, 2001.)

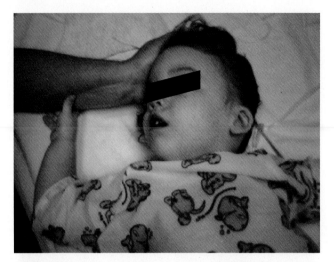

Figure 29-17 Ill-appearing child. This child appears weak and clingy, but alert and reactive. Her ill appearance is the result of a mucocutaneous form of mycoplasma infection. (Courtesy of Evan J. Weiner, MD.)

TABLE **29-4**	**Familiar Medically Important Viruses**
Infection/disease	**Common or Typical Name**
Adult T-cell Lymphoma, AIDS	Retroviridae HIV
	Human papilloma virus
Cervical cancer	Herpes simplex virus HSV2
Common warts, plantar warts	Human papilloma virus
Oral herpes	Herpes simplex virus 1
Chicken pox and shingles	Varicella zoster virus
Hepatitis B	Hepatitis B virus
Poliomyelitis	Poliovirus
Common cold	Human rhinovirus A
Gastroenteritis (one type)	Norovirus
Rubella	Rubella virus
Influenza	Influenza A and B
Measles	Rubeola virus
Respiratory trace infections (one type)	Respiratory syncytial virus
Rabies	Rabies virus
Smallpox	Smallpox (variola vera)

can be seen only with an electron microscope, not the usual microscope found in the medical office. They require a living host for survival and replication and are referred to as *parasites*. Because viruses are not susceptible to antibiotics, most are extremely difficult to treat. Antiviral therapies are being developed for many of the viruses.

Viruses are identified by morphology, replication, host, and disease caused. When a virus enters a cell, it lives in the cell to make copies of itself. Viral diseases are detected by changes in how the host cells look and function. For a list of familiar diseases and the responsible common viral name, see Table 29-4.

PATIENT EDUCATION

WHAT DO I NEED TO KNOW ABOUT THE FLU SHOT?

People get flu shots for protection from getting the flu. Although the flu shot does not always provide total protection, it's worth getting.

Influenza is a respiratory infection that can cause serious complications, particularly to young children and older adults. Flu shots are the most effective way to prevent influenza and its complications. The Centers for Disease Control and Prevention (CDC) now recommends that everyone age 6 months or older be vaccinated annually against influenza.

Here are the answers to common questions about flu shots.

When should I get a flu shot?
September through mid-November is when the vaccine is usually available and also when flu begins to be identified in the population. It takes up to 2 weeks to build immunity after a flu shot.

Why do you get the flu shot every year?
Influenza that is active one season can be different by the next season. Health officials use information about flu from all over the world to determine what the flu vaccine needs to during the next season. The vaccine usually lasts in the body about 6 months after receiving a flu shot.

Should everyone get a flu vaccine?
The CDC now recommends vaccinations for everyone age 6 months or older. Vaccination is important for people with conditions that could lead to complications from the flu, including:

- Pregnant women
- Older adults
- Young children

Chronic medical conditions can also increase your risk of influenza complications. Examples include:

- Asthma
- Cerebral palsy
- Chronic obstructive pulmonary disease
- Cystic fibrosis
- Epilepsy
- HIV/AIDS
- Kidney or liver disease
- Muscular dystrophy
- Obesity
- Sickle cell disease

Who should not have the flu shot?
Do not get a flu shot if you:

- Have had a bad reaction to the vaccine in the past
- Are allergic to chicken eggs
- Have a fever that day

 CHECKPOINT QUESTION

11. What diseases are caused by viruses?

Eukaryotic Microorganisms

Eukaryotic cells contain a nucleus, whereas prokaryotic cells have no nucleus. All bacteria are prokaryotic. Many eukaryotic organisms are human pathogens. Eukaryotic pathogens include the groups fungi, algae, protozoans, and parasites.

Fungi

Mycology is the study of fungi. Infectious fungi are small organisms like bacteria with the potential to produce disease in susceptible hosts. Some fungi are microscopic, but many can be seen without the aid of a microscope. They usually become pathogenic when the host's normal flora cannot defend against them.

Diseases caused by fungal infections are **mycoses.** They are classified by the amount of tissue involved and the route of entry into the body. These are:

- **Superficial**—skin, hair, nails, only
- **Subcutaneous**—the dermis, subcutaneous tissue or adjacent structures
- **Systemic**—infection of the internal organs
- **Opportunistic**—infection only in the immunocompromised

Human fungal infections are usually limited to conditions such as candidiasis (thrush) and dermatophyte skin infections such as athlete's foot. Figure 29-18 is a picture

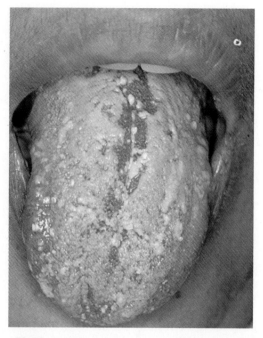

Figure 29-18 Oral candidiasis. These curdlike lesions can easily be removed with gauze. (From Goodheart HP, MD. Goodheart's Photoguide of Common Skin Disorders, 2nd Edition. Philadelphia: Lippincott Williams & Wilkins, 2003.)

of the tongue of a patient with oral candidiasis (thrush). Figure 29-19 is a picture of a patient with candidiasis of the web spaces of the fingers. If a patient does not have normal immunity, normally nonpathogenic fungi can cause potentially fatal infections. Today's common travel in foreign countries transports unusual fungi into this country. Examples include histoplasmosis, blastomycosis, coccidiomycosis and paracoccidiodomycosis.

- *Histoplasmosis.* This is caused by *Histoplasma capsulatum. H. capsulatum* is common in many parts

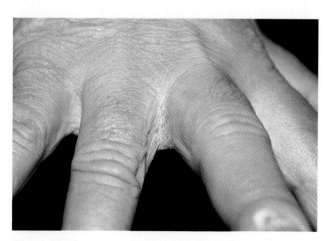

Figure 29-19 Cutaneous candidiasis. Candidal infection of the web spaces of the fingers is present. (From Goodheart HP, MD. Goodheart's Photoguide of Common Skin Disorders, 2nd Edition. Philadelphia: Lippincott Williams & Wilkins, 2003.)

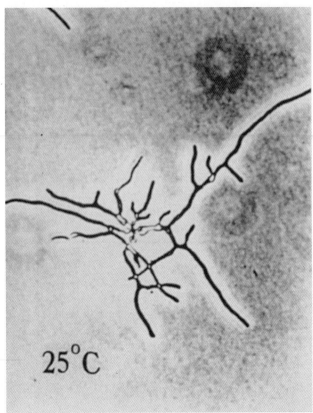

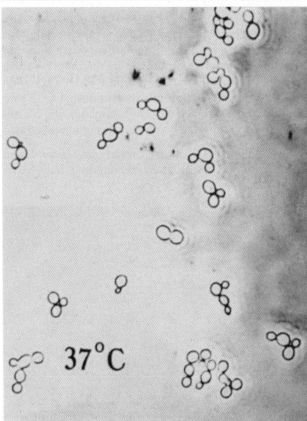

Figure 29-20 Photomicrographs illustrate the fungus *Histoplasma capsulatum* grown at 25°C (*top*) and at 37°C (*bottom*). (From Engelkirk P. Burton's Microbiology for the Health Professions. 8th ed. Baltimore: Lippincott Williams & Wilkins, 2007.)

of the world including the United States. It spreads through contaminated soil and is usually asymptomatic (Figs. 29-20 and 29-21). The lungs are the main site of infection. The symptoms of pulmonary infection can resemble those of tuberculosis.

- *Opportunistic fungi.* These fungi grow where they have the opportunity, as in patients with weak immune systems. Because of the weak immune systems, other fungi that are normally not pathogenic, such as *Fusarium* (Fig. 29-22) or *Penicillium* (Fig. 29-23), may cause infections.
- *Aspergillosis.* This is the name of several diseases caused by the mold *Aspergillus*. It occurs world-wide. The organism can infect the lungs, inner ear, sinuses, and, rarely, the eye.
- *Candidiasis. C. albicans*, a part of the normal human flora, can grow and spread in patients having reduced immunity (Fig. 29-24).
- *Cryptococcosis.* The yeast *Cryptococcus neoformans* can cause systemic infection. When inhaled, the organism causes subacute meningitis or pulmonary infection. The disease can affect a healthy person and is found globally. *C. neoformans* is commonly found in pigeon droppings.
- *Pneumocystis.* This is an infection of the lung caused by *Pneumocystis jiroveci*. The organism is a common cause of fatal pneumonia in AIDS patients.

Protozoa and Helminths

Parasitology is the study of protozoa and helminths. Parasites cause foodborne or waterborne illness. Although some parasites use a permanent host, others move through different animal or human hosts. Parasites disrupt the host's nutrient absorption, causing weakness and disease.

Parasites are often excreted in the feces of the human or animal they are currently infesting. They may be transmitted from host to host through contaminated food and water, or by oral exposure to anything that has touched the feces of an infected person or animal.

Some common parasites and their related diseases or symptoms include:

- *Entamoeba:* diarrhea, dysentery, and liver and lung disorders. Figure 29-25 diagrams the life cycle of *Entamoeba histolytica*.
- *Giardia:* giardiasis, diarrhea, and malabsorption of nutrients. Figure 29-26 is a scanning electron micrograph of *Giardia intestinalis*.
- *Trichomonas:* trichomoniasis, vaginitis, and urinary tract infection. Figure 29-27 is a trophozoite phase of the parasite *Trichomona vaginalis*. This phase is often seen in the urine of patients with vaginitis.
- *Plasmodium:* malaria.
- *Toxoplasma:* toxoplasmosis and fetal abnormalities. Figure 29-28 is a toxoplasmic lesion in the brain.

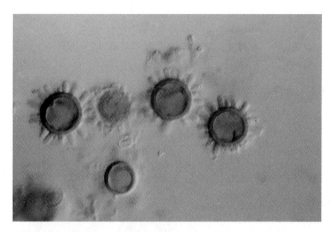

Figure 29-21 Microscopic appearance of the mold phase of *H. capsulatum*. (From McClatchey KD. Clinical Laboratory Medicine. 2nd ed. Philadelphia: Lippincott Williams & Wilkins, 2002.)

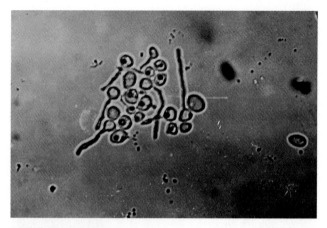

Figure 29-24 *Candida albicans* (original magnification ×3600). (From McClatchey KD. Clinical Laboratory Medicine. 2nd ed. Philadelphia: Lippincott Williams & Wilkins, 2002.)

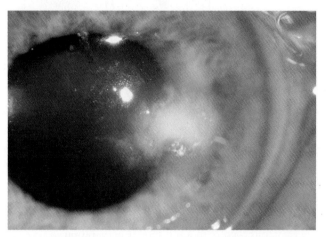

Figure 29-22 This corneal ulcer in a patient using extended wear soft contact lenses was caused by a filamentous fungal organism, *Fusarium*. (From Tasman W, Jaeger E. The Wills Eye Hospital Atlas of Clinical Ophthalmology, 2e. Lippincott Williams & Wilkins, 2001.)

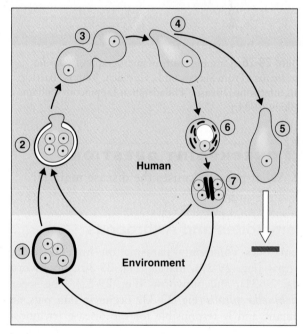

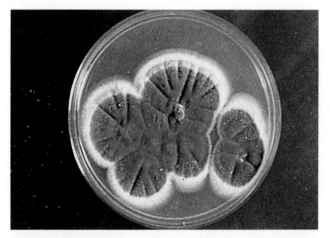

Figure 29-23 Colonies of a *Penicillium* species. Although penicillin is derived from *Penicillium*, this mold can also cause infections in immunosuppressed patients. (Koneman's Color Atlas and Textbook of Diagnostic Microbiology, 6th ed. Philadelphia: Lippincott Williams & Wilkins, 2006.)

Figure 29-25 Life cycle of *E. histolytica*. Humans acquire amebic infection by oral ingestion of the cyst form of the parasite (1). Viable cysts may be ingested from the external environment, from the stool of other infected persons, or from the stools of the patients themselves (the arrow from 7 to 2). In the upper GI tract, the parasite excysts after passing through the stomach (2), replicates (3), and transforms to the potentially pathogenic trophozoite form (4), which is typically found in the large intestine. Trophozoites die rapidly when they are shed into the external environment (5). When conditions in the GI tract are unfavorable, trophozoites transform into cysts (6–7), which can remain dormant for long periods of time in the host and the environment. (From Engleberg NC, Dermody T, DiRita V. Schaecter's Mechanisms of Microbial Disease, 4th Edition. Baltimore: Lippincott Williams & Wilkins, 2007.)

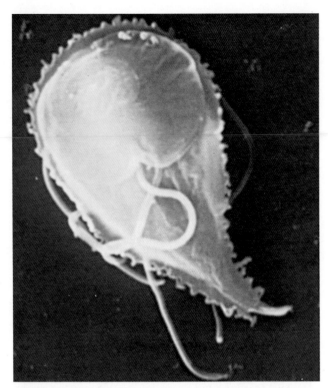

Figure 29-26 Scanning electron micrograph of *Giardia intestinalis*. (From Sherwood L. Gorbach, John G. Bartlett, etal. Infectious Diseases. Philadelphia: Lippincott Williams & Wilkins, 2004.)

 CHECKPOINT QUESTION

12. What parasite causes the disease malaria?

Nematodes and Arthropods

Nematodes commonly parasitic on humans include *Ascaris* (Fig. 29-29), filarias (Fig. 29-30), hookworms (Fig. 29-31), and pinworms (Fig. 29-32). The species *Trichinella spiralis* (Fig. 29-33), occurs in rats, pigs, and humans and is responsible for the disease trichinosis. The patient may be exposed to the *Trichinella spiralis* by eating undercooked pork. Infestations of nematodes cause gastrointestinal (GI) obstruction and bronchial damage.

Arthropods that cause discomfort and/or disease in humans include mites (Fig. 29-34), lice (Fig. 29-35), ticks, and fleas (Fig. 29-36) along with bees, spiders, wasps, mosquitoes, and scorpions (Fig. 29-37). All may cause injury by their bites or stings, and several are also capable of transmitting disease by their bite or sting.

 CHECKPOINT QUESTION

13. Which parasite is the cause of the disease trichinosis?

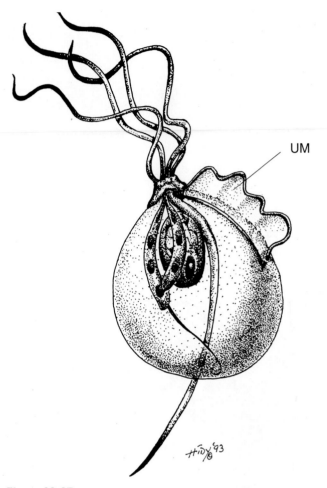

UM

Figure 29-27 *T. vaginalis* trophozoite, 7 to 23 μm long by 5 to 15 μm wide. *T. vaginalis* trophozoites are easy to recognize in a wet mount preparation. Their flagella and undulating membrane cause them to be constantly in motion. (From Paul G. Engelkirk, Gwendolyn R. W. Burton, Burton's Microbiology for the Health Sciences, Eighth Edition. Philadelphia: Lippincott Williams & Wilkins, 2007.)

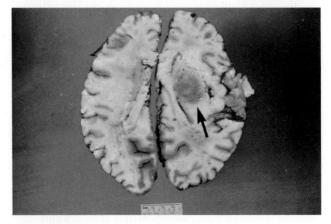

Figure 29-28 A cross section of the brain of a patient with AIDS shows a toxoplasmic lesion (*arrow*).

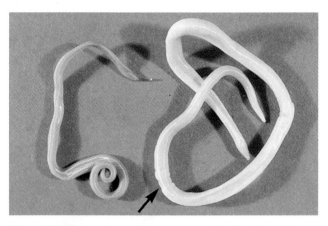

Figure 29-29 Female and male worms of *A. lumbricoides.*

COG **Infections of Body Systems**

Besides recognizing organisms by morphology, it is important to recognize the body system they most commonly affect. This discussion of infections of body systems is not comprehensive; however, representative organisms and conditions are included.

Integumentary

When burns, puncture wounds, surgery, or bites break the skin surface, bacteria can invade and spread via blood or lymph, causing infection. Bacterial skin infections are very common, and they can range from annoying to deadly. The most common bacterial infections of the skin are caused by either *S. aureus* or a form of *Streptococcus.* Bacterial infections of skin include:

- Cellulitis—infection of the deeper layers of the skin, the dermis and the subcutaneous tissue.
- **Folliculitis**—an infection in the hair follicle (Fig. 29-38) distinguishes folliculitis, furuncles, and carbuncles.
- Hot tub folliculitis—an infection of the hair follicles caused by the bacteria *Pseudomonas aeruginosa.* This

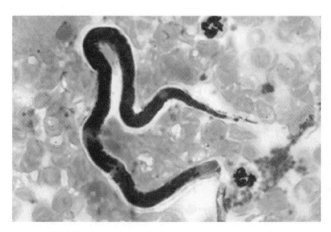

Figure 29-30 *Filaria.* (From Sun T. Parasitic Disorders, 2nd Edition. Baltimore: Williams & Wilkins, 1998. fig. 37.3.)

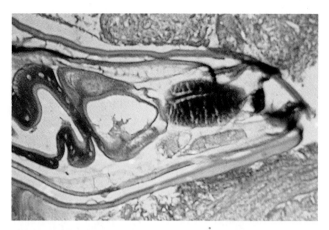

Figure 29-31 An intestinal tissue specimen shows a longitudinal section of a hookworm.

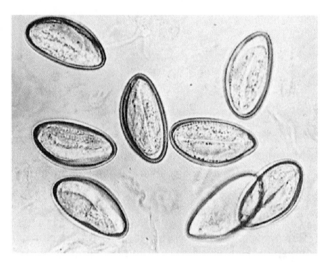

Figure 29-32 Nematodes: *Enterobius vermicularis,* pinworm ova. (From Koneman EW, et al. Color Atlas and Textbook of Diagnostic Microbiology, 5th Edition. Philadelphia: Lippincott, 1997.)

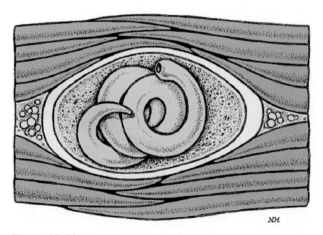

Figure 29-33 Nematode: *T. spiralis,* pork worm, causes of trichinosis; larva encysted in human muscle. (From Neil O. Hardy. Wesport, CT. From Stedman's Medical Dictionary, 27th Edition. Baltimore: Lippincott Williams & Wilkins, 2000.)

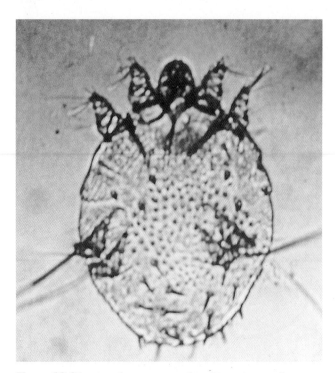

Figure 29-34 Mite that causes scabies (*Sarcoptes scabiei*).

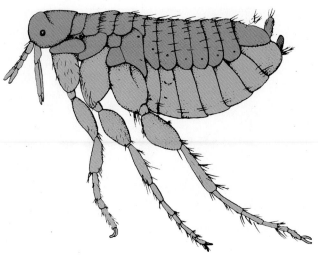

Figure 29-36 Flea (*Pulex irritans*).

bacteria is found in contaminated whirlpools, hot tubs, water slides, physiotherapy pools, and loofah sponges.

- A **furuncle**—an infection of the pilosebaceous unit. The pilosebaceous unit consists of the hair shaft, the hair follicle, the sebaceous gland, and the **erector pili muscle**, which causes the hair to stand up when it contracts.
- A **carbuncle**—a collection of multiple infected hair follicles. It is a serious abscess. A carbuncle is actually several furuncles that are packed together.
- **Impetigo**—a bacterial infection of the top layer of the skin (Fig. 29-39).

- **Erythrasma**—a bacterial skin infection occurring where skin touches skin, like between toes, in armpits, or groin.

 CHECKPOINT QUESTION

14. Name two bacteria most commonly responsible for infections of the skin.

Viral infections commonly result in skin lesions and rashes. Some viruses lie dormant in the host's cells and reactivate up to years later. Viral infections of the skin may also be chronic.

Common viral skin infections include:

- *Warts:* Papilloma viruses cause skin cells to multiply producing a benign growth called a *wart*. Warts are spread by direct contact.
- *Smallpox (variola):* Smallpox is transmitted by the respiratory route and moved to the skin by the bloodstream. Pustules expand; scab; and leave deep, pitted scars. Patients experience severe pain. Death usually

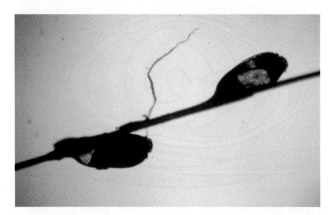

Figure 29-35 Head lice. The nits are attached to the hair shaft. (From Goodheart HP, MD. Goodheart's Photoguide of Common Skin Disorders, 2nd Edition. Philadelphia: Lippincott Williams & Wilkins, 2003.)

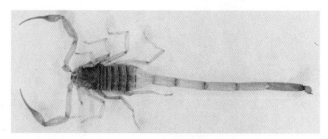

Figure 29-37 Scorpion (*Centruroides exilicauda*). (From Fleisher GR, MD, Ludwig S, MD, Baskin MN, MD. Atlas of Pediatric Emergency Medicine. Philadelphia: Lippincott Williams & Wilkins, 2004.)

Superficial folliculitis
• Erythema
• Pustule
• Single-follicle
  involvement

Deep folliculitis
• Extensive follicular
  involvement

Furuncle
• Red, tender nodule
  surrounding a follicle
• Single draining point

Carbuncle
• Deep follicular abscesses
  of several follicles
• Several draining points

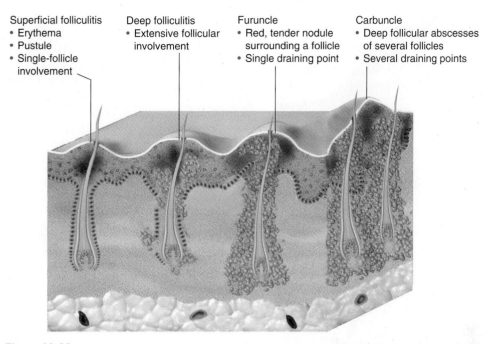

Figure 29-38 Distinguishing folliculitis, furuncles, and carbuncles. (Provided by Anatomical Chart Co.)

occurs during the second week. Smallpox is a potential agent in bioterrorism (Fig. 29-40).

• *Chicken pox and shingles:* The varicella zoster virus is transmitted by the respiratory system and moves to the skin, causing a rash. After having the chicken pox virus, it can remain dormant in nerve cells and later reappear as shingles. Shingles (Herpes zoster) is a painful rash following the path of the affected nerves (Fig. 29-41).

• *Cold sores:* Herpes simplex virus (HSV) infection results in cold sores. The HSV-1 virus remains

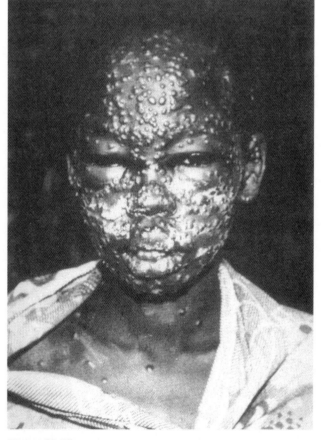

Figure 29-40 Smallpox, eastern Zaire, 1968. (Image from Rubin E MD and Farber JL MD. Pathology, 3rd Edition. Philadelphia: Lippincott Williams & Wilkins, 1999.)

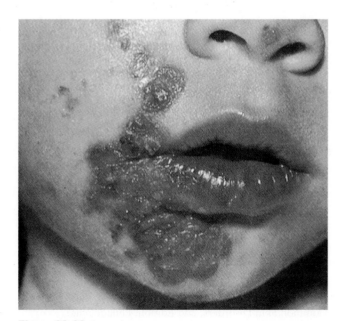

Figure 29-39 Impetigo.

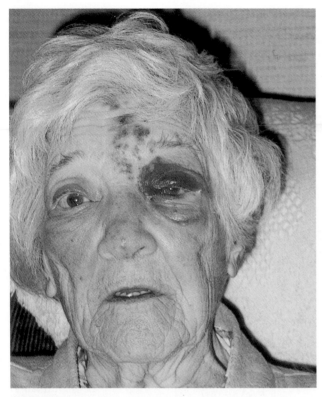

Figure 29-41 Herpes zoster (shingles). (From Brunner & Suddarth's Textbook of Medical-Surgical Nursing.)

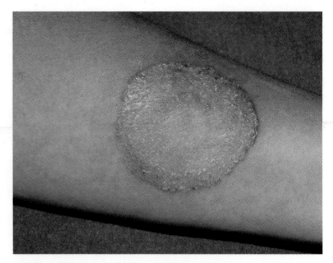

Figure 29-42 Tinea corporis. (From Goodheart HP, MD. Goodheart's Photoguide of Common Skin Disorders, 2nd Edition. Philadelphia: Lippincott Williams & Wilkins, 2003.)

dormant in nerve cells, and cold sores recur when the virus is activated. Herpes encephalitis results when HSVs move to the brain.

- *Genital herpes:* Genital herpes is a sexually transmitted disease (STD) caused by HSV-1 or HSV-2. Most genital herpes is caused by HSV-2. Most individuals have no or only minimal signs or symptoms from HSV-1 or HSV-2 infection. When signs do occur, they typically appear as one or more blisters on or around the genitals or rectum. The blisters break, leaving tender ulcers (sores) that may take 2 to 4 weeks to heal. The infection can stay in the body indefinitely.
- *Measles (rubeola):* Measles is caused by the rubeola virus and transmitted by the respiratory route. Vaccinations are available. The virus incubates in the respiratory tract and lesions appear on the skin. Complications of measles include middle ear infections, pneumonia, and encephalitis.
- *Rubella and congenital rubella syndrome:* Rubella is transmitted by the respiratory route. A red rash may appear, but the disease can be asymptomatic. Rubella can affect a fetus when a woman becomes infected with rubella during the first trimester of her pregnancy. Damage includes stillbirth, deafness, eye cataracts, heart defects, and mental retardation. Vaccination with live rubella virus provides immunity.

- *Cutaneous mycoses:* Cutaneous mycoses infect the outer layers of skin, hair, and nails, and do not invade living tissues. The fungi are called *dermatophytes.* Common conditions caused by dermatophytes are:
  - *Tinea corporis*—small lesions occurring anywhere on the body (Fig. 29-42).
  - *Tinea pedis ("athlete's foot")*—infection between the toes and on the soles of feet (Fig. 29-43).
  - *Tinea unguium (onychomycosis)*—infection of the fingernails and toenails (Fig. 29-44).
  - *Tinea capitis*—infection on the head (Fig. 29-45).
  - *Tinea cruris ("jock itch")*—infection of the groin, perineum or perianal area.
  - *Tinea barbae*—ringworm of the bearded areas of the face and neck (Fig. 29-46).

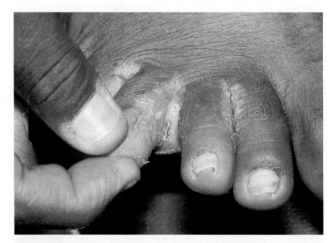

Figure 29-43 Interdigital tenia pedis (toe web infection). (From Goodheart HP, MD. Goodheart's Photoguide of Common Skin Disorders, 2nd Edition. Philadelphia: Lippincott Williams & Wilkins, 2003.)

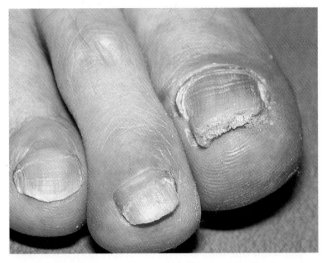

Figure 29-44 Onychomycosis. (From Goodheart HP, MD. Goodheart's Photoguide of Common Skin Disorders, 2nd Edition. Philadelphia: Lippincott Williams & Wilkins, 2003.)

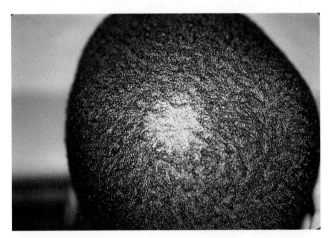

Figure 29-45 Tinea capitis. Circumscribed area of hair loss with scaliness of scalp. (Courtesy of George A. Datto, III, MD.)

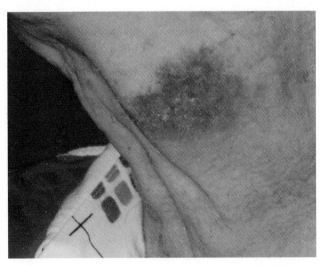

Figure 29-46 Tinea barbae. (From Dale Berg and Katherine Worzala, Atlas of Adult Physical Diagnosis. Philadelphia: Lippincott Williams & Wilkins, 2006.)

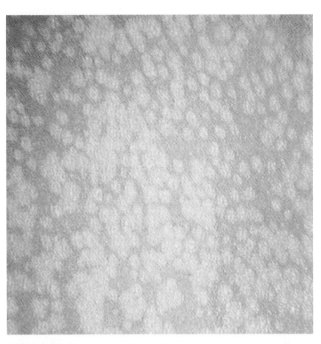

Figure 29-47 Tinea versicolor: close-up view of hypopigmented macules on the back.

- *Tinea versicolor*—characterized by a blotchy discoloration of skin that may itch (Fig. 29-47).

WHAT IF?

What if your patient asks you how to prevent cutaneous mycoses such as tinea pedis?

Explain to your patient that tinea pedis is a common fungal infection. Then offer the following suggestions, which can aid prevention:

- Practice good basic hygiene.
- Thoroughly dry between the toes.
- Do not share footwear.
- Use antifungal powder between the toes and in shoes.
- Wear foot protection when using public showers.

CHECKPOINT QUESTION

15. Name the virus that causes chicken pox.

Respiratory System

Upper Respiratory Infections

- The *common cold* is commonly a viral infection.
- *Sinusitis* is commonly a viral infection.
- *Pharyngitis* is commonly caused by *Streptococcus pyogenes*.

Lower Respiratory Infections

- *Bronchitis* is commonly a viral infection.
- *Bronchiolitis* is commonly a viral infection.
- *Pneumonia* can be viral, bacterial, or fungal. The most common bacterial agent is *Streptococcus pneumoniae* (Fig. 29-48).
- *Nosocomial infections* are infections contracted in a healthcare setting. Nosocomial pneumonias and pneumonias in immunosuppressed patients are usually caused by such agents as Gram-negative organisms and *Staphylococcus* species.

 CHECKPOINT QUESTION

16. Pharyngitis is most commonly caused by what organism?

Gastrointestinal System

Acute gastroenteritis is the second cause of death worldwide. Other intraabdominal infections are relatively common and present dilemmas in diagnosis and management.

- Helicobacter pylori: *H. pylori* is a gram-negative rod that attaches to epithelial cells in the stomach. It damages mucus-secreting cells, promoting an acute and chronic inflammatory response.
- *Food poisoning:* Because of processed foods and dining away from home, food poisoning is an important problem in the United States. Symptoms range from gastroenteritis to life-threatening paralysis or colitis. Bacterial food poisoning can be caused by many different species. Some of them are:
  - *S. aureus*
  - *E. coli*

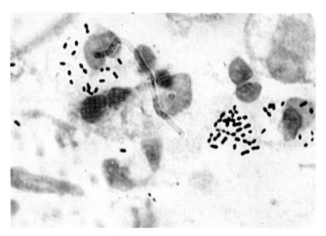

Figure 29-48 Gram-positive *S. pneumoniae* in a Gram-stained smear of a pus-containing sputum. Note the diplococci. (From Koneman's Color Atlas and Textbook of Diagnostic Microbiology, 6th ed. Philadelphia: Lippincott Williams & Wilkins, 2006.)

- *Salmonella* species
- *Shigella* species
- *Viruses:* Viral gastroenteritis is one of the most common human infections. Common viruses causing gastroenteritis are:
  - Rotaviruses
  - Caliciviruses
  - Noroviruses
- *Infections of the gallbladder:* These infections that cause abdominal pain spread into the biliary tract. Some of the potential bacterial pathogens include:
  - *E. coli*
  - *Streptococci*
  - *Staphylococci*
  - *Clostridium* species
- *Common bile duct obstruction:* This may result from parasitic infestation with *Ascaris lumbricoides*.
- *Acute diverticulitis:* Tiny perforations of diverticula cause contamination of the peritoneal cavity by *Bacteroides* species, *E. coli*, and *Enterococci*. The result is often a small abscess that may expand and then rupture. This leads to fecal contamination of the peritoneal cavity.
- *Peritonitis:* Infectious peritonitis is most commonly caused by *E. coli*.

 CHECKPOINT QUESTION

17. Why is understanding food processing important in the United States?

Nervous System

The central nervous system (CNS) is protected from infection, but it is very susceptible to infection.

- *Meningitis:* Meningococcal meningitis tends to occur in epidemics. An example is outbreaks in college dorms. *Pneumococcus* species and *H. influenzae* are common causes. Meningitis is often seen in patients that have had recent otitis or upper respiratory infection.
- *Encephalitis:* Infection of the brain is most commonly viral. Viruses commonly seen are polio, rabies, herpes zoster, and arboviruses.
- *Rabies:* The rabies virus enters the body through the bite of an infected dog, fox, vole, bat, or other wild animal. The viral infection that mainly involves the cervical cord, the brainstem, and the temporal lobes. The period between the bite and the symptoms of the disease may be up to a year.
- *Herpes zoster:* The varicella zoster virus primarily affects spinal and cranial nerves.
- *Cytomegalovirus:* Cytomegalovirus is a member of the herpes virus family. It causes eye and brain damage in utero.

- *Tick paralysis:* Wood ticks are common in underbrush. The tick's toxin may result in severe weakness. The weakness may be so severe that respiratory paralysis causes death.
- *Tetanus: Clostridium tetani* enters a wound, and its toxin blocks nerve impulses in the motor nerves. Patients develop pain, stiffness, and spasms of the muscles, especially in the jaw.
- *Botulism: Clostridium botulinum* toxin is most commonly found in improperly canned foods. It attaches to motor nerve endings. Treatment includes ventilatory support and specific antiserum
- *Toxoplasmosis:* Toxoplasmosis may occur as a congenital infection or in immunosuppressed patients. Children born with toxoplasmosis may be stillborn or have significant mental and neurologic damage.
- *Lyme disease:* The spirochete *Borrelia burgdorferi* is transmitted by a tick. The tick bite site develops a small red spot spreading outward from tick bite. The center of the spot is clear. Fatigue and a generally unwell feeling are the first symptoms. Early diagnosis is important because treatment with oral antibiotics may be effective then.

PATIENT EDUCATION

PATIENT SCENARIO #1

A 23-year-old white female came to the medical office on August 11, 2012. Her temperature was 99.5°F. She complained of fatigue, tender joints, a headache, a stiff neck, and a backache. The physician noticed a circular "rash" on her right arm about 5 inches in diameter, with a bright-red leading edge and a dim center in the form of a "bull's eye."

The patient gave the following history: She is a graduate student in the wildlife program at the nearby university. She was in the field for 3 weeks in the Smoky Mountains during June. She tracks small mammals in the field and studies their behavior. She complained of a large number of biting flies, mosquitoes, and ticks in the area. She felt well until about 2 weeks after returning home.

- What is your best diagnosis of this case?
  The best diagnosis is Lyme disease.
- What features are critical to a potential diagnosis?
  The key symptom is the "bull's eye" rash. Also of note is the low grade fever, joint pain, and aching. The exposure to ticks is likewise a strong indicator.

CHECKPOINT QUESTION

18. What bacterial cause of meningitis is most common in children up to age 2 years?

Genitourinary System

- *Urinary tract infections (UTIs):* Infectious diseases of the urinary tract include:
  - *Cystitis.* The most common bacteria causing cystitis is *E. coli.*
  - *Nephritis.* Infection of the kidney usually starts with cystitis. The bacteria move up the ureters into the bladder and then to the kidneys. *E.coli* is the most common cause.
  - *Urethritis.* Pathogens are usually transmitted to the urethra sexually. The most common causes of urethritis are *Chlamydia trachomatis* and *Neisseria gonorrhoeae.*
- *Genital tract infections:* Infectious diseases of the genital tract include:
  - *Cervicitis* is an infection of the **cervix** (the part of the uterus that opens into the vagina).
  - *Endometritis* is an infection of the **endometrium** (the inner layer of the uterine wall).
  - *Pelvic inflammatory disease (PID)* is an infection of the fallopian tubes. PID is caused by *N. gonorrhoeae,* and *C. trachomatis.*
  - *Vaginitis* is an infection of the vagina. The three most common infectious agents are:
    - *Candida albicans* (a yeast)
    - *Trichomonas vaginalis* (a protozoan)
    - Bacteria: *Mobiluncus* and *Gardnerella*

CHECKPOINT QUESTIONS

19. What two bacteria are responsible for urethritis?
20. What are the two bacterial causes of PID?

Reproductive System

There is crossover between the GU system when discussing infectious diseases of the reproductive system. Items covered previously in this chapter will be noted.

Bacterial Diseases of the Reproductive Systems

Most diseases of the reproductive system are STDs.

- *Gonorrhea:* Gonorrhea is caused by the Gram-negative diplococcus *N. gonorrhoeae.* Gonorrhea is the most common reportable communicable disease in the United States. Women may not have symptoms until the infection spreads to the uterus and uterine tubes. Men's symptoms are painful urination and pus discharge. **Ophthalmia neonatorum** is an eye infection acquired by infants passing through the birth canal of a mother infected with *N. gonorrhoeae.*
- *Pelvic inflammatory disease:* PID is discussed earlier in this chapter.
- *Syphilis:* The spirochete *Treponema pallidum* is the cause of syphilis (Fig. 29-49). The disease is transmitted

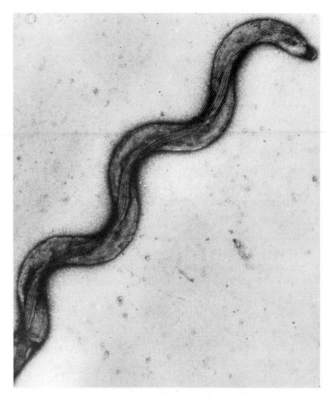

Figure 29-49 Electron photomicrograph of *T. pallidum*. (Courtesy of Dr. E. M. Walker, Department of Microbiology and Immunology, UCLA School of Medicine, Los Angeles, CA.)

by direct contact. In the primary stage the patient develops a primary lesion at the site of the infection. In the secondary stage, the patient has a widely disseminated rash on skin and mucous membranes. The rash actually contains the spirochetes. The second stage is so mild, it also is not noticed by the patient. This stage ends with a dormant period. Tertiary lesions can appear on many organs at least 10 years after the secondary lesions heal. Cardiovascular syphilis weakens the aorta. Neurosyphilis symptoms, range from dementia to loss of voluntary motor movement.

 CHECKPOINT QUESTIONS

21. What is the most common reportable communicable disease in the United States?
22. Name the spirochete that causes syphilis.

Host Defense Mechanisms

Defenses against infectious organisms are natural barriers and immune responses.

- Intact, healthy skin bars invading microorganisms. Exceptions include human papillomavirus and some parasites.

- Mucous membranes are covered in secretions with antimicrobial properties.
- The respiratory tract has upper airway filters protecting the lungs. Coughing also helps remove organisms.
- Protection in the GI tract includes the acidic pH of the stomach. Peristalsis facilitates removal of microorganisms. Normal bowel flora can inhibit pathogens.
- GU tract barriers are the length of the urethra in men and the acid pH of the vagina in women.

Physical Methods of Control

- *Temperature:* Change from an organism's optimal growth temperature will slow down or stop growth altogether.
  - A simple method of dry heat sterilization is to expose the object to a direct flame or electric heat. Dry heat is less effective than moist or wet heat. Dry heat takes higher temperatures. An advantage of hot-air sterilization is its use on substances that would be damaged by steam.
  - Moist heat is more effective in controlling or killing microbial growth because it needs lower temperatures and shorter periods of time. It requires an autoclave or special equipment.
  - Cold temperatures control some microbial growth but do not disinfect or sterilize.
- *Desiccation:* This inhibits microbial growth by removing the water required for survival.
- *Filtration:* This is separating solids from fluid or gas using filters. Filters must have pores small enough to keep the microorganisms from flowing in with the fluid or gas.

 CHECKPOINT QUESTION

23. What happens to an organism when the temperature of its surroundings changes?

Chemical Methods of Control

- *Disinfectants and antiseptics:* Disinfectants cannot be used on living surfaces. Antiseptics are used on living tissue. No chemical works in all circumstances. No chemical agent sterilizes because there are resistant organisms that survive the treatment.
- *Antimicrobial agents:* These include a variety of chemical compounds. These compounds attack cell function. Safety must be considered as some of the agents are chemical hazards to humans.

 COG Fecal Blood Testing

Because stool specimens are tested in microbiology, the stool test for blood is usually performed in microbiology as well. The fecal test for blood is performed in the microbiology department. Stool may be tested for blood for several reasons. Blood in stool is abnormal, but the cause may be simple or serious. Visible blood likely results from lesions in the lower colon or hemorrhoids. Blood in stool is not always visible. Blood that is not visible is called *occult*. For that reason, the test is often called "stool for occult blood." This test is waived and often performed by medical assistants. See Procedure 29-8.

Positive occult blood tests are confirmed with a colonoscopy. The colonoscopy can identify abnormal tissue. The scope is inserted and passed through the colon to the very lowest part of the small intestine. As it passes, the physician can stop and take pictures and samples of abnormal tissue. The specimens are sent to the laboratory for histology and pathology testing and examination. The pathologist reports the final diagnosis of the biopy specimens.

COG The Immune System

The immune system is the mechanism for identifying and destroying pathogens. For pathogens, it is a set of barriers. Immunology is the study of the actions of the immune system. **Immunity** is the response to foreign bodies. Antigens and antibodies interact to form complexes during an immune reaction.

Antigens and Antibodies

Antigens are substances foreign to the body. They cause the body to begin the production of antibodies. Pathogens are among the substances recognized by the body as antigens. *Antibodies* are proteins produced by the body in response to a specific antigen. Each antibody combines with only one antigen; this is called **specificity**.

Because an antibody has a particularly strong attraction for its antigen, little antigen need be present in a sample for the antibody to find it; this is referred to as *sensitivity*. An antibody is named by using its specific antigen's name and adding the prefix *anti-*. In hepatitis, for instance, if the antigen is hepatitis A, then the antibody's name is antihepatitis A. If the antigen is hepatitis B, then the antibody is antihepatitis B. If the antigen is a bacteria, like *Streptococcus*, then the antibody's name is antistreptococcal antigen.

Diseases Caused by the Immune System

Diseases caused by the immune system occur when there are problems with the immune reaction. The problem may be that the response is faulty, that it is too much, or that it is too little.

- *Allergies and hypersensitivity reactions:* An allergen is a substance that is usually not harmful. This would be substances like pollen, mold, dust, cat dander, foods, insect stings, insect bites, certain foods, or medicines. The allergy comes when the immune system overacts and produces antibodies against these substances that are not pathogens.
- *Autoimmune diseases:* These diseases occur when the body cannot distinguish between its own antigens and outside antigens. This causes the body to fight its own tissues.
  - *Myasthenia gravis* causes the patient to develop autoantibodies to attack neuromuscular function. The early stages involve the patient's eye and throat muscles. Later there is complete loss of muscle function followed by death.
  - *Multiple sclerosis (MS)* causes patient cells to attack the central nervous system. Triggers considered as causes of MS have been viral infection, environmental factors, or genetic predisposition.
  - *Graves hyperthyroidism* is caused when autoantibodies bind to thyroid cells. This stimulates thyroid activity. The result is a goiter.
  - *Systemic lupus erythematosus (SLE)* is caused by autoantibodies damaging many body systems. The classic symptom of SLE is the characteristic "butterfly rash" across the checks and nose. SLE can destroy organs requiring organ transplants.
  - Rheumatoid arthritis is an autoimmune disease that causes gradual debilitating damage to the joints. Treatment includes anti-inflammatory agents or immunosuppressive drugs.
- *Immune deficiency diseases:* Acquired immunodeficiency syndrome (AIDS) is caused by human immunodeficiency virus. Once the disease progresses, symptoms vary because the infections that follow are by opportunistic organisms.

 CHECKPOINT QUESTION

24. How do autoimmune diseases occur?

COG Immunological Testing Principles

Immunology testing uses the binding of a specific antibody to its specific antigen. The antigen is detected by use of a solution containing the antibody. Or, the antibody is detected by using a solution containing the antigen. The way that an antigen-antibody reaction is identified is by detection of the complex of the antigen and antibody.

Immunoassay test kits include reagents to extract the antigen from the specimen. The extraction is dripped onto the test strip or cartridge. The drops react with reagents in the test strip or cartridge. If the extracted specimen contains the antigen, a color change (usually

---

BOX 29-6

TIPS FOR PERFORMING IMMUNOASSAYS

1. Follow the times exactly.
2. Add reagents in correct order.
3. Use reagents only with other reagents from the same kit.
4. Use the exact amount of reagents stated in directions.
5. Ensure that reagents and samples are at room temperature.
6. Ensure that reagents have not expired.

BOX 29-8

IMMUNOASSAY TROUBLESHOOTING TIPS

If an immunoassay control is not producing an acceptable result, try the following:

1. Reread the procedure to be sure a step was not omitted.
2. Check the labels of reagents to be sure the correct reagents were added in the correct order.
3. Visually check reagents for signs of contamination, such as cloudiness or color change.
4. Repeat the test with a new bottle of control.
5. Repeat the test with a new kit or reagent.
6. Call the manufacturer for assistance.

---

blue or red) will indicate a positive result. Accuracy of testing is dependent upon following the specific manufacturer's instructions (Box 29-6).

Box 29-7 lists all of the CLIA-waived tests based on immunological testing principles.

Immunoassay reagents are manufactured as kits. These kits contain all of the reagents and often supplies, such as pipettes, tubes, and cups, needed to perform tests on a given number of samples. The kits must be stored at the temperature recommended on the kit box or package insert. Some kits are stored at room temperature, and some are stored in the refrigerator. It is important to follow the manufacturer's directions. If the kits are stored improperly, the reagents may deteriorate, and false results may be obtained.

Each kit package is marked with a lot number and expiration date. All reagents with the same lot number were made at the same time in the same manufacturing facility. The expiration date is the day past which the reagents are no longer guaranteed to perform correctly.

Reagents from kits with different lot numbers should not be used together. The manufacturer will not guarantee that they will work correctly when components from different lots are mixed. Reagents should never be used past their expiration date. A list of corrective actions for immunology assays is in Box 29-8. The box describes actions to take if an immunoassay control is not producing an acceptable result.

The date of opening the box and the initials of the worker who opened it should also be written on the box when the kit is opened and used for the first time. Some kits have a new expiration date, starting from the day the kit is opened. Always read the package insert for details about storing and handling the reagents and supplies. There may be specific specimen collection guidelines indicated on each kit. Be sure to read and follow the manufacturer's instructions.

Waived Tests Based on Immunological Test Principles

There are many immunoassay test kits available today, and the number is growing. This is an area of CLIA-waived testing that is making an increasing number of diagnostic test results available in the physician's office. The three most common immunoassays will be discussed here.

- *Infectious mononucleosis:* Infectious mononucleosis is caused by the Epstein-Barr virus. The symptoms are fever, sore throat, and swollen lymph glands. Because these symptoms are common to several illnesses, the immunoassay test is useful for a differential diagnosis (Procedure 29-12). False-negative results can occur early in the disease before antibodies are produced.
- *Pregnancy test:* The test for pregnancy (Procedure 29-13) is based on the detection of the hormone

---

BOX 29-7

WAIVED TESTS BASED ON IMMUNOLOGICAL TESTING PRINCIPLES

Streptococcus, group A (microbiology)
Helicobacter pylori (microbiology)
Urine HCG
Infectious mononucleosis
Influenza A/B (virology)
Respiratory syncytial virus (virology)
Adenovirus (virology)
HIV-1 and HIV-2 antibodies
Ovulation test (luteinizing hormone)
Follicle-stimulating hormone

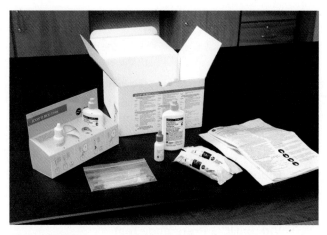

Figure 29-50 Pregnancy test kit.

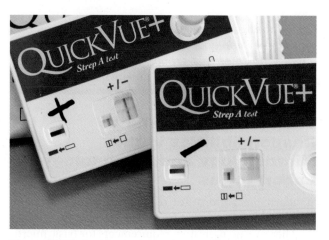

Figure 29-52 Positive and negative rapid strep test results.

human chorionic gonadotropin (HCG). Today's tests are sensitive enough to determine pregnancy before the first missed menses. A pregnancy test is frequently used to rule out pregnancy before a medical procedure that might harm the fetus (Fig. 29-50). A urine specimen that is too dilute can give a false-negative reaction. The first morning urine specimen is the most likely to contain HCG if the patient is pregnant. Certain tumors (testicular and some fibroids) produce HCG and can cause a false-positive result.

• *Group A streptococcus:* Group A streptococcus (*Streptococcus pyogenes*) is one of the most common bacterial causes of sore throat and upper respiratory tract infections. Because of the need for rapid diagnosis to begin appropriate treatment, many immunoassay kits are available to test quickly for group A beta-hemolytic streptococcus or *S. pyogenes* (Fig. 29-51). If the test result is positive, treatment can begin at once.

Group A strep infection can be diagnosed by bacterial culture or immunoassay for the antigenic presence of the bacteria (Fig. 29-52). (See Procedure 29-14.) If

improper technique is used in collecting the throat swab or an inadequate specimen is obtained, a false-negative result can occur. Culture testing is considered more sensitive and should be used to confirm negative immunoassay test results.

CHECKPOINT QUESTIONS

25. What virus is the cause of infectious mononucleosis?
26. What is the result of improper specimen collection technique on a group A strep test?

PATIENT EDUCATION

PATIENT SCENARIO #2

A 5-year-old male arrived a medical office with his mother. He was brought in because he had a fever and had complained of a sore throat for about 24 hours. On physical examination, the patient had a fever of 102.3°F, and he had considerable swelling and drainage of the pharynx. His tonsils were enlarged and coated with a white, patchy exudate. He had a red throat.

• What would be a presumptive diagnosis for this child?
  A presumptive diagnosis for this child would be strep throat.
• Why?
  The fever and enlarged tonsils with white patches are signs.
• What diagnostic testing would be indicated to follow this exam?
  Group A *Streptococcus*
• How would the test results be interpreted?

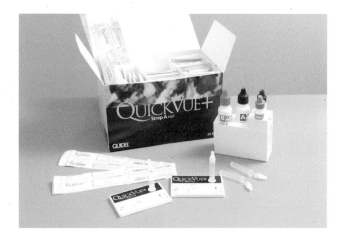

Figure 29-51 Rapid strep test kit.

(continued)

A positive test result indicates the presence of group A *Streptococcus*, whereas a negative test result indicates that group A strep is not present and is not the cause of the patient's sore throat.

The Medical Assistant's Responsibilities in the Microbiology and Immunology Laboratories

Standard precautions are required in all areas of the physician's office laborotory or any laboratory.

There are no pretesting requirements for basic microbiology procedures. Procurement of a patient specimen must be documented in the patient's chart. You must follow laboratory policies on the documentation of test results. Procedures will involve methods for retaining test results in the laboratory and also documenting the test results in the patient's chart.

As a medical assistant, you may perform microbiology and immunology procedures approved for your scope of practice once you are trained and documented to be proficient by a medical technologist or a physician.

español SPANISH TERMINOLOGY

Voy a hacerle un cultivo de garganta.
I am going to swab your throat.

Por favor eche su cabeza hacia atrás.
Please tilt your head back.

Voy a tomar una muestra de su nariz.
I am going to swab inside your nose.

Tosa flema de su pecho.
Cough up phlegm from your chest.

MEDIA MENU

- **Student Resources on thePoint**
  - **Animation: Immune Response**
  - **Video: Collecting a Throat Specimen (Procedure 29-1)**
  - **Video: Testing Stool Specimen for Occult Blood: Guaiac Method (Procedure 29-8)**
  - **Video: Preparing a Smear for Microscopic Evaluation (Procedure 29-9)**
  - **Video: HCG Pregnancy Test (Procedure 29-13)**
  - **Video: Rapid Group A Strep Testing (Procedure 29-14)**
  - **CMA/RMA Certification Exam Review**
- **Internet Resources**

  CLIA Tests Waived by FDA
  http://www.accessdata.fda.gov/scripts/cdrh/cfdocs/cfClia/testswaived.cfm

  MedlinePlus Health Information from the National Library of Medicine
  http://medlineplus.gov

  Microbiology Microbes Bacteria Information and Links
  http://www.microbes.info

  American College of Allergy, Asthma and Immunology (ACAAI)
  http://www.acaai.org

  Atlas of Microbiology
  www.medmaster.net/atlasofmicrobiol.html

  Bacterial Morphology
  http://nhscience.lonestar.edu/biol/wellmeyer/bacteria/bacmorph.htm

PSY PROCEDURE 29-1: **Collect a Throat Specimen**

Purpose: Obtain a throat specimen for rapid strep testing or culture
Equipment: Tongue blade, light source, sterile specimen container and swab, PPE, hand sanitizer, surface sanitizer, biohazard transport bag (if to be sent to the laboratory for analysis)

Steps	Reasons
1. Wash your hands.	Handwashing aids infection control.
2. Assemble the equipment and supplies.	Equipment must be readily accessible for the procedure to be done.
3. Put on PPE.	Following standard precautions prevents the transmission of infectious microorganisms.
4. **AFF** Greet and identify the patient. Explain the rationale of the performance of the collection to the patient	Identifying the patient prevents errors in treatment.
5. **AFF** If the patient is hearing impaired, you need to speak clearly and distinctly in front of the patient's face.	Speaking clearly and distinctly to the patient's face will assist the patient in understanding spoken instructions. Have an easy-to-read instruction guide for the patient to follow and point out where there are questions. If the patient can sign and you cannot, have someone proficient in sign language assist you in instructing the patient.
6. **AFF** Use active listening to observe patients' body language and detect a lack of understanding of instructions. Obtain assistance when you realize that you are not able to communicate with the patient.	Someone else in the office may have experience with sign language or may be more effective helping your patient understand.
7. **AFF** Leave time for the patient to ask questions.	Display sensitivity to patient feelings in collecting specimens.
8. **AFF** Display empathy for the patient and family.	Offer this in a timely manner so as not to extend the discomfort of expectation of the procedure.
9. Have the patient sit with a light source directed in the throat.	Enhancing visualization of specimen site improves accuracy of sampling.
10. **AFF** Demonstrate awareness of the patient's territorial boundaries.	As you position yourself for enhanced vision, you may be closer than the patient finds comfortable. Attempt to respect this comfort zone.
11. Carefully remove the sterile swab from the container. If performing both the rapid strep and culture or confirming negative results with a culture, swab with two swabs held together. **Step 11.** Carefully remove the sterile swab from the container.	Swabbing with two swabs at once eliminates discomfort to the patient of having to perform the procedure twice.
12. Have the patient say "Ah" as you press down on the midpoint of the tongue with the tongue depressor. If the tongue depressor is placed too far forward, it will not be effective; if it is placed too far back, the patient will gag unnecessarily.	Saying "Ah" raises the uvula to avoid contaminating the specimen and decreases the gag reflex.

(continued)

PSY **PROCEDURE 29-1:**   **Collect a Throat Specimen** *(continued)*

Steps	**Reasons**
13. Swab the mucous membranes, especially the tonsillar area, the crypts, and the posterior pharnx in a "figure 8" motion. Turn the swab to expose all of its surfaces to the membranes. Avoid touching teeth, sides of mouth, and uvula.	Pathogens must be collected with a twisting motion for maximum collection. Touching the areas noted to avoid will contaminate the specimen with normal flora and inhibit testing accuracy.

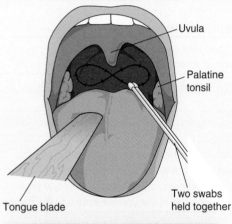

Uvula

Palatine tonsil

Tongue blade

Two swabs held together

Step 13A. Technique for obtaining a throat sample.

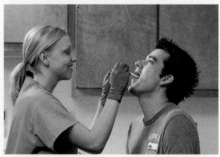

Step 13B. Avoid touching areas that will contaminate the specimen.

14. Maintain the tongue depressor position while withdrawing the swab from the patient's mouth.	Keeping the tongue down prevents contaminating the swab with normal flora.

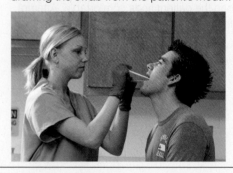

Step 14. Withdraw the swab with the tongue depressor still in position.

15. Follow the instructions on the specimen container for transferring the swab or processing the specimen in the office using a commercial kit. Label the specimen with the patient's name, the date and time of collection, and the origin of the material.	Improper handling of the specimen will compromise test results. Improper labeling will result in test delay and require the patient to have the procedure repeated.
16. Properly dispose of the equipment and supplies in a biohazard waste container. Remove PPE and wash your hands.	This prevents the spread of microorganisms.

PSY PROCEDURE 29-1: **Collect a Throat Specimen *(continued)***

Steps	Reasons
17. Route the specimen or store it appropriately until routing can be completed.	Delay in transport to the testing site or improper storage will compromise test results.
18. Document the procedure.	Procedures that are not documented are considered to have not been performed.
19. Sanitize the work area.	Sanitation aids in infection control.

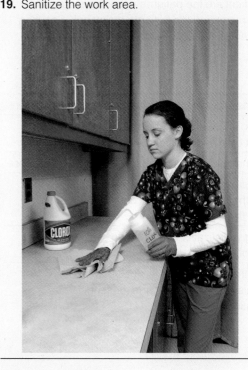

Step 19. Sanitize the work area.

Charting Example:

11/20/2012 10:30 AM Throat specimen obtained, Dx code ###.## per Dr. Lewis.
Rapid strep test negative, specimen to reference lab for C&S —————————— M. Mohr, CMA

Note: The medical assistant may sign his or her name in the patient record using only the "CMA" credential if the office has a signature log denoting the entire credential as "CMA(AAMA)."

PSY PROCEDURE 29-2: **Collecting a Nasopharyngeal Specimen**

Purpose: This test is used to evaluate nasopharyngeal secretions for the presence of pathogenic organisms
Equipment: Penlight, tongue blade, sterile flexible swab, transport media, PPE, hand sanitizer, surface sanitizer, biohazard transport bag (if to be sent to the laboratory for analysis)

Steps	Reasons
1. Wash your hands.	Handwashing aids infection control.
2. Assemble the equipment and supplies.	Equipment must be readily accessible for the procedure to be done.
3. Put on PPE.	Following standard precautions prevents the transmission of infectious microorganisms.

(continued)

PSY **PROCEDURE 29-2:** **Collecting a Nasopharyngeal Specimen** *(continued)*

Steps	Reasons
4. **AFF** Greet and identify the patient. Explain the rationale of the performance of the collection to the patient.	Identifying the patient prevents errors in treatment.
5. **AFF** If your patient is developmentally challenged, have the individual who transported the patient to the office assist you with communicating with the patient. The developmentally challenged patient may struggle if you have to proceed with something he or she does not understand. Have another medical assistant available to help you should extra support be necessary to support the patient.	Two issues in working with a developmentally challenged patient are the patient's understanding and physically managing the patient's resistance. Securing help is safer for you and the patient.
6. **AFF** Leave time for the patient to ask questions.	Display sensitivity to patient feelings in collecting specimens.
7. **AFF** Display empathy for the patient and family.	Offer this in a timely manner so as not to extend the discomfort of expectation of the procedure.
8. Position the patient with his head tilted back.	Tilting the head improves access to the interior of the nose.
9. **AFF** Demonstrate awareness of the patient's territorial boundaries.	As you position yourself for enhanced vision, you may be closer than the patient finds comfortable. Attempt to respect this comfort zone.
10. Using a penlight, inspect the nasopharyngeal area.	Enhancing visualization of specimen site improves accuracy of sampling.
11. Gently pass the swab through the nostril and into the nasopharynx, keeping the swab near the septum and floor of the nose. Rotate the swab quickly, and then remove it and place it in the transport media. **Step 11.** Gently swab within the nostril.	Do not let the swab touch the sides of the patient's nostril or his or her tongue to prevent specimen contamination.
12. Label the specimen with the patient's name, the date and time of collection, and the origin of repeated.	Improper labeling will result in test delay and require the patient to have the procedure specimen.
13. Properly dispose of the equipment and supplies in a biohazard waste container. Remove PPE and wash your hands.	This prevents the spread of microorganisms.
14. Route the specimen or store it appropriately until routing can be completed.	Delay in transport to the testing site or improper storage will compromise test results.
15. Document the procedure.	Procedures not documented are considered not performed.
16. Sanitize the work area.	Sanitation aids in infection control.

Charting Example:

11/20/2012 10:30 AM Nasopharyngeal specimen obtained, Dx code ###.## per Dr. Lewis. Specimen to reference lab for C&S —————————————————————————————————— M. Mohr, CMA

Note: The medical assistant may sign his or her name in the patient record using only the "CMA" credential if the office has a signature log denoting the entire credential as "CMA(AAMA)."

PSY **PROCEDURE 29-3:**   **Collecting a Wound Specimen**

Purpose: This test is used to evaluate wound exudate for the presence of pathogenic organisms
Equipment: Sterile swab, transport media, PPE, hand sanitizer, surface sanitizer, biohazard transport bag
(if to be sent to the laboratory for analysis)

Steps	Reasons
1. Wash your hands.	Handwashing aids infection control.
2. Assemble the equipment and supplies.	Equipment must be readily accessible for the procedure to be done.
3. Put on PPE.	Following standard precautions prevents the transmission of infectious microorganisms.
4. **AFF** Greet and identify the patient. Explain the procedure.	Identifying the patient prevents errors in treatment.
5. **AFF** If your patient is struggling with dementia, be prepared to gently repeat yourself as necessary until you have collected your specimen. You may have to physically adjust your patient as necessary to collect the specimen. Be gentle but remember to speak to the patient as an adult.	The patient may forget what you just explained. He or she may have some trouble understanding immediately after you explained it. The patient may recognize when being spoken to rudely or as a child.
6. If dressing is present, remove it and dispose of it in biohazard container. Assess the wound by observing color, odor, and amount of exudate. Remove contaminated gloves and put on clean gloves.	Thorough visualization of specimen site improves accuracy of sampling.
7. Use the sterile swab to sample the exudate. Saturate swab with exudate, avoiding the skin edge around the wound.	Skin around the wound will contain normal flora that may inhibit growth of the pathogen.

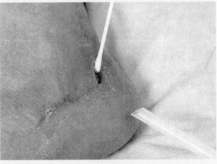

Step 7. Saturate swab with exudate.

Steps	Reasons
8. Avoid skin edge around wound.	Normal skin flora may contaminate specimen and compromise viability of pathogens in specimen.
9. Place swab back into container and crush the ampule of transport medium.	Fastidious bacteria may require transport medium to maintain viability.

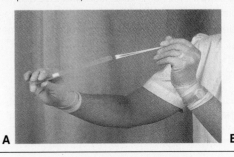

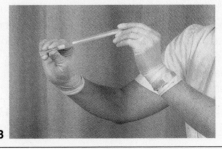

Step 9. (A) Place swab in culturette tube. **(B)** Crush the ampule of media at the bottom of the tube.

(continued)

PSY PROCEDURE 29-3: Collecting a Wound Specimen *(continued)*

Steps	Reasons
10. Label the specimen with the patient's name, the date and time of collection, and the origin of specimen.	Improper labeling will result in test delay and require the patient to have the procedure repeated.
11. Route the specimen or store it appropriately until routing can be completed.	Delay in transport to the testing site or improper storage will compromise test results.
12. Clean the wound and apply a sterile dressing using sterile technique.	A sterile dressing protects the wound from infection.
13. Properly dispose of the equipment and supplies in a biohazard waste container. Remove PPE and wash your hands.	This prevents the spread of microorganisms.
14. Document the procedure.	Procedures not documented are considered not performed.
15. Sanitize the work area.	Sanitation aids in infection control.

Charting Example:

11/20/2012 10:30 AM Wound specimen obtained from right heel, Dx code ###.## per Dr. Lewis.
Specimen to reference lab for C&S —————————————————————— M. Mohr, CMA

Note: The medical assistant may sign his or her name in the patient record using only the "CMA" credential if the office has a signature log denoting the entire credential as "CMA(AAMA)."

PSY PROCEDURE 29-4: Collecting a Sputum Specimen

Purpose: This test is used to evaluate sputum for the presence of disease
Equipment: Sterile specimen container, PPE, hand sanitizer, surface sanitizer, biohazard transport bag.

Steps	Reasons
1. Wash your hands.	Handwashing aids infection control.
2. Assemble the equipment and supplies.	Equipment must be readily accessible for the procedure to be done.
3. Put on PPE.	Following standard precautions prevents the transmission of infectious microorganisms.
4. **AFF** Greet and identify the patient. Explain the procedure.	Identifying the patient prevents errors in treatment. Explanations will help gain compliance and ease anxiety.
5. **AFF** If English is not your patient's primary language, you will need to have someone available to translate. Often someone who speaks English will accompany the patient to the office. If this is not the case, use the assistance of someone else in the office who speaks the patient's language. Some offices subscribe to a telephone translation service.	Providing support for communication with ESL and non-English speaking patients reduces fear and helps them understand ways to help with accurate specimen collection.
6. Provide the patient with a cup of water and instruct him or her to rinse his or her mouth with water.	Rinsing the mouth reduces contamination of sputum specimen with normal mouth flora.

PSY PROCEDURE 29-4: **Collecting a Sputum Specimen (continued)**

Steps	Reasons
7. Ask the patient to cough deeply, using the abdominal muscles as well as the accessory muscles to bring secretions from the lungs and not just the upper airways.	The desired specimen should contain pathogens and epithelial cells from the lining of the lower res- respiratory tract.
8. Ask the patient to expectorate directly into the specimen container without touching the inside and without getting sputum on the outsides of the container. About 5–10 mL is sufficient for most sputum studies.	Touching the inside of the container will contaminate the container and specimen. Sputum on the outside of the container may be hazardous.
9. Handle the specimen container according to standard precautions. Cap the container immediately and put it into the biohazard bag for transport to the laboratory. Fill out a laboratory requisition slip to accompany the specimen.	The specimen is a biohazard, and capping the container immediately eliminates the danger of spreading microorganisms. A laboratory requisition will tell the laboratory personnel the type of specimen and the specific tests ordered.
10. Label the specimen with the patient's name, the date and time of collection, and the origin of the specimen.	Improper labeling will result in test delay and require the patient to have the procedure repeated.
11. Route the specimen to the laboratory.	Delay in transport to the testing site will compromise test results. The pathogens may either proliferate, causing overgrowth, or die, causing a false-negative result.
12. Properly dispose of the equipment and supplies in a biohazard waste container. Remove PPE and wash your hands.	This prevents the spread of microorganisms.
13. Document the procedure.	Procedures not documented are considered not performed.
14. Sanitize the work area.	Sanitation aids in infection control.

Charting Example:

11/20/2012 10:30 AM Moderate amount of thick, yellow sputum, Dx code ###.## per Dr. Lewis.
Specimen to reference lab for C&S ———————————————————————— M. Mohr, CMA

Note: The medical assistant may sign his or her name in the patient record using only the "CMA" credential if the office has a signature log denoting the entire credential as "CMA(AAMA)."

PSY PROCEDURE 29-5: Collecting a Stool Specimen

Purpose: This test is used to evaluate stool for pathogens and/or blood

Equipment: Specimen container dependent on test ordered (sterile container or Para-Pak Collection System for C&S or ova and parasites; test kit or slide for occult blood testing; see laboratory procedure manual), tongue blade or wooden spatula, PPE, hand sanitizer, surface sanitizer, biohazard transport bag, Para-Pak stool collection containers

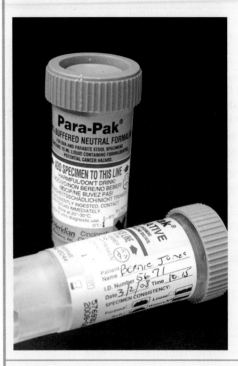

Para-Pak stool collection containers.

Steps	Reasons
1. Wash your hands.	Handwashing aids infection control.
2. Assemble the equipment and supplies.	Equipment must be readily accessible for the procedure to be done.
3. **AFF** Greet and identify the patient. Explain the procedure. Explain any dietary, medication, or other restrictions necessary for the collection. (These restrictions and instructions for the patient are detailed earlier in this chapter in the Patient Education box titled, *Patient Preparation for Fecal Occult Blood Testing*.) Instruct patient to defecate and return specimen to the laboratory.	Identifying the patient prevents errors in treatment. Explanations will help gain compliance and ease anxiety. Noncompliance with preparation for specimen collection may cause false-positive results and unnecessary follow-up testing.
4. **AFF** If you are in a significantly different generation than the patient, you will need to take extra precautions with communication. First, remember that collecting a stool specimen is embarrassing for most patients. Watch the patient's facial expressions to note if he or she is understanding your instructions. This is one of the times you may find that your patient does not understand professional terminology.	Patients prefer not to hear repeated instructions openly discussing body functions. Follow up with enough questions to validate the patient's understanding.

PSY PROCEDURE 29-5: **Collecting a Stool Specimen** *(continued)*

Steps	Reasons
5. When obtaining a stool specimen for C&S or ova and parasites, the patient should collect an amount of the first and last portion of the stool after the bowel movement with the wooden spatula or tongue blade and place it in the specimen container without contaminating the outside of the container. Fill Para-Pak until fluid reaches "fill" line, and recap the container.	Touching the inside of the container will contaminate the container and specimen. Stool on the outside of the container may be hazardous. The specimen is a biohazard, and capping the container immediately eliminates the danger of spreading microorganisms.
6. Upon receipt of the specimen, you should put on gloves and place the specimen into the biohazard bag for transport to the reference laboratory. Fill out a laboratory requisition slip to accompany the specimen.	A laboratory requisition will tell the laboratory personnel the type of specimen and the specific tests ordered.
7. Label the specimen with the patient's name, the date and time of collection, and the origin of the specimen.	Improper labeling will result in test delay and require the patient to have the procedure repeated.
8. Transport the specimen to the laboratory or store the specimen as directed. Refer to the laboratory procedure manual since some samples require refrigeration; others are kept at room temperature, and some must be placed in an incubator at a laboratory as soon as possible after collecting.	Improper storage and/or delay in transport to the testing site will compromise test results.
9. Properly dispose of the equipment and supplies in a biohazard waste container. Remove PPE and wash your hands.	This prevents the spread of microorganisms.
10. Document the procedure including patient instructions.	Procedures not documented are not considered to be performed.
11. Sanitize the work area.	Sanitation aids in infection control.

Charting Example:

11/20/2012 10:30 AM Patient instructed on preparation for and collection of stool for occult blood. Patient demonstrated understanding and will return specimen to lab upon completion. Dx code ###.## per Dr. Lewis.——————————————————————————— M. Mohr, CMA
11/21/2012 8:00 AM Patient delivered stool specimen to the laboratory——————————————— M. Mohr, CMA

Note: The medical assistant may sign his or her name in the patient record using only the "CMA" credential if the office has a signature log denoting the entire credential as "CMA(AAMA)."

PSY PROCEDURE 29-6: **Collecting Blood for Culture**

Purpose: This test is used to evaluate blood for pathogens
Equipment: Specimen container depends on testing site (yellow-top sodium polyanethol sulfonate vacutainer tubes or aerobic and anaerobic blood culture bottles), blood culture skin prep packs (or 70% isopropyl alcohol wipes and povidone-iodine solution swabs or towelettes), venipuncture supplies (see Chapter 26), PPE, hand sanitizer, surface sanitizer

Steps	Reasons
1. Wash your hands.	Handwashing aids infection control.
2. Assemble the equipment and supplies, checking expiration dates.	Expired collection or culture supplies must be discarded.

(continued)

Steps	Reasons
3. Put on PPE.	Following standard precautions prevents the transmission of infectious microorganisms.
4. **AFF** Greet and identify the patient. Explain the procedure. Verify that the patient has not started antibiotic therapy. If therapy has started, document antibiotic, strength, dose, duration, and time of last dose.	Identifying the patient prevents errors in treatment. Antibiotic therapy can cause false-negative test results.
5. **AFF** If the patient is hearing impaired, you need to speak clearly and distinctly in front of the patient's face. You should have an easy-to-read instruction guide for the patient to follow and point out where he or she has questions. If the patient can sign and you cannot, have someone proficient in sign language assist you in instructing the patient.	Speaking clearly and distinctly to the patient's face will assist the patient in understanding spoken instructions.
6. Using skin preparation kits or supplies, apply alcohol to venipuncture site and allow to air dry. Apply povidone-iodine prep in progressively increasing concentric circles without wiping back over skin that is already prepped. Let stand for at least 1 minute and allow the site to air dry. Do not touch skin following preparation. **Step 6.** Swab the antecubital space of the arm using a povidone-iodine swab, cleaning in progressively increasing circles.	The povidone-iodine reduces false-positive culture results from skin contaminants. Touching the site following preparation may reintroduce contaminants.
7. Wipe bottle stoppers with povidone-iodine solution.	Bottle tops require decontamination to prevent specimen contamination.
8. Perform venipuncture as described in Procedure 26-1.	
9. Fill bottles or tubes according to the specific laboratory procedure. Invert each 8–10 times as soon as collected. If using culture bottles, fill the aerobic bottle first.	Inversion mixes blood with media. Collecting the aerobic bottle first removes any residual air in the needle to avoid contaminating the anaerobic bottle.
10. Complete venipuncture. Use an isopropyl alcohol wipe to remove residual povidone-iodine from skin. Label the specimen with the patient's name, the date and time of collection, and the origin of specimen.	Leaving iodine solution on skin can cause irritation.
11. Remove gloves and wash hands. In preparation for the second collection 30 minutes after the first, put on new gloves and repeat Steps 5–9 at a second venipuncture site.	A minimum of 30 mL of blood should be collected between the two venipunctures.. Using two collection sites increases success of isolating pathogen if present.
12. Label the specimens with the patient's name and the date and time of collection.	Improper labeling will result in specimen rejection by the testing laboratory.

PSY PROCEDURE 29-6: Collecting Blood for Culture *(continued)*

Steps	Reasons
13. Properly dispose of the equipment and supplies in a biohazard waste container. Remove PPE and wash your hands.	This prevents the spread of microorganisms.
14. Document the procedure.	Procedures not documented have not been performed.
15. Sanitize the work area.	Sanitation aids in infection control.

Charting Example:

11/20/2012 10:30 AM Blood culture specimens collected from antecubital area of left and right arms,

Dx code ###.## per Dr. Lewis. ———————————————————— M. Mohr, CMA

Note: The medical assistant may sign his or her name in the patient record using only the "CMA" credential if the office has a signature log denoting the entire credential as "CMA(AAMA)."

PSY PROCEDURE 29-7: Collecting Genital Specimens for Culture

Purpose: This test is used to evaluate for pathogens
Equipment: Specimen container depends on testing requested (bacterial, viral, and *Chlamydia* specimens require different media), PPE, hand sanitizer, surface sanitizer

Steps	Reasons
1. Wash your hands.	Handwashing aids infection control.
2. Assemble the equipment and supplies, checking expiration dates.	Expired collection or culture supplies must be discarded.
3. Put on PPE.	Following standard precautions prevents the transmission of infectious microorganisms.
4. Your role will be to assist the physician in the collection and handling of these specimens. Be sure to verbally verify patient identification.	Identifying the patient prevents errors in treatment.
5. **AFF** Be sensitive to indications that the patient is uncomfortable with your perception of her. Be reassuring with a gentle, professional demeanor. Be aware of your body language.	
6. **AFF** Assist the physician with patients having communication problems. Secure assistance as it is necessary.	
7. Accept specimens from the physician, securing them in the appropriate medium follow the instructions for that particular medium.	Isolating the pathogen is necessary to the appropriate environment for transport and culture.

(continued)

PSY PROCEDURE 29-7: **Collecting Genital Specimens for Culture (continued)**

Steps	Reasons
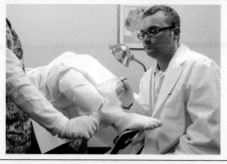	
	Step 7. Physician places swab into culturette tube in the medical assistant's gloved hand.
8. Label the specimen with the patient's name, the date and time of collection, and the origin of specimen.	Improper labeling will result in specimen rejection by the testing laboratory.
9. Repeat Steps 6 and 7 for each specimen.	Multiple specimens may be collected.
10. Store specimens per procedure instructions until transport. Transport to testing facility as soon as possible.	Improper storage and/or delay in transport to the testing site will compromise test results.
11. Properly dispose of the equipment and supplies in a biohazard waste container. Remove PPE and wash your hands.	This prevents the spread of microorganisms.
12. Document the procedure.	Procedures not documented are not performed.
13. Sanitize the work area.	Sanitation aids in infection control.

Charting Example:

> *11/20/2012 10:30 AM Vaginal specimens collected for C&S, herpes, and Chlamydia and referred to reference lab, Dx code ###.## per Dr. Lewis. —————————————————————————————— M. Mohr, CMA*

Note: The medical assistant may sign his or her name in the patient record using only the "CMA" credential if the office has a signature log denoting the entire credential as "CMA(AAMA)."

 PSY PROCEDURE 29-8: **Testing Stool Specimen for Occult Blood: Guaiac Method**

Purpose: Test stool for occult blood in a sample obtained by the patient using a test kit and brought or mailed into the office

Equipment: Gloves, patient's labeled specimen pack, developer or reagent drops, PPE, hand sanitizer, surface sanitizer, contaminated waste container

Steps	Reasons
1. Wash your hands and put on clean examination gloves.	Handwashing aids infection control. Follow standard precautions when handling stool specimens.
2. Assemble the supplies and verify the patient identification on the patient's prepared test pack. Check the expiration date on the developing solution.	Proper identification prevents errors. Solution that has expired may yield inaccurate results.

PSY PROCEDURE 29-8: **Testing Stool Specimen for Occult Blood: Guaiac Method (continued)**

Steps	Reasons
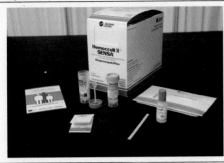	**Step 2.** Assemble the supplies and check expiration dates.
3. Open the test window on the back of the pack and apply one drop of the developer or testing reagent to each window according to manufacturer's directions. Read the color change within the specified time, usually 60 seconds.	Following the manufacturer's instructions ensures accurate results.
4. Apply one drop of developer as directed on the control monitor section or window of the pack. Note whether the quality control results are positive or negative as appropriate. If results are acceptable, patient results may be reported. If results are not acceptable, notify the physician.	Patient test results cannot be reported if quality control (QC) results are not acceptable.
5. Properly dispose of the test pack and gloves. Wash your hands.	Follow standard precautions throughout the procedure.
6. Record the procedure.	Procedures not documented are not performed.
7. Sanitize the work area.	Sanitation aids in infection control.

Charting Example:

> 3/28/2012 3:00 PM Occult blood slides ×3 returned to office via mail; testing performed Dx ###.## per Dr. Franklin; findings positive. Dr. Franklin notified———————————————————————————— J. Smith, RMA

Note: The medical assistant may sign his or her name in the patient record using only the "CMA" credential if the office has a signature log denoting the entire credential as "CMA(AAMA)."

 PSY PROCEDURE 29-9: **Preparing a Smear for Microscopic Evaluation**

Purpose: To aid in the identification of microorganisms in a specimen
Equipment: Specimen, Bunsen burner, slide forceps, slide, sterile swab or inoculating loop, pencil or diamond-tipped pen, PPE, hand sanitizer, surface sanitizer, contaminated waste container

Steps	Reasons
1. Wash your hands.	Handwashing aids infection control.
2. Assemble the equipment.	Equipment must be readily accessible to perform the procedure.
3. Label the slide with the patient's name and the date on the frosted edge with a pencil.	Labeling will ensure proper identification. Pencil markings will not rinse off during staining.

(continued)

PSY **PROCEDURE 29-9:** **Preparing a Smear for Microscopic Evaluation (continued)**

Steps	Reasons
4. Put on PPE.	Always comply with standard precautions.
5. Hold the edges of the slide between the thumb and index finger. Starting at the right side of the slide and using a rolling motion of the swab, gently and evenly spread the material from the specimen over the slide. The material should fill the area center of the slide within half an inch of each end.	Spread the material thinly to avoid obscuring the slide with too much material. Rolling ensures that as much of the specimen as possible is deposited on the slide. Sweeping the loop accomplishes the same purpose. Confining the specimen to within half an inch of the edges avoids of each contaminating the gloves.

Step 5. The material should thinly fill the center of the slide.

Steps	Reasons
6. Do not rub the material vigorously over the slide.	Doing so may destroy fragile microorganisms.
7. Dispose of the contaminated swab or disposable inoculating loop in a biohazard container.	The swab and the loop contain body fluid and are biohazardous.
8. Allow the smear to air dry in a flat position for at least half an hour. Do not blow on the slide or wave it about in the air. Heat should not be applied until the specimen has been allowed to dry. Some specimens (e.g., Pap smear) require a fixative spray.	The cells will dry slowly at room temperature. If you blow on the slide, you may contaminate the specimen with bacteria from your mouth. Fixative may be sprayed from 4–6 inches to protect the cells from contaminants or to keep them from becoming dislodged. Heat at this point may destroy the microorganisms.
9. Hold the dried smear slide with the slide forceps. Pass the slide quickly through the flame of a bunsen burner or safety match three or four times. The slide has been fixed properly when the back of the slide feels slightly warm to the back of the gloved hand. *Caution:* Any excess heat will distort and probably destroy the specimen material on the slide.	Passing the slide through the heat kills the microorganisms and attaches them firmly to the slide so they do not wash off during staining and are not dislodged during viewing. Excessive heat may distort the specimen cells. It should not feel uncomfortably hot.
10. Properly dispose of the equipment and supplies in a biohazard waste container. Remove PPE and wash your hands.	This prevents the spread of microorganisms.
11. Document the procedure.	Procedures not documented have not been performed.
12. Sanitize the work area.	Sanitation aids in infection control.

Charting Example:

07/23/2012 10:00 AM Specimen taken from nostril and prepared as a direct smear Dx. ###.## per Dr. York

——

———— B. White, RMA

PSY PROCEDURE 29-10: Performing a Gram Stain

Purpose: To aid in the identification of pathogens in a specimen

Equipment: Crystal violet stain, staining rack, Gram iodine solution, wash bottle with distilled water, alcohol-acetone solution, counterstain (e.g., safranin), absorbent (bibulous) paper pad, specimen smear on glass slide labeled with a pencil or diamond-tipped pen (as prepared in Procedure 29-9), Bunsen burner, slide forceps, stopwatch or timer, PPE, hand sanitizer, surface sanitizer, contaminated waste container

Steps	Reasons
1. Wash your hands.	Handwashing aids infection control.
2. Assemble the equipment.	Equipment must be readily accessible to perform the procedure.
3. Make sure the specimen is heat-fixed to the labeled slide and the slide is at room temperature (see Procedure 29-9).	Instructions for performing this step are detailed in Procedure 29-9.
4. Put on PPE.	
5. Place the slide on the staining rack with the smear side up.	The staining rack collects the dye as it runs off the slide for disposal.
6. Flood the smear with crystal violet. Time for 60 seconds.	Add dye for the appropriate amount of time to provide a good stain.

Step 6. Flood the smear with crystal violet.

Steps	Reasons
7. Hold the slide with slide forceps. A. Tilt the slide to an angle of about 45° to drain the excess dye. B. Rinse the slide with distilled water for about 5 seconds and drain off excess water.	Washing the slide stops the staining process.
8. Replace the slide on the slide rack. Flood the slide with Gram iodine solution for 60 seconds.	The iodine acts as a mordant and fixes, or binds, the crystal violet to the Gram-positive bacteria. The stain will be permanent in the receptive Gram-positive cells after it is fixed with the iodine solution.
9. Using the forceps, tilt the slide at a 45° angle to drain iodine solution. With the slide tilted, rinse the slide with distilled water from the wash bottle for about 5 to 10 seconds. Slowly and gently wash with the alcohol-acetone solution until no more stain runs off.	The alcohol-acetone removes the crystal violet stain from the Gram-negative bacteria. The Gram-positive bacteria retain the purple dye. If the process is carried on too long or too vigorously, dye may leach out of the Gram-positive bacteria and lead to incorrect findings.
10. Immediately rinse the slide with distilled water for 5 seconds and return the slide to the rack.	Rinsing stops the decolorizing.
11. Flood with safranin or suitable counterstain for 60 seconds.	The Gram-negative bacteria stain pink or red with the counterstain.

(continued)

PSY PROCEDURE 29-10: **Performing a Gram Stain** *(continued)*

Steps	Reasons
12. Drain the excess counterstain from the slide by tilting it at a 45° angle. Rinse the slide with distilled water for 5 seconds to remove the counterstain. Gently blot the smear dry with bibulous paper. Take care not to disturb the smeared specimen. Wipe the back of the slide clear of any solution. It may be placed between the pages of a bibulous paper pad and gently pressed to remove excess moisture.	Moisture or excess solution may obscure the specimen and hinder identification.

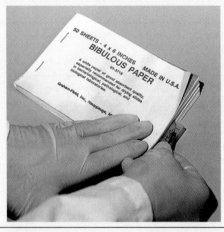

Step 12. Gently blot smear dry with bibulous paper.

Steps	Reasons
13. Properly dispose of the equipment and supplies in a biohazard waste container. Remove PPE and wash your hands.	This prevents the spread of microorganisms.
14. Document the procedure.	Procedures not documented have not been performed.
15. Sanitize the work area.	Sanitation aids in infection control.

Note: Results may be misinterpreted if a reagent is defective or near expiration or if the timing is not as directed. The bacteria may overstain, or color may leach from the cells if care is not taken to observe the time limits. The results will not be accurate if the specimen was not heated properly (killing the bacteria) or was not incubated long enough or if the general technique was not performed correctly. Prepared smears of known Gram-positive and Gram-negative organisms are processed with the patient's specimen for quality control.

Charting Example:

07/23/2012 10:10 AM Slide of patient's specimen Gram stained and submitted to Dr. York to review. Dx. ###.##——————

——B. White, RMA

Note: The medical assistant may sign his or her name in the patient record using only the "CMA" credential if the office has a signature log denoting the entire credential as "CMA(AAMA)."

PSY PROCEDURE 29-11: Inoculating a Culture

Purpose: To introduce a portion of a specimen into the culture medium for growth and replication of microorganisms and to produce isolated colonies

Equipment: Specimen on a swab or loop, china marker or permanent laboratory marker, sterile or disposable loop, Bunsen burner, labeled Petri dish of culture medium (the patient's name should be on the side of the plate containing the medium because it is always placed upward to prevent condensation from dripping onto the culture), PPE, hand sanitizer, surface sanitizer, contaminated waste container.

Steps	Reasons
1. Wash your hands.	Handwashing aids infection control.
2. Assemble the equipment.	Equipment must be readily accessible to perform the procedure.
3. Put on PPE.	Use PPE for protection from biohazards.
4. Label the medium side of the plate with the patient's name, identification number, source of specimen, time collected, time inoculated, your initials, and date.	Because culture incubation may take 24–72 hours, dating ensures that the plate is read at the proper time. Labeling the medium side will prevent misplacing culture.

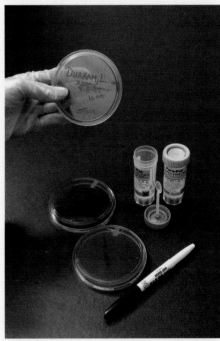

Step 4. Correctly labeled specimen plate.

5. Remove the Petri plate from the cover (the Petri plate is always stored with the cover down), and place the cover on the work surface with the opening up. Do not open the cover unnecessarily.	Each time the cover is removed, there is a chance of contamination. Having the cover's opening upward avoids contamination from the work surface.
6. Using a rolling and sliding motion, streak the specimen swab across one fourth of the plate, starting at the top and working to the center. Dispose of the swab in a biohazard container. The specimen will spread in gradually thinning colonies of bacteria.	

(continued)

PSY PROCEDURE 29-11: Inoculating a Culture *(continued)*

Steps	Reasons

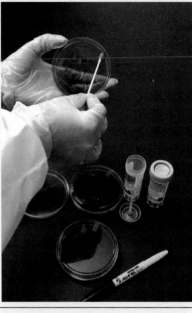

Step 6. Use a rolling and sliding motion to apply specimen to plate.

7. Use a disposable loop.	The loop is the tool for spreading the specimen.
8. Turn the plate a quarter turn from its previous position. Pass the loop a few times in the original inoculum, and then across the medium approximately a quarter of the surface of the plate. Do not enter the originally streaked area after the first few sweeps.	The loop draws into the clean surface a bit of the specimen that was streaked in the first part of the procedure.

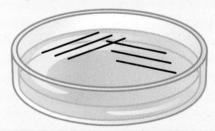

Step 8. Streak lightly from the original inoculum across the next quarter of the plate.

9. Turn the plate another quarter turn so that now it is 180° to the original smear. Working in the previous manner, draw the loop at right angles through the most recently streaked area. Again, do not enter the originally streaked area after the first few sweeps.	The loop pulls out gradually thinning bits of the specimen to isolate colonies. Large groups of colonies close together are more difficult to identify than isolated colonies.

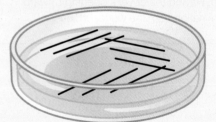

Step 9. Streak the third quadrant of the plate.

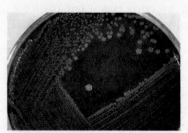

Pale yellow colonies of *Staphylococcus aureus*. Colonies demonstrate growth of the microbe on a properly streaked plate.

PSY PROCEDURE 29-11: Inoculating a Culture (continued)

Steps	Reasons
FOR QUANTITATIVE CULTURES: A. Streak the plate with the specimen from side to side across the middle. 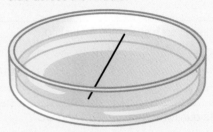	
	Step 9A. Streak the plate from one side to the other in a straight line across the middle.
B. Streak the entire plate back and forth across the initial inoculate. This allows bacteria to grow in a way that colonies can be counted. 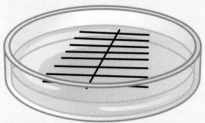	
	Step 9B. Streak the entire plate from side to side over the original inoculum.
10. Properly dispose of the equipment and supplies in a biohazard waste container. Remove PPE and wash your hands.	This prevents the spread of microorganisms.
11. Document the procedure.	Procedures not documented have not been performed.
12. Sanitize the work area.	Sanitation aids in infection control.

Charting Example:

7/14/2012 9:15 AM Swab specimen taken of (L) heel wound, transferred to culture medium for incubation.

To be read 7/16/08. Dx. ###.## per Dr. Brehmer. ———————————————— *G. Gray, RMA*

PSY PROCEDURE 29-12: Mononucleosis Testing

Purpose: To determine the presence or absence of infectious mononucleosis
Equipment: Patient's labeled specimen (whole blood, plasma, or serum, depending on the kit), CLIA-waived mononucleosis kit (slide or test strip), stopwatch or timer, PPE, hand sanitizer, surface sanitizer, contaminated waste container

Steps	Reasons
1. Wash your hands.	Handwashing aids infection control.
2. Verify that the names on the specimen container and the laboratory form are the same.	Patient identification is critical in accurate reporting.
3. Assemble the equipment and ensure that the materials in the kit and the patient specimen are at room temperature.	Equipment must be reasily accessible to perform the procedure.

PSY PROCEDURE 29-12:   **Mononucleosis Testing (continued)**

Steps	Reasons
4. Label the test pack or test strip (depending on type of kit) with the patient's name, positive control, and negative control. Use one test pack or strip per patient and control.	This ensures accurate testing.
5. Aspirate the patient's specimen using the transfer pipette and place instructed volume on the sample well of the test pack or dip test strip labeled with the patient's name. Volume instructions may be found in the kit package insert.	This adds the patient's specimen for testing.
6. Sample the positive and negative controls as directed in Step 5.	This satisfies quality assurance (QA) and QC standards.
7. Set timer for incubation period indicated in package insert.	Timing is critical for an accurate test result.
8. Read reaction results at the end of incubation period.	Waiting the appropriate amount of time ensures that testing is complete.
9. Verify the results of the controls before documenting the patient's results. Log the QC and patient information on the worksheet.	This satisfies documentation of QC and the patient's results.
10. Properly dispose of the equipment and supplies in a biohazard waste container.	Using a biohazard container for disposal of biohazards provents potential exposure.
11. Remove PPE and wash your hands	This prevents the spread of microorganisms.
12. Document the procedure.	Procedures not documented have not been performed.
13. Sanitize the work area.	Sanitation aids in infection control.

Note: Kits vary with the manufacturer; read instructions carefully before beginning. Controls for test kits may be performed at different intervals depending on laboratory protocol. Follow procedures to ensure quality.

Charting Example:

04/23/2012 10:00 AM Mono test performed, Dx ###.## per Dr. Scott. Results negative ———————— S. Miller, CMA

Note: The medical assistant may sign his or her name in the patient record using only the "CMA" credential if the office has a signature log denoting the entire credential as "CMA(AAMA)."

 PSY PROCEDURE 29-13:   **HCG Pregnancy Test**

Purpose: To detect the production of HCG to determine pregnancy
Equipment: Patient's labeled specimen (plasma, serum, or urine depending on the kit), HCG pregnancy kit (test pack and transfer pipettes or test strip; kit contents will vary by manufacturer), HCG positive and negative control (different controls may be needed when testing urine), timer, PPE, hand sanitizer, surface sanitizer, contaminated waste container

Steps	Reasons
1. Wash your hands.	Handwashing aids infection control.
2. Assemble the equipment.	Equipment must be readily accessible to perform the procedure.

PSY PROCEDURE 29-13: HCG Pregnancy Test (continued)

Steps	Reasons
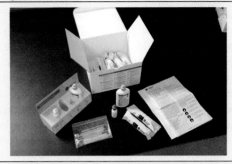 **Step 2.** Assembled equipment from an HCG test kit.	
3. Verify that the names on the specimen container and the laboratory form are the same.	This validates the identity of the specimen.
4. Label the test pack or strip (depending on type of kit) with the patient's name, positive control, and negative control. Use one test pack or strip per patient and control.	Identifying the test pack or strip removes confusion about the specimen added to that pack or strip.
5. Note in the patient's information and in the control log whether you are using urine, plasma, or serum. Be sure that the kit and controls are at room temperature.	The specimen type may influence the interpretation of the test result.
6. Aspirate the patient's specimen using the transfer pipette and place volume indicated in kit package insert on the sample well of the test pack or dip test strip labeled with the patient's name.	Apply the specimen for test measurement.
7. Sample the positive and negative controls as directed in Step 6.	This satisfies QA and QC standards.
8. Set timer for incubation period indicated in package insert.	CLIA requires performing the procedure as instructed by the manufacturer.
9. Read reaction results at the end of incubation period.	Waiting the appropriate amount of time ensures that testing is complete.
10. Verify the results of the controls before documenting the patient's results. Log controls and patient information on the worksheet.	This satisfies QA and QC standards.
11. Properly dispose of the equipment and supplies in a biohazard waste container.	Disposing biohazards appropriately reduces the risk of exposure.
12. Remove PPE and wash your hands.	This prevents the spread of microorganisms.
13. Document the procedure.	Procedures not documented have not been performed.
14. Sanitize the work area.	Sanitation aids in infection control.

Note: Kits vary with the manufacturer; read instructions carefully before beginning. Controls for test kits may be performed at different intervals depending on laboratory protocol. Perform at least the minimum controls required in the product information to ensure quality. Your office protocol may require more frequent QC testing.

Charting Example:

12/14/2012 9:30 AM HCG test performed on urine, dx ###.## per Dr. Schanzer. Positive result reported to doctor

———————————————————————————————— J. Simpson, CMA

Note: The medical assistant may sign his or her name in the patient record using only the "CMA" credential if the office has a signature log denoting the entire credential as "CMA(AAMA)."

PSY PROCEDURE 29-14: **Rapid Group A Strep Testing**

Procedure Note: To validate negative rapid group A strep results, set up a culture on beta-strep agar with the addition of a bacitracin disk to the first quadrant. Check the plate after 24 hours for presence of beta-hemolytic colonies. If beta-hemolytic colonies are present, the patient is positive for group A strep. A culture is more sensitive than a rapid immunoassay test. The culture procedure is not CLIA waived and cannot be performed by medical assistants. This additional step will require that a second swab be collected or that the agar plate be inoculated before the swab is used for the rapid test.

Purpose: To determine the presence of *Streptococcus pyogenes* in the specimen

Equipment: Patient's labeled throat specimen, group A strep kit (controls may be included, depending on the kit), timer, PPE, hand sanitizer, surface sanitizer, contaminated-waste container

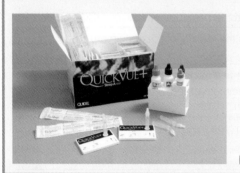
Rapid strep kit.

Steps	**Reasons**
1. Wash your hands.	Handwashing aids in infection control.
2. Verify that the names on the specimen and the laboratory form are the same.	Patient identification is critical for accurate reporting.
3. Label one extraction tube with the patient's name, one for the positive control, and one for the negative control. **Step 3.** Label extraction tubes for patient and each control.	Labeling tubes reduces identification errors.
4. Follow the directions for the kit. Add the appropriate reagents and drops to each of the extraction appropriate test-tubes. Avoid splashing, and use the correct number of drops.	Following the manufacturer's instructions exactly will ensure that you adhere to the guidelines.
5. Insert the patient swab into the labeled extraction tube.	

PSY PROCEDURE 29-14: **Rapid Group A Strep Testing** *(continued)*

Steps	Reasons
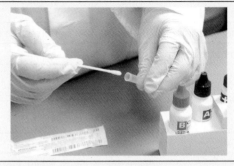 **Step 5.** Insert patient swab into labeled extraction tube.	
6. Add the appropriate controls to each of the labeled extraction tubes.	This begins the chemical reaction and provides the proper dilution factor for proper control results.
7. Set the timer for the appropriate time to ensure accuracy.	Timing ensures accuracy.
8. Add the appropriate reagent and drops to each of the extraction tubes.	
9. Use the swab to mix the reagents. Then press out any excess fluid on the swab against the inside of the tube.	This maximizes the volume of the extraction solution for testing.
10. Add three drops from the well-mixed extraction tube to the sample window of the strep A test unit or dip the test stick labeled with the patient's name. Do the same for each control.	
11. Set the timer for the time indicated in the kit package insert.	Timing the test is required for an accurate result.
12. A positive result appears as a line in the result window within 5 minutes. The strep A test unit or strip has an internal control; if a line appears in the control window, the test is valid. 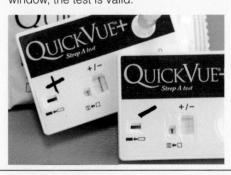 **Step 12.** Picture of positive- and negative-control packs.	These are the instructions for interpreting the test results.
13. Read a negative result at exactly 5 minutes to avoid a false negative.	Waiting a full 5 minutes will avoid false-negative results.
14. Verify results of the controls before recording or reporting test results. Log the controls and the patient's information on the worksheet.	This satisfies QA and QC standards.
15. Properly dispose of the equipment and supplies in a biohazard waste container.	Disposing biohazards appropriately reduces the possibility of infection.

(continued)

PSY PROCEDURE 29-14: **Rapid Group A Strep Testing** *(continued)*

Steps	Reasons
16. Remove PPE and wash your hands.	This prevents the spread of microorganisms.
17. Document the procedure.	Procedures not documented have not been performed.
18. Sanitize the work area.	Sanitation aids in infection control.

Note: Kits vary with the manufacturer; read instructions carefully before beginning. Controls for test kits may be performed at different intervals depending on laboratory protocol. Follow procedures to ensure quality.

Charting Example:

05/22/2012 11:15 AM Group A rapid strep test performed, dx code ###.##, per Dr. Harrison. Positive result reported to physician ——————————————————————————— B. White, CMA

Note: The medical assistant may sign his or her name in the patient record using only the "CMA" credential if the office has a signature log denoting the entire credential as "CMA(AAMA)."

- Most microbiology specimens for culture in a physicians' office laboratory are referred to a reference laboratory. To identify the correct method for collecting and transporting these specimens, the medical assistant refers to the reference laboratory's specimen manual. The medical assistant must follow the guidelines listed in the charts to identify the correct methods for the specific specimen being referred. The result of a laboratory test is only as good as the specimen.

- Label the specimen according to laboratory procedure. The minimum requirements are patient's first and last name, date and time of collection, and the identification of the collector. Some laboratories require additional labeling information. All information must be included. If the specimen is not fully and correctly labeled, the laboratory may be required to dispose of the specimen and cancel the request.

- Handle all specimens as if infectious. Follow standard precautions.

- Explaining the rationale behind the instructions for a a procedure will encourage the patient to specifically follow the details of the instructions.

- Care must be taken to transport or process the specimen as soon as possible so the organisms do not die. The sooner the specimen is processed, the sooner the pathogen can be identified and treatment can begin. Some microorganisms, such as N. gonorrhoeae, are very fragile and must be cultured under controlled conditions as quickly as possible. For the most reliable results, laboratory tests should be performed on fresh specimens within 1 hour after collection. When this is not possible, the specimen must be stored properly to preserve the physical and chemical properties necessary for accurate diagnosis. Specimens should never be subjected to extreme temperature changes.

- Media support the growth of microorganisms for identification. The microorganism will multiply for diagnosis of disease when it is provided an environment for optimal growth. The medium provides nutrients, moisture, and the proper pH. The inoculated media are incubated in an incubator with the temperature set between 20° and 40° C. The temperature and darkness are maintained by an incubator. The incubator maintains optimal temperature, humidity and other conditions such as the carbon dioxide and oxygen content of the atmosphere inside.

- To observe microorganisms with a microscope, the specimen requires preparation on a slide and staining. The primary stain used in the microbiology lab is the Gram stain. CLIA regulations allow the medical assistant to prepare the Gram stain to be read and reported by the physician. It is beyond the scope of practive for a medical assistant to perform the microscopic evaluation of the stained smear.

- When microorganisms are unable to grow in the presence of one or more antimicrobial drugs, they are said to be susceptible to that drug. Susceptibility testing determines the potential of an antimicrobial agent to be effective in inhibiting growth of an organism. The name of the technique is the Kirby-Bauer method.

- The presence of pathogenic bacteria is considered a positive culture. A culture that is reported as "no growth in 24 hours" will be incubated another 24 hours to confirm there is no growth. A culture that is reported as "no growth in 24 or 48 hours" usually indicates that there is no infection.

- Diseases caused by Rickettsia species include Rocky Mountain spotted fever.

- Mycoplasma that are pathogenic to humans cause atypical pneumonia and GU infections

- Viruses cause influenza, infectious hepatitis, rabies, polio, and AIDS.

- Diseases caused by fungi are mycoses. In healthy patients, they are limited to conditions such as candidiasis (thrush) and dermatophyte skin infections such as athlete's foot. In the immunocompromised host, normally mild or nonpathogenic fungi can cause potentially fatal infections.

- Parasitology is the study of protozoa, helminths, nematodes, and arthropods. Parasites can be identified as causes of foodborne or waterborne illness in the United States. Parasites are organisms that derive nourishment and protection from other living organisms known as hosts.

- The most common bacterial infections of the skin are caused by either S. aureus or a form of Streptococcus.

- In the respiratory system, the common cold and sinusitis are commonly viral infections. Acute gastroenteritis is the second cause of death worldwide. Food poisoning is caused by toxin-producing strains of E. coli and increasing drug resistance among Salmonella, Shigella, and other common bacteria.

- Pneumococcal meningitis is common in patients with an infection at another site such as the ears or chest, in patients with immunologic deficiency, and in alcoholics. H. influenzae infection is common in children up to age 2 years.

- The most common bacteria causing cystitis is E. coli.

- The immune system is the biological mechanism for identifying and destroying pathogens within a larger organism. An antibody is named by using its specific antigen's name and adding the prefix *anti-*. In hepatitis for instance, if the antigen is hepatitis A, then the antibody's name is antihepatitis A. Diseases caused by the immune system occur when there are problems with the immune reaction.

- An allergen is a substance that is usually not harmful. This would be substances like pollen or mold. The allergy comes when the immune system overacts and produces antibodies against these substances that are not pathogens. Autoimmune diseases occur when the body cannot distinguish between its own antigens and outside antigens. This causes the body to fight its own tissues.

- In immunology, the substance to be tested is identified or the amount present (quantity) is measured using the binding of a specific antibody to its specific antigen. If the extracted specimen contains the antigen, a color change (usually blue or red) will indicate a positive result.

Warm Ups — for Critical Thinking

1. You are asked to give a brief talk to a group of elementary school children on microbiological life forms. Develop an age-appropriate discussion of this topic. How would you make it possible for the children to correlate the presence of microbes with the need to wash their hands?

2. Write a policy that explains how to care for media and how to transport specimens.

3. Create a patient education brochure for streptococcal pharyngitis infections. Include information about what it is, how it is transmitted, signs and symptoms, and the testing procedure.

4. In performing an immunoassay, your controls do not give acceptable results. How would you resolve this problem and provide results for the patient?

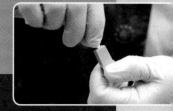

Outline

Learning Outcomes

Cognitive Domain

1. Spell and define the key terms
2. List the common electrolytes and explain the relationship of electrolytes to acid–base balance
3. Describe the nonprotein nitrogenous compounds and name conditions with abnormal values
4. List and describe the substances commonly tested in liver function assessment
5. Explain thyroid function and the hormone that regulates the thyroid gland
6. Describe how an assessment for a myocardial infarction is made with laboratory tests
7. Describe how pancreatitis is diagnosed with laboratory tests
8. Describe glucose use and regulation and the purpose of the various glucose tests

9. Describe the function of cholesterol and other lipids and their correlation to heart disease

Psychomotor Domain

Note: AAMA/CAAHEP 2008 Standards are italicized.

1. Perform blood glucose testing (Procedure 30-1)
2. Perform blood cholesterol testing (Procedure 30-2)
3. Perform routine maintenance of a glucose meter (Procedure 30-3)
4. *Use medical terminology, pronouncing medical terms correctly, to communicate information*
5. *Perform within scope of practice*

6. *Practice within the standard of care of a medical assistant*
7. *Screen test results*
8. *Analyze charts, graphs, and/or tables in the interpretation of health care results*
9. *Distinguish between normal and abnormal test results*
10. *Practice standard precautions*
11. *Perform handwashing*

Affective Domain

Note: AAMA/CAAHEP 2008 Standards are italicized.

1. *Distinguish between normal and abnormal test results*

ABHES Competencies

1. Perform CLIA-waived tests that assist with diagnosis and treatment
2. Perform chemistry testing
3. Perform routine maintenance of clinical equipment safely
4. Screen and follow up patient test results
5. Use standard precautions

Key Terms

acidosis	bile	endocrine	lipoproteins
alkalosis	buffer systems	enzyme	metabolism
amylase	catabolism	exocrine	urea
atherosclerosis	creatinine	ions	
azotemia	electrolyte	jaundiced	
bicarbonate	electrolyte balance	lipase	

Clinical chemistry is the science of using the chemical analysis of body fluids to obtain information about the clinical condition of the body. Some of the chemicals in body fluids include electrically charged atoms called **ions** (K$^+$, Na$^+$, Cl$^-$), proteins, liver enzymes, and lipids. Measuring these chemicals can help the physician access organ function and understand the patient's health status.

Only a few specific chemistry tests may be performed in the physician office laboratory (POL). Most of the tests done on patients are done in the chemistry laboratory so there is a lot to know about this specialty. Specimen collection, reporting, and follow-up of the patient is the responsibility of the medical assistant. Normal ranges included in this may vary from laboratory to laboratory. Different laboratories use different reagents, temperatures, and analyzers resulting in the differences in normal values.

Many chemistry tests are grouped according to body system. These are called *panels* or *profiles* and are described in Chapter 24. A summary of the common chemistry tests is presented in Table 30-1.

COG Electrolytes, Fluid Balance, and Acid–Base Balance

The job of kidneys is to get rid of waste, maintain fluid balance, and maintain acid–base balance. When the kidneys begin to fail, waste products build up in the blood. The patient becomes edematous, and the acid–base balance is upset. The physician may order tests for electrolytes, blood urea nitrogen (BUN), and creatinine. These tests and a urinalysis inform the physician of the health of the kidneys.

Minerals are necessary for the normal functioning cells. The body needs large quantities of

- Calcium
- Chloride
- Magnesium
- Phosphate
- Potassium
- Sodium

Bone, muscle, heart, and brain function depend on these minerals.

TABLE 30-1	Common Chemistry Panel Tests			
Test	**Body Function**	**Normal Values**	**Causes of Increase**	**Causes of Decrease**
BUN	Metabolic byproduct	7–18 mg/dL	Kidney disease, kidney obstruction, dehydration	Liver failure, malnutrition
Calcium	Structural element for bones, teeth, muscles	8.6–10.0 mg/dL	Hyperparathyroidism, hyperthyroidism, Addison disease, bone cancer, multiple myeloma, other malignancies	Hypoparathyroidism, renal failure
Chloride	Acid–base balance, component of stomach acid	98–107 mmol/L	Dehydration, Cushing syndrome, hyperventilation	Severe vomiting, diarrhea, severe burns, pyloric obstruction, heat exhaustion
Cholesterol	Building block for cell membranes, steroid hormones, bile acids	140–200 mg/dL	Atherosclerosis, heart disease, certain liver diseases with obstruction, hypothyroidism	Liver disease, hyperthyroidism, malabsorption syndrome
Creatinine	Metabolic byproduct	Men: 0.6–1.2 mg/dL Women: 0.5–1.1 mg/dL	Kidney disease, muscle disease	Muscular dystrophy
Glucose (fasting)	Energy source	70–110 mg/dL	Diabetes mellitus, Cushing syndrome, liver disease	Excessive insulin, Addison disease, bacterial sepsis, hypothyroidism
Phosphorus	Used in bone, endocrine processes	2.7–4.5 mg/dL	Renal disease, hypoparathyroidism, hypocalcemia, Addison disease	Hyperparathyroidism, bone disease
Potassium	Acid–base balance	3.4–5.0 mmol/L	Kidney disease, cell damage, Addison disease	Diarrhea, starvation, severe vomiting, severe burns, some liver diseases
Sodium	Fluid balance	135–145 mmol/L	Dehydration, Cushing syndrome, diabetes insipidus	Severe burns, diarrhea, vomiting, Addison disease
Triglycerides	Energy source; lipid deposits for stored energy, organ support	67–157 mg/dL	Atherosclerosis, liver disease, poorly controlled diabetes, pancreatitis	Malnutrition
Uric acid	Metabolic byproduct	Men: 3.5–7.2 mg/dL Women: 2.6–6.0 mg/dL	Renal failure, gout, leukemia, eclampsia	Drug therapy to lower uric acid levels

Minerals are an essential part of a healthy diet. To keep healthy mineral levels, the best choice is to eat a balanced diet containing a variety of foods. Restrictive diets may not provide enough minerals. For example, a vegetarian diet may not provide enough iron. The body needs a smaller amount of iron than some of the other minerals, but the body uses iron many ways.

Electrolytes and Fluid Balance

Electrolytes are minerals in the body that have an electrical charge. An **electrolyte** is any substance containing ions. Ions carry electricity through the body. The body needs electricity for fluid balance, acid–base balance, and for nerves to function. Fluid levels need to be stable.

CHECKPOINT QUESTION

1. Why does the body need electrolytes?

The body moves electrolytes to the cells through the bloodstream. If the body needs more fluid in the cells, it raises the electrolyte concentration in the cells. To keep fluid balance, the electrolytes must be at the right levels. Having electrolytes at the right levels is called **electrolyte balance.** The kidneys keep the electrolytes at the right levels by filtering the electrolytes when the blood flows through them. The kidneys move the excess electrolytes into the urine.

When kidneys cannot keep the electrolytes stable, disease develops. Conditions that can destabilize electrolytes include becoming dehydrated; taking certain drugs; and having certain heart, kidney, or liver disorders.

Sodium

The body has water inside the cells and outside the cells. Sodium is the major electrolyte outside the cell. Normal serum levels are 135 to 145 mmol/L. The level of sodium in the body depends on three things: how much water is drunk, how much water the kidneys allow into the urine, and if the kidney is healthy. See Table 30-2 for sodium reference ranges.

Because sodium is the major electrolyte outside the cell, it causes the most problems when its level is not stable. *Hyponatremia* is the term when the sodium level is too low. Hyponatremia can result from vomiting, diarrhea, burns, and kidney failure. Symptoms of hyponatremia are gastrointestinal (GI) and neurological.

Hypernatremia is the term when the sodium level is too high. Hypernatremia can result from profuse sweating, diarrhea, burns, and diabetes insipidus. When the body senses hypernatremia, healthy kidneys retain water to dilute the sodium in the body.

Potassium

Potassium is the major positive electrolyte inside the cell. Normal potassium levels are 3.4 to 5.0 mmol/L (Table 30-3). Potassium's job in the body is to support contraction of skeletal and cardiac muscles.

Hypokalemia is the term when the potassium level is too low. Hypokalemia occurs with GI or urinary losses.

TABLE **30-2**	Reference Ranges for Sodium
Measure	**Range**
Serum, plasma	135–145 mmol/L
24-hour urine	40–220 mmol/day, varies with diet
Spinal fluid	138–150 mml/L

TABLE **30-3**	Reference Ranges for Potassium
Measure	**Range**
Plasma, serum	3.4–5.0 mmol/L
24-hour urine	25–125 mmol/day

Symptoms of hypokalemia are weakness, fatigue, and constipation.

When the level is extremely low, it becomes difficult for the patient to breathe.

Hyperkalemia is the term when the potassium level is too high. The primary causes of hyperkalemia are high blood pressure and poor kidney function. Poor venipuncture techniques make the potassium level appear to be high, when it really is not. Venipuncture techniques that cause red blood cells (RBCs) to lyse result in falsely elevated potassim levels. Those venipuncture techniques include a traumatic venipuncture, or the tourniquet left on the arm too long or applied too tightly. Symptoms of hyperkalemia are muscle weakness, numbness, mental confusion, and cardiac arrhythmias.

Chloride

To carry the electricity in the body, some electrolytes have positive charges and some have negative charges. Chloride is the major electrolyte outside the cell that carries a negative charge. The normal range for chloride is 98 to 107 mmol/L.

Hypochloremia is the term used when the chloride level is too low. *Hyperchloremia* is the term used when the chloride level is too high. Stable chloride levels are important to maintain acid–base balance. Chloride can be made unstable if the patient is suffering diabetic ketoacidosis and metabolic acidosis.

Bicarbonate

Bicarbonate is an electrolyte with a negative charge. Bicarbonate is formed when carbon dioxide dissolves in the blood. It is reported from the laboratory as carbon dioxide. Normal carbon dioxide levels are 22 to 29 mmol/L. Bicarbonate is the most important electrolyte used in acid–base balance. The body's normal pH range is 7.35 to 7.45. The kidneys and lungs coordinate maintaining acid–base balance. Carbon dioxide is exhaled and also excreted through the kidneys.

 CHECKPOINT QUESTIONS

2. List the common electrolytes.
3. What is the primary electrolyte used by the renal and respiratory systems to regulate acid–base balance?

Magnesium

Magnesium is an electrolyte inside the cell. Magnesium carries a positive charge. Normal magnesium levels range from 1.2 to 2.1 mEq/L. Magnesium's jobs in the body are cardiovascular, metabolic, and neuromuscular function.

Hypomagnesemia is the term used when the magnesium level is too low. Hypomagnesemia is seen in patients experiencing a long-term severe illness. Hypomagnesemia is a result of GI disorders and possible laxative abuse. Hypomagnesemia can result from loss through the kidneys. The effects of hypomagnesemia are cardiovascular, neuromuscular, and psychiatric.

Hypermagnesemia is the term used when the magnesium level is too high. The cause of hypremagnesemia is poor excretion due to kidney failure. Early symptoms of hypermanesemia are low blood pressure, irregular heartbeat, nausea, vomiting, and fatigue.

Calcium

Calcium carries a positive charge. Calcium normal levels are 8.6 to 10.0 mg/dL. Three hormones work in conjunction to regulate calcium levels. The hormones are parathyroid hormone, vitamin D, and calcitonin. Most of the body's calcium is in the bone.

Again, *hypo-* and *hyper-* designate low and high calcium levels, respectively. Symptoms of *hypocalcemia* include muscle cramps and cardiac arrhythmia. *Hypercalcemia* is primarily due to hyperparathyroidism or malignancies.

Phosphorus

Phosphorus is the major negative electrolyte inside the cell. Normal levels are 2.7 to 4.5 mg/dL. Most of the body's phosphorus is in the bone. The body uses phosphorus to build its genetic material.

Hypo- and *hyper-* designate low and high phosphorus levels, respectively. *Hypophosphatemia* results from inadequate absorption from the diet, GI losses, electrolyte shifts, and endocrine disorders. *Hyperphosphatemia* results from hypocalcemia, hypoparathyroidism, and kidney disease.

Acid–Base Balance

It is necessary for acidity or alkalinity to be stable in the blood. The body's balance between acidity and alkalinity is referred to as *acid–base balance*. When the levels of the electrolytes carrying *positive* charges rise, so does the body's *alkalinity*. These ions can come from increased intake of acid foods and beverages or from decreased elimination in the urine. When the levels of the electrolytes carrying *negative* charges rise, so does the body's *acidity*. When acidity goes up, alkalinity comes down. When alkalinity goes up, acidity goes down. Because the acid levels and base levels are dependent on **metabolism**,

imbalances show up when an organ or body system is not functioning well.

Understanding the mechanisms the body uses to control the acid–base balance helps in grasping the concept.

Role of the Lungs: Carbon dioxide (bicarbonate), is one factor to consider in the control of blood pH. As we inhale oxygen, we exhale carbon dioxide from the lungs. Carbon dioxide is mildly acidic. Carbon dioxide is considered a waste product of oxygen metabolism. As the blood picks up the carbon dioxide waste from the cells, it carries it to the lungs, where it is exhaled. As the pH measurement gets lower, the acidity is becoming higher. As carbon dioxide accumulates in the blood, the pH of the blood gets lower. To control the carbon dioxide level, the brain controls the speed and depth of breaths. As more carbon dioxide is exhaled the pH comes up and the blood is less acid.

Role of the Kidneys: Positive and negative ions (acids and bases) are excreted by the kidneys.

Buffer Systems: Lungs change pH rapidly. Kidneys change pH slowly. The body manages the changes using a **buffer system**. The buffer system keeps the changes balanced. In addition to regular acids and bases that are primary to acid–base balance, the body has other weak acids and weak bases. When weak acids and bases are in balance, the body's pH is normal at 7.4. Carbonic acid is an important weak acid. The corresponding weak base is bicarbonate ions. Both of these are types of dissolved carbon dioxide.

Acidosis and Alkalosis: Acid–base balance can be out of balance two ways.

- **Acidosis:** The blood pH is below 7.4. The cause is either too much acid or too little base.
- **Alkalosis:** The blood pH is above 7.4. The cause is either too much base or too little acid.

Acidosis and alkalosis indicate a serious problem. There are two categories of acidosis and two categories of alkalosis. The categories for both are either *metabolic* or *respiratory*, depending on their cause. The metabolic causes for acidosis and alkalosis involve the kidneys. The respiratory causes for acidosis and alkalosis are breathing disorders.

The common cause of metabolic acidosis is either kidney disease or kidney failure. In these diseases, the kidneys do not excrete enough acid and do not produce enough bicarbonate. The lungs cannot work quickly enough to make up for the acidosis coming from the kidneys. Chronic obstructive pulmonary disease (COPD) can cause respiratory acidosis. An example of COPD is emphysema.

 CHECKPOINT QUESTION

4. What kind of acid–base balance state results from renal failure?

The common cause of metabolic alkalosis is emptying of the stomach contents. Vomiting results in a loss of the hydrochloric acid in the stomach. Another cause of alkalosis is taking too much antacid medication. The common cause of respiratory alkalosis is hyperventilation. Chronic respiratory alkalosis is a result of hyperventilation. Hyperventilation may be the result of anxiety, high fever, or an overdose of aspirin (an acidic compound).

 CHECKPOINT QUESTION

5. How does vomiting impact metabolic alkalosis?

TABLE 30-4	Causes of Elevated BUN Concentrations
Pre-renal	Congestive heart failure Corticosteroid therapy Dehydration Increased protein **catabolism** Shock, hemorrhage
Renal	Acute and chronic renal failure Glomerular nephritis
Post-renal	Urinary tract obstruction

COG Nonprotein Nitrogenous Compounds

There are about 15 nonprotein nitrogenous (NPN) compounds in the body. Physicians most commonly request three NPN compounds for evaluating kidney function: BUN, **creatinine**, and uric acid.

Urea

This measurement is requested from the laboratory as BUN. **Urea** is the waste product from the body's metabolism of protein. Metabolizing protein releases nitrogen. Nitrogen is converted to ammonia. Ammonia is a very strong base; it has a high pH. It is important to the body to metabolize ammonia quickly because it raises the pH so high. Because urea is neither acidic nor basic, the body is comfortable using it to dispose of the nitrogen formed from protein metabolism. Normal BUN levels are 7 to 18 mg/dL. Measuring BUN is important to measure for

- evaluating renal function,
- evaluating hydration,
- diagnosising renal disease, and
- evaluating for adequate dialysis.

Poor kidney function causes the body to retain BUN in the blood. This results in abnormal BUN levels in the blood. Retention of BUN results in **azotemia**, abnormally high levels of nitrogen-containing compounds. (Table 30-4). This condition results in damage to all the parts of the kidneys and obstruction of urine flow.

 CHECKPOINT QUESTION

6. What is azotemia?

Creatinine

Creatinine is a waste product from making the energy that muscles use to function. Normal range for creatinine

is 0.5 to 1.2 mg/dL. Creatinine is a laboratory test with results that vary from laboratory to laboratory. When the kidneys are healthy, urinary excretion of creatinine is the same as the amount produced in the body. Daily creatinine excretion is fairly stable. Creatinine is more specific than BUN for assessing kidney function.

The creatinine level is abnormally high when kidneys are diseased. Measurement of creatinine concentration is used to determine sufficiency of kidney function, the severity of kidney damage, and to monitor the progression of kidney disease.

A healthy kidney filters creatinine to keep its secretion equal to its production. A test called *creatinine clearance* measures this filtering ability. A 24-hour urine sample is collected for a creatinine clearance because excretion of creatinine varies throughout the day. (See Chapter 28 for 24-hour urine collection instructions.) To calculate the body's ability get rid of a substance requires measuring how much of that substance is removed. For the creatinine clearance, the clearance of creatinine is measured from urine in 24 hours. The creatinine clearance test requires that a blood sample be drawn during the 24 hours the patient is collecting the urine. The blood value is used to measure how much creatinine was cleared during the 24 hours. The medical assistant must remember that the test requires the blood specimen to be drawn during the 24-hour collection. Arranging the blood collection is critical to the completion of the procedure.

 CHECKPOINT QUESTION

7. What body organ is monitored by measuring creatinine?

Uric Acid

Uric acid is another waste product from breaking down protein. It is disposed via the kidneys. For men, the normal range is 3.5 to 7.2 mg/dL, and for women, it is 2.6 to 6.0 mg/dL. Elevated levels are usually a result of diet and are more clinically significant than low levels.

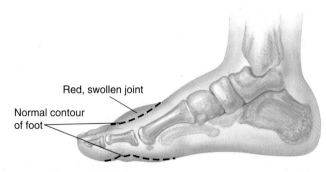

Figure 30-1 Gout of the foot.

The most uric acid the serum can hold is 6.8 mg.dl. When the level rises higher than 6.8 mg.cl, uric acid crystals may form in body tissues. This condition is called *gout* (Fig. 30-1). The reasons physicians order a uric acid test are to confirm diagnosis and monitor treatment of gout, to assist in the diagnosis of kidney stones, and to detect kidney disease.

CHECKPOINT QUESTION

8. What are the three primary NPN compounds?

WHAT IF?

What if a patient is diagnosed with gout and asks you about dietary restrictions?

Always speak to the physician to determine whether the patient has any other medical conditions that warrant a special diet. Most patients with gout are prescribed a low-protein diet. Foods that are high in protein are liver, kidneys, sardines, and anchovies. Diet and medications can often keep gout under control.

Ammonia

The body converts ammonia to urea to maintain acid–base balance. The normal range for ammonia is 15–45 mcg/dL.

Ammonia is a key factor in these conditions:

- Severe liver disease is the most common cause of abnormal ammonia levels. When the liver is severely diseased, it cannot remove ammonia from the circulation, so the ammonia cannot be converted to urea. Elevated ammonia levels are neurotoxic and are often associated with encephalopathy.
- Reye syndrome is most commonly seen in children. It often follows the use of aspirin to treat viral infection. Reye syndrome results in fatty infiltrates into the liver. The fatty liver does not function to convert the ammonia to urea so that it can be excreted. Reye syndrome may be fatal if ammonia levels remain high.

COG Liver Function Assessment

The liver takes nutrients from the digestive system and processes them. The liver stores the processed nutrients and sends them to different parts of the body in the right form and quantity. The liver regulates the level of sugars in the blood. It manufactures **bile** to break down fats in the stomach. It helps remove toxins, drugs, and hormones from our bloodstream.

Liver function tests are sometimes referred to as *LFTs*. LFTs are a combination of blood tests that give an assessment of liver function. Liver damage can be the result of many abnormalities in the body. An abnormal liver test result does not give a specific diagnosis. The results of several liver function tests and other factors of a patient's case must be evaluated by a physician. Blood tests for liver assessment include:

- Bilirubin
- AST (aspartate aminotransferase)
- ALT (alanine aminotransferase)
- ALP (alkaline phosphatase)
- LD (lactate dehydrogenase)

One abnormal test result can cause a concern about the patient's liver function, but there are other causes besides the liver that can make these same test results abnormal. Some of the examples are listed in Table 30-5. When several of the liver test results are out of the normal range (reference interval [RI]), the source of the abnormal results becomes the liver.

An **enzyme** is a protein produced by living cells that speeds up chemical reactions. The liver has many enzymes including AST, ALT, ALP, and LD. Reference ranges for enzyme tests are the most sensitive to deviation among laboratories. In evaluating patient results, always compare them to the RIs for the laboratory that performed the test. They will be listed on the result report.

TABLE 30-5	Nonhepatic Sources of Abnormalities for Select Laboratory Tests	
Test	**Nonhepatic Source**
Bilirubin	RBCs (e.g., hemolysis, intra-abdominal bleed, hematoma)
AST	Skeletal muscle, cardiac muscle
LDH	Heart, RBCs
ALP	Bone, first-trimester placenta, kidneys, intestines

ALT and AST are two of the most useful measures of liver function. In addition to liver disease, high AST levels are seen in acute muscle injury. A common cause of increase in AST and ALT levels is fatty liver disease seen most often in those with obesity, diabetes, or elevated blood lipid levels. Fatty liver is also seen in those who drink alcohol. Approximate reference intervals for ALT and AST are 6 to 37 U/L and 5 to 30 U/L, respectively.

ALP is present in the bones, liver, intestines, kidneys, and placenta. ALP in the blood is primarily from the liver and bone. Levels of ALP rise in bone and liver disorders. RIs vary with age. High levels of ALP are considered normal during periods of bone growth, such as childhood growth spurts and third-trimester pregnancy. An approximate reference interval for ALP is 30 to 95 U/L. ALP is elevated due to bile duct obstruction and primary biliary cirrhosis.

Gamma glutamyl transpeptidase (GGT) is an enzyme produced in bile ducts. It is elevated in bile duct illness. The GGT test may be elevated due to any type of liver disease. In addition to liver disease, drugs and alcohol cause increased levels of GGT.

 CHECKPOINT QUESTION

9. What are the five primary liver function tests?

Bilirubin Level Elevations

Bilirubin is produced by the normal breakdown of hemoglobin. The liver and spleen remove worn-out RBCs from the blood. These cells break down, and hemoglobin is released. Hemoglobin breaks down to bilirubin. The bilirubin travels to the liver via the blood. The liver extracts the bilirubin and conjugates it. The conjugated bilirubin is excreted into bile. The bile moves to the intestines and is eliminated. This happens so quickly that the amount of conjugated bilirubin that stays in the blood is tiny. If the conjugated bilirubin is increased in the blood, it is due to liver disease. Conjugated bilirubin is the only form of bilirubin that can appear in urine, so finding a positive urine bilirubin result is also due to liver disease. Bilirubin is yellow-orange; if excess amounts settle into the skin and sclera, it makes the patient appear yellow (**jaundiced**).

The laboratory can also measure another type of bilirubin called *unconjugated bilirubin*. This is useful when all the liver test results are normal, except the total bilirubin. When the total bilirubin level is elevated, and more than 90% is unconjugated, liver disease is not indicated.

 CHECKPOINT QUESTION

10. What are the two types of bilirubin measured in the laboratory?

COG Thyroid Function and Thyroid Hormones

The thyroid gland is a small gland, weighing less than one ounce. It has two lobes that lie along the trachea and are joined together by a narrow band of thyroid tissue, known as the *isthmus*.

Thyroid cells are the only cells in the body that can absorb iodine. These cells use iodine to make the hormones triiodothyronine (T_3) and thyroxine (T_4). The bloodstream carries T_3 and T_4 throughout the body where they control metabolism. Metabolism is the conversion of oxygen and calories to energy. The thyroid hormones regulate metabolism in all of the cells in the body.

The thyroid gland is directed by the pituitary gland, a small gland the size of a peanut at the base of the brain. When the levels of T_3 and T_4 decrease, the pituitary gland is activated to produce thyroid-stimulating hormone (TSH) (Fig. 30-2). TSH activates the thyroid

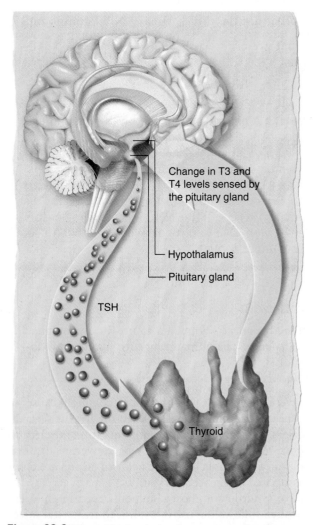

Change in T3 and T4 levels sensed by the pituitary gland

Hypothalamus

Pituitary gland

TSH

Thyroid

Figure 30-2 Thyroid-stimulating hormone production.

TABLE 30-6	Thyroid Function Tests	
Test	**Common Name**	**RI**
Serum T_4	T_4	4.6–12 ug/dl
Free T_4	FT_4	0.7–1.9 ng/dl
Serum T_3	T_3	80–180 ng/dl
Thyroid Stimulating Hormone	TSH	0.5-5.0 µU/mL

gland to manufacture and secrete T_3 and T_4. This production raises the T_3 and T_4 blood levels. When the pituitary senses that the T_3 and T_4 are increasing, it stops its TSH production. If the thyroid gland is malfunctioning, it cannot be activated regardless of the amount of TSH secreted. TSH levels may be quite high in cases such as this. The TSH reference interval is 0.5 to 5.0 µU/mL.

Table 30-6 lists thryoid tests and their RIs.

CHECKPOINT QUESTIONS

11. Which gland produces TSH?
12. What are the jobs of T_3 and T_4?

COG Cardiac Markers and Myocardial Infarction

No one test is completely sensitive and specific for myocardial infarction (MI). Comparison of timing with patient symptoms and electrocardiograms (EKGs) is important. Creatine kinase (CK) is a simple test measured by many laboratory instruments. CK is elevated in MI. MI is not the only condition that causes abnormal CK levels. Most of the CK is located in skeletal muscle.

Creatine Kinase MB Fraction

CK has three parts: MM, MB, and BB. The *MM fraction* is present in both cardiac and skeletal muscle. The *MB fraction* is much more specific for cardiac muscle, whereas less than 2% in skeletal muscle is MB. The *BB fraction* (found in brain, bowel, and bladder) is not routinely measured.

The CKMB fraction increases within 3 to 4 hours following MI. CKMB indicates heart involvement when it is ≥6% of the total CK result.

Troponins

Troponin I and T are contained in cardiac muscle. They are released into the bloodstream with myocardial injury. Troponins will begin to rise following MI within 3 to 12 hours. Troponin levels are the best indicator of MI.

Myoglobin

Myoglobin is a protein found in skeletal and cardiac muscle. It is used to evaluate the size of muscle injury. The rise in myoglobin can help to determine the size of an infarction. A negative myoglobin can help to rule out myocardial infarction.

B-Type Natriuretic Peptide

B-type natriuretic peptide (BNP) is released from the myocardium in response to excessive stretching of heart muscle cells. BNP is a marker for heart failure. BNP levels indicate the severity of the symptoms and the prognosis in congestive heart failure. The level of BNP in the blood decreases when the heart failure condition is stable. BNP levels can be elevated even if the patient has no symptoms. BNP levels predict heart failure, atrial fibrillation, and stroke.

Waived testing is available to make BNP levels easily available for patient treatment. See Figure 30-3.

C-Reactive Protein

C-reactive protein (CRP) is elevated in cases of inflammation. Since inflammation is part of MI, CRP is tested to predict the diagnosis of MI.

CHECKPOINT QUESTION

13. What is the most specific test for MI?

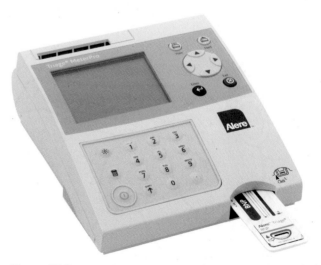

Figure 30-3 Alere Triage BNP. Waived testing instrument for measuring B-type natriuretic peptide. (Courtesy Alere Inc., Waltham, MA).

Pancreas

Pancreatic Enzymes

The pancreas is located behind the liver and mostly on the right side of the body. Two major digestive enzymes are secreted by the pancreas. **Lipase** helps in the digestion of fats. **Amylase** breaks down starch into sugar.

Pancreatitis is an inflammation of the pancreas. It can either be acute or chronic. Acute pancreatitis has a sudden onset and needs immediate medical intervention. It is most often caused by alcoholism and/or gallstones. Chronic pancreatitis is usually caused by long-term alcohol abuse; 25% of cases of pancreatitis have no known cause.

Amylase is greatly increased in pancreatitis. The salivary glands also produce amylase. Blood amylase levels may be elevated due to pancreatitis or in salivary gland diseases. Lipase levels also rise with pancreatitis and stay elevated longer than do amylase levels.

CHECKPOINT QUESTION

14. What are the two enzymes that are elevated in pancreatitis?

Pancreatic Hormones

The pancreas is both an **exocrine** and **endocrine** organ (Fig. 30-4). Endocrine glands release hormones into the blood in order to cause a response from another organ in the body. Exocrine glands release enzymes through ducts and include mammary glands, salivary glands, sweat glands, and glands that secrete digestive enzymes into the stomach and intestine.

The pancreas makes two endocrine hormones that are important in diabetes. The pancreas makes insulin. Insulin is the hormone responsible for controlling the amount of glucose in the blood. When there is more glucose in the blood than the body actually needs, insulin causes liver, muscle, and fat tissue to take up the extra glucose.

The pancreas also makes glucagon. Glucagon works the opposite of insulin. The pancreas releases glucagon when the blood sugar drops too low. Glucagon stimulates the liver, muscle, and fat to release stored glucose to make it available for energy. Both of these hormones come from the endocrine part of the pancreas known as the *islets of Langerhans*. These islets are made up of alpha and beta cells. Alpha cells secrete glucagon and beta cells secrete insulin.

Diabetes is a condition in which insulin is either low or does not exist. Insulin can also be present but not function. In type 1 diabetes, the pancreas no longer makes insulin. Daily injections of insulin are required to digest sugar. Type 2 diabetes usually develops later in life, and its symptoms are low insulin levels and high blood sugar.

Type 2 diabetes is a result of genetics and lifestyle factors. In type 2 diabetes the body builds up a tolerance to insulin. Higher and higher levels of insulin are needed to maintain a normal blood sugar. Eventually the pancreas cannot keep up with demand unless a change is made in lifestyle. At this point, a patient with type 2 diabetes will also require insulin injections.

 Glucose and Its Regulation

Physiology

Glucose is a primary energy source for the body. When foods are metabolized, nutrients including glucose enter the bloodstream. The two hormones produced in the pancreas, insulin and glucagon, regulate glucose levels in the blood.

CHECKPOINT QUESTION

15. What are the two hormones secreted by the pancreas that maintain blood glucose stability?

 Blood Glucose Testing

The glucose reflectance photometer (glucose meter) is an accurate, waived procedure to measure a patient's blood glucose level. Glucose meters are sold under several names, including Accu-Chek™, Ascensia™, and One Touch™, among others (Fig. 30-5). Testing includes application of whole blood to a reagent strip, which is read optically by the instrument after a designated time (Procedure 30-1). The amount of color change correlates with glucose concentration, and the value is measured and reported. Each type of blood glucose meter requires

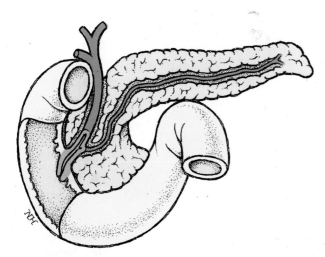

Figure 30-4 The pancreas.

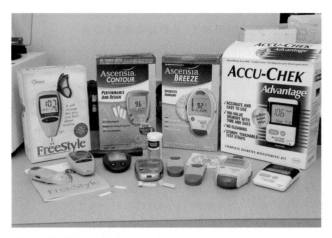

Figure 30-5 Various blood glucose monitoring systems.

proper maintenance and storage. Use Procedure 30-3 to maintain the glucose meter.

It is important to time the specimen collection for the desired length of fasting or the desired time since the last meal.

- *Fasting Glucose.* A fasting blood sugar (FBS) level requires the patient to fast 8 to 12 hours. Procedure 30-1 describes obtaining an FBS level using a glucose meter. The FBS is used to detect either diabetes mellitus or hypoglycemia. The American Diabetes Association's (ADA) cutoff point for normal fasting blood glucose levels is 100 mg/dL. A value of 100 mg/dL or above indicates a diagnosis of prediabetes. Prediabetes occurs when a person's glucose levels are higher than normal but not yet high enough for a diagnosis of diabetes. Studies indicate that many people in the prediabetic range go on to develop diabetes within 10 years. Further testing by a 2-hour postprandial (PP) glucose test confirms the diagnosis.

    An FBS level of 45 mg/dL equates to hypoglycemia. Hypoglycemic symptoms include sweating, weakness, dizziness, headache, trembling, and lethargy.
- *Random Glucose.* The use of a random glucose level is for screening. It does not result in a diagnosis. A random glucose is just that—done any time and not dependent on fasting or meals. Because the collection time is random, the reference interval varies from less than 130 mg/dL to less than 180 mg/dL.
- *Two-Hour PP Glucose.* A 2-hour PP glucose test is diagnostic of diabetes. It is also the tool used to monitor insulin therapy and to screen for diabetes. Timing of the specimen collection is extremely important for this test result. "Good control" of diabetes has been defined as a 2-hour PP value of less than 140 mg/dL.
- *Oral Glucose Tolerance Test.* The ADA does not encourage the use of the glucose tolerance test (GTT) to diagnose diabetes. For those situations in which

it is still used, the procedure should begin with effective patient preparation. For 3 days prior to the test, the patient should be mobile and eating a normal to high-carbohydrate diet. The patient should fast for 10 to 16 hours prior to starting the test. The GTT should be performed in the morning because of diurnal variations in glucose levels. In preparation for the test and during the test, the patient should not exercise, smoke, or consume anything other than water.

The patient is given 100 g of glucose in a flavored solution. Then blood glucose levels are checked on a time schedule to determine how the body metabolizes the glucose. The first step of the GTT is to check the fasting glucose. Blood is obtained 30 minutes, 1, 2, and 3 hours after the glucose has been consumed. Blood samples must be drawn on time. Urine specimens may also be collected on the same time table. Blood samples are drawn and processed for testing.

Numerous methods are used to interpret the values obtained from a GTT. The criteria proposed by the National Diabetes Data Group and the World Health Organization and endorsed by the ADA recommend a diagnosis of diabetes if the fasting glucose level is greater than 110 mg/dL and the 2-hour measurement is equal to or above 155 mg/dL. See Figure 30-6 for a graph of various glucose tolerance responses.

- *Glucose Tolerance Testing in Obstetric Patients.* A lack of glucose tolerance has been frequently noted among pregnant patients in the second and third trimesters. This lack of glucose tolerance is called *gestational diabetes.* Because gestational diabetes endangers the fetus, the pregnant patient's glucose level must be monitored. The screening method used for this purpose is to administer a 50 g glucose liquid, and draw blood 1 hour later. If the value exceeds 155 mg/dL, a GTT is indicated for a diagnosis of

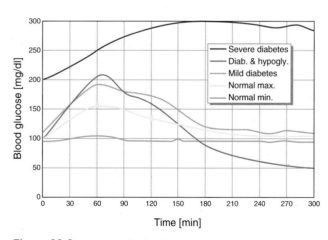

Figure 30-6 GTT graphs by disease severity.

gestational diabetes. This screen is usually done during the second trimester.

- *Hemoglobin A1C.* The test for regulating glucose long term is hemoglobin A1C. The goal for a diabetic patient is to keep a steady glucose level below the cut off levels for diabetes. The physiology of glucose makes this type of measurement possible. Glucose molecules attach to the RBCs circulating in the blood. RBCs have a life span of about 120 days. The hemoglobin A1C is a test that measures just the glucose that is attached to hemoglobin molecules. This glucose result gives the physician a picture of the patient's glucose levels over the past 3 months.

 CHECKPOINT QUESTIONS

16. What type of glucose measurement provides confirmation of a diagnosis of diabetes?
17. Is the oral GTT the test of choice for the diagnosis of diabetes?
18. Why is hemoglobin A1C the best test for monitoring diabetic patients?

The maintenance procedure for a glucose meter is also used to solve problems with the meter. Meters can suddenly begin to report very high glucose levels. Measuring and evaluating the control solution should be the first step of troubleshooting the problem. Performing the maintenance procedure and rechecking the controls will often resolve the problem. If the control fails, another vial of test strips should be evaluated with the control to validate proper function of the meter. If the patient or medical assistant cannot identify the problem, the technical service number on the package insert should be used to seek assistance. The weakness of glucose meters is that they are not 100% accurate in comparison to a regular laboratory measurement of blood glucose.

The glucose meter should not be stored in a place that gets too hot or cold. The meter should never be left in a location that can reach temperatures of over 100° F or less than 60° F. This can cause the meter to malfunction. Store test strips at room temperature, away from any humidity, in a tightly sealed container. Dispose of test strips that have gone beyond their expiration date. Expired test strips do not give dependable test results. Test strips should be labeled for use on the glucose meter in use.

The meter must be handled in a manner that prevents getting blood on the meter instead of the strip. Blood contamination leads to meter failure and inaccurate test results. Patient instructions should include that food or other substances on the hands can transfer to the meter, causing the meter to malfunction.

 PATIENT EDUCATION

USING A GLUCOSE METER

Many diabetic patients routinely monitor glucose levels at home. You can help reinforce use of this procedure and help the patient get familiar with the analyzer. Instruct the patient to adhere to the manufacturer's instructions. Here are points to stress:

- Teach patients about the need to test and document glucose levels regularly.
- Instruct the patient in maintaining a quality control record for the instrument using control materials within the expiration date and as directed by the manufacturer.
- Offer instructions in the proper technique for obtaining a blood sample (e.g., cleanse the area well before beginning and do not milk the finger).
- Caution patients against self-regulating with insulin. Have patients call the physician if glucose levels are abnormal.
- Alert patients to the signs and symptoms of high and low glucose levels and the treatments for each.
- Most pharmacies and surgical supply stores that sell glucose meters will teach patients how to use them. The strips for glucose meters are expensive and may be covered by certain insurance companies if the physician clearly documents the need.

COG ## Cholesterol and Other Lipids

Physiology

Lipoproteins are substances composed of lipids and proteins. Cholesterol and lipoproteins have long been implicated in heart disease. But, these same compounds are important building blocks of our bodies and in proper quantities are vital to health maintenance. They are a component of every cell membrane and of the myelin sheath around the nerves. They also cushion and support organs. Point-of-care testing instruments provide cholesterol levels on the spot (Figs. 30-7 and 30-8).

Atherosclerosis is a buildup of plaques in the arteries. The plaques are formed from cholesterol. Blood can be tested for cholesterol. High cholesterol levels build up the layers of plaque that can lead to narrowed or blocked arteries throughout the body. High cholesterol levels do not cause any signs or symptoms, so a cholesterol test is an important tool. High cholesterol levels

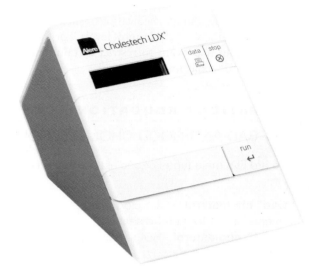

Figure 30-7 Alere Cholestek LDX (Courtesy Alere Inc., Waltham, MA).

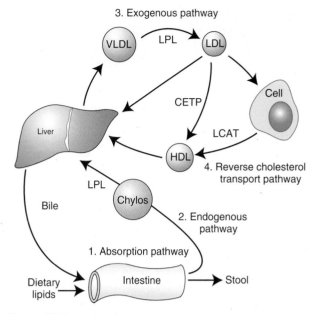

Figure 30-9 Diagram of major lipoprotein metabolism pathways.

CHECKPOINT QUESTION

19. What product of cholesterol is used by the intestine to digest fats?

Blood Cholesterol Testing

Lipid profiles will include the measurement of four types of fats (lipids) in blood:

- *Total cholesterol.* Total cholesterol is composed primarily of HDL and LDL.
- *High-density lipoprotein (HDL) cholesterol.* HDL carries LDL cholesterol away from the cells to be excreted, thus reducing the risk of atherosclerosis. HDL carries cholesterol from the cell back to the liver to be excreted in bile. High levels of HDL have a part in reducing the risk of heart disease. Low levels of HDL correlate with increased risk of heart disease.
- *Low-density lipoprotein (LDL) cholesterol.* LDL is often called "bad" cholesterol. LDL transports cholesterol from the liver to the walls of arteries. Plaques form, causing the affected vessel to thicken and become more rigid. Circulation to the organs and other areas normally supplied by these arteries is reduced. Atherosclerosis is the major cause of coronary heart disease, angina pectoris, MI, and other cardiac disorders. As LDL values rise above the normal range (see Table 30-7), the risk of heart disease increases.
- *Triglycerides.* Triglycerides are formed from calories ingested but not used. Triglycerides are stored in fat

are a significant risk factor for heart disease. Figure 30-9 is a diagram of the body's major lipoprotein metabolism pathways.

Bile acids, partly formed by cholesterol, are produced in the liver, stored in the gallbladder, and released into the intestine as needed for the digestion of fats. Vitamin D is formed from cholesterol at the skin's surface during exposure to sunlight. Various hormones, such as cortisol, testosterone, and estrogen, are also synthesized from cholesterol. Only in proportions over what is necessary for cell maintenance and other body functions should cholesterol be considered a health hazard. The ideal range for cholesterol is less than 200 mg/dL (as recommended by the American Heart Association) (Table 30-7). Anyone with a cholesterol level above 200 mg/dL is considered to be at risk for developing atherosclerosis.

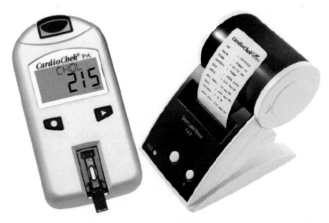

Figure 30-8 CCPA CardioChek Cholesterol Meter (Courtesy Polymer Technology Systems, Inc., Indianapolis, IN).

TABLE 30-7	Adult Reference Intervals for Lipids
Analyte	**Reference Interval**
Total cholesterol	<200 mg/dL
HDL cholesterol	>40 mg/dL
LDL cholesterol	<130 mg/dL
Triglyceride	<150 mg/dL

cells. Causes of elevated triglyceride levels are eating too many sweets or drinking too much alcohol as well as unmanaged glucose levels in people with diabetes. The normal range is less than 150 mg/dL (see Table 30-7). Triglycerides are a risk factor in heart disease.

All adults age 20 years or older should have a cholesterol test once every 5 years. Measurement should begin while the patient is healthy so that there is an established baseline for comparison with age. An acute illness, a heart attack or severe stress can affect cholesterol levels.

Cholesterol testing is very important in patients who:

- Have a family history of high cholesterol or heart disease
- Are overweight
- Are physically inactive
- Have diabetes
- Eat a high-fat diet

These factors increase the risk of developing high cholesterol and heart disease.

CHECKPOINT QUESTION

20. List the four tests that are included in a lipid panel.

Fasting is required to obtain dependable results of lipid testing. The object of the test is to evaluate how the body handles fat intake. A regular diet should be maintained until preparation time for the test. The patient should fast for 9 to 12 hours before the test. Encourage the patient to drink water in the time leading up to the test but avoid any other food or beverages. There are several items patients may question: coffee the morning of the test, chewing gum, and breath mints. These items are restricted during fasting.

CHECKPOINT QUESTION

21. Can the patient drink water while fasting?

The physician may have other requirements in addition to fasting. Some medications, such as birth control pills, can increase cholesterol levels. For this reason the physician may want to restrict certain items in preparation for the specimen collection.

PATIENT EDUCATION

BAD AND GOOD CHOLESTEROL

There are two main types of cholesterol that affect health:

- **"Bad" cholesterol**: LDLs clog arteries and put patients at risk for heart disease.
- **"Good" cholesterol**: HDLs help remove bad cholesterol from the body.

Controlling diet and getting plenty of exercise are great ways to help get bad cholesterol down and get good cholesterol up. This well-known saying helps remember which is the "bad" or "good" cholesterol: Keep **LDL** **l**ow and keep **HDL** **h**igh.

How do you know if your bad cholesterol is high? Many people don't. *People with high LDL cholesterol usually do not have any symptoms.* That is why it is so important for adults to get a cholesterol screening at least every 5 years.

COG Lead

The Centers for Disease Control names lead poisoning the number one environmental threat to children. Lead poisoning is entirely preventable. Lead has been prohibited in paint, so children living in older homes are at a greater risk for lead poisoning. Lead poisoning can cause learning problems and serious illness. If young children live in the home and a parent works with lead, they should be tested. Bloodborne lead crosses the placenta, exposing the fetus to the toxic effects of lead.

CHECKPOINT QUESTION

22. How does exposure to lead affect children?

Lead affects all organs and functions of the body to varying degrees. The frequency and severity of symptoms among exposed individuals depends upon the amount of exposure. Symptoms of lead poisoning in children include:

- irritability or behavioral problems
- pica (eating of nonnutritious things such as dirt and paint chips)
- difficulty concentrating
- weight loss
- abdominal pain

- vomiting or nausea
- pallor (pale skin) from anemia
- seizures

Lead limits RBCs' ability to carry oxygen. This results in anemia. Most lead moves to the bone. Lead can interfere with the production of blood cells and the absorption of calcium that bones need to grow healthy and strong. Calcium is essential for strong bones and teeth, muscle contraction, and nerve and blood vessel function.

A blood test is necessary to diagnose lead poisoning. A waived testing instrument is available that is within the scope of practice for a medical assistant (Fig. 30-10). Many children with lead poisoning do not show signs of being sick, so it is important to eliminate lead risks at home. For children, a level of 10 mcg/dL or greater is considered unsafe. The typical level for U.S. adults is less than 10 mcg/dL.

CHECKPOINT QUESTION

23. What does lead do to RBCs?

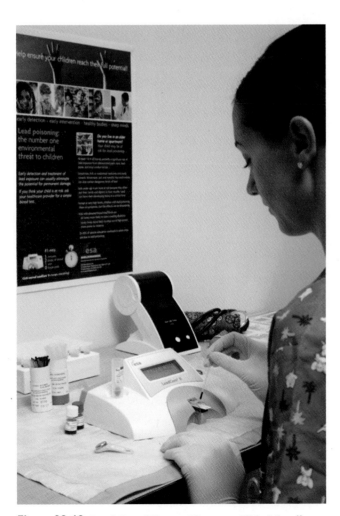

Figure 30-10 Lead Care II in use (Courtesy ESA, Magellan Biosciences, Chelmsford, MA).

WHAT IF?

What if your patient asks how to protect children from lead exposure?
   Reducing the Risk of Lead Exposure in the Home

- **Old plumbing might be lined with lead.** Copper pipes and lead solder were used in homes built prior to 1970. If you live in a home built before 1970, you may want to get your water tested. The local health department can suggest a laboratory that will test water for lead content. Take precautions to limit exposure. If the water from the cold faucet has not been run for several hours, let cold water run for 30 seconds before drinking it. Hot water absorbs more lead than cold water. Do not use hot tap water for meals.
- **Keep your home and your family clean.** Wash hands and toys frequently. Keep dusty surfaces clean with a wet cloth.
- **Eat regular meals with adequate amounts of calcium and iron.** Eating regular meals is helpful because lead is absorbed more during periods of fasting.

COG Responsibilities of the Medical Assistant in the Chemistry Laboratory

As with all of the laboratory specialties, the medical assistant must perform within scope of practice, practicing within the standard of care of a medical assistant. Some of these standards are:

- Running only CLIA (Clinical Laboratory Improvements Amendment)-waived tests
- Screening test results
- Analyzing charts, graphs, and/or tables in the interpretation of health care results
- Distinguishing between normal and abnormal test results

español
SPANISH TERMINOLOGY

Por favor, lávese las manos.
   Please wash your hands.

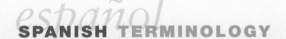

MEDIA MENU

- **Student Resources on thePoint**
  - **Video: Performing a Glucose Test (Procedure 30-1)**
  - **Video: Performing Routine Maintenance of a Glucose Meter (Procedure 30-3)**
  - **CMA/RMA Certification Exam Review**
- **Internet Resources**

  American Diabetes Association
  http://www.diabetes.org

  American Heart Association
  http://www.americanheart.org

  World Health Organization
  http://www.who.int/en

  National Diabetes Information Clearinghouse
  http://www.diabetes.niddk.nih.gov

PSY PROCEDURE 30-1: **Perform Blood Glucose Testing**

Standard: This task should take about 10 minutes.
Purpose: To determine the level of glucose in the blood for diagnosis and treatment of hypoglycemia and hyperglycemia
Equipment: Glucose meter, glucose reagent strips, control solutions, capillary puncture device, alcohol pad, gauze, paper towel, adhesive bandage, personal protective equipment (PPE), hand sanitizer, surface sanitizer, contaminated waste container

Steps	Purpose
1. Wash your hands. Put on gloves.	Handwashing and PPE aid infection control.
2. Assemble the equipment and supplies.	
3. Review the instrument manual for your glucose meter.	Following the manufacturer's instructions ensures accurate testing.
4. Turn on the instrument and verify that it is calibrated.	Calibration of the glucose meter is essential for accurate test results.
5. Perform the test on the quality control (QC) material. Record results. Determine whether QC is within control limits. If yes, proceed with patient testing. If no, take corrective action and recheck controls. Document corrective action. Proceed with patient testing when acceptable QC results are obtained.	For waived testing, CLIA requires that quality control procedures be performed in compliance with the manufacturer's instructions.
6. Remove one reagent strip, lay it on the paper towel, and recap the container.	The paper towel will serve as a disposable work surface and will absorb excess blood added to the strip. The strips are sensitive to humidity and will deteriorate if allowed to absorb moisture.
7. **AFF** Greet and identify the patient. Explain the procedure. Ask for and answer any questions.	Help the patient feel at ease in an unfamiliar environment.
8. Have the patient wash hands in warm water.	Sugar residues on hands can falsely elevate glucose results if the strip is touched. Washing removes sugar residues from the skin, and the warm water stimulates blood flow.
9. Cleanse the selected puncture site (finger) with alcohol. **Step 9.** Cleanse the selected puncture site with alcohol.	Alcohol removes bacteria from the site.
10. Perform a capillary puncture, following the steps described in Chapter 26. Wipe away the drop of blood.	The first drop of blood is contaminated with tissue fluid and will produce erroneous test first results.

(continued)

PSY **PROCEDURE 30-1:** **Perform Blood Glucose Testing (continued)**

Steps	Purpose

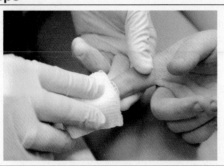

Step 10. Wipe away the first drop of blood.

11. Turn the patient's hand palm down and gently squeeze the finger to form a large drop of blood.	Gentle squeezing obtains a blood specimen without diluting the sample with tissue fluid.

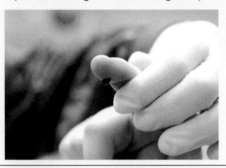

Step 11. Turn the patient's hand palm down and gently squeeze the finger to form a large drop of blood.

12. Bring the reagent strip up to the finger and touch the pad to the blood. Do not touch the finger. Completely cover the pad or fill the chamber with blood.	The entire pad must be covered or testing chamber filled for accurate reading. There is no chance of contamination by oils or other testing residue remaining on the finger if this surface is not touched.

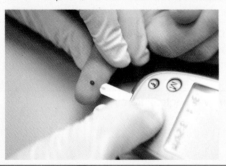

Step 12. Touch the pad to the blood. Do not touch the finger.

13. Insert reagent strip into analyzer, while applying pressure to the puncture wound with gauze. The meter will continue to incubate the strip and measure the reaction.	This allows time for the reaction.

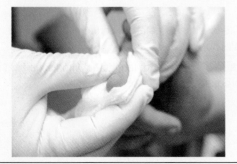

Step 13. Apply pressure to puncture wound with gauze.

PSY PROCEDURE 30-1: **Perform Blood Glucose Testing** *(continued)*

Steps	Purpose
14. The instrument reads the reaction strip and displays the result in milligrams per deciliter. 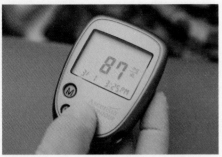	The reaction is now complete. The color change is photo-optically measured and reported in milligrams per deciliter.
	Step 14. Record the reading from the instrument display.
15. Apply a small adhesive bandage to the patient's fingertip.	The bandage will protect the puncture site.
16. Properly care for or dispose of equipment and supplies.	Remove biohazards from the work space.
17 Clean the work area. Remove PPE and wash hands.	Washing hands is the key step in standard precautions.

Note: These are generic instructions for using a glucose meter. Refer to the manufacturer's instructions for instructions specific to the particular instrument.

Charting Example:

02/12/2012 10:00 AM. Capillary puncture left middle finger for glucose DX ###.## per Dr. Miller.
Glucose tested with meter. Results: 60 mg/dL. Dr. Miller notified. ———————————————— *M. Miller, CMA*

Note: The medical assistant may sign his or her name is the patient record using only the "CMA" credential if the office has a signature log denoting the entire credential as "CMA(AAMA)."

PSY PROCEDURE 30-2: **Perform Blood Cholesterol Testing**

Standard: This task should take about 10 minutes.
Purpose: To determine the level of cholesterol in the blood for diagnosis and treatment of lipid disorders
Equipment: Cholesterol meter and supplies or test kit, control solutions, capillary puncture equipment or blood specimen as indicated by manufacturer, PPE, hand sanitizer, surface sanitizer, contaminated waste container

Steps	Purpose
1. Wash your hands. Put on gloves	Handwashing and PPE aid infection control.
2. Assemble the equipment and supplies.	
3. Review the instrument manual for your cholesterol meter or kit.	Following the manufacturer's instructions ensures accurate testing.

(continued)

PSY PROCEDURE 30-2: Perform Blood Cholesterol Testing (continued)

Steps	Purpose
4. Perform the test on the quality control material. Record results. Determine whether QC is within control limits. If yes, proceed with patient testing. If no, take corrective action and recheck controls. Document corrective action. Proceed with patient testing when acceptable QC results are obtained.	For waived testing, CLIA requires that quality control procedures be performed in compliance with the manufacturer's instructions.
5. Follow manufacturer's instructions in using a patient specimen obtained by capillary puncture or from vacutainer a tube.	CLIA requires that the manufacturer's instructions be followed on all procedures.
6. Follow manufacturer's instructions for applying the sample to the testing device and inserting the device into the analyzer. Record results.	A written record is required for all laboratory test results.
7. Properly care for or dispose of equipment and supplies.	Remove biohazards from the work space.
8. Clean the work area. Remove PPE, and wash your hands.	Washing hands it the key factor of standard precautions.

Note: These are generic instructions for performing cholesterol testing. Refer to the manufacturer's manual or package insert for instructions specific to the particular instrument or test kit.

02/12/2012 10:00 AM Cholesterol test performed. Dx ###.## per Dr. Peters. Results: 274 mg/dL. Dr. Peters notified.

———————————————————————————————————— M. Miller, CMA

 ## PSY PROCEDURE 30-3: Perform Routine Maintenance of a Glucose Meter

Standard: This task should take about 20 minutes.
Purpose: To comply with manufacturers' and CLIA guidelines for maintaining equipment in optimum functional condition
Equipment: Glucose meter, maintenance and testing supplies, manufacturer's manual for glucose analyzer, control solutions, PPE, hand sanitizer, surface sanitizer, contaminated waste container

Steps	Purpose
1. Wash your hands. Put on gloves.	Handwashing and PPE aid infection control.
2. Assemble the equipment and supplies.	
3. Review the instrument manual for your glucose meter.	Following the manufacturer's instructions for instrument maintenance is a CLIA requirement.
4. Perform the maintenance procedures listed in the manufacturer's instructions. Document the performance of these procedures in the instrument maintenance log.	CLIA requires that all instrument maintenance procedures included in the manufacturer's instructions be performed and documented.

PSY PROCEDURE 30-3: | **Perform Routine Maintenance of a Glucose Meter** *(continued)*

Steps	Purpose
5. Perform the test on the quality control material. Record results. Determine whether QC is within control limits. If yes, maintenance was successful and the instrument is ready for patient testing. If no, take corrective action and recheck controls. Document corrective action. Instrument is available for patient testing when acceptable QC results are obtained.	For waived testing, CLIA requires that quality control procedures be performed in compliance with the manufacturer's instructions.
6. Properly care for or dispose of equipment and supplies.	Remove biohazards from the work space.
7. Clean the work area. Remove PPE and wash your hands.	Washing hands is the key factor of standard precautions.

Note: These are generic instructions for performing maintenance of a glucose analyzer. Refer to the manufacturer's manual for instructions specific to the particular instrument.

- Clinical chemistry is the science of using the chemical analysis of body fluids to obtain information regarding the clinical condition of the body.

- The kidneys rid the body of waste products and help maintain fluid balance and acid-base balance. When the kidneys begin to fail, waste products build up in the blood. The patient becomes edematous, and the acid–base balance is upset. To assess renal function, the physician may order tests for serum measurements of electrolytes, BUN, creatinine, and other components.

- Electrolytes are minerals in the body that have an electric charge. These minerals are ions (chemicals that carry an electrical charge) in blood, urine, and body fluids. They may be positively charged or negatively charged.

- Electrolytes, particularly sodium, help the body maintain fluid balance. Fluid balance means that there are normal fluid levels in these compartments. How much fluid a compartment contains depends on the concentration of electrolytes in it.

- If electrolyte concentration ⇑ (is high) then fluid moves into that compartment.

- If electrolyte concentration ⇓ (is low) then fluid moves out of that compartment.

- The acid–base system is extremely sensitive and cannot tolerate large pH fluctuations. The body's normal pH range is 7.35 to 7.45, very slightly basic (neutral = 7.0). The renal and respiratory systems work to regulate acid–base balance. Measurement of carbon dioxide is considered more useful for pH balance assessment than for measuring renal function, but it also aids in the overall assessment of renal function.

- The determination of NPN substances in the blood has traditionally been used to monitor renal function. Physicians most commonly request three NPN compounds for laboratory measurement: BUN, creatinine, and uric acid.

- The liver works to keep the body's internal chemistry in balance. It takes nutrients from the digestive system and processes them. The liver stores the processed nutrients and sends them to different parts of the body in the right form and quantity. The liver regulates the level of sugars in the blood.

- Thyroid cells make T_3 and T_4. T_3 and T_4 are then released into the blood stream and are transported throughout the body where they control metabolism. Every cell in the body depends upon thyroid hormones for regulation of their metabolism.

- There are several laboratory tests available to measure the amounts of the various cardiac markers in the blood. No one test is completely sensitive and specific for MI. Comparison of timing with patients symptoms and EKGs are important.

- The pancreas makes two competing endocrine hormones that play an important role in diabetes. The pancreas makes insulin, the hormone responsible for controlling the amount of glucose in the blood. The pancreas also makes glucagon. Glucagon is released when the blood sugar drops too low. It stimulates the liver to convert stored glucose (glycogen) into glucose available for energy.

- Two major digestive enzymes are secreted by the pancreas. Lipase helps in the digestion of fats. Pancreatic amylase breaks down starch into sugar; starches are simply long chains of sugars.

- Glucose is a primary energy source for the body. For glucose to be used for stored energy in the form of glycogen, it must be brought into the cells. Insulin brings the glucose used for energy into cells for immediate use or for storage. By facilitating glucose storage, insulin keeps glucose levels down, thereby maintaining a stable blood level.

- For diagnostic usefulness, the time a blood sample is taken for glucose testing must be related to the length of fasting or to the time of the previous meal.

- A cholesterol test can help determine the risk of atherosclerosis. Bile acids, partly formed by cholesterol, are produced in the liver, stored in the gallbladder, and released into the intestine as needed for the digestion of fats. Vitamin D is formed from cholesterol at the skin's surface during exposure to sunlight.

- Children get lead poisoning from lead-based paint. Children living in older homes are at a greater risk for lead poisoning. Lead poisoning in children is especially dangerous because it can cause learning problems and serious illness.

1. A patient with edema is told by her physician to restrict her salt intake. Why may this help improve her condition?

2. A patient with diabetes gave herself too much insulin by mistake. Would you expect her glucose to be very high or very low? Why?

3. A patient's glucose level is repeatedly normal at routine office visits, but she continues to have worsening side effects of hyperglycemia. What test might the physician request that would reflect her glucose levels over a period of weeks?

4. A medical assistant draws a red-top tube for a number of chemistry tests. Unfortunately, the tube is left on the counter for several hours before being centrifuged and refrigerated. Which chemistries may be affected by this? Why?

5. A physician needs to evaluate a patient's kidney function. Which chemistry measurements will the physician request? Which of these measurements is least impacted by the patient's diet?

6. Describe three ways cholesterol is beneficial to the body.

Appendix A

Key English-to-Spanish Health Care Phrases

Although English is the major language spoken in North America, a variety of languages are used in certain areas. Prominent among them is Spanish, representing Spain, the Caribbean Islands, Central and South America, and the Philippines. Rapport can be more easily established, and the patient and family will be at ease and feel more relaxed, if someone on the staff speaks their language. Some health care facilities, especially in areas with a large population of Spanish-speaking people, provide interpreters. In smaller hospitals or smaller communities this may not be possible.

It is to your advantage to learn the second most prominent language in your community. For this reason, the following table of English-to-Spanish phrases has been prepared. Instructions for using it are simple. Look for the phrase in English in the first column of the table. The second column gives the phrase in Spanish. You can write this or point to it. The third column gives a phonetic pronunciation. The syllable in each word to be accented is printed in italic type. Even if you are not proficient in English-to-Spanish, your Spanish-speaking patients will appreciate your trying to converse in their language. Begin with "Buenos días. ¿Cómo se siente?" And remember "por favor."[a]

Introductory Phrases

please[a]	por favor	por fah-*vor*
thank you	gracias	*grah*-see-ahs
good morning	buenos días	*bway*-nos *dee*-ahs
good afternoon	buenas tárdes	*bway*-nas *tar*-days
good evening	buenas noches	*bway*-nas *noh*-chays
my name is	mi nombre es	me *nohm*-bray ays
yes/no	si/no	see/no
What is your name?	¿Cómo se llama?	¿Koh-moh say *jah*-mah?
How old are you?	¿Cuántos años tienes?	¿*Kwan*-tohs ahn-yos tee-*aynj*ays?
Do you understand me?	¿Me entiende?	¿Me ayn-tee-*ayn*-day?
Speak slower.	Habla más despacio.	*Ah*-blah mahs days-*pah*-see-oh
Say it once again.	Repítalo, por favor.	Ray-*pee*-tah-loh, por fah-*vor*
How do you feel?	¿Cómo se siente?	¿*Koh*-moh say see-*ayn*-tay?
good	bien	bee-ayn
bad	mal	*mah*l
physician	médico	*may*-dee-koh
hospital	hospital	*ooh*-spee-tall
midwife	comadre	koh-*mah*-dray
native healer	curandero	ku-ren-*day*-roh

From Rosdahl, C.B. [1995]. *Textbook of Basic Nursing*, 6th ed. Philadelphia: J.B. Lippincott.
[a]You should begin or end any request with the word PLEASE (POR FAVOR).

General

zero	cero	*se*-roh
one	uno	*oo*-noh
two	dos	dohs
three	tres	trays
four	cuatro	*kwah*-troh
five	cinco	*sin*-koh
six	seis	says
seven	siete	see-*ay*-tay
eight	ocho	oh-choh
nine	nueve	new-*ay*-vay
ten	diez	*dee*-ays
hundred	ciento, cien	see-*en*-toh, see-*en*
hundred and one	ciento uno	see-*en*-toh *oo*-noh
Sunday	domingo	doh-*ming*-goh
Monday	lunes	*loo*-nays
Tuesday	martes	*mar*-tays
Wednesday	miércoles	mee-*er*-cohl-ays
Thursday	jueves	*hway*-vays
Friday	viernes	vee-*ayr*-nays
Saturday	sábado	*sah*-bah-doh
right	derecho	day-*ray*-choh
left	izqierdo	ees-kee-*ayr*-doh
early in the morning	temprano por la mañana	tehm-*prah*-noh por lah mah-*nyah*-na
in the daytime	en el dìa	ayn el *dee*-ah
at noon	a mediodía	ah meh-dee-oh-*dee*-ah
at bedtime	al acostarse	al ah-kos-*tar*-say
at night	por la noche	por la *noh*-chay
today	ñoy	oy
tomorrow	mañana	mah-*nyah*-nah
yesterday	ayer	ai-*yer*
week	semana	say-*may*-nah
month	mes	mace

Parts of the Body

the head	la cabeza	la kah-*bay*-sah
the eye	el ojo	el *o*-hoh
the ears	los oídos	lohs o-*ee*-dohs
the nose	la nariz	la nah-*reez*
the mouth	la boca	lah *boh*-kah
the tongue	la lengua	la *len*-gwah
the neck	el cuello	el koo-*eh*-joh
the throat	la garganta	lah gar-*gan*-tah
the skin	la piel	la pee-el
the bones	los huesos	lohs hoo-*ay*-sos
the muscles	los músculos	lohs *moos*-koo-lohs
the nerves	los nervios	lohs *nayhr*-vee-ohs
the shoulder blades	las paletillas	lahs pah-lay-*tee*-jahs
the arm	el brazo	el *brah*-soh
the elbow	el codo	el *koh*-doh
the wrist	la muñeca	lah moon-*yeh*-kah
the hand	la mano	lah *mah*-noh
the chest	el pecho	el *pay*-choh

the lungs	los pulmones	lohs puhl-*moh*-nays
the heart	el corazón	el koh-rah-*son*
the ribs	las costillas	lahs kohs-*tee*-jahs
the side	el flanco	el *flahn*-koh
the back	la espalda	lay ays-*pahl*-dah
the abdomen	el abdomen	el ahb-*doh*-men
the stomach	el estómago	el ays-*toh*-mah-goh
the leg	la pierna	lah pee-ehr-nah
the thigh	el muslo	el *moos*-loh
the ankle	el tobillo	el toh-*bee*-joh
the foot	el pie	el *pee*-ay
urine	urino	u-*re*-noh

Diseases

allergy	alergia	ah-*layr*-hee-ah
anemia	anemia	ah-*nay*-mee-ah
cancer	cancer	kahn-sayr
chickenpox	varicela	vah-ree-*say*-lah
diabetes	diabetes	dee-ah-bay-tees
diphtheria	difteria	deef-*tay*-ree-ah
German measles	rubéola	roo-*bay*-oh-lah
gonorrhea	gonorrea	gun-noh-*ree*-ah
heart disease	enfermedad del corazón	ayn-*fayr*-may-*dahd* dayl koh-rah-*sohn*
high blood pressure	presión alta	pray-see-*ohn* al-ta
influenza	gripe	*gree*-pay
lead poisoning	envenenamiento con plomo	ayn-vay-nay-nah-mee-*ayn*-toh kohn *ploh*-moh
liver disease	enfermedad del hígado	ayn-*fayr*-may-dahd del *ee*-gah-doh
measles	sarampión	sah-rahm-pee-*ohn*
mumps	paperas	pah-*pay*-rahs
nervous disease	enfermedades nerviosa	ayn-fayr-may-*dahd*-days nayr-vee-oh-sah
pleurisy	pleuresía	play-oo-ray-*see*-ah
pneumonia	pulmonía	pool-moh-*nee*-ah
rheumatic fever	reumatismo (fiebre reumatica)	ray-oo-mah-*tees*-moh (fee-*ay*-bray ray-oo-*mah*-tee-kah)
scarlet fever	escarlatina	ays-kahr-lah-*tee*-nah
syphilis	sífilis	*see*-fee-lees
tuberculosis	tuberculosis	too-*bayr*-koo-lohs-sees

Signs and Symptoms

Do you have stomach cramps?	¿Tiene calambres en el estómago?	¿Tee-*ay*-nay kah-*lahm*-brays ayn el ays-*toh*-mah-goh?
chills?	escalofrios?	ays-kah-loh-*free*-ohs?
an attack of fever	un ataque de fiebre?	oon ah-*tah*-kay day fee-*ay*-bray?
hemorrhage?	hemoragia?	ay-moh-*rah*-hee-ah?
nosebleeds?	hemoragia por la nariz?	ay-moh-*rah*-hee-ah por-lah nah-*rees*?
unusual vaginal bleeding?	hemoragia vaginal fuera de los periodos?	ay-moh-*rah*-hee-ah *vah*-hee-nahl foo-*ay*-rah day lohs pay-ree-oh-dohs?
hoarseness?	ronquera?	rohn-*kay*-rah?
a sore throat?	le duele la garganta?	lay doo-*ay*-lay lah gahr-*gahn*-tah?

Does it hurt to swallow?	¿Le duele al respirar?	*Lay* doo-*ay*-lay ahl trah-gar?
Have you any difficulty in breathing?	¿Tiene difficultad al respirar?	Tee-*ay*-nay dee-fee-kool-*tahd* ahl rays-*pee*-rahr?
Does it pain you to breathe?	¿Le duele la cabeza?	*Lay* doo-*ay*-lay ahl rays-*pee*-rahr?
How does your head feel?	¿Cómo siente la cabeza?	*Koh*-moh see-*ayn*-tay lah kah-*bay*-sah?
Is your memory good?	¿Es buena su memoria?	Ays *bway*-nah soo may-*moh*-ree-ah?
Have you any pain the head?	¿Le duele al tragar?	*Lay* doo-*ay*-lay lah Kah-*bay*-sah?
Do you feel dizzy?	¿Tiene usted vértigo?	Tee-ay-nay ood-*stayd vehr*-tee-goh?
Are you tired?	¿Está usted cansado?	Ay-*stah* ood-*stayd* kahn-*sah*-doh?
Can you eat?	¿Puede comer?	*Pway*-day koh-*mer*?
Have you a good appetite?	¿Tiene usted buen apetito?	Tee-*ay*-nay ood-*stayd* bwayn ah-pay-*tee*-toh?
How are your stools?	¿Cómo son sus heces fecales?	*Kog*-moh sohn soos *bay*-says fay-*kal*-ays?
Are they regular?	¿Son regulares?	Sohn ray-goo-*lah*-rays?
Are you constipated?	¿Está estreñido?	Ay-*stah* ays-trayn-*yee*-do?
Do you have diarrhea?	¿Tiene diarrea?	Tee-*ay*-nay dee-ah-*ray*-ah?
Have you any difficulty passing water?	¿Tiene dificultad en orinar?	Tee-*ay*-nay dee-fee-kool-*tahd* ayn oh-ree-*nahr*?
Do you pass water involuntarily?	¿Orina sin querer?	*Oh-ree*-nah seen kay-rayr?
How long have you felt this way?	¿Desde cuándo se siente asi?	*Days*-day *Kwan*-doh say see-*ayn*-tay ah-see?
What diseases have you had?	¿Qué enfermedades ha tenido?	*Kay* ayn-fer-may-*dah*-days hah tay-*nee*-doh?
Do you hear voices?	¿Tiene los voces?	Tee-*ay*-nay los *vo*-ses?

Examination

Remove your clothing.	Quítese su ropa.	*Key*-tay-say soo *roh*-pah.
Put on this gown.	Pongáse la bata.	Phon-*gah*-say lah *bah*-tah.
We need a urine specimen.	Es necesário una muestra de su orina.	Ays nay-*say*-sar-ee-oh oo-nah moo-*ay*-strah day oh-*ree*-nah.
Be seated.	Siéntese.	See-*ayn*-tay-say.
Recline.	Acuestése.	Ah-*cways*-tay-say.
Sit up.	Siéntese.	See-*ayn*-tay-say.
Stand.	Parése.	*Pah*-ray-say.
Bend your knees.	Doble las rodíllas.	*Doh*-blay lahs roh-*dee*-yahs.
Relax your muscles.	Reláje los músculos.	Ray-*lah*-hay lohs *moos*-koo-lohs.
Try to . . .	Atente . . .	Ah-*tayn*-tay . . .
Try again.	Atente ótra vez.	Ah-*tayn*-tay *oh*-tra vays.
Do not move.	No se muéva.	Noh say moo-*ay*-vah.
Turn on (or to) your left side.	Voltese a su lado izquierdo.	Vohl-*tay*-say ah soo *lah*-doh is-key-ayr-doh.
Turn on (or to) your right side.	Voltése a su ládo derécho.	Vohl-*tay*-say ah soo *lah*-doh day-*ray*-choh.
Take a deep breath.	Respíra profúndo.	Ray-*speer*-rah pro-*foon*-doh.
Hold your breath.	Deténga su respiración.	Day-*tayn*-gah soo ray-speer-ah-see-*ohn*.
Don't hold your breath.	No deténga su respiración.	Noh day-tayn-gah soo ray-speer-ah-see-*ohn*.
Cough.	Tosa.	*Toh*-sah.
Open your mouth.	Abra la boca.	*Ah*-brah lah *boh*-kah.

Show me . . .	Enséñeme . . .	Ayn-*sayn*-yay-may . . .
Here?	¿Aqui?	¿Ah-*kee*?
There?	¿Allí?	¿Ah-*jee*?
Which side?	¿En qué lado?	¿Ayn kay *lah*-doh?
Let me see your hand.	Enséñeme la mano.	Ayn-*sehn*-yay-may lah *mah*-noh.
Grasp my hand.	Apriete mi mano.	Ah-*pree*-it-tay mee *mah*-noh.
Raise your arm.	Levante el brazo.	Lay-*vahn*-tay el *brah*-soh.
Raise it more.	Más alto.	Mahs *ahl*-toh.
Now the other.	Ahora el otro.	Ah-*oh*-rah el *oh*-troh.

Treatment

It is necessary.	Es necesario.	Ays neh-say-*sah*-ree-oh.
An operation is necessary.	Una operación es necesaria.	Oo-nah oh-peh-rah-see-*ohn* ays neh-say-*sah*-ree-ah.
a prescription	una receta	*oo*-na ray-say-tah
Use it regularly.	Tómelo con regularidad.	*Toh*-may-loh kohn ray-goo-*lah*-ree-dad.
Take one teaspoonful three times daily (in water).	Toma una cucharadita tres veces al dia, con agua.	*Toh*-may oo-na koo-chah-rah-*dee*-tah trays *vay*-says ahl *dee*-ah, kohn ah-gwah.
Gargle.	Haga gargaras.	*Ah*-gah gar-*gah*-rahs.
Use injection.	Use una inyección.	*Oo*-say oo-nah in-*yek*-see-ohn.
oral contraceptives	una pildora	*oo*-nah peel-*doh*-rah
a pill	una pastilla	*oo*-nah pahs-*tee*-yah
a powder	un polvo	oon *pohl*-voh
before meals	antes de las comidas	*ahn*-tays day lahs koh-*mee*-dahs
after meals	despues de las comidas	*days*-poo-ehs day lahs koh-mee-dahs
every day	todos los día	*toh*-dohs lohs *dee*-ah
every hour	cada hora	*kah*-dah *oh*-rah
Breathe slowly—like this (in this manner).	Respire despacio—asi.	Rays-*pee*-ray days-*pah*-see-oh—ah-*see*.
Remain on a diet.	Estar a dieta.	Ays-*tar* a dee-*ay*-tah.

General

How do you feel?	¿Cómo se siénte?	¿*Koh*-moh say see-*ayn*-tay?
Do you have pain?	¿Tiéne dolor?	¿Tee-*ay*-nay doh-*lorh*?
Where is the pain?	¿Adónde es el dolor?	¿Ah-*dohn*-day ays ayl doh-*lorh*?
Do you want medication for your pain?	¿Quiére medicación para su dolor?	¿Kay-*ay*-ray may-dee-kah see-*ohn* *pak*-rah soo doh-*lorh*?
Are you comfortable?	¿Está confortáble?	¿Ay-*stah* kohn-for-*tah*-blay?
Are you thirsty?	¿Tiéne sed?	¿Tee-*ay*-nay sayd?
You may not eat/drink.	No cóma/béba.	Noh *koh*-mah/bay-*bah*.
You can only drink water.	Solo puede tomar agua.	Soh-loh *pway*-day toh-mar *ah*-gwah.
Apply bandage to . . .	Ponga una vendaje a . . .	*Pohn*-gah oo-nah vehn-*dah*-hay ah . . .
Apply ointment.	Aplíquese unguento.	Ah-*plee*-kay-say oon-goo-*ayn*-toh.
Keep very quiet.	Estese muy quieto.	Ays-*tay*-say moo-ay key-*ay*-toh.
You must not speak.	No debe hablar.	Noh *day*-bay ha-*blahr*
It will be uncomfortable.	Séra incomódo.	*Say*-rah een-koh-*moh*-doh.
It will sting.	Va ardér.	Vah ahr-*dayr*.
You will feel pressure.	Vá a sentír presión.	Vah ah sayn-*teer* pray-see-*ohn*.
I am going to . . .	Voy a . . .	Voy ah . . .
Count (take) your pulse.	Tomár su púlso.	*Toh*-marh soo *pool*-soh.

Take your temperature.	Tomár su temperatúra.	Toh-*marh* soo taym-pay-rah-*too*-rah.
Take your blood pressure.	Tomar su presión.	Toh-*mahr* soo pray-see-*ohn*.
Give you pain medicine.	Dárle medicación para dolór.	*Dahr*-lay may dee-kah-see-*ohn* pah-rah doh-*lohr*.
You should (try to) . . .	Trate de . . .	*Tray*-tay day . . .
Call for help/assistance.	Llamar para asisténcia.	Yah-*marh* pah-rah ah-sees-*tayn*-see-ah.
Empty your bladder.	Orinar.	Oh-ree-*narh*.
Do you still feel very weak?	¿Se siente muy débil todavía?	¿Say see-*ayn*-tay moo-ee *day*-beel toh-dah-*vee*-ah?
It is important to . . .	Es importánte que . . .	Ays eem-por-*tahn*-tay Kay . . .
Walk (ambulate).	Caminar.	Kah-mee-*narh*.
Drink fluids.	Beber líquidos.	Bay-*bayr lee*-kay-dohs.

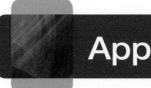

Appendix B

Abbreviations and Symbols

Abbreviations and symbols that appear in red font are considered "Dangerous Abbreviations" and should not be used.

Abbreviation or Symbol	Meaning	Abbreviation or Symbol	Meaning
ā	before	BCC	basal cell carcinoma
A	anterior; assessment	BD	bipolar disorder
A&P	auscultation and percussion	b.i.d.	twice a day
A&W	alive and well	BKA	below-knee amputation
AB	abortion	BM	bowel movement
ABG	arterial blood gas	BMP	basic metabolic panel
a.c.	before meals	BP	blood pressure
ACE	angiotensin-converting enzyme	BPH	benign prostatic hypertrophy; benign prostatic hyperplasia
ACS	acute coronary syndrome		
ACTH	adrenocorticotropic hormone	BRP	bathroom privileges
AD	right ear	BS	blood sugar
ad lib.	as desired	BUN	blood urea nitrogen
ADH	antidiuretic hormone	Bx	biopsy
ADHD	attention-deficit/hyperactivity disorder	c̄	with
		C	Celsius; centigrade
AIDS	acquired immunodeficiency syndrome	C&S	culture and sensitivity
		CABG	coronary artery bypass graft
AKA	above-knee amputation	CAD	coronary artery disease
alb	albumin	Cap	capsule
ALS	amyotrophic lateral sclerosis	CAT	computed axial tomography
ALT	alanine aminotransferase (enzyme)	CBC	complete blood count
		cc	cubic centimeter
a.m.	morning	CC	chief complaint
amt	amount	CCU	coronary (cardiac) care unit
ANS	autonomic nervous system	CF	cystic fibrosis
AP	anterior-posterior	CHF	congestive heart failure
APKD	adult polycystic kidney disease	CIN	cervical intraepithelial neoplasia
Aq	water	CIS	carcinoma in situ
AS	left ear	cm	centimeter
ASD	atrial septal defect	CMP	comprehensive metabolic panel
AST	aspartate aminotransferase (enzyme)	CNS	central nervous system
		c/o	complains of
AU	both ears	CO	cardiac output
AV	atrioventricular	CO_2	carbon dioxide
Ⓑ	bilateral	COPD	chronic obstructive pulmonary disease
BAEP	brainstem auditory evoked potential		
		CP	cerebral palsy; chest pain
BAER	brainstem auditory evoked response	CPAP	continuous positive airway pressure

Abbreviation or Symbol	Meaning
CPD	cephalopelvic disproportion
CPR	cardiopulmonary resuscitation
CSF	cerebrospinal fluid
CSII	continuous subcutaneous insulin infusion
CT	computed tomography
CTA	computed tomographic angiography
cu mm or mm³	cubic millimeter
CVA	cerebrovascular accident
CVS	chorionic villus sampling
CXR	chest x-ray
d	day
D&C	dilation and curettage
D&E	dilation and evacuation
DC	discharge; discontinue; doctor of chiropractic
DDS	doctor of dental surgery
DJD	degenerative joint disease
DKA	diabetic ketoacidosis
DO	doctor of osteopathy
DPM	doctor of podiatric medicine
dr	dram
DRE	digital rectal exam
DTR	deep tendon reflex
DVT	deep vein thrombosis
Dx	diagnosis
ECG	electrocardiogram
echo	echocardiogram
ECT	electroconvulsive therapy
ECU	emergency care unit
ED	erectile dysfunction
EDC	estimated date of confinement
EDD	estimated date of delivery
EEG	electroencephalogram
EGD	esophagogastroduodenoscopy
EKG	electrocardiogram
EMG	electromyogram
ENT	ear, nose, and throat
EPS	electrophysiologic study
ER	emergency room
ERCP	endoscopic retrograde cholangiopancreatography
ESR	erythrocyte sedimentation rate
ESWL	extracorporeal shock wave lithotripsy
ETOH	ethyl alcohol
EUS	endoscopic ultrasonography
F	Fahrenheit
FBS	fasting blood sugar
Fe	iron
FH	family history
fl oz	fluid ounce

Abbreviation or Symbol	Meaning
FS	frozen section
FSH	follicle-stimulating hormone
Fx	fracture
g	gram
GAD	generalized anxiety disorder
GERD	gastroesophageal reflux disease
GH	growth hormone
GI	gastrointestinal
gm	gram
gr	grain
gt	drop
gtt	drops
GTT	glucose tolerance test
GYN	gynecology
h	hour
H&H	hemoglobin and hematocrit
H&P	history and physical
HAV	hepatitis A virus
HBV	hepatitis B virus
HCT or Hct	hematocrit
HCV	hepatitis C virus
HD	Huntington disease
HEENT	head, eyes, ears, nose, and throat
HGB or Hgb	hemoglobin
HIV	human immunodeficiency virus
hpf	high-power field
HPI	history of present illness
HPV	human papillomavirus
HRT	hormone replacement therapy
h.s.	hour of sleep
HSV-1	herpes simplex virus type 1
HSV-2	herpes simplex virus type 2
Ht	height
HTN	hypertension
Hx	history
I&D	incision and drainage
ICD	implantable cardioverter defibrillator
ICU	intensive care unit
ID	intradermal
IM	intramuscular
IMP	impression
IOL	intraocular lens
IP	inpatient
IUD	intrauterine device
I.V.	intravenous
IVP	intravenous pyelogram
IVU	intravenous urogram
JCAHO	Joint Commission on Accreditation of Healthcare Organizations
kg	kilogram

Abbreviation or Symbol	Meaning
KUB	kidneys, ureters, bladder
L	liter
Ⓛ	left
L&W	living and well
LASIK	laser-assisted in situ keratomileusis
lb	pound
LEEP	loop electrosurgical excision procedure
LH	luteinizing hormone
LLETZ	large-loop excision of transformation zone
LLQ	left lower quadrant
LP	lumbar puncture
lpf	low-power field
LTB	laryngotracheobronchitis
LUQ	left upper quadrant
m	meter
ⓜ	murmur
MCH	mean corpuscular (cell) hemoglobin
MCHC	mean corpuscular (cell) hemoglobin concentration
MCV	mean corpuscular (cell) volume
MD	medical doctor; muscular dystrophy
mg	milligram
MI	myocardial infarction
ml or mL	milliliter
mm	millimeter
mm³ or cu mm	cubic millimeter
MPI	myocardial perfusion image
MRA	magnetic resonance angiography
MRI	magnetic resonance imaging
MRSA	methicillin resistant *Staphylococcus aureus*
MS	multiple sclerosis; musculoskeletal
MSH	melanocyte-stimulating hormone
MUGA	multiple-gated acquisition (scan)
MVP	mitral valve prolapse
NAD	no acute distress
NCV	nerve conduction velocity
NG	nasogastric
NK	natural killer (cell)
NKA	no known allergy
NKDA	no known drug allergy
noc.	night
NPO	nothing by mouth
NSAID	nonsteroidal antiinflammatory drug
NSR	normal sinus rhythm

Abbreviation or Symbol	Meaning
O	objective
O_2	oxygen
OA	osteoarthritis
OB	obstetrics
OCD	obsessive-compulsive disorder
OCP	oral contraceptive pill
OD	right eye; doctor of optometry
OH	occupational history
OP	outpatient
OR	operating room
ORIF	open reduction, internal fixation
OS	left eye
OU	both eyes
oz	ounce
p̄	after
P	plan; posterior; pulse
PA	posterior-anterior
PACU	postanesthetic care unit
$PaCO_2$	partial pressure of carbon dioxide
PaO_2	partial pressure of oxygen
Pap	Papanicolaou (smear)
PAR	postanesthetic recovery
p.c.	after meals
PCI	percutaneous coronary intervention
PD	panic disorder
PDA	patent ductus arteriosus
PE	physical examination; pulmonary embolism; polyethylene
PEFR	peak expiratory flow rate
per	by or through
PERRLA	pupils equal, round, and reactive to light and accommodation
PET	positron emission tomography
PF	peak flow
PFT	pulmonary function testing
pH	potential of hydrogen
PH	past history
PI	present illness
PID	pelvic inflammatory disease
PIH	pregnancy-induced hypertension
p.m.	after noon
PLT	platelet
PMH	past medical history
PMN	polymorphonuclear (leukocyte)
PNS	peripheral nervous system
p.o.	by mouth
post-op or postop	postoperative
PPBS	postprandial blood sugar

Abbreviation or Symbol	Meaning	Abbreviation or Symbol	Meaning
PR	per rectum	SpGr	specific gravity
pre-op or preop	preoperative	SQ	subcutaneous
p.r.n. or prn	as needed	SR	systems review
PSA	prostate-specific antigen	$\overline{ss}$	one-half
PSG	polysomnography	STAT	immediately
pt	patient	STD	sexually transmitted disease
PT	physical therapy; prothrombin time	SUI	stress urinary incontinence
		suppos	suppository
PTCA	percutaneous transluminal coronary angioplasty	SV	stroke volume
		Sx	symptom
PTH	parathyroid hormone	T	temperature
PTSD	posttraumatic stress disorder	T_3	triiodothyronine
PTT	partial thromboplastin time	T_4	thyroxine
PUD	peptic ulcer disease	T&A	tonsillectomy and adenoidectomy
PV	per vagina	tab	tablet
PVC	premature ventricular contraction	TAB	therapeutic abortion
		TB	tuberculosis
Px	physical examination	TEDS	thromboembolic disease stockings
q	every		
q.d.	every day, daily	TEE	transesophageal echocardiogram
qh	every hour	TIA	transient ischemic attack
q2h	every 2 hours	t.i.d.	three times a day
q.i.d.	four times a day	TM	tympanic membrane
q.o.d.	every other day	TMR	transmyocardial revascularization
qt	quart	tPA or TPA	tissue plasminogen activator
R	respiration	Tr	treatment
®	right	TSH	thyroid-stimulating hormone
RA	rheumatoid arthritis	TURP	transurethral resection of the prostate
RBC	red blood cell; red blood count		
RLQ	right lower quadrant	TV	tidal volume
R/O	rule out	Tx	treatment; traction
ROM	range of motion	UA	urinalysis
ROS	review of symptoms	UCHD	usual childhood diseases
RP	retrograde pyelogram	URI	upper respiratory infection
RRR	regular rate and rhythm	US or U/S	ultrasound
RTC	return to clinic	UTI	urinary tract infection
RTO	return to office	VC	vital capacity
RUQ	right upper quadrant	VCU or VCUG	voiding cystourethrogram
Rx	recipe; prescription		
$\overline{s}$	without	V/Q	ventilation/perfusion
S	subjective	VS	vital signs
SA	sinoatrial	VSD	ventricular septal defect
SAB	spontaneous abortion	VT	tidal volume
SAD	seasonal affective disorder	w.a.	while awake
SC	subcutaneous	WBC	white blood cell; white blood count
SCA	sudden cardiac arrest		
SCC	squamous cell carcinoma	WDWN	well developed, well nourished
SH	social history	wk	week
Sig:	instruction to patient	WNL	within normal limits
SLE	systemic lupus erythematosus	Wt	weight
SOB	shortness of breath	x	times; for
SPECT	single-photon emission computed tomography	x-ray	radiography
		y.o. or y/o	year old

Abbreviation or Symbol	Meaning	Abbreviation or Symbol	Meaning
yr	year	O-	lying
♀	female	×	times; for
♂	male	>	greater than
#	number; pound	<	less than
°	degree; hour	ĭ	one
↑	increase; above	ĭĭ	two
↓	decrease; below	ĭĭĭ	three
✔	check	ĭv	four
Ø	none; negative	I, II, III, IV, V, VI, VII, VIII, IX, and X	uppercase Roman numerals 1–10
♀	standing		
♀	sitting		

From Willis MC. Medical Terminology: The Language of Health Care. 2nd ed. Baltimore: Lippincott Williams & Wilkins; 2006.

Sample Medical Reports

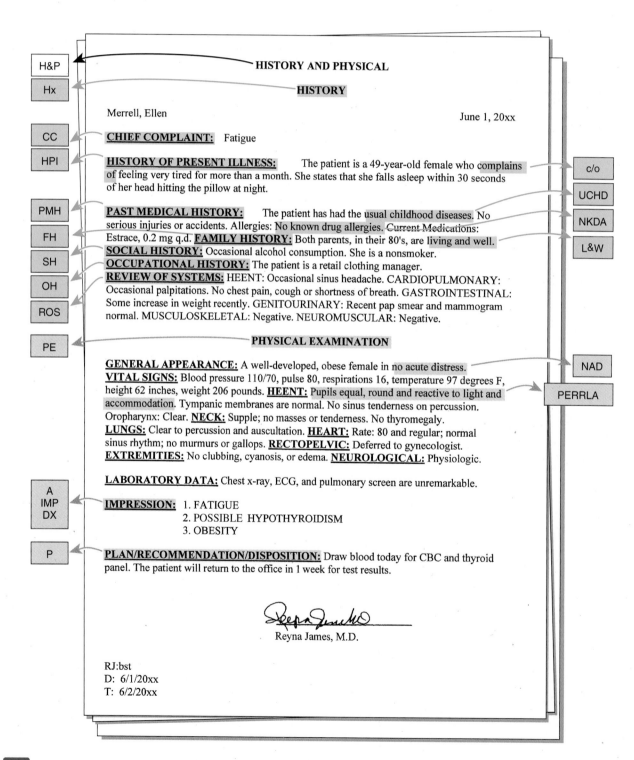

H&P

Hx

HISTORY AND PHYSICAL

HISTORY

Merrell, Ellen
June 1, 20xx

CC

CHIEF COMPLAINT: Fatigue

HPI

HISTORY OF PRESENT ILLNESS: The patient is a 49-year-old female who complains of feeling very tired for more than a month. She states that she falls asleep within 30 seconds of her head hitting the pillow at night.

c/o

PMH

PAST MEDICAL HISTORY: The patient has had the usual childhood diseases. No serious injuries or accidents. Allergies: No known drug allergies. Current Medications: Estrace, 0.2 mg q.d. **FAMILY HISTORY:** Both parents, in their 80's, are living and well.
SOCIAL HISTORY: Occasional alcohol consumption. She is a nonsmoker.
OCCUPATIONAL HISTORY: The patient is a retail clothing manager.
REVIEW OF SYSTEMS: HEENT: Occasional sinus headache. CARDIOPULMONARY: Occasional palpitations. No chest pain, cough or shortness of breath. GASTROINTESTINAL: Some increase in weight recently. GENITOURINARY: Recent pap smear and mammogram normal. MUSCULOSKELETAL: Negative. NEUROMUSCULAR: Negative.

UCHD

NKDA

L&W

FH

SH

OH

ROS

PE

PHYSICAL EXAMINATION

GENERAL APPEARANCE: A well-developed, obese female in no acute distress.
VITAL SIGNS: Blood pressure 110/70, pulse 80, respirations 16, temperature 97 degrees F, height 62 inches, weight 206 pounds. **HEENT:** Pupils equal, round and reactive to light and accommodation. Tympanic membranes are normal. No sinus tenderness on percussion. Oropharynx: Clear. **NECK:** Supple; no masses or tenderness. No thyromegaly.
LUNGS: Clear to percussion and auscultation. **HEART:** Rate: 80 and regular; normal sinus rhythm; no murmurs or gallops. **RECTOPELVIC:** Deferred to gynecologist.
EXTREMITIES: No clubbing, cyanosis, or edema. **NEUROLOGICAL:** Physiologic.

NAD

PERRLA

LABORATORY DATA: Chest x-ray, ECG, and pulmonary screen are unremarkable.

A
IMP
DX

IMPRESSION: 1. FATIGUE
2. POSSIBLE HYPOTHYROIDISM
3. OBESITY

P

PLAN/RECOMMENDATION/DISPOSITION: Draw blood today for CBC and thyroid panel. The patient will return to the office in 1 week for test results.

Reyna James, M.D.

RJ:bst
D: 6/1/20xx
T: 6/2/20xx

CENTRAL MEDICAL CENTER

211 Medical Center Drive • Central City, US 90000-1234 • PHONE: (012) 125-6784 • FAX: (012) 125-9999

OPERATIVE REPORT

DATE OF OPERATION: June 3, 20xx.

PREOPERATIVE DIAGNOSIS: Chronic tonsillitis.

POSTOPERATIVE DIAGNOSIS: Frequent, recurrent tonsillitis.

SURGEON: Patrick Rodden, M.D.

ASSISTANT SURGEON: None

ANESTHESIOLOGIST: Robert Jung, M.D.

ANESTHESIA: General.

SURGERY PERFORMED: Tonsillectomy.

DESCRIPTION OF OPERATION: After general anesthesia induction, with intubation, the McGivor mouth gag and tongue retractor were utilized for exposure of the oropharynx. Local anesthetic consisting of 6mL of 0.5% Xylocaine with 1:100,000 epinephrine was utilized. Tonsillectomy was carried out using dissection and air technique. The right tonsillectomy electrocoagulation Bovie suction was utilized for hemostasis. Examination of the nasopharynx was normal.

The patient tolerated the procedure well and went to the recovery room in good condition.

P. Rodden MD

PATRICK RODDEN, M.D.

JR:as
D: 6/3/20xx
T: 6/4/20xx

OPERATIVE REPORT	
	PT. NAME: PERRON, CARLEEN
	ID NO: 672894017
	ROOM NO: 312
	ATT. PHYS: PATRICK RODDEN, M.D.

CENTRAL MEDICAL CENTER

211 Medical Center Drive • Central City, US 90000-1234 • PHONE: (012) 125-6784 • FAX: (012) 125-9999

PATHOLOGY REPORT

PATIENT: PERRON, CARLEEN
           28 Y (FEMALE)

DATE RECEIVED: June 3, 20xx.   DATE REPORTED: June 4, 20xx

GROSS:

Received are two tonsils each 2.5 cm in greatest diameter.

MICROSCOPIC:

The sections show deep tonsilar crypts associated with follicular lymphoid hyperplasia. No bacterial granules are seen.

DIAGNOSIS:

CHRONIC LYMPHOID HYPERPLASIA OF RIGHT AND LEFT TONSILS.

MARY NEEDHAM, M.D.

MN:gds

D: 6/4/20xx
T: 6/5/20xx

CENTRAL MEDICAL CENTER

211 Medical Center Drive • Central City, US 90000-1234 • PHONE: (012) 125-6784 • FAX: (012) 125-9999

DISCHARGE SUMMARY

DATE OF ADMISSION: 10/25/20xx   DATE OF DISCHARGE: 10/29/20xx

ADMITTING DIAGNOSIS:
Left ureteropelvic junction obstruction.

DISCHARGE DIAGNOSIS:
Left ureteropelvic junction obstruction.

PROCEDURE PERFORMED:
Left dismembered pyeloplasty and placement of stent.

BRIEF SUMMARY:
The patient is a 19-year-old male who was admitted to the hospital a month ago with left pyelonephritis. He was found to have a left ureteropelvic junction obstruction. The patient was brought to the hospital at this time for repair of the moderately to severely obstructed left kidney. A preoperative urine culture was sterile. The patient underwent the procedure without complication. A double-J stent was placed. The Jackson-Pratt drain was removed on the second postoperative day because of minimal drainage. The patient initially had urinary retention, but this resolved by the third postoperative day. He was doing fine at the time of discharge. His condition on discharge is good.

INSTRUCTIONS TO THE PATIENT:
1) Regular diet. 2) No heavy lifting, straining, or driving an automobile for six weeks from the day of surgery. He should also keep the incision relatively dry this week. 3) Follow up in my office in three weeks. 4) It is anticipated the stent will remain indwelling for six weeks and then will be removed cystoscopically at that time. 5) Discharge medication is Tylenol #3, 1-2 q 4 h p.r.n. pain.

L. Zlatkin, M.D.
L. Zlatkin, M.D.

LZ:mr

D: 10/29/20xx
T: 10/30/20xx

DISCHARGE SUMMARY	PT. NAME: MERCIER, CHARLES F.
	ID NO: IP-392689
	ROOM NO: 444
	ATT. PHYS: L.ZLATKIN, M.D.

CENTRAL MEDICAL CENTER

211 Medical Center Drive • Central City, US 90000-1234 • PHONE: (012) 125-6784 • FAX: (012) 125-9999

OPERATIVE REPORT

DATE: December 7, 20xx

PREOPERATIVE DIAGNOSIS: Congenital left ureteropelvic junction obstruction status post pyeloplasty. Indwelling left ureteral stent.

POSTOPERATIVE DIAGNOSIS: Congenital left ureteropelvic junction obstruction status post pyeloplasty. Indwelling left ureteral stent, removed

OPERATION: Cystoscopy, removal of left ureteral stent, and left retrograde pyelogram.

PROCEDURE: The patient was identified, was placed on the operating table, and was administered a general anesthetic. He was placed in the lithotomy position, and a KUB was obtained. The genitalia were prepped and draped in a sterile fashion. After reviewing the KUB, it was noted at this time that the position of the stent was normal. Cystoscopy was performed with a #22 French cystoscope. The stent was identified coming from the left ureteral orifice, and the end was grasped with forceps and removed through the cystoscope. A #8 French cone-tipped ureteral catheter was then placed in the left ureteral orifice and passed to 10 cm. Then, 20 cm^3 of contrast was injected into a left collecting system. A film was exposed, and this showed patency without extravasation at the left ureteropelvic junction. There was some filling of calyces and partial filling of the dilated renal pelvis. A drainage film was subsequently obtained showing complete emptying of the pelvis and partial emptying of the mid and distal ureters. Dilated calyces were noted in the kidney. The patient was allowed to awaken and was returned to the recovery room in satisfactory condition. There were no intraoperative complications. He had no bleeding. The patient did receive 1 gm Ancef one-half hour prior to the onset of the procedure.

L. Zlatkin, M.D.

LZ:mr
D: 12/07/20xx
T: 12/08/20xx

OPERATIVE REPORT	PT. NAME: MERCIER, CHARLES F.
	ID NO: OP-912689
	ROOM NO: ASC
	ATT. PHYS: L.ZLATKIN, M.D.

CENTRAL MEDICAL GROUP, INC.
Department of Internal Medicine

201 Medical Center Drive • Central City, US 90000-1234 • PHONE: (012) 125-8888 • FAX: (012) 125-3434

PATIENT: COHEN, SARA E. DATE: April 8, 20xx

HISTORY

CHIEF COMPLAINT: Epigastric distress

HISTORY OF PRESENT ILLNESS: This 33-year-old Caucasian female comes in because of excessive burping, epigastric distress and nausea for several weeks. Coffee makes it worse. She complains that it is worse at night when lying down. She gets an acid-like taste in her mouth. She has tried antacids, to no avail.

PAST MEDICAL HISTORY: The patient states that she had the usual childhood diseases. She has had no serious medical illnesses and has been involved in no accidents. Family History: There is some diabetes on her mother's side. Her mother is 52 and has hypertension. Her father, age 56, is living and well. She has a sister who is anemic and a brother who has ulcers. Social History: The patient discontinued smoking ten years ago. Drinks alcohol socially. Allergies: NKDA. Current Medications: Medications at this time consist of Entex, Guaifed, birth control pills, iron and vitamin supplements.

REVIEW OF SYSTEMS: HEENT: Chronic sinusitis. She sees an ENT specialist and an allergist. Respiratory: Negative. Cardiac: Occasional flutters. Gastrointestinal: As stated above. Genitourinary: Occasional infections. Pap smear is up-to-date and negative. She has had no mammogram at this point. Neuromuscular: Negative.

PHYSICAL EXAMINATION

GENERAL APPEARANCE: Reveals a well-developed, well-nourished female in no acute distress.

VITAL SIGNS: Blood Pressure: 120/80. Pulse: 76 and regular.

HEENT: Head normocephalic. Eyes: Pupils are equal, round, and reactive to light and accommodation. Fundi are benign. Ears, nose and throat are negative. NECK: No thyromegaly. No carotid bruits.

CHEST: Clear to percussion and auscultation. BREASTS: Reveal no masses. HEART: Normal sinus rhythm. No murmurs.

ABDOMEN: Liver, spleen and kidneys could not be felt. Femorals pulsate well, no bruits.

EXTREMITIES: No edema. Pulses are good and equal.

PELVIC & RECTAL EXAMS: Deferred to gynecologist.

NEUROLOGIC EXAM: Physiologic.

IMPRESSION: 1. PROBABLE PEPTIC ULCER DISEASE WITH GASTROESOPHAGEAL REFLUX.
2. POSSIBLE GALLBLADDER DISEASE.

PLAN: Patient started on Pepcid 40 mg, 1 at night. She is given Gaviscon tablets so she can carry them with her. Schedule routine lab work and upper GI series. If negative, schedule ultrasound of the gallbladder.

D. Everley, M.D.

DE:mc
D: 4/8/20xx
T: 4/9/20xx

CENTRAL MEDICAL GROUP, INC.
Department of Otorhinolaryngology
201 Medical Center Drive • Central City, US 90000-1234 • PHONE: (012) 125-8888 • FAX: (012) 125-3434

Patient: Perron, Carleen   DATE: February 17, 20xx

Referring Physician: C. Camarillo, M.D.

CONSULTATION

REASON FOR CONSULTATION: This 28-year-old white female presents with a one week history of upper respiratory infection (URI), sinusitis, and some periorbital headaches in recent weeks. She also has expectorated yellow-green mucus occasionally and has had a history of tonsillitis.

MEDICATIONS: None. **ALLERGIES:** No known allergies (NKA). **SURGERIES:** None. **HOSPITALIZATIONS:** None.

PAST MEDICAL HISTORY/REVIEW OF SYSTEMS: Cardiopulmonary: There is no history of angina, dyspnea, hemoptysis, emphysema, asthma, chronic obstructive pulmonary disease (COPD), hypertension, or heart murmurs. Cardiovascular: There is no history of high blood pressure. Renal: There is no history of dysuria, polyuria, nocturia, hematuria, or cystoliths. Gastrointestinal: There is no history of gallbladder disease, hepatitis, pancreatitis, or colitis. Musculoskeletal: There is no history of arthritis. Endocrine: There is no history of diabetes. Hematologic: There is no history of anemia, blood transfusion, or easy bruising. Gynecological: The patient states her menses are regular, and the start of her last menstrual cycle occurred 15 days ago.

FAMILY HISTORY: The patient states her maternal grandmother has diabetes.

SOCIAL HISTORY: The patient is single and has no children. She denies smoking tobacco. She denies drinking alcoholic beverages. She denies taking drugs.

CHILDHOOD DISEASES: The patient has had the usual childhood diseases.

OTOLARYNGOLOGIC EXAMINATION: Otoscopy: Tympanic membranes (TMs) are dull and slightly congested. Sinuses: There is maxillary fullness. Rhinoscopic examination reveals mild nasoseptal deviation (NSD). Pharynx: There is moderate inflammation; no exudates. Oropharynx: No masses. Nasopharynx: No masses. Larynx: Clear. Neck: Supple. Cervical Adenopathy: There is mild adenopathy.

IMPRESSION:
1. MAXILLARY SINUSITIS.
2. PHARYNGITIS.
3. CHRONIC TONSILLITIS.

DISPOSITION:
1. Warm salt water gargle (WSWG).
2. Ery-Tab 333, #24, 1 t.i.d. p.c.
3. Robitussin.
4. Return to office (RTO) in one week.

P. Rodden MD

PATRICK RODDEN, M.D.

JR:ti
D: 2/17/20xx
T: 2/18/20xx   9:50 a.m.

CENTRAL MEDICAL GROUP, INC.

Department of Otorhinolaryngology

201 Medical Center Drive • Central City, US 90000-1234 • PHONE: (012) 125-8888 • FAX: (012) 125-3434

PROGRESS NOTES

Patient: PERRON, CARLEEN

03/30/20xx

S: The patient presents with a sore throat × 2 weeks.

O: Sinus exam: Maxillary and frontal congestion. Hypopharynx/adenoids: No inflammation.

A: Recurrent pharyngitis/sinusitis × 2 weeks.

P: 1)   Ceftin 250 mg, #21, 1 t.i.d. p.o. p.c.

     2)   Entex LA, #30, 1 b.i.d. p.o.

     3)   Warm salt water gargle.

P Rodden MD
PATRICK RODDEN, M.D.

05/25/20xx

S: Recurrent sore throat every month.

O: Recurrent tonsillitis, cryptic tonsillitis. Sinus exam: Maxillary and frontal congestion. Neck: Supple; no masses. Hypopharynx/Adenoids: No inflammation. Paranasal Sinus X-ray: Bilateral frontal and maxillary sinusitis.

A: Recurrent tonsillitis, 8-10 times per year. Chronic maxillary and frontal sinusitis.

P: 1)   Tonsillectomy discussed with the patient. The risks of general and local anesthesia, as well as the surgical procedure, were discussed with the patient. The consent form was signed.

     2)   An admitting order was given to the patient for CBC, UA, and basic metabolic panel to be done one day prior to being admitted.

     3)   Ceftin 250 mg, #21, 1 t.i.d. p.o. p.c.

     4)   Entex LA, #30, 1 b.i.d. p.o.

     5)   Flonase nasal inhaler, 2 sprays each nostril b.i.d.

     6)   Warm salt water gargle.

P Rodden MD
PATRICK RODDEN, M.D.

CENTRAL MEDICAL CENTER

211 Medical Center Drive • Central City, US 90000-1234 • PHONE: (012) 125-6784 • FAX: (012) 125-9999

X-RAY REPORT

LUMBOSACRAL SPINE:
Multiple views reveal no evidence of fracture. There is slight lumbar spondylosis with slight lipping and minimal bridging. The disc spaces appear maintained except for slight narrowing at L4-L5 and L5-S1. There is also a Grade I spondylolisthesis of L5 on S1 and evidence of spondylolysis at L5 on the left. There is also slight dextroscoliosis in the lumbar region and slight increased lordosis in the lumbosacral region. The bony architecture is unremarkable except for eburnation between the articulating facets at L5-S1. The SI joints appear unremarkable. Incidentally noted are slight osteoarthritic changes involving both hips.

CONCLUSION: 1.   Slight lumbar spondylosis with hypertrophic lipping and slight narrowing of the L4-L5 and L5-S1 disc spaces, rule out discogenic disease. If clinically indicated, CT of the lumbosacral spine may prove helpful in further evaluation.

2.   Grade I spondylolisthesis of L5 on S1 with evidence of spondylolysis at L5 on the left.

3.   Slight dextroscoliosis in the lumbar region and slight increased lordosis in the lumbosacral region.

M. Volz MD
M. Volz, M.D.

MV:ti

D: 10/19/20xx
T: 10/20/20xx

X-RAY REPORT	PT. NAME:	DORN, JAY F.
	ID NO:	RL-483091
	ATT. PHYS:	T. LIGHT, M.D.

Medical reports courtesy of Willis M. Medical Terminology: A Programmed Learning Approach to the Language of Health Care. 2nd ed. Baltimore: Lippincott Williams & Wilkins, 2007; and Willis MC. Medical Terminology: The Language of Health Care. 2nd ed. Baltimore: Lippincott Williams & Wilkins; 2006.

Appendix D

Metric Measurements

Unit	Abbreviation	Metric Equivalent	U.S. Equivalent
Units of Length			
kilometer	km	1000 meters	0.62 miles; 1.6 km/mile
meter*	m	100 cm; 1000 mm	39.4 inches; 1.1 yards
centimeter	cm	1/100 m; 0.01 m	0.39 inches; 2.5 cm/inch
millimeter	mm	1/1000 m; 0.001 m	0.039 inches; 25 mm/inch
micrometer	μm	1/1000 mm; 0.001 mm	
Units of Weight			
kilogram	kg	1000 g	2.2 lb
gram*	g	1000 mg	0.035 oz; 28.5 g/oz
milligram	mg	1/1000 g; 0.001 g	
microgram	μg, mcg	1/1000 mg; 0.001 mg	
Units of Volume			
liter*	L	1000 mL	1.06 qt
deciliter	dL	1/10 L; 0.1 L	
milliliter	mL	1/1000 L; 0.001 L	0.034 oz; 29.4 mL/oz
microliter	μL	1/1000 mL; 0.001 mL	

*Basic unit.

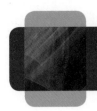

Appendix E

Celsius–Fahrenheit Temperature Conversion Scale

Celsius to Fahrenheit

Use the following formula to convert Celsius readings to Farenheit readings:

$$°F = 9/5 × °C + 32$$

For example, if the Celsius reading is 37°:

$$°F = (9/5 × 37) + 32$$
$$= 66.6 + 32$$
$$= 98.6°F \text{ (normal body temperature)}$$

Fahrenheit to Celsius

Use the following formula to convert Fahrenheit readings to Celsius readings:

$$°C = 5/9(°F − 32)$$

For example, if the Fahrenheit reading is 68°:

$$°C = 5/9(68 − 32)$$
$$= 5/9 × 36$$
$$= 20 °C \text{ (a nice spring day)}$$

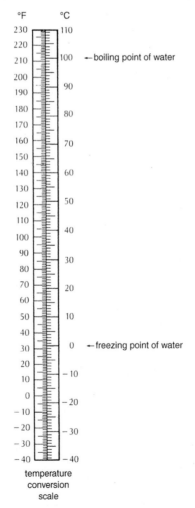

temperature
conversion
scale

From Memmler RL, Cohen BJ, Wood, DL. The Human Body in Health and Disease. 10th ed. Baltimore: Lippincott Williams & Wilkins; 2005.

Appendix F

Laboratory Tests

TABLE 1	Routine Urinalysis	
Test	**Normal Value**	**Clinical Significance**
General characteristics and measurements		
Color	Pale yellow to amber	Color change can be due to concentration or dilution, drugs, metabolic or inflammatory disorders
Odor	Slightly aromatic	Foul odor typical of urinary tract infection; fruity odor in uncontrolled diabetes mellitus
Appearance (clarity)	Clear to slightly hazy	Cloudy urine occurs with infection or after refrigeration; may indicate presence of bacteria, cells, mucus, or crystals
Specific gravity	1.003–1.030 (first morning catch; routine is random)	Decreased in diabetes insipidus, acute renal failure, water intoxication; increased in liver disorders, heart failure, dehydration
pH	4.5–8.0	Acid urine accompanies acidosis, fever, high protein diet; alkaline urine in urinary tract infection, metabolic alkalosis, vegetarian diet
Chemical determinations		
Glucose	Negative	Glucose present in uncontrolled diabetes mellitus, steroid excess
Ketones	Negative	Present in diabetes mellitus and in starvation
Protein	Negative	Present in kidney disorders, such as glomerulonephritis, acute kidney failure
Bilirubin	Negative	Breakdown product of hemoglobin; present in liver disease or in bile blockage
Urobilinogen	0.2–1.0 Ehrlich units/dL	Breakdown product of bilirubin; increased in hemolytic anemias and in liver disease; remains negative in bile obstruction
Blood	Negative	Detects small amounts of blood cells, hemoglobin, or myoglobin; present in severe trauma, metabolic disorders, bladder infections
Nitrite	Negative	Product of bacterial breakdown of urine; positive result suggests urinary tract infection and needs to be followed up with a culture of the urine
Microscopic		
Red blood cells	0–3 per high-power field	Increased because of bleeding within the urinary tract from trauma, tumors, inflammation, or damage within the kidney
White blood cells	0–4 per high-power field	Increased in infection of the kidney or bladder

TABLE 1	Routine Urinalysis *(continued)*	
Test	**Normal Value**	**Clinical Significance**
Renal epithelial cells	Occasional	Increased number indicates damage to kidney tubules
Casts	None	Hyaline casts normal; large number of abnormal casts indicates inflammation or a systemic disorder
Crystals	Present	Most are normal; may be acid or alkaline
Bacteria	Few	Increased in infection of urinary tract or contamination from infected genitalia
Others	Any yeasts, parasites, mucus, spermatozoa, or other microscopic findings would be reported here	

TABLE 2	Complete Blood Count (CBC)	
Test	**Normal Value***	**Clinical Significance**
Red blood cell (RBC) count	Men: 4.6–6.2 million/µL Women: 4.2–5.4 million/µL	Decreased in anemia; increased in dehydration, polycythemia
Hemoglobin (Hb)	Men: 13–18 g/dL Women: 12–16 g/dL	Decreased in anemia, hemorrhage, hemolytic reactions; increased in dehydration, heart and lung disease
Hematocrit (Hct)	Men: 45%–52% Women: 37%–48%	Decreased in anemia; increased in polycythemia, dehydration
Red blood cell (RBC) indices follow below:		These values, calculated from the RBC count, HGB, and HCT, give information valuable in the diagnosis and classification of anemia
Mean corpuscular volume (MCV)	80–95 µL/red cell	Measures the average size or volume of each RBC: small size (microcytic) in iron-deficiency anemia; large size (macrocytic) typical of pernicious anemia
Mean corpuscular hemoglobin (MCH)	27–31 pg/red cell	Measures the weight of hemoglobin per RBC; useful in differentiating types of anemia in a severely anemic patient
Mean corpuscular hemoglobin concentration (MCHC)	32–36 g/dL	Defines the volume of hemoglobin per RBC; used to determine the concentration of hemoglobin per RBC
White blood cell (WBC) count	4300–10,800µL	Increased in leukemia and in response to infection, inflammation, and dehydration; decreased in bone marrow suppression
Platelets	200,000–400,000/µL	Increased in many malignant disorders; decreased in disseminated intravascular coagulation (DIC) or toxic drug effects; spontaneous bleeding may occur at platelet counts below 20,000 µL
Differential (peripheral blood smear)		A stained slide of the blood is needed to perform the differential. The percentages of the different WBCs are estimated, and the slide is microscopically checked for abnormal characteristics in WBCs, RBCs, and platelets.

(continued)

TABLE 2	Complete Blood Count (CBC) *(continued)*	
Test	**Normal Value***	**Clinical Significance**
WBCs		
Segmented neutrophils (SEGs, POLYs)	40%–74%	Increased in bacterial infections; low numbers leave person very susceptible to infection
Immature neutrophils (BANDs)	0%–5%	Increased when neutrophil count increases
Lymphocytes (LYMPHs)	20%–40%	Increased in viral infections
Monocytes (MONOs)	3%–8%	Increased in specific infections
Eosinophils (EOs)	0%–6%	Increased in allergic disorders and parasite infestation
Basophils (BASOs)	0%–1%	Increased in allergic disorders

*Values vary depending on instrumentation and type of test.

TABLE 3	Blood Chemistry Tests	
Test	**Normal Value**	**Clinical Significance**
Basic panel: An overview of electrolytes, waste product management, and metabolism		
Blood urea nitrogen (BUN)	7–18 mg/dL	Increased in renal disease and dehydration; decreased in liver damage and malnutrition
Carbon dioxide (CO_2) (includes bicarbonate)	22–29 mmol/L	Useful to evaluate acid-base balance by measuring total carbon dioxide in the blood; elevated in vomiting and pulmonary disease; decreased in diabetic acidosis, acute renal failure, and hyperventilation
Chloride (Cl)	98–107 mmol/L	Increased in dehydration, hyperventilation, and congestive heart failure; decreased in vomiting, diarrhea, and fever
Creatinine	0.5–1.2 mg/dL	Produced at a constant rate and excreted by the kidney; increased in kidney disease
Glucose	Fasting: 70–100 mg/dL Random: 85–125 mg/dL	Increased in diabetes and severe illness; decreased in insulin overdose or hypoglycemia
Potassium (K)	3.4–5.0 mmol/L	Increased in renal failure, extensive cell damage, and acidosis; decreased in vomiting, diarrhea, and excess administration of diuretics or IV fluids
Sodium (Na)	135–145 mmol/L	Increased in dehydration and diabetes insipidus; decreased in overload of IV fluids, burns, diarrhea, or vomiting
Additional blood chemistry tests		
Alanine amino-transferase (ALT)	6–47 U/L*	Used to diagnose and monitor treatment of liver disease and to monitor the effects of drugs on the liver; increased in myocardial infarction

TABLE 3	Blood Chemistry Tests (continued)	
Test	**Normal Value**	**Clinical Significance**
Albumin	2.5–5.7 g/dL	Albumin maintains osmotic pressure in blood; decreased in liver disease and kidney disease
Albumin–globulin ratio (A/G ratio)	>1	Low A/G ratio signifies a tendency for edema because globulin is less effective than albumin at holding water in the blood
Alkaline phosphatase (ALP)	30–95 U/L*	Enzyme of bone metabolism; increased in liver disease and metastatic bone disease
Amylase	<180 U/L*	Used to diagnose and monitor treatment of acute pancreatitis and to detect inflammation of the salivary glands
Aspartate amino-transferase (AST)	5–30 U/L*	Enzyme present in tissues with high metabolic activity; increased in myocardial infarction and liver disease
Bilirubin, total	<1.5 mg/dL	Breakdown product of hemoglobin from red blood cells; increased when excessive red blood cells are being destroyed or in liver disease
Calcium (Ca)	8.6–10.0 mg/dL	Increased in excess parathyroid hormone production and in cancer; decreased in alkalosis, elevated phosphate in renal failure, and excess IV fluids
Cholesterol	<200 mg/dL	Screening test used to evaluate risk of heart disease; levels of 200 mg/dL or above indicate increased risk of heart disease and warrant further investigation
Creatine phospho-kinase (CPK or CK)	130–250 U/L*	Elevated enzyme level indicates damage to cardiac or skeletal muscle; when elevated, the specific fraction CKMB is tested for specific presence of cardiac muscle damage
Gamma-glutamyltransferase (GGT)	Men: 6–26 U/L Women: 4–18 U/L*	Used to diagnose liver disease and to test for chronic alcoholism
Globulins	2.3–3.5 g/dL	Proteins active in immunity; help albumin keep water in blood
Iron, serum (Fe)	40–60 µg/dL	Decreased in iron deficiency and anemia; increased in hemolytic conditions
High-density lipoproteins (HDLs)	>40 mg/dL	Used to evaluate the risk of heart disease
Lactate dehydrogenase (LDH or LD)	95–200 U/L*	Enzyme released in many kinds of tissue damage, including myocardial infarction, pulmonary infarction, and liver disease
Lipase	<60 U/L*	Enzyme used to diagnose pancreatitis
Low-density lipoproteins (LDLs)	<130 mg/dL	Used to evaluate the risk of heart disease
Magnesium (Mg)	1.2–2.1 mEq/L	Vital in neuromuscular function; decreased levels may occur in malnutrition, alcoholism, pancreatitis, diarrhea
Phosphorus (inorganic)	2.7–4.5 mg/dL	Evaluated in response to calcium; main store is in bone; elevated in kidney disease; decreased in excess parathyroid hormone
Protein, total	6–8 g/dL	Increased in dehydration, multiple myeloma; decreased in kidney disease, liver disease, poor nutrition, severe burns, excessive bleeding

(continued)

TABLE 3	Blood Chemistry Tests *(continued)*	
Test	**Normal Value**	**Clinical Significance**
Serum glutamic oxalacetic transaminase (SGOT)		See Aspartate aminotransferase (AST)
Serum glutamic pyruvic trans-aminase (SGPT)		See Alanine aminotransferase (ALT)
Thyroxin (T4)	4.0–12.0 µg/dL (may vary by test method)	Screening test of thyroid function; increased in hyperthyroidism; decreased in myxedema and hypothyroidism
Thyroid-stimulating hormone (TSH)	0.5–5.0 mU/L	Produced by pituitary to promote thyroid gland function; elevated when thyroid gland is not functioning
Triglycerides	<150 mg/dL	An indication of ability to metabolize fats; increased triglycerides and cholesterol indicate high risk of atherosclerosis
Uric acid	Men: 3.5–7.2 mg/dL Women: 2.6–6.0 mg/dL	Produced by breakdown of ingested purines in food and nucleic acids; elevated in kidney disease, gout, leukemia

*Varies significantly by test method.
Compare patient results to normal range printed on laboratory report.
Adapted from Memmler RL, Cohen BJ, Wood DL. The Human Body in Health and Disease. 10th ed. Baltimore: Lippincott Williams & Wilkins; 2005.

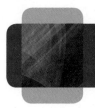

Appendix G

Body Systems and Laboratory Testing

System	Organs	Diseases	Laboratory Tests
Body Systems and Laboratory Testing			
Cardiovascular	Heart Blood vessels (i.e., arteries, capillaries, veins)	Coronary artery disease Ischemic heart disease	Cholesterol Triglycerides LDL HDL
		Myocardial infarction	Sodium Potassium CKMB Troponin Myoglobin
		Rheumatic fever Rheumatic heart disease	WBC count Hemoglobin Hematocrit Streptococcal antibody level
Circulatory	Heart, Blood vessels	Arteriosclerosis	Cholesterol Triglycerides LDL HDL
		Anemias	RBC count Hemoglobin Hematocrit MCV MCHC WBC count Reticulocyte count Platelet count Bone marrow studies
		Agranulocytosis	WBC count Bone marrow studies Blood cultures Urine culture Oral culture
		Polycythemia	RBC count Hemoglobin Hematocrit WBC count Platelet count

(continued)

Body Systems and Laboratory Testing (continued)

System	Organs	Diseases	Laboratory Tests
Digestive	Mouth	Oral tumor	Biopsy
		Herpes simplex (cold sores)	Viral cultures
		Thrush	Microscopic evaluation of lesion scrapings RBC count Hemoglobin Hematocrit Iron TIBC HIV
		Necrotizing periodontal disease	Throat culture
		Oral leukoplakia	Biopsy
		Oral cancer	Biopsy
	Esophagus	Gastroesophageal reflux disease	Biopsy
		Esophageal cancer	Biopsy
	Stomach	Peptic ulcer	*Helicobacter pylori* antibodies Fecal occult blood Hemoglobin Hematocrit Serum albumin Transferrin
		Gastritis	Biopsy WBC count Fecal occult blood
		Gastric cancer	Biopsy
	Liver	Cirrhosis of the liver	AST ALT Total bilirubin
		Hepatitis A	Hepatitis A antibody IgM Hepatitis B core antibody IgM Hepatitis B surface antigen Hepatitis C virus antibody Albumin Total protein ALP ALT AST Total bilirubin Direct bilirubin Prothrombin time Urinalysis

System	Organs	Diseases	Laboratory Tests
		Hepatitis B	Hepatitis A antibody IgM Hepatitis B core antibody IgM Hepatitis B surface antigen Hepatitis C virus antibody Albumin Total protein ALP ALT AST Total bilirubin Direct bilirubin Prothrombin time Urinalysis
		Heptitis C	Albumin Total protein ALP ALT AST Total bilirubin Direct bilirubin Hepatitis C virus RNA test Hepatitis C virus antibody
		Cancer of the liver	Alpha-fetoprotein Biopsy
	Gallbladder	Cholelithiasis Cholecystitis	Total bilirubin WBC count Total bilirubin
	Pancreas	Pancreatitis	Serum amylase Serum lipase WBC count Hematocrit Glucose
		Pancreatic cancer	CA 19-9 Biopsy
	Small intestine Large intestine	Gastroenteritis	Stool culture Fecal occult blood Stool WBCs Electrolytes
		Acute appendicitis	CBC Urinalysis
		Crohn disease (any portion of the gastrointestinal tract from mouth to anus) Ulcerative colitis	CBC Serum albumin Electrolytes Fecal occult blood Hemoglobin WBC count Stool culture Biopsy
		Intestinal obstruction	Electrolytes WBC count

Body Systems and Laboratory Testing (continued)

System	Organs	Diseases	Laboratory Tests
Endocrine	Hypothalamus	Hypothalamic disease	TSH Prolactin Cortisol ACTH Testosterone Growth hormone
	Pituitary	Gigantism	Growth hormone Insulin-like growth factor
		Acromegaly	Growth hormone
		Hypopituitarism	Thyrotropin Adrenocorticotropic hormone Gonadotropin
		Dwarfism	Growth hormone
		Diabetes insipidus	Urinalysis Osmolality Antidiuretic hormone
	Thyroid	Goiter	Thyrotropin T_3 T_4
		Hashimoto thyroiditis Hyperthyroidism	TSH T_3 T_4 TSH Thyroid-stimulating hormone
		Hypothyroidism	T_3 T_4 TSH
		Cretinism	T_4 TSH
		Myxedema	Total T_4 Total T_3 Free T_4 TSH
		Thyroid cancer	Biopsy Calcitonin Carcinoembryonic antigen
	Parathyroids	Hyperparathyroidism	Serum-intact parathyroid hormone Calcium Phosphorus ALP

Body Systems and Laboratory Testing *(continued)*

System	Organs	Diseases	Laboratory Tests
		Hypoparathyroidism	Calcium Phosphorus Parathyroid hormone
	Adrenals	Cushing syndrome	Free cortisol
		Addison disease	Blood cortisol Urine cortisol Sodium Fasting glucose CBC Hematocrit
	Pancreas	Diabetes mellitus	Fasting glucose Urinalysis Insulin
		Gestational diabetes	Urine glucose Fasting glucose Oral glucose tolerance tests Two-hour postprandial glucose Glycated hemoglobin
		Hypoglycemia	Glucose
	Pineal body	Seasonal affective disorder	Seratonin Melatonin
	Ovaries	Menopause	FSH Estrogen
		Polycystic ovary syndrome	Estrogen FSH Luteinizing hormone Testosterone 17 Hydroxyketosteroids Fasting glucose Glucose tolerance Insulin resistance Cholesterol Triglycerides HDL LDL Serum HCG Prolactin T_4 TSH
	Testes	Epididymitis	Urinalysis Urine culture WBC count
Excretory	Small and large intestines	Diverticulitis	Fecal occult blood CBC
	Rectum Anus	Colorectal cancer	Fecal occult blood Biopsy

(continued)

Body Systems and Laboratory Testing *(continued)*

System	Organs	Diseases	Laboratory Tests
Immune	Bone marrow	Leukemia	Peripheral blood smear Bone marrow aspiration
		Anemia	CBC Peripheral blood smear Bone marrow aspiration
		Lymphoma	Biopsy CBC ALP
	Thymus gland	Myasthenia gravis	Acetylcholine receptor antibodies
		DiGeorge anomaly (thymic hypoplasia or aplasia)	T-cell count Chromosome studies
	Spleen	Splenomegaly	Albumin Total protein ALP ALT AST Total bilirubin Direct bilirubin
	Lymph nodes	Lymphadenopathy	CBC
		Lymphadenitis	WBC count Throat culture Sputum culture
		Lymphoma	Lymph node biopsy CBC ESR Bone marrow aspirate Albumin Total protein ALP ALT AST Total bilirubin Direct bilirubin BUN Creatinine
Integumentary	Skin	Herpes zoster (shingles)	Vesicle scrapings culture Varicella-zoster antibodies
		Impetigo	Gram stain
		Cellulitis	Blood culture
		Tinea cruris (jock itch)	Lesion culture
		Decubitus ulcers	Culture and sensitivity
	Hair	Alopecia (baldness)	CBC T_4 TSH
		Folliculitis	Culture of purulent material

Body Systems and Laboratory Testing *(continued)*

System	Organs	Diseases	Laboratory Tests
	Nails	Deformed or discolored nails	Comprehensive metabolic profile
		Paronychia	Exudate culture
	Sweat glands	Sweat gland abscess	Culture
Lymphatic	Ducts and lymph nodes	See "Lymph nodes" in the *Immune system*	
	Palatine tonsil	Tonsillitis	WBC count Throat culture
	Thymus gland	See "Thymus gland" in the *Immune system*	
Muscular	Muscles (smooth, cardiac, and skeletal)	Muscle tumors	Core needle biopsy
		Muscular dystrophy	Muscle biopsy CK
		Polymyositis	CK Aldolase AST ALT Lactate dehydrogenase Muscle biopsy
Nervous	Brain	Epilepsy	Comprehensive metabolic panel
	Spinal cord	Meningitis	CSF levels of WBCs, protein, and glucose CSF culture
	Nerves	Guillain-Barré syndrome	CSF protein
Reproductive	Male (penis and testes)	Klinefelter syndrome	Serum and urine gonadotropin Semen analysis Chromosome studies
	Female (vagina)	Vaginitis	Wet prep KOH prep Culture
		Vaginal cancer	Pap smear Biopsy
		Trichomoniasis	Wet prep Urinalysis
	Uterus	Endometrial cancer	Biopsy CBC Urinalysis Creatinine BUN Albumin Total protein ALP ALT AST Total bilirubin Direct bilirubin
	Ovaries	Ovarian cancer	CA 125

(continued)

Body Systems and Laboratory Testing (continued)

System	Organs	Diseases	Laboratory Tests
Respiratory	Nose	Leishmaniasis	Biopsy
		Epistaxis	Platelet count
	Pharynx	Pharyngitis	CBC
	Larynx	Tumors of the larynx	Biopsy
	Trachea	Sarcoidosis	Biopsy Serum angiotensin-converting enzyme
	Bronchi	Hemoptysis	PT PTT
		Bronchiectasis	Sputum culture
	Alveoli	Fibrosing alveolitis	Biopsy
	Bronchioles	Cystic fibrosis	CF transmembrane conductance regulator Sweat chloride
	Lungs	Pneumonia	Sputum culture Blood culture
		Pulmonary abscess	Sputum culture Blood culture
		Legionellosis	WBC count ALP ALT AST ESR Sputum culture
		Respiratory syncytial virus	Respiratory syncytial virus
		Pneumonia Pulmonary tuberculosis	Sputum culture
		Lung cancer	Sputum cytology
Skeletal	Bone	Paget disease (osteitis deformans)	Bone marrow biopsy ALP Urine hydroxyproline
		Bone tumors	ALP Serum calcium Bone marrow evaluation Biopsy
		Osteomalacia and rickets	Comprehensive metabolic panel Vitamin D level ESR
	Bone marrow	Leukemia	See *Immune system*
		Anemia	See *Circulatory system*
		Lymphoma	See *Immune system*

Body Systems and Laboratory Testing (continued)

System	Organs	Diseases	Laboratory Tests
	Joints	Gout	Microscopy of synovial joint fluid Serum uric acid
	Teeth	Dental diseases	Dental treatment
	Ligaments	Orthopedics	
	Cartilage	Costochondritis	WBC count
Urinary	Kidneys	Chronic glomerulonephritis	Urinalysis Renal biopsy BUN Creatinine
		Nephrotic syndrome (nephrosis)	Urinalysis with microscopic evaluation Serum albumin Cholesterol Triglyceride HDL LDL Renal biopsy
		Acute renal failure	Urinalysis BUN Creatinine Potassium
		Chronic renal failure	BUN Creatinine Potassium Hematocrit Urinalysis
		Pyelonephritis	Clean-catch urinalysis Blood culture Urine culture
	Ureter	Ureteral obstruction (renal calculi)	Urinalysis Renal calculi analysis
	Urethra	Urethritis	Clean-catch urinalysis with microscopic evaluation Urine culture
Sensory	Sense of sight	Ophthalmology	
	Sense of hearing	Cancer of the ear	Biopsy
	Sense of feeling	Vitamin B_{12} deficiency	Vitamin B_{12} Serum folate CBC
	Sense of smell	Anosmia	Neurology evaluation
	Sense of taste	Loss from gingivitis	Throat culture
		Loss from strep throat	Rapid strep test Throat culture

(continued)

Body Systems and Laboratory Testing *(continued)*

System	Organs	Diseases	Laboratory Tests
		Sjögren syndrome	Antithyroglobulin antibody Rheumatoid arthritis test Antinuclear antibody test
	Sense of balance	Vitamin B_{12} deficiency Hypoglycemia Audiology evaluation	See "Sense of feeling" Glucose

Note: Lists are representative, not comprehensive.

LDL, low-density lipoprotein; HDL, high-density lipoprotein; CKMB, creatine kinase-MB (muscle, brain); CK, creatine kinase; WBC, white blood cell; RBC, red blood cell; MCV, mean corpuscular volume; MCHC, mean corpuscular hemoglobin concentration; TIBC, total iron-binding capacity; HIV, human immunodeficiency virus; AST, aspartate aminotransferase; ALT, alanine aminotransferase; ALP, alkaline phosphatase; FSH, follicle-stimulating hormone; IgM, immunoglobulin M; CBC, complete blood count; T_3, triiodothyronine; T_4, thyroxine; TSH, thyroid-stimulating hormone; HCG, human chorionic gonadotropin; ESR, erythrocyte sedimentation rate; BUN, blood urea nitrogen; CSF, cerebrospinal fluid; KOH, potassium hydroxide; PT, prothrombin time; PTT, partial thromboplastin time; CF, cystic fibrosis.

Glossary

A

abdominal regions divisions of the abdomen into nine regions by two horizontal and two vertical lines; used to identify specific locations.

ablation removal or excision of a part; laser ablation is destruction/removal of tissue by use of laser.

abortion termination of pregnancy or products of conception prior to fetal viability and/or 20 weeks of gestation.

accreditation a nongovernmental professional peer review process that provides technical assistance and evaluates educational programs for quality based on pre-established academic and administrative standards.

acidosis condition in which there is too much acid in the body.

acquired immunodeficiency syndrome (AIDS) a cluster of disorders caused by HIV that specifically destroys cell-mediated immunity.

acromegaly a disorder marked by progressive enlargement of the head, face, hands, and feet, due to excessive secretion of growth hormone after puberty.

acrosome the superior surface of the head of the spermatozoon.

activities of daily living (ADL) activities usually performed in the course of the day, i.e., bathing, dressing, feeding oneself.

acute abrupt in onset.

Addison disease partial or complete failure of the adrenal cortex functions, causing general physical deterioration.

adenosine triphosphate (ATP) the energy currency used by the body; breaking down the phosphate bond of the compound releases high energy potential.

adhesion occurs when platelets stick across the injured surface.

adipose of or pertaining to fat.

adjustment a change in a posted account.

adnexa any part added to a main structure; an accessory part.

advance directive a statement of a patient's wishes regarding health care prior to a critical medical event.

aerobe microorganism that requires oxygen to live and reproduce.

aerosol suspended particles in gas or air.

afebrile body temperature not elevated above normal.

afferent carrying impulses towards the center.

agglutination clumping of cells due to the presence of antibodies called *agglutinins*.

albumin because it is a small molecule, one of the first proteins able to pass through the kidneys into the urine when there are kidney problems.

aliquots portions of the original patient specimen that have been placed into a separate container to be routed to the appropriate laboratory work station for testing

alkalosis condition in which the blood has too much base, resulting in an increase in blood pH.

allergen any substance that causes manifestations of an allergy, usually a protein to which the body has built antibodies.

allergy acquired abnormal response to a substance (allergen) that does not ordinarily cause a reaction.

alopecia baldness.

alpha-fetoprotein substance produced by the embryonic yolk sac.

alveolar–capillary membrane the structure in the lung fields through which oxygen and carbon dioxide diffuse during the respiratory process.

amenorrhea condition of not menstruating, without menses.

Americans with Disabilities Act (ADA) a law designed to meet the needs of people with physical and mental challenges.

amino acids building blocks of protein.

ammonia a common metabolic waste product.

amniocentesis puncture of the amniotic sac in order to remove fluid for testing.

amphiarthroses slightly movable joints.

ampule small glass container that must be broken at the neck to aspirate the solution into the syringe.

amylase an enzyme secreted by the pancreas into the intestines to aid in digestion; also secreted by the salivary glands.

anabolism the constructive phase of metabolism, when smaller molecules are converted to large ones.

anacusis complete hearing loss.

anaerobe bacterium that requires the absence of oxygen for growth and reproduction.

analyte substance or constituent for which a laboratory conducts testing.

anaphylactic shock severe allergic reaction within minutes to hours after exposure to a foreign substance.

anaphylaxis severe allergic reaction that may result in death.

anatomic position a position used for reference in which the subject is standing erect, facing forward, feet are slightly apart and pointing forward, and the hands are down at the sides with palms forward and thumbs outward.

anatomy the study of the structure of the body.

anchor holding a vein in place so that it does not roll.

anencephaly a neural tube defect in developing fetuses.

aneroid sphygmomanometer that measures blood pressure without using mercury.

aneurysm local dilation in a blood vessel wall.

angina pectoris paroxysmal chest pain usually caused by a decrease in blood flow to the heart muscle due to coronary artery occlusion.

angiotensin a substance occurring in the blood that works with renin to affect the blood pressure, usually increasing the pressure by vasoconstriction.

anions chemicals that carry a negative charge.

anisocytosis blood abnormality in which red blood cells are not equal in size (aniso = unequal).

ankylosing spondylitis stiffening of the spine with inflammation.

anorexia loss of appetite.

anovulation condition of not ovulating.

antagonism mutual opposition or contrary action with something else; opposite of synergism.

antagonist any muscle that opposes the action of the prime mover to balance movement. (Example: When the biceps contract and pull the forearm upward, the triceps oppose the motion and relax.)

antecubital space inner surface of the bend of the elbow where the major veins for venipuncture are located.

antepartum period of time prior to labor.

anthropometric pertaining to measurements of the human body.

antibiotic a drug that inhibits or destroys pathogenic microorganisms.

antibody a complex glycoprotein produced by B lymphocytes in response to an antigen.

anticoagulant a chemical compound introduced to the blood or blood sample to prevent clotting. Anticoagulants suppress the function of clotting factors normally present in blood.

antigen protein markers on cells that cause formation of antibodies and react specifically with those antibodies.

antihistamine medication that opposes the action of a histamine.

antiseptic any substance that inhibits the growth of bacteria; used on skin before any procedure that breaks the integumentary barrier.

anuria failure of the kidneys to produce urine.

apnea the absence of respirations.

apothecary system of measurement old system that uses grains, minims, and drams.

appendicular skeleton the parts of the skeleton added to the axial skeleton, including the shoulder and pelvic girdles and all of the bones of the upper and lower extremities.

applicator device for applying local treatments and tests.

approximate bring tissue surfaces as close as possible to their original positions.

arachnoid web-like membrane covering the brain and spinal cord.

arrector pili involuntary muscle attached to the hair follicle that, when contracted, causes "goose bumps."

arteriole a small arterial branch that joins a capillary to an artery.

arthrogram x-ray of a joint.

arthroplasty surgical repair of a joint.

arthroscopy examination of the inside of a joint through an arthroscope.

artifact activity recorded in an electrocardiogram caused by extraneous activity such as patient movement, loose lead, or electrical interference.

artifactual something added to a substance or structure, not belonging to it; in medicine, generally implies a negative connotation.

ascites accumulation of serous fluid in the peritoneal cavity.

asepsis a state of being sterile; a condition free from germs, infection, and any form of life, including spore forms.

aspiration drawing in or out by suction; as in breathing objects into the respiratory tract or suctioning substances from a site.

assault an attempt or threat to touch another person without his or her consent.

assessment process of gathering information about the patient and the presenting condition.

asymmetry lack or absence of symmetry; inequality of size or shape on opposite sides of the body.

asymptomatic without any symptoms.

atelectasis collapsed lung fields; incomplete expansion of the lungs, either partial or complete.

atherosclerosis buildup of fatty plaque on the interior lining of arteries.

atraumatic without injury; may pertain to treatments or instruments that are not likely to cause further damage.

atria (plural) the upper chamber of each half of the heart; the atria receive blood from the great vessels (singular: atrium).

atrioventricular (AV) node located on the floor of the right atrium on or close to the septum; receives the electrical impulse from the sinoatrial node after it is transmitted through the upper half of the heart; transmits the impulse to the bundle of His.

attenuated diluted or weakened; pertaining to reduced virulence of a pathogenic microorganism.

aura a visual or other sensory warning experienced before an impending seizure.

auscultation act of listening for sounds within the body, usually with a stethoscope, such as to evaluate the heart, lungs, intestines, or fetal heart tones.

autoclave appliance used to sterilize medical instruments with steam under pressure.

autoimmunity condition in which the immune system attacks its own host's body.

autonomic self-controlling, spontaneous.

autonomous existing or functioning independently.

axial skeleton the bones forming the main skeleton around which the appendicular skeleton moves, including bones of the head, thorax, and trunk.

axon part of the neuron that transmits impulses away from the cell body.

azidothymidine (AZT) a drug used to treat AIDS by blocking the growth of the virus after it enters the T-cell lymphocyte.

azotemia from the Latin *azote* meaning nitrogen, plus -emia, meaning blood; the condition of having excessive amounts of nitrogen in the blood.

B

Babinski reflex reflex (dorsiflexion of the great toe and extension and fanning of the other toes upon stroking the sole of the foot) exhibited normally by infants. This reflex is abnormal in children and adults.

bacilli rod-shaped or cylindrical organisms.

bactericidal substance that kills or destroys bacteria.

bacteriology the science and study of bacteria.

bacteriuria the presence of bacteria in urine.

band younger, less mature neutrophil.

bandage noun, a soft material applied to a body part to hold a dressing in place, immobilize a body part, or aid in controlling bleeding; verb, to apply a wrapping material for treatment.

barrier precautions any device, including PPE, that provides an obstacle to minimize the risk of infection with bloodborne pathogens.

Bartholin glands small mucous glands bilaterally in the vaginal vestibule.

basal ganglia pertaining to the gray matter in the cerebral hemispheres.

basal metabolic rate the amount of energy used in a unit of time to maintain vital functions by a fasting, resting subject.

basic pH nonacidic pH 8–12.

baseline original or initial measure with which other measurements will be compared.

basophil a type of leukocyte.

B cells lymphoid stem cells from the bone marrow that migrate to and become mature antigen-specific cells in the spleen and lymph nodes.

Benedict reaction the copper reduction test for measuring glucose.

benign not cancerous or malignant.

bevel the angled point of the needle cut on a slant to ease skin penetration.

bias formation of an opinion without foundation or reason; prejudice.

bicarbonate the dissolved form of carbon dioxide; it combines with water to make carbonic acid, H_2CO_3. Carbonic acid loses one of its hydrogen (H) ions to then form bicarbonate, HCO_3^-.

bile a bitter, yellow-green secretion of the liver stored by the gallbladder; derived from bilirubin, cholesterol, and other substances. Emulsifies fats in the small intestine so they can be further digested and absorbed.

biliary obstruction blockage of one of the bile ducts (the tubes leading from liver and gallbladder into duodenum); common causes include cysts, tumors, and stones.

bilirubin formed during the breakdown of hemoglobin.

bilirubinuria bilirubin in the urine.

bimanual pertaining to the use of both hands; an examination performed with both hands.

biohazard biological agent that has the capacity to harm humans.

biohazard symbol icon on the label for specimens containing potential biological agents.

biohazardous describing a substance that is a risk to the health of living organisms.

biohazardous waste infectious waste or biomedical waste; any waste containing infectious materials or potentially infectious substances such as blood.

biological agent bacteria, viruses, fungi, other microorganisms, and their toxins.

biotransform convert the molecules of a substance from one form to another, as in medications within the body.

blister a collection of fluid in or beneath the epidermis; a vesicle.

block a type of letter format in which the date, subject line, closing, and signature are justified to the right margin; all other lines are justified left.

blood cultures specimens drawn to culture the blood for pathogens.

blood urea nitrogen (BUN) blood test to determine the amount of nitrogen in blood in the form of urea, a waste product normally excreted in urine.

bloodborne pathogens viruses that can be spread through direct contact with blood or body fluids from an infected person.

body fluids any of the fluids that accumulate in the compartments of the body, such as the blood plasma, and the intracellular and extracellular spaces.

body mass index (BMI) a measurement of an individual's ratio of fat to lean body mass. It is calculated by using the following formula: [weight (pounds) ÷ height (inches) 2] × 703. A BMI over 30 is considered obese.

body mechanics using the correct muscles and posture to complete a task safely and efficiently.

boil an abscess of the subcutaneous tissues of the skin; a furuncle.

bolus a mobile mass, for instance, a mass of food that passes into the upper gastrointestinal tract in one swallow, or a dose of medication injected intravenously.

bore diameter of the interior of a needle.

bradycardia heart rate of less than 60 beats per minute.

bradykinesia abnormally slow voluntary movements.

Braxton-Hicks contractions uterine contractions during pregnancy.

"breathing the syringe" pull back the plunger to about halfway up the barrel, then push it back; makes the plunger move more smoothly and reduces the tendency to jerk when it is first pulled after insertion into the vein.

broth liquid media is most often poured into glass tubes or bottles.

bruit abnormal sound or murmur in the blood vessels during auscultation.

buccal describing medication administered between the cheek and gum of the mouth.

buffer extra time to accommodate emergencies, walk-ins, and other demands on the provider's daily time schedule that are not considered direct patient care.

buffer system system that guards against sudden shifts in acidity and alkalinity depending on the body's own naturally occurring weak acids and weak bases.

bulla large blister or vesicle.

BUN *see* blood urea nitrogen.

bundle of His a band of specialized cardiac muscle fibers that receives the electrical impulse from the atrioventricular node and transmits it through right and left branches to the Purkinje fibers.

bursae small sacs filled with clear synovial fluid that surround some joints.

butterfly winged infusion set.

byte a unit of symbolic transfer; each character equals one byte.

C

calibrated marked in units of measurement, as a thermometer calibrated in Celsius.

calibration the standardization of any measuring instrument or testing procedure.

callus in the musculoskeletal system, a deposit of new bone tissue that forms between the healing ends of broken bones; in the integumentary system, a thickened area of the epidermis caused by pressure or friction.

calorie a unit of heat content or energy. The amount of heat necessary to raise 1 g of water from 14.5 to 15.5°C (small calorie).

calyx (plural, calyces) a cuplike collecting structure of the kidney.

cancellous   porous, spongy bone inside the medulla of the bone, usually filled with marrow.

carbohydrates   chemical elements in food that convert to sugar, providing energy.

carbuncle   infection of interconnected group of hair follicles or several furuncles forming a mass.

cardiac cycle   period from the beginning of one heartbeat to the beginning of the next; includes systole and diastole.

cardiac output   the amount of blood ejected from either ventricle per minute, either to the pulmonary or to the systemic circulation.

cardinal signs   usually, vital signs; signifies their importance in assessment.

cardiogenic shock   type of shock in which the left ventricle fails to pump enough blood for the body to function.

cardiomegaly   enlarged heart muscle.

cardiomyopathy   any disease affecting the myocardium.

carina   a ridge-like structure; that part of the trachea that projects from the lower end of the trachea.

carrier   person infected with a microorganism but without signs of disease; a company that assumes the risk of an insurance company.

cassette   light-proof holder in which x-ray film is exposed.

catabolism   the destructive phase of metabolism in which larger molecules are converted into smaller molecules.

catabolize   to break down fats.

cataracts   progressive loss of transparency of the lens of the eye, resulting in opacity and loss of sight.

catheterization   procedure for introducing a flexible tube into the body; urinary catheterization is for removal of urine from the bladder.

cations   chemicals that carry a positive charge.

cautery   means, device, or agent that destroys or coagulates tissue; may be electrical current, freezing or burning agent, or chemical solution (caustic).

cell   the most basic unit of all living organisms.

cellulitis   inflammation or infection of the skin and deeper tissues that may result in tissue destruction if not treated properly.

Celsius, centigrade (C)   a temperature scale on which 0 degrees is the freezing point of water and 100 degrees is the boiling point of water at sea level.

Centers for Disease Control and Prevention (CDC)   U.S. federal agency under the Department of Health and Human Services that works to protect public health and safety. CDC provides information to enhance health decisions.

Centers for Medicare and Medicaid Services (CMS)   government department that mandates the use of panels defined by the American Medical Association (AMA) for national standardization of nomenclature and testing.

centesis   surgical puncture made into a cavity.

centrifugation   process of separating blood or other body fluid cells from liquid components using a centrifuge.

cephalalgia   headache.

cerebellum   located in the posterior part of the brain, responsible for balance and muscle coordination.

cerebrovascular accident (CVA)   ischemia of the brain due to an occlusion of the blood vessels supplying the brain, resulting in varying degrees of debilitation.

cerebrum   largest part of the brain, divided into two hemispheres; responsible for thought processes, sensory and motor functions, speech, writing, memory, and emotions.

Certificate of Waiver (CW)   one of four types of certificates issued under CLIA; certifies the laboratory to perform waived testing.

cerumen   yellowish or brownish wax-like secretion in the external ear canal; earwax.

cervix   the part of the uterus that opens into the vagina.

Chadwick sign   sign of early pregnancy in which the vaginal, cervical, and vulvar tissues develop a bluish violet color.

chain-of-custody procedure   accurate written record to track the possession, handling, and location of chain-of-custody samples and data from collection through reporting.

challenge   a method of testing a patient's sensitivity or response to a substance by introducing it into the body and watching its effects.

chancre   a hard ulcer that appears 2 to 3 weeks after exposure to syphilis, near the site of infection.

Chemical Hygiene Plan (CHP)   a part of the Occupational Safety and Health Administration's HazCom standard.

chemical name   exact chemical descriptor of a drug.

chlamydia   a parasitic microorganism with properties common to bacteria but unable to sustain life without a host, in the manner of a virus.

chronic obstructive pulmonary disease (COPD)   progressive, irreversible condition with diminished respiratory capacity.

chronological order   placing in the order of time; usually the most recent is placed foremost.

chyle   milky, fatty product of digestion absorbed through the small intestines and returned to circulation by the lymphatics.

chyme   the thick, semi-liquid mass of ingested food mixed with gastric juices as it passes from the stomach.

cilia   hair-like projections on cells that either propel the cell or objects that come in contact with the cell.

circumcision   surgical removal of the prepuce.

clarification   explanation; removal of confusion or uncertainty.

CLIA certification   required by any group that performs even one test, including a waived test on materials derived from the human body for the purpose of providing information for the diagnosis, prevention, or treatment of any disease or impairment of, or the assessment of the health of, human beings to meet certain federal requirements. See Clinical Laboratory Improvement Amendments.

climacteric period   menopause; developmental phase in which a woman's reproductive ability ceases.

clinical   pertaining to direct patient care (e.g., nonadministrative tasks that a medical assistant will perform).

clinical chemistry   the study of the presence and measurement of substances in blood.

clinical diagnosis   a diagnosis based only on the patient's clinical symptoms.

Clinical Laboratory Improvement Amendments (CLIA)   guidelines established by Congress in 1988 to standardize and improve laboratory testing.

Clinical and Laboratory Standards Institute (CLSI)   a committee appointed to establish rules to ensure the safety, standards, and integrity of all testing performed on human specimens.

Clinitest™   most common test for reducing sugars.

cloning   genetically identical replication of cells, an organ, or an organism in the laboratory.

coagulate   change from a liquid to a solid or semi-solid mass.

coagulation   the study of the blood's ability to clot.

coagulopathies   diseases associated with abnormal blood clotting functions.

cocci   spherical bacteria.

collagen   protein substance that gives structure to the connective tissue.

colpocleisis   surgery to occlude the vagina.

colporrhaphy   suturing of the vagina.

colposcopy   visual examination of the vagina and cervix under magnification.

Commission on Office Laboratory Accreditation (COLA)   works to support the health care industry by providing knowledge and resources for maintaining quality laboratory operations.

competency assessment   evaluation of a person's ability to perform a test and to use a testing device.

complete blood count (CBC)   the CBC is a frequently ordered laboratory test consisting of white blood cell count and differential, red blood cell count, hemoglobin, hematocrit, erythrocyte indices, and platelet count.

computed tomography (CT)   a diagnostic procedure that uses x-rays to produce cross-sectional views of internal body structures.

concussion   injury to the brain due to trauma.

confidentiality   protection of patient data from unauthorized personnel.

confirmatory test   an additional, more specific test performed to rule out or confirm a preliminary test result to provide a final result.

congenital anomaly   abnormality, either structural or functional, present at birth.

congestive heart failure   condition in which the heart cannot pump effectively.

conjugated bilirubin   bilirubin that does dissolve into the bloodstream.

consent   an agreement between a patient and physician to do a given medical procedure.

contracture   abnormal shortening of muscles around a joint caused by atrophy of the muscles and resulting in flexion and fixation.

contraindication   situation or condition that prohibits the prescribing or administering of a drug or medication.

contrast medium   substance ingested or injected into the body to facilitate imaging of internal structures.

control   a device or solution used to monitor the test to ensure correct test results.

contusion   collection of blood in tissues after an injury; a bruise.

convoluted tubules   the twisted portion of the nephron that connects the glomerulus to the collecting tubules; consists of a proximal and a distal portion connected by the loop of Henle.

convulsion   sudden, involuntary muscle contraction of a voluntary muscle group.

corpora cavernosa   the erectile bodies of the penis or clitoris.

corpus spongiosum   erectile tissue around the male urethra.

corticoid   any of the hormonal steroid substances obtained from the adrenal cortex.

cortisol   a naturally occurring steroidal hormone that regulates metabolism and acts as an anti-inflammatory agent.

coumarin   an anticoagulant prescribed for persons likely to form blood clots, such as valve replacement recipients; also called *Coumadin* (trade name) or *warfarin*.

cranium   the portion of the skull that encloses the brain.

creatinine   a breakdown product of creatine that aids in delivering energy to cells.

cretinism   severe congenital hypothyroidism; signs include dwarfism, low intelligence, puffy features, dry skin, macroglossia, and poor muscle tone.

critical values   considered to be life-threatening test results.

cryosurgery   the surgical destruction of tissue using freezing temperature with liquid nitrogen or carbon dioxide.

cryptorchidism   one or both testicles that have not moved into the scrotum before birth. Also known as *undescended testicles*.

cul-de-sac   blind pouch or cavity, as in the cul-de-sac that lies between the rectum and the posterior uterus.

culdocentesis   surgical puncture and aspiration of fluid from the vaginal cul-de-sac for diagnosis or therapy.

culture   a laboratory process whereby microorganisms are grown in a special medium often for the purpose of identifying a causative agent in an infectious disease; also means the way of life, including commonly held beliefs, of a group of people.

curettage   scraping of a body cavity, such as the uterus.

Cushing syndrome   a disorder resulting from increased adrenocortical secretion of cortisol.

CW testing site   location where CLIA-waived testing takes place. See *Clinical Laboratory Improvement Amendments* and *Certificate of Waiver*.

cyanotic   a bluish discoloration of the skin due to the lack of oxygen.

cystocele   herniation of the urinary bladder into the vagina.

cystoscopy   direct visualization of the urinary bladder through a cystoscope inserted through the urethra.

cytogenetics   a type of cytology in which the genetic structure of the cells obtained from tissue, blood, or body fluids, such as amniotic fluid, are examined or tested for chromosome deficiencies related to genetic disease.

cytology   Study of the microscopic structure of cells.

D

deciduous   to fall or shed; deciduous teeth: the set of 20 teeth appearing during infancy and shedding during childhood.

decongestant   substance that reduces congestion or swelling.

degenerative joint disease (DJD)   also known as osteoarthritis; arthritis characterized by degeneration of the bony structure of the joints, usually noninflammatory.

deglutition   the act of swallowing.

dehiscence   separation or opening of the edges of a wound.

demeanor   the way a person looks, behaves, and conducts himself or herself.

dementia   progressive organic mental deterioration with loss of intellectual function.

demographic   relating to the statistical characteristics of populations.

dendrite   part of the neuron that transmits impulses toward the cell body.

dental cavities   holes in the teeth.

dentin the main component of the tooth structure, surrounds the inner pulp and lies just below the enamel.

Department of Health and Human Services (HHS) U.S. government's agency for protecting the health of all Americans and providing essential human services.

depolarization progressive wave of stimulation causing contraction of the myocardium.

dermatophytosis fungal infection of the skin.

dermis layer of skin under the epidermis.

desiccation inhibits microbial growth by removing the water required for metabolism.

detoxification clearing of drugs from the body and treating the withdrawal symptoms.

dextrocardia the condition of having the heart in the right side of the thoracic cavity.

diabetes insipidus a disorder of metabolism characterized by polyuria and polydipsia; caused by a deficiency in antidiuretic hormone (ADH) or an inability of the kidneys to respond to ADH.

diagnosis identification of a disease or condition by evaluating physical signs and symptoms, health history, and laboratory tests; a disease or condition identified in a person.

diagnostic test medical test performed to aid in the diagnosis or detection of disease.

dialysis removal of waste in blood not filtered by kidneys by passing fluid through a semipermeable barrier that allows normal electrolytes to remain, either with a machine with circulatory access or by passing a balanced fluid through the peritoneal cavity.

diaphoresis profuse sweating.

diaphragmatic excursion the movement of the diaphragm during respiration.

diarthroses freely movable joints; also called *synovial joints*.

diastole relaxation phase of the cardiac cycle.

dideoxycytidine (ddC) a drug used to treat AIDS by blocking the growth of the virus after it enters the T-cell lymphocytes.

dideoxyinosine (ddI) a drug used to treat AIDS by blocking the growth of the virus after it enters the T-cell lymphocytes.

diencephalon part of the brain lying beneath the hemispheres, containing the thalamus and hypothalamus.

differential diagnosis a diagnosis made by comparing the patient's symptoms to two or more diseases that have similar symptoms.

differential stain staining process which uses more than one chemical stain to better differentiate between different microorganisms or structures/cellular components of a single organism.

diluent specified liquid used to reconstitute powder medications for injection

diplococci spherical cocci in pairs.

direct microscopic examination examination of a patient specimen using a microscope; a type of nonwaived testing.

disease definite pathologic process having a distinctive set of symptoms and course of progression.

disinfectant a chemical that can be applied to objects to destroy microorganisms; will not destroy bacterial spores.

disinfection killing or rendering inert most but not all pathogenic microorganisms.

distal away from the origin.

diuretics substances that promote the formation and excretion of urine.

diurnal variation variation over a 24-hour period.

documentation the process of recording patient information.

donor one who contributes something to another.

dowager's hump exaggerated cervical curve with prominence of the top thoracic vertebrae found in some osteoporotic elderly women; a type of kyphosis.

dressing a covering applied directly to a wound to apply pressure, give support, absorb secretions, protect from trauma or microorganisms, stop or slow bleeding, or hide disfigurement.

drug any substance that may modify one or more of the functions of an organism.

dura mater the outer covering of the brain.

durable power of attorney a legal document giving another person the authority to act on one's behalf.

duress the act of compelling or forcing someone to do something that they do not want to do.

dwarfism (endocrine or pituitary) abnormal underdevelopment of the body with extreme shortness but normal proportions; achondroplastic dwarfism is an inherited growth disorder characterized by shortened limbs and a large head but almost normal trunk proportions.

dysmenorrhea painful menstruation.

dyspareunia painful coitus or sexual intercourse.

dysphagia inability to swallow or difficulty in swallowing.

dysphasia difficulty speaking.

dysphonia impairment of voice; hoarseness.

dyspnea difficulty breathing.

dysuria painful or difficult urination.

E

ecchymosis characteristic black and blue mark that results from blood as it accumulates under the skin.

eczema superficial dermatitis.

edema an accumulation of fluid within the tissues.

edematous describes a swollen area due to excess tissue fluid.

efferent carrying impulses away from the center.

elastin protein substance that gives elasticity and flexibility to the connective tissues.

electrocardiography procedure that produces a record of the electrical activity of the heart.

electrode medium for conducting or detecting electrical current.

electrolyte balance having electrolytes in the right concentrations in order to maintain fluid balance among the compartments.

electrolytes certain chemical substances dissolved in the blood and having numerous basic functions such as conducting electrical currents; the principal electrolytes are sodium, potassium, chloride, and bicarbonate.

electromyography recording of electrical nerve transmission in skeletal muscles.

element a substance that cannot be separated or broken down into substances with properties other than its own; a primary substance.

embolus mass of matter (thrombus, air, fat globule) freely floating in the circulatory system.

emergency medical services (EMS) a group of health care providers working as a team to care for sick or injured patients before they arrive at the hospital.

empathy   the ability to understand or to some extent share what someone else is feeling.

encounter form   a preprinted statement that lists codes for basic office charges and has sections to record charges incurred in an office visit, the patient's current balance, and next appointment.

endemic   a disease that occurs continuously in a particular population but has a low mortality; used in contrast to epidemic.

endocarditis   inflammation of the inner lining of the heart.

endocardium   the innermost part of the heart wall; it lines the heart chamber and covers the connective tissue skeleton of the heart valves.

endocrine   system of glands which secrete a type of hormone directly into the bloodstream to regulate the body.

endocrinologist   a physician who specializes in disorders of the endocrine system.

endogenous   having its origin within an organism.

endometrium   the inner layer of the uterine wall.

endorphins   chemicals that are often called the body's "natural painkillers" that tend to produce a euphoria, or "good feeling." Release of endorphins is often caused by physical movement or exercise.

endotracheal tube   a large instrument usually inserted through the mouth (may use the nose) and into the trachea to the point of the tracheal division to deliver oxygen under pressure.

enumerated   counted.

enuresis   bed wetting.

enzyme   a protein that begins (catalyzes) a chemical reaction.

eosinophil   a type of leukocyte increased in allergic reactions and parasitic infections.

epicardium   the inner or visceral layer of the pericardium that forms the outermost layer of the heart wall.

epidermis   outer layer of the skin.

epiglottis   the leaf-like flap that closes down over the glottis during swallowing.

epiphyseal end plate   a thin layer of cartilage at the end of long bones where new growth takes place.

episiotomy   incision of the perineum to accommodate vaginal delivery of fetus.

erectile dysfunction   the inability of a male to get and keep an erection. May also be referred to as *impotence* or *ED*.

erector pili muscle   muscle that causes the hair to stand up when it contracts.

ergonomic   describes a workstation designed to prevent work-related injuries and to promote work efficiency.

ergonomics   the study of human physical characteristics and their environment to minimize the risk for injury through the use of appropriate adaptive equipment.

erythema   redness of the skin.

erythematous   characterized by redness (erythema).

erythrasma   bacterial skin infection occuring where skin touches skin, like between toes, in armpits, or groin.

erythrocyte   a red blood cell.

erythrocyte indices   three measurements (mean cell volume, mean cell hemoglobin, and mean cell hemoglobin concentration) that indicate the size of the red blood cell and how much hemoglobin the red blood cell holds.

erythrocyte sedimentation rate   measures the rate in millimeters per hour at which red blood cells settle out in a tube.

erythropoietin   a hormone produced mainly by the kidney in response to lowered oxygen levels; stimulates the production of red blood cells to increase blood oxygen levels.

essential amino acids   amino acids nutritionally required by an organism and that must be supplied in its diet (i.e., cannot be synthesized by the organism).

ethylene oxide   gas used to sterilize surgical instruments and other supplies.

etiology   cause of disease.

eunuchoidism   deficient production of male hormone by the testes, resulting in loss of the secondary male characteristics.

eustachian tubes   a mucous membrane-lined tube between the nasopharynx and the middle ear bilaterally that equalizes the internal and external otic air pressure.

euthanasia   allowing a patient to die with minimal medical interventions.

evacuated tube   a type of blood collection tube that is sealed with a premeasured, partial vacuum. The tube receives the patient's blood during venipuncture.

evaluation   the process of indicating how well the patient or person is progressing toward a particular goal; to appraise; to determine the worth or quality of something or someone.

exocrine   glands that release enzymes through ducts, including mammary glands, salivary glands, sweat glands, and glands that secrete digestive enzymes into the stomach and intestine.

exogenous   having its origin outside of the organism; its opposite is endogenous.

exophthalmia   abnormal protrusion of the eyeballs.

exophthalmic goiter   abnormal protrusion of the eyeballs accompanied by goiter.

exposure control plan   written plan required by the Occupational Safety and Health Administration that outlines an employer's system for preventing infection.

exposure risk factors   conditions that tend to put employees at risk for contact with biohazardous agents such as bloodborne pathogens.

external control   monitors the test from applying the specimen to result interpretation; controls the performance of the test.

extracellular   outside of the cell.

extraocular   outside the eye, as in extraocular eye movement.

eyewashes   used to irrigate and flush the eyes following a hazardous exposure.

F

familial   referring to a disorder that tends to occur more often in a family than would be anticipated solely by chance.

fascia   fibrous membrane tissue that covers and supports the muscles and joins the skin with underlying tissue.

fast   to abstain from eating or drinking anything but water; often done before a medical test or procedure.

febrile   having an above-normal body temperature.

Federal Register   official daily publication of the federal government; includes rules, proposed rules, notices of federal agencies and organizations, executive orders and other presidential documents.

fibrinolysis   normal body process that keeps naturally occurring blood clots from growing and causing problems; the normal breakdown of clots.

film   raw material on which x-rays are projected through the body; prior to processing, it does not contain a visible image (similar to photographic film).

fixative   a chemical substance used to bind, fix, or stabilize specimens of tissue to slides for later examination.

flagella   hair-like extremity of a bacterium or protozoan; used to facilitate movement.

flanges   extensions on the sides of the rim of the needle holder to aid in tube placement and removal.

fluorescein angiography   intravenous injection of fluorescent dye; photographing blood vessels of the eye as dye moves through them.

fluoroscopy   special x-ray technique for examining a body part by immediate projection onto a fluorescent screen.

folate   a salt of folic acid; it acts to help enzymes that build structures such as blood cells.

folliculitis   inflammation of hair follicles.

Food and Drug Administration (FDA)   responsible for protecting and promoting public health through the regulation and supervision of blood transfusions, medical devices, and other medically and nonmedically related products.

for cause   drug screening required by an employer following a questionable event.

forced expiratory volume (FEV)   volume of air forced out of the lungs.

forceps   surgical instrument used to grasp, handle, compress, pull, or join tissues, equipment, or supplies.

fulgurate   destroy tissue by electrodessication.

full-thickness burn   burn that has destroyed all skin layers.

furuncle   infection in a hair follicle or gland; characterized by pain, redness, and swelling with necrosis of tissue in the center.

G

gait   manner or style of walking.

galactosuria   condition in newborns lacking an enzyme that metabolizes galactose; increased levels of galactose appear in the blood and urine (if proper therapy is not initiated, mental retardation and other difficulties will occur).

gastroenteritis   inflammation of the gastrointestinal tract caused by bacteria or viruses.

gauge   diameter of a needle lumen.

gauze sponges   pads that come in multiple sizes depending open their use in various clinical areas.

gel separator   a nonreacting substance located in an evacuated tube that forms a physical barrier between the cells and serum or plasma after the specimen has been centrifuged.

generic name   official name given to a drug whose patent has expired.

germicide   chemical that kills most pathogenic microorganisms; disinfectant.

gerontologist   specialist who studies aging.

gestation   period of time from conception to birth; usually 37–41 weeks.

gestational diabetes   a disorder characterized by an impaired ability to metabolize carbohydrates, usually due to insulin deficiency, occurring in pregnancy and usually disappearing after delivery.

gigantism   excessive size and stature caused most frequently by hypersecretion of the human growth hormone (HGH).

gingiva   the gums; the mucous membrane–covered tissues that support the teeth.

glaucoma   abnormal increase in the fluid in the eye, usually as a result of obstructed outflow, resulting in degeneration of the intraocular components and blindness.

glomerulus   a small cluster of blood vessels within the Bowman capsule.

glucose oxidase   very specific testing method for measuring glucose.

glycosuria   the presence of glucose in the urine.

goiter   an enlargement of the thyroid gland.

gonads   a generic term referring to the sex glands of both sexes, either ovaries or testes.

goniometer   instrument used to measure the angle of joints for range of motion.

Goodell sign   softening of the cervix early in pregnancy.

Gram negative   describes bacteria that lose the purple color of the Gram stain when exposed to the ethyl alcohol and appear pink.

Gram positive   describes bacteria that keep the purple color of the Gram stain even when exposed to the ethyl alcohol.

Gram stain   primary stain used in the microbiology lab.

granulocytes   white blood cells that have visible granules when stained.

Graves disease   pronounced hyperthyroidism with signs of enlarged thyroid and exophthalmos.

gravid   pregnant.

gravida   pregnant woman.

gravidity   pregnancy.

grief   great sadness caused by loss.

gross hematuria   large amount of blood in the urine.

guaiac   substance used in laboratory tests for occult blood in the stool.

gyri   the convolutions of the brain tissue.

H

Hashimoto thyroiditis   diffuse infiltration of the thyroid gland with lymphocytes, resulting in diffuse goiter and hypothyroidism.

HCFA   see Health Care Financing Administration.

Health Care Financing Administration (HCFA)   a federal agency that regulates health care financing and the procedural classification (Volume 3 of the ICD-9-CM coding book).

Health Insurance Portability and Accountability Act (HIPAA)   federal law, originally passed as the Kassebaum Kennedy Act, that requires all health care settings to ensure privacy and security of patient information. Also requires health insurance to be accessible for working Americans and available when changing employment.

heat cramps   type of hyperthermia that causes muscle cramping resulting from high-sodium heat exhaustion; hyperthermia resulting from physical exertion in heat without adequate fluid replacement.

heat exhaustion a type of hyperthermia that causes an altered mental status due to inadequate fluid replacement.

heat stroke most serious type of hyperthermia; body is no longer able to compensate for elevated temperature.

hemachromatosis disorder that increases the amount of iron in patients' blood to dangerous levels.

hematemesis vomiting blood or bloody vomitus.

hematocrit the percentage of red blood cells in whole blood.

hematology the study of blood and blood-forming tissues.

hematoma blood clot that forms at an injury site.

hematopoiesis blood cell production; also known as *hemopoiesis*.

hematuria blood in the urine.

hemoconcentration decrease in the volume of plasma in blood causing an increase in blood components. Can be caused by excessive application of the tourniquet.

hemoglobin the functioning unit of the red blood cell.

hemoglobinuria presence of free hemoglobin in urine.

hemolysis rupture of erythrocytes with the release of hemoglobin into the plasma or serum causing the specimen to appear pink or red in color.

hemolytic anemia a disorder characterized by premature destruction of the red cells; this may be brought on by an infectious process, inherited red cell disorders, or as a response to certain drugs or toxins.

hemoptysis coughing up blood from the respiratory tract.

hemostasis process that results in control of bleeding after an injury.

hemostat surgical instrument with slender jaws used for grasping blood vessels.

heparin a naturally occurring anticoagulant given to prevent clot formation.

hepatomegaly enlarged liver.

hepatotoxin substance that can damage the liver.

hereditary referring to traits or disorders that are transmitted from parent to offspring.

hernia protrusion of an organ through the muscle wall of the cavity that normally surrounds it.

herpes simplex infection caused by the herpes simplex virus.

herpes zoster infection caused by reactivation of varicella zoster virus, which causes chickenpox.

hiatus an opening or gap; hiatal hernia: a protrusion of part of the stomach upward through the diaphragm.

HIPAA see Health Insurance Portability and Accountability Act.

hirsutism abnormal or excessive growth of hair in women.

histamine substance found normally in the body in response to injured cells, producing the inflammatory process: dilation of capillaries, increased gastric secretions, and contraction of smooth muscles.

histology study of the microscopic structure of tissue.

homeopathic referring to an alternative type of medicine in which patients are treated with small doses of substances that produce similar symptoms and use the body's own healing abilities.

homeostasis maintaining a constant internal environment by balancing positive and negative feedback.

hordeolum an infection of any of the lacrimal glands of the eyelids, causing redness, swelling, and pain.

hormone a substance that is produced by an endocrine gland and travels through the blood to a distant organ or gland where it acts to modify the structure or function of that gland or organ.

human chorionic gonadotropin (hCG) hormone secreted by the placenta and found in the urine and blood of a pregnant female.

human immunodeficiency virus (HIV) virus that causes acquired immunodeficiency syndrome (AIDS); the immune system begins to fail, leading to life-threatening opportunistic infections.

humidifier appliance that increases the moisture content in the air.

hydrocele a fluid-filled sac surrounding one or both testicles that results in swelling of the scrotum.

hydrogen ion hydrogen that is missing an electron and therefore readily binds with substances having extra electrons; it is an important constituent of acids.

hypercalcemia an excessive amount of calcium in the blood.

hyperchromia increased hemoglobin in red blood cells.

hyperextend extend beyond the normal range of motion.

hyperglycemia an increase in blood sugar, as in diabetes mellitus.

hyperopia farsightedness.

hyperosmolarity a condition of having increased numbers of dissolved substances in the plasma.

hyperplasia excessive proliferation of normal cells in the normal tissue arrangement of an organism.

hyperpnea abnormally deep, gasping breaths.

hyperpyrexia dangerously high temperature, 105° to 106°F.

hypersensitivities the immune system responds inappropriately or too intensely to harmless compounds.

hypertension morbidly high blood pressure.

hyperventilation a respiratory rate that greatly exceeds the body's oxygen demands.

hyperthermia general condition of excessive body heat.

hypochromia red blood cells appearing paler with more area of central pallor.

hypoglycemia deficiency of sugar (glucose) in the blood.

hypopnea shallow respirations.

hypothalamus part of the diencephalon; activates and controls the peripheral nervous system, endocrine system, and certain involuntary functions.

hypothermia below-normal body temperature.

hypovolemic shock shock caused by loss of blood or other body fluids.

hysterosalpingogram radiograph of the uterus and fallopian tubes after injection with a contrast medium.

hysteroscopy visual examination with magnification of the uterus.

I

iatrogenic a condition caused by treatment or medical procedures.

idiopathic unknown etiology.

immune globulins proteins produced by plasma cells in response to foreign antigens; provide immediate antibody protection for a few weeks to a few months.

immunity lack of susceptibility to a disease.

immunization   act or process of rendering an individual immune to specific disease.

immunodeficiency   parts of the immune system fail to provide an adequate response.

immunohematology   the study of blood typing and compatibility testing for transfusion.

immunology   the study of antigen–antibody reactions.

impetigo   highly infectious skin infection causing erythema and progressing to honey-colored crusts.

implementation   the process of initiating and carrying out an action such as a teaching plan or patient treatment.

impotence   inability to achieve or maintain an erection.

incontinence   inability to control elimination, either urine or feces or both.

indices (singular, index)   numbers expressing a property or ratio.

induration   hardened area at the injection site after an intradermal screening test for tuberculosis.

infarction   death of tissues due to lack of oxygen.

infection   invasion by disease-producing microorganisms.

infiltration   leakage of intravenous fluids into surrounding tissues.

informed consent   a statement of approval from the patient for the physician to perform a given procedure after the patient has been educated about the risks and benefits of the procedure; also referred to as expressed consent.

inguinal   pertaining to the regions of the groin.

insertion   a place of attachment, usually the freely movable portion of a muscle.

inspection   visual examination.

insufflator   device for blowing air, gas, or powder into a body cavity.

insula   fifth lobe of the cerebrum.

insulin-dependent diabetes mellitus   a deficiency in insulin production that leads to an inability to metabolize carbohydrates.

interaction   effects, positive or negative, of two or more drugs taken by a patient.

interferon   group of proteins released by white blood cells and fibroblasts when the invading microorganism is a virus.

intermittent   occurring at intervals.

internal control   control built into the testing device.

interosseous   between bones.

interstitial   the spaces between the cells.

intertrigo   rash of the body folds.

intracellular   inside of the cell.

intraocular pressure   pressure within the eyeball.

intrauterine pregnancy (IUP)   pregnancy located in the uterus.

intravascular coagulation   clot formation within the vessels; strands of fibrin may form from one wall of the vessel to the other and shear red cells as they pass by.

intravenous pyelogram (IVP)   radiography using contrast medium to evaluate kidney function.

intrinsic   found within a structure.

introitus   vaginal orifice.

iodine   an element that is an essential micronutrient used in the thyroid gland to manufacture its hormones; present in seafood, foods grown in iodized soil, iodized salt, and some dairy products.

ion   an atom or group of atoms that has become electrically charged by the loss or gain of one or more electrons.

iontophoresis   introduction of various chemical ions into the skin by means of electrical current.

ischemia   decrease in oxygen to tissues.

isolate   separate from any other microorganisms present.

J

jaundiced   bilirubin settles into the skin and sclera, making the patient appear yellow.

K

Kaposi sarcoma   cancer of the skin that is extremely rare except in AIDS patients.

Kegel exercises   isometric exercises in which the muscles of the pelvic floor are voluntarily contracted and relaxed while urinating.

keratin   a tough, insoluble protein substance of the stratum corneum, hair, and nails.

keratoses (senile)   premalignant overgrowth or thickening of the upper layer of epithelium or horny layer of the skin.

keratosis   skin condition characterized by overgrowth and thickening.

ketoacidosis   acidosis accompanied by an accumulation of ketones in the body.

ketones   the end products of fat and protein metabolism.

kinesics   a form of nonverbal communication including gestures, body movements, and facial expressions.

Kirby-Bauer method   manual technique for sensitivity testing.

kit   a packaged set containing test devices, instructions, reagents, and supplies needed to perform a test and generate results.

Krebs cycle   a sequence of reactions within cells that metabolizes sugars and other energy sources, such as carbohydrates, proteins, and fats, into carbon dioxide, water, and adenosine triphosphate.

kyphosis (dowager's hump)   abnormally deep dorsal curvature of the thoracic spine; also known as *humpback* or *hunchback*.

L

laboratory   a place where research, investigation, or scientific testing takes place.

laboratory procedure manual   Clinical Laboratory Improvement Amendments regulations require each laboratory to have its own procedure manual describing how to perform every test in the laboratory.

laparoscopy   process of viewing the internal abdominal cavity and its contents through a specialized endoscope.

laparotomy   incision of the abdominal cavity.

laryngectomy   surgical removal of the larynx.

laser ablation   destruction or removal of tissue by use of laser.

lead   electrode or electrical connection attached to the body to record electrical impulses in the body, especially the heart or brain.

lentigines   brown skin macules occurring after exposure to the sun; freckles; tan or brown macules found on elderly skin after prolonged sun exposure; also known as *liver spots*.

leukocyte   a white blood cell.

leukocyte esterase an enzyme present in leukocytes; a reagent strip test that is positive for leukocyte esterase can identify a urinary tract infection.

leukocytosis abnormal increase of leukocytes (white blood cells).

leukopenia diminished numbers of leukocytes.

leukoplakia white, thickened patches on the oral mucosa or tongue that are often precancerous.

ligament a flexible band of tissue that holds joints together.

lightening the descent of the fetus in the pelvis.

lipase any of several enzymes that begin the breakdown of fats in the digestive tract.

lipids any of the free fatty acids (fats) in the body.

lipoproteins a substance made up of a lipid and a protein.

lithotripsy crushing of a stone with sound waves.

lochia uterine discharge following childbirth, composed of some blood, mucus, and tissue.

loop of Henle a portion of the renal tubule that is shaped like a U and consisting of a thick ascending and thin descending vessels.

lordosis abnormally deep ventral curve at the lumbar flexure of the spine; also known as swayback.

lubricant agent that reduces friction.

Luer adapter a device for connecting a syringe or evacuated holder to the needle to promote a secure fit.

lumen bore; hollow interior of a needle.

lymphedema obstruction of the lymphatic system.

lymphocyte a type of leukocyte.

lyse to cause disintegration; i.e., destruction of adhesions or the breakdown of red blood cells.

M

macrocytosis abnormally large red blood cells with a mean corpuscular volume above 95 fL.

macrophage a monocyte that has left the circulation and settled and matured in tissue; macrophages process antigens and present them to T cells, activating the immune specific response.

macule small, flat discoloration of the skin.

magnetic resonance imaging imaging technique that uses a strong magnetic field.

malaise general feeling of illness without specific signs or symptoms.

malignant cancerous.

malocclusion abnormal contact between the teeth in the upper and lower jaw.

manipulation skillful use of the hands in diagnostic procedures.

Mantoux intradermal injection screening test for tuberculosis.

masticate the act of chewing or grinding, as in chewing food.

material safety data sheet (MSDS) a detailed record of all characteristics and protection required from a hazardous substance.

media a Petri plate containing a solid nutrient gel for growing bacteria from culture specimens.

mediastinum the mid-portion of the thoracic cavity containing the heart, the great vessels, the upper esophagus, and the trachea.

medical asepsis removal or destruction of microorganisms.

medical history record containing information about a patient's past and present health status.

medulla oblongata part of the brain that controls breathing, heart rate, and blood pressure.

meiosis the cell division specific to sperm and ova that results in 23 chromosomes rather than 46 (23 pairs).

melanin dark pigment that gives color to the skin, hair, and eyes.

melanocyte cell that produces melanin.

melena black, tarry stools caused by digested blood from the gastrointestinal tract.

menarche onset of first menstruation.

meninges membranes of the spinal cord and brain.

meningocele meninges protruding though the spinal column.

meniscus the curved upper surface of a liquid in a container.

menorrhagia excessive bleeding during menstruation.

menses menstruation; bloody discharge monthly or cyclically in the female when fertilization has not occurred.

mensuration the act or process of measuring.

metabolic acidosis an acidic condition of the body caused when excess acids are produced in the body's fluids (as in the metabolism of fats instead of glucose) or when the body's natural bicarbonates are lost or diminished.

metabolism sum of chemical processes that result in growth, energy production, elimination of waste, and body functions performed as digested nutrients are distributed; conversion of oxygen and calories to energy.

methicillin-resistant Staphylococcus aureus a strain of Staphylococcus aureus bacteria that is resistant to many antibiotics used to treat Staphylococcus skin infections. Commonly abbreviated MRSA.

metric system system of measurement that uses grams, liters, and meters.

metrorrhagia irregular uterine bleeding.

microalbumin tiny bits of albumin that appear in the urine in early kidney disease.

microbiology the study of pathogen identification and antibiotic susceptibility determination.

microcytosis red blood cells are smaller than usual.

microhematuria the amount of blood in the urine is so small that the color of the specimen is not affected.

microorganisms microscopic living organisms.

micturition also known as *voiding* or *urination*.

midbrain part of the brainstem, responsible for relaying messages.

migraine type of severe headache, usually unilateral; may appear in clusters.

minerals inorganic substances (such as sodium, potassium, calcium, phosphorus, magnesium, iron, iodine, fluorine, zinc, copper, cobalt, and chromium) used in the formation of hard and soft body tissue; necessary for muscle contraction, nerve conduction, and blood clotting.

monocyte a type of leukocyte.

monosaccharide a simple sugar that cannot be broken down further.

mordant a substance used to fix, or bind, dyes or stains.

morphology description of the structural characteristics of blood cells.

mourning to demonstrate signs of grief; grieving.

multipara woman who has given birth to more than one viable fetus.

multisample needle used with the evacuated tube method of blood collection because multiple tubes of blood can be drawn during a multitube draw without removing the needle from the vein. The end of the needle that penetrates the stopper of the tube has a retractable rubber sleeve that covers it when the tube is removed and prevents leaks during tube changes.

muscular dystrophies a group of genetically transmitted diseases characterized by progressive atrophy of skeletal muscles.

mycology the science and study of fungi.

mycoses diseases caused by fungi.

myelofibrosis a disorder in which bone marrow tissue develops in abnormal sites such as the liver and spleen; signs include immature cells in the circulation, anemia, and splenomegaly.

myelogram invasive radiologic test in which dye is injected into the spinal fluid.

myelomeningocele protrusion of the spinal cord through the spinal defect; spina bifida.

myocardial infarction (MI) death of cardiac muscle due to lack of blood flow to the muscle; also known as heart attack.

myocarditis inflammation of the myocardial layer of the heart.

myocardium the middle layer of the walls of the heart, composed of cardiac muscle.

myofibrils a slender light/dark strand of muscle tissue in striated muscle.

myoglobin protein found in skeletal and cardiac muscle; very sensitive indicator of muscle injury.

myopia nearsightedness.

myringotomy incision into the tympanic membrane to relieve pressure.

myxedema the most severe form of hypothyroidism; signs include edema of the extremities and the face.

N

nasal septum wall or partition dividing the nostrils.

nebulizer device for administering respiratory medications as a fine inhaled spray.

needle disposal unit container for the disposal of used needles, lancets, and other sharp objects in a puncture-resistant, leak-proof disposable container.

needle holder type of surgical forceps used to hold and pass suture through tissue.

negative stress stress that does not allow for relaxation periods.

neonatologist physician who specializes in the care and treatment of newborns.

neoplasm abnormal growth of new tissue; tumor.

nephron the portion of the kidney responsible for the production of urine.

nephrostomy placement of a catheter in the kidney pelvis to drain urine from an obstructed kidney.

neurogenic shock shock that results from dysfunction of nervous system following spinal cord injury.

neuron a nerve cell.

neurotransmitter chemical needed to transmit a message between synapses.

neutral pH pH = 7, neither an acid or a base.

neutrophil the most abundant leukocyte and the main granulocyte.

nitrite a factor used to assess the presence of bacteria in urine.

nitrogenous pertaining to or containing nitrogen, usually the end-product of protein metabolism.

nitroprusside a compound that reacts with ketones to produce a purple reaction.

nocturia excessive urination at night.

noncompliance the patient's inability or refusal to follow prescribed orders.

non–insulin-dependent diabetes mellitus (NIDDM) a type of diabetes in which patients do not require insulin to control the blood sugar.

nonwaived testing complex tests that do not meet the Clinical Laboratory Improvements Amendments' criteria for waiver and require training and specific quality measures to ensure the accuracy and reliability of test results.

normal flora microorganisms normally found in the body; also known as *resident flora*.

normal value acceptable range as established for an age, a population, or a sex; variations usually indicate a disorder.

nosocomial infection infection acquired in a medical setting, generally presumed to be in a hospital setting but may also refer to the medical office.

NPO patient must have nothing by mouth after midnight until the procedure is done; patient cannot have water.

nuclear medicine branch of medicine that uses radioactive isotopes to diagnose and treat disease.

nulligravida a woman who has never been pregnant.

nullipara a woman who has never given birth to a viable fetus.

nutrition the study of food and how it is used for growth, nourishment, and repair.

O

obligate to require; a parasite that has no choice but to attach to a living organism.

obligate intracellular parasite requires a living host for replication and survival.

obstipation extreme constipation.

obturator smooth, rounded, removable inner portion of a hollow tube, such as an anoscope, that allows for easier insertion.

occult hidden or concealed from observation.

Occupational Safety and Health Administration (OSHA) the federal agency that oversees working conditions, with the mission to protect employees from work-related hazards.

olecranon fossa the depression in the posterior surface of the humerus that allows the arm to extend by receiving the olecranon process.

olecranon process the proximal end of the ulna that becomes the point of the elbow that fits into the olecranon fossa.

oligomenorrhea scanty menstruation.

oliguria scanty urine production.

oncology the medical treatment of cancer.

oophorectomy excision of an ovary.

ophthalmia neonatorum eye infection acquired by infants passing through the birth canal of a mother infected with *Neisseria gonorrhoeae*.

ophthalmic describing medication instilled into the eye.

ophthalmologist physician who specializes in treatment of disorders of the eyes.

ophthalmoscope lighted instrument used to examine the inner surfaces of the eye.

opportunistic infection infection resulting from a defective immune system that cannot defend against pathogens normally found in the environment.

optician specialist who grinds lenses to correct errors of refraction according to prescriptions written by optometrists or ophthalmologists.

optometrist specialist who can measure for errors of refraction and prescribe lenses but who cannot treat diseases of the eye or perform surgery.

order of draw guidelines for proper tube sequence to reduce cross-contamination from one tube to the next and to prevent tissue thromboplastin contamination on specimens for coagulation testing. Carryover of additives and/or tissue thromboplastin can cause erroneous test results.

organ any part that is made up of cells and tissues that cause it to perform its specified function in conjunction with a body system.

origin the source or starting point; (muscle) the more fixed end of a muscle, usually the proximal end.

orthopnea inability to breathe lying down; the patient usually has to sit upright to breathe.

OSHA see Occupational Safety and Health Administration.

osteoporosis abnormal porosity of the bone, most often found in the elderly, predisposing the affected bony tissue to fracture.

otic describing medication instilled into the ear.

otolaryngologist physician who specializes in treatment of diseases and disorders of the ears, nose, and throat.

otoscope instrument used for visual examination of the ear canal and tympanic membrane.

over-the-counter (OTC) available without a prescription; includes herbal and vitamin supplements.

ovulation the periodic rupture of the mature ovum from the ovary.

ovum (plural, ova) the female reproductive cell; sex cell or egg.

P

Paget disease degenerative bone disease usually in older persons with bone destruction and poor repair.

palliative easing symptoms without curing.

palmar the palm surface of the hand.

palpate to examine by feeling or pressing, used in diagnostic procedures such as vein location for phlebotomy.

palpation technique in which the examiner feels the texture, size, consistency, and location of parts of the body with the hands.

palpitations feeling of an increased heart rate or pounding heart that may be felt during an emotional response or a cardiac disorder.

panels laboratory tests organized into standard groups to effectively evaluate disease processes or organ systems.

panic value critical limits defining the boundaries of the life-threatening values of laboratory test results.

Papanicolaou (Pap) test or smear smear of tissue cells examined for abnormalities including cancer, especially of the cervix; named for George N. Papanicolaou, a physician, anatomist, and cytologist.

papilla (plural, papillae) a small nipple-shaped projection.

papillae lingua the taste buds.

parameters values used to describe or measure a set of data representing a physiologic function or system.

parasite organism that derives nourishment and protection from other living organisms known as hosts.

parasitology the science and study of parasites.

parasympathetic the part of the autonomic nervous system involved in periods free from stress.

parenteral describing medication administered by any method other than orally.

parity pregnancy that resulted in a viable birth.

partial-thickness burn burn that involves epidermis and varying levels of the dermis.

pathogens disease-causing microorganisms.

patient education active participation of the patient in a process that will yield a change in behavior.

peak level the highest serum level of a free or unbound drug in a patient based on a dosing schedule that is usually measured about 60 minutes after the end of an infusion.

pediatrician physician who specializes in the care of infants, children, and adolescents.

pediatrics specialty of medicine that deals with the care of infants, children, and adolescents.

pediculosis infestation with parasitic lice.

percussion striking with the hands to evaluate the size, borders, consistency, and presence of fluid or air.

percutaneous transluminal coronary angioplasty (PTCA) procedure that improves blood flow through a coronary artery by pressing the plaque against the wall of the artery with a balloon on a catheter, allowing for more blood flow.

pericarditis inflammation of the sac that covers the heart.

pericardium the double-layered serous, membranous sac that encloses the heart and the origins of the great vessels.

peripheral pertaining to or situated away from the center.

peristalsis contraction and relaxation of involuntary muscles of the alimentary canal producing wavelike movement of products through the digestive system.

PERRLA abbreviation used in documentation to denote pupils equal, round, reactive to light, and accommodation if all findings are normal; refers to the size and shape of the pupils, their reaction to light, and their ability to adjust to distance.

personal protective equipment (PPE) equipment used to protect a person from exposure to blood or other body fluids.

pessary device that supports the uterus when inserted into the vagina.

petri plate a shallow glass or plastic dish with a lid to hold solid media for cultures.

pH abbreviation for potential hydrogen; pH is a scale representing the relative acidity or alkalinity of a substance in which 7.0 is neutral; numbers lower than 7.0 are acidic, and numbers above 7.0 are basic.

phagocyte a cell that has the ability to ingest and destroy particular substances such as bacteria, protozoa, cells, and cell debris by ingesting them.

phagocytosis the process by which certain cells engulf and dispose of microorganisms; to eat or ingest.

pharmacodynamics study of how drugs act within the body.

pharmacokinetics study of the action of drugs within the body from administration to excretion.

pharmacology   study of drugs and their origins, natures, properties, and effects upon living organisms.

phimosis   narrowing or tightening of the prepuce that prevents retraction over the glans penis.

phonophoresis   ultrasound treatment used to force medications into tissues.

phosphates   compounds containing phosphorus and oxygen; they are very important in living organisms, especially for the transfer of genetic information.

physician office laboratory (POL)   laboratory in a medical office.

physiology   the study of the function of the body.

pia mater   thin vascular covering that adheres to the surface of the brain.

pilosebaceous unit   consists of the hair shaft, the hair follicle, the sebaceous gland, and the erector pili muscle which causes the hair to stand up when it contracts.

placebo   an inert substance given as a medicine for its suggestive effect; an inert compound identical in appearance to material being tested in experimental research, which may or may not be known to the physician and/or patient, administered to distinguish between drug action and suggestive effect of the material under study.

planes   a point of reference made by a straight cut through the body at any given angle.

planning   the process of using information gathered during the assessment phase to organize learning or patient care objectives in order to accomplish the specific learning or treatment goal.

plasma   top liquid layer of a blood specimen if the specimen was anticoagulated and not allowed to clot.

platelets   thrombocytes.

pleura   the serous membrane enclosing the lungs (visceral pleura: the layer that covers the lungs most closely; parietal pleura: the layer that follows the contours and lines the chest wall, the diaphragm, and the mediastinum).

poikilocytosis   abnormal variations in the shapes of red blood cells (*poikilo* = variation).

point-of-care testing (POC or POCT)   testing at the point where patient care is given.

polychromosia   some red blood cells (RBCs) have a blue color; bluish RBCs are more immature cells.

polycythemia vera   a condition that causes an elevated hematocrit.

polydipsia   excessive thirst.

polymenorrhea   abnormally frequent menstrual periods.

polyphagia   abnormal hunger.

polyuria   excessive excretion and elimination of urine.

pons   part of the brainstem, responsible for communication with the central nervous system.

positive feedback   an increase in function in response to a stimulus.

positive stress   stress that allows a person to perform at peak levels and then relax afterward.

positron emission tomography (PET)   computerized radiography using radioactive substances to assess metabolic or physiologic functions within the body rather than anatomic structures.

postexposure testing   laboratory tests that may be performed after a person comes into contact with a biohazard.

postural hypotension   sudden drop in blood pressure upon standing.

potentiation   describes the action of two drugs taken together in which the combined effects are greater than the sum of the independent effects.

precision   test results are similar when test is repeated.

preexisting condition   medical problem treated by a physician before an insurance plan's effective date. A third-party payer may exclude coverage for preexisting conditions.

prepuce   a fold of skin that forms a cover.

presbyacusis   (also: presbycusis) loss of hearing associated with aging.

presbyopia   vision change (farsightedness) associated with aging.

present illness   a specific account of the chief complaint, including time frames and characteristics.

preservative   substance that delays decomposition.

primary diagnosis   the condition or chief complaint that brings a person to a medical facility for treatment.

primary survey   an initial assessment of an emergency patient for life-threatening problems.

prime mover   the muscle most responsible for the desired muscle action or movement.

primigravida   a woman who is pregnant for the first time.

primipara   a woman who has given birth to one viable infant.

probing   digging with the needle to locate a vein.

problem-oriented medical record (POMR)   a common method of compiling information that lists each problem of the patient, usually at the beginning of the folder, and references each problem with a number throughout the folder.

procedure manual   handbook that contains test methods and other information needed to perform testing, is suggested by the United States Department of Health and Human Services (HHS) and the Centers for Disease Control and Prevention (CDC) as a valuable resource for Certificate of Waiver sites.

product insert   written product information usually supplied by the manufacturer with each test kit or test system containing instructions and critical details for performing the test; also referred to as the package insert.

proficiency testing   program to assess tests and the testers' performance by providing challenge samples to test as if they were patient specimens.

prophylaxis   prevention of development of a disease or condition.

prostate-specific antigen   normal protein produced by the prostate that usually elevates in the presence of prostate cancer.

prosthesis   any artificial replacement for a missing body part, such as false teeth or an artificial limb.

protected health information (PHI)   individually identifiable personal health information as defined by the Health Insurance Portability and Accountability Act. Information that can be linked to a particular individual by name, code, or number is PHI.

proteinuria   the presence of large quantities of protein in the urine; usually a sign of renal dysfunction.

prothrombin time (PT)   test that monitors a patient's blood clotting time.

provider-performed microscopy (PPM)   direct examination of a patient specimen using a microscope; a type of nonwaived testing.

proxemic   having to do with the degree of physical closeness tolerated by humans.

pruritus   itching.

psoriasis   chronic skin disorder that appears as red patches covered by thick, dry, silvery scales.

psychogenic   of psychological origin.

psychomotor   describes a physical task.

psychosocial   relating to mental and emotional aspects of social encounters.

puerperium   period of time (about 6 weeks) from childbirth until reproductive structures return to normal.

Purkinje fibers   extensions of the bundle of His that branch through the myocardium to end the transmission of the electrical impulse and cause the ventricles to contract.

purulent   describes drainage that is white, green, or yellow; characteristic of an infection.

pyosalpinx   pus in the fallopian tube(s).

pyrexia   body temperature of 102°F or higher rectally or 101°F or higher orally.

pyuria   pus in the urine.

Q

quadrants   a division of the abdomen into four equal parts by one horizontal and one vertical line dissecting at the umbilicus.

qualitative   has positive or negative results; not a specified amount.

quality assessment   plan for ensuring the quality of all areas of the laboratory's technical and support functions.

quality assurance (QA)   an evaluation of health care services as compared to accepted standards.

quality control (QC)   method to evaluate the proper performance of testing procedures, supplies, or equipment in a laboratory.

quality improvement   a plan that allows an organization to scientifically measure the quality of its product and service.

quantification   the process of ascertaining the amount of something.

quantitative   the measuring of an amount.

quantitative test   quantity measured and reported in a number value.

Queckenstedt test   test to determine presence of obstruction in the cerebrospinal fluid flow performed during a lumbar puncture.

R

radiograph   processed film that contains a visible image.

radiographer   technical specialist who works to assist the radiologist in the performance of procedures and who is responsible for producing routine examination images for the radiologist to interpret.

radiography   art and science of producing diagnostic images with x-rays.

radiologist   physician who specializes in radiology; performs some procedures and interprets images to provide diagnostic information.

radiology   branch of medicine including diagnostic and therapeutic applications of x-rays.

radiolucent   permitting the passage of x-rays.

radionuclide   radioactive material with a short life that is used in small amounts in nuclear medicine studies.

radiopaque   not permeable to passage of x-rays.

range of motion (ROM)   range in degrees of angle through which a joint can be extended and flexed.

ratchet   notched mechanism, usually at the handle end of an instrument, that clicks into position to maintain tension on the opposing blades or tips of the instrument.

reagent   a substance used to react in a certain manner in the presence of specific chemicals to obtain a diagnosis.

recommended dietary allowance (RDA)   the amount of a nutrient most people need each day to stay healthy.

reconstitution   adding water to bring a material back to its liquid state.

rectocele   herniation of the rectum into the vaginal area.

rectovaginal   pertaining to the rectum and vagina.

reducing sugars   sugars other than glucose.

reduction   correcting a fracture by realigning the bones; may be closed (corrected by manipulation) or open (requires surgery).

reference interval   a range established for test results assumed to be typical for a population asymptomatic for disease processes.

referral laboratory   a large facility in which thousands of tests of various types are performed each day.

reflux   a return or backward flow of fluid.

refraction   bending of light rays that enter the pupil to reflect exactly on the fovea centralis, the area of greatest visual acuity.

relapsing fever   fever that returns after extended periods of being within normal limits.

remittent   fluctuating.

renal cortex   the portion of the kidney that contains the structures that form urine.

renal medulla   the inner portion of the kidney that contains the collecting structures.

renal pelvis   the funnel-shaped upper portion of the ureters that collects urine from the kidneys.

renal pyramids   situated in the renal medulla, part of the collecting structures.

renin   enzyme formed in the kidney that works with angiotensin to affect the blood pressure.

repolarization   the active process of restoring the cardiac fibers to the resting (polarized) state; re-establishment of the electrical polarized state in a muscle or nerve fiber following contraction or conduction of a nerve impulse.

reportable range   the very lowest and highest value the manufacturer has documented the test can determine.

resident flora   microorganisms normally found in the body; also known as normal flora.

resistance   body's immune response to prevent infections by invading pathogenic microorganisms.

resistant   describes organisms that grow even in the presence of an antimicrobial agent.

respiration   the exchange of oxygen and carbon dioxide (external respiration: the exchange between the alveoli and the bloodstream; internal respiration: the exchange between the cells and the bloodstream).

restrain   control or confine movement.

retinal degeneration   pathologic changes in the cell structure of the retina that impair or destroy its function, resulting in blindness.

retrograde pyelogram an x-ray of the urinary tract using contrast medium injected through the bladder and ureters; useful in diagnosing obstructions.

retroperitoneal the space behind the peritoneal cavity that contains the kidneys.

retrovirus virus containing reverse transcriptase, which allows the viral cell to replicate its DNA in the DNA of the host cell, thereby taking over the substance of the cell.

Rickettsia organism that is smaller than bacteria, larger than viruses.

ringworm lay term for tinea, a group of fungal diseases.

risk factors any issue that possesses a safety or liability concern for an organization.

Romberg test test for inability to maintain body balance when eyes are closed and feet are together; indication of spinal cord disease.

rugae ridges or folds in the skin or mucous membranes that allow for expansion of a part.

rule of nines the most common method of determining the extent of burn injury; the body surface is divided into sections of 9% or multiples of 9%.

S

salpingectomy excision of the fallopian tube.

salpingo-oophorectomy surgical excision of both the fallopian tube and the ovary.

sanitation maintenance of a healthful, disease-free environment.

sanitization processes used to lower the number of microorganisms on a surface by cleansing with soap or detergent, water, and manual friction.

sanitize reduce the number of microorganisms on a surface by use of low-level disinfectant practices.

scale a thin, dried flake of skin.

scalpel small, pointed knife with a convex edge for surgical procedures.

scissors sharp instrument composed of two opposing cutting blades, held together by a central pin on which the blades pivot.

sclera white fibrous tissue that covers the eye.

sclerotherapy use of chemical agents to treat esophageal varices to produce fibrosis and hardening of the tissue.

scoliosis lateral curve of the spine, usually in the thoracic area, with a corresponding curve in the lumbar region, causing uneven shoulders and hips.

screening a preliminary procedure, such as a test or exam, to detect the more characteristic signs of a disorder.

sebaceous gland oil gland.

seborrhea overproduction of sebum by the sebaceous glands.

sebum fatty secretion of the sebaceous gland.

sediment the cells and other particulate matter that collect in the bottom of the tube when a urine sample is centrifuged.

seizure abnormal discharge of electrical activity in the brain, resulting in involuntary contractions of voluntary muscles.

senility general mental deterioration associated with aging.

sensitive describes organisms that are inhibited by an antimicrobial agent.

sensitivity susceptibility to a certain substance.

sensitivity testing testing to determine the antibiotic that will most effectively inhibit the pathogen.

sentinel event an unexpected death or serious physical or psychological injury to a patient in a health care facility.

septic shock shock that results from general infection in the bloodstream.

septicemia presence of pathogenic bacteria in the blood.

serration groove, either straight or crisscross, etched or cut into the blade or tip of an instrument to improve its bite or grasp.

serum top liquid layer of a blood specimen if the specimen was allowed to clot.

sesamoid resembling the shape of a sesame seed.

sharps container a rigid, leak-proof, plastic container used to discard disposable sharp devices in a manner to reduce needlesticks.

shift a situation in which quality control results make an obvious change in performance levels.

shock lack of oxygen to individual cells of the body.

sick-child visit a pediatric visit for the treatment of illness or injury.

sickle cell anemia a condition in which the patient has both copies of the gene for hemoglobin S; the red cells become sickle shaped and nonflexible causing obstruction of small vessels and capillaries. Necrosis due to tissue hypoxia occurs beyond the obstruction. Most commonly seen in African-Americans.

signs objective indications of disease or bodily dysfunction as observed or measured by the health care professional.

sinoatrial (SA) node considered the pacemaker of the heart, located in the upper portion of the right atrium; a specialized group of cells that initiate the electrical impulse of the heart.

smears materials that have been dried on glass slides.

smegma a cheesy secretion of the sebaceous glands in either the labia or the prepuce.

SOAP a style of charting that includes subjective, objective, assessment, and planning notes.

sound long instrument for exploring or dilating body cavities or searching cavities for foreign bodies.

specialty a subcategory of medicine, such as pediatrics, studied after completion of medical school.

specific gravity density of a liquid, such as urine, compared with water.

specificity relating to a definite result.

specimen a small portion of anything used to evaluate the nature of the whole; samples, such as blood or urine, used to evaluate a patient's condition.

speculum instrument that enlarges and separates the opening of a cavity to expose its interior for examination.

spherocytosis red blood cells showing no area of central pallor.

sphygmomanometer device used to measure blood pressure.

spicules sharp points.

spina bifida occulta, spina bifida congenital defect in the spinal column caused by lack of union of the vertebrae.

spinal pertaining to the spine.

spirochete long, flexible, motile microorganisms.

splint device used to immobilize a sprain, strain, fracture, or dislocated limb.

spore bacterial life form that resists destruction by heat, drying, or chemicals. Spore-producing bacteria include botulism and tetanus.

staghorn stone formation in the renal pelvis that fills the chamber and assumes the shape of the calyces.

standard precautions usual steps to prevent injury or disease.

staphylococci spherical microorganism found in grapelike clusters.

STAT immediately.

status asthmaticus asthma attack that is not responsive to treatment.

stereotyping to place in a fixed mold, without consideration of differences.

sterile field a specific area, such as within a tray or on a sterile towel, that is considered free of microorganisms.

sterilization process, act, or technique for destroying micro-organisms using heat, water, chemicals, or gases.

stoma an opening to the surface; suggests that it is surgically created.

stomatitis inflammation of the mucous membranes of the mouth.

strabismus a misalignment of eye movements usually caused by muscle incoordination.

stratum corneum outer layer of the epidermis.

Streptococcus genus of bacteria commonly implicated in infections of the skin.

stress a factor that induces body tension; can be positive or negative.

stratum germinativum innermost layer of the epidermis.

striated having a striped appearance with alternating light and dark bands.

subcutaneous beneath the skin.

sublingual describing medication administered under the tongue.

substrate an underlying layer; a substance acted upon, as by an enzyme or reagent.

sudoriferous gland sweat gland.

sulci a groove in the brain tissue.

sulfosalicylic acid an acid used to test for protein.

superficial describes fungal infections limited to skin, hair, and nails.

superficial burn burn limited to the epidermis.

supernatant the urine that rises above the sediment when the tube of urine is centrifuged.

surgical asepsis destruction of organisms before they enter the body.

surgical pathology the primary subspecialty of anatomic athology. Studies are performed on tissue and body fluid specimens from aspirations, autopsies, biopsies, organ removal, and other procedures to identify or evaluate the effects of cancer and other diseases.

surrogate mother a woman who carries a baby to term for another female who is unable to carry a pregnancy to term.

susceptibility testing determines the potential of an anti-microbial agent to be effective in inhibiting growth of an organism.

sustained fever fever that is constant or not fluctuating.

swab *noun*, stick topped with cotton or other absorbent man-made fiber for cleaning areas, applying treatments, or obtaining specimens; *verb*, to wipe with a swab.

swaged needle metal needle fused to suture material.

symmetry equality in size or shape or position of parts on opposite sides of the body.

sympathetic the part of the autonomic nervous system involved in stress reaction.

sympathy feeling sorry for or pitying someone.

symptoms subjective indications of disease or bodily dysfunction as sensed by the patient.

synapse the junction of two neurons.

synarthroses immovable joints.

syncope sudden fall in blood pressure or cerebral hypoxia resulting in loss of consciousness.

synergism harmonious action of two agents, such as drugs or organs, producing an effect that neither could produce alone or that is greater than the total effects of each agent operating by itself.

synergist muscles that work together for more efficient movement.

syringe used for the phlebotomy of fragile veins because the vacuum can be applied slowly and gently, rather than all at once as with vacuum tubes.

systemic describes an infection of the internal organs.

systole contraction phase of the cardiac cycle.

T

T cells lymphoid cells from bone marrow that migrate to the thymus gland where they mature into differentiated lymphocytes that circulate between blood and lymph.

tachycardia heart rate of more than 100 beats per minute.

tactile pertaining to the sense of touch.

Tamm-Horsfall mucoprotein mucoprotein that cements urinary casts together.

taut pull skin gently so that there is no give or slack.

teleradiology use of computed imaging and information systems to transmit diagnostic images to distant locations.

tendons tough, flexible fibers that bind muscle to bone.

tetany severe cramping, convulsions, or muscle spasms due to an abnormality of calcium metabolism.

thalamus part of the diencephalon, responsible for sorting messages.

thalassemia a hemolytic anemia caused by deficient hemoglobin synthesis; more commonly found in those of Mediterranean heritage.

therapeutic having to do with treating or curing disease; curative.

therapeutic phlebotomy phlebotomy done as part of the patient's treatment for certain blood disorders.

therapeutic range test result range the physician wants for the patient.

thoracentesis surgical puncture into the pleural cavity for aspiration of serous fluid or for injection of medication.

threshold the least amount of something that produces a response.

thrombocytes platelets in the blood.

thrombocytopenia decreased platelets.

thrombocytosis increased platelets.

thromboplastin a complex substance found in blood and tissues that aids the clotting process.

thrombosed veins that lack resilience, feel like rope or cord and roll easily.

thrombosis blood clotting inside a blood vessel.

thyrotoxicosis excess quantities of thyroid hormone in the tissues.

tidal volume amount of air inhaled and exhaled during a normal respiration.

tine test   skin test for exposure to tuberculosis, involves pricking the skin with sharp tines coated with the tuberculin bacillus.

tinnitus   an extraneous noise heard in one or both ears, described as whirring, ringing, whistling, roaring, etc.; may be continuous or intermittent.

titer   measure of the amount of an antibody in serum.

tomography   procedure in which the x-ray tube and film move in relation to each other during exposure, blurring out all structures except those in the focal plane.

tonometry   measurement of intraocular pressure using a tonometer.

tonsils   a small mass of lymphoid tissue; includes the palatine, nasopharyngeal, and lingual tonsils.

tonus   the steady, partial contraction of skeletal muscles that allows the body to remain upright.

topical   describing medication applied directly to the skin or mucous membranes.

total testing process   multistep process that begins and ends with the needs of the patient.

toxicology   the study of the presence and measurement of drugs in the blood.

toxoid   toxin treated to destroy its toxicity but still capable of inducing formation of antibodies.

trace minerals   minerals needed by the body only in small amounts.

tracheostomy   permanent surgical stoma in the neck with an indwelling tube.

tracheotomy   incision into the trachea below the larynx to circumvent a blockage superior to this point; suggests an emergency situation and a reversible procedure.

trade name   name given to a medication by the company that owns the patent.

transient flora   microorganisms that do not normally reside in a given area; transient flora may or may not produce disease.

transient ischemic attack (TIA)   acute episode of cerebrovascular insufficiency, usually a result of narrowing of an artery by atherosclerotic plaques, emboli, or vasospasm; usually passes quickly but should be considered a warning for predisposition to cerebrovascular accidents.

transillumination   passage of light through body tissues for the purpose of examination.

transition   passing from one place or activity to another.

traumatic   causing or relating to tissue damage.

trend   when control results progressively increase or decrease over time.

triage   sorting of patients into categories based on their level of sickness or injury to ensure that life-threatening medical conditions are treated immediately.

trigone   the triangle formed in the base of the bladder by the entrance of the two ureters and the exit of the urethra.

trough level   the lowest serum level of a free or unbound drug remaining in the patient's circulation; drawn just prior to the next drug dose.

truss   a device that presses against a hernia to keep it in place.

turbid   cloudy.

turbidity   cloudiness.

turbinates   mucous membrane–covered conchae, the three scroll-shaped bones that project into the nasal cavity bilaterally from the lateral walls; each covers a sinus meatus.

turgor   normal tension in a cell or the skin; normal skin turgor resists deformation and will resume its former position after being grasped or pulled.

tympanic membrane   thin, semitransparent membrane in the middle ear that transmits sound vibrations; the eardrum.

tympanic thermometer   device for measuring the temperature using the blood flow through the tympanic membrane, or eardrum.

U

ultrasound   imaging technique that uses sound waves to diagnose or monitor various body structures.

unitized test device   a self-contained test device to which a specimen is added directly and in which all steps of the testing process occur. A unitized device is used for a single test and must be discarded after testing.

universal precautions   controlling infection by treating all human blood and certain human body fluids as if known to be infectious for HIV, hepatitis B virus, hepatitis C virus, and other bloodborne pathogens.

upper respiratory infection (URI)   infection of the nasopharynx, throat, and bronchi.

urea   the final product of protein metabolism in the body and the main nitrogenous component in the urine.

uremic frost   a frost-like deposit of uremic compounds on the skin of patients whose kidneys are no longer functional.

ureterostomy   surgical opening to the outside of the body from the ureter to facilitate drainage of urine from an obstructed kidney.

ureters   the pair of tubes designed to carry urine from the kidneys to the bladder.

urethra   the short tube that carries urine from the bladder to the outside of the body.

urethral meatus   the external opening of the urethra.

uric acid   a byproduct of protein metabolism present in the blood and excreted by the kidneys.

urinalysis   examination of the physical, chemical, and microscopic properties of urine.

urinary frequency   the urge to urinate occurring more often than is required for normal bladder elimination.

urine dipstick   urine reagent test strip.

urobilinogen   the chemical that results when bacterial action converts bilirubin when it is secreted in the bile.

urticaria   hives.

V

vaccine   suspension of infectious agents or some part of them; given to establish resistance to an infectious disease.

values   established ideals of life, conduct, customs, etc., of an individual person or members of a society.

varicella zoster   viral infection manifested by characteristic rash of successive crops of vesicles that scab before resolution; also called *chicken pox*.

vasopressin   a hormone formed in the hypothalamus and transported to the posterior lobe of the pituitary through the hypothalamo-hypophyseal tract. It has an antidiuretic and a pressor effect that elevates the blood pressure.

vector (biological) a living, nonhuman carrier of disease, usually an arthropod; (mechanical) a carrier of disease that does not support growth; examples include contaminated inanimate objects.

ventricle either of the two lower chambers of the heart that, when filled with blood, contract to propel it into the arteries.

venule the small vessel that joins a capillary to a vein.

verruca wart.

vertigo sensation of whirling of oneself or the environment; dizziness.

vesicle skin lesion that appears as a small sac containing fluid; a blister.

viable capable of growing and living.

vial glass or plastic container sealed at the top by a rubber stopper.

villus (plural, villi) tiny, almost microscopic projections in the mucous membrane of the small intestines.

virology the science and study of viruses.

virulent highly pathogenic and disease-producing; describes a microorganism.

virus a harmful invader that can damage your computer.

visualization a relaxation technique that allows the mind to wander and the imagination to run free and focus on positive and relaxing situations.

vitiligo depigmentation of patches of the skin.

vulva external genitalia of females.

W

waived test determined by Clinical Laboratory Improvement Amendments to be so simple that there is little risk of error.

WBC differential 100 white blood cells (WBCs) are counted, tallied according to type, and reported as percentages.

well-child visit visit to the medical office for administration of immunizations and evaluation of growth and development.

Western blot specific confirmatory antibody test for presence of HIV in blood.

whole blood blood containing all its cellular components.

whorls a spiral arrangement, as in the ridges on the finger that make up a fingerprint.

X

x-rays invisible electromagnetic radiation waves used in diagnosis and treatment of various disorders.

Y

yolk sac a structure that develops in the inner zygotic cell mass and supplies nourishment for the embryo until the seventh week when the placenta takes over the function.

Index

Page numbers in *italics* denote figures; those followed by a t denote tables.

A

AAMA (*see* American Association of Medical Assistants)
AAP (*see* American Academy of Pediatrics)
AAPCC (American Association of Poison Control Centers), 257
Abbreviations
    for medication administration, 193, 194t
    table of, 783t–787t
Abdomen
    assessing in emergency care, 230
    physical examination, 110
Abdominal hernia, 417
ABG (Arterial blood gases), 370
Abortion, spontaneous, 482
Abrasion, 252
Abruptio placentae, 490
Absence seizures, 434
Abuse
    child, 536
    elder, *554,* 554–555
Academy of Pediatrics (AAP), 522
Acetest, 677, 678
Achilles reflex, 111
Acidosis, 757
Acne vulgaris, 280
ACOG (American College of Obstetricians and Gynecologists), 475
Acromegaly, 512, *512*
ACS (American Cancer Society), 112
ACTH (adrenocorticotropic hormone), 511
Activities of daily living (ADL), 553
ADA (American Diabetes Association), 763
Addiction, 21
Addison's disease, 511, *511*
ADH (antidiuretic hormone), 513
ADHD (attention deficit hyperactivity disorder), 539–540
Adhesive capsulitis (frozen shoulder), 312–313
Adhesive skin closures, 147, *149*
Adjustment knob, microscope, 581
ADL (activities of daily living), 553
Administration routes, buccal, 199–200, *200*
Adrenal gland disorder
    Addison's disease, 511, *511*
    Cushing's syndrome, 511–512, *512*
Adrenergic blocking agents, 179, 180t
Adrenergics, 179, 180t
Adrenocorticotropic hormone (ACTH), 511
Adson forceps, 127, *128*
Adverse reactions, 185, 186t
AED (*see* Automatic external defibrillator)
Aerobes, 28, 696
Afebrile, 66
AFP (Alpha-fetoprotein), 490
Agar, 702
Age
    blood pressure and, 77
    body temperature and, 68
    effect on pharmacodynamics, 184–185
    variations in pulse rate by, 71, 73t
    variations in respiration by, 74t

Aging (*see also* Geriatrics)
    coping with, 552–553
AHFS (American Hospital Formulary Service), 187
AIDS prevention, 456
Air pollution, 18–19
Airbags, 19
Airway
    accessing in emergency care, 247
    opening with head tilt–chin lift method, 247–248, *248*
    opening with jaw thrust method, 248, *249*
    procedure for managing foreign body obstruction, 266–267
Alanine aminotransferase (ALT), 759
ALARA concept, 235
Albinism, 282, *282*
Albuterol, 365
Alcohol
    consumption, 18
    disinfectant, 34t
    substance abuse, 21
Alcohol wipes, 623
Alcoholism, 553
Aldosterone, 505t
Aliquots, 572
Alkaline phosphatase (ALP), 759
Alkalinity, 757
Alkalosis, 757
Allergens, 256
Allergic reactions, 256–257
Allergic rhinitis, 344
Allergies, drug, 186
Allergies reactions, 723
Alligator biopsy, 126t
Allis tissue forceps, 127, *128*
Alopecia, 281
ALP (Alkaline phosphatase), 759
Alpha-fetoprotein (AFP), 490
ALT (Alanine aminotransferase), 759
Alzheimer's disease, 562, 563t
AMA (*see* American Medical Association)
Amenorrhea, 475
American Academy of Pediatrics (AAP), 522
American Association of Medical Assistants (AAMA), CPR certification, 245
American Association of Poison Control Centers (AAPCC), 257
American Cancer Society (ACS), 112
American College of Obstetrics and Gynecology (ACOG), 475
American Diabetes Association (ADA), 763
American Heart Association, CPR certification and training by, 245
American Medical Association (AMA), 579
    laboratory test panels, 579, 579t
American Red Cross, 245
American Safety and Health Institute, CPR certification and training by, 245
Amino acids, essential, 5
Amniocentesis, 490
Amphetamines, 21

Ampules, 200–201, *202*
Amputation injury, 252
Amylase, 762
Amyotrophic lateral sclerosis (ALS), 434
Anabolism, 5
Anaerobes, 28, 696
Analgesics, 179, 180t
Anaphylactic reactions (anaphylaxis), 186, 256–257
Anaphylactic shock, 251
Anatomic and surgical pathology department, 575
Anemia, 392–393
    folate deficiency, 652t
    hemoglobin determination, 392, 651
    iron deficiency, 205, 649
    sickle cell, 651
Anesthesia, local anesthetics, 147, *147*
Aneurysm, 392, *393*
Angina pectoris, 383
Angiocatheter, 208
Anisocytosis, 654
Ankle reflex, *441*
Ankylosing spondylitis, 308
Anorexia, 413
Anoscope, 105, *105*
Anoscopy, 417, 423
ANS (Autonomic nervous system), 430
Antacids, 179, 180t
Antagonism, 185
Antecubital space, 624
Antecubital vein, 625, *625*
Anthelmintics, 179, 180t
Anthropometric measurements
    baseline, 65
    height, 65–66, *66,* 81
    weight, 65, *66,* 79–80
Anti-inflammatory agents, 179, 179t
Antianginal agents, 179, 180t
Antianxiety agents, 179, 180t
Antiarrhythmics, 179, 180t
Antibiotics
    action, 179, 180t
    sensitivity testing, 705–706, *708*
Antibodies, 723
Anticholinergics, for Parkinson's disease, 561
Anticoagulants, 179, 180t, 574, 617
Anticonvulsants, 179, 180t
Antidepressants, 179, 180t
Antidiarrheals, 179, 180t
Antidiuretic hormone (ADH), 513
Antiemetic agents, 179, 180t
Antifungals, 179, 180t
Antigen, 574
Antihistamines, 179, 180t, 562
Antihypertensives, 179, 502t
Anti-inflammatory agents, 179, 180t
Antimicrobial agents, 722
Antineoplastic agents, 179, 180t
Antipsychotics, 179, 180t
Antipyretics, 179, 180t
Antiseptics, 623, 722